Companion CD Contents

W9-APK-160

One NCLEX® Examination Review Questions

- Drug Action: Pharmaceutic, Pharmacokinetic, and Pharmacodynamic Phases
- Nursing Process and Client Teaching
- Principles of Drug Administration, Medications, and Calculations
- Transcultural and Genetic Considerations
- Drug Interaction and Over-the-Counter Drugs, Herbal Therapy with Nursing Implications
- Pediatric Pharmacology, Geriatric Pharmacology
- Vitamin and Mineral Replacement
- Fluid and Electrolyte Replacement
- Nutritional Support
- Adrenergics and Adrenergic Blockers
- Cholinergics and Anticholinergics
- Central Nervous System Stimulants
- Central Nervous System Depressants
- Drugs for Pain Management: Nonnarcotic and Narcotic Analgesics
- Anticonvulsants
- Drugs for Neurologic Disorders: Parkinsonism and Alzheimer's Disease
- Drugs for Neuromuscular Disorders: Myasthenia Gravis, Multiple Sclerosis, and Muscle Spasms
- Antipsychotics, Anxiolytics, Antidepressants, and Mood Stabilizer
- Antiinflammatory Drugs
- Antibacterials: Penicillins, Cephalosporins, Macrolides, Tetracyclines, Aminoglycosides, Fluoroquinolones, and Sulfonamides
- Antitubercular Drugs, Antifungal Drugs, Peptides, and Metronidazole
- Antiviral, Antimalarial, and Anthelmintic Drugs
- HIV and AIDS-Related Agents
- Vaccines
- Anticancer Drugs
- Biologic Response Modifiers
- Drugs for Common Upper Respiratory Disorders
- Drugs for Acute and Chronic Lower Respiratory Disorders
- Cardiac Glycosides, Antianginals, and Antidysrhythmics
- Diuretics
- Antihypertensive Drugs
- Anticoagulants, Antiplatelets, and Thrombolytics
- Antilipidemics and Peripheral Vasodilators
- Drugs for Gastrointestinal Tract Disorders
- Antiulcer Drugs
- Drugs for Disorders of the Eye and the Ear
- Drugs for Dermatologic Disorders
- Endocrine Pharmacology: Pituitary, Thyroid, Parathyroids, and Adrenals
- Antidiabetic Drugs
- Drugs Related to Women's Health and Disorders
- Drugs Related to Male Reproductive Disorders

Two Pharmacology Animations

- Nursing, Medical, and Pharmacology Domains
- Client Noncompliance
- Agonists/Antagonists
- Receptor Interaction
- Passive Diffusion
- Impact of Surface Area
- Overview of Pharmacokinetics: Oral Administration
- Distribution: Fat- vs. Water-Soluble Drugs
- Cytochrome P-450 Drug Metabolism
- Half-Life of Intravenously Administered Ampicillin
- Drug Movement Through the Body
- Normal Electrophysiology
- Renin-Angiotensin in Control of Blood Pressure
- Time to Steady State
- Time to Steady State: Starting and Stopping Drug

Three IV Therapy Checklists

- Administering Bolus Medication Through Continuous IV
- Administering Medication Through an Intermittent IV (Saline Lock)
- Adding Medication to an Intravenous Bag, Bottle, or Volume Control Set
- Administering Medication via a Piggyback or Secondary Set
- Changing the Container of an Existing Intravenous Solution

Four Medication Errors Checklists

- Interpreting Medication Orders
- Transcribing Medication Orders
- Reviewing Medication Orders
- Preparing Medications
- Administering Medications
- Assessing Client Response
- Appropriate Documentation of Medication Administration
- Procedural Safeguards

Five Drug Calculation Problems

- Oral Medication Administration: Solid
- Oral Medication Administration: Liquid
- Injectable Medication (IM) Administration
- Intravenous Medication Administration
- Intermittent IV Administration
- IV Infusion Pump Administration
- Direct IV Injection Administration
- Pediatric Medication Administration
- Pediatric Intramuscular Administration
- Pediatric Intravenous Administration
- Pediatric IV Infusion Pump Rate

Six Electronic Calculators

- Body Mass Index (BMI)
- Body Surface Area (BSA)—Adults
- Body Surface Area (BSA)—Pediatric
- Fluid Deficit
- Sodium Deficit
- IV Infusion Rate
- Calculated Serum Osmolality
- Predicted Peak Flow (PPF) Females
- Predicted Peak Flow (PPF) Males
- Glomerular Filtration Rate (MDRD)

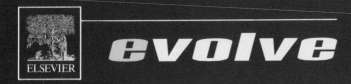

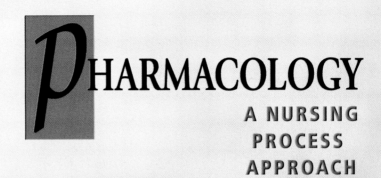

PHARMACOLOGY

A NURSING
PROCESS
APPROACH

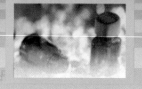
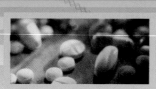
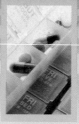
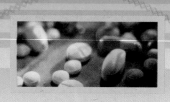
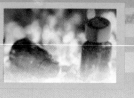

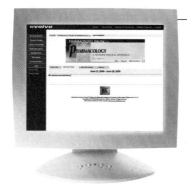
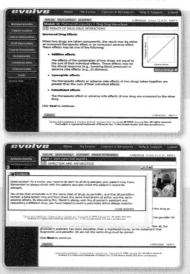
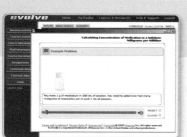
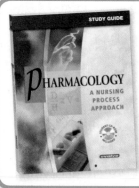

PHARMACOLOGY

$$\frac{D}{H} \times V =$$

5TH EDITION

A NURSING PROCESS APPROACH

Joyce LeFever Kee, MS, RN
Associate Professor Emerita
School of Nursing
College of Health Sciences
University of Delaware
Newark, Delaware

Evelyn R. Hayes, PhD, APRN, BC
Professor
School of Nursing
College of Health Sciences
University of Delaware
Newark, Delaware

Linda E. McCuistion, PhD, RN, ANP, CNS
Professor
Division of Nursing
Our Lady of Holy Cross College
New Orleans, Louisiana

SAUNDERS

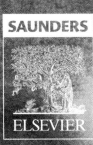

ELSEVIER

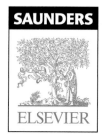

11830 Westline Industrial Drive
St. Louis, MO 63146

PHARMACOLOGY: A NURSING PROCESS APPROACH
Copyright © 2006, Elsevier Inc.

ISBN-13: 978-0-7216-3927-7
ISBN-10: 0-7216-3927-5

Previous editions copyrighted 1993, 1997, 2000, and 2003.

ISBN-13: 978-0-7216-3927-7
ISBN-10: 0-7216-3927-5

Executive Publisher: Robin Carter
Developmental Editor: Deanna Davis
Publishing Services Manager: Jeff Patterson
Project Manager: Clay S. Broeker
Designer: Teresa McBryan

Printed in the United States of America

Last digit is the print number: 9 8 7 6 5 4 3 2 1

Meet the Authors

Joyce LeFever Kee

Evelyn R. Hayes

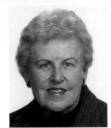

Joyce LeFever Kee received her Bachelor of Science and Master of Science degree in Nursing from the University of Maryland and earned 36 post-graduate credits from the University of Delaware. She was a distinguished faculty educator at the University of Maryland for 4 years and at the University of Delaware for 27 years. The subjects she taught included pharmacology, pathophysiology, fluid and electrolyte imbalances, and medical-surgical nursing in the classroom and clinical areas. She had taught in the undergraduate and graduate programs at the University of Delaware. She retired as Associate Professor Emerita from the University of Delaware.

Joyce is a member of the Sigma Theta Tau Nursing Honor Society and Phi Kappa Phi Honor Society. She received the Excellence in Teaching Award from and was inducted into the Mentor's Circle at the University of Delaware.

Joyce gave numerous lectures and presentations throughout the United States from 1970 to 1990. She has written various subject articles, particularly on fluid and electrolytes, laboratory and diagnostic tests, and research projects, in the *American Journal of Nursing, Nursing Clinics of North America, Nursing Journal*, and *Critical Care Quarterly*. She has participated in several research studies on "Identification of Hypertensive Young Adults."

Joyce has authored and co-authored several text and reference books, including *Fluids and Electrolytes with Clinical Applications* (2004), seventh edition, *Handbook of Fluid, Electrolyte, and Acid-Base Imbalances* (2004), second edition, *Pharmacology: A Nursing Process Approach* (2006), fifth edition, with ancillaries including Companion CD for students, Instructor's Resource CD-ROM, and Study Guide, *Clinical Calculations in General and Specialty Areas* (2004) fifth edition, with Instructor's Manual, Testbank, and CD, *Laboratory and Diagnostic Tests with Nursing Implications* (2005), seventh edition, and *Handbook of Laboratory and Diagnostic Tests with Nursing Implications* (2004), fifth edition.

Joyce and her husband enjoy traveling to various countries, including Australia, New Zealand, China, Japan, Great Britain, Russia, Greece, Italy, France, Turkey, Egypt, Spain, South America, Scandinavian countries, Mexico, the Caribbean islands, and others. They enjoy snorkeling, swimming, and playing golf.

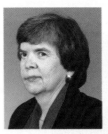

Evelyn (Lyn) R. Hayes received her Bachelor of Science in Nursing from Cornell University—New York Hospital School of Nursing; an MPH in Public Health Nursing from the University of North Carolina, School of Public Health in Chapel Hill, North Carolina; and a PhD in Higher Education from Boston College. In addition, she completed a Post Master's Certificate as Family Nurse Practitioner at the University of Massachusetts at Amherst and is a certified family nurse practitioner. She has valuable practice experience in acute care institutions and in the community. Currently she is Professor in the School of Nursing, College of Health Sciences, at the University of Delaware. In this role she has had teaching responsibilities at both the undergraduate and graduate levels and experience with distance learning. She also serves as Associate Director, UD Nursing Center. Lyn has consulted with faculty in Taiwan and Panama.

A strong advocate of health promotion, Lyn served as Project Director and co-investigator of a U.S. Public Health Service grant Promoting Health Lifestyles in Delaware.

As author, co-author, and collaborative team member, she has published in multiple journals. General areas of interest include smoking cessation in teens and young adults, comprehensive geriatric assessments, and preparing students for perceived threats in the community with recent publications in *Public Health Nursing, Journal of Nursing Education*, and *Nurse Educator*; the use of research based protocols in nursing practice in *Clinical Nurse Specialist*; and issues related to prenatal care in *Journal of Perinatal Education* and *Applied Nursing Research*.

Throughout her career, Lyn has held member and leadership positions at various levels within the University of Delaware as well as professional and community organizations. She has ably provided long-term service and leadership to Sigma Theta Tau International, American Nurses Association, National League for Nursing Accrediting Commission (NLNAC), and the Delaware Nurses Association.

Now a retired colonel in the United States Army Reserve, Lyn's last two assignments were as Principal Reservist to Deputy Commander for Nursing, Walter Reed Army Medical Center, Washington, D.C., and Moncrief Army Community Hospital, Fort Jackson, South Carolina. She also is a frequent traveler, both for pleasure and business. When at her home base, she enjoys being creative with crafts and spending time with friends.

Linda E McCuistion

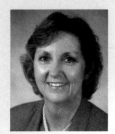

Dr. Linda E. McCuistion received a Diploma of Nursing from the Lutheran Hospital School of Nursing in Fort Wayne, Indiana; BSN from William Carey College in Hattiesburg, Mississippi; MN from Louisiana State University Medical Center; and a PhD in Curriculum and Instruction from the University of New Orleans. She is licensed as an Advanced Practice Nurse and has 35 years of nursing experience, including acute care and home health nursing. Currently, Linda is a Professor in the Division of Nursing at Our Lady of Holy Cross College in New Orleans, Louisiana. She received an Endowed Professorship Award in 2000 and 2003.

Linda has served as a past president, vice-president, and faculty advisor of the Sigma Theta Tau International Honor Society in Nursing, Xi Psi chapter-at-large. She is a past associate editor of the *NODNA Times*, which is the New Orleans District Nurses' Association newsletter. She is a member of Phi Delta Kappa and The American Society of Hypertension.

To ease the transition of new nursing graduates into the workforce, Linda has held the role as coordinator for the Graduate Plus Internship Program, a preceptorship program for new nursing graduates in the state of Louisiana. She has served as a legal nurse consultant and as a member of a medical review panel. Linda is a past Advisory Board Member, Consultant, and Reviewer of a software preparation company for the state licensure examination. She has served as an Advisory Board member for a School for Surgical Technicians. Linda has also served as a consultant to improve the quality of nursing care and to assist acute care facilities in preparation for accreditation.

Linda was chosen as a "Great One Hundred Nurse" by the New Orleans District Nurses' Association in 1993. She is also listed in the 2005/2006 Edition of the Empire Who's Who Executive and Professional Registry.

Linda has given numerous lectures and presentations regionally and nationally on a variety of nursing topics, particularly hypertension, orthopedic assessment, arthritis, multiple organ dysfunction syndrome, Alzheimer's disease, and intravenous workshops. She has published articles in nursing journals and authored many chapters in several nursing textbooks including *Pharmacotherapeutics: Clinical Decision-Making in Nursing* (1999), *Saunders Manual of Medical-Surgical Nursing: A Guide for Clinical Decision-Making* (2002), and the *Real World Nursing Survival Guide: Pathophysiology* (2002). She is author, co-author of many chapters, and co-editor of the *Real World Nursing Survival Guide: Pharmacology* (2002).

Linda enjoys cruises to the Caribbean and traveling to Europe, Aruba, and across the United States. When at home, she enjoys visiting family and friends, playing golf, and writing.

Contributors

Joseph I. Boullata, PharmD, BCNSP
Professor of Pharmacy Practice
School of Pharmacy
Temple University
Philadelphia, Pennsylvania
Appendix D: Herb-Drug Interactions

Robin Webb Corbett, PhD, RN, C
Associate Professor
East Carolina University
School of Nursing
Greenville, North Carolina
Chapters 51, 52, and 53

Sandra Elliott, CNM, MSN
Instructor
University of Delaware
Newark, Delaware
President
Woman to Woman Health Care
Milford, Delaware
Chapters 54 and 56

Judith W. Herrman, PhD, RN
Assistant Chair/Faculty
University of Delaware
Newark, Delaware
Staff Development Instructor
Alfred I. DuPont Hospital for Children
Wilmington, Delaware
Chapter 10

Kathleen J. Jones, RN-C, MS, ANP
Adult Nurse Practitioner
Walter Reed Army Medical Center
Washington, DC
Chapter 55

Robert Kizior, BS, RPh
Education Coordinator
Department of Pharmacy
Alexian Brothers Medical Center
Elk Grove Village, Illinois
Chapter 34

Paula Klemm, DNSc, RN, OCN
Associate Professor
University of Delaware, School of Nursing
Newark, Delaware
Chapter 36

Anne E. Lara, RN, MS, AOCN, APRN, BC
Manager
Siemens Medical-Health Services
Malvern, Pennsylvania
Chapter 37

Linda Laskowski-Jones, RN, MS, APRN, BC, CCRN, CEN
Director
Trauma, Emergency and Aeromedical Services
Christiana Care Health System
Christiana Hospital
Newark, Delaware
Chapter 57

Patricia Graber O'Brien, MA, MSN, APRN, BC
Instructor
University of New Mexico
Certified Clinical Research Coordinator
Lovelace Scientific Resources
Albuquerque, New Mexico
Chapter 8

Laura K. Williford Owens, PharmD
Assistant Professor
Department of Pharmacy Practice
Campbell University School of Pharmacy
Buies Creek, North Carolina
Chapters 51, 52, and 53

Lisa Ann Plowfield, PhD, RN
Professor and Chairperson
School of Nursing
University of Delaware
Newark, Delaware
Chapter 34

Larry Purnell, PhD, RN, FAAN
Professor
University of Delaware
Newark, Delaware
Chapter 6

Lynette M. Wachholz, MN, APRN, IBCLC
Clinical Faculty
University of Washington Department of Family and Child Nursing
Seattle, Washington
Pediatric Nurse Practitioner and Lactation Consultant
The Everett Clinic
Everett, Washington
Chapter 35

Reviewers

Nancy Balkon, PhD, ANP-C
Clinical Associate Professor
School of Nursing
Stony Brook University
Stony Brook, New York

Rebecca A. Cappo, RN, MSN
Instructor
Allied Health Technology
Lenape Technical School
Ford City, Pennsylvania

Jennifer Chan, PharmD
Clinical Assistant Professor
Pharmacotherapy
University of Texas at Austin
College of Pharmacy
San Antonio, Texas

Doris Dennison, MSN, NP, ACNP
Clinical Instructor
Wayne State University
College of Nursing
Detroit, Michigan

Robert Ekas, Jr., PhD
Pharmaceutical Medical Liaison
Bristol-Myers Squibb
New Orleans, Louisiana

Alice Gardner, PhD
Assistant Professor of Pharmacology and Toxicology
Pharmaceutical Sciences
Massachusetts College of Pharmacy
Worcester, Massachusetts

Shirley Garick, PhD, RN
Associate Professor of Nursing
Nursing College of Health and Behavioral Sciences
Texas A & M University
Texarkana, Texas

Margaret Gingrich, RN, MSN
Professor of Nursing
Hamsburg Area Community College
Mechanicsburg, Pennsylvania

Andrea Knesek, MSN, BSN, BC
Faculty
Department of Nursing
Macomb Community College
Warren, Michigan

Georgiana Leavesley, RN, MSN, PhD
Division of Nursing
Our Lady of Holy Cross College
New Orleans, Louisiana

Brenda Pavill, RN, PhD, IBCLC
Associate Professor
Nursing Department
College Misericordia
Dallas, Pennsylvania

Roberta J. Secrest, PhD, PharmD, RPh
Eli Lilly and Company
Indianapolis, Indiana

Wanda C. Wagner, RN, MSN
Division of Nursing
Our Lady of Holy Cross College
New Orleans, Louisiana

Michele Welch, MSN, RN
Senior Director of Study Delivery
Astra Zeneca
Wilmington, Delaware

In Loving Memory of My Parents
Esther B. and Samuel H. LeFever

Joyce LeFever Kee

To My Parents
Margaret and Justin Hayes
for their ever-present love and confidence

Evelyn R. Hayes

To Dr. Gerald DeLuca for expert guidance
and my mother, Pauline E. Schmidt

Linda E. McCuistion

Preface

The fifth edition of *Pharmacology: A Nursing Process Approach* is written for students in a variety of nursing programs who can benefit from its presentation of the principles of pharmacology in a straightforward, student-friendly manner. It focuses on need-to-know content and it helps students learn to administer drugs safely and eliminate medication errors through extensive practice in dosage calculation and careful application of the nursing process.

Organization

Pharmacology: A Nursing Process Approach is organized into **17 units** and **57 chapters.** Unit One is an overview of the principles of pharmacology from the unique perspective of nursing. The unit begins with chapters on drug action, the nursing process and client teaching, and principles of drug administration. Unit Two, Chapter 4: Medications and Calculations—a comprehensive review of drug dosage calculation for adults and children—is a unique strength of this book. This extensive unit—tabbed for quick reference—consists of six sections:

- Section 4A: Systems of Measurement with Conversion
- Section 4B: Methods for Calculation
- Section 4C: Calculations of Oral Dosages
- Section 4D: Calculations of Injectable Dosages
- Section 4E: Calculations of Intravenous Fluids
- Section 4F: Pediatric Drug Calculations

Unit Two presents **six methods of dosage calculation, color-coded to identify each method:**

- Method 1: Basic Formula
- Method 2: Ratio and Proportion
- Method 3: Fractional Equation
- Method 4: Dimensional Analysis (expanded in this edition)
- Method 5: Body Weight
- Method 6: Body Surface Area

Integral to Unit Two are its **clinical practice problems,** featuring **80 actual drug labels in full color,** which provide extensive practice in real-world dosage calculations. With this wide array of practice problems in a variety of health care settings, the chapter eliminates the need to purchase a separate dosage calculation book. In addition, color photographs illustrate the equipment used to deliver medications. The accompanying Study Guide and **new Companion CD** included with the text provide additional practice problems with answers, a review of need-to-know mathematics, printable checklists, and more.

Unit Three covers contemporary issues in pharmacology, including the changing drug approval process (Chapter 5), drug interactions and over-the-counter drugs (Chapter 7), a **new chapter dedicated to discussion of drugs of abuse**

(Chapter 8), and more. The book promotes a global approach toward client care with a separate transcultural considerations chapter (Chapter 6), updated and expanded for the fifth edition. An expanded chapter on herbal therapy (Chapter 9) discusses client self-treatment with herbal products and its nursing implications. Lifespan issues are addressed in chapters on pediatric and geriatric pharmacology (Chapters 10 and 11).

Unit Four addresses nutrition and fluids and electrolytes, with separate chapters covering vitamin and mineral replacement (Chapter 14), fluid and electrolyte replacement (Chapter 15), and nutritional support (Chapter 16).

Units Five through Seventeen are the core of *Pharmacology: A Nursing Process Approach* and cover the drug families that students will need to understand in order to practice effectively. Each drug family chapter includes a chapter outline, learning objectives, a list of key terms, at least one Prototype Drug Chart, a drug table, and an extensive Nursing Process section.

The **Prototype Drug Charts**—over 100 throughout the fifth edition—are a unique tool that students can use to view the many facets of a prototype drug through the lens of the nursing process. Each of these charts includes Drug Class, Trade Names, Contraindications, Dosage, Drug-Lab-Food Interactions, Pharmacokinetics, Pharmacodynamics, Therapeutic Effects/Uses, Side Effects, and Adverse Reactions. With these charts, students can see how the steps of the Nursing Process correlate with these key aspects of drug information and therapy.

The **drug tables** are a quick reference to routes, dosages, uses, and considerations for the most commonly prescribed medications for a given class. They provide drug names (generic, trade, and Canadian), dosages, uses and considerations, pregnancy categories, pharmacodynamics, and pharmacokinetics.

The **Nursing Process sections**—redesigned for this edition—provide a convenient summary of how to assess a client, develop nursing diagnoses, determine and follow through with the plan of care, and evaluate the outcomes of your efforts. The Nursing Process sections also include highlighted **culturally sensitive content (denoted with a ⊕ symbol), nursing interventions,** suggestions for **client teaching,** and **new herbal information ( ).**

New to this Edition

The fifth edition of *Pharmacology: A Nursing Process Approach* features several significant new components.

As noted previously, **dimensional analysis** content has been expanded in Chapter 4. In addition, each of the six methods of calculation—basic formula, ratio and proportion, fractional equation, dimensional analysis, body weight, and body surface area—are **consistently highlighted with a unique color**, making it easier to facilitate quick location of the appropriate method for review.

With herbal therapies now seen more in mainstream health care, an understanding of drug-herb interactions is becoming critical. To address this need, this edition includes over **30 Herbal Alert boxes** throughout the drug family chapters. Herbal Alert boxes provide a convenient overview of herbs that interact with drug groups, either by enhancing or inhibiting drug actions. In addition, we have expanded herbal information in the Nursing Process sections (identified with an herbal interactions icon, as mentioned previously). Also added is a new herb-drug interaction appendix, which compliments the drug-drug interaction list already provided.

Because of the ever-expanding number of drugs available, pharmacology can be an overwhelming subject. To help students grasp essential content without becoming overwhelmed, we have divided several units and chapters into multiple smaller chapters. The result is **a revised layout of chapters and units which will be more user-friendly:**

- New Unit Five, Autonomic Nervous System Agents: discusses adrenergics/adrenergic blockers and cholinergics/anticholinergics
- Drugs for Pain Management: retitled for clarity of content and expanded to include discussion of pain as the fifth vital sign
- Drugs for Neurologic Disorders and Drugs for Neuromuscular Disorders: divided into two chapters for easier location of content
- New Unit Seven, Psychiatric Agents: containing discussion on antipsycholytics/anxiolytics and antidepressants/mood stabilizers
- Cardiac Glycosides, Antianginals, and Antidysrhymics: retitled for clarity of content
- Circulatory disorders divided into two chapters for easier location of content: Anticoagulants, Antiplatelets, and Thrombolytics, and Antilipidemics and Peripheral Vasodilators
- Expanded appendix section: now including information on alcohol- and sugar-free products, the most frequently prescribed drugs, herb-drug interaction list, and drugs as weapons of bioterrorism

Also new to this edition, we have provided **expanded unit introductions,** with illustrated overviews of anatomy and physiology. Drug information has been updated throughout, including the **latest FDA-approved drugs in all categories. A quick reference to selected drug interactions** is provided in Appendix C.

Abbreviations used throughout the text have been revised thoroughly to be consistent with the **newest JCAHO guidelines**. This compliance is part of a refined focus toward the prevention of medication errors, which is discussed in detail in Chapter 3 and seen in the **new Preventing Medication Error boxes** now found through-

out the text. The commonly used abbreviations appendix has been thoroughly revised to reflect JCAHO guidelines.

Additional Features

Throughout this edition, we have retained and enhanced a variety of popular features that teach students the fundamental principles of pharmacology as well as the role of the nurse in drug therapy:

- **Coverage of Pathophysiology.** Relevant pathophysiology is included in Units Five through Seventeen. Understanding the pathophysiology of disease processes is foundational to understanding the rationale for drug therapy.
- **Nursing Process.** In addition to the revised and expanded Nursing Process content and inclusion of the nursing process in the Prototype Drug Charts, each chapter includes clearly delineated coverage of all five steps of the nursing process, with the following headings: Assessment, Nursing Diagnoses, Planning, Nursing Interventions, and Evaluation.
- **Client Teaching.** Under Nursing Interventions, we include client and family teaching information. This content has been expanded in the fifth edition and now includes helpful **teaching tips** that relate to general information, self-administration, diet, side effects, and cultural considerations.
- **Cultural Considerations.** In addition to an entire chapter discussing general cultural considerations in drug therapy (expanded from the fourth edition), this text includes Cultural Considerations in the Nursing Interventions sections of the Nursing Process.
- **Critical Thinking Case Studies.** Each chapter concludes with a clinical scenario, followed by a series of critical thinking questions. These exercises challenge students to carefully consider the scenario and apply their knowledge and analytical skills to respond to the situations. Answers are provided only in the Instructor's Manual, to encourage thorough consideration before seeking expert feedback.
- **Study Questions.** At the end of each chapter, a series of Study Questions provides students with an immediate review and reinforces the objectives of the chapter. Students can scan the content of the chapter to confirm their answers.
- **Electronic Resources boxes, new to this edition,** provide internet and other database resource information for more in-depth researching of the material discussed within each chapter.

Additional Teaching and Learning Resources

The fifth edition of *Pharmacology: A Nursing Process Approach* is the core of a complete teaching and learning package for nursing pharmacology. Additional components of this package include resources for students, resources for both students and faculty members, and resources just for faculty members.

For Students

A comprehensive *Study Guide* provides more than 1800 study questions and answers, including clinically based situational practice problems, more than 160 drug calculation problems and questions (many with actual drug labels), and critical thinking exercises to help students master textbook content. Question formats include multiple-choice, matching, word searches, crossword puzzles, and completion exercises. Answers—with detailed math solutions and rationales, where appropriate—are provided at the end of the Study Guide.

For Both Students and Faculty

A completely updated website (*http://evolve.elsevier.com/KeeHayes/pharmacology/*) provides additional resources for students and faculty, including content updates, answers to frequently asked questions, information on drugs recently approved or withdrawn by the FDA, case studies, suggestions for using the book in various programs, and teaching tips. The site is updated periodically to keep both faculty members and students informed of the latest information in nursing pharmacology.

A **new Companion CD** is now provided in the back of each fifth edition text, a valuable *free* learning tool including NCLEX-style review questions, animations, IV therapy and medication error checklists, drug calculation problems, and electronic calculators for applying various formulas used in the text.

All faculty and students using *Pharmacology: A Nursing Process Approach*, fifth edition, are entitled to free basic-level access to *Mosby's Drug Consult Internet Edition*, a resource with information on new drug approvals, new indications for existing drugs, and drug safety notices. To access this resource, log on to *mosbysdrugconsult.com*.

Just for Faculty Members

An *Instructor's Electronic Resource CD-ROM* is available for faculty members. This "IER" includes a complete Instructor's Manual that contains learning objectives,

chapter outlines, and teaching strategies to promote critical thinking. The Instructor's Manual also provides a basic math test with answers. Faculty members can incorporate their own materials into the Instructor's Manual or simply print chapters out as provided.

The IER contains a thoroughly revised and expanded Test Bank featuring almost 1000 NCLEX-style questions in ExamView format, with nursing process step, cognitive level, rationale, and cross-referencing to related content in the text.

Also included is an Electronic Image Collection containing 150 images, and a collection of more than 300 PowerPoint text slides. **New to the fifth edition are unique interactive slides**, presenting questions or case studies to provoke further thought during class time. These electronic images and PowerPoint slides can be imported into any electronic lecture presentation or printed on transparency acetates.

Pharmacology Online, **a unique new library of online assets** including case studies, video and clips, interactive learning activities, animations, image collection, PowerPoint presentations, test bank, drug calculation review, and much more, is now available for faculty who want to find a wealth of course-building resources in one convenient location. *Pharmacology Online* will enable you to build a web-enhanced nursing pharmacology course corresponding to the fifth edition text.

Also available for faculty is the *Elsevier ePharmacology Update*. Prepared by Evelyn Salerno, PharmD, this full-color, quarterly newsletter provides current and well-documented information on new drugs, drug warnings, medication errors, and more.

It is our hope that *Pharmacology: A Nursing Process Approach* and its comprehensive ancillary package will serve as a dynamic resource for teaching nursing students the basic principles of pharmacology and their vital role in drug therapy.

Joyce LeFever Kee

Evelyn R. Hayes

Linda E. McCuistion

Acknowledgements

We wish to extend our sincere appreciation to the many professionals who assisted in the preparation of the fifth edition of *Pharmacology: A Nursing Process Approach* by reviewing chapters and offering suggestions.

We wish to especially thank the authors of the new chapters and the original authors and those who updated the established chapters: Larry D. Purnell, PhD, RN, FAAN; Patricia S. Lincoln, BSN, RN; Robert Kizior, BS, RPh; Judith W. Herrman, PhD, RNC; Lynette M. Wachholz, MN, APRN, IBCLC; Anne E. Lara, RN, MS, AOCN, APRN, BC; Jane Purnell Taylor, RN, MS; Linda Goodwin, RNC, MEd; Nancy C. Sharts-Hopko, RN, PhD, FAAN; Kathleen J. Jones, RN-C, MS, ANP; Linda Laskowski-Jones, RN, MS, APRN, BC, CCRN, CEN; Ronald J. LeFever, RN, RPh; Patricia Graber O'Brien, MA, MSN, APRN, BC; Lisa A. Plowfield, PhD, RN; Paula Klemm, DNSc, RN, OCN; Robin Webb Corbett, PhD, RN, C; Laura K. Williford Owens, PharmD; and Sandra Elliott, CNM, MSN.

Of course, we are deeply indebted to the many clients and students we have had throughout our many years of professional nursing practice. From them we have learned many fine points about the role of therapeutic pharmacology in nursing practice.

Our deepest appreciation goes to pharmaceutical companies for permission to use their drug labels. Pharmaceutical companies that extended their courtesy to this book include:

Abbott Laboratories	Mead Johnson
American Home Products	Pharmaceuticals
Lederale Laboratories	E. R. Squibb and Sons, Inc.
American Regent	**DuPont/Merck**
Luitold Pharmaceuticals	**Pharmaceuticals**
Astra Zeneca	**Eli Lilly and Company**
Pharmaceuticals	**Elkins-Sinn, Inc.**
Bayer Corporation Inc.	A subsidiary of A. H. Robins
Bristol-Myers Squibb Co.	**Glaxo-SmithKline**
Apothecon Laboratories	**Marion Merrell Dow, Inc.**

McNeilab, Inc.	**SmithKline Beecham**
McNeil Consumer	**Pharmaceutical**
Products Co.	**Warner-Lambert**
Ortho-McNeil	**Consumer Health**
Pharmaceutical	**Products**
Merck and Co., Inc.	Parke-Davis
Mylan Pharmaceuticals	**Wyeth-Ayerst Laboratories**
Pfizer Inc.	

We extend our sincere thanks to the companies and publishers who gave us permission to use photographs, illustrations, and other materials in the text. These include:

American Association of	**F. A. Davis**
Critical-Care Nursing	**IMED Corporation**
Appleton & Lange	**Medical Letter, Inc.**
Baxter Healthcare Corp.	**MiniMED, Inc.**
Becton-Dickinson Division	**Prentice Hall Health**
Ciba-Geigy	**Pyxis System**
Pharmaceuticals	**Wyeth-Ayerst Laboratories**
Elsevier, Inc.	
Mosby, Inc.	
W.B. Saunders	

Our sincere and deepest thanks to the staff at Elsevier, especially Robin Carter, Executive Publisher, Nursing Books; Deanna Davis, Developmental Editor, Nursing; Clay Broeker, Project Manager; and Jeff Patterson, Publishing Services Manager, for their suggestions and assistance. Also, thanks to Don Passidomo, librarian at the Department of Veterans Affairs, Wilmington, Delaware, for his help with library research.

Appreciation and love go out to my husband, Edward D. Kee (JLK), to my parents, Margaret K. and Justin F. Hayes (ERH), and to Robert Ekas, Jr. (LEM), for their support.

Joyce LeFever Kee

Evelyn R. Hayes

Linda E. McCuistion

Contents

Sixteen

Reproductive and Gender-Related Agents, 791

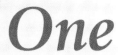

One

A Nurse's Perspective of Pharmacology

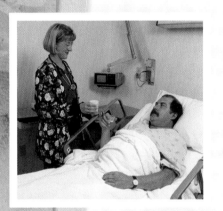

Assessing a client's response to drug therapy is an ongoing nursing responsibility. To adequately assess, plan, intervene, and evaluate drug effects, the nurse needs to have knowledge of the pharmaceutic, pharmacokinetic, and pharmacodynamic phases of drug action, all of which are described in Chapter 1, Drug Action: Pharmaceutic, Pharmacokinetic, and Pharmacodynamic Phases. A drug chart organizes specific drug data needed for preparation and application of the nursing process (see Chapter 2, Nursing Process and Client Teaching). Client teaching, also discussed in Chapter 2, is essential to promote client and family adherence to the drug regimen and therapy.

Along with understanding the three phases of drug action, the nursing process, and client teaching, two other important functions in nursing practice include application of drug administration principles and calculation of drug doses. Chapter 3, Principles of Drug Administration, contains basic learning material for the administration of medications. It describes the "ten rights" in drug administration, drug orders, drug distribution, drug charts, drug administration guidelines, and drug administration routes (with illustrated parenteral sites).

Chapter 3 and Unit Two may be used for drug administration and calculation in place of a nursing fundamentals text or a drug calculation text.

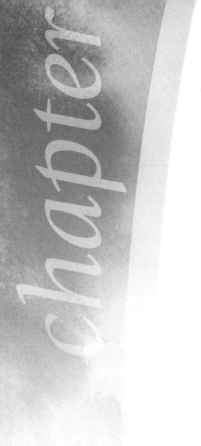

1

Drug Action: Pharmaceutic, Pharmacokinetic, and Pharmacodynamic Phases

ELECTRONIC RESOURCES *evolve*

Additional information can be found on the companion website at *http://evolve.elsevier.com/KeeHayes/pharmacology/* or on the companion CD-ROM, which includes:
- *NCLEX-style examination review questions*
- *Pharmacology animations*
- *Medication error and IV therapy checklists*
- *Medication calculation problems*
- *Electronic calculators*

OBJECTIVES

- Differentiate the three phases of drug action.
- Identify the two processes that occur before tablets are absorbed into the body.
- Describe the four processes of pharmacokinetics.
- Explain the meaning of *pharmacodynamics, dose response, maximal efficacy,* the *receptor,* and *nonreceptors* in drug action.
- Define the terms *protein-bound drugs, half-life, therapeutic index, therapeutic drug range, side effects, adverse reaction,* and *drug toxicity.*
- Check drugs for half-life, percentage of protein-binding effect, therapeutic range, and side effects in a drug reference book.
- Describe the nursing implications of pharmacokinetics and pharmacodynamics.

TERMS

active absorption	excipients	onset of action	rate limiting
adverse reactions	first-pass effect	passive absorption	receptors
agonists	free drugs	peak action	side effects
antagonists	half-life ($t^1/_2$)	peak drug level	tachyphylaxis
bioavailability	high therapeutic index	pharmaceutic phase	therapeutic index (TI)
creatinine clearance (CL_{cr})	ligand-binding domain	pharmacodynamics	therapeutic range (thera-
disintegration	loading dose	pharmacogenetics	peutic window)
dissolution	low therapeutic index	pharmacokinetics	time-response curve
distribution	metabolism	pinocytosis	toxic effects
duration of action	nonselective drugs	placebo effect	toxicity
elimination	nonspecific drugs	protein-binding effect	trough level

Introduction

A drug taken by mouth goes through three phases—pharmaceutic (dissolution), pharmacokinetic, and pharmacodynamic—as drug actions occur. In the pharmaceutic phase, the drug becomes a solution so that it can cross the biologic membrane. When the drug is administered parenterally by subcutaneous (subQ), intramuscular (IM), or intravenous (IV) routes, there is no pharmaceutic phase. The second phase, the pharmacokinetic phase, is composed of four processes: absorption, distribution, metabolism (or biotransformation), and excretion (or elimination). In the pharmacodynamic phase, a biologic or physiologic response results.

Pharmaceutic Phase

Approximately 80% of drugs are taken by mouth. The **pharmaceutic phase** (dissolution) is the first phase of drug action. In the gastrointestinal (GI) tract, drugs need to be in solution so they can be absorbed. A drug in solid form (tablet or capsule) must disintegrate into small particles to dissolve into a liquid, a process known as *dissolution*. Drugs in liquid form are already in solution. Figure 1–1 displays the pharmaceutic phase of a tablet.

Tablets are not 100% drug. Fillers and inert substances, generally called **excipients**, are used in drug preparation to allow the drug to take on a particular size and shape and to enhance drug dissolution. Some additives in drugs, such as the ions potassium (K) and sodium (Na) in penicillin potassium and penicillin sodium, increase the absorbability of the drug. Penicillin is poorly absorbed by the GI tract because of gastric acid. However, by making the drug a potassium or sodium salt, penicillin can then be absorbed. An infant's gas-

tric secretions have a higher pH (alkaline) than those of adults; therefore infants can absorb more penicillin.

Disintegration is the breakdown of a tablet into smaller particles. **Dissolution** is the dissolving of the smaller particles in the GI fluid before absorption. **Rate limiting** is the time it takes the drug to disintegrate and dissolve to become available for the body to absorb it. Drugs in liquid form are more rapidly available for GI absorption than are solids. Generally, drugs are both disintegrated and absorbed faster in acidic fluids with a pH of 1 or 2 rather than in alkaline fluids. Both the very young and the elderly have less gastric acidity; therefore drug absorption is generally slower for those drugs absorbed primarily in the stomach.

Enteric-coated drugs resist disintegration in the gastric acid of the stomach, so disintegration does not occur until the drug reaches the alkaline environment of the small intestine. Enteric-coated tablets can remain in the stomach for a long time; therefore their effect may be delayed in onset. Enteric-coated tablets or capsules and sustained-release (beaded) capsules *should not be crushed*. Crushing would alter the place and time of absorption of the drug.

Food in the GI tract may interfere with the dissolution and absorption of certain drugs. However, food can also enhance absorption of other drugs; thus some drugs should be taken with food. Some drugs irritate the gastric mucosa, so fluids or food may be necessary to dilute drug concentration and to act as protectants.

Pharmacokinetic Phase

Pharmacokinetics is the process of drug movement to achieve drug action. The four processes are absorption, distribution, metabolism (or biotransformation), and excretion (or elimination). The nurse applies knowledge of pharmacokinetics when assessing the client for possible adverse drug effects. The nurse communicates assessment findings to members of the health care team in a timely manner to promote safe and effective drug therapy for the client.

Absorption

Absorption is the movement of drug particles from the GI tract to body fluids by passive absorption, active absorption, or pinocytosis. Most oral drugs are absorbed into the

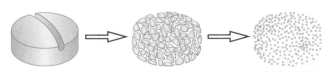

TABLET   **DISINTEGRATION**   **DISSOLUTION**

FIGURE 1–1 The two pharmaceutic phases are disintegration and dissolution.

surface area of the small intestine through the action of the extensive mucosal villi. Absorption is reduced if the villi are decreased in number because of disease, drug effect, or the removal of small intestine. Protein-based drugs, such as insulin and growth hormones, are destroyed in the small intestine by digestive enzymes. **Passive absorption** occurs mostly by diffusion (movement from higher concentration to lower concentration). With the process of diffusion, the drug does not require energy to move across the membrane. **Active absorption** requires a carrier, such as an enzyme or protein, to move the drug against a concentration gradient. Energy is required for active absorption. **Pinocytosis** is a process by which cells carry drug across their membrane by engulfing the drug particles (Figure 1–2).

The GI membrane is composed mostly of lipid (fat) and protein, so drugs that are lipid soluble pass rapidly through the GI membrane. Water-soluble drugs need a carrier, either enzyme or protein, to pass through the membrane. Large particles pass through the cell membrane if they are nonionized (no positive or negative charge). Weak acid drugs, such as aspirin, are less ionized in the stomach, and they pass through the stomach lining easily and rapidly. Certain drugs, such as calcium carbonate and many of the antifungals, need an acidic environment to achieve greater drug absorption; thus food can stimulate the production of gastric acid. Hydrochloric acid destroys some drugs, such as penicillin G; therefore a large oral dosage of penicillin is needed to offset the partial dose loss. Drugs administered by many routes do not pass through the GI tract or liver, including parenteral drugs, eyedrops, eardrops, nasal sprays, respiratory inhalants, transdermal drugs, and sublingual drugs.

REMEMBER: Drugs that are lipid soluble and nonionized are absorbed *faster* than water-soluble and ionized drugs.

Blood flow, pain, stress, hunger, fasting, food, and pH affect drug absorption. Poor circulation as a result of shock, vasoconstrictor drugs, or disease hampers absorption. Pain, stress, and foods that are solid, hot, and fatty can slow gastric emptying time, so the drug remains in the stomach longer. Exercise can decrease blood flow by causing more blood to flow to the peripheral muscle, thereby decreasing blood circulation to the GI tract.

Drugs given IM are absorbed faster in muscles that have more blood vessels, such as the deltoid, than in those that have fewer blood vessels, such as the gluteal. Subcutaneous tissue has fewer blood vessels, so absorption is slower in such tissue.

Some drugs do *not* go directly into the systemic circulation following oral absorption but pass from the intestinal lumen to the liver via the portal vein. In the liver, some drugs may be metabolized to an inactive form, which may then be excreted, thus reducing the amount of active drug. Some drugs do not undergo metabolism at all in the liver, and others may be metabolized to drug metabolite, which may be equally or more active than the original drug. The process in which the drug passes to the

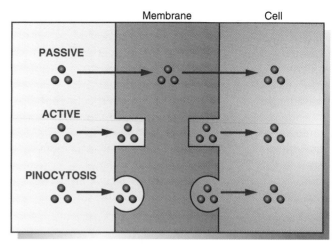

FIGURE 1–2 The three major processes for drug absorption through the gastrointestinal membrane are passive absorption, active absorption, and pinocytosis.

liver first is called the **first-pass effect,** or hepatic first pass. Examples of drugs with first-pass metabolism are warfarin (Coumadin) and morphine. Lidocaine and some nitroglycerins are *not* given orally because they have extensive first-pass metabolism and therefore most of the dose would be destroyed.

Bioavailability is a subcategory of absorption. It is the percentage of the administered drug dose that reaches the systemic circulation. For the oral route of drug administration, bioavailability occurs after absorption and hepatic drug metabolism. The percentage of bioavailability for the oral route is always less than 100% but for the intravenous route it is usually 100%. Oral drugs that have a high first-pass hepatic metabolism may have a bioavailability of only 20% to 40% on entering systemic circulation. To obtain the desired drug effect, the oral dose could be three to five times larger than the drug dose for IV use.

Factors that alter bioavailability include (1) the drug form (e.g., tablet, capsule, sustained-release, liquid, transdermal patch, rectal suppository, inhalation), (2) route of administration (e.g., oral, rectal, topical, parenteral), (3) GI mucosa and motility, (4) food and other drugs, and (5) changes in liver metabolism caused by liver dysfunction or inadequate hepatic blood flow. A decrease in liver function or a decrease in hepatic blood flow can increase the bioavailability of a drug but only if the drug is metabolized by the liver. Less drug is destroyed by hepatic metabolism in the presence of liver disorder.

With some oral drugs, rapid absorption increases the bioavailability of the drug and can cause an increase in drug concentration. Drug toxicity may result. Slow absorption can limit the bioavailability of the drug, thus causing a decrease in drug serum concentration.

Distribution

Distribution is the process by which the drug becomes available to body fluids and body tissues. Drug distribution is influenced by blood flow, its affinity to the tissue,

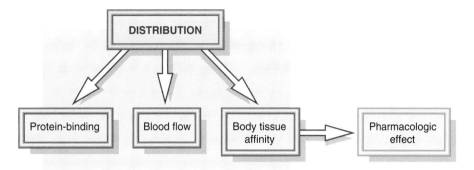

FIGURE 1–3 Drug distribution.

and the **protein-binding effect** (Figure 1–3). In addition, volume of drug distribution (Vd) is dependent on drug dose and its concentration in the body. Drugs with a larger volume of drug distribution have a longer half-life (see Metabolism, or Biotransformation, later in this chapter), and thus these drugs stay in the body longer.

As drugs are distributed in the plasma, many are bound to varying degrees (percentages) with protein (primarily albumin). Drugs that are greater than 89% bound to protein are known as *highly protein-bound drugs;* drugs that are 61% to 89% bound to protein are *moderately highly protein-bound;* drugs that are 30% to 60% bound to protein are *moderately protein-bound;* and drugs that are less than 30% bound to protein are *low protein-bound drugs.* Table 1–1 lists selected highly protein-bound drugs and moderately highly protein-bound drugs. The portion of the drug that is bound is inactive because it is not available to receptors, and the portion that remains unbound is free, active drug. Only **free drugs** (drugs not bound to protein) are active and can cause a pharmacologic response. As the free drug in the circulation decreases, more bound drug is released from the protein to maintain the balance of free drug.

When two highly protein-bound drugs are given concurrently, they compete for protein-binding sites, thus causing more free drug to be released into the circulation. In this situation, drug accumulation and possible drug toxicity can result. Also, a low protein level decreases the number of protein-binding sites and can cause an increase in the amount of free drug in the plasma. Drug overdose may then result. Drug dose is prescribed according to the percentage in which the drug binds to protein.

With some health conditions that result in a low serum protein level, excess free or unbound drug goes to nonspecific tissue binding sites until needed and excess free drug in the circulation does not occur.

Some drugs bind with a specific protein component such as albumin or globulin. Most anticonvulsants bind primarily to albumin. Some basic drugs, such as antidysrhythmics (e.g., lidocaine, quinidine), bind mostly to globulins.

Clients with liver or kidney disease or who are malnourished may have an abnormally low serum albumin level. This results in fewer protein-binding sites, which, in turn, leads to excess free drug and eventually to drug toxicity. The elderly are more likely to have hypoalbuminemia.

Checking the protein-binding percentage of all drugs administered to a client is important to avoid possible drug toxicity. The nurse should also check the client's plasma protein and albumin levels because a decrease in plasma protein (albumin) decreases protein-binding sites, permitting more free drug in the circulation. Depending on the drug, the result could be life threatening.

Abscesses, exudates, body glands, and tumors hinder drug distribution. Antibiotics do not distribute well at abscess and exudate sites. In addition, some drugs accumulate in particular tissues, such as fat, bone, liver, muscle, and eye tissues.

Metabolism, or Biotransformation

Drugs can be metabolized in both the GI tract and liver; however, the liver is the primary site of **metabolism.** Most drugs are inactivated by liver enzymes and are then converted or transformed by hepatic enzymes to inactive metabolites or water-soluble substances for excretion. A large percentage of drugs are lipid soluble; thus the liver metabolizes the lipid-soluble drug substance to a water-soluble substance for renal excretion. However, some drugs are transformed into active metabolites, causing an increased pharmacologic response. Liver diseases, such as cirrhosis and hepatitis, alter drug metabolism by inhibiting the drug-metabolizing enzymes in the liver. When the drug metabolism rate is decreased, excess drug accumulation can occur, which can lead to toxicity.

The **half-life (t½)** of a drug is the time it takes for one half of the drug concentration to be eliminated. Metabolism and elimination affect the half-life of a drug. For example, with liver or kidney dysfunction, the half-life of the drug is prolonged and less drug is metabolized and eliminated. When a drug is taken continually, drug accumulation may occur. Table 1–1 gives the half-life of selected drugs.

A drug goes through several half-lives before more than 90% of the drug is eliminated. If the client takes 650 mg of aspirin and the half-life is 3 hours, it takes 3 hours for the first half-life to eliminate 325 mg, 6 hours for the second half-life to eliminate an additional 162 mg, and so on until the sixth half-life (or 18 hours), when 10 mg of aspirin is left in the body (Table 1–2). A short half-life is considered to be 4 to 8 hours, and a long one is 24 hours or longer. If the drug has a long half-life (such as digoxin at

Table 1–1

Protein-Binding and Half-Life of Drugs

Drug	Protein-Bound (%)	Half-Life (t½) (h)
Highly Protein-Bound Drugs (>89%)		
amitriptyline	97	40
chlorpromazine	95	30
diazepam	98	30-80
dicloxacillin	95	0.5-1
digitoxin	90	8
furosemide	95	1.5
ibuprofen	98	2-4
lorazepam	92	15
piroxicam	99	30-86
propranolol	92	4
rifampin	89	2
sulfisoxazole	85-95	4.5-7.5
valproic acid	92	15
Moderately Highly Protein-Bound Drugs (61%-89%)		
erythromycin	70	3
nafcillin	86	2-20
phenytoin	88	10-40
quinidine	70	6
trimethoprim	70	11
Moderately Protein-Bound Drugs (30%-60%)		
aspirin	49	0.25-2
lidocaine	50	2
meperidine	56	3
pindolol	40	3-4
theophylline	60	9
ticarcillin	45-65	1-1.5
Low Protein-Bound Drugs (<30%)		
amikacin	4-11	2-3
amoxicillin	20	1-1.5
atenolol	6-16	6-7
cephalexin	10-15	0.5-1.2
digoxin	25	36
neostigmine bromide	15-25	1-1.5
terbutaline sulfate	25	3-11
timolol maleate	<10	3-4
tobramycin sulfate	10	2-3

h, Hour; >, greater than; <, less than.

36 hours), it takes several days for the body to completely eliminate the drug.

By knowing the half-life, the time it takes for a drug to reach a steady state of serum concentration can be computed. Administration of the drug for three to five half-lives saturates the biologic system to the extent that the intake of drug equals the amount metabolized and excreted. An example is digoxin, which has a half-life of 36 hours with normal renal function. It would take approximately 5 days to 1 week (three to five half-lives) to reach a steady state for digoxin concentration. Steady-state serum concentration is predictive of therapeutic drug effect. The half-life of drugs is also discussed under Pharmacodynamic Phase.

Excretion, or Elimination

The main route of drug **elimination** is through the kidneys (urine). Other routes include hepatic metabolism, bile, feces, lungs, saliva, sweat, and breast milk. The kidneys filter free, unbound drugs; water-soluble drugs; and drugs that are unchanged. Protein-bound drugs cannot be filtered through the kidneys. Once the drug is released from the protein, it is a free drug and is eventually excreted in the urine. The lungs eliminate volatile drug substances and products metabolized to carbon dioxide (CO_2) and water (H_2O).

The urine pH influences drug excretion. Urine pH varies from 4.5 to 8. Acid urine promotes elimination of weak base drugs, and alkaline urine promotes elimination of weak acid drugs. Aspirin, a weak acid, is excreted rapidly in alkaline urine. If a person takes an overdose of aspirin, sodium bicarbonate may be given to change the urine pH to alkaline to help potentiate excretion of the drug. Large quantities of cranberry juice can decrease urine pH, causing an acid urine and thus inhibiting the elimination of aspirin.

With a kidney disease that results in decreased glomerular filtration rate (GFR) or decreased renal tubular secretion, drug excretion is slowed or impaired. Drug accumulation with possible severe adverse drug reactions can result. A decrease in blood flow to the kidneys can also alter drug excretion.

The most accurate test to determine renal function is **creatinine clearance (CL$_{cr}$)**. Creatinine is a metabolic byproduct of muscle that is excreted by the kidneys. Creatinine clearance varies with age and gender. Lower values are expected in elderly and female clients because of their decreased muscle mass. A decrease in renal GFR results in

Table 1–2

Half-Life of 650 mg of Aspirin

Number t½	Time of Elimination (h)	Dosage Remaining (mg)	Percentage Left
1	3	325	50
2	6	162	25
3	9	81	12.5
4	12	40	6.25
5	15	20	3.1
6	18	10	1.55

h, Hour; *t*½, half-life.

an increase in serum creatinine level and a decrease in urine creatinine clearance.

With renal dysfunction either in the elderly or as a result of kidney disorders, drug dosage usually needs to be decreased. In these cases, the creatinine clearance needs to be determined to establish appropriate drug dosage. When the creatinine clearance is decreased, drug dosage likewise may need to be decreased. Continuous drug dosing according to a prescribed dosing regimen could result in drug toxicity.

The creatinine clearance test consists of a 12- or 24-hour urine collection and a blood sample. Normal creatinine clearance is 85 to 135 ml/min. This rate decreases with age because aging decreases muscle mass and results in a decrease in functioning nephrons. Elderly clients may have a creatinine clearance of 60 ml/min. For this reason, drug dosage in the elderly may need to be decreased. See Chapter 11, Geriatric Pharmacology, for further explanation of drug dosing in the elderly.

Pharmacodynamic Phase

Pharmacodynamics is the study of drug concentration and its effects on the body. Drug response can cause a primary or secondary physiologic effect, or both. The primary effect is desirable, and the secondary effect may be desirable or undesirable. An example of a drug with a primary and secondary effect is diphenhydramine (Benadryl), an antihistamine. The primary effect of diphenhydramine is to treat the symptoms of allergy, and the secondary effect is a central nervous system depression that causes drowsiness. The secondary effect is undesirable when the client drives an automobile, but at bedtime it could be desirable because it causes mild sedation.

Dose Response and Maximal Efficacy

Dose response is the relationship between the minimal versus the maximal amount of drug dose needed to produce the desired drug response. Some clients respond to a lower drug dose, whereas others need a high drug dose to elicit the desired response. Lehne (2001) states that the drug dose is usually graded to achieve the desired drug response.

All drugs have a maximum drug effect (maximal efficacy). For example, morphine and propoxyphene hydrochloride (Darvon) are prescribed to relieve pain. The maximum efficacy of morphine is greater than propoxyphene hydrochloride, regardless of how much propoxyphene hydrochloride is given. Propoxyphene hydrochloride has a lower maximum efficacy than morphine. The pain relief with the use of propoxyphene hydrochloride is not as great as it is with morphine.

Onset, Peak, and Duration of Action

One important aspect of pharmacodynamics is knowing the drug's onset, peak, and duration of action. **Onset of action** is the time it takes to reach the minimum effective concentration (MEC) after a drug is administered. **Peak action** occurs when the drug reaches its highest blood or plasma

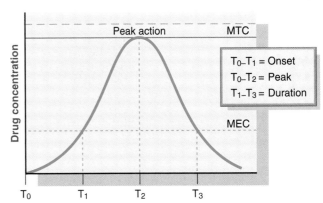

FIGURE 1–4 The time-response curve evaluates three parameters of drug action: (1) onset, (2) peak, and (3) duration. *MEC*, Minimum effective concentration; *MTC*, minimum toxic concentration.

concentration. **Duration of action** is the length of time the drug has a pharmacologic effect. Figure 1–4 illustrates the areas in which onset, peak, and duration of action occur.

Some drugs produce effects in minutes, but others may take hours or days. A **time-response curve** evaluates three parameters of drug action: the onset of drug action, peak action, and duration of action. Figure 1–4 indicates these parameters by using T (time) with subscripts (e.g., T_0, T_1, T_2, T_3).

It is necessary to understand the time response in relationship to drug administration. If the drug plasma or serum level decreases below threshold or MEC, adequate drug dosing is *not* achieved; too high a drug level, above the minimum toxic concentration (MTC), can result in toxicity.

Receptor Theory

Most **receptors**, protein in structure, are found on cell membranes. Drug-binding sites are primarily on proteins, glycoproteins, proteolipids, and at enzymes. Lehne (1998) states that there are four receptor families: (1) cell membrane-embedded enzymes, (2) ligand-gated ion channels, (3) G protein–coupled receptor systems, and (4) transcription factors. The term *ligand-binding domain* is the site on the receptor in which drugs bind.

- *Cell membrane–embedded enzymes.* The **ligand-binding domain** for drug binding is on the cell surface. The drug activates the enzyme (inside the cell), and a response is initiated.
- *Ligand-gated ion channels.* The drug spans the cell membrane and, with this type of receptor, the channel opens, allowing for the flow of ions into and out of the cells. The ions are primarily sodium and calcium.
- *G protein–coupled receptor systems.* There are three components to this receptor response: (1) the receptor, (2) G protein that binds with guanosine triphosphate (GTP), and (3) the effector that is either an enzyme or an ion channel. The system works as follows:

$$\text{drug} \xrightarrow{\text{activates}} \text{receptor} \xrightarrow{\text{activates}} \text{G protein} \xrightarrow{\text{activates}} \text{effector}$$

- *Transcription factors.* Transcription factors are on the deoxyribonucleic acid (DNA) in the cell nucleus and not on the surface of the cell membrane. Activation of re-

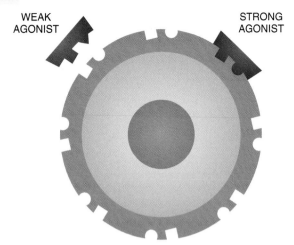

WEAK AGONIST   STRONG AGONIST

FIGURE 1–5 Two drug agonists attach to the receptor site. The drug agonist that has an exact fit is a strong agonist and is more biologically active than the weak agonist.

ceptors through the transcription factors is prolonged. With the first three receptor groups, activation of the receptors is rapid.

Drugs act through receptors by binding to the receptor to produce (initiate) a response or to block (prevent) a response. The activity of many drugs is determined by the ability of the drug to bind to a specific receptor. The better the drug fits at the receptor site, the more biologically active the drug is. It is similar to the fit of the right key in a lock. Figure 1–5 illustrates a drug binding to a receptor.

Agonists and Antagonists

Drugs that produce a response are called **agonists**, and drugs that block a response are called **antagonists.** Isoproterenol (Isuprel) stimulates the beta$_1$ receptor, and so it is an agonist. Cimetidine (Tagamet), an antagonist, blocks the histamine (H$_2$) receptor, thus preventing excessive gas-

tric acid secretion. The effects of an antagonist can be determined by the inhibitory (I) action of the drug concentration on the receptor site. I$_{50}$ indicates that the drug is effective in inhibiting receptor response in 50% of persons.

Nonspecific and Nonselective Drug Effects

Almost all drugs, agonists and antagonists, lack specific and selective effects. A receptor produces a variety of physiologic responses, depending on where in the body that receptor is located. Cholinergic receptors are located in the bladder, heart, blood vessels, lungs, and eyes. A drug that stimulates or blocks the cholinergic receptors affects all anatomic sites of location. Drugs that affect various sites are **nonspecific drugs** and have properties of nonspecificity. Bethanechol (Urecholine) may be prescribed for postoperative urinary retention to increase bladder contraction. This drug stimulates the cholinergic receptor located in the bladder, and urination occurs by strengthening bladder contraction. Because bethanechol affects the cholinergic receptor, other cholinergic sites are also affected. The heart rate decreases, blood pressure decreases, gastric acid secretion increases, the bronchioles constrict, and the pupils of the eye constrict (Figure 1–6). These other effects may be either desirable or harmful. Drugs that evoke a variety of responses throughout the body have a nonspecific response.

Drugs may act at different receptors. Drugs that affect various receptors are **nonselective drugs** or have properties of nonselectivity. Chlorpromazine (Thorazine) acts on the norepinephrine, dopamine, acetylcholine, and histamine receptors, and a variety of responses result from action at these receptor sites (Figure 1–7). Epinephrine acts on the alpha$_1$, beta$_1$, and beta$_2$ receptors.

Drugs that produce a response but do *not* act on a receptor may act by stimulating or inhibiting enzyme activity or hormone production.

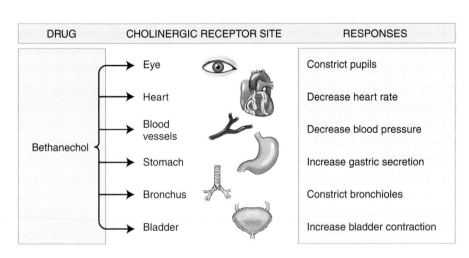

DRUG	CHOLINERGIC RECEPTOR SITE	RESPONSES
Bethanechol	Eye	Constrict pupils
	Heart	Decrease heart rate
	Blood vessels	Decrease blood pressure
	Stomach	Increase gastric secretion
	Bronchus	Constrict bronchioles
	Bladder	Increase bladder contraction

FIGURE 1–6 Cholinergic receptors are located in the bladder, heart, blood vessels, stomach, bronchi, and eyes.

DRUG	RECEPTOR	SITES	RESPONSES

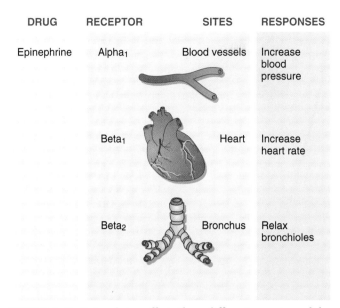

Epinephrine	Alpha₁	Blood vessels	Increase blood pressure
	Beta₁	Heart	Increase heart rate
	Beta₂	Bronchus	Relax bronchioles

FIGURE 1-7 Epinephrine affects three different receptors: alpha, beta₁, and beta₂.

Categories of Drug Action

The four categories of drug action include (1) stimulation or depression, (2) replacement, (3) inhibition or killing of organisms, and (4) irritation. In drug action that stimulates, the rate of cell activity or the secretion from a gland increases. In drug action that depresses, cell activity and function of a specific organ are reduced. Replacement drugs, such as insulin, replace essential body compounds. Drugs that inhibit or kill organisms interfere with bacterial cell growth (e.g., penicillin exerts its bactericidal effects by blocking the synthesis of the bacterial cell wall). Drugs also can act by the mechanism of irritation (e.g., laxatives irritate the inner wall of the colon, thus increasing peristalsis and defecation).

Drug action might last hours, days, weeks, or months. The length of action depends on the half-life of the drug; therefore the half-life is a reasonable guide for the determination of drug dosage intervals. Drugs with a short half-life, such as penicillin G (2 hours), are given several times a day. Drugs with a long half-life, such as digoxin (36 hours), are given once a day. If a drug with a long half-life is given two or more times a day, drug accumulation in the body and drug toxicity are likely to result. If there is liver or renal impairment, the half-life of the drug increases. In these cases, high doses of the drug or too-frequent dosing can result in drug toxicity.

Therapeutic Index and Therapeutic Range (Therapeutic Window)

The safety of drugs is a major concern. The **therapeutic index (TI)** estimates the margin of safety of a drug through the use of a ratio that measures the effective (therapeutic or

concentration) dose (ED) in 50% of persons or animals (ED_{50}) and the lethal dose (LD) in 50% of animals (LD_{50}) (Figure 1-8). The closer the ratio is to 1, the greater the danger of toxicity.

$$TI = \frac{LD_{50}}{ED_{50}}$$

In some cases the ED may be 25% (ED_{25}) or 75% (ED_{75}).

Drugs with a **low therapeutic index** have a narrow margin of safety (Figure 1-9, *A*). Drug dosage might need adjustment, and plasma (serum) drug levels need to be monitored because of the small safety range between ED and LD. Drugs with a **high therapeutic index** have a wide margin of safety and less danger of producing toxic effects (Figure 1-9, *B*). Plasma (serum) drug levels do not need to be monitored routinely for drugs with a high TI.

The **therapeutic range (therapeutic window)** of a drug concentration in plasma should be between the minimum effective concentration in the plasma for obtaining desired drug action and the minimum toxic concentration, the toxic effect. When the therapeutic range is given, it includes both protein-bound and unbound portions of the drug. Drug reference books give many plasma (serum) therapeutic ranges of drugs. If the therapeutic range is narrow, such as for digoxin (0.5 to 2 ng/ml), the plasma drug level should be monitored periodically to avoid drug toxicity. Monitoring the therapeutic range is not necessary if the drug is *not* considered highly toxic. Table 1-3 lists the therapeutic ranges and toxic levels for anticonvulsants.

Peak and Trough Levels

Peak drug level is the highest plasma concentration of drug at a specific time. If the drug is given orally, the peak time might be 1 to 3 hours after drug administration. If the drug is given IV, the peak time might occur in 10 minutes.

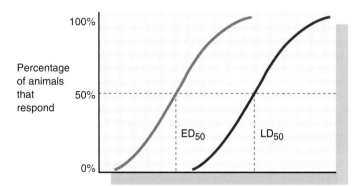

FIGURE 1-8 The therapeutic index measures the margin of safety of a drug. It is a ratio that measures the effective therapeutic dose and the lethal dose.

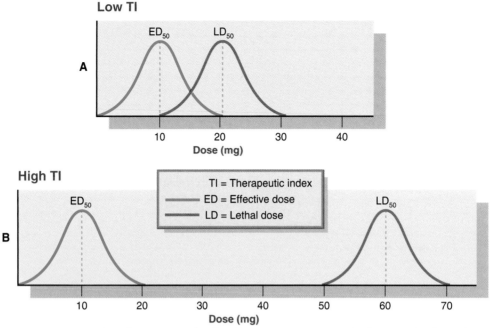

FIGURE 1–9   A, A low therapeutic index drug has a narrow margin of safety, and the drug effect should be closely monitored. B, A high therapeutic index drug has a wide margin of safety and carries less risk of drug toxicity.

Table 1-3

Anticonvulsants: Therapeutic Ranges and Toxic Levels

Drug	Therapeutic Range (mcg/ml)	Toxic Level (mcg/ml)
carbamazepine	6-12	>12-15
ethosuximide	40-80	>80-100
phenytoin	10-20	>30
primidone	5-10	>12-15
valproic acid	50-100	>100

>, Greater than.

A blood sample should be drawn at the proposed peak time, according to the route of administration.

The **trough level** is the lowest plasma concentration of a drug, and it measures the rate at which the drug is eliminated. Trough levels are drawn immediately before the next dose of drug is given, regardless of route of administration. Peak levels indicate the rate of absorption of the drug, and trough levels indicate the rate of elimination of the drug. Peak and trough levels are requested for drugs that have a narrow therapeutic index and are considered toxic, such as the aminoglycoside antibiotics (Table 1–4). If either the peak or trough level is too high, toxicity can occur. If the peak is too low, no therapeutic effect is achieved.

Loading Dose

When immediate drug response is desired, a large initial dose, known as the **loading dose,** of drug is given to achieve a rapid minimum effective concentration in the plasma. After a large initial dose, a prescribed dosage per day is ordered. Digoxin, a digitalis preparation, requires a loading dose when first prescribed. *Digitalization* is the process by which the minimum effective concentration level for digoxin is achieved in the plasma within a short time.

Table 1-4

Aminoglycoside Antibiotics: Peak and Trough Levels

Drug	Peak (mcg/ml)	Trough (mcg/ml)	Toxic Peak Level (mcg/ml)	Toxic Trough Levels (mcg/ml)
amikacin	15-30	5-10	>35	>10
gentamicin	5-10	<2	>12	>2
tobramycin	5-10	<2	>12	>2

>, Greater than; <, less than.

Side Effects, Adverse Reactions, and Toxic Effects

Side effects are physiologic effects not related to desired drug effects. All drugs have side effects, desirable or undesirable. Even with a correct drug dosage, side effects occur and are predicted. Side effects result mostly from drugs that lack specificity, such as bethanechol (Urecholine). In some health problems, side effects may be desirable, such as the use of diphenhydramine HCl (Benadryl) at bedtime when its side effect of drowsiness is beneficial. At times, however, side effects are called adverse reactions. The terms *side effects* and *adverse reactions* might be used interchangeably. Some side effects are expected as part of drug therapy. The occurrence of these expected but undesirable side effects is not a reason to discontinue therapy. The nurse's role includes teaching clients to report any side effects, of which many can be managed with dosage adjustments, changing to a different drug in the same class of drugs, or implementing other interventions. It is important to know that the occurrence of side effects is one of the primary reasons clients stop taking the prescribed medication. **Adverse reactions** are more severe than side effects. They are a range of untoward effects (unintended and occurring at normal doses) of drugs that cause mild to severe side effects, including anaphylaxis (cardiovascular collapse). Adverse reactions are always undesirable. Adverse effects must always be reported and documented because they represent variances from planned therapy.

Toxic effects, or **toxicity,** of a drug can be identified by monitoring the plasma (serum) therapeutic range of the drug. However, for drugs that have a wide therapeutic index, the therapeutic ranges are seldom given. For those drugs with a narrow TI, such as aminoglycoside antibiotics and anticonvulsants, the therapeutic ranges are closely monitored. When the drug level exceeds the therapeutic range, toxic effects are likely to occur from overdosing or drug accumulation.

Pharmacogenetics

Pharmacogenetics is the effect of a drug action that varies from a predicted drug response because of genetic factors or hereditary influence. Because people have different genetic makeup, they do not always respond identically to a drug dosage or planned drug therapy. Genetic factors can alter the metabolism of the drug in converting its chemical form to an inert metabolite; thus the drug action can be enhanced or diminished. Some persons are less or more sensitive to drugs and their drug actions because of genetic factors. For example, African Americans do not respond as well as whites to some classes of antihypertensive medications.

Tachyphylaxis

Drug tolerance to a frequently repeated administration of a certain drug is known as **tachyphylaxis.** Drug categories that can cause tachyphylaxis include narcotics, barbiturates, laxatives, and psychotropic agents. For example, drug tolerance to narcotics can result in decreased pain relief for the client. If the nurse does not recognize the development of drug tolerance, the client's request for more pain medication might be interpreted as drug-seeking behavior associated with addiction. Prevention of tachyphylaxis should always be part of the therapeutic regimen.

Placebo Effect

A **placebo effect** is a psychologic benefit from a compound that may not have the chemical structure of a drug effect. The placebo is effective in approximately one third of persons who take a placebo compound. Many clinical drug studies involve a group of subjects who receive a placebo. The nurse can increase the therapeutic effect of the drug (narcotics for pain management) but violate the truth-telling ethical principle if he or she presents a nontherapeutic drug as a therapeutic agent. Hence it is required that participants in drug trials be told from the start that they might receive a placebo.

Summary

The phases of drug action are pharmaceutic, pharmacokinetic, and pharmacodynamic. Figure 1–10 illustrates these three phases for drugs given orally, but drugs given by injection are involved only in the pharmacokinetic and pharmacodynamic phases. Nurses should be aware that tablets must disintegrate and go into solution (the pharmaceutic phase) to be absorbed.

To avoid toxic effects, the nurse needs to know the half-life, protein-binding percentage, normal side effects, and therapeutic ranges of the drug. This information can be obtained from drug reference books.

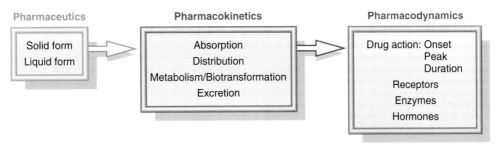

FIGURE 1–10 The three phases of drug action.

Nursing Process

ASSESSMENT

■ Recognize that drugs in liquid form are absorbed faster than those in solid form.

■ Assess for signs and symptoms of drug toxicity when giving two drugs that are highly protein bound. The drugs compete for protein-binding sites, and displacement of drugs occurs. More free drug is in circulation because there are not enough protein-binding sites. Too much of a free drug can result in drug toxicity.

■ Identify side effects of drugs that are nonspecific (same receptor at different tissue and organ sites). For example, when atropine is the drug to be administered, assess for tachycardia, dry mouth and throat, constipation, urinary retention, and blurred vision. If nonspecific drugs are given in large doses or at frequent intervals, many side effects are likely to occur.

■ Check peak levels and trough levels of drugs that have a narrow therapeutic range, such as aminoglycosides. If the trough level is high, toxic effects can result.

NURSING INTERVENTIONS

■ Advise client not to eat fatty food before ingesting an enteric-coated tablet because fatty foods decrease absorption rate.

■ Check the drug literature for the protein-binding percentage of the drug. Drugs with a high protein-binding effect have a large portion of drug bound to protein, which causes the drug to become inactive until it is released from the protein. The portion not bound to protein is free and active drug.

■ Report to the health care provider if drugs with a long half-life (e.g., greater than 24 hours) are given more than once a day. Some drugs with a long half-life, such as the anticoagulant warfarin (Coumadin), can be more dangerous than others and should be monitored frequently.

■ Monitor the therapeutic range of drugs that are more toxic or have a narrow therapeutic range, such as digoxin.

Cultural Considerations

• Be aware that individuals from some cultures metabolize drugs differently than the general population.

• Assess for adverse effects that may result from this variation in metabolism.

EVALUATION

■ Evaluate the determinants that affect drug therapy according to Figure 1–11.

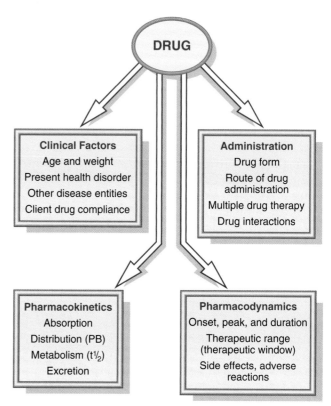

FIGURE 1–11 Determinants that affect drug therapy.

WEBSITES

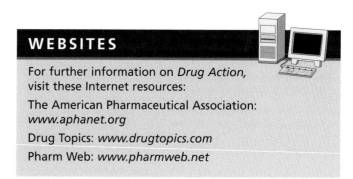

For further information on *Drug Action,* visit these Internet resources:

The American Pharmaceutical Association: *www.aphanet.org*

Drug Topics: *www.drugtopics.com*

Pharm Web: *www.pharmweb.net*

Study Questions

1. What are the three phases of drug action?

2. What are the two processes that a tablet undergoes before it is absorbed? Describe each process.

3. What is the purpose of pharmacokinetics? Name the four processes involved in pharmacokinetics, and describe each.

4. Explain the term *first-pass effect* or *hepatic metabolism* of the drug. What effect does first-pass have on drug bioavailability and activity?

5. What is the purpose of pharmacodynamics? What is the role of receptors in this phase? Of what importance is the location of the receptor? Differentiate between nonspecific and nonselective drug responses.

6. Define the following terms: *bioavailability, protein-bound drugs, half-life, therapeutic index, therapeutic drug range, therapeutic window, side effects, adverse reaction,* and *toxicity.* What are the implications of these terms to your nursing practice?

7. A drug that is 75% protein bound is considered to be _____ protein bound.

8. What are the nursing implications of pharmacokinetics and pharmacodynamics?

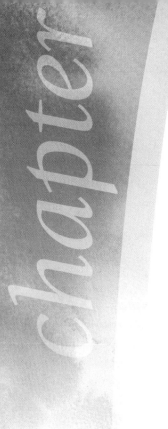

2 Nursing Process and Client Teaching

ELECTRONIC RESOURCES

Additional information can be found on the companion website at *http://evolve.elsevier.com/KeeHayes/pharmacology/* or on the companion CD-ROM, which includes:
- *NCLEX-style examination review questions*
- *Pharmacology animations*
- *Medication error and IV therapy checklists*
- *Medication calculation problems*
- *Electronic calculators*

OUTLINE

OBJECTIVES

- Differentiate the steps of the nursing process and their purpose in relation to drug therapy.
- Identify the components of a goal.
- State at least eight principles for health teaching related to drug therapy plans.
- Describe at least six culturally sensitive health teaching tips.
- Discuss the nurse's role related to drug therapy plans.

TERMS

assessment
culturally sensitive
evaluation

goal setting
holistic nursing approach
implementation

nursing diagnosis
planning

Introduction

Nurses have a significant role in the management of drug therapy. Influences on this role include technology, increased longevity of the citizenry, and survival of persons with multiple and varied biopsychosocial needs. Variables in drug therapy are numerous and, at times, unknown. A **holistic nursing approach** to care is crucial to the success of drug therapy initiation, maintenance, and evaluation.

This chapter explores the use of the nursing process as it relates to drug therapy. Careful detail to each step of the process fosters the client's success with the prescribed medication regimen. Considerations for the use of over-the-counter (OTC) drugs and herbal remedies are explored in Chapters 7, Drug Interaction and Over-the-Counter Drugs, and 9, Herbal Therapy with Nursing Implications, respectively.

Nursing Process

The four steps of the nursing process are assessment (including nursing diagnosis), planning, implementation, and evaluation. Each step is discussed as it relates to health teaching in drug therapy.

Assessment

Assessment, the first step of the nursing process, is particularly important because the data provided by the assessment form the basis on which care is planned, implemented, and evaluated. Data collection involves both subjective and objective information.

Subjective Data

The components listed below are reflective of subjective data:

Current health history, including any problems with swallowing

Client symptoms as verbalized by client

Current medications
  Dosage, frequency, route, prescribing health care provider, if any
  Client knowledge about drug and its side effects and for what diagnosis and symptoms the client is taking the drug
  Client expectation and perception of drug effectiveness
  Client knowledge about what effects or drug reactions to report to health care provider
  Client compliance with regimen and reasons for deviations. Are deviations based on valid data/rationale and clinically sound?
  Drug allergies or reactions, both past and present; also food and dye intolerance and reactions
  OTC drugs
  Herbal remedies

Street drugs. If used, what is their frequency of use?
Alcohol consumption
Smoking

Past health history
  Past illnesses, major injuries, and drug therapy, including reactions
  Medications saved from previous use; how stored; expiration date
  Street drugs

Client's environment
  Client's language and communication needs
  History of compliance with drug therapy as prescribed (i.e., were prescriptions filled and finished?)
  Does client read and follow instructions from the health care provider and the pharmacy?
  Client knowledge of specific drug storage requirements, if any
  Availability, willingness, and ability to administer or assist in the administration of medications. This information is essential for third-party payment for continued home visits or for admission to an extended care facility.
  Household members, neighbors, friends, and their roles; ages of household members
  Learning style preferences
  First language, if other than English
  Readiness to learn
  Activities of daily living (ADLs) capabilities
  Dietary patterns, cultural and economic influences, safety
  Financial resources (drugs can be expensive)
  Mental status

REMEMBER: Clients, even those who do not intend to withhold information, do not always tell all about their medications. Therefore, in addition to asking about prescription drugs, ask specifically about vitamin, herbal, oral contraceptive, aspirin or acetaminophen, and antihistamine or decongestant use. Also identify caffeine and nicotine use. Ask to see the contents of the medicine chest at home (or other storage area for medications), and ask whether a pharmacist is used as a consultant.

Objective Data

The components listed below are reflective of objective data:
  Gross and fine motor control, hand joint range of motion, and muscle strength decreases can interfere with client's ability to open medication containers. Visual impairment can limit a client's ability to read labels and correctly measure dosages.

Laboratory tests	Baseline data for future
Diagnostic studies	comparisons
Physical assessment	

Data collection should focus on symptoms and those organs most likely to be affected by drug therapy. For example, if a drug is nephrotoxic, the client's creatinine clearance should be assessed. Assess major body systems for any signs of reaction or interaction of drugs or ineffectiveness of therapy.

Based on assessment data, the nurse must identify high-risk clients (those likely to have adverse reactions). The client's health history, physical assessment, and laboratory test results are sources of these data. The client's attitudes and values about taking medication are very important in planning intervention to support the client's decision to adopt health behaviors related to taking medications. Emphasis is on assessing the client's social support system, for it is this special support system that promotes the taking of medication as prescribed or notifying the health care provider if a problem arises.

Enhancing client compliance with the drug therapy regimen is an essential component of health teaching. The client and family response to the following three questions provides the nurse with critical information unique to each client's teaching situation.

1. What things help you take your medicine as prescribed?
2. What things prevent you from taking your medicine as prescribed?
3. What would you do or what do you do if you forgot to take a dose of medication?

Frequently cited factors for noncompliance include forgetfulness, knowledge deficit, side effects, low self-esteem, depression, lack of trust in the health care system, family problems, language barriers, high cost of medications, anxiety, value systems (religious and other), and lack of motivation. The nurse's role is critical to drug therapy. The nurse is most often the one person who follows the client most closely and the one who is frequently first to assess the client's response to drugs. The nurse applies knowledge of pharmacology to anticipate drug responses in the individual client.

Nursing Diagnosis

A **nursing diagnosis** is made based on the analysis of the assessment data. More than one applicable nursing diagnosis may be generated, and a nursing diagnosis may be actual or potential. The registered nurse formulates nursing diagnoses and uses them, with the assistance of others, to guide the development of a care plan. A list of nursing diagnoses accepted by the North American Nursing Diagnosis Association (NANDA) is presented in Box 2–1.

Common nursing diagnoses related to drug therapy include the following:

- Deficient knowledge about drug action, administration, and side effects related to cultural/language barrier or speech articulation problem.
- Pain (acute or chronic) related to hesitancy in taking prescribed pain medications due to fear of addiction.
- Ineffective health maintenance related to not having recommended preventive care
- Ineffective protection related to effects of anticoagulant medication on clotting mechanism

- Ineffective therapeutic regimen management
- Noncompliance related to forgetfulness
- Risk for injury related to side effects of drug, such as dizziness and drowsiness
- Ineffective therapeutic regimen management related to lack of finances or health care coverage to purchase medications

Use of the nursing diagnosis is beneficial to the client because it facilitates the development of an individualized care plan. The abnormal data collected during the assessment serve as the defining characteristics (for actual problem) or risk factors (for high risk for problem) to support the appropriate nursing diagnosis for each client.

Planning

The **planning** phase of the nursing process is characterized by **goal setting** or expected outcomes. Planning also includes development of nursing interventions that will be used to assist the client in meeting the outcome. Implementation occurs once the nursing interventions are actually put into action. Effective goal setting has the following qualities:

- Client-centered; clearly states the expected change
- Acceptable to both client and nurse (dependent on client's decision-making ability)
- Realistic and measurable
- Shared with other health care providers
- Realistic deadlines
- Identifies components for evaluation

Examples of a goal are (1) E.C. (the client) will independently administer prescribed dose of insulin by the end of the fourth session of instruction; (2) D.Z. (the client) will prepare a medication recording sheet that correctly reflects prescribed medication schedule within 3 days.

Implementation

The **implementation** phase includes the nursing actions/interventions necessary to accomplish the established goals or expected outcomes. Client education and teaching are key nursing responsibilities during this phase. In most practice settings, administration of drugs and assessment of drug effectiveness are also important nursing responsibilities (see Chapter 3, Principles of Drug Administration).

Client Teaching

Client education is an ongoing process. Teaching is more effective in an environment free of distractions, and the information should be tailored to the client's interests and level of understanding. Assessment data suggest the complexity, number, and length of teaching sessions that may be required. Be sensitive to the client's motivation to learn, attention span, and level of frustration. Readiness to learn is paramount. Readiness should be assessed first, *before* information is presented to the client. Use a positive approach; for example, "This narcotic is usually effective for the relief of the type of pain you have." Be an *active* listener and observer. The inclusion of a family member or friend in the teaching plan is an excellent idea. Assessment data guide the

BOX 2–1

NANDA-Approved Nursing Diagnoses: 2005-2006

Activity intolerance
Activity intolerance, risk for
Adjustment, impaired
Airway clearance, ineffective
Allergy response, latex
Allergy response, latex, risk for
Anxiety
Anxiety, death
Aspiration, risk for
Attachment, impaired parent/infant/child, risk for
Autonomic dysreflexia
Autonomic dysreflexia, risk for
Body image, disturbed
Body temperature, imbalanced, risk for
Bowel incontinence
Breastfeeding, effective
Breastfeeding, ineffective
Breastfeeding, interrupted
Breathing pattern, ineffective
Cardiac output, decreased
Caregiver role strain
Caregiver role strain, risk for
Comfort, impaired
Communication, verbal, impaired
Communication, readiness for enhanced
Conflict, decisional (specify)
Conflict, parental role
Confusion, acute
Confusion, chronic
Constipation
Constipation, perceived
Constipation, risk for
Coping, ineffective
Coping, readiness for enhanced
Coping, community, ineffective
Coping, community, readiness for enhanced
Coping, defensive
Coping, family, compromised
Coping, family, disabled
Coping, family, readiness for enhanced
Death syndrome, sudden infant, risk for
Denial, ineffective
Dentition, impaired
Development, delayed, risk for
Diarrhea
Disuse syndrome, risk for
Diversional activity, deficient
Energy field, disturbed
Environmental interpretation syndrome, impaired
Failure to thrive, adult
Falls, risk for
Family processes: alcoholism, dysfunctional
Family processes, interrupted
Fatigue
Fear
Feeding pattern, infant, ineffective
Fluid balance, readiness for enhanced
Fluid volume, deficient
Fluid volume, excess
Fluid volume, deficient, risk for
Fluid volume, imbalanced, risk for
Gas exchange, impaired
Grieving

Grieving, anticipatory
Grieving, dysfunctional
Grieving, risk for dysfunctional
Growth and development, delayed
Growth disproportionate, risk for
Health maintenance, ineffective
Health-seeking behaviors
Home maintenance, impaired
Hopelessness
Hyperthermia
Hypothermia
Identity, personal, disturbed
Incontinence, urinary, functional
Incontinence, urinary, reflex
Incontinence, urinary, stress
Incontinence, urinary, total
Incontinence, urinary, urge
Incontinence, urinary, urge, risk for
Infant behavior, disorganized
Infant behavior, disorganized, risk for
Infant behavior, organized, readiness for enhanced
Infection, risk for
Injury, risk for
Injury, perioperative positioning, risk for
Intracranial adaptive capacity, decreased
Knowledge, deficient
Knowledge of (specify), readiness for enhanced
Lifestyle, sedentary
Loneliness, risk for
Memory, impaired
Mobility, bed, impaired
Mobility, physical, impaired
Mobility, wheelchair, impaired
Nausea
Neglect, unilateral
Noncompliance
Nutrition, readiness for enhanced
Nutrition: less than body requirements, imbalanced
Nutrition: more than body requirements, imbalanced
Nutrition: more than body requirements, risk for imbalanced
Oral mucous membrane, impaired
Pain, acute
Pain, chronic
Parenting, readiness for enhanced
Parenting, impaired
Parenting, impaired, risk for
Peripheral neurovascular dysfunction, risk for
Poisoning, risk for
Post-trauma syndrome
Post-trauma syndrome, risk for
Powerlessness
Powerlessness, risk for
Protection, ineffective
Rape-trauma syndrome
Rape-trauma syndrome: compound reaction
Rape-trauma syndrome: silent reaction
Religiosity, impaired
Religiosity, readiness for enhanced
Religiosity, risk for impaired
Relocation stress syndrome
Relocation stress syndrome, risk for
Role performance, ineffective
Self-care deficit, bathing/hygiene

Continued

BOX 2–1

NANDA-Approved Nursing Diagnoses: 2005-2006—cont'd

Self-care deficit, dressing/grooming
Self-care deficit, feeding
Self-care deficit, toileting
Self-concept, readiness for enhanced
Self-esteem, chronic low
Self-esteem, situational low
Self-esteem, situational low, risk for
Self-mutilation
Self-mutilation, risk for
Sensory perception, disturbed
Sexual dysfunction
Sexuality patterns, ineffective
Skin integrity, impaired
Skin integrity, impaired, risk for
Sleep deprivation
Sleep patterns, disturbed
Sleep, readiness for enhanced
Social interaction, impaired
Social isolation
Sorrow, chronic
Spiritual distress
Spiritual distress, risk for
Spiritual well-being, readiness for enhanced
Suffocation, risk for

Suicide, risk for
Surgical recovery, delayed
Swallowing, impaired
Therapeutic regimen management, effective
Therapeutic regimen management, ineffective
Therapeutic regimen management, readiness for enhanced
Therapeutic regimen management, community, ineffective
Therapeutic regimen management, family, ineffective
Thermoregulation, ineffective
Thought processes, disturbed
Tissue integrity, impaired
Tissue perfusion, ineffective
Transfer ability, impaired
Trauma, risk for
Urinary elimination, readiness for enhanced
Urinary elimination, impaired
Urinary retention
Ventilation, spontaneous, impaired
Ventilatory weaning response, dysfunctional
Violence, other-directed, risk for
Violence, self-directed, risk for
Walking, impaired
Wandering

nurse to the appropriate persons to be included. This other person may (1) act as a psychologic support, (2) actually administer all or part of the drug therapy, (3) observe the effectiveness and side effects of drug therapy, and (4) implement other changes, such as food shopping or instituting new methods of food preparation. Provide simple written materials appropriate for individual client needs. The client and family need to have the appropriate information (e.g., telephone number, e-mail) to reach the health care provider for questions and concerns. Health care providers need to be available to provide timely responses.

Client teaching is a complex activity. As such, it might be helpful for the nurse to use an outline format. Suggested headings related to pharmacotherapeutics include the following:

- *General.* Instruct the client to take the drug as prescribed. Compliance is of utmost importance because discontinuing the drug before the course is completed may result in relapse or future ineffectiveness of the drug. Do not adjust dose, frequency, or time of day taken unless directed by the health care provider. Advise women contemplating pregnancy to check first with their health care provider before taking prescription, OTC medications, or herbal products. Advise clients to consult with their health care provider about laboratory tests such as liver enzymes, blood urea nitrogen (BUN), creatinine, and electrolytes, which should be monitored when taking drugs such as antifungal agents.
- *Self-administration.* Instruct the client on the administration of the drug according to the prescribed route, such as eyedrops or nose drops, subcutaneous insulin injec-

tions, suppositories, swish-and-swallow suspensions, and metered-dose inhalers with and without spacers. Include demonstration and return demonstration in the instructions when appropriate, and give written instructions for the sighted client and audio instructions for the visually impaired. Instruct more than one person, when possible, because this aids in reinforcement and retention of information. It also provides a "backup" if the client is unable to self-administer the drug.
- *Diet.* Instruct clients about what foods to include in their diet and what foods to avoid. For example, advise clients to eat foods rich in potassium (e.g., bananas) when taking most diuretics, unless they are on a potassium chloride (KCl) supplement, and to avoid large amounts of green, leafy vegetables if taking warfarin (Coumadin) preparations.
- *Side effects.* Instruct the client to report immediately to the designated health care provider—usually a nurse, physician, or pharmacist—if he or she experiences unusual symptoms. Also, give the client instructions that help minimize any side effects, such as avoiding direct sunlight when there is risk of photosensitivity or sunburn. Inform the client of any expected changes in the color of urine or stool. Advise the client who has dizziness caused by orthostatic hypotension to rise slowly from a sitting to a standing position.
- *Cultural considerations.* Be alert to client and family cultural expectations. For example, *time* may not be viewed as important; therefore this may affect the client's adherence to taking medications at specific time intervals during the day to ensure therapeutic blood levels of the medication.

BOX 2–2

Culturally Sensitive Health Teaching Tips

- Flexibility in timing appointments may be necessary for those who have a circular sense of time, such as American Indian/Alaskan Natives and some Hispanic/Latino populations, rather than the dominant culture's linear sense of time.
- Make reminder calls for appointments, and encourage the client about the importance of timeliness.
- When language barriers exist, use videos and literature in the client's preferred language; with pictures of that group may help compliance with health interventions.
- Decrease language barriers by decoding the jargon of the health care environment for those with language difficulties and for those who are not in the health care field.
- Failing to allow adequate time for information processing may result in an inaccurate response or no response. Allow time for people to respond to questions, especially for those who have language barriers. Speak clearly and slowly, giving time for translation. Obtain an interpreter if necessary.
- Although more traditional and older individuals in some cultures do not maintain eye contact, the acculturated and more educated usually do maintain eye contact. Do not assume that lack of eye contact means the client is not listening or does not care. It might indicate respect.
- Do not misunderstand loud voice volume as necessarily reflecting anger among some African Americans and Arabs, who may be merely expressing their thoughts in a dynamic manner.
- When translation is needed, discuss the ethnicity of the interpreter as well as the language desired. Provide an interpreter with the same ethnic background and gender if possible, especially with sensitive topics. Do not rely on family members, who may not fully disclose because of honor or shame.
- Speak slowly and clearly with exaggerated mouthing or using a loud voice volume, which changes the tone of words. Even though the client may appear to understand the fundamentals of the English language, provide an interpreter if in doubt.
- Do not give directions such as take one "blue" pill at a specified time. Instead, provide the name and dosage of the medication.

- Ask open-ended questions and have clients demonstrate, rather than verbalize, their understanding of treatments. Because politeness and saving face may prevail, do not assume that a positive response means a definite *yes*.
- Use simple and clear instructions. Ask family members to assist with translation only if an interpreter is not available. Do not use compound sentences.
- Do not take offense from a casual touch on the arm or shoulder or if clients stand closer than that to which you are accustomed. Do not assume that prolonged eye contact is a sign of anger.
- Health care workers should ask indirectly whether the Asian client understands instructions and should have the client or family member do a return demonstration of a procedure or repeat an instruction rather than question his or her comprehension. Speak clearly and slowly. Allow time to respond to questions, giving time for translating the dialect into English. Asking if the person understands may elicit a positive response because of cultural reluctance to say no.
- Many ethnocultural groups from countries outside the United States, and some people from within the United States as well, may be accustomed to not taking all their medications as ordered or use medicines prescribed for other people. Emphasize that medications need to be taken as prescribed, medications are ordered specifically for each ailment, unused drugs should be discarded, and use of medications by individuals other than the intended may have serious consequences.
- When offering a prescription, instructions, or pamphlets to Asians and Pacific Islanders, use both hands, which shows respect.
- To establish trust among Hispanics/Latinos or Appalachians, it is necessary to demonstrate an interest in the client's family and other personal matters, to drop hints instead of giving orders, and to solicit the client's opinions and advice.
- Some individuals may respond better to verbal instructions and education with reinforcement from videos rather than printed communications.

Adapted from Purnell, L., Paulanka, B.: *A guide to culturally competent health care,* Philadelphia, 2004, FA Davis.

The nurse applies knowledge of cultural considerations to individualize a teaching plan. For example, respect for health care providers is a value among many Asian cultures and the client will adopt communication behaviors that demonstrate that respect. This behavior includes not making eye contact, not asking questions, and not disagreeing with the nurse or physician. The client may nod in agreement when the nurse asks whether he or she understands what the nurse is teaching even if he or she does not understand. In this situation, it is better for the nurse to have the client do a return demonstration or repeat what he or she has learned.

NOTE: See Chapter 6, Transcultural and Genetic Considerations, for comprehensive discussion. Cultural content is found throughout the text and in the Nursing Process boxes sections within each chapter. Also see Box 2–2, Culturally Sensitive Health Teaching Tips.

A teaching plan with interventions that involve stimulation of several senses and active participation by the client enhances learning. Inclusion of return demonstrations by the client and others, when applicable, gives the nurse important feedback about the client's learning and gives the client confidence in carrying out the regimen or selected aspects of the regimen. Additional teaching tips include the following:

- Establish a trusting relationship.
- Incorporate interventions that involve stimulation of several senses.
- Actively involve the client.
- Provide written instructions in addition to other teaching aids.
- Use colorful charts and graphs.
- Consider using a variety of media, including compact discs and videos.

- Encourage questions from the client and family; provide time for this. Do not rush.
- Use materials and language appropriate to the client's level of understanding; access computerized drug information system with client information sheets on medications in different languages and appropriate reading levels.
- Space instruction over several sessions if appropriate.
- Review community resources related to the client's nursing diagnosis.
- Support multiagency collaboration in the mobilization of resources.
- Identify clients at risk for nonadherence with regimen. Alert health care provider and pharmacist so they can develop a plan to minimize the number of drugs and times administered.
- Evaluate client's understanding of medication regimen on regular basis.
- Empower client to take responsibility for managing medications.

A client teaching session is shown in Figure 2–1. The use of teaching drug cards is helpful. These cards provide information about a specific drug or drug group. They may be developed by the health care provider or obtained from drug manufacturers. Audiocassettes and videotapes are available from many drug companies. Group classes are useful for clients with certain diagnoses or who require certain drugs. A variety of formats can be developed. Be creative! Helpful components for the teaching drug cards include the following:

- Name of drug
- Reason for taking drug
- Dose amount
- Specific times to take the drug
- What specific things should or should not be done while taking the medication; for example, tablets may or may not be crushed or may be taken with or without food
- Possible side effects of medication
- Possible adverse effects of medication; when to notify health care provider

In addition to the individualized component of the teaching drug card, there are some general helpful and healthful points to remember. Box 2–3 presents these points.

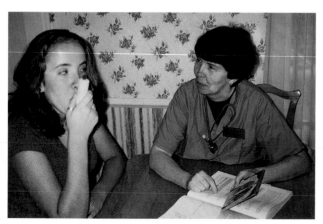

FIGURE 2–1   Client teaching session.

BOX 2–3

Helpful and Healthful Points to Remember

- Take medication as prescribed by your health care provider. If you have questions, call.
- Keep medication in the original labeled container, and store as instructed.
- Keep all medicines **out of reach** of children. Remind grandparents and visitors to monitor their purses and luggage when visiting.
- **Before** using any over-the-counter (OTC) drugs, check with your health care provider. This includes use of aspirin, laxatives, and so on. Pharmacists are good resources to ask before buying or using a product.
- Bring all medications with you when you visit the health care provider.
- Know why you are taking each medication and under what circumstances to notify the health care provider.
- Alcohol may alter the action and absorption of the medication. Use of alcoholic beverages is discouraged around the time you take your medications and is absolutely contraindicated with certain medications.
- Smoking tobacco also alters the absorption of some medications (e.g., theophylline-type drugs, tranquilizers, antidepressants, and pain medications). Consult your health care provider or pharmacist for specific information.

Many people take multiple medications simultaneously several times each day, which presents a challenge to the client, his or her family, and the nurse. This complex activity can be segmented into several simple tasks, which include the following:

- Preparation of 1 day's or 1 week's supply of medication. The day's medication can be put in one container. Sorting of a day's supply allows the client and nurse to see at a glance what medications have and have not been taken. Keep in mind that a missing pill may have been dropped and not actually taken. A variation in accomplishing this task is to take a day's medication and sort or package the pills according to the time each is to be taken. Multicompartment dispensers (available at local drug or variety stores) or an egg carton may help some clients sort their drugs.
- A recording sheet may be helpful. The client or a family member marks when each medication is taken. The sheet is designed to meet the client's individual needs; for example, the time can be noted by the client or could be entered before hand, with the client marking when each dose is taken. A generic format follows:

	DOSAGE	DAY OF WEEK						
MEDICATION	(mg daily)	S	M	T	W	T	F	S
Captopril (Capoten)	12.5							
Digoxin	0.25							
Furosemide (Lasix)	40							

- Figure 2–2 shows a nurse reviewing a medication record with her client. Alternatives to recording sheets are also

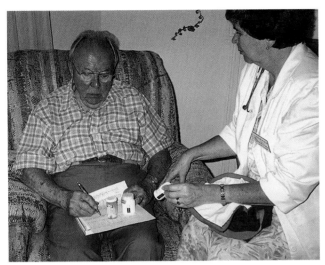

FIGURE 2–2 A client records his medications on a schedule sheet.

available. Mechanical alarm reminder devices may be helpful to some clients.

- A combination of daily supply and recording may be helpful. Consider color coding. Visual acuity, manual dexterity, and mental processes have a major effect on which system works best for each client.

Throughout the teaching plan, the nurse promotes client independence. The nurse should not lose sight of the goals or outcomes and become immersed in the intervention process (e.g., teaching a client with short-term memory loss). Box 2–4 presents suggestions for a checklist for health teaching in drug therapy.

BOX 2–4

Checklist for Health Teaching in Drug Therapy

- Comprehensive drug and health history
- Reason for medication therapy
- Expected results
- Side effects and adverse reactions
- When to notify health care provider or pharmacist
- Drug-drug, drug-food, drug-laboratory, drug-environment interactions
- Required changes in activities of daily living (ADLs)
- Demonstration of learning; may take several forms, such as listening, discussing, or return demonstration of psychomotor skills (insulin administration)
- Medication schedule, associated with ADLs and drug level of action as appropriate
- Recording system
- Discussion and monitoring of access to financial resources, medication, and associated equipment
- Development and support of backup system
- Community resources

Evaluation

The effectiveness of health teaching about drug therapy and attainment of goals are addressed in the **evaluation** phase of the nursing process. The time at which the evaluation of a goal occurs is dependent on the time frame specified in the statement of a goal. Evaluation should be ongoing and related to progress as well as to attainment of the final goal.

If goals are not met, the nurse (in collaboration with client, when possible) needs to determine the reasons for this and revise the plan accordingly. This includes additional assessment data and the setting of new goals. If the goals are met, the plan of care has been completed.

To complete the care for any current client, follow these recommendations:
- Review with the client and family the need for follow-up care, if required.
- Encourage choices in ADLs.
- Refer the client to community resources as necessary.

Figure 2–3 shows a nurse meeting with a client and his spouse to review his therapeutic regimen.

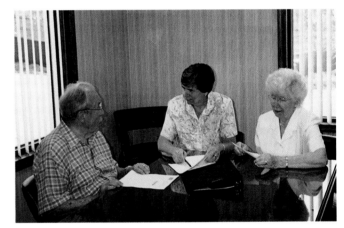

FIGURE 2–3 A nurse reviews the therapeutic regimen with a client and his spouse.

WEBSITES

For further information on *Nursing Process and Client Teaching*, visit these Internet resources:

National Library of Medicine: *www.nlm.nih.gov*

Centers for Disease Control and Prevention: *www.cdc.gov*

Client Handouts in Spanish: *www.advancefornurses.com* (click on "Spanish Patient Handouts" in the left bar under "Resources & Events")

Study Questions

1. What are the steps of the nursing process and the primary purpose of each step?

2. Explain how the nursing process relates to administration of medications.

3. What are the essential components of a goal? Write a goal that incorporates all the essential components. How and when would you know if a goal or outcome is realistic for client?

4. What is the basis of a nursing diagnosis?

5. List at least five principles of health teaching about drug therapy regimens.

6. Describe at least six health teaching strategies that demonstrate cultural sensitivity.

7. Identify at least two ways to organize multiple medications taken on a daily basis.

8. List three ways to evaluate whether a client is compliant with a drug therapy regimen.

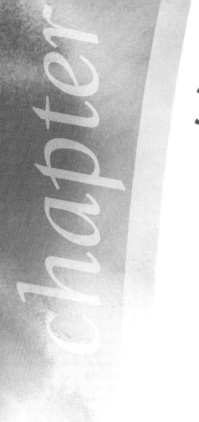

3 Principles of Drug Administration

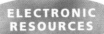 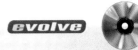

ELECTRONIC RESOURCES

Additional information can be found on the companion website at *http://evolve.elsevier.com/KeeHayes/pharmacology/* or on the companion CD-ROM, which includes:
- *NCLEX-style examination review questions*
- *Pharmacology animations*
- *Medication error and IV therapy checklists*
- *Medication calculation problems*
- *Electronic calculators*

OUTLINE

OBJECTIVES

- Describe the "five-plus-five rights" of drug administration.
- List safety guidelines for drug administration.
- Describe factors that modify drug response.
- Differentiate routes of administration.
- Identify the various sites for parenteral therapy.
- Explain the equipment and technique used in parenteral therapy.
- Explain the method for charting medications.
- Describe the nursing interventions related to administration of medications by various routes.

TERMS

absorption	intravenous	right client	subcutaneous
buccal	JCAHO medication error	right documentation	sublingual
canister	meniscus	right dose	suppositories
cumulative effect	metabolism (biotransfor-	right drug	tolerance
distribution	mation)	right evaluation	topical
informed consent	metered-dose inhaler	right route	toxicity
inhalation	(MDI)	right time	transdermal
instillations	parenteral	right to education	unit dose method
intradermal	pharmacogenetics	right to refuse	Z-track technique
intramuscular	right assessment	spacers	

Introduction

Administration of medications is a basic activity in nursing practice. As a result of the transition from hospitals and institutions to community-based services, an increasing number of nurses are practicing in a variety of settings. Nurses therefore must be knowledgeable about the specific drugs and their administration, client response, drug interactions, client allergies, and related resources.

Nurses are accountable for the safe administration of medications. Nurses must know all the components of a drug order and question those orders that are not complete, unclear, give a dosage outside the recommended range, or are contraindicated by client allergy or laboratory test results. Nurses are legally liable if they give a prescribed drug and the dosage is incorrect or the drug is contraindicated for the client's health status. In some health care settings, medical students write drug orders; these orders must be countersigned by an attending or staff physician or other prescribing health care provider before they are considered official. Once the drug has been administered, the nurse becomes liable for the predicted effects of that drug. Drug references (e.g., *United States Pharmacopeia [USP], National Formulary [NF], Physicians' Desk Reference [PDR]*, and *American Hospital Formulary* drug reference handbook), human resources (e.g., pharmacists), and technology resources (Micromedix, Pyxis, Palm Pilot Epocrates) must be consulted when the nurse is unsure about the expected therapeutic effect, contraindications, dosage, potential side effects, or adverse reactions and interactions of a medication.

This chapter describes selected, essential content related to the administration of medications, a multifaceted activity. Selected content areas include the "rights" of drug administration, factors that modify drug response, guidelines for various routes of administration, and related nursing implications.

The "Five-Plus-Five Rights" of Drug Administration

To provide safe drug administration, the nurse should practice the "rights" of drug administration. The traditional five rights are (1) the *right client*, (2) the *right drug*, (3) the *right dose*, (4) the *right time*, and (5) the *right route*. Experience indicates that five additional rights are essential to professional nursing practice: (1) the *right assessment*, (2) the *right documentation*, (3) the *client's right to education*, (4) the *right evaluation*, and (5) the *client's right to refuse*.

The **right client** can be ensured by checking the client's identification bracelet and by having the client state her or his name. Some clients answer to any name or are unable to respond, so client identification should be verified *each* time a medication is administered. In the event of a missing identification bracelet, the nurse *must* verify the client's identity *before* any drug administration.

Nursing implications include the following:
- Verify client by checking the identification bracelet. Some facilities put the client's photo on his or her health record.
- Distinguish between two clients with the same last name; have warnings highlighted in a bright color on identification (ID) tools, such as med cards, bracelet, or Kardex.
- Some institutions have ID bracelets coded for allergy status. Be aware of this policy.

When clients do not wear ID bands (e.g., schools, occupational health departments, outpatient departments, health care provider offices), the nurse also has the responsibility of accurately identifying the individual when administering a medication.

The **right drug** means that the client receives the drug that was prescribed. Medication orders may be prescribed by a physician (MD), dentist (DDS), podiatrist (DPM), or licensed health care provider, such as an advanced practice registered nurse (APRN), with authority from the state to order medications. Prescriptions may be written on a prescription pad and filled by a pharmacist at a drug store or hospital pharmacy (Figure 3–1). For institutionalized clients, the drug orders may be written on "order sheets" and signed by the duly authorized person (Figure 3–2). A telephone order (TO) or verbal order (VO) for medication must be cosigned by the prescribing health care provider within 24 hours. The nurse must comply with the institution's policy regarding a TO, which sometimes requires that two licensed practitioners listen to and sign the order.

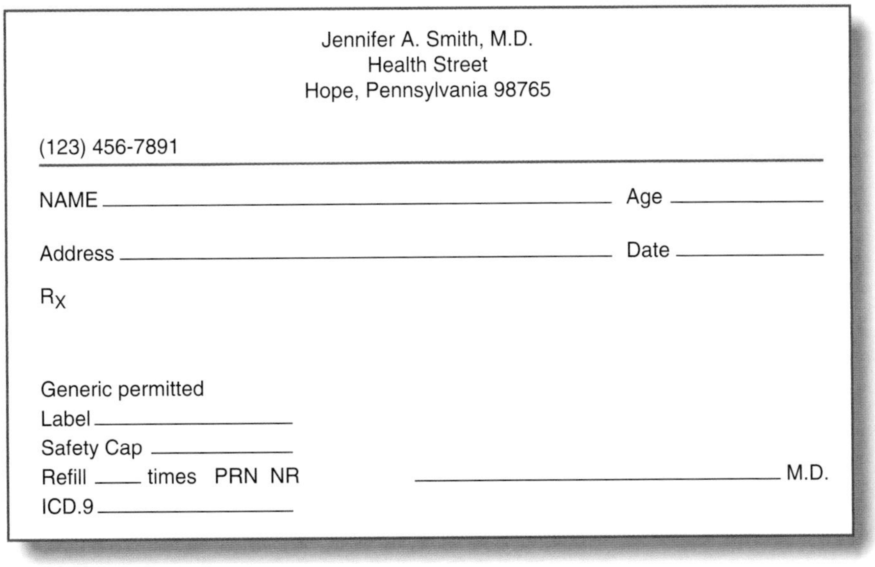

Jennifer A. Smith, M.D.
Health Street
Hope, Pennsylvania 98765

(123) 456-7891

NAME ______ Age ______

Address ______ Date ______

Rx

Generic permitted
Label ______
Safety Cap ______
Refill ____ times PRN NR ______ M.D.
ICD.9 ______

FIGURE 3–1 Example of prescription pad medication order.

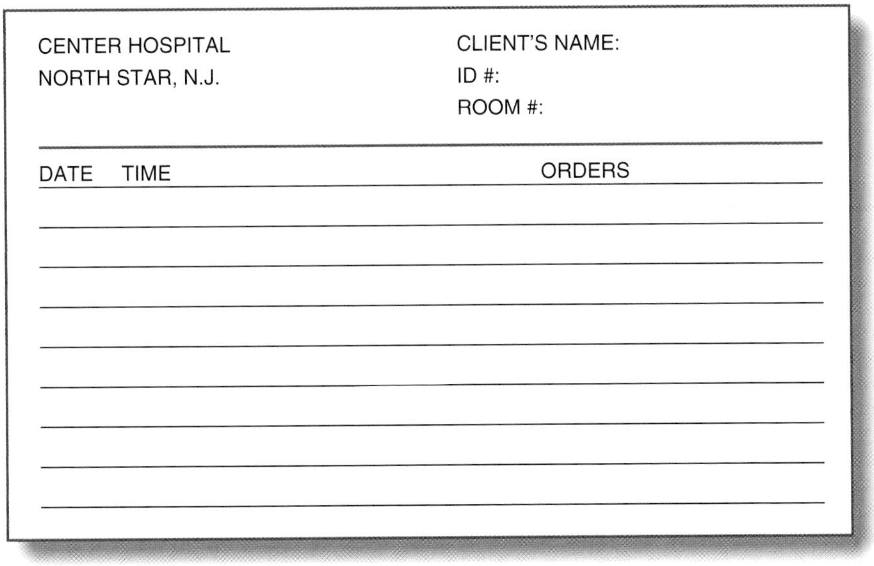

CENTER HOSPITAL
NORTH STAR, N.J.

CLIENT'S NAME:
ID #:
ROOM #:

DATE	TIME	ORDERS

FIGURE 3–2 Example of client's order form.

The use of computerized order systems has added speed and a safety feature to the order process. Orders can be written from virtually any location and sent via modem. The computer will not process the order unless all the information is included. Also, there is no need to worry about illegible orders or signatures. The same benefits are available for nurses to record the medications given or refused. In general, the same information is documented in both written and computerized systems.

The components of a drug order are as follows:

- Date and time the order is written
- Drug name (generic preferred)
- Drug dosage
- Route of administration
- Frequency and duration of administration (e.g., × 7 days, × 3 doses)
- Any special instructions for withholding or adjusting dosage based on nursing assessment, drug effectiveness, or laboratory results
- Physician or other health care provider's signature or name if TO or VO
- Signatures of licensed practitioners taking TO or VO

Although the nurse's responsibility is to follow an appropriate order, if any one of the components is missing, the drug order is incomplete and the drug should not be administered. Clarification of the order must be done in a timely manner; the health care provider is usually contacted and the conversation content documented. The following is an example of a drug order and its interpretation:

6/4/05 10:10A Lasix 40 mg, PO, daily (signature). (Give 40 mg of Lasix by mouth daily.)

To avoid drug error, the drug label should be read three times: (1) at the time of contact with the drug bottle or container, (2) before pouring the drug, and (3) after pouring the drug. The first dose, one-time, and "as needed" (PRN) medication orders should be checked against original orders. Nurses should be aware that certain drug names sound alike and are spelled similarly. Examples are digoxin and digitoxin; quinidine and quinine; Keflex and Kantrex; Demerol and dicumarol; and Percocet and Percodan. More specifically, Percocet contains oxycodone and acetaminophen, whereas Percodan contains oxycodone and aspirin. A client may be allergic to aspirin, so it is important that this client receive Percocet. **Read the labels carefully.**

Nursing implications include the following:

- Check that the medication order is complete and legible. If the order is not complete or legible, notify the nurse manager and health care provider.
- Know the reason for which the client is to receive the medication.
- Check the drug label three times before administration of the medication.
- Know the date the medication was ordered and any ending date (e.g., for controlled substances and antibiotics and for limited or a specific number of doses). Some agencies have "automatic stop orders," which are generally facility specific. Examples of such orders include controlled drugs that need to be renewed every 48 hours, anticoagulants and antibiotics to be renewed after 7 days, and cancellation of all medications when the client goes to surgery.

The following are the four categories of drug orders:

1. Standing
2. One-time (single)
3. PRN
4. STAT (at once)

Table 3-1 summarizes the drug order categories with examples of each.

The **right dose** is the dose prescribed for a particular client. In most cases, this dose is within the recommended range for the particular drug. Nurses must calculate each drug dose accurately, considering the variables: drug availability and the prescribed drug dose. In selected situations, such as pediatrics, the client's weight range must also be considered, such as 3 mg per kilogram of body weight daily. See Chapter 4, Medications and Calculations, for drug calculations.

Before calculating a drug dose, the nurse should have a general idea of the answer based on a knowledge of the basic formula or ratios and proportions. Calculation of drug doses should be rechecked if a fraction of a dose or an extremely large dose has been calculated. Consultation with a peer or a pharmacist should occur whenever doubt exists.

The stock drug method and unit dose method are the two most frequently used methods of drug distribution. Table 3-2 describes these methods and the advantages and disadvantages of each.

In the traditional stock drug method, the drugs are dispensed to all clients from the same containers. In the **unit dose method,** drugs are individually wrapped and labeled for single doses. The unit dose method is popular in many institutions and community settings. Unit dosing has eliminated many drug dosage errors.

Automation of medication administration, introduced more than a decade ago, is promoted as saving time and decreasing costs associated with the administration of medications. Some features include a link to the pharmacy information system and current clinical client data. In addition, the ability to collect information automatically about charting and recording of medication is available. An activity report menu is a popular feature. Flexible dose modes are available, including single dose, multidose, and multiple medications. Pyxis is an example of automated medication-dispensing technology (Figure 3-3). It assists the nurse in correctly and quickly administering medications. Thus this technology has the potential to improve client care by promoting accurate and quick access to medications.

The nursing implications include the following:

- Calculate the drug dose correctly. When in doubt, the drug dose should be recalculated and checked by another nurse. In many settings, the first nurse to administer the particular drug to the client must calculate the dose according to the stated formulary doses and sign in the nurse's signature space once the safety parameter has been established. In some settings, two registered nurses (RNs) are required to check dosage for specific medications such as insulin and heparin.

Table 3-1

Categories of Drug Orders

Category	Description	Examples
Standing orders	May be an ongoing order or may be given for a specific number of doses or days	Digoxin 0.25 mg PO daily
		Colace 100 mg PO daily, PRN
	May have special instructions to base administration on laboratory values	Digoxin, maintain blood level of 0.5-2.0 ng/ml
	May include PRN orders	
One-time or single orders	Given once and usually at a specific time	Versed 2 mg IM at 7 AM on 10/5/05
PRN orders	Given at the client's request and nurse's judgment concerning need and safety	Tylenol 650 mg q3 to 4h PRN for headache
STAT orders	Given once, immediately	Morphine sulfate 2 mg IV STAT

IM, Intramuscular; *IV,* intravenous; *PO,* by mouth; *PRN,* as needed; *STAT,* immediately.

Table 3–2

Drug Distribution Methods

Stock Method	Unit Dose Method
Description	
Drugs are stored on unit and dispensed to all clients from the same container	Drugs are packaged in doses for 24 h by the pharmacy
Advantages	
Always available	Saves time for nurse; no dose calculation required
Cost-efficiency of large quantities	Billed for specific doses
	More accountability
	Less chance for contamination and error
Disadvantages	
Drug errors are more prevalent with multiple "pourers"	Potential delay in receiving drug
More risk of abuse by health care workers	Not immediately replaceable if contaminated
Less accountability for amount used; unable to track usage	More expensive
Increased opportunity for contamination (multiple pourers challenge aseptic/sterile status)	

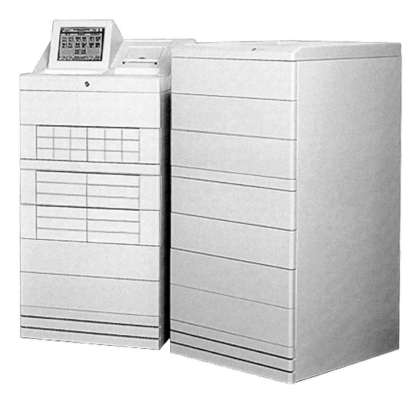

FIGURE 3–3 Computerized medication management system. (Courtesy Pyxis Corp., San Diego, Calif.)

• Check the *PDR, American Hospital Formulary,* drug package insert, or other drug references for recommended range of specific drug doses.

The **right time** is the time at which the prescribed dose should be administered. Daily drug dosages are given at specified times during a day, such as twice a day (b.i.d.), three times a day (t.i.d.), four times a day (q.i.d.), or every 6 hours (q6h), so that the plasma level of the drug is maintained. When the drug has a long half-life ($t\frac{1}{2}$), the drug is given once a day. Drugs with a short half-life are given several times a day at specified intervals (see Chapter 1, Drug Action: Pharmaceutic, Pharmacokinetic, and Pharmacodynamic Phases). Some drugs are given before meals, and others are given with meals or with food.

Many nursing settings currently use military time (a 24-hour clock). For example, 2 AM is 0200, 2 PM is 1400, 6:10 AM is 0610, and 5:30 PM is 1730. AM hours correlate with the traditional clock; 12 hours are added for the PM hours (Figure 3–4). Military time has the advantages of reducing administration errors and decreasing documentation.

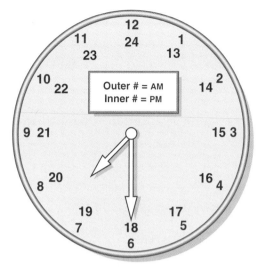

FIGURE 3–4 Military time.

Nursing implications include the following:

- Administer drugs at the specified times. Drugs may be given 0.5 hour before or after the time prescribed if the administration interval is >2 hours. Refer to agency policy.
- Administer drugs that are affected by foods, such as tetracycline, before meals.
- Administer drugs that can irritate the stomach (gastric mucosa), such as potassium and aspirin, with food.
- The drug administration schedule may sometimes be adjusted to fit the schedule of the client's lifestyle, activities, tolerances, or preferences.
- It is the nurse's responsibility to check whether the client is scheduled for any diagnostic procedures, such as endoscopy or fasting blood tests, that would contraindicate the administration of medications. Determine per policy whether the medication should be given after the test is completed.
- Check the expiration date. Discard the medication or return it to the pharmacy (depending on policy) if the date has passed.
- Antibiotics should be administered at even intervals (e.g., q8h rather than t.i.d.) throughout a 24-hour period so therapeutic blood levels are maintained.

The **right route** is necessary for adequate or appropriate absorption. The more common routes of absorption include oral (by mouth): liquid, elixir, suspension, pill, tablet, or capsule; **sublingual** (under tongue for venous absorption); **buccal** (between gum and cheek); via feeding tube; topical (applied to the skin); **inhalation** (aerosol sprays); instillation (in nose, eye, ear); suppository (rectal, vaginal); and four parenteral routes: intradermal, subcutaneous (subQ), intramuscular (IM), and intravenous (IV).

Nursing implications include the following:

- Assess the client's ability to swallow before the administration of oral medications.
- Do not crush or mix medications in other substances before consultation with a pharmacist. Do not mix medications with sweet substance to "trick" children into taking medications. Do not mix medications in an infant's formula feeding.
- Use aseptic technique when administering drugs. Sterile technique is required with the parenteral routes.
- Administer the drugs at the appropriate sites.
- Stay with the client until oral drugs have been swallowed.
- If it is necessary to combine medication with another substance, explain this to the client.

The **right assessment** requires that appropriate data be collected before administration of the drug. Examples of assessment data may include measuring the apical heart rate before the administration of digitalis preparations or serum blood sugar levels before the administration of insulin.

The **right documentation** requires that the nurse immediately record the appropriate information about the drug administered. This includes (1) the *name* of the drug, (2) the *dose,* (3) the *route* (injection site if applicable), (4) the *time* and *date,* and (5) the nurse's *initials* or *signature.* Documentation of the client's response to the medication is required with a variety of medications, such as (1) narcotics (how effective was the pain relief?), (2) nonnarcotic analgesics, (3) sedatives, (4) antiemetics, and (5) unexpected reactions to the medication, such as gastrointestinal (GI) irritation or signs of skin sensitivity. A delay in charting could result in forgetting to chart the medication or in another nurse's administration of the drug because she or he thought the drug was not given.

To assist in the accurate and timely recording of drugs administered, many health care facilities use a graphic format or computerized systems (Figure 3–5).

The **right to education** requires that the client receive accurate and thorough information about the medication and how it relates to his or her particular situation. Client teaching also includes therapeutic purpose, possible side effects of the drug, any dietary restrictions or requirements, skill of administration, and laboratory monitoring. This right is a principle of **informed consent,** which is based on the individual having the knowledge necessary to make a decision.

The **right evaluation** requires that the effectiveness of the medication be determined by the client's response to the medication. Evaluation in this context asks, "Did the medication do for the client what it was supposed to do?" It is also appropriate to determine the extent of side effects and adverse reactions, if any.

The client has the **right to refuse** the medication. Clients can and do refuse to take a medication. It is the nurse's responsibility to determine, when possible, the reason for the refusal and to take reasonable measures to facilitate the client's taking the medication. Explain to the client the risk of refusing to take the medication, and reinforce the reason for the medication. When a medication is refused, this refusal must be documented immediately. The nurse manager, primary nurse, or health care provider should be informed when the omission may pose a

```
6SB   -7530-01      W J M C   DEVELOPMENT   HOSP #6
      09:00 AM  SCHEDULED MEDICATIONS DUE   6SB   (QJB$$N)      PAGE 001
                                            ISSUED:  07:47 AM 02/12/05


   6116A  MARILYN, MARILYN          0001393300      0215500019   GIV NGIV


   U  (ADVIL, MOTRIN, NUPRIN, RUFEN) IBUPROFEN TAB 400MG
         DOSE: #1, PO
      BID-PC (08/06/02 06PM-..)


   U  (DELTASONE, METICORTEN, ORASONE) PREDNISONE TAB 5MG
         DOSE: #1, PO
      QD-AM/Q24H (08/07/02 09AM-..)


   U  (FERGON) FERROUS GLUC TAB 320MG
         DOSE: #1, PO
      (URINE AND STOOL MAY DARKEN) BID/Q12H (12/06/02 09PM-..)


   U  (LANOXIN) DIGOXIN TAB 0.25MG
         DOSE: #1, PO
      QD-AM/Q24H HOLD FOR HR < 50 (01/15/04 09AM-..)


         ALLERGIES: CEPHALORSPORINS, PENICILLIN,
         MORPHINE, GENTAMICIN SULFATE, IODINE,
         PENICILLIN, SHELLFISH, POISON IVY/OAK,
         ANIMAL DANDER/HAIR, BEE STINGS


   * * * * * * * * * * * * * * * * * * * * * * * * * * * * * * * * * * * *
```

A

UNIVERSITY HOSPITAL

CLIENT'S NAME:
ID #:
ROOM #:

Nurse's Signature/Title		Initials
Evelyn Hayes	RN	EH
Joyce Kee	RN	JK
Rodney Brown	LPN	RB
Jody Smith	LPN	JS

Allergies: *Codeine*

Continuing Medical Record

Date Order	Stop Date	Medication/Dosage/Route/Frequency	Time	Date 8/14	8/15	Initials 8/16	8/17
8/14		Digoxin 0.125 mg po qd 0900	0900	EH	EH	JK	
EH				AR=74	AR=70	AR=70	
8/14		Capoten 12.5 mg po bid	0900	EH	EH	JK	
EH			2100	RB	RB	RB	
8/15	8/22	Amoxicillin 250 mg po q6h	0600	✕	✕	JS	
EH	LD 0600	x7d	1200		EH	JK	
1100			1800		RB	RB	
			2400		JS	JS	

One-Time/PRN/STAT Medications

Date	Medication/Dosage/Route/Frequency	Time/Initials	Reason	Result
8/14	Nitroglycerin 1/150 gr sublingual PRN	1600 EH	Chest pain	Relief of pain
	Chest pain			

B

FIGURE 3–5 Medication record. A, Computerized; B, written format.

specific threat to the client, such as with insulin. Follow-up is also required when a change is expected in the laboratory test values, such as with insulin and warfarin (Coumadin).

All medication errors are serious or potentially serious. A medication error may involve one or more of the following: administration of the wrong medication or IV fluid; the incorrect dose or rate; administration to the wrong client, by the incorrect route, at the incorrect schedule interval; administration of known allergic drug or IV fluid; omission of dose or discontinuation of medication or IV fluid that was not discontinued.

The Institute of Medicine (IOM) report of 1999, *To Err is Human: Building A Safer Health Care System,* spurred work on identifying system changes to decrease errors. More than 100,000 medication errors were reported by hospitals nationwide in 2001. A medication error may be defined as "any preventable event that may cause or lead to inappropriate medication use or harm to a patient." Medication errors may occur throughout the cycle; one national report included 39% related to ordering, 12% transcribing, 11% preparing, and 38% administering.

A major factor affecting medication errors is the increase in the number of drugs; from 3000 in 1990 to more than 17,000 in 2000. Other contributing causes include violation of "10 rights"; lack of drug knowledge; memory lapses; transcription, dispensing, or delivery problems; inadequate monitoring; distractions; staff being overworked; lack of standardization; confusing packaging prescription; equipment failures; inadequate client history; and poor interdepartmental communication.

In response to the escalating number of medication errors causing human deaths and costing billions of dollars, in 2002 the Food and Drug Administration (FDA) proposed a rule titled *Bar Code Label Requirements for Human Drug Products and Blood;* this has increased the prominence of this coding. At a minimum the bar code would contain the drug's national drug code that "uniquely identifies the drug, its strength, and its dosage form". A revision to this rule eliminates blood and blood products that have had bar codes since 1985. Once the rule is published in the *Federal Registry,* companies have 3 years to comply. The FDA reports that in hospitals with bar coding, a 71% to 86% decrease in the rate of medication errors has resulted. Most staff embraces bar coding once they are proficient with its use. Further, they note that bar coding is a tool but not a substitute for critical thinking.

Computerized prescriber order entry (CPOE) systems interact with laboratory, pharmacy, and client data. This integrated system of client data is the basis for the success of bar coding. The FDA posits that the bar coding rule will have hospitals act on investing in the required technologies. With bar coding, the client's medication administration record (MAR), a part of the database that is encoded in the client's wristband, is accessible to the nurse using a handheld device. After scanning the client's wristband, the nurse would see the individual's MAR on the device. To administer a medication, the nurse would first scan the drug's

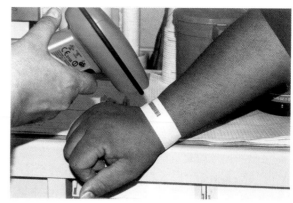

FIGURE 3–6   Bar code reader used to scan the client's wristband.

bar code, the number of the client's medical record, and his or her ID badge code. The client's MAR would then be updated accordingly. Figure 3–6 shows a nurse scanning a client's wristband. The nurse receives verification on the handheld device of "5 rights", warnings, and clinical alerts (e.g., drug is discontinued or not ordered for client). As part of their 2004 National Patient Safety Goals, the Joint Commission on Accreditation of Healthcare Organizations (JCAHO) announced that all accredited organizations must **not use** the following abbreviations, acronyms, and symbols:

- U (for unit)
- IU (for international unit)
- QD (for every day)
- QOD (for every other day)
- Trailing zero and lack of leading zero; never write a zero by itself after a decimal point (e.g., 5.0 mg), and always use a zero before a decimal point (e.g., 0.5 mg).
- MS and MSO_4

Please see the JCAHO website at end of this chapter for detailed safety information.

Watch for Safe Medication Administration boxes throughout the text.

The nurse must be ever vigilant about safety in medication administration. Actions to create a culture of safety include:

- Use drug references and visit *www.ISMP.org* regularly.
- Contact the health care provider; do not guess about the order. Document clarification.
- Double-check all calculated doses.
- Use leading zero (0.5); do **not** use trailing zero (5.0).
- Avoid verbal orders; if you must take them, repeat out loud to confirm.
- Scan bar code at the point-of-care.
- Include the pharmacist on client rounds.
- Use a computerized prescriber order entry (CPOE).
- Avoid dangerous abbreviations (e.g., HCT: hydrocortisone or hydrochlorothiazide?)
- **Consistently think critically**

Several resources address medication errors and their prevention; two of these resources follow. A current database of medication errors and "near misses" will assist all health care personnel to identify, implement, and evaluate strategies to prevent medication errors. It is strongly suggested that one report list (which will be held confidential) errors or "near misses" to the FDA at (800) 23-ERROR. The National Coordinating Council for Medication Error Reporting and Prevention (NCCMERP) specializes in medication errors from an interdisciplinary perspective; contact them at (800) 822-8772.

Medication Self-Administration

Self-administration (SAM) of medication is a common practice in the home and in many community-based settings, such as the workplace. However, SAM is relatively new to clients and staff in institutional settings. In practical terms, SAM means that the nurse gives the client a packet of appropriate medications and instructions that are kept at the bedside and the client takes home on discharge. The client is responsible for taking the medications according to the instructions when he or she feels they are needed. The client has a key role in his or her care and exercises control associated with taking selected medications. SAM helps clients to manage medications during the hospital stay and prepares them to keep as comfortable as possible at home. For example, see Chapter 51, Drugs Associated with the Female Reproductive Cycle I: Pregnancy and Preterm Labor, and Chapter 52, Drugs Associated with the Female Reproductive Cycle II: Labor, Delivery, and the Preterm Neonate, for a detailed description of SAM for the maternity client.

Special Considerations: Factors That Modify Drug Response

The pharmacologic response to a drug is complex. Nurses must be mindful of the number and variety of factors that influence an individual's response to a drug. (See Chapter 7, Drug Interaction and Over-the-Counter Drugs; Chapter 10, Pediatric Pharmacology; and Chapter 11, Geriatric Pharmacology for detailed descriptions of influencing factors.) Examples of factors that modify drug responses include the following:

- *Absorption.* A major variable in absorption is the route of administration of the drug. Oral absorption takes place as drug particles move from the GI tract (stomach and small intestine) to body fluids. Any GI disturbances (e.g., vomiting or diarrhea) affect drug absorption.
- *Distribution.* Protein binding is a major modifier of drug distribution in the body. Propranolol (Inderal) is 90% protein bound. Another factor is the blood-brain barrier, which allows only lipid-soluble drugs (e.g., general anesthetics, barbiturates) to enter into the brain and cerebrospinal fluid. Compounds that are strongly ionized and poorly soluble in fat are barred from entry into the brain. Neoplastic agents are examples of drugs that do not cross the blood-brain barrier. The placental barrier is

a membrane that, for the most part, keeps the blood of the mother and fetus separate. However, both lipid-soluble and lipid-insoluble drugs can diffuse across the placenta. Some drugs have teratogenic effects if taken during the first trimester of pregnancy; that is, they may induce aberrant development of fetal organs or body systems. This is especially true if the drugs are taken during the fourth through eighth weeks of gestation.

- *Metabolism (biotransformation).* The liver is the primary organ for drug metabolism. All infants, especially neonates and low-birth-weight infants, have immature liver and kidney function. Influences on liver function, such as the aging process and chronic liver disease, also affect the metabolism of a medication.
  - *Excretion.* The main route of drug excretion is via the kidney. Through the normal aging process and chronic disease or kidney failure, there is a decrease in the functioning cells of the kidney, resulting in decreased excretion of drugs. Bile, feces, respiration, saliva, and sweat are also routes of drug excretion.
  - *Age.* Infants and the elderly are more sensitive to drugs. The elderly are hypersensitive to barbiturates and central nervous system (CNS) depressants. Such clients have poor absorption through the GI tract because of decreased gastric secretion. Infant doses are calculated based on weight in kilograms rather than on biologic or gestational age.
  - *Body weight.* Drug doses (e.g., of antineoplastics) may be ordered according to body weight. Obese persons may need increased drug doses, and very thin persons may need decreased doses.
- *Toxicity.* This term refers to the *first adverse symptoms* that occur at a particular dose. Toxicity is more prevalent in persons with liver or renal impairment and in the very young and old.
- *Pharmacogenetics.* This term refers to the influence of genetic factors on drug response. If a parent has an adverse reaction to a drug, the child may also. Some genetic factors are associated with ethnicity.
  - *Route of administration.* Drugs administered by IV act more rapidly than those administered by mouth.
  - *Time of administration.* The presence or absence of food in the stomach can affect the action of some drugs.
  - *Emotional factors.* Suggestive comments about the drug and its side effects may influence its effects.
  - *Preexisting disease state.* Liver, kidney, heart, circulatory, and GI disorders are examples of preexisting states that can affect a response to a drug. For example, persons with diabetes should not be given elixirs or syrups that contain sugar.
  - *Drug history.* Be aware that past use of the same or different drugs may reduce or intensify the effects of the drug.
- *Tolerance.* The ability of a client to respond to a particular dose of a certain drug may diminish after days or weeks of repeated administration. A combination of

drugs may be given to decrease or delay the development of tolerance for a specific drug.

- *Cumulative effect.* This occurs when the drug is metabolized or excreted more slowly than the rate at which it is being administered.
  - *Drug-drug interaction.* The effects of a combination of drugs may be greater than, equal to, or less than the effects of a single drug. Some drugs may compete for the same receptor sites. An adverse reaction may lead to toxicity or complications, such as anaphylaxis.
  - *Food-drug interaction.* The effects of selected foods may speed, delay, or prevent absorption of specific drugs.

Guidelines for Drug Administration

General guidelines for drug administration are listed in Boxes 3–1 and 3–2. These guidelines are summarized as the *do*'s and *dont*'s of drug administration. Nurses should follow these guidelines to enhance safety when administering medications. Application of the nursing process to medication administration is presented later in this chapter.

Forms and Routes for Drug Administration

A variety of forms and routes are used for the administration of medications, including sublingual, buccal, oral (tablets, capsules, liquids, suspensions, elixirs), transdermal, topical, instillation (drops and sprays), inhalations, nasogastric and gastrostomy tubes, suppositories, and parenteral (Figure 3–7). A brief description of each follows.

Tablets and Capsules

- Oral medications are *not* given to clients who are vomiting, lack a gag reflex, or who are comatose. Clients who gag may need a brief rest before proceeding with further intake of medications.
- Do not mix with a large amount of food or beverage or with contraindicated food. Clients may not be able to

---

BOX 3–1

Guidelines for Correct Administration of Medications

Preparation

1. Wash hands before preparing medications.
2. Check for drug allergies; check the assessment history and Kardex.
3. Check medication order with health care provider's orders, Kardex, medicine sheet, and medicine card.
4. Check label on drug container three times.
5. Check expiration date on drug label, card, Kardex; use only if date is current.
6. Recheck drug calculation of drug dose with another nurse.
7. Verify doses of drugs that are potentially toxic with another nurse or pharmacist.
8. Pour tablet or capsule into the cap of the drug container. With unit dose, open packet at bedside after verifying client identification.
9. Pour liquid at eye level. Meniscus, the lower curve of the liquid, should be at the line of desired dose (see Figure 3–8).
10. Dilute drugs that irritate gastric mucosa (e.g., potassium, aspirin), or give with meals.

Administration

11. Administer only drugs that you have prepared. Do not prepare medications to be administered by another.
12. Identify the client by ID band or ID photo.
13. Offer ice chips to numb taste buds when giving bad-tasting drugs.
14. When possible, give bad-tasting medications first, followed by pleasant-tasting liquids.
15. Assist the client to an appropriate position, depending on the route of administration.
16. Provide only liquids allowed on the diet.
17. Stay with the client until the medications are taken.
18. Administer no more than 2.5 to 3 ml of solution intramuscularly at one site. Infants receive no more than 1 ml of solution intramuscularly at one site and no more

than 1 ml subcutaneously. Never recap needles (universal precautions).
19. When administering drugs to a group of clients, give drugs last to clients who need extra assistance.
20. Discard needles and syringes in appropriate containers.
21. Drug disposal is dependent on agency policy and state law. For example, discard drugs in the sink or toilet, not in the trash can. Controlled substances must be returned to the pharmacy. Some disposals need signatures of witnesses.
22. Discard unused solutions from ampules.
23. Appropriately store (some require refrigeration) unused stable solutions from open vials.
24. Write date and time opened and your initials on label.
25. Keep narcotics in a double-locked drawer or closet. Medication carts must be locked at all times when a nurse is not in attendance.
26. Keys to the narcotics drawer must be kept by the nurse and not stored in a drawer or closet.
27. Keep narcotics in a safe place, out of reach of children and others in the home.
28. Avoid contamination of one's own skin or inhalation to minimize chances of allergy or sensitivity development.

Recording

29. Report drug error immediately to client's health care provider and to the nurse manager. Complete an incident report.
30. Charting: record drug given, dose, time, route, and your initials.
31. Record drugs promptly after given, especially STAT doses.
32. Record effectiveness and results of medication administered, especially PRN medications.
33. Report to health care provider and record drugs that were refused with reason for refusal.
34. Record amount of fluid taken with medications on input and output chart.

ID, Identification; *PRN*, as needed; *STAT*, immediately.

eat all the food and will not get the full dose of medication. Do not mix in infant formula.

- Enteric-coated and timed-release capsules *must* be swallowed whole to be effective.
- Administer irritating drugs *with food* to decrease GI discomfort.

- Administer drugs on an empty stomach if food interferes with medication absorption.
- Drugs given sublingually (placed under tongue) or buccally (placed between cheek and gum) remain in place until fully absorbed. No food or fluids should be taken while the medication is in place.
- Encourage the use of child-resistant caps. The Consumer Public Safety Commission has ordered a redesign of these caps because the current caps are difficult for elderly clients to use. This has contributed to a safety hazard for children and others because many people, in an effort to have easy access to their medications, leave the caps off. The new design requires a person to lightly squeeze the two side bottle tabs and turn the cap. Non–child-resistant caps are available on request.

Liquids

- There are several forms of liquid medication, including elixirs, emulsions, and suspensions.
- Read the labels to determine whether dilution or shaking is required.
- The **meniscus** is at the line of desired dose (Figure 3–8).
- Many liquids require refrigeration once reconstituted.

Transdermal

- **Transdermal** medication is stored in a patch placed on the skin and absorbed through skin, thereby having systemic effect. Widespread use of such patches began in the 1980s. Patches for cardiovascular drugs, neoplastic drugs, hormones, drugs to treat allergic reactions, and insulin are in production or being developed. Transdermal drugs provide more consistent blood levels and avoid GI absorption problems associated with oral products (Figure 3–9).
- A common question is whether to cut the patches in half. A nurse might suggest the purchase of patches with a lower dosage rather than cutting the patch and guessing the dose the client will receive. However, depending on the client's situation and the type of patch, it may be appropriate to cut the patch. If the drug is embedded in a *matrix patch* and diffuses into the skin (e.g., Climara, Vivelle, Nicotrol, Nitro-Dur, and Testoderm), the drug is spread over the entire surface of the patch and probably may be cut. Clients must be alert for underdosing or overdosing. The drug is pooled in a *reservoir patch* and is released via a semipermeable membrane (e.g.,

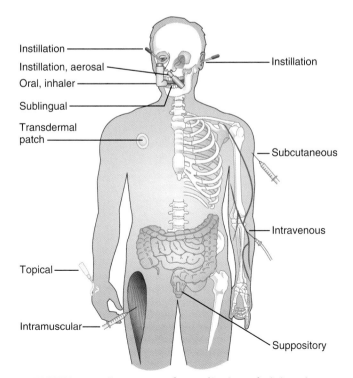

FIGURE 3–7 Some routes for medication administration.

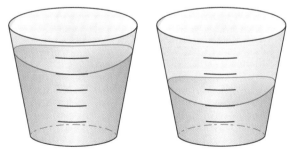

FIGURE 3–8 To read the meniscus, locate the lowest fluid mark.

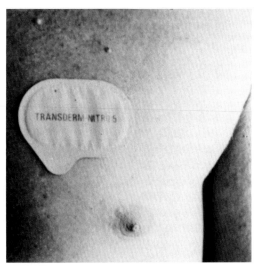

FIGURE 3–9 Transdermal nitroglycerin patch. (Courtesy Summit Pharmaceuticals, Novartis, East Hanover, NJ.)

Catapres-TTS, Duragesic, Estraderm, Transderm-Scōp, Transderm-Nitro, Androderm). These patches should not be cut because too much drug may be released. However, it is possible to peel back the protective layer halfway. Advise clients to secure the patch with tape, being careful not to apply it too tightly, which could alter the drug delivery. For legal and financial reasons, manufacturers do not recommend cutting the patches. Remember to remove temporarily a patch with any metallic component before magnetic resonance imaging (MRI) is performed to avoid skin burns. Many patches have a foil backing to prevent leakage.

Topical

- **Topical** medications can be applied to the skin in a number of ways, such as with a glove, tongue blade, or cotton-tipped applicator. A nurse should never apply a topical medication without first protecting his or her own skin.
- Use appropriate technique to remove the medication from the container, and apply it to clean, dry skin, when possible. Do not contaminate the medication in a container; instead use gloves or an applicator.
- Do not "double dip." Gloves and applicators that come in contact with a client should not be reinserted into the container. Estimate the amount needed, and remove it from the container or use a fresh sterile applicator each time the container is entered.

PREVENTING MEDICATION ERRORS

Safety alert:

- Remember to remove foil-backed patches before magnetic resonance imaging (MRI) is performed to prevent burns.

- Observe sterile technique when the skin is broken. Take precautions to avoid medication stains.
- Use firm strokes if the medication is to be rubbed in.

Instillations

Instillations are liquid medications usually administered as drops, ointment, or sprays in the following forms:
- Eyedrops (Box 3–3, Figure 3–10)
- Eye ointment (Box 3–4, Figure 3–11)
- Eardrops (Box 3–5, Figure 3–12)
- Nose drops and sprays (Box 3–6, Figures 3–13 and 3–14)

BOX 3–3

Administration of Eye Drops

1. WASH HANDS.
2. Instruct client to lie or sit down and to look up toward ceiling.
3. Remove any discharge by gently wiping out from inner canthus. Use separate cloth for each eye.
4. Gently draw skin down below the affected eye to expose the conjunctival sac.
5. Administer the prescribed number of drops into the center of the sac. Medication placed directly on the cornea can cause discomfort or damage. Do not touch eyelids or eyelashes with dropper. Self-administration of drops is enhanced with the use of Drop-eze, a cuplike device that holds the eyelids open.
6. Gently press on the lacrimal duct with sterile cotton ball or tissue for 1 to 2 min after instillation to prevent systemic absorption through lacrimal canal.
7. Client should keep eyes closed for 1 to 2 minutes following application to promote absorption.

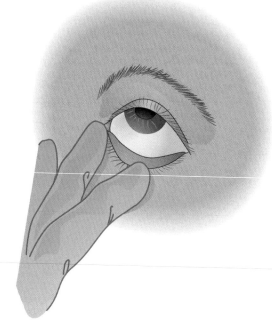

FIGURE 3–10 To administer eyedrops, gently pull down the skin below the eye to expose the conjunctival sac.

BOX 3–4

Administration of Eye Ointment

1. WASH HANDS.
2. Instruct client to lie or sit down and to look up toward ceiling.
3. Remove any discharge by gently wiping out from inner canthus. Use separate cloth for each eye.
4. Gently draw skin down below the affected eye to expose the conjunctival sac.
5. Squeeze strip of ointment (about ¼ inch unless stated otherwise) onto conjunctival sac. Medication placed directly on cornea can cause discomfort or damage.
6. Instruct client to close eyes for 2 to 3 minutes.
7. Instruct client to expect blurred vision for a short time. Apply at bedtime, if possible.

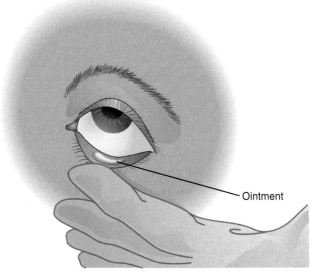

Ointment

FIGURE 3–11 To administer eye ointment, squeeze a ¼-inch-wide strip of ointment onto the conjunctival sac.

BOX 3–5

Administration of Eardrops

1. WASH HANDS.
2. Medication should be at room temperature.
3. Client should sit up with head tilted slightly toward the unaffected side. To straighten the external ear canal for better visualization and to facilitate drops reaching the affected area, see Figure 3–12.
4. *Child:* pull down and back on auricle. After 3 years of age, same as adult.
   Adult: pull up and back on auricle.
5. Instill prescribed number of drops.
6. Take care not to contaminate dropper.
7. Have client maintain position for 2 to 3 minutes.

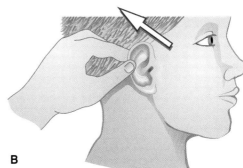

A

B

FIGURE 3–12 To administer eardrops, straighten the external ear canal by pulling down (A) on the auricle in children or pulling back on the auricle in adults (B).

BOX 3–6

Administration of Nose Drops and Sprays

1. Have client blow nose.
2. Have client tilt head back for drops to reach frontal sinus and tilt head to affected side to reach ethmoid sinus.
3. Administer the prescribed number of drops or sprays. Some sprays have instructions to close one nostril, tilt head to closed side, and hold breath or breathe through nose for 1 minute.
4. Have client keep head tilted backward for 5 minutes after instillation of drops.

Inhalations

- Handheld nebulizers deliver a very fine-sized particle spray of medication.
- Handheld metered-dose devices are a convenient method of administration for these medications. See Figure 3–15.
- **Spacers** are devices used to enhance the delivery of medications from the **metered-dose inhaler (MDI)**. Figure 3–15 illustrates the distribution of medication with and without a spacer. Aero Chamber (distributed by For-

est Pharmaceuticals, St. Louis) and Inspirease (distributed by Key Pharmaceuticals, Kenilworth, NJ) are examples of available spacers.
- The preferred client position is semi- or high Fowler's.
- Teach the client correct use of equipment.
- Nebulizer (aerosol) changes a liquid medication into a fine mist.
- MDIs are hand-held devices that deliver medications to oropharyngeal and lower respiratory tracts. See Box 3–7 for the correct use of an inhaler and Figure 3–16 to monitor the amount of medication in the **canister.**

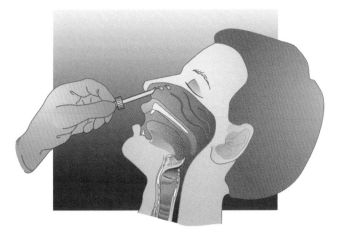

FIGURE 3–13   Administering nose drops.

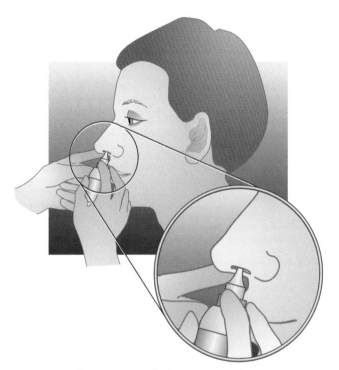

FIGURE 3–14   Administering nasal spray.

BOX 3–7

Correct Use of Metered-Dose Inhaler

1. Insert the medication canister into the plastic holder.
2. Shake the inhaler well before using. Remove cap from mouthpiece.
3. Breathe out through the mouth. Open mouth wide and hold the mouthpiece 1 to 2 inches from the mouth. Do *not* put mouthpiece in the mouth unless using a spacer. Discuss techniques with the health care provider.
4. With mouth open, take slow, deep breath through mouth and at same time push the top of the medication canister once. Autohalers (e.g., Maxair) do not require coordination of pushing down top of canister and taking deep breath. With the autohaler in upright position, raise lever and shake. Inhale deeply through mouthpiece with steady, moderate force, which triggers the release of medicine, making a "click" sound and puffing out the medicine. Continue to take deep breaths.
5. Hold breath for a few seconds; exhale slowly through pursed lips.
6. If a second dose is required, wait 2 minutes and repeat the procedure by first shaking the canister in the plastic holder with the cap on.
7. If the inhaler has not been used recently or when it is first used, "test spray" before administering the metered dose.
8. If a glucocorticoid inhalant is to be used with a bronchodilator, wait 5 minutes before using the inhaler containing the steroid.
9. Teach client to monitor pulse rate.
10. Caution against overuse, because side effects and tolerance may result.
11. Teach client to monitor amount of medication remaining in the canister (see Figure 3–15). Advise the client to ask his or her health care provider or pharmacist to estimate when a new inhaler will be needed based on dosing schedule. A common practice of placing the canister in water to determine the amount of drug remaining is not appropriate for all inhalers; ask health care provider or pharmacist.
12. Instruct client to avoid smoking.
13. Teach client to do daily cleaning of the equipment, including (1) wash hands; (2) take apart all washable parts of equipment and wash with warm water; (3) rinse; (4) place on clean towel and cover with another clean towel to air dry; and (5) store in a clean plastic bag when *completely* dry. It is a good idea to have two sets of washable equipment to make this process easier.

FIGURE 3–15   Distribution of medication with and without a spacer.

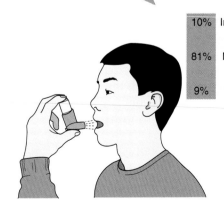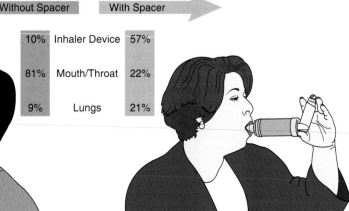

Without Spacer		With Spacer
10%	Inhaler Device	57%
81%	Mouth/Throat	22%
9%	Lungs	21%

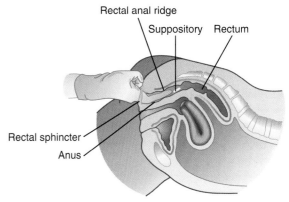

FIGURE 3-17 Inserting a rectal suppository.

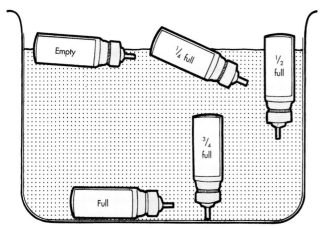

FIGURE 3-16 Measure the amount of medication remaining in an inhaler canister by immersion in water. (From Lilley L, Harrington S, Snyder J: *Pharmacology and the nursing process*, ed 4, St Louis, 2005, Mosby.)

Nasogastric and Gastrostomy Tubes

- Check for proper placement of tube.
- Pour drug into syringe without plunger or bulb, release clamp, and allow medication to flow in properly, usually by gravity.
- Flush tubing with 50 ml of water or prescribed amount. (Refer to agency policy for exact amount.)
- Clamp tube and remove syringe.

Suppositories

Rectal Suppositories

- Medications administered as **suppositories** or enemas can be given rectally for local and systemic absorption. The numerous small capillaries in the rectal area promote absorption.
- The foil around the suppository is removed, and the suppository may be lubricated before insertion. When medications such as antipyretics and bronchodilators are given, the client must be reminded to retain the medication and not to expel it.
- Suppositories tend to soften at room temperature and therefore need to be refrigerated.
- Explain the procedure to the client, and provide privacy.
- Use a glove for insertion.
- Instruct the client to lie on left side and breathe through the mouth to relax the anal sphincter.
- Apply a small amount of water-soluble lubricant to the tip of the unwrapped suppository, and gently insert the suppository beyond the internal sphincter (Figure 3-17).
- Have the client remain on his or her side for 20 minutes after insertion.

- If indicated, teach clients how to self-administer suppositories, and observe a return demonstration for effectiveness.

Vaginal Suppositories

Vaginal suppositories are similar to rectal suppositories. They are generally inserted into the vagina with an applicator (Figure 3-18). Wear gloves. The client should be in the lithotomy position. After insertion of the medication, provide the client with a sanitary pad.

Parenteral

Safety is always a special concern with **parenteral** medication. Thus manufacturers have responded with safety features in an effort to decrease or eliminate needlestick injuries and the possible transfer of blood-borne diseases, such as hepatitis and human immunodeficiency virus (HIV). (Figure 3-19 shows examples of safety needles.) Nursing implications for administration of parenteral medications are at the end of this section.

There are multiple types of parenteral routes, including **intradermal, subcutaneous, intramuscular,** Z-track tech-

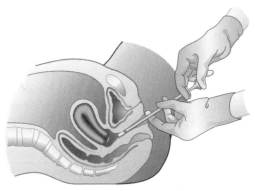

FIGURE 3-18 Inserting a vaginal suppository.

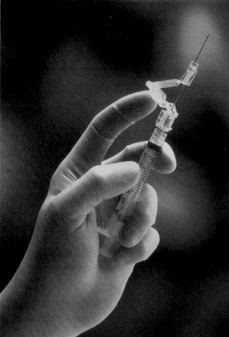

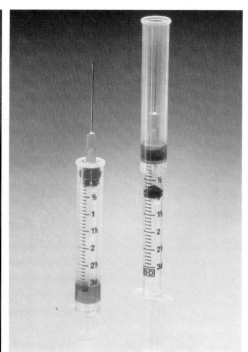

FIGURE 3–19 Safety needles. (Courtesy Becton Dickinson and Company, Franklin Lakes, NJ.)

nique, and **intravenous.** A description of each follows with special considerations noted for the pediatric client.

Intradermal

Action

- Local effect
- A small amount is injected so that volume does not interfere with wheal formation or cause a systemic reaction.
- Used for observation of an inflammatory (allergic) reaction to foreign proteins. Examples include tuberculin testing, testing for drug and other allergic sensitivities, and some immunotherapy for cancer.

Sites

Locations are chosen so that an inflammatory reaction can be observed. Preferred areas are lightly pigmented, thinly keratinized, and hairless, such as the ventral midforearm, clavicular area of the chest, and scapular area of the back (Figure 3–20).

Equipment

- Needle: 26 to 27 gauge
- Syringe: 1 ml calibrated in 0.01-ml increments (usually 0.01 to 0.1 ml injected)

Technique

- Cleanse the area using a circular motion; observe sterile technique.
- Hold the skin taut.
- Insert the needle, bevel up, at a 10- to 15-degree angle; the outline of the needle under the skin should be visible (Figure 3–21).
- Inject the medication slowly to form a wheal (blister or bleb).

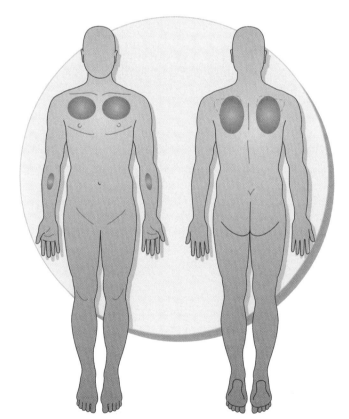

FIGURE 3–20 Common sites for intradermal injection.

- Remove the needle slowly; do not recap.
- Do *not* massage the area; also instruct the client not to do so.
- Mark the area with a pen, and ask the client not to wash it off until read by a health care provider.
- Assess for allergic reaction in 24 to 72 hours; measure the diameter of local reaction. For tuberculin, measure

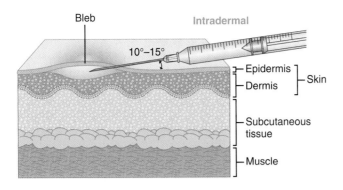

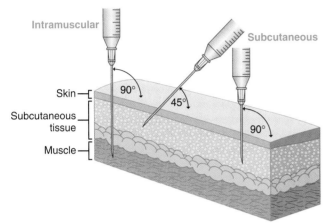

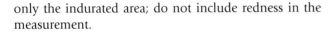

FIGURE 3–21 Needle-skin angle for intradermal, subcutaneous, and intramuscular injections.

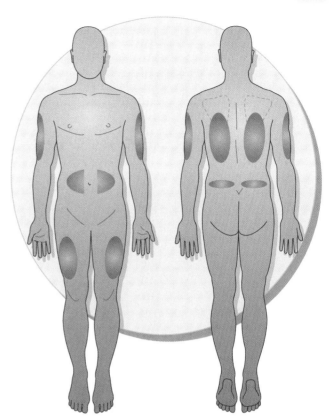

FIGURE 3–22 Common sites for subcutaneous injections.

only the indurated area; do not include redness in the measurement.

Subcutaneous

Action

- Systemic effect
- Sustained effect; absorbed mainly through capillaries; usually slower in onset than with the IM route
- Used for small doses of nonirritating, water-soluble drugs

Sites

Locations for subQ injection are chosen for adequate fat-pad size and include the abdomen, upper hips, upper back, lateral upper arms, and lateral thighs (Figure 3–22).

Equipment

- Needle: 25 to 27 gauge, $1/2$ to $5/8$ inches in length
- Syringe: 1 to 3 ml (usually 0.5 to 1.5 ml injected)
- Insulin syringe measured in units for use with insulin only

Technique

- Cleanse the area with a circular motion using sterile technique.
- Pinch the skin.
- Insert the needle at an angle appropriate to body size: 45 to 90 degrees (45 degrees for those with little subQ tissue) (see Figure 3–21).

- Release the skin.
- Aspirate, except with heparin.
- Inject the medication slowly.
- Remove the needle quickly; do not recap.
- Gently massage the area unless contraindicated, as with heparin.
- Apply gentle pressure to the injection site if the client is on anticoagulant therapy to prevent bleeding or oozing into the tissue and subsequent bruising and tissue damage.
- Apply bandage if needed.

Intramuscular

Action

- Systemic effect
- Usually more rapid effect of drug than with the subQ route
- Used for irritating drugs, aqueous suspensions, and solutions in oils

Sites

Locations are chosen for adequate muscle size and minimal major nerves and blood vessels in the area. Locations include ventrogluteal, dorsogluteal, deltoid, and vastus lateralis (pediatrics). A section on each site is shown in the diagrams of the sites (Figures 3–23 through 3–26) and includes the volume of drug administered, needle size, angle of injection, client position, site location, advantages and disadvantages of site, and additional considerations, if any. Clients with low weight should be evaluated for sites with

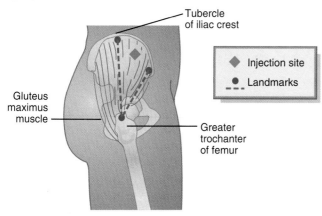

FIGURE 3–23   Ventrogluteal injection site.

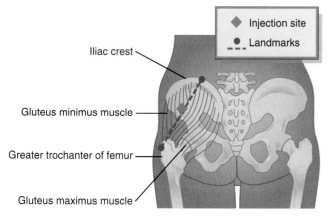

FIGURE 3–24   Dorsogluteal injection site.

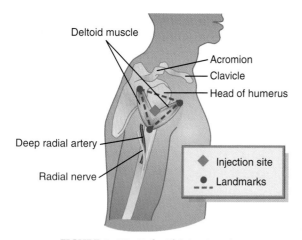

FIGURE 3–25   Deltoid injection site.

adequate muscle. The ventrogluteal is the preferred site for adults and infants older than 7 months.

Equipment

Needle: 20 to 23 gauge; 18 gauge for blood products; 1 to 1.5 inches in length

Technique

- Same as for subQ injection, with two exceptions: flatten the skin area using the thumb and index finger and in-

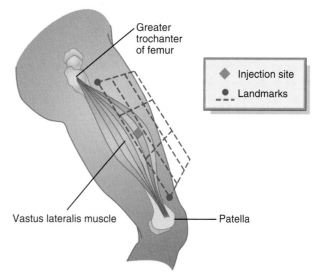

FIGURE 3–26   Vastus lateralis injection site in children.

ject between them; insert the needle at a 90-degree angle into the muscle (see Figure 3–21)
- Syringe: 1 to 3 ml (usually 0.5 to 1.5 ml injected)

Preferred Intramuscular Injection Sites

Table 3–3 presents the four sites, client position, advantages, and disadvantages of each injection site. Diagrams of each injection site with associated landmarks are presented in Figures 3–23 through 3–26.

- *Ventrogluteal* (see Figure 3–23). Volume of drug administered is 1 to 3 ml, with a 20- to 23-gauge, 1.25- to 2.5-inch needle. Slightly angle the needle toward the iliac crest.
- *Dorsogluteal* (see Figure 3–24). Volume of drug administered is 1 to 3 ml; 5 ml gamma globulin with 18- to 23-gauge, 1.25- to 3-inch needle. Place the needle at a 90-degree angle to the skin with the client prone.
- *Deltoid* (see Figure 3–25). Volume of drug administered is 0.5 to 1 ml, with a 23- to 25-gauge, $5/8$- to 1.5-inch needle. Place the needle at a 90-degree angle to the skin or slightly toward acromion.
- *Vastus lateralis* (see Figure 3–26). Volume of drug administered is <0.5 ml in infants (max = 1 ml), 1 ml pediatrics, 1 to 1.5 ml adults (max = 2 ml). Direct the needle at the knee at a 45- to 60-degree angle to the frontal, sagittal, and horizontal planes of the thigh.

Z-Track Injection Technique

The **Z-track technique** prevents medication from leaking back into the subQ tissue. It is frequently advised for medications that cause visible and permanent skin discolorations (e.g., iron dextran). The gluteal site is preferred. While following the medication's order policy and aseptic technique, draw up the medication. Replace the first needle with a second needle of appropriate gauge and length to penetrate muscle tissue and deliver the medication to the selected site. Removal of the first needle prevents the medication that is adhering to the needle shaft from being taken into the subQ tissue. If removal is not possible,

Table 3–3

Intramuscular Injection Sites: Client Position, Advantages, and Disadvantages

Site	Client Position	Advantages	Disadvantages
Ventrogluteal	Supine lateral	Anatomic landmarks well defined Muscle mass suited for deep IM or Z-track injections Free of major nerves	In the event of hypersensitivity reaction, medication absorption cannot be delayed by tourniquet
Dorsogluteal	Prone	Muscle mass suited for deep IM or Z-track injections	Requires correct/accurate site and technique to avoid injury to major nerves and vascular structures In the event of hypersensitivity reaction, medication absorption cannot be delayed by tourniquet
Deltoid	Lateral, prone, sitting, supine	Readily accessible In the event of hypersensitivity reaction, medication absorption can be delayed by tourniquet	Small muscle mass; limited to small volume doses Close to nerves; requires accurate technique
Vastus lateralis	Sitting, supine	Good site for infants Size acceptable for multiple injections Free of major nerves	Special attention required to avoid sciatic nerve or femoral structures if long needle is used

IM, Intramuscular.

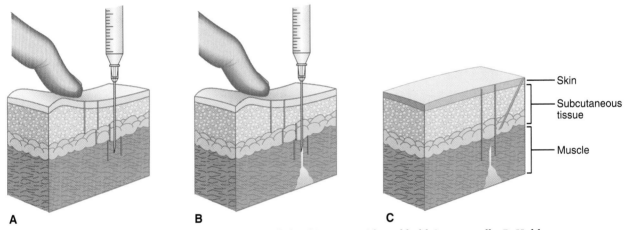

A   **B**   **C**

FIGURE 3–27   Z-track injection. A, Pull the skin to one side and hold; insert needle. B, Holding skin to side, inject medication. C, Withdraw needle and release skin. This technique prevents medication from entering subcutaneous tissue.

gently wipe the needle with a sterile source; this does present a chance for contamination and also for "self-sticks." Consider having the medication prepared in the pharmacy.

The Z-track injection technique is presented in Figure 3–27.

Intravenous

Action

• Systemic effect
• More rapid than the IM or subQ routes

Sites

Accessible peripheral veins (e.g., cephalic or cubital vein of arm; dorsal vein of hand) are preferred (Figure 3–28). When possible, ask the client of his or her preference.

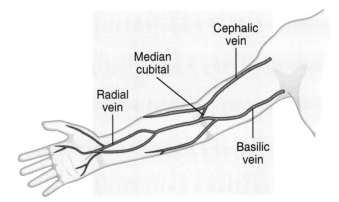

FIGURE 3–28   Common sites for intravenous administration.

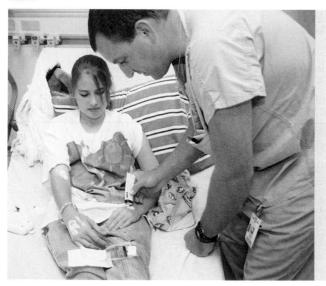

FIGURE 3–29 Applied to the skin at the site of injection, eutectic mixture of local anesthetics cream reduces the pain of needle or catheter insertion and reduces the child's distress. (From Bowden V, Dickey S, Greenberg C: *Children and their families: the continuum of care*, Philadelphia, 1998, Saunders.)

Avoid needless restriction. In newborns, the veins of the feet, lower legs, and head may also be used after the previous sites have been exhausted.

Equipment
- Needle
  Adults: 20 to 21 gauge; 1 to 1.5 inches
  Infants: 24 gauge; 1 inch
  Children: 22 gauge; 1 inch
  Larger bore for viscous drugs, whole blood or fractions; large volume for rapid infusion
- Electronic IV delivery device, an infusion controller, or pump
- Patient-controlled analgesia (PCA) system, if ordered
- Eutectic mixture of local anesthetics (EMLA), if appropriate (Figure 3–29)

Technique
- Apply a tourniquet.
- Cleanse the area using aseptic technique.
- Insert butterfly or a catheter, and feed up into the vein until blood returns. Remove tourniquet.
- Stabilize the needle and dress site.
- Monitor the flow rate, distal pulses, skin color and temperature, and insertion site.
- Consult agency policy regarding the addition of medications to bottle or bag, piggyback technique, and IV push.

Nursing Implications for Administration of Parenteral Medications

Sites
- Ventrogluteal site is preferred for IM injections in adults and infants older than 7 months.

- Do not use the dorsogluteal site for IM injections in children. For infants younger than 7 months, the vastus lateralis is preferred.

Equipment
- Use a needle size and syringe appropriate to the client's needs.
- The syringe size should approximate the volume of medication to be administered.
- Use the tuberculin syringe for amounts <0.5 ml.
- Use the filter needle to draw up the medication from a glass vial or ampule. Change the needle before administration to prevent tissue irritation from any medication left on the needle.

Technique
- Explain to the client what is going to be done. Gain the client's cooperation. Allow the client time to cooperate, if possible.
- Demonstrate empathy and concern for every client and his or her family, as well as using proper technique.
- Allay anxiety. Encourage expression of feelings.
- Position the client.
- Administer medication only via the ordered route.
- Inspect the skin before each injection.
- Inject medication slowly to minimize tissue damage.
- Do not administer injections if sites are inflamed, edematous, or lesioned (e.g., moles, birth marks, scars).
- Rotate the injection site to enhance absorption of the drug (e.g., insulin). Document the injection site.
- Observe the client for drug effectiveness. Report any untoward reactions immediately.

Developmental Needs of Pediatric Clients

Anticipate developmental needs. Examples of needs associated with administration of medications include the following (refer to Chapter 10, Pediatric Pharmacology, for additional examples):
- Stranger anxiety (infant): Maintain a nonthreatening approach and move slowly.
- Hospitalization, illness, or injury may be viewed as punishment (3 to 6 years old): Allow control where appropriate; obtain child's view of situation; encourage positive relationships and expression of feelings in acceptable manner and activities. Include the family or a support person if appropriate.
- Fear of mutilation (3 to 6 years old): Explain the procedures carefully; use less intrusive routes whenever possible, such as the oral route; allow children to give "play injections" to a doll or stuffed animal.

Technologic Advances

Advances in drug administration therapy continue to enhance safety, increase accessibility to sites, promote client mobility, and improve client adherence. Examples of these advances include the following:

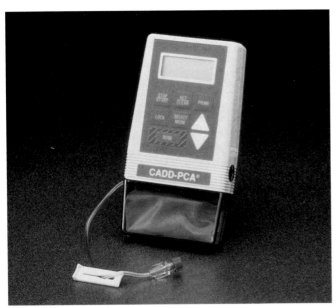

FIGURE 3–30 A patient-controlled analgesia system. (Courtesy SIMS Deltec, Inc., St. Paul, Minn.)

- Pain-free delivery of insulin through patch.
- PCA infusion machine that scans Abbott drugs (Figure 3–30). Drug name and concentration are automatically entered when syringe is inserted (Abbott Laboratories).
- Data from medication administration record (MAR) are displayed on handheld device that is updated with each prescriber's medication entry. This device, compatible with most computerized documentation systems, signals when a new medication order is received, is linked to infusion pump, and the nurse is alerted about future doses (Baxter Health Care Corps).
- An infusion pump with a scanner is used so that after reading the IV bag label the nurse scans the medication; then the nurse and client ID band & information regarding infusion are programmed into the pump (B. Braun Medical Inc.).

Nursing Process

Overview of Medication Administration

ASSESSMENT

■ Obtain appropriate vital signs and relevant laboratory test results for future comparisons and evaluation of the therapeutic response.
■ Obtain drug history, including drug allergies.
■ Identify high-risk clients for reactions.
■ Assess client's capability to follow therapeutic regimen.

POTENTIAL NURSING DIAGNOSES

■ Risk for injury related to possible adverse reaction.

■ Ineffective individual/family therapeutic regimen management related to knowledge deficit, economic difficulties, or complexities of the regimen.

PLANNING

■ Identify goals.
■ Promote therapeutic response and prevent or minimize adverse reactions.
■ Identify strategies to promote adherence.
■ Identify interventions.

NURSING INTERVENTIONS

■ Prepare equipment and environment; wash hands.
■ Check for allergies and other assessment data.
■ Check drug label three times; check expiration date.
■ Be certain of drug calculation; verify dose with another RN as necessary.
■ Pour liquids at eye level.
■ Keep all drugs stored properly, especially related to temperature, light, and moisture.
■ Avoid contact with topical and inhalation preparations.
■ Verify client identification.
■ Administer only drugs that you have prepared.
■ Assist client to desired position.
■ Discard needles and syringes in "sharps" container.
■ Follow policy related to discarding drugs and controlled substances.
■ Report drug errors immediately.
■ Document all appropriate information in a timely manner.
■ Record effectiveness of drugs administered and reason for any drugs refused.

Client Teaching

General
- Emphasize safety.
- Monitor client's physical abilities regularly as needed.
- Keep or store medications in original labeled containers with child-resistant caps when needed.
- Provide client or family with written instructions (or audio instructions if visually impaired) about the drug regimen.
- Advise client or family about the expected therapeutic effect and length of time to achieve a therapeutic response from the medication and the expected duration of treatment.
- Instruct client or family about possible drug-laboratory test interaction.
- Advise client of nonpharmacologic measures to promote therapeutic response.
- Encourage client or family to have adequate supply of necessary medications available.
- Caution against the use of OTC preparations including herbal remedies without *first* contacting the health care provider.

- Reinforce the importance of follow-up appointments with health care providers.
- Encourage client to wear Medic-Alert band with medications or allergies indicated.
- Reinforce that community resources are available and need to be mobilized according to the client or family needs.

Diet

- Advise client or family about possible drug-food interactions.
- Advise client or family what foods are contraindicated.
- Instruct regarding alcohol use.

Self-Administration

- Instruct client or family regarding drug dose and dosing schedule.
- Instruct client or family on all psychomotor skills related to the drug regimen.
- Provide client or family with contact person and telephone number for questions and concerns.

Side Effects

- Instruct client or family about general side effects and adverse reactions of the medications.
- Advise client or family when and how to notify health care provider.

Cultural Considerations

- Assess personal beliefs of clients or family.

- Modify communications to meet cultural needs of client or family.
- Communicate respect for culture and cultural practices of client or family.

EVALUATION

- Evaluate effectiveness of medications administered.
- Identify expected time frame of desired drug response; consider modification of therapy as needed.
- Determine client satisfaction with regimen.

WEBSITES

For further information on *Principles of Drug Administration,* visit these Internet resources:

U.S. Food and Drug Administration (FDA): The FDA issues bar code regulations: *http://www.fda.gov/oc/initiatives/barcode-sadr/fs-barcode.html*

National Coordinating Council for Medication Error Reporting and Prevention (NCC MERP): *http://www.nccmerp.org/*

Joint Commission on Accreditation of Healthcare Organizations: *http://www.jcaho.org/*

The Institute for Safe Medication Practice: *http://www.ismp.org*

Study Questions

1. What is the meaning of the "rights" of medication administration to your nursing practice? What precautions must be taken to ensure them?

2. List 10 safety guidelines for safe administration of medications.

3. Describe how bar coding promotes safety in medication administration.

4. What are the nursing implications for each route of medication administration?

5. What is the preferred angle of needle insertion for each type of parenteral injection?

6. What are the essential items to be charted for the administration of each medication? What should be recorded when an ordered medication is not given?

7. What should be done when a client refuses to take a medication?

8. Describe at least 10 factors that modify client response to a drug.

9. List at least three nursing interventions specific to the pediatric client associated with the administration of medications.

10. List six abbreviations that are not to be used in ordering or documentation according to JCAHO requirements.

Two

Medications and Calculations

Unit Two (Chapter 4), Medications and Calculations, provides practice in the calculation of drug dosages. The chapter is divided into six sections; systems of measurement, four methods for calculating drug dosages, orals, intramuscular, intravenous, and pediatric drug calculations. Though the sections in Chapter 4 are condensed, there are many practice problems.

This unit is thorough and could be used by students in place of the purchase of a drug calculation text. It may also serve as a review of drug calculation in preparing for state boards or for nurses in practice settings.

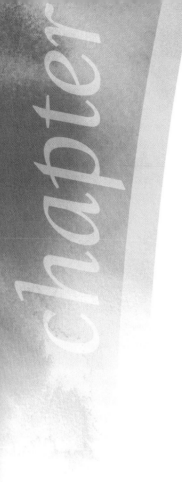

4 Medications and Calculations

Overview

This chapter on medications and calculations is subdivided into six sections: (A) systems of measurement with conversion; (B) methods for calculation; (C) calculations of oral dosages; (D) calculations of injectable dosages; (E) calculations of intravenous (IV) fluids; and (F) pediatric drug calculations. The nurse may proceed independently through Sections A to F to practice and master calculation of drug dosages during the fundamental nursing or pharmacology course. This chapter also serves as a review of drug calculation for nurses in practice settings.

Numerous drug labels are used in the drug calculation problems to familiarize the nurse with important information on a drug label. That information is then used in correctly calculating the drug dose.

Six calculation methods are explained. Four are general methods: (1) basic formula, (2) ratio and proportion, (3) fractional equation, and (4) dimensional analysis. The nurse should select one of these general methods for the calculation of drug dosages. The other two methods are used to individualize drug dosing by body weight and body surface area. Each of the calculation methods has a color-coded icon that identifies the method used in the chapters.

The drug calculation charts in Tables 4A–4 and 4B–1 may be used in the clinical setting. Abbreviations for drug dosing are found in Appendix H. The nurse might find it helpful to review Chapter 3, Principles of Drug Administration.

Keeping in mind that the goal is to prepare and administer medications in a safe and correct manner, the following recommendations are offered:

- **Think.** Focus on each step of the problem. This applies to simple *and* difficult problems.
- **Read accurately.** Pay particular attention to the location of the decimal point and to the operation to be done, such as conversion from one system of measurement to another.
- **Picture the problem.**
- **Identify an expected range for the answer.**
- **Seek to understand the problem.** Do not merely master the mechanics of how to do it. Ask for help when unsure of the calculation.

Section 4A SYSTEMS OF MEASUREMENT WITH CONVERSION

OBJECTIVES

- Name the three systems of measurement.
- Convert measurement within the metric system, larger units to smaller units, and smaller units to larger units.
- Convert measurements within the apothecary system, larger units to smaller units, and smaller units to larger units.
- Convert measurements within the household system, larger units to smaller units, and smaller units to larger units.
- Convert metric, apothecary, and household measurements among the three systems of measurement as appropriate.

TERMS

apothecary system
dram
grain
gram

household measurement
liter
meter

metric system
minim
ounce

Introduction

Three systems of measurement—metric, apothecary, and household—are used to measure drugs and solutions. The metric system, developed in the late eighteenth century, is the internationally accepted system of measure. It is replacing the apothecary system, which dates back to the Middle Ages and had been used in England since the seventeenth century. Household measurement is commonly used in community and home settings in the United States.

Metric System

The **metric system** is a decimal system based on the power of 10. The basic units of measure are **gram** (g, gm, G, Gm) for weight; **liter** (l, L) for volume; and **meter** (m, M) for linear measurement, or length. Prefixes indicate the size of the units in multiples of 10. Table 4A–1 gives the metric units of measure in weight (gram), volume (liter), and length (meter) in larger and smaller units that are commonly used.

Kilo is the prefix used for larger units (e.g., kilometer), and *milli, centi, micro,* and *nano* are the prefixes for smaller units (e.g., millimeter). The prefix stands for a specific degree of mag-

Table 4A–1

Metric Units of Measurements

Unit	Names and Abbreviations	Measurements
Gram (weight)	1 kilogram (kg, Kg)	1000 g
	1 gram (g, gm, G, Gm)	1 g
	1 milligram (mg)	0.001 g
	1 microgram (mcg)	0.000001 g
	1 nanogram (ng)	0.000000001 g
Liter (volume)	1 kiloliter (kl, KL)	1000 L
	1 liter (L, l)	1 L
	1 milliliter (ml)	0.001 L
Meter (length)	1 kilometer (km)	1000 m
	1 meter (m, M)	1 m
	1 centimeter (cm)	0.01 m
	1 millimeter (mm)	0.001 m

NOTE: 1 ml (milliliter) = 1 cc (cubic centimeter). Values are the same in drug and fluid therapy.
1 mg (milligram) = 1000 mcg (micrograms).

nitude; for instance, kilo stands for thousands, milli for one thousandth, centi for one hundredth, and so on. Because the difference between degrees of magnitude is always a multiple of 10, converting from one magnitude to another is relatively easy.

Conversion Within the Metric System

The metric units most frequently used in drug notation are the following:

$$1 \text{ g} = 1000 \text{ mg}$$
$$1 \text{ L} = 1000 \text{ ml}$$
$$1 \text{ mg} = 1000 \text{ mcg}$$

To be able to convert a quantity, one of the values must be known, such as gram or milligrams, liter or milliliters, and milligrams or micrograms. Gram, liter, and meter are larger units; milligram, milliliter, and millimeter are smaller units.

Metric Conversion

A. When converting *larger* units to smaller units in the metric system, move the decimal point one space to the *right* for each degree of magnitude change.
Note: This does *not* apply to micro and nano units.

EXAMPLE   Change 1 gram to milligrams.
Grams are three degrees of magnitude *greater* than milligrams (see Table 4A–1). Move the decimal point three spaces to the right.

$$1 \text{ g} = 1.000 \text{ mg} \quad \text{or} \quad 1 \text{ g} = 1000 \text{ mg}$$

B. When converting *smaller* units to larger units in the metric system, move the decimal point one space to the *left* for each degree of magnitude of change.

EXAMPLE   Change 1000 milligrams to grams.
Milligrams are three degrees of magnitude *smaller* than grams. Move the decimal point three spaces to the left.

$$1000 \text{ mg} = 1\,000. \text{ g} \quad \text{or} \quad 1000 \text{ mg} = 1 \text{ g}$$

REMEMBER: When changing *larger* units to smaller units, move the decimal point to the *right*, and when changing *smaller* units to larger units, move the decimal point to the *left*.

PRACTICE
PROBLEM 1

METRIC CONVERSION	
Larger to Smaller Units	**Smaller to Larger Units**
1. Change 2 g to mg	4. Change 1500 mg to g
2. Change 0.5 (½) g to mg	5. Change 3 g to kg
3. Change 2.5 L to ml	6. Change 500 ml to L

Apothecary System

The apothecary system of measurement was the common system used by most practitioners before the universal acceptance of the International Metric System. Now all pharmaceuticals are manufactured using the metric system, and the apothecary system is no longer included on any drug labels. All medication should be prescribed and calculated using metric measures, but occasionally the use of the fluid ounce or grains is found. For those rare circumstances, nurses should have a general understanding of the apothecary system.

The **apothecary system** uses Roman numerals instead of Arabic numbers to express the quantity. The Roman numeral is placed after the symbol or abbreviation for the unit of measure. The Roman numerals are written in lowercase letters; for example, gr x stands for 10 grains. The letters $\overline{\text{ss}}$ indicate one half; for example, gr $\overline{\text{ss}}$ stands for ½ grain.

Table 4A-2

Apothecary Equivalents in Weights and Fluid Volume

Dry Weight			Fluid Volume*		
Larger Units		**Smaller Units**	**Larger Units**		**Smaller Units**
1 ounce (oz)	=	480 grains (gr)	1 quart (qt)	=	2 pints (pt)
1 ounce (oz)	=	8 drams (3)	1 pint (pt)	=	16 fluid ounces (fl oz, fl3, or f3)
1 dram (3)	=	60 grains (gr)	1 fluid ounce	=	8 fluid dram (fl dr, fl3, or f3)
1 scruple	=	20 grains (gr)	1 fluid dram	=	60 minims (min, or ♏)
			1 minim	=	1 drop (gt)

*Fluid volume units are more commonly used than dry weight units and thus should be remembered.

In the apothecary system, the unit of weight is the **grain** (gr), and the units of fluid volume are the **ounce** (fluidounce, or $f3$), the **dram** (fluidram, or $f3$), and the **minim** (min, or ♏). Drams and minims are used infrequently.

In clinical practice, ounce and dram are more frequently used for measurement of fluid volume than for dry weights. Therefore, when writing fluid volume, the word fluid (f) in front of an ounce or dram is usually dropped. Table 4A-2 gives the apothecary equivalent of larger and smaller units of measure in dry weight and fluid volume.

Your nursing program may have you omit the apothecary system. If so, study only the metric system and the household system in this section and the following sections of the Unit.

Apothecary Conversion

A. When converting a *larger* unit to a smaller unit, *multiply* the measurement that is requested by the basic equivalent value.

EXAMPLE

1. 3 Fluidounces (fl3, fl oz) = _____ fluid dram ($f3$, fl dr).
   The equivalent value is 1 $f3$ (1 fl oz) = 8 $f3$ (8 fl dr).

$$3\ f3\ (3\ \text{fl oz}) \times 8\ f3\ (8\ \text{fl dr}) = \underline{24}\ f3\ (\text{fl dr})$$

B. When converting a *smaller* unit to a larger unit, *divide* the requested number by the basic equivalent value.

EXAMPLE

1. 8 fluidounces ($f3$) = _____ pint (pt).
   The equivalent value is 1 pt = 16 $f3$.

PRACTICE PROBLEM 2

APOTHECARY CONVERSION

Larger to Smaller Units

1. Change 3 qt to pt
2. Change 1.5 pt to $f3$

Smaller to Larger Units

3. Change 3 pt to qt
4. Change 32 $f3$ to qt

Household System

Household measurement is not as accurate as the metric system because of the lack of standardization of spoons, cups, and glasses. The measurements are approximate. A teaspoon (t) is considered to be equivalent to 5 ml according to the official *United States Pharmacopeia*. Milliliters (ml) is the same as cubic centimeters (cc) in value (Figure 4A-1). Three teaspoons equal 1 tablespoon (T). Ounces (oz) are fluid ounces in the household measurement system; the

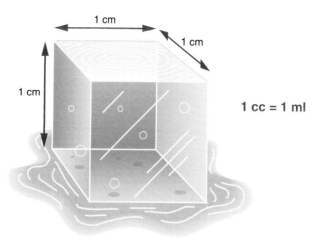

1 cc = 1 ml

FIGURE 4A–1 One cubic centimeter (cc) equals one milliliter (ml).

Table 4A–3

Household Equivalents in Fluid Volume

1 measuring cup	=	8 ounces (oz)
1 medium-size glass (tumbler size)	=	8 ounces (oz)
1 coffee cup (c)	=	6 ounces (oz) (varies with cup size)
1 ounce (oz)	=	2 tablespoons (T)
1 tablespoon (T)	=	3 teaspoons (t)
1 teaspoon (t)	=	60 drops (gtt)*
1 drop (gt)*	=	1 minim (min, or ♍)

*Varies with viscosity of liquid and dropper opening.

word "fluid" in front of ounce is usually not used. One milliliter of water fills a cubic centimeter exactly.

Table 4A–3 gives the household equivalents in fluid volume. The measurements with asterisks are frequently used in drug therapy and should be remembered.

Household Conversion

A. When converting *larger* units to smaller units within the household system, *multiply* the requested number by the basic equivalent value.

EXAMPLE

Change 2 glasses of water to ounces.
   The equivalent value is 1 medium-sized glass = 8 oz.

$$2 \text{ glasses} \times 8 \text{ oz} = \underline{16} \text{ oz}$$

PRACTICE
PROBLEM 3

HOUSEHOLD CONVERSION

REMEMBER: To change *larger* units to smaller units, *multiply* the requested number of units by the basic equivalent value. To change *smaller* units to larger units, *divide* the requested number of units by the basic equivalent value. Refer to Table 4A-3 as needed.

Larger to Smaller Units

1. Change 3 oz to T
2. Change 5 T to t
3. Change 3 coffee cups to oz

Smaller to Larger Units

4. Change 3 T to oz
5. Change 16 oz to a measuring cup
6. Change 12 t to T

PRACTICE PROBLEM 4

SUMMARY: METRIC, APOTHECARY, AND HOUSEHOLD MEASUREMENTS

Metric System: Refer to Table 4A–1 as needed.
1. 2 g = _____ mg
2. 1.2 kg = _____ g
3. 5 mg = _____ mcg
4. 2.5 L = _____ ml
5. 500 mg = _____ g
6. 10,000 mcg = _____ mg
7. 2400 mg = _____ g
8. 1500 ml = _____ l

Apothecary System: Refer to Table 4A–2 as needed.
1. 5 qt = _____ pt
2. 2 pt = _____ f$\bar{3}$
3. f$\bar{3}$v = _____ f3
4. 1.5 pt = _____ f$\bar{3}$
5. 8 f$\bar{3}$ = _____ pt
6. 3 pt = _____ qt
7. 12 f3 = _____ f$\bar{3}$
8. 32 f$\bar{3}$ = _____ qt

Household System: Refer to Table 4A–3 as needed.
1. 5 glasses = _____ oz
2. 3 T = _____ t
3. 2 c = _____ oz
4. 4 oz = _____ T
5. 15 t = _____ T
6. 5 T = _____ oz

Conversion Among the Metric, Apothecary, and Household Systems

Drug doses are usually ordered in metric units (grams, milligrams, liters, or milliliters), but some health care providers still use the apothecary units of measurement (grain) when prescribing medication. To calculate drug doses, the same unit of measure (grams, milligrams, or grains) must be used. The nurse needs to be familiar with the three systems of measure and their equivalents (Table 4A–4). Note that the metric and apothecary equivalents are approximate; thus the equivalents should be rounded off to a whole number, for example, 1 g = 15.432 gr, or 1 g = 15 gr.

Table 4A–4

Approximate Metric, Apothecary, and Household Equivalents

	Metric System		Apothecary System	Household System
Weight	1 kg;	1000 g	2.2 lb	2.2 lb
	*1 g;	1000 mg	15 (16) gr	
	0.5 g;	500 mg	7 $^1/_2$ gr	
	0.3 g;	300 (325) mg	5 gr	
	0.1 g;	100 mg	1$^1/_2$ gr	
	*0.06 g;	60 (65) mg	1 gr	
	0.03 g;	30 (32) mg	$^1/_2$ gr	
	0.01g	10 mg	$^1/_6$ gr	
		0.6 mg	$^1/_{100}$ gr	
		0.4 mg	$^1/_{150}$ gr	
		0.3 mg	$^1/_{200}$ gr	
Volume	1 L; 1000 ml (cc)		1 qt; 32 oz (f$\bar{3}$)	1 qt
	0.5 L; 500 ml		1 pt; 16 oz (f$\bar{3}$)	1 pt
	0.24 L; 240 ml		8 $\bar{3}$ (f$\bar{3}$)	1 glass
	0.18 L; 180 ml		6 $\bar{3}$ (f$\bar{3}$)	1 c
	*30 ml		1 $\bar{3}$ (f$\bar{3}$); 8 f3	2 T; 6 t
	15 ml		$^1/_2$ $\bar{3}$ (f$\bar{3}$); 4 f3	1 T; 3 t
	†5 ml			1 t
	4 ml		1 $\bar{3}$; 60 m (min)	1 t
	1 ml		15 (16) m	15-16 gtt
Height/Distance	2.54 cm		1 in	1 in
	25.4 mm		1 in	1 in

*Equivalents commonly used for computing conversion problems by ratio.
†5 ml = 1 t (teaspoon); official *United States Pharmacopeia* measurement.
$\bar{3}$, dram; f3, *fluid dram*; f$\bar{3}$, *fluid ounce*; m, minim; *cc*, cubic centimeter; *cm*, centimeter; *g*, gram; *gr*, grain; *gtt*, drops; *in*, inch; *kg*, kilogram; *L*, liter; *lb*, pound; *mg*, milligram; *ml*, milliliter; *mm*, millimeter; *pt*, pint; *qt*, quart; *T*, tablespoon; *t*, teaspoon.

SECTION A

Some authorities indicate that it is easier to convert to the unit used on the bottle or container. The answer is in the system of the drug to be dispensed. If the label on the bottle reads in milligrams and the order is in grains, the conversion should be from grains to milligrams.

EXAMPLE   Order: Compazine spansule gr ¼.
Available: Compazine spansule 15 mg. Convert grains to milligrams, gr ¼ = 15 mg.

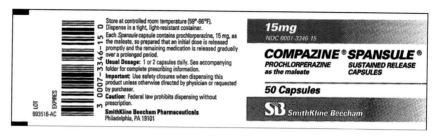

Metric, Apothecary, and Household Equivalents

Conversion to one unit of measure is essential in the administration of drugs. With discharge teaching for a client who requires liquid medication(s) at home, the nurse may find it necessary to convert metric to household measurements. Table 4A–4 gives the metric and apothecary equivalents by weight, and the metric, apothecary, and household equivalents by volume.

ANSWERS TO PRACTICE PROBLEMS

1   METRIC CONVERSION

1. 2.0 g = 2.000 mg   or   2.0 g = 2000 mg

   The gram is three degrees of magnitude greater than the milligram, so the decimal point is moved three spaces to the right.

2. 0.5 g = 0.500 mg   or   0.5 g = 500 mg

   The gram is three degrees of magnitude greater than the milligram, so the decimal point is moved three spaces to the right.

3. 2.5 L = 2.500 ml   or   2.5 L = 2500 ml

   The liter is three degrees of magnitude greater than the milliliter, so the decimal point is moved three spaces to the right.

4. 1500 mg = 1 500. g   or   1500 mg = 1.5 g

   The milligram is three degrees of magnitude smaller (less) than the gram, so the decimal point is moved three spaces to the left.

5. 3 g = 003. kg   or   3 g = .003 kg

   The gram is three degrees of magnitude smaller than the kilogram, so the decimal point is moved three spaces to the left.

6. 500 ml = 500. L   or   500 ml = 0.5 L

   The milliliter is three degrees of magnitude smaller than the liter, so the decimal point is moved three spaces to the left.

2   APOTHECARY CONVERSION

1. 3 qt × 2 pt = 6 pt;
   the equivalent value is 1 qt = 2 pt

2. 1.5 pt × 16 = 24 f℥;
   the equivalent value is 1 pt = 16 f℥

3. 3 pt = 1.5 qt;
   the equivalent value is 1 qt = 2 pt; 3 pt ÷ 2 = 1.5 qt

4. 32 f℥ = 2 pt or 1 qt;
   the equivalent values are 1 pt = 16 f℥ or 1 qt = 2 pt

3   HOUSEHOLD CONVERSION

1. 3 oz = <u>6</u> T;
   the equivalent value is 3 oz × 2 = 6 T

2. 5 T = <u>15</u> t;
   the equivalent value is 1 T = 3 t

3. 3 c = <u>18</u> oz;
   the equivalent value is 1 c = 6 oz

4. 3 T = <u>1½</u> oz;
   the equivalent value is 3 T ÷ 2 = 1½ or 1.5 oz

5. 16 oz = <u>2</u> c;
   the equivalent value is 1 measuring cup = 8 oz

6. 12 t = <u>4</u> T;
   the equivalent value is 1 T = 3 t

4   SUMMARY: METRIC, APOTHECARY, AND HOUSEHOLD MEASUREMENTS

Metric

1. 2000 mg (1 g = 1000 mg)
   2 × 1000 mg = 2000 mg
   or 2 000 mg
   (three spaces to the right)

2. 1200 g

3. 5000 mcg (1 mg = 1000 mcg)

4. 2500 ml

5. 0.5 g (1000 mg = 1 g)
       500 ÷ 1000 = 0.5
          or 500 g = 0.5 g
   (three spaces to the left)

6. 10 mg

7. 2.4 g

8. 1.5 L

Apothecary

1. 10 pt

2. 32 f℥

3. 40 f℥ (v = 5 [Roman numeral])

4. 24 f℥

5. ½ pt

6. 1½ qt

7. 1½ f℥

8. 1 qt

Household

1. 40 oz

2. 9 t

3. 12 oz

4. 8 T

5. 5 T

6. 2½ oz

SECTION B

Section 4B   METHODS FOR CALCULATION

OBJECTIVES

- Select a formula—the basic formula, the ratio-and-proportion method, fractional equation, or dimensional analysis—for calculating drug dosages.

- Convert all measures to the same system and same unit of measure within the system before calculating drug dosage.

- Calculate drug dosage using one of the general formulas.
- Calculate drug dosage according to body weight and body surface area.
- List meanings for abbreviations used in drug therapy.

TERMS

basic formula (BF)	body weight (BW)	fractional equation (FE)
body surface area (BSA)	dimensional analysis (DA)	ratio and proportion (RP)

Introduction

The four general methods for the calculation of drug doses are the (1) basic formula, (2) ratio and proportion, (3) fractional equation, (4) and dimensional analysis. These methods are used to calculate oral and injectable drug doses. The nurse should select one of the methods to calculate drug doses and use that method consistently.

For drugs that require individualized dosing, calculation by body weight (BW) or by body surface area (BSA) may be necessary. In the past, these two methods (5) and (6), have been used for the calculation of pediatric dosage and for drugs used in the treatment of cancer (antineoplastic drugs). BW and BSA methods of calculation are especially useful for individuals whose BW is low, who are obese, or who are older adults.

Before calculating drug doses, all units of measure must be converted to a single system (see Section 4A). It is most helpful to convert to the system used on the drug label. If the drug is ordered in grains (gr) and the drug label gives the dose in milligrams (mg), then convert grains to milligrams (the measurement on the drug label) and proceed with the drug calculation. Table 4B–1 gives the metric and apothecary conversions most frequently used for dry and liquid measurements.

Again, if your nursing program prefers to use only the metric system for drug calculations, it will not be necessary for you to learn the conversion between metric and apothecary; however, conversion within the metric system—grams and milligrams—should be studied and remembered.

Table 4B–1

Metric and Apothecary Conversions

Metric		Apothecary
Grams (g)	**Milligrams (mg)**	**Grains (gr)**
1	1000	15
0.5	500	$7\frac{1}{2}$
0.3	300 (325)	5
0.1	100	$1\frac{1}{2}$
0.06	60 (64)	1
0.03	30 (32)	$\frac{1}{2}$
0.015	15 (16)	$\frac{1}{4}$
0.010	10	$\frac{1}{8}$
0.0006	0.6	$\frac{1}{100}$
0.0004	0.4	$\frac{1}{150}$
0.0003	0.3	$\frac{1}{200}$

Liquid (Approximate)		
30 ml (cc)	=	1 oz ($f\tilde{3}$) = 2 tbsp (T) = 6 tsp (t)
15 ml (cc)	=	0.5 oz = 1 T = 3 t
1000 ml (cc)	=	1 quart (qt) = 1 liter (L)
500 ml (cc)	=	1 pint (pt)
5 ml (cc)	=	1 tsp (t)
4 ml (cc)	=	1 fl dr ($f\tilde{3}$)
1 ml (cc)	=	15 minims ($\mathfrak{m}$) = 15 drops (gtt)

cc, Cubic centimeter; *f3*, fluid dram; *f3*, fluid ounce; *ml*, milliliter; *tbsp*, tablespoon; *tsp*, teaspoon.

Interpreting Oral And Injectable Drug Labels

Pharmaceutical companies usually label their drugs with the brand name of the drug in large letters and the generic name in smaller letters. The dose per tablet, capsule, or liquid (for oral and injectable doses) is printed on the drug label. Two examples of drug labels are given below, the first for an oral drug and the second for an injectable drug.

EXAMPLE 1
ORAL DRUG

Tagamet is the brand (trade) name, cimetidine is the generic name, and the dose is 200 mg/tablet.

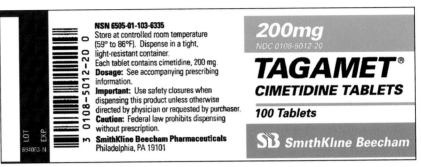

EXAMPLE 2
INJECTABLE DRUG

Compazine is the brand (trade) name, prochlorperazine is the generic name, and the dose is 5 mg/ml injectable.

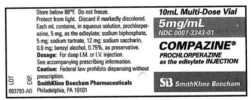

Method 1: Basic Formula (BF)

The **basic formula** is easy to recall and is most frequently used in calculating drug dosages. The basic formula is the following:

$$\frac{D}{H} \times V = A$$

where D is the desired dose (i.e., drug dose ordered by the health care provider),
   H is the on-hand dose (i.e., drug dose on label of container [bottle, vial]),
   V is the vehicle (i.e., drug form in which the drug comes [tablet, capsule, liquid]), and
   A is the amount calculated to be given to the client.

EXAMPLES

1. Order: cefaclor (Ceclor) 0.5 g PO b.i.d.
   Available:

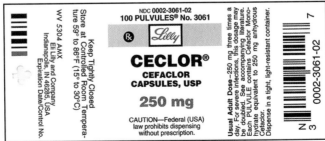

   a. The unit of measure that is ordered (grams) and the unit on the bottle (milligrams) are from the same system of measurement, the metric system. Conversion to the same unit is necessary to work the problem. Because the bottle is in milligrams, convert grams to milligrams.

To convert grams (large value) to milligrams (smaller value), move the decimal point three spaces to the right (see Section 4A: Conversion Within the Metric System).

0.5 g = 0.500 mg or 500 mg

b. $\dfrac{D}{H} \times V = \dfrac{500 \text{ mg}}{250 \text{ mg}} \times 1 \text{ capsule} = \dfrac{500}{250} = 2 \text{ capsules}$

2. Order: codeine gr i̇ (1) PO STAT
Available:

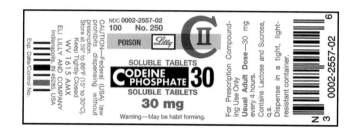

a. Grains must be converted to milligrams before the drug dose can be calculated (see Table 4A–4 or 4B–1). 1 gr = 60 mg

b. $\dfrac{D}{H} \times V = \dfrac{60 \text{ mg}}{30 \text{ mg}} \times 1 \text{ tablet} = \dfrac{60}{30} = 2 \text{ tablets}$

Method 2: Ratio and Proportion (RP)

The **ratio-and-proportion** method is the oldest method currently used in the calculation of drug dosages. The formula is the following:

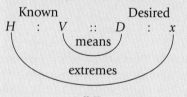

Known   Desired
H : V :: D : x
        means
       extremes

x =

where *H* is the drug on hand (available),
V is the vehicle or drug form (tablet, capsule, liquid),
D is the desired dose (as ordered),
x is the unknown amount to give, and
:: stands for "as" or "equal to."

Multiply the means and the extremes. Solve for *x*; *x* is the divisor.

EXAMPLES

1. Order: amoxicillin (Amoxil) 100 mg PO q.i.d.
Available:

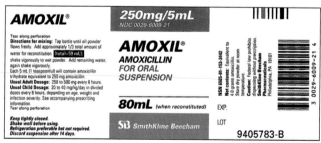

a. Conversion is not needed because both are expressed in the same unit of measure.

b.
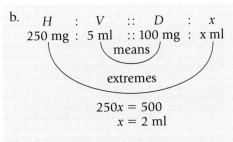

$$250x = 500$$
$$x = 2 \text{ ml}$$

Answer: amoxicillin 100 mg = 2 ml

2. Order: aspirin/ASA gr *x* q4h PRN
   Available: aspirin 325 mg/tablet
   a. Convert to one system and unit of measure. Change grains to milligrams (see Table 4A-4 or 4B-1).

   b.
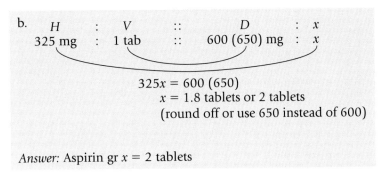

$$325x = 600 \text{ (650)}$$
$$x = 1.8 \text{ tablets or 2 tablets}$$
(round off or use 650 instead of 600)

Answer: Aspirin gr *x* = 2 tablets

Method 3: Fractional Equation (FE)

The **fractional equation** method is similar to ratio and proportion except it is written as a fraction.

$$\frac{H}{V} = \frac{D}{X} \qquad \frac{H}{V} \qquad \frac{\text{dosage on hand}}{\text{Vehicle}} = \frac{D}{X} \quad \frac{\text{desired dosage}}{\text{unknown}}$$

Cross-multiply and solve for *x*.

EXAMPLES

Order: ciprofloxacin (Cipro) 500 mg PO q12h
Available:

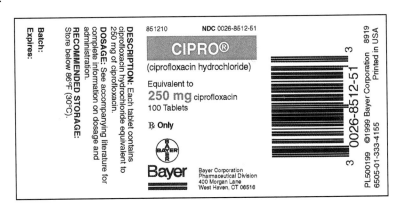

How many tablet(s) should the client receive per dose?

Answer:

$$\frac{H}{V} = \frac{D}{X} \qquad \frac{250 \text{ mg}}{1 \text{ ml}} = \frac{500 \text{ mg}}{X \text{ ml}}$$

Cross-multiply and solve for *x*.

$$250 \, x = 500$$
$$x = 2 \text{ tablets of Cipro per dose}$$

Method 4: Dimensional Analysis (DA)

The **dimensional analysis** method (also called *factor labeling* or the *label factor method*) calculates dosages using three factors:

1. *Drug label factor:* The form of the drug dose *(V)* with the equivalence in units *(H)*; for example, 1 capsule = 500 mg.

2. *Conversion factor (C):* It will help to memorize the following common conversions:

1 g = 1000 mg	1 g = 15 gr
1000 mg = 15 gr	1 gr = 60 mg

3. *Drug order factor:* The dosage desired *(D)*.

These three factors are set up in an equation that allows the units to be cancelled, resulting in the correct units for delivery.

$$V = \frac{V \text{ (vehicle)} \times \quad C \text{ (H)} \quad \times D \text{ (desired)}}{H \text{ (on hand)} \times \quad C \text{ (D)} \quad \times \quad 1}$$

(drug label)   (conversion factor)   (drug order)

With dimensional analysis, the conversion factor is built into the equation and is included when the units of measurements of the drug order and drug container differ. If the two are of the same units of measurement, the conversion factor is eliminated from the equation.

EXAMPLES   Order: acetaminophen (Tylenol) gr xv, PO, PRN
Available:

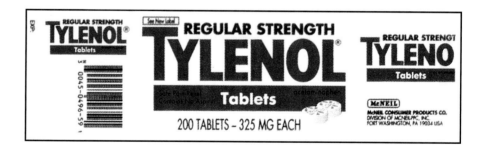

Factors: 325 mg = 1 tablet (from drug label)
15 gr/1 (from drug order)
Conversion factor: 1000 mg = 15 gr
How many tablet(s) should be given? _____

$$\text{tab} = \frac{1 \text{ tab} \times 1000 \text{ mg} \times 15 \text{ gr}}{325 \text{ mg} \times 15 \text{ gr} \times 1} = \frac{1000}{325} = 3.07 \text{ tab or 3 tab}$$

Method 5: Body Weight (BW)

The **body weight (BW)** method of calculation allows for the individualization of the drug dose and involves the following three steps:

1. Convert pounds to kilograms if necessary (lb ÷ 2.2=kg).
2. Determine drug dose per BW by multiplying as follows:

   drug dose × body weight = client's dose per day

3. Follow the basic formula, ratio and proportion, or dimensional analysis method to calculate the drug dosage.

EXAMPLES

1. Order: fluorouracil (5-FU), 12 mg/kg/day IV, not to exceed 800 mg/day. The adult weighs 132 lb.
   a. Convert pounds to kilograms by dividing the number of pounds by 2.2 (1 kg = 2.2 lb).

   $$132 \div 2.2 = 60 \text{ kg}$$

   b. mg × kg = client's dose

   $$12 \times 60 = 720 \text{ mg IV/day}$$

   Answer: fluorouracil 12 mg/kg/day = 720 mg

2. Order: cefaclor (Ceclor) 20 mg/kg/day in three divided doses. The child weighs 31 lb. Available:

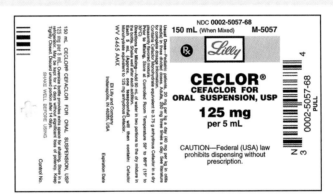

   a. Convert pounds to kilograms.

   $$31 \div 2.2 = 14 \text{ kg}$$

   b. 20 mg × 14 kg = 280 mg/day

   $$280 \text{ mg} \div 3 \text{ divided doses} = 93 \text{ mg/dose}$$

   c. BF: $\dfrac{D}{H} \times V' = \dfrac{93}{125} \times 5 = \dfrac{465}{125} = 3.7$ ml   or   DA: ml $= \dfrac{5 \text{ ml} \times 93 \text{ mg}}{125 \text{ ml} \times 1} =$

   $$\dfrac{465}{125} = 3.7 \text{ ml}$$

   or: RP: H : V :: D : x

   $$125 \text{ mg} : 5 \text{ ml} :: 93 \text{ mg} : x \text{ ml}$$
   $$125x = 465$$
   $$x = \dfrac{465}{125} = 3.7 \text{ ml}$$

   Answer: cefaclor 20 mg/kg/day = 3.7 ml per dose

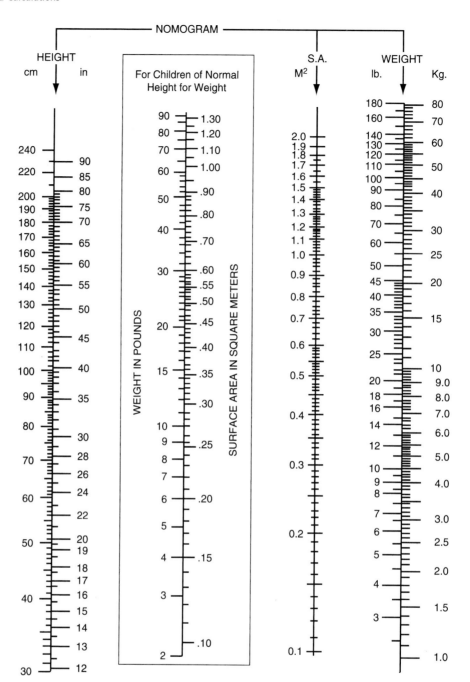

FIGURE 4B–1 West nomogram for infants and children. Directions: *(1)* Find height. *(2)* Find weight. *(3)* Draw a straight line that connects the height and weight. *(4)* Where the line intersects on the surface area column is the body surface area (m²). (Modified from data by Boyd E, West CD. In Behrman RE, Vaughan VC, editors: *Nelson textbook of pediatrics,* ed 14, Philadelphia, 1992, Saunders.)

Method 6: Body Surface Area (BSA)

The **body surface area (BSA)** method is considered the most accurate way to calculate the drug dose for infants, children, older adults, and clients who are on antineoplastic agents or whose BW is low. The BSA, in square meters (m²), is determined by where the person's height and weight intersect the nomogram scale (Figures 4B–1 [children] and 4B–2 [adults]). To calculate the drug dosage using the BSA method, multiply the drug dose ordered by the number of square meters.

$$100 \text{ mg} \times 1.8 \text{ m}^2 \text{ (BSA)} = 180 \text{ mg/day}$$

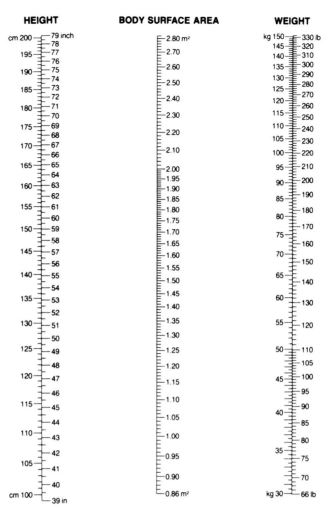

HEIGHT	BODY SURFACE AREA	WEIGHT

FIGURE 4B–2 Nomogram of body surface area for adults. Directions: *(1)* Find height. *(2)* Find weight. *(3)* Draw a straight line that connects the height and weight. *(4)* Where the line intersects on the body surface area column is the body surface area (m²). (From Deglin JH, Vallerand AH, Russin A: *Davis's drug guide for nurses*, ed 2, Philadelphia, 1991, FA Davis; Lentner C, editor: *Geigy scientific tables*, ed 8, vol 1, Basel, Switzerland, 1981, Ciba-Geigy, pp. 226–227.)

EXAMPLES

1. Order: cyclophosphamide (Cytoxan) 100 mg/m²/day, IV
   Available:

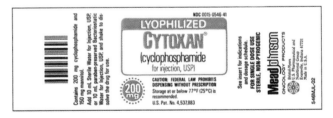

   Client is 70 inches tall and weighs 160 lb.
   a. 70 inches and 160 lb intersect the nomogram scale at 1.97 m² (BSA).
   b. 100 mg × 1.97 = 197 mg.

   Answer: Administer cyclophosphamide 197 mg or 200 mg/day.

2. Order: mephenytoin (Mesantoin) 200 mg/m² PO in three divided doses. Child is 42 inches tall and weighs 44 lb.
   a. 42 inches and 44 lb intersect the nomogram scale at 0.8 m².
   b. 200 mg × 0.8 = 160 mg/day or 50 mg (53) t.i.d.

   Answer: Administer mephenytoin 50 mg t.i.d.

BSA with the Square Root

BSA can be calculated by using the square root and a fractional formula of height and weight divided by a constant. Now that calculators are readily available, research has shown that this method results in fewer errors than drawing intersecting lines on a nomogram,
The formula for BSA using the square root is

$$BSA = \sqrt{\frac{\text{height (inches)} \times \text{wt (lbs)}}{3131 \text{ (constant)}}}$$

EXAMPLE

Order: melphalon (Alkeran) 16 mg/m^2 q 2 weeks. Client is 68 inches tall and weights 172 pounds. Use the BSA inches and pounds formula.

a. $BSA = \sqrt{\dfrac{68 \text{ in} \times 172 \text{ lb}}{3131}}$

$BSA = \sqrt{\dfrac{11696}{3131}}$

$BSA = \sqrt{3.73}$

$BSA = 1.9 \text{ m}^2$

b. 16 mg $\times$ 1.9 m^2 = 30.4 mg/m^2 or 30 mg/m^2.
Client should receive 30 mg every 2 weeks.

PRACTICE PROBLEM 1

Additional practice problems are given in Sections 4C and 4D (calculation of oral and injectable dosages).

DRUG DOSAGE USING BASIC FORMULA, RATIO AND PROPORTION, OR FRACTIONAL EQUATION

Solve the problem and determine the drug dose given the following:
1. Order: cimetidine (Tagamet) 0.4 g PO, q6h
   Available:

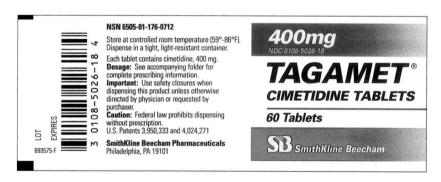

How many tablet(s) of Tagamet should the client receive? _____
2. Order: doxycycline hyclate (Vibra-Tab), PO, initially 200 mg; then 50 mg, PO, b.i.d.
   Drug available:

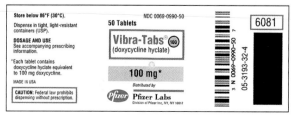

a. How many tablet(s) would you give as the initial dose? _____

b. How many tablets would you give for *each* dose after the initial dose? _____

3. Order: phenobarbital gr ½ PO, t.i.d.

   Available: phenobarbital 15-mg tablet

   How many tablet(s) should the client receive? _____

4. Order: hydrochlorothiazide (HydroDIURIL) 25 mg PO, daily

   Available:

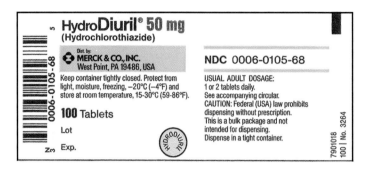

How many tablet(s) should the client receive? _____

5. Order: cefadroxil (Duricef) 500 mg PO, b.i.d.

   Available:

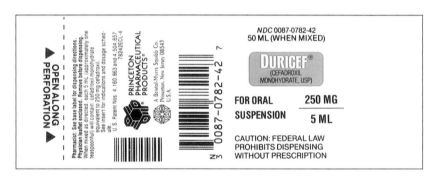

How many milliliters should the client receive? _____

6. Order: dicloxacillin 100 mg PO, q8h

   Available: dicloxacillin 62.5 mg/5 ml

   How many milliliters should the client receive? _____

7. Order: meperidine (Demerol) 35 mg IM STAT

   Available:

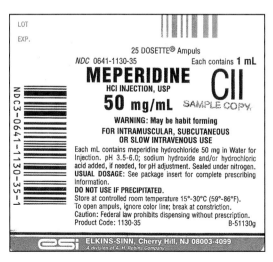

How many milliliters should the client receive? _____

8. Order: atropine sulfate gr $^1/_{200}$ SC on call
   Available: atropine sulfate 0.4 mg/1 ml

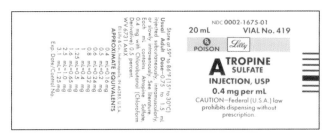

How many milliliters should the client receive? _____

DRUG DOSAGE USING DIMENSIONAL ANALYSIS (FACTOR LABELING)

9. Order: ampicillin (Principen) 50 mg/kg/day PO in four divided doses (q6h). Client weighs 88 pounds, or 40 kg (88 ÷ 2.2 = 40 kg).
   Available:

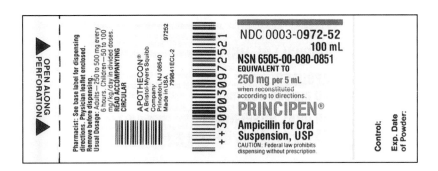

Factors: 250 mg = 5 ml (drug label)
Conversion factor: none (both are in milligrams)
a. How many milligrams per day should the client receive? _____
b. How many milligrams per dose should the client receive? _____
c. How many milliliters should the client receive per dose? _____

10. Order: Codeine gr i (1) PO, STAT
    Available:

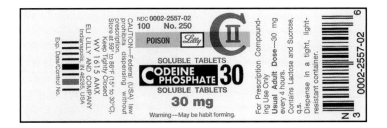

Factors: 30 mg = 1 tablet (drug label)
Conversion factor: 1 gr = 60 mg
How many tablet(s) should be given? _____

11. Order: Ciprofloxacin (Cipro) 0.5 g, PO, b.i.d.
Available:

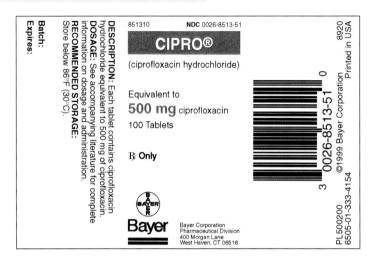

How many tablets should the client receive per dose? _____

PRACTICE PROBLEM 3

DRUG DOSAGE USING BODY WEIGHT

12. Order: sulfisoxazole (Gantrisin) 50 mg/kg/day PO in four divided doses (q6h). Child weighs 44 lb.
How many mg should the client receive per day? _____ Per dose? _____

13. Order: albuterol (Proventil) 0.1 mg/kg/day PO in four divided doses. Client weighs 86 lb.
How many mg should the client receive per dose? _____

14. Order: cefprozil (Cefzil) 15 mg/kg/day PO in two divided doses. Child weighs 33 lb.
Available:

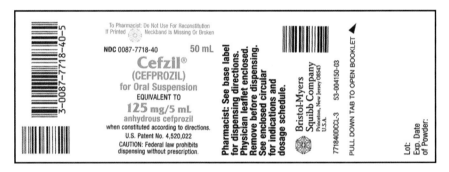

a. How many milligrams should be given per day? _____
b. How many milliliters should the child receive per dose? _____

PRACTICE PROBLEM 4

DRUG DOSAGE USING BODY SURFACE AREA

15. Client is 62 inches tall and weighs 130 lb. What is the BSA? _____

16. Order: bleomycin sulfate 20 units/m^2 IV. Client is 70 inches tall and weighs 160 lb.
How many unit(s) should the client receive? _____

17. Order: sulfisoxazole (Gantrisin) 2 g/m^2 in four divided doses. Child is 50 inches tall and weighs 60 lb.
Available: sulfisoxazole 500 mg/5 ml
a. What is the child's BSA? _____
b. How many gram(s) should the child receive per day? _____
c. How many milliliters should the child receive per dose? _____

ANSWERS TO PRACTICE PROBLEMS

1   DRUG DOSAGE USING BASIC FORMULA, RATIO AND PROPORTION, OR FRACTIONAL EQUATION

1. a. Convert grams to milligrams by moving the decimal point three spaces to the right.

$$0.4 \text{ g} = 0.400 \text{ mg}$$

   b. BF: $\dfrac{D}{H} \times V = \dfrac{400 \text{ mg}}{400 \text{ mg}} \times 1 \text{ tablet} = 1 \text{ tablet}$

2. a. Initially:

     BF: $\dfrac{D}{H} \times V = \dfrac{\overset{2}{\cancel{200}}}{\underset{1}{\cancel{100}}} \times 1 = 2 \text{ tablets}$

   or

   RP: $H \quad : \quad V \quad :: \quad D \quad : x$
       $100 \text{ mg} : 1 \text{ tab} :: 200 \text{ mg} : x$
            $100x = 200$
               $x = 2 \text{ tablets}$

   or

   FE (cross-multiply):

$$\frac{100}{1} \times \frac{200}{x} =$$

           $100x = 200$
             $x = 2 \text{ tablets}$

   or

   DA: No conversion factor

$$\text{Tablet(s)} = \frac{1 \times \overset{2}{\cancel{200}}}{\underset{1}{\cancel{100}} \times 1} = 2 \text{ tablets}$$

   b. Daily: RP: $H \quad : \quad V \quad :: \quad D \quad : x$
         $100 \text{ mg} : 1 \text{ tab} :: 500 \text{ mg} : x$
             $100x = 50$
               $x = \frac{1}{2} \text{ tablet}$

   or

   DA: No conversion factor

$$\text{Tablet(s)} = \frac{1 \text{ tab} \times \overset{1}{\cancel{50 \text{ mg}}}}{\underset{2}{\cancel{100 \text{ mg}}} \times 1} = \frac{1}{2} \text{ tablet}$$

3. a. Convert grains to milligrams. Table 4A–4 or 4B–1 gives 30 mg = $\frac{1}{2}$ gr, or 60 mg = 1 gr

     $60 \text{ mg} \quad : 1 \text{ gr} :: x \text{ mg} : \frac{1}{2} \text{ gr}$
            $x = 60 \times 0.5 \; (\frac{1}{2})$
            $x = 30 \text{ mg}$

   b. RP: $H \quad : V :: \quad D \quad : x$
        $15 \text{ mg} : 1 :: 30 \text{ mg} : x$
           $15x = 30$
            $x = 2 \text{ tablets}$

4. $\frac{1}{2}$ tablet

5. 10 ml

6. FE: $\dfrac{H}{V} = \dfrac{D}{x} \quad \dfrac{62.5 \text{ mg}}{5 \text{ ml}} = \dfrac{100 \text{ mg}}{x \text{ ml}}$
                       $62.5x = 500$
                          $x = 8 \text{ ml}$

7. 0.7 ml

8. a. The drug label shows 0.4 mg = 1 ml. Change $\frac{1}{200}$ gr to milligrams (see Table 4A–4 or 4B–1). $\frac{1}{200}$ gr = 0.3 mg

   b. BF: $\dfrac{D}{H} \times V = \dfrac{0.3}{0.4} \times 1 \text{ ml} = 0.4\overline{)0.3.0}^{\;0.75} = 0.75 \text{ ml}$

   or

     RP: $H \quad : \quad V \quad :: \quad D \quad : x$
        $0.4 \text{ mg} : 1 \text{ ml} :: 0.3 \text{ mg} : x$
             $0.4x = 0.3 = 0.75 \text{ ml}$

2   DRUG DOSAGE USING DIMENSIONAL ANALYSIS (FACTOR LABELING)

9. a. 50 mg/kg/day = 50 × 40 = 2000 mg
   b. 2000 mg ÷ 4 = 500 mg per dose

   c. $\text{ml} = \dfrac{5 \text{ ml} \times 500 \cancel{\text{mg}}}{250 \cancel{\text{mg}} \times 1} = \dfrac{10}{1} = 10 \text{ ml}$

10. $\text{Tablets} = \dfrac{1 \text{ tablet} \times \overset{2}{\cancel{60 \text{ mg}}} \times 1 \cancel{\text{gr}}}{\underset{1}{\cancel{30 \text{ mg}}} \times 1 \cancel{\text{gr}} \times 1} = 2 \text{ tablets}$

11. $\text{tab} = \dfrac{1 \text{ tab} \times \overset{2}{\cancel{1000 \text{ mg}}} \times 0.5 \cancel{\text{g}}}{\underset{1}{\cancel{500 \text{ mg}}} \times 1 \cancel{\text{g}} \times 1} = 1 \text{ tablet}$

3   DRUG DOSAGE USING BODY WEIGHT

12. a. 44 lb ÷ 2.2 kg = 20 kg
  b. 50 mg × 20 kg = 1000 mg/day
    1000 ÷ 4 times a day = 250 mg q.i.d., or q6h
13. a. 86 ÷ 2.2 = 39 kg
  b. 0.1 mg × 39 = 3.9 mg, or 4 mg
    4 ÷ 4 = 1 mg q6h

14. 33 ÷ 2.2 = 15 kg
  15 mg × 15 = 225 mg/day
  225 ÷ 2 times a day = 112.5 mg, q12h per dose

$$\frac{D}{H} \times = \frac{112.5}{125} \times 5\ ml = \frac{562.5}{125} = 4.5\ ml\ q12h$$

  a. Administer cefprozil 225 mg/day
  b. Administer 112.5 mg = 4.5 ml, q12h

4   DRUG DOSAGE USING BODY SURFACE AREA

15. 1.65 m²
16. a. Client's height and weight intersect the nomogram scale at 1.97 m².
  b. 20 Unit × 1.97 = 39.4 or 39 Unit
17. a. Height and weight intersect the nomogram scale at 0.98 m².

  b. 2 g × 0.98 = 1.96 g, or 2 g/day

  c. 5 ml (convert grams to milligrams.
    0.5 g = 0.500 mg)

Section 4C CALCULATIONS OF ORAL DOSAGES

OUTLINE

Objectives
Terms
Introduction
Tablets, Capsules, and Liquids
Interpreting Oral Drug Labels

Drug Differentiation
Calculation for Tablet, Capsule, and Liquid Doses
Body Weight and Body Surface Area
Drugs Administered Via Nasogastric Tube

OBJECTIVES

- Calculate oral dosages from tablets, capsules, and liquids with selected formula.
- Calculate oral medications according to body weight and body surface area.
- Calculate the amount of tube feeding solution needed for dilution according to the percentage ordered.

TERMS

body surface area (BSA)
capsules
enteric-coated
sustained-release
tablets
tube feeding

Introduction

Eighty percent of all drugs consumed are given orally. Oral drugs are available in tablet, capsule, powder, and liquid form. The written abbreviation for drugs given orally is P.O. or PO (*per os,* or *by mouth*). Oral medications are absorbed by the gastrointestinal (GI) tract, mainly from the small intestine.

Oral medications have the following advantages: (1) the client frequently can take oral medications without assistance, (2) the cost of oral medications is usually less than when given via other routes (e.g., parenteral), and (3) oral medications are easy to store. The disadvantages include (1) variation in absorption as a result of food in the GI tract and pH variation of GI secretions, (2) irritation of the gastric mucosa by certain drugs (e.g., potassium chloride), and (3) destruction or partial inactivation of the drugs by liver enzymes. This section discusses oral dosages for adults; Section 4F discusses oral dosages for children.

Tablets, Capsules, and Liquids

Tablets come in different forms and drug strengths. Most tablets are scored and thus can be readily broken when half of the drug amount is needed. **Capsules** are gelatin shells that contain powder or time-release pellets (beads). **Sustained-release** (pellet) capsules *should not* be crushed and diluted, because the medication will be absorbed at a much faster rate than indicated by the manufacturer. Many medications that are in tablet form are also available in liquid form. When the client has difficulty taking tablets, the liquid form of the medication is given. The liquid form can be in a suspension, syrup, elixir, or tincture. Some liquid medications that irritate the stomach, such as potassium chloride, are diluted. The tincture form is always diluted.

Enteric-coated (hard shell) tablets *must not* be crushed, because the medication could irritate the gastric mucosa. Enteric-coated drugs pass through the stomach into the small intestine where the drug's coating dissolves and then absorption occurs. Oral drugs (tablets, capsules, liquids) that irritate the gastric mucosa should be taken with 5 to 8 ounces of fluids or taken with food. Figure 4C–1 shows the different forms of tablets and capsules.

Liquid medications are poured into a medicine cup that is calibrated in ounces, teaspoons, tablespoons, and milliliters. Figure 4C–2 shows the markings on a medicine cup.

Interpreting Oral Drug Labels

Pharmaceutical companies usually label their drugs with the brand (trade) name of the drug in large letters and the generic name in smaller letters. The dose per tablet, capsule, or liquid is often printed under the drug name.

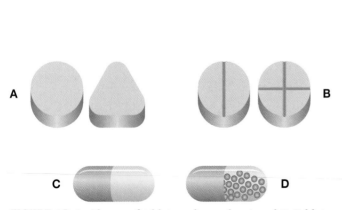

FIGURE 4C–1 Shapes of tablets and capsules. A and B, Tablets; C and D, capsules.

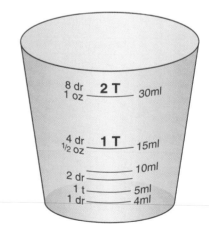

FIGURE 4C–2 Medicine cup for liquid measurement. (From Kee JL, Marshall SM: *Clinical calculations*, ed 5, Philadelphia, 2004, Saunders, p. 115.)

EXAMPLE

Ceftin is the brand (trade) name, and cefuroxime axetil is the generic name. The dose is 125 mg/5 ml (oral suspension).

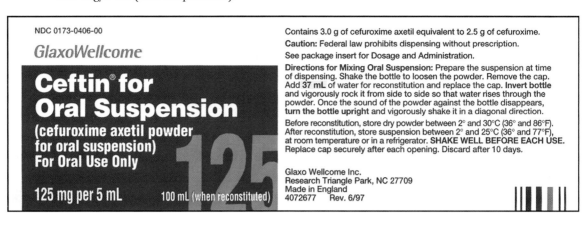

Drug Differentiation

Preventing Medication Errors

Some drugs' spelling, look alike or sound alike but have different chemical drug structures and are prescribed for different health problems. When ordering drugs make sure the spelling of the drug is correct and be extremely careful when administering drugs whose names look alike. Caution: Physicians' hand writing of drug names.

EXAMPLE 1
QUINIDINE AND QUININE

Quinidine is an antiarrhythmic drug, and quinine is an antimalarial drug. Read drug label three times before pouring the drug.

EXAMPLE 2
CELEBREX, CELEXA, AND CEREBYX

All three drugs are brand drugs and have a similar spelling. Celebrex (celecoxib) is an analgesic, a cyclo-oxygenase 2 (COX-2) inhibitor; Celexa (citalopram) is an antidepressant, a selective serotonin reuptake (SSR) inhibitor; and Cerebyx (fosphenytoin sodium) is an anticonvulsant.

EXAMPLE 3
PERCODAN AND PERCOCET

Percodan contains oxycodone and aspirin, and Percocet contains oxycodone and acetaminophen. A client may be allergic to aspirin or should not take aspirin because of a stomach ulcer; therefore it is important that the client take Percocet. *Read the drug labels carefully.*

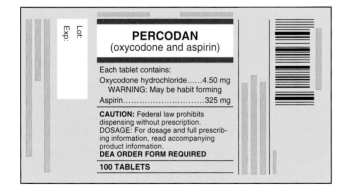

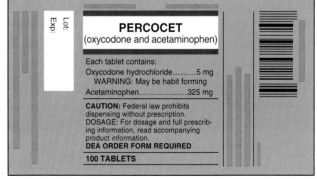

EXAMPLE 4
HYDROXYZINE AND HYDRALAZINE

Hydroxyzine is an antianxiety drug, and hydralazine is an antihypertensive drug.

Calculation For Tablet, Capsule, And Liquid Doses

When calculating oral dosages, choose one of the methods for calculation from Section 4B.

EXAMPLES
1. Order: diltiazem (Cardizem) 60 mg PO, b.i.d.
   Available:

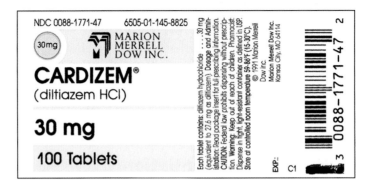

a. BF: $\dfrac{D}{H} \times V = \dfrac{60}{30} \times 1 = 2$ tablets

b. RP:

H	:	V	::	D	:	x
30 mg	:	1 tab	::	60 mg	:	x tab

$$30x = 60$$

$$x = 2 \text{ tablets}$$

Answer: diltiazem (Cardizem) 60 mg = 2 tablets

c. FE: $\dfrac{H}{V} = \dfrac{D}{x}$ $\dfrac{30}{1} \times \dfrac{60}{x}$ (cross multiply) $= 30x = 60$

$$x = 2 \text{ tablets}$$

d. DA: tab $= \dfrac{1 \text{ tab} \times \overset{2}{\cancel{60}} \text{ mg}}{\underset{1}{\cancel{30}} \text{ mg} \times 1} = 2$ tablets

Conversion is not needed.

2. Order: codeine phosphate 1 gr PO, STAT
   Available: See the conversion Tables 4A–4 or 4B–1.

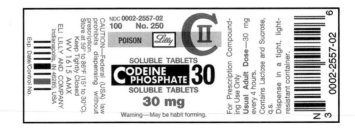

a. BF: gr 1 = 60 mg

$\dfrac{D}{H} \times V = \dfrac{60}{30} \times 1 = 2$ tablets

b. FE: $\dfrac{H}{v} = \dfrac{D}{x}$ $\dfrac{30}{1} = \dfrac{60}{x} =$

$$30x = 60$$
$$x = 2 \text{ tablets}$$

c. DA: tablet $= \dfrac{1 \times \overset{2}{\cancel{60}} \text{ mg} \times 1 \text{ gr}}{\underset{1}{\cancel{30}} \text{ mg} \times 1 \text{ gr} \times 1} = 2$ tablets

Answer: codeine 1 gr = 2 tablets

3. Order: clarithromycin (Biaxin) 100 mg, PO q6h
   Available:

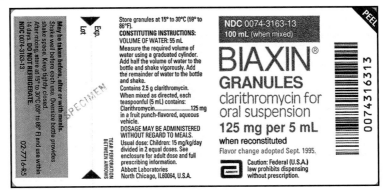

How many milliliters should the client receive per dose? _____

a. BF: $\dfrac{D}{H} \times V = \dfrac{100}{\underset{25}{\cancel{125}}} \times \overset{1}{\cancel{5}} = 4$ ml

or

b. RP: H : V :: D : V
   125 : 5 :: 100 : x
   $$125x = 500$$
   $$x = 4 \text{ ml}$$

or

c. DA: ml $\dfrac{5 \text{ ml} \times \overset{4}{\cancel{100}} \text{ mg}}{\underset{5}{\cancel{125}} \text{ mg} \times 1} = \dfrac{20}{5} = 4$ ml

PRACTICE PROBLEM 1

ORAL MEDICATIONS

Solve the drug problems for *x*, the unknown amount of drug to be given. See Sections 4A and 4B for the conversion tables, methods of conversion, and the method chosen to solve the drug problems.

1. Order: doxepin HCl (Sinequan) 30 mg PO, at bedtime.
   Available:

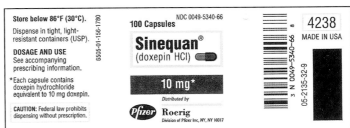

How many capsule(s) should the client receive? _____

2. Order: lisinopril (Zestril) 5 mg PO, daily.
   Available:

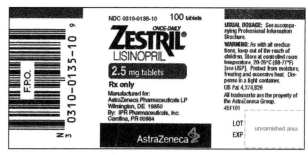

How many tablets should the client receive? _____

3. Order: aspirin gr *x* STAT
   Available: aspirin 325 mg tablet
   How many tablet(s) of aspirin should the nurse give? _____

4. Order: digoxin (Lanoxin) 0.5 mg PO, daily.
   Available:

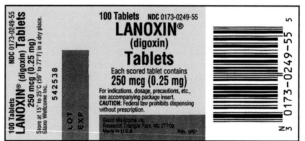

How many tablet(s) should the nurse administer? _____

5. Order: nitroglycerin (Nitrostat) $\frac{1}{150}$ gr sublingual STAT
   Available:

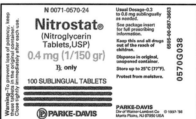

How many sublingual tablet(s) should the client take? _____

6. Order: bethanechol Cl (Urecholine) 20 mg PO, t.i.d.
   Available:

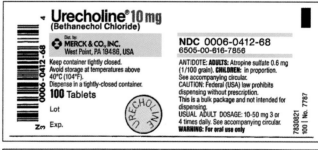

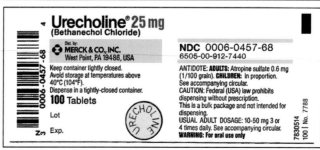

a. Which Urecholine bottle should the nurse select? _____

b. How many tablet(s) should the client receive per dose? _____

7. Order: amoxicillin clavulanate (Augmentin) 500 mg PO, b.i.d.

Available:

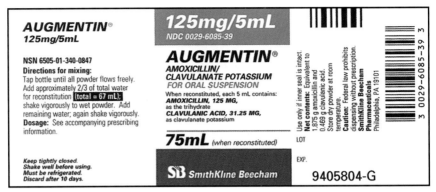

How many milliliters should the client receive per dose? _____

8. Order: cefadroxil (Duricef) 500 mg PO, b.i.d.

Available:

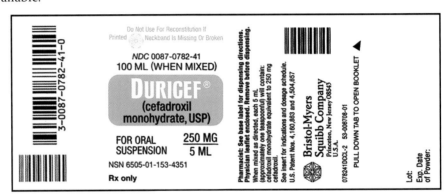

How many milliliters should the client receive per dose? _____

9. Order: prazosin (Minipress) 10 mg PO, daily.

Available: prazosin 1-mg, 2-mg, and 5-mg tablets

Which tablet should be selected and how much should be given? _____

10. Order: carbidopa-levodopa (Sinemet) 12.5–125 mg PO, b.i.d.

Available: Sinemet 25- to 100-, 25- to 250-, 10- to 100-mg tablets

Which tablet should be selected and how much should be given? _____

Additional Dimensional Analysis

11. Order: omeprazole (Prilosec) 20 mg PO, daily.

Available:

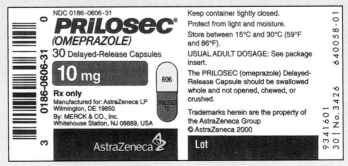

Factors: 10 mg = 1 capsule (drug label)

Conversion factor: none (both are in milligrams)

How many capsule(s) should the client receive? _____

12. Order: amoxicillin (Amoxil) 0.1 g PO, q8h
    Available:

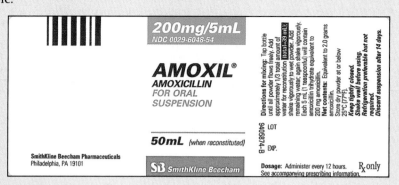

Factors: 200 mg = 5 ml
Conversion factor: 1000 mg = 1 g
How many milliliters should the client receive per dose? _____

Body Weight And Body Surface Area

Calculating the drug dosage for adults by body weight (BW) and body surface area (BSA) is used mostly when administering drugs to treat cancer (antineoplastic drugs). These two individualized methods are also used frequently to calculate drug dosages for children. Examples and practice problems for pediatrics are given in Section 4F.

To use the body weight method, convert the person's weight in pounds to kilograms (kg). To convert, divide pounds by 2.2 to equal kilograms. To use the **body surface area (BSA)** method, the person's weight and height and a nomogram are needed. (See Sections 4B and 4F). Daily requirements are usually divided into two to four doses per day.

EXAMPLE

Order: cyclophosphamide (Cytoxan) 2 mg/kg PO daily. Client weighs 143 lb.
How much does the client weigh in kilograms? _____ How many milligrams (mg) should the client receive? _____

Answer: 143 lb ÷ 2.2 = 65 kg

2 mg × 65 = 130 mg of cyclophosphamide daily

PRACTICE
PROBLEM 2

BODY WEIGHT

1. Order: valproic acid (Depakene) 8 mg/kg/day in four divided doses. Client weighs 165 lb.
   How much Depakene should be administered per dose? _____
2. Order: cyclophosphamide (Cytoxan) 4 mg/kg/day. Client weighs 176 lb.
   How much Cytoxan should the client receive per day? _____

Drugs Administered Via Nasogastric Tube

Oral medications can be administered through a nasogastric tube but should *not* be mixed with the entire **tube feeding** solution. Mixing the medications in a large volume of tube feeding solution decreases the amount of drug the client receives for a specific time. The medication (NOT time-released or sustained-release capsules and psyllium hydrophilic mucilloid [Metamucil]) should be diluted in 1 ounce (30 ml) of warm water unless otherwise instructed, administered through the tube, and followed with extra water to ensure that the drug reaches the stomach and is not left in the tube.

ANSWERS TO PRACTICE PROBLEMS

1 **ORAL MEDICATIONS USING BASIC FORMULA, RATIO AND PROPORTION, FRACTIONAL EQUATION, OR DIMENSIONAL ANALYSIS**

1. 3 capsules of Sinequan

2. 2 tablets of Zestril

3. Convert grains to milligrams. See Tables 4A–4 or 4B–1.
   5 gr = 300, or 325 mg; thus 10 gr = 650 mg (approximate value)

   a. BF: $\dfrac{D}{H} \times V = \dfrac{650}{325} \times 1 = 2$ tablets

   or

   b. RP: $H \ : \ V \ :: \ D \ : \ x$
   325 mg : 1 tab :: 650 mg : x tab
   $325x = 650$
   $x = 2$ tablets

   c. DA: tab $= \dfrac{1 \ \times 1000 \ \text{mg} \times \overset{2}{\cancel{10}} \ \text{gr}}{325 \ \text{mg} \times \ \underset{3}{\cancel{15}} \ \text{gr} \ \times \ 1} =$

   $\dfrac{2000}{975} = 2.05$ or 2 tab

4. 2 tablets

   a. BF: $\dfrac{D}{H} \times V = \dfrac{0.5}{0.25} \times 1 = 0.25\sqrt{0.50\,0} = 2$ tablets

   or

   b. RP: $H \ : \ V \ :: \ D \ : \ x$
   0.25 mg : 1 tab :: 0.5 mg : x tab
   $0.25x = 0.5 = 2$ tablets

   c. DA: tab $= \dfrac{1 \ \times 0.5 \ \text{mg}}{0.25 \ \text{mg} \times \ 1} = 2$ tablets

5. 1 sublingual tablet
   Convert grains to milligrams. $1/150$ gr = 0.4 mg

6. a. Select Urecholine 10 mg bottle.

   b. BF: $\dfrac{D}{H} \times V = \dfrac{20 \text{ mg}}{10 \text{ mg}} \times 1 \text{ tab} = \dfrac{20}{10}$
   = 2 tablets
   or
   DA: tab $= \dfrac{1 \ \times 20 \ \text{mg}}{10 \ \text{mg} \times \ 1} = 2$ tablets
   no conversion needed

7. 20 ml of Augmentin suspension

8. 10 ml of cefadroxil

   a. BF: $\dfrac{D}{H} \times V = \dfrac{500}{250} \times 5 = \dfrac{2500}{250} = 10$ ml

   b. FE: $\dfrac{H}{V} = \dfrac{D}{x} = \dfrac{250 \text{ mg}}{5 \text{ ml}} = \dfrac{500 \text{ mg}}{x \text{ ml}}$
   $250x = 2500$
   $x = 10$ ml

   c. DA: ml $= \dfrac{5 \text{ ml} \ \times 5\overset{2}{\cancel{00}} \ \text{mg}}{2\underset{1}{\cancel{50}} \ \text{mg} \times \ 1} = 10$ ml

9. Select 5-mg tablets. Give two tablets.

10. Select 25–250 mg strength. Give half a tablet.

11. 2 capsules

   capsules $= \dfrac{1 \text{ cap} \ \times \overset{2}{\cancel{20}} \ \text{mg}}{\underset{1}{\cancel{10}} \ \text{mg} \times \ 1} = 2$ capsules

12. 2.5 ml per dose

   ml $= \dfrac{5 \text{ ml} \ \times 1\overset{5}{\cancel{000}} \ \text{mg} \times 0.1 \text{ g}}{\underset{1}{\cancel{200}} \ \text{mg} \times \ 1 \text{ g} \ \times \ 1}$
   = 2.5 ml per dose

2 **BODY WEIGHT**

1. 75 kg; 150 mg/dose; 600 mg/day

2. 80 kg; 320 mg/day

Section 4D CALCULATIONS OF INJECTABLE DOSAGES

OBJECTIVES

- Describe the difference between vials and ampules.
- Describe the types of syringes and needles and their uses.
- Explain how to administer intradermal, subcutaneous, and intramuscular injections.
- Calculate dosage of drugs for subcutaneous and intramuscular injections.
- Identify the amount of insulin dosage with the use of an insulin syringe.
- Explain the methods for mixing two insulins in one insulin syringe and for mixing two injectable drugs in one syringe.
- Describe the procedure for the preparation and calculation of medications in powdered form for injectable use.

TERMS

ampule	insulin syringe	parenteral
bevel	intradermal	subcutaneous (subQ)
diluent	intramuscular (IM)	tuberculin syringe
gauge	lumen	vial

Introduction

When medications cannot be taken by mouth because of (1) an inability to swallow, (2) a decreased level of consciousness, (3) an inactivation of the drug by gastric juices, or (4) a desire to increase the effectiveness of the drug, the parenteral route may be the route of choice. **Parenteral** medications are administered intradermally (under the skin), subcutaneously (into the fatty tissue), intramuscularly (IM, within the muscle), and intravenously (IV, in the vein). IV injectables are discussed in Section 4E. The injectables in this section include intradermal, subQ (including insulin and heparin), and IM from prepared liquid and reconstituted powder in vials and ampules. Prefilled drug cartridges (syringes) are also discussed.

This section is divided into five parts: (1) injectable preparations, (2) intradermal injections, (3) subQ injections, (4) insulin injections, and (5) IM injections. For the four latter parts, examples and practice problems to solve for the correct dosage are provided.

Injectable Preparations

The appropriate drug container (vial or ampule) and the correct selection of needle and syringe are essential in the preparation of the prescribed drug dose. The route of administration is part of the medication order.

Vials and Ampules

A **vial** is usually a small glass container with a self-sealing rubber top. Some are multiple-dose vials, and when properly stored, they can be used over time. An **ampule** is a glass container with a tapered neck for snapping open and using only once. Drugs that deteriorate readily in liquid form are packaged in powder form in vials and ampules for storage. Once the dry form of the drug is reconstituted (usually with sterile water, bacteriostatic water, or saline), the drug is used immediately or must be refrigerated. Check the accompanying drug circular for specific storage length and other instructions. The person reconstituting the drug should write on the label when the drug is to be discarded and include her or his initials. Usually a vial should be used within 96 hours.

Drug labels on vials and ampules provide the following information: (1) generic and brand name of the drug, (2) drug dose in weight (milligrams, grams, milliequivalents) and amount (milliliters), (3) expiration date, and (4) directions about administration. If the drug is in powdered form, mixing instructions and dose equivalents (e.g., milligrams equal milliliters) may be given. Figure 4D–1 is a diagram of a vial and ampule.

Syringes

The syringe is composed of a barrel (outer shell), plunger (inner part), and the tip where the needle joins the syringe (Figure 4D–2). Syringes are available in various types and sizes, the most common of which are the 3-ml and 5-ml tuberculin, insulin, and metal and plastic syringes for prefilled cartridges. Glass syringes may be used in the operating room and on special instrument trays. The tip of the syringe and inside of the plunger should remain sterile.

The 3-ml syringe is calibrated in tenths (0.1 ml) and minims. The amount of fluid in the syringe is determined by the black rubber end of the plunger (the inner end of the plunger) that is closest to the tip (Figure 4D–3). REMEMBER: Milliliter (ml) and cubic centimeter (cc) may be used interchangeably. An advance in safety needle technology is the SafetyGlide shielding hypodermic needle (Figure 4D–4). This type of needle reduces needlestick injuries.

The 5-ml syringe is calibrated in 0.2-ml marks. A 5-ml syringe is usually used when the fluid needed is more than 2.5 ml. It is frequently used when reconstituting the dry drug form with

SECTION D

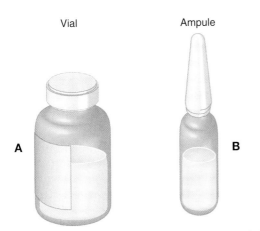

FIGURE 4D–1 **A,** Vial. **B,** Ampule. (From Kee JL, Marshall SM: *Clinical calculations,* ed 5, Philadelphia, 2004, Saunders, p. 148.)

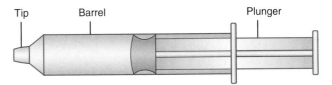

FIGURE 4D–2 Parts of a syringe. (From Kee JL, Marshall SM: *Clinical calculations,* ed 5, Philadelphia, 2004, Saunders, p. 149.)

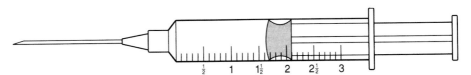

FIGURE 4D–3 A 3-ml syringe. (From Kee JL, Marshall SM: *Clinical calculations,* ed 5, Philadelphia, 2004, Saunders, p. 149.)

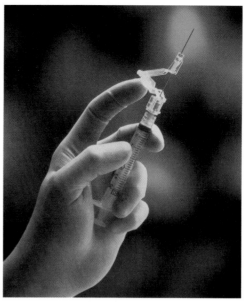

FIGURE 4D–4   SafetyGlide needle. (Courtesy Becton-Dickinson Division, Franklin Lakes, NJ.)

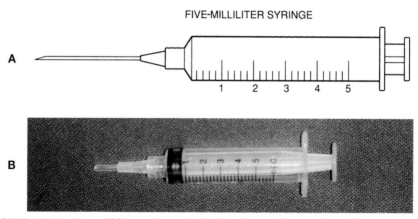

FIGURE 4D–5   Five-milliliter syringes: **A,** 5-ml syringe with 0.2-ml markings; **B,** needleless 5-ml BD syringe that can penetrate a rubber-top vial.

sterile bacteriostatic water or saline. The needleless syringes are used primarily for intermittent infusion therapy to irrigate the intermittent infusion device for maintaining patency and to administer IV medication through the IV tubing device. See intermittent infusion adapters/devices in Section E. Figure 4D–5 shows the 5-ml syringe and 5-ml needleless syringe.

The **tuberculin syringe** is a 1-ml slender syringe with markings in tenths (0.1) and hundredths (0.01). It is also marked in minims (Figure 4D–6). This syringe is used when the amount of drug solution to be administered is less than 1 ml and for pediatric and heparin dosages. The tuberculin syringe is also available in a 0.5-ml syringe. Figure 4D–7 illustrates the 0.5-ml and 1-ml tuberculin syringes.

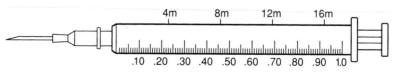

FIGURE 4D–6   Tuberculin syringe. (From Kee JL, Marshall SM: *Clinical calculations,* ed 5, Philadelphia, 2004, Saunders, p. 151.)

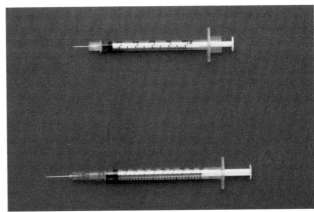

FIGURE 4D–7 Two types of tuberculin syringes. (Courtesy Becton-Dickinson Division, Franklin Lakes, NJ.)

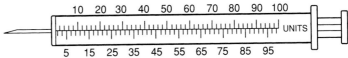

FIGURE 4D–8 Insulin syringe. (From Kee JL, Marshall SM: *Clinical calculations*, ed 5, Philadelphia, 2004, Saunders, p. 152.)

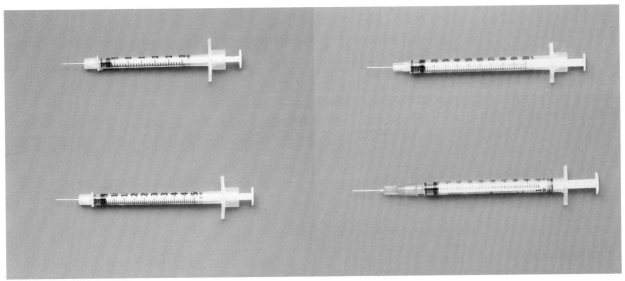

FIGURE 4D–9 Various types of insulin syringes. (Courtesy Becton-Dickinson Division, Franklin Lakes, NJ.)

The **insulin syringe** has the capacity of 1 ml; however, insulin is measured in units, and insulin dosage *must not* be calculated in milliliters. Insulin syringes are calibrated as 2-unit marks, and 100 units equal 1 ml (Figure 4D–8). *Insulin syringes must be used for the administration of insulin.*

Insulin syringes are available as low-dose insulin syringes. The 1-ml insulin syringe may be purchased with a permanent attached needle or a detachable needle (Figure 4D–9).

Prefilled Drug Cartridges and Syringes

Many injectable drugs are packaged in prefilled, disposable cartridges. The disposable cartridge is placed into a Tubex injector or a reusable metal or plastic holder. Usually the prefilled cartridge contains 0.1 to 0.2 ml of excess drug solution. Based on the amount of drug to be administered, the excess solution must be expelled before administration. Figure 4D–10, *A*, illustrates the Carpuject syringe; Figure 4D–10, *B*, shows the Tubex syringe.

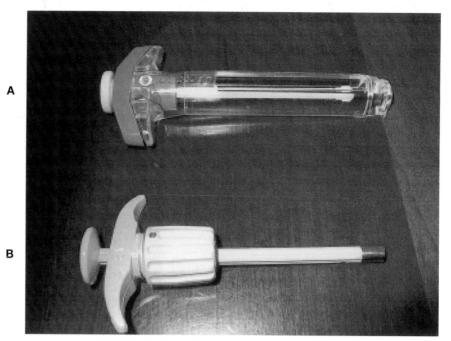

A

B

FIGURE 4D–10 **A,** Carpuject syringe. **B,** Tubex syringe.

Needles

Needle size has two components: **gauge** (diameter of the lumen) and length. The larger the gauge number, the smaller the diameter of the **lumen**, and the smaller the gauge, the larger the diameter of the lumen. The most common gauge numbers of needles range from 18 to 26. Needle length varies from $^3/_8$ inch to 2 inches. Table 4D–1 lists the needle gauges and lengths for use in subcutaneous and IM injections.

When choosing the needle length for an IM injection, the size of the client and the amount of fatty tissue must be considered. A client with minimal fatty (subQ) tissue may need a needle length of 1 inch. For an obese client, the length of the needle for an IM injection would be 1.5 to 2 inches.

Many insulin syringes and prefilled cartridges have permanently attached needles. With other syringes, the needle can be changed to the desired needle size. Needle gauge and length are indicated on the syringe package or on the top cover of the syringe. It appears as gauge/length; for example, 20 g/1$^1/_2$.

Figure 4D–11 illustrates the parts of a needle.

Table 4D-1		
Needle Size and Length		
Type of Injection	**Needle Gauge**	**Needle Lengths (Inches)**
Intradermal	25, 26	$^3/_8$, $^1/_2$, $^5/_8$
Subcutaneous	23, 25, 26	$^3/_8$, $^1/_2$, $^5/_8$
Intramuscular	19, 20, 21, 22	1, 1$^1/_2$, 2

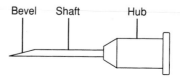

FIGURE 4D–11   Parts of a needle.

Angles for Injections

For injections, the needle enters the skin at different angles. Intradermal injections are given at a 10- to 15-degree angle, subQ injections at a 45- to 90-degree angle, and IM injections at a 90-degree angle. Figure 3–21 illustrates the angles for intradermal, subQ, and IM injections.

PRACTICE PROBLEM 1

SYRINGES AND NEEDLES

Think through and answer each question. Correct answers are given at the end of the section.
1. To mix 4 ml of bacteriostatic water in a vial with a powdered drug, which size syringe should be used?
2. To give 0.4 ml of drug solution subQ, what type of syringe should be used?
3. Meperidine (Demerol) is available in a prefilled cartridge. Half of the drug solution is used. Should the remaining solution in the cartridge be saved for future use?
4. Which has the larger needle lumen, a 21-gauge needle or a 26-gauge needle?
5. Which needle has a length of ⅝ inch, a 21-gauge needle or a 25-gauge needle?
6. Which needle is used for an IM injection, a 20-gauge needle with a 1.5-inch length or a 25-gauge needle with a ⅝-inch length?

Interpreting Injectable Drug Labels

Drugs for injections are stored in liquid and powder form in vials and ampules. If the drug is in liquid form, the drug dose with its equivalent in milliliters is printed on the drug label. However, drugs in powder form must be reconstituted (i.e., changed to liquid form before use). Usually the instructions for reconstitution are given on the drug label and drug instructions. If this is not the case, consult a pharmacist or the drug circular.

EXAMPLE

Nafcillin sodium is the generic name; there is no brand (trade) name. The drug is for IM or IV administration. Instructions on the drug label read: "When reconstituted with 6.6 ml of diluent, each vial contains 8 ml of solution."

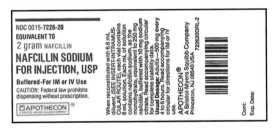

Intradermal Injections

An **intradermal** injection is usually used for skin testing to diagnose the cause of an allergy or to determine the presence of a microorganism. The choice of syringe for intradermal testing is the tuberculin syringe with a 25-gauge needle.

The inner portion of the forearm is frequently used for diagnostic testing because there is less hair in the area and the test results are more visible. The upper back may also be used as a testing site. The needle is inserted with the **bevel** pointing upward at a 10- to 15-degree angle. Do not aspirate. Test results are read 48 to 72 hours after the intradermal injection. A reddened or raised area is a positive reaction.

Subcutaneous Injections

Drugs injected into the **subcutaneous (subQ)** or fatty tissue are absorbed slowly because there are fewer blood vessels in fatty tissue. The amount of drug solution administered subQ is generally 0.5 to 1 ml at a 45-, 60-, or 90-degree angle. Drug solutions that irritate fatty tissues are given IM because they can cause sloughing of the subQ tissue.

The two types of syringes used for subQ injections are the tuberculin syringe (1 ml), calibrated in 0.1 ml and 0.01 ml, and the 3-ml syringe, calibrated in 0.1 ml. The needle gauge commonly used is 25 or 26, and the length is $3/8$ to $5/8$ inch. Insulin is also administered subQ and is discussed later in this section.

Calculations: Subcutaneous Injections

To calculate dosages for subQ injections, use the basic formula of $D/H \times V$, the ratio-and-proportion method, fractional equation, or dimensional analysis (see Section 4B). Heparin is a drug frequently administered subQ. It can be given at a 60- to 90-degree angle, depending on the amount of fatty tissue. The skin is lifted, and the heparin solution is injected into the subQ tissue. Do not aspirate or massage the injected site, because massage could cause small-vessel damage and bleeding.

Units should be written out as a word and not abbreviated as "U" only. When U is written, it may appear as O, and thus the client could receive a higher dose of the drug.

EXAMPLE

Order: heparin 2500 units subQ
Available: heparin 10,000 Units/ml in multiple-dose vial (10 ml)

Basic Formula:
$$\frac{D}{H} \times V = \frac{2500 \text{ units}}{10000 \text{ units}} \times 1 \text{ ml} = \frac{25}{100} = 0.25 \text{ ml}$$

Ratio-and-Proportion Method:

$$
\begin{array}{ccccccc}
H & : & V & :: & D & : & x \\
10,000 \text{ units} & : & 1 \text{ ml} & :: & 2500 \text{ units} & : & x \text{ ml}
\end{array}
$$

$$10,000x = 2500$$
$$x = \frac{25}{100} = 0.25 \text{ ml}$$

Fractional Equation:
$$\frac{H}{V} = \frac{D}{x} \qquad \frac{10,000 \text{ units}}{1 \text{ ml}} = \frac{2500 \text{ units}}{x \text{ ml}}$$
$$10,000x = 2500$$
$$x = 0.25 \text{ ml}$$
Answer: Heparin 2500 units = 0.25 ml

Dimensional Analysis:
$$ml = \frac{1 \text{ ml}}{10,000 \text{ units} \times} \times \frac{2,500 \text{ units}}{1} = 1/4 \text{ or } 0.25 \text{ ml}$$

PRACTICE
PROBLEM 2

SUBCUTANEOUS INJECTIONS

Use the formula chosen for the calculation of drug dosages from Section 4B. The same formula should be used when calculating oral, subQ, IM, insulin, and IV dosages. Refer to conversion Tables 4A–4 or 4B–1 as needed.

EXAMPLE

1. Order: heparin 7500 units subQ
   Available:

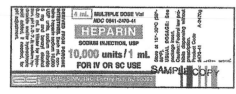

How many milliliters should the client receive? _____

2. Order: atropine sulfate 0.5 mg subQ
   Available:

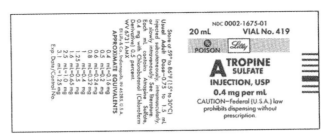

How many milliliters should the client receive? _____
3. Order: epinephrine (Adrenalin) 0.2 mg subQ, STAT
   Available: epinephrine 1 mg/ml (1:1000) in ampule
   What type of syringe should be used? _____

Insulin Injections

Insulin is prescribed and measured in United States Pharmacopeia (USP) units. Most insulins are produced in concentrations of 100 units/ml. Insulin should be administered with an insulin syringe, which is calibrated to correspond with the 100 units of insulin. Insulin bottles and syringes are color-coded to avoid error. The 100 units/ml (or U-100) insulin bottle and the 100 units/ml syringe are coded orange. Administering insulin with a tuberculin syringe *should be avoided*.

Administration of medication requires attention to detail, and insulin is no exception. Insulin is ordered in units. For example, if the prescribed insulin dosage is 30 units, withdraw 30 units from a bottle of 100 units of insulin using a 100-unit calibrated insulin syringe (Figure 4D–12).

Insulin is administered subQ at a 45-, 60-, or 90-degree angle into the subQ tissue. The subQ absorption rate of insulin is slower because there are fewer blood vessels in the fatty tissue than in muscular tissue. The angle for administering insulin depends on the amount of fatty tissue. For an obese person, the angle may be 90 degrees; for a very thin person, the angle may be 45 to 60 degrees.

Types of Insulins

Insulins are clear (regular or crystalline insulin) and cloudy (NPH, Lente) because of the substances protamine and zinc, which are used to prolong the action of insulin in the body. Only clear (regular) insulin can be given IV as well as subQ. The source of insulin is beef, pork, beef-

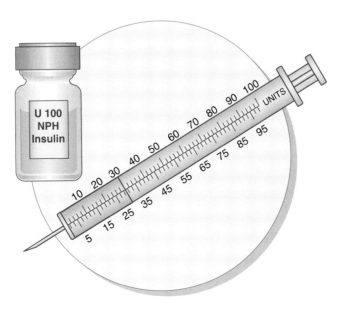

FIGURE 4D–12 Bottle of U 100 insulin and a U 100 calibrated insulin syringe. (From Kee JL, Marshall SM: *Clinical calculations*, ed 5, Philadelphia, 2004, Saunders, p. 159.)

SECTION D

pork, and human (Humulin). Some individuals are allergic to beef insulin, so pork insulin is used because it has biologic properties similar to those of human insulin. Currently, Humulin insulin is more commonly used.

Insulin is categorized as (1) fast-acting (regular and lispro [Humalog]), (2) intermediate-acting (Humulin N, Humulin L, NPH, Lente), and (3) long-acting (Humulin U, Lantus). Commercially premixed combination insulins, Humulin 70/30 and Humulin 50/50, are popular for the client with diabetes who mixes fast-acting and intermediate-acting insulins. Humulin 70/30 and Humalog 75/25 come in prefilled disposable pens. Chapter 50, Antidiabetic Drugs, discusses the various types of insulins and preparations and their peak and duration times. The new long-acting insulin is Lantus, an insulin glargine that is an analogue of human insulin. Lantus is the first long-acting recombinant DNA (rDNA) human insulin for clients with type 1 and type 2 diabetes mellitus. It is usually administered at bedtime; incidence of nocturnal hypoglycemia is not as common with Lantus as with other insulins. It is administered with an insulin pen.

A, Fast-acting insulins.

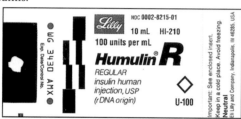
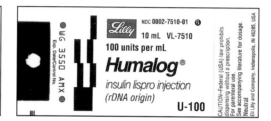

B, Intermediate acting insulins.

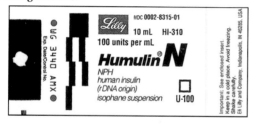
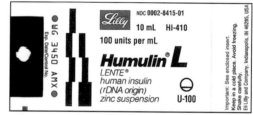

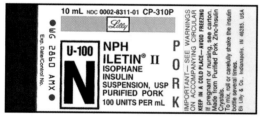
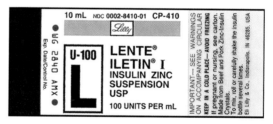

C, Long-acting insulin.

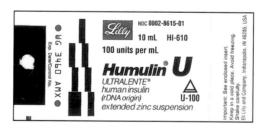

D, Selected combinations of insulins.

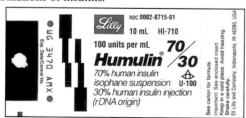
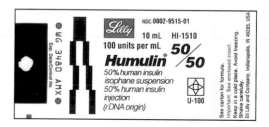

E, Selected insulins for pen injections.

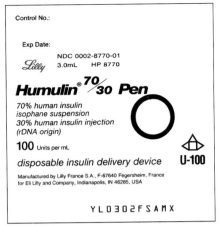
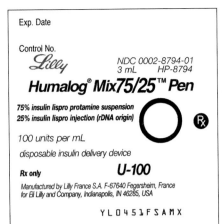

Mixing Insulins

Regular insulin is frequently mixed with insulin containing protamine (NPH) and zinc (Lente). The following is an example of a method for mixing insulin.

EXAMPLE   Order: regular insulin 10 units and NPH insulin 35 units subQ q 7:00 AM
      Available: regular insulin 100 units/ml and NPH insulin 100 units/ml. Insulin syringe: 100 units/ml

Method

1. Clean the rubber tops of the insulin bottles.
2. Draw up 35 units of air and inject into the NPH insulin bottle. Avoid letting the needle contact the NPH insulin solution. Withdraw the needle.
3. Draw up 10 units of air and inject into the regular insulin bottle.
4. First, withdraw 10 units of regular insulin. Regular insulin is always drawn up first.
5. Insert needle into NPH bottle and withdraw 35 units of NPH insulin. The total is 45 units.
6. Administer the two insulins immediately after mixing. Do *not* allow the insulin mixture to stand, because unpredicted physical changes may occur. Unpredicted changes are more common with protamine insulins, such as NPH, than with Lente insulin.

PRACTICE
PROBLEM 3

INSULINS

Indicate on the insulin syringe the amount of insulin that should be withdrawn for each type of insulin.

1. Order: NPH insulin 45 units subQ
   Available: NPH insulin 100 units/ml and insulin syringe 100 units/ml

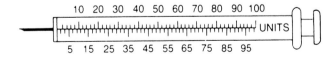

2. Order: regular insulin 15 units and NPH insulin 25 units subQ
   Available: regular insulin 100 units/ml and NPH insulin 100 units/ml, and insulin syringe 100 units/ml

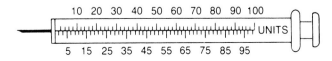

3. Order: regular insulin 6 units and Lente insulin 40 units
    Available: regular insulin 100 units/ml and Lente insulin 100 units/ml, and insulin syringe 100 units/ml

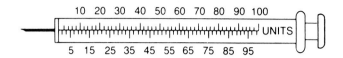

Intramuscular Injections

Muscle has more blood vessels than fatty tissue, so medications given by **intramuscular (IM)** injection are absorbed more rapidly than those given by subQ injection. The volume of solution for an IM injection is 0.5 to 3 ml, with the average being 1 to 2 ml. A volume of drug solution greater than 3 ml causes increased muscle tissue displacement and possible tissue damage. Occasionally 5 ml of selected drugs, such as magnesium sulfate, may be injected into a large muscle, such as the dorso-gluteal. A dose greater than 3 ml is usually divided and given at two different sites.

The needle gauges for IM injections that contain thick solutions are 19 and 20, and 20 and 21 for thin solutions. IM injections are administered at a 90-degree angle. The needle length depends on the amount of adipose (fat) and muscle tissues; the average needle length is 1.5 inches.

The discussion on IM injections is divided into three subsections: (1) drug solutions for injection, (2) powdered drug reconstitution, and (3) mixing injectable drugs. An example is given for each subsection, and practice problems follow.

Sites of IM injections are shown in Chapter 3, Principles of Drug Administration.

Drug Solutions for Injection

Commercially premixed drug solutions are stored in vials and ampules for ready use. The drug label on the container gives the drug dose by weight and its equivalent in milliliters.

EXAMPLE   Order: gentamicin (Garamycin) 50 mg IM
            Available: gentamicin 80 mg/2 ml in a vial

a. BF: $\dfrac{D}{H} \times V = \dfrac{50}{80} \times 2 = \dfrac{100}{80} = 1.25$ ml

b. RP:
$$H \quad : \quad V \quad :: \quad D \quad : \quad x$$
$$80 \text{ mg} \quad : \quad 2 \text{ ml} \quad :: \quad 50 \text{ mg} \quad : \quad x \text{ ml}$$

$$80x = 100$$
$$x = \dfrac{100}{80} = 1.25 \text{ ml}$$

c. FE: $\dfrac{H}{V} = \dfrac{D}{x}$ $\dfrac{80 \text{ mg}}{2 \text{ ml}} = \dfrac{50 \text{ mg}}{x}$
$$80x = 100$$
$$x = 1.25 \text{ ml}$$

d. DA: ml $= \dfrac{2 \text{ ml} \times 50 \text{ mg}}{80 \text{ mg} \times 1} = \dfrac{100}{80} = 1.25$ ml

Powdered Drug Reconstitution

Certain drugs lose their potency in liquid form; therefore manufacturers package these drugs in powdered form. They are reconstituted using a **diluent** (bacteriostatic water or saline) before administration. The drug label or the instructional insert (accompanying pamphlet) frequently gives the type and amount of diluent to use. If the type and amount of diluent are not on the drug label or in the instructional insert, contact the pharmacist.

Usually manufacturers determine the amount of diluent to mix with the drug powder to yield 1 to 2 ml/dose. The powdered drug occupies space; therefore the volume of the drug solution is increased. Once the powdered drug has been reconstituted, the unused drug solution should be dated and initialed on the drug label. Unused drug solutions in vials are refrigerated and may be used for 48 hours to 1 week according to the manufacturer's recommendation. Unused drug solutions in ampules are discarded.

EXAMPLE   Order: cefotetan disodium (Cefotan) 0.5 g IM, q12h
Available (NOTE: Circular states to add 2.6 ml of diluent to yield 3 ml of drug.):

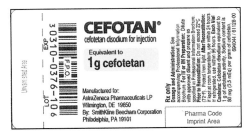

Add 2.6 ml of diluent; 1 g of cefotetan disodium = 3 ml

BF: $\dfrac{D}{H} \times V = \dfrac{0.5}{1} \times 3 \text{ ml} = 1.5 \text{ ml} = 0.5 \text{ g of cefotetan disodium}$

DA: $\text{ml} = \dfrac{3 \text{ ml} \times 0.5 \cancel{g}}{1 \cancel{g} \times 1} = 1.5 \text{ ml}$

No conversion is needed.

Mixing Injectable Drugs

Drugs mixed together in the same syringe must be compatible to prevent precipitation. To determine drug compatibility, check drug reference texts or with a pharmacist. When in doubt about compatibility, do *not* mix drugs.

The three methods used for mixing drugs are (1) mixing two drugs in the same syringe from two vials, (2) mixing two drugs in the same syringe from one vial and one ampule, and (3) mixing two drugs in a prefilled cartridge from a vial.

Method 1: Mixing Two Drugs in the Same Syringe from Two Vials

1. Draw air into the syringe to equal the amount of solution to be withdrawn from the first vial, and inject the air into the first vial. Do *not* allow the needle to come into contact with the solution. Remove the needle.
2. Draw air into the syringe to equal the amount of solution to be withdrawn from the second vial. Invert the second vial, and inject the air. Withdraw the desired amount of solution from the second vial.
3. Change the needle, unless the entire volume in the first vial will be used.
4. Invert the first vial, and withdraw the desired amount of solution.

Method 2: Mixing Two Drugs in the Same Syringe from One Vial and One Ampule

1. Inject air into the vial.
2. Remove the desired amount of solution from the vial.
3. Withdraw the desired amount of solution from the ampule.

Method 3: Mixing Two Drugs in a Prefilled Cartridge from a Vial

1. Check the drug dose and the amount of solution in the prefilled cartridge. If a smaller dose is needed, expel the excess solution.
2. Draw air into the cartridge to equal the amount of solution to be withdrawn from the vial. Invert the vial, and inject the air.
3. Withdraw desired amount of solution from the vial. Be sure that the needle remains in the fluid, and do *not* take more solution than needed.

SECTION D

EXAMPLE
**MIXING DRUGS
IN THE SAME
SYRINGE**

Order: meperidine (Demerol) 25 mg and atropine sulfate 0.4 mg IM
   Available: meperidine in a Tubex cartridge labeled 50 mg/ml
   Atropine sulfate in a multidose vial labeled 0.4 mg/ml
   How many milliliters of each drug should be given, and how are they mixed? _____

1. Meperidine dose

a. $\dfrac{D}{H} \times V = \dfrac{25}{50} \times 1 = \dfrac{25}{50} = 0.5$ ml

b.
$$H \quad : \quad V \quad :: \quad D \quad : \quad x$$
$$50\ mg \quad : \quad 1\ ml \quad :: \quad 25\ mg \quad : \quad x\ ml$$

$$50x = 25$$
$$x = \dfrac{1}{2} = 0.5\ ml$$

2. Atropine dose:
   The label indicates 0.4 mg = 1 ml

Answer: Give meperidine 0.5 ml and atropine 1 ml.

Procedure

Mix two drugs in the cartridge with one drug from a vial and the other drug in the prefilled cartridge.
1. Check the drug dose and volume on the prefilled cartridge.
2. Expel 0.5 ml and any excess drug solution (meperidine) from the cartridge (0.5 ml remains in the cartridge). Have another nurse witness the waste of a narcotic.
3. Draw 1 ml of air into the cartridge, and inject the air into the vial that contains the atropine.
4. Withdraw 1 ml of atropine from the vial into the meperidine solution in the cartridge.

**PRACTICE
PROBLEM 4**

INTRAMUSCULAR INJECTIONS

1. Order: cefazolin (Ancef) 500 mg IM, q6h
   Available:

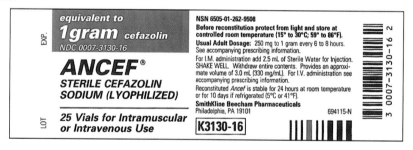

   How many milliliters should be given? _____
2. Order: atropine sulfate 0.3 mg IM, STAT
   Available: atropine sulfate

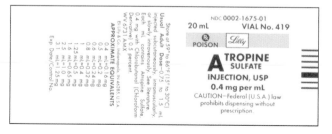

   How many milliliters (ml) of atropine should be given? _____

SECTION D

3. Order: oxacillin 250 mg IM q6h
   Available: (Drug label states to add 2.7 ml of diluent = 3 ml of drug solution)

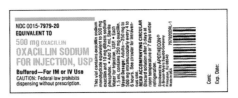

How many milliliters should be given? ____ After the drug is reconstituted, how long can it be refrigerated? ____

4. Order: digoxin 0.25 mg IM q.d.
   Available: digoxin 0.5 mg/2 ml

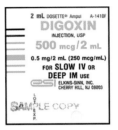

How many milliliters should be given? ____What should be done with the excess digoxin solution? ____ (Usually parenteral digoxin is administered IV.)

5. Order: chlorpromazine (Thorazine) 50 mg IM, STAT
   Available:

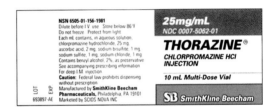

How many milliliters should be given? ____ Can the vial be used again? ____

6. Order: meperidine 60 mg and hydroxyzine (Vistaril) 25 mg, IM. These two drugs are compatible.
   Available: Hydroxyzine 100 mg/2 ml in vial

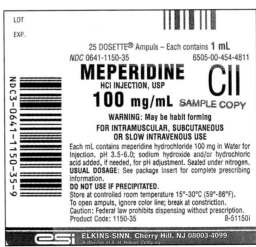

How many milliliters of meperidine and how many of hydroxyzine should be given? ____

Explain how the two drugs would be mixed.

7. Order: morphine SO$_4$ 6 mg IM q4h, PRN
   Available:

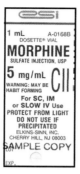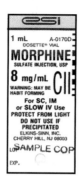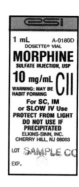

a. Which morphine vial should be selected? _____
   Explain _____
b. How many milliliters of morphine should be administered per dose? _____
   Explain _____

8. Order: ampicillin 250 mg q6h IM
   Available:

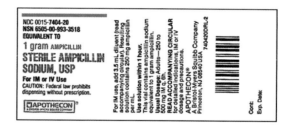

a. How many milliliters of diluent should be added to the ampicillin vial? _____
b. How many milliliters of ampicillin should the client receive per dose? _____
c. How many milligrams should the client receive per day? _____

Additional Dimensional Analysis (Refer to Section 4B as needed.)

9. Order: tobramycin 60 mg IM q8h. The adult client weighs 180 pounds.
   Dose parameter: 3 mg/kg/day in three divided doses
   Available:

1 box • 25 vials • 2 mL   NDC 0003-2725-10

Equivalent to 80 mg TOBRAMYCIN/2 mL (40 mg/mL)
TOBRAMYCIN
Sulfate Injection USP
For INTRAMUSCULAR or INTRAVENOUS use
Must dilute for IV use

□APOTHECON®
A BRISTOL-MYERS SQUIBB COMPANY

TOBRAMYCIN Sulfate Injection USP
Each mL contains 40 mg tobramycin (as sulfate), 0.1 mg edetate disodium, 3.2 mg sodium metabisulfite, and 5 mg phenol, as a preservative, in Water for Injection. pH 3.0-6.5; sulfuric acid and, if necessary, sodium hydroxide have been added for pH adjustment. Sealed under nitrogen.
Usual Dosage: Read accompanying package insert for dosage and IV dilution.
Store at controlled room temperature 15°-30° C (59°-86° F).
Caution: Federal law prohibits dispensing without prescription.

APOTHECON®
A Bristol-Myers Squibb Co.
Princeton, NJ 08540
Made in USA   C1640 / P2510

Factors: 80 mg = 2 ml (drug label)
Conversion factor: none (both are in milligrams)
a. How many kilograms does the client weigh? _____
b. How many milligrams should the client receive per day? _____
c. Is the drug dose within safe parameter? _____
d. How many milliliters should the client receive per dose? _____

10. Order: Cefobid 500 mg IM, q12h

   Available (NOTE: Instructions state to add 1.6 ml of diluent to the vial; drug liquids in 1 g = 2 ml.):

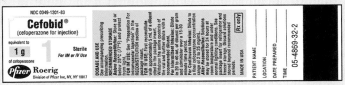

   Factors: 1 g = 2 ml (drug label and after reconstitution)

   Conversion factor: 1000 mg = 1 g

   How many milliliters should the client receive per dose? _____

11. Order: meperidine (Demerol) 35 mg and promethazine (Phenergan) 10 mg, IM.

   Drugs available: meperidine 50 mg/ml in an ampule; promethazine 25 mg/ml in an ampule.

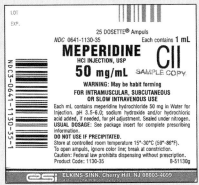

   a. How many milliliters of meperidine would you give? _____

   b. How many milliliters of promethazine would you give? _____

   c. Explain how the two drugs would be mixed.

   _____

ANSWERS TO PRACTICE PROBLEMS

1   SYRINGES AND NEEDLES

1. 5-ml syringe
2. Tuberculin syringe (1 ml)
3. No, it should be discarded in the sink or toilet and witnessed by another RN or LPN, according to policy.

4. 21-gauge needle
5. 25-gauge needle
6. 20-gauge needle 1.5 ($1\frac{1}{2}$) inches in length

2   SUBCUTANEOUS INJECTIONS

1. 0.75 ml
2. The drug label reads: 1.25 ml = 0.5 mg of atropine. Also, under the word *"atropine,"* it reads 0.4 mg/ml

   a. BF: $\dfrac{D}{H} \times V = \dfrac{0.5}{0.4} \times 1 = 1.25$ ml

b. RP: $H \ : \ V \ :: \ D \ : \ x$

   0.4 mg $: 1$ ml $:: 0.5$ mg $: x$ ml

   $0.4x = 0.5$

   $x = \dfrac{0.5}{0.4} = 1.25$ ml

c. DA: ml $= \dfrac{1 \text{ ml} \ \times 0.5 \ \cancel{mg}}{0.4 \ \cancel{mg} \times \quad 1} = 1.25$ ml

   Answer: atropine sulfate 0.5 mg = 1.25 ml

3. A tuberculin syringe should be used.

a. $\dfrac{D}{H} \times V = \dfrac{0.2}{1.0} \times 1 = 1.0\overset{0.2}{\sqrt{0.20}} = 0.2$ ml

b. $\begin{array}{ccccccc} H & : & V & :: & D & : & x \\ 1.0\text{ mg} & : & 1\text{ ml} & :: & 0.2\text{ mg} & : & x\text{ ml} \end{array}$

$1.0x = 0.2$

$x = \dfrac{0.2}{1.0} = 0.2$ ml

Answer: epinephrine 0.2 mg = 0.2 ml

---

3   INSULINS

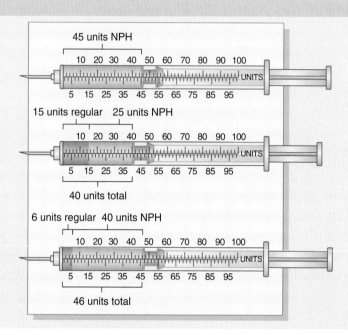

45 units NPH

10 20 30 40 50 60 70 80 90 100 UNITS
5 15 25 35 45 55 65 75 85 95

15 units regular   25 units NPH

10 20 30 40 50 60 70 80 90 100 UNITS
5 15 25 35 45 55 65 75 85 95

40 units total

6 units regular 40 units NPH

10 20 30 40 50 60 70 80 90 100 UNITS
5 15 25 35 45 55 65 75 85 95

46 units total

SECTION D

4   INTRAMUSCULAR INJECTIONS USING BASIC FORMULA, RATIO AND PROPORTION, FRACTIONAL EQUATION, OR DIMENSIONAL ANALYSIS

1. Instructions on the drug label read: add 2.5 ml of sterile water. The drug solution equals 3.0 ml (drug powder is equal to 0.5 ml).
Change 1 g to mg. 1 g = 1000 mg *or*
Change 500 mg to g. 500 mg = 0.500 g (0.5 g)

a. BF: $\dfrac{D}{H} \times V = \dfrac{0.5}{1\text{ g}} \times 3$ ml = 1.5 ml

b. RP: $\begin{array}{ccccccc} H & : & V & :: & D & : & x \\ 1000\text{ mg} & : & 3\text{ ml} & :: & 500\text{ mg} & : & x\text{ ml} \end{array}$
$\quad\quad\quad\quad 1000x = 1500$
$\quad\quad\quad\quad\quad\quad x = 1.5$ ml

c. DA: $\text{ml} = \dfrac{3\text{ ml} \times \quad 1\,\cancel{g} \quad \times \overset{1}{\cancel{500}}\text{ mg}}{1\,\cancel{g} \times \underset{2}{\cancel{1000}}\text{ mg} \times \quad 1} = \dfrac{3}{2}$

$\quad\quad\quad = 1.5$ ml

Answer: cefazolin 500 mg = 1.5 ml

2. The atropine drug label is marked as 0.4 mg/ml. The approximate equivalent of 0.3 mg is 0.8 ml as marked on the label. If the 0.3 mg = 0.8 ml is unknown, the problem may be calculated using 0.4 mg = 1 ml.

BF: $\dfrac{D}{H} \times V = \dfrac{0.3}{0.4} \times 1 = \dfrac{0.3}{0.4} = 0.75$, or 0.8 ml

3. For oxacillin sodium, the drug label indicates that 2.7 ml of sterile water should be added to the vial containing 500 mg of drug. The total volume would be 3.0 ml.

a. BF: $\dfrac{D}{H} \times V = \dfrac{250}{500} \times 3.0 = \dfrac{750}{500} = 1.5$ ml

b. FE: $\dfrac{H}{V} = \dfrac{D}{x} \quad \dfrac{500\text{ mg}}{3\text{ ml}} = \dfrac{250\text{ mg}}{x\text{ ml}}$

$\quad\quad\quad\quad 500\,x = 750$
$\quad\quad\quad\quad\quad\quad x = 1.5$ ml

c. DA: $\text{ml} = \dfrac{3\text{ ml} \times \overset{1}{\cancel{250}}\text{ mg}}{\underset{2}{\cancel{500}}\text{ mg} \times \quad 1} = 1.5$ ml

No conversion is needed.

Answer: Oxacillin 250 mg = 1.5 ml. It can be refrigerated for 96 h after it has been reconstituted.

4. BF: $\dfrac{D}{H} \times V = \dfrac{0.25}{0.50} \times 2 = \dfrac{0.50}{0.50} = 1$ ml

Withdraw 1 ml from the ampule. Discard the remaining 1 ml of digoxin solution.

5. Thorazine 50 mg = 2 ml. Yes, the vial can be used for multiple doses.

6. Meperidine 60 mg = 0.6 ml; hydroxyzine 25 mg = 0.5 ml

Meperidine

BF: $\dfrac{D}{H} \times V = \dfrac{60}{100} \times 1 = \dfrac{60}{100} = 0.6$ ml

Hydroxyzine

BF: $\dfrac{D}{H} \times V = \dfrac{25}{100} \times 2 = \dfrac{50}{100} = 0.5$ ml

PROCEDURE

a. Withdraw 0.5 ml of hydroxyzine from the vial.

b. Meperidine is in a dosette ampule. Withdraw 0.6 ml of meperidine solution into the syringe containing hydroxyzine.

c. Total amount of the two drug solutions is 1.1 ml. Administer IM.

7. a. Morphine vials 8 mg/ml and 10 mg/ml. Morphine 5 mg/ml vial could not be used because it is a single-vial dose.

b. *Morphine 8 mg/ml*

BF: $\dfrac{D}{H} \times V = \dfrac{6\ \text{mg}}{8\ \text{mg}} \times 1\ \text{ml} = \dfrac{6}{8} = 0.75$ ml

Morphine 10 mg/ml

BF: $\dfrac{D}{H} \times V = \dfrac{6\ \text{mg}}{10\ \text{mg}} \times 1\ \text{ml} = \dfrac{6}{10} = 0.6$ ml

8. a. 3.5 ml of diluent (3.5 ml diluent + 0.5 ml of powdered drug = 4 ml of 1 g of ampicillin)

b. 1 ml = 250 mg (1 g or 1000 mg = 4 ml)

c. 250 mg × 4 (q6h) = 1000 mg or 1 g/day

9. a. The client weighs 180 pounds, or 81.8 kg.

b. 245.4 mg per day

c. The dose if safe, 180 mg per day, which is below the dose parameter for the client's weight.

d. 1.5 ml per dose

DA: $\text{ml} = \dfrac{2\ \text{ml} \times \overset{3}{\cancel{60}}\ \cancel{\text{mg}}}{\underset{4}{\cancel{80}}\ \cancel{\text{mg}} \times 1} = \dfrac{6}{4} = 1.5$ ml

10. 1 ml per dose

DA: $\text{ml} = \dfrac{2\ \text{ml} \times 1\ \cancel{g} \times \overset{1}{\cancel{500}}\ \cancel{\text{mg}}}{1\ \cancel{g} \times \underset{2}{\cancel{1000}}\ \cancel{\text{mg}} \times 1} = \dfrac{2}{2} = 1$ ml

11. a. *meperidine:*

DA: $\text{ml} = \dfrac{1\ \text{ml} \times \overset{7}{\cancel{35}}\ \cancel{\text{mg}}}{\underset{10}{\cancel{50}}\ \cancel{\text{mg}} \times 1} = \dfrac{7}{10} = 0.7$ ml

b. *promethazine*

DA: $\text{ml} = \dfrac{1\ \text{ml} \times \overset{2}{\cancel{10}}\ \text{mg}}{\underset{5}{\cancel{25}}\ \text{mg} \times 1} = \dfrac{2}{5} = 0.4$ ml

c. Procedure: 1. Obtain 0.7 ml of meperidine from the ampule and 0.4 ml of promethazine from the ampule.

2. Discard the remaining solutions within the ampules.

Section 4E CALCULATIONS OF INTRAVENOUS FLUIDS

OUTLINE

Objectives

Terms

Introduction

Continuous Intravenous Administration
Intravenous Sets
Calculating Intravenous Flow Rate
Mixing Drugs for Continuous Intravenous Administration

Intermittent Intravenous Administration

Secondary Intravenous Sets Without IV Pumps

Intermittent Infusion Adapters/Devices

SASH Procedure

Direct Intravenous Injections

Electronic Intravenous Regulators

Patient-Controlled Analgesia
Client Teaching

Calculating Flow Rates for Intravenous Drugs

SECTION E

OBJECTIVES

- Describe the differences between continuous intravenous infusion and intermittent intravenous infusion.
- Define macrodrip and microdrip sets, keep vein open (KVO), and to keep open (TKO).
- Calculate intravenous flow rate using one of the given formulas.
- Explain how intravenous drug solutions administered by secondary set are calculated.
- Differentiate between volumetric and nonvolumetric intravenous regulators and pump electronic regulators.

TERMS

bolus
drop factor
electronic intravenous (IV)
    regulators
IV piggyback (IVPB)
keep vein open (KVO)

macrodrip set
microdrip (minidrip) set
nonvolumetric regulator
patient-controlled analgesia
    (PCA)
primary IV line set

SASH procedure
secondary IV line set
to keep open (TKO)
volumetric regulator

Introduction

Intravenous (IV) fluid therapy is used to administer fluids that contain water, dextrose, vitamins, electrolytes, and drugs. Today an increasing number of drugs are administered by the IV route for direct absorption and fast action. Some drugs are given by IV push **(bolus).** Many drugs administered IV irritate the veins, so these drugs are diluted in 50 to 100 ml of fluid. Other drugs are delivered in a large volume of fluid over a specific period, such as 4 to 8 hours.

Two methods are used to administer IV fluids and drugs: continuous IV infusion and intermittent IV infusion. Continuous IV infusion replaces fluid loss, maintains fluid balance, and serves as a vehicle for drug administration. Intermittent IV infusion is used primarily to give IV drugs.

Nurses have an important role in the preparation and administration of IV solutions and IV drugs. The nursing functions and responsibilities during drug preparation include the following:

- Knowing IV sets and their drop factors
- Calculating IV flow rates
- Mixing and diluting drugs in IV fluids
- Gathering equipment
- Knowing the drugs and the expected and untoward reactions

Nursing responsibilities continue with assessment of the client for effectiveness and untoward effects of the therapy and assessment of the IV site.

Continuous Intravenous Administration

When IV solutions are required, the health care provider orders the type and amount of IV solution in liters over a 24-hour period or in milliliters per hour. The nurse calculates the IV flow rate according to the drop factor, the amount of fluids to be administered, and the time period.

Intravenous Sets

Various IV infusion sets are marketed by Abbott, Cutter, McGaw, and Travenol. The **drop factor,** the number of drops per milliliter, is normally printed on the packaging cover of the IV set. A set that delivers large drops per milliliter (10 to 20 gtt/ml) is called a **macrodrip set,** and one with small drops per milliliter (60 gtt/ml) is called a **microdrip (minidrip) set.** Examples of drop factors, macrodrip sets, and microdrip sets are listed in Table 4E–1.

In most instances, the nurse has the choice of using either the macrodrip or microdrip set. If the IV rate is to infuse at 100 ml/hour or more, the macrodrip set is usually used. If the infu-

Table 4E–1

Intravenous Sets

Manufacturer	Drops (gtt/ml)
Macrodrip Sets	
Abbott	15
Cutter	20
McGaw	15
Travenol	10
Microdrip Sets	
Travenol	60
Minidrip sets	60

sion rate is less than (<) 100 ml/hour or the client is a child, the microdrip set is preferred. Slow drip rates of <100 ml/hour make macrodrip adjustment difficult.

At times, IV fluids are given at a slow rate to **keep vein open (KVO)**, also called **to keep open (TKO).** The reasons for ordering KVO include a suspected or potential emergency situation for rapid administration of fluids and drugs and the need for an open line to give IV drugs at specified hours. For KVO, a microdrip set (60 gtt/ml) and a 250-ml IV bag may be used. KVO is usually regulated to deliver 10 ml/hour.

Calculating Intravenous Flow Rate

Three different methods may be used to calculate IV flow rate (drops per minute, gtt/min). The nurse should select one method, memorize it, and consistently use it to calculate IV flow rate. Method II is usually the preferred method.

Method I: Three-Step

1. $\dfrac{\text{Amount of solution}}{\text{Hours to administer}} = \text{milliliters/hour (ml/h)}$

2. $\dfrac{\text{Milliliters per hour}}{60 \text{ minutes}} = \text{milliliters/minute (ml/min)}$

3. Milliliters per minute × drops per milliliter of IV set = drops/minute (gtt/min)

Method II: Two-Step

1. $\dfrac{\text{Amount of fluid}}{\text{Hours to administer}} = \text{milliliters/hour (ml/h)}$

2. $\dfrac{\text{Milliliters per hour} \times \text{Drops per milliliter (IV set)}}{60 \text{ minutes}} = \text{drops/minute (gtt/min)}$

If the milliliters per hour is known, then use Step 2 to determine the drops per minute.

Method III: One-Step

1. $\dfrac{\text{Amount of fluid} \times \text{Drops per milliliter (IV set)}}{\text{Hours to administer} \times \text{Minutes per hour (60)}} = \text{drops/minute (gtt/min)}$

Mixing Drugs for Continuous Intravenous Administration

Drugs such as potassium chloride and vitamins are frequently added to the IV solution bag for continuous IV infusion. Drugs should be added to the bag or bottle immediately before administering the IV fluid. Inject the drug into the rubber stopper on the IV bag or bottle and rotate the bag several times to ensure that the drug is dispersed throughout the solution (Figure 4E–1). *Do not add the drug while the infusion is running unless the bag is rotated.* A drug solution injected into an upright infusing IV solution concentrates the drug into the lower portion of the IV bag, preventing it from dispersing evenly. The client receives a concentrated drug solution, which may be harmful, for example, if the drug is potassium chloride. If

SECTION E

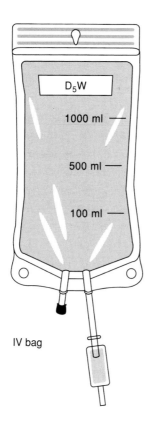

D_5W

1000 ml —

500 ml —

100 ml —

IV bag

FIGURE 4E–1 Intravenous bag. (From Kee JL, Marshall SM: *Clinical calculations*, ed 5, Philadelphia, 2004, Saunders, p. 201.)

Table 4E–2

Abbreviations of Solutions

Intravenous Solutions	Abbreviations
5% Dextrose in water	D_5W, 5% D/W
10% Dextrose in water	$D_{10}W$, 10% D/W
0.9% Sodium chloride, normal saline solution	0.9% NaCl, NSS
0.45% Sodium chloride, ½ normal saline solution	0.45% NaCl, ½ NSS
5% Dextrose in 0.9% sodium chloride	D_5NSS, 5% D/NSS, 5% D/0.9% NaCl
5% Dextrose in 0.45% sodium chloride or 5% Dextrose in ½ normal saline solution	D_5/ ½ NSS, 5% D/½ NSS
Lactated Ringer's solution	LR

drugs are injected into the IV bag before use, the bag should be refrigerated to maintain drug potency.

There are various nutrients (e.g., dextrose) and electrolytes in commercially prepared IV solutions. The commonly used solutions are 5% dextrose in water (D_5W), normal saline (NSS), one-half normal saline (½ NSS), and lactated Ringer's (LR). Abbreviations for these types of solutions are listed in Table 4E–2.

EXAMPLE

Order: 1000 ml of 5% dextrose in water (D_5W) with potassium chloride (KCl) 20 mEq in 8 h

Available: 1000 ml of 5% dextrose in water

Potassium chloride 40 mEq/20 ml ampule

IV set labeled 10 gtt/ml

Drug calculation: Use the basic formula, the ratio-and-proportion method, fractional equation, or dimensional analysis (refer to Section 4B if needed).

a. BF: $\dfrac{D}{H} \times V = \dfrac{20}{40} \times 20 = \dfrac{400}{40} = 10$ ml of KCl

b. RP:

$$H \quad : \quad V \quad :: \quad D \quad : \quad x$$
$$40 \text{ mEq} \quad : \quad 20 \text{ ml} \quad :: \quad 20 \text{ mEq} \quad : \quad x \text{ ml}$$

$$40x = 400$$
$$x = 10 \text{ ml of KCl}$$

c. DA: $\text{ml} = \dfrac{20 \text{ ml} \times \overset{1}{\cancel{20}} \text{ mEq}}{\underset{2}{\cancel{40}} \text{ mEq} \times 1} = 10$ ml of KCL

The calculation of IV flow rate is described using the three methods outlined previously. However, it is strongly recommended that only one method be selected to determine IV flow rate.

Method I

1. $\dfrac{1000 \text{ ml}}{8\text{h}} = 125$ ml/h

2. $\dfrac{125 \text{ ml}}{60 \text{ min}} = 2.0\text{–}2.1$ ml/min

3. $2.1 \times 10 = 21$ gtt/min

Method II

1. $1000 \div 8 = 125$ ml/h

2. $\dfrac{125 \text{ ml/h} \times \overset{1}{\cancel{10}} \text{ gtt/ml}}{\underset{6}{\cancel{60}} \text{ min}} = \dfrac{125}{6} = 20\text{–}21$ gtt/min

Method III

1. $\dfrac{1000 \text{ ml} \times \overset{1}{\cancel{10}} \text{ gtt/ml}}{8 \text{ h} \times \underset{6}{\cancel{60}} \text{ min}} = \dfrac{1000}{48} = 20$ or 21 gtt/min

PRACTICE PROBLEM 1

CONTINUOUS INTRAVENOUS FLOW RATES

Select one of the three methods to calculate IV flow rate.
1. Order: 1000 ml of D$_5$/$^1/_2$ NSS to infuse over 12 h
   Available: macrodrip set with 10 gtt/ml and a microdrip set with 60 gtt/ml
   a. Should a macrodrip or microdrip IV set be used? _____
   b. Calculate the IV flow rate in drops per minute according to the IV set that was selected. _____

2. Order: 3 L of IV solutions to infuse over 24 h
   1 liter of D$_5$W and 2 liters of D$_5$/$^1/_2$ NSS
   a. One liter is equal to how many milliliters? _____
   b. Each liter should infuse for how many hours? _____
   c. The institution uses a set with a drop factor of 15 gtt/ml. How many drops per minute should the client receive? _____

3. Order: 250 ml of D$_5$W to KVO
   a. What type of IV set should be used? _____
   b. Determine how many drops per minute the client should receive. _____

4. Order: 1000 ml of D$_5$/$^1/_2$ NSS, 1 vial of multiple vitamin (MVI), and 10 mEq of KCl (potassium chloride) in 10 h
   Available: 1000 ml of D$_5$/$^1/_2$ NSS
   Macrodrip set: 15 gtt/ml; microdrip set: 60 gtt/ml
   MVI: 5 ml vial
   KCl: 20 mEq/20 ml vial
   a. How many milliliters of KCl should be injected into the IV bag? _____
   b. How many drops per minute should the client receive using the macrodrip set and microdrip set? _____

Intermittent Intravenous Administration

Some IV drugs are prescribed to be administered three to six times a day in a small volume of IV fluid (50 to 100 ml of D_5W or NSS 0.9% sodium chloride). The drug solution is usually infused over a period of 15 minutes to 1 hour. Separate tubing for IV drugs, the **secondary IV line set,** is inserted into a port (rubber stopper) of the IV connector on the continuous, or **primary IV line set.** This type of IV administration is called *intermittent IV therapy.*

Secondary Intravenous Sets Without IV Pumps

Two IV sets available to administer IV drugs are (1) the calibrated cylinder (chamber) with tubing, such as the Buretrol, Volutrol, and Soluset; and (2) the secondary IV set, which is similar to a regular IV set except the tubing is shorter (Figure 4E–2). The secondary IV line set is used mostly to infuse small volumes—50, 100, 250 ml and for children's IV solution. The chamber of the Buretrol, Volutrol, and Soluset holds 150 ml of solution. Medication is injected into the chamber and then diluted with solution. These methods of administering IV drugs are referred to as **IV piggyback (IVPB).**

Drugs for IV infusion are diluted before infusion. Clinical agencies frequently have their own protocols for dilutions; the pharmacist and the drug circular are also resources for infusion guidelines. Guidelines and protocols help to prevent drug and fluid incompatibility.

When using the Buretrol, 15 to 20 ml of IV solution should be added to flush the drug out of the IV line once the infusion is completed.

Intermittent Infusion Adapters/Devices

When continuous IV fluid infusion is to be discontinued and intermittent drug therapy is to begin, an adapter is attached to the IV catheter or needle where the IV tubing was disconnected. Adapters have ports (stoppers) where needles, needleless, or IV tubing can be inserted as needed to continue drug therapy. The use of adapters increases the client's mobility by not hav-

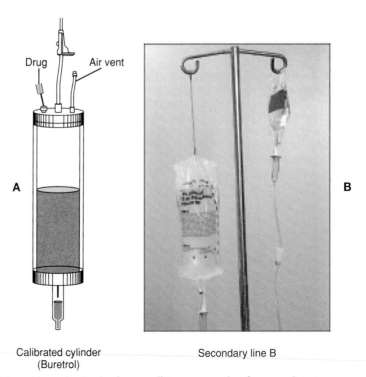

FIGURE 4E–2   A, The calibrated cylinder (Buretrol) is an example of a secondary intravenous (IV) device. **B,** An example of a secondary line containing medication. The primary IV bag is 6 inches below the secondary IV bag. **(A,** From Kee JL, Marshall SM: *Clinical calculations,* ed 5, Philadelphia, 2004, Saunders. **B,** From Leahy JM, Kizilay PE: *Foundations of nursing practice: a nursing process approach,* Philadelphia, 1998, Saunders.)

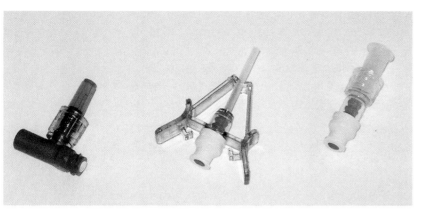
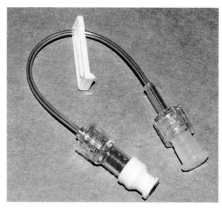

FIGURE 4E–3   Needleless infusion devices. Medication in a needleless syringe can be inserted into a needleless infusion device. (From Kee JL, Marshall SM: *Clinical calculations,* ed 5, Philadelphia, 2004, Saunders, p. 194.)

ing an IV line "tagging along" and is cost-effective because less IV tubing, solution, and equipment are needed. See Figure 4E–3 for examples of needleless infusion devices.

SASH Procedure

The adapter may have short tubing, which is called the *heparin lock.* IV catheters and needles with adapters are kept free of blood clots by administering low doses of heparin or saline after each drug infusion. In some institutions, this is known as the **SASH procedure.** SASH stands for the following:

S = Solution (saline) flush (2 ml)
A = Administer drug into rubber stopper
S = Solution (saline) flush (2 ml)
H = Heparin 1 : 100 solution (1 ml) (NOTE: may or may not be used.)

Before any drug is given, the IV tubing and adapter are flushed with 2 ml of saline solution to clear the line of heparin solution and to assess for IV patency. After the drug is administered, a 2-ml saline flush is given, followed by a low dose of heparin. In Figure 4E–4, the nurse is using the SASH procedure.

Direct Intravenous Injections

Medications that are given by the IV injection route are calculated in the same manner as medications for intramuscular (IM) injection. This route is often referred to as *IV push.* Clinically, it is the preferred route for clients with poor muscle mass or decreased circulation or for a drug that is poorly absorbed from the tissues. Medications administered by this route have a rapid onset of action, and calculation errors can have serious, even fatal, consequences. Drug information inserts must be read carefully, and attention must be given to the amount of drug that

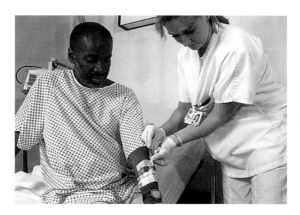

FIGURE 4E–4   To clear the line, the nurse performs the SASH procedure. (From Leahy JM, Kizilay PE: *Foundations of nursing practice: a nursing process approach,* Philadelphia, 1998, Saunders.)

can be given per minute. If the drug is pushed into the bloodstream at a faster rate than specified in the drug literature, adverse reactions to the medication are likely to occur.

EXAMPLE   Order: Lasix 80 mg, IV, STAT.
      Drug available: Lasix 10 mg/ml. IV infusion not to exceed 40 mg/min.
a. RP: H : V :: D : x
     10 mg : 1 ml :: 80 mg : x
         $10x = 80$
           $x = 8$ ml of Lasix

or

DA: ml $= \dfrac{1 \text{ ml} \times \overset{8}{\cancel{80}} \text{ mg}}{\underset{1}{\cancel{10}} \text{ mg} \times 1} = 8$ ml of Lasix

b. known drug : known minutes :: desired drug : desired minutes
    40 mg   :   1 min   ::   80 mg   : x
                    $40x = 80$
                     $x = 2$ min

Electronic Intravenous Regulators

Pumps are **electronic intravenous (IV) regulators** used in hospitals and some community settings. The electronic IV regulators are set to deliver a prescribed rate of IV solution. If the flow rate is obstructed, an alarm sounds.

IV pumps deliver IV solution against resistance. The flow rate is set in milliliters per hour. Pumps do not recognize infiltration. The alarm does not sound until the pump has exerted its maximum pressure to overcome resistance.

IV pumps are recommended for use with all central lines, such as femoral and subclavian sites, and peripheral lines. Ongoing nursing assessment is essential when using electronic IV regulators.

There are two types of flow control for electronic IV regulators: volumetric and nonvolumetric regulators. A **volumetric regulator** delivers a specific volume of fluid at a specific rate, in milliliters per hour. A **nonvolumetric regulator** is designed to infuse at a drop rate in drops per minute. To determine whether the machine is volumetric or nonvolumetric, check to see whether the panel display is calibrated for ml/hour or gtt/minute. Figure 4E–5 shows double pump regulator. There are various electronic IV regulators for the administration of IV fluids and drugs (Figure 4E–6).

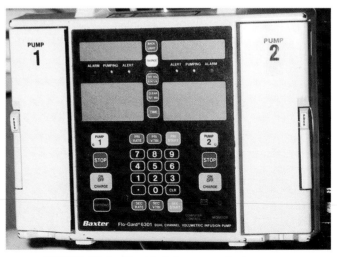

FIGURE 4E–5   Double intravenous Baxter pump.

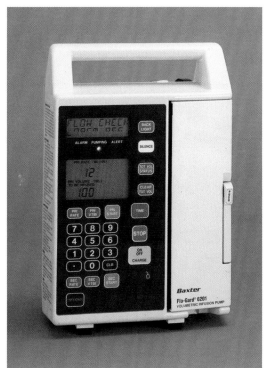 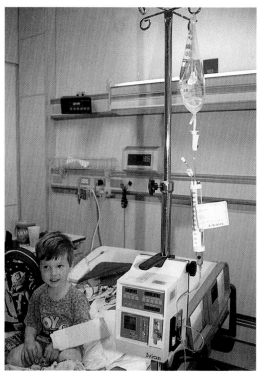

FIGURE 4E–6 **A,** Flo-Gard volumetric infusion pump. (Courtesy Baxter Healthcare Corp., Deerfield, Ill.) **B,** Buretrol with an electronic IV regulator for IV drug administration. (From Bowden VR, Dickey SB, Greenberg CS: *Children and their families: a continuum of care,* Philadelphia, 1998, Saunders.)

Patient-Controlled Analgesia

Patient-controlled analgesia (PCA) is another method used to administer drugs IV. The objective of PCA is to provide a uniform serum concentration of drug(s), thus avoiding drug peaks and valleys. This method is designed to meet the needs of clients who require at least 24 to 48 hours of regular IM narcotic injections.

Several reasons for the use of PCA include (1) effective pain control without the client feeling over-sedated, (2) considerable reduction in the amount of narcotic used (approximately one-half that of IM delivery), and (3) clients' feelings of having greater control over their pain.

There are choices available in the delivery of PCA. The pump is programmed to administer the prescribed medication (1) at client demand, (2) continuously, and (3) continuously and supplemented by client demand. Figure 4E–7 shows examples of PCA infusion pumps.

The health care provider's order must include the following:
- Drug ordered
- Loading dose: administered by the health care provider to obtain baseline serum concentration of analgesic
- PCA dose: amount to be administered each time client activates the button
- Lockout interval: time during which PCA cannot be administered
- Dose limit: the maximum amount the client can receive during a specified time

Client Teaching
- Inform the client that the pain should be tolerable, not necessarily absent.
- Advise the client of the pump's safety features, including the alarms.
- Instruct the client in the use of the control button (medication administered when button is *released*).
- Instruct the client to report any side effects or adverse reactions to the medication.
- Have naloxone (Narcan) easily accessible.

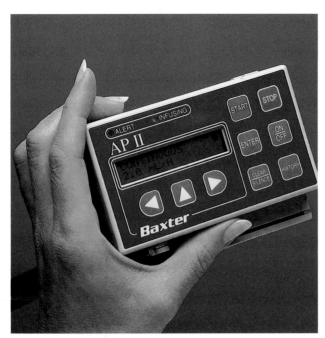

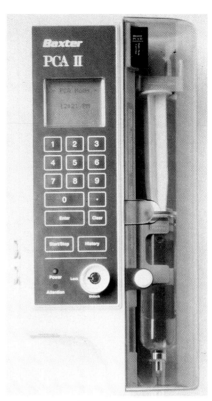

FIGURE 4E–7 Two examples of patient-controlled analgesic (PCA) infusion pumps. (From Monahan FD, Neighbors M: *Medical-surgical nursing,* ed 2, Philadelphia, 1998, Saunders, p. 152. Courtesy Baxter Healthcare Corp., Deerfield, Ill.)

Calculating Flow Rates For Intravenous Drugs

IV drug infusion rates depend on the drug dosing instructions, which indicate the amount of solution for dilution, and the length of infusion time. The nurse must first calculate the drug dose from the health care provider's order, then calculate the flow rate.

1. *Secondary Sets:* To find drops per minute for IV drugs, use calibrated cylinders (Buretrol, Volutrol), 50- to 250-ml bag (Add-A-Line), or any nonvolumetric regulator.

$$\frac{\text{Amount of solution} \times \text{Drops per milliliter of the set}}{\text{Minutes to administer}} = \text{Drops/minute (gtt/min)}$$

2. *Volumetric Regulators:* To find milliliters per hour

$$\text{Amount of solution} \div \frac{\text{Minutes to administer}}{60 \text{ minutes/hour}} = \text{Milliliters/hour (ml/h)}$$

Problems for calculating IV drug dosage and IV flow rate in drops per minute and in milliliters per hour are given below.

EXAMPLE   Order: ceftazidime (Fortaz) 1.5 g IV q6h
Available:

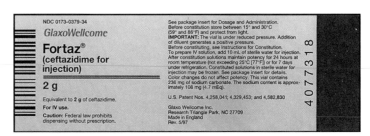

NDC 0173-0379-34

GlaxoWellcome

Fortaz®
(ceftazidime for
injection)

2 g

Equivalent to **2 g** of ceftazidime.

For IV use.

Caution: Federal law prohibits dispensing without prescription.

See package insert for Dosage and Administration.
Before constitution store between 15° and 30°C (59° and 86°F) and protect from light.
IMPORTANT: The vial is under reduced pressure. Addition of diluent generates a positive pressure.
Before constituting, see Instructions for Constitution.
To prepare IV solution, add 10 mL of sterile water for injection. After constitution solutions maintain potency for 24 hours at room temperature (not exceeding 25°C [77°F]) or for 7 days under refrigeration. Constituted solutions in sterile water for injection may be frozen. See package insert for details.
Color changes do not affect potency. This vial contains 236 mg of sodium carbonate. The sodium content is approximately 108 mg (4.7 mEq).

U.S. Patent Nos. 4,258,041; 4,329,453; and 4,582,830

Glaxo Wellcome Inc.
Research Triangle Park, NC 27709
Made in England
Rev. 5/97

4077318

Set and solution: Cylinder set with drop factor of 60 gtt/ml; 500 ml of D_5W.
Instruction: Dilute ceftazidime 1.5 g in 100 ml of D_5W and infuse over 30 minutes.

1. Calculate drug dosage according to drug label.
2. Calculate drops per minute for drug solution.
3. Calculate milliliters per hour using volumetric pump rate.

Answer

1. Drug Calculation
Drug label states to add 10 ml of sterile water (2 g = 10 ml)

$$\text{BF:} \quad \frac{D}{H} \times V = \frac{1.5 \text{ g}}{2.0 \text{ g}} \times 10 \text{ ml} = \frac{15}{2} = 7.5 \text{ ml of ceftazidime}$$

$$\text{DA:} \quad \text{ml} = \frac{10 \text{ ml} \times 1.5 \text{ g}}{2.0 \text{ g} \times 1} = \frac{15}{2} = 7.5 \text{ ml}$$

2. IV Flow Calculation (Secondary Set)

$$\frac{\text{Amount of Solution} = \text{Drops per milliliter (set)}}{\text{Minutes to administer}} = \frac{100 \text{ ml} \times \overset{2}{\cancel{60}} \text{ gtt}}{\underset{1}{\cancel{30}} \text{ min}} = 200 \text{ gtt/min}$$

Inject 7.5 ml of ceftazidime in 100 ml of D_5W in the cylinder chamber.

Regulate IV flow rate to 200 gtt/min. It may be impossible to count 200 gtt/min. Instead of using the cylinder chamber, the nurse may use a secondary set that has a larger drop factor or a regulator. If the cylinder set is the only available secondary IV set, then the 200 gtt/min may be approximated.

3. Volumetric Pump Rate

$$\text{Amount of Solution} \div \frac{\text{Minutes to administer}}{60 \text{ minutes per hour}} = 100 \text{ ml} + 7.5 \text{ ml (drug)} \div \frac{30 \text{ min}}{60 \text{ min}}$$

$$\text{(invert the divisor and multiply)} \qquad = 107.5 \text{ ml} \times \frac{\overset{2}{\cancel{60}}}{\underset{1}{\cancel{30}}} = 215 \text{ ml/h}$$

Set volumetric rate at 215 ml/h to deliver drug in 30 min.

**PRACTICE
PROBLEM 2**

INTERMITTENT INTRAVENOUS SET

Solve the IV drug problems by (1) calculating the drug dosage according to the drug label or information given and (2) calculating drops per minute for the drug solution.

1. Order: kanamycin (Kantrex) 15 mg/kg/day in three divided doses (q8h) IV. Client weighs 50 kg.
   Available:

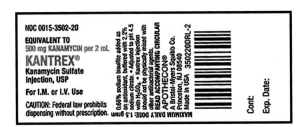

How many milliliters of kanamycin should the client receive per dose? _____
Set and solution: Cylinder set with a drop factor of 60 gtt/ml; 500 ml D_5W.
Instruction: Dilute the drug in 75 ml of D_5W and infuse over 30 min.

2. Order: cefamandole (Mandol) 500 mg IV q6h
   Available: cefamandole (Mandol) is in powdered form in a vial

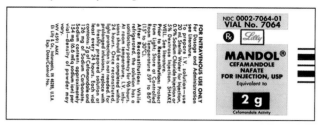

For reconstitution: Add 6.6 ml of diluent = 8 ml of drug solution (2 g = 8 ml).
Set and solution: Secondary set with 100 ml D$_5$W. Drop factor is 15 gtt/ml.
Instruction: Dilute drug solution in 100 ml of D$_5$W and infuse over 30 min.

3. Order: tobramycin (Nebcin) 50 mg IV q8h
   Drug parameters: 3 mg/kg/day in three divided doses. Client weighs 65 kg.
   Available:

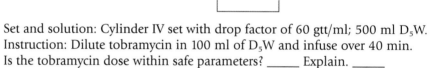

Set and solution: Cylinder IV set with drop factor of 60 gtt/ml; 500 ml D$_5$W.
Instruction: Dilute tobramycin in 100 ml of D$_5$W and infuse over 40 min.
Is the tobramycin dose within safe parameters? _____ Explain. _____

4. Order: ampicillin 500 mg IV q6h
   Available: Add 4.5 ml of diluent = 5 ml (2 g = 5 ml)

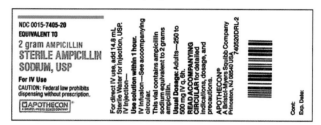

Convert grams to milligrams.
Set and solution: Cylinder set with drop factor of 60 gtt/ml; 500 ml of D$_5$W.
Instruction: Dilute ampicillin in 50 ml of D$_5$W and infuse over 15 min.
Determine the volumetric pump rate for this problem in addition to the drug and IV flow calculations.

5. Order: ticarcillin (Ticar) 750 mg IV q6h
   Available:

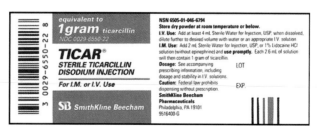

How many milliliters should be given per dose? _____
Set and solution: Cylinder IV set with drop factor of 60 gtt/ml; 500 ml D$_5$W.
Instruction: Dilute ticarcillin in 20 ml of D$_5$W and infuse over 30 min.

6. Order: digoxin 400 mcg (0.40 mg) IV b.i.d. × 1 day. Client weighs 75 kg.
   Drug parameter: 10 to 15 mcg/kg/day (1 mg) in divided doses
   Available:

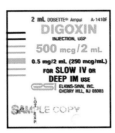

Instruction: Administer digoxin diluted in 4 ml of D_5W or 0.9% saline solution (NaCl) by direct IV injection over 5 or more minutes.
   a. Is the drug dose within safe drug parameter? _____
   b. How many milliliters of drug should the client receive per dose? _____

7. Order: diltiazem (Cardizem) 0.25 mg/kg IV bolus (direct IV) over 2 min. Client weighs 178 lb.
   Available:

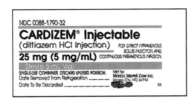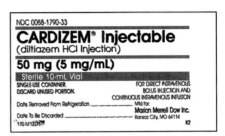

   a. Which Cardizem vial should be chosen? _____Why? _____
   b. How many milligrams should the client receive? _____
   c. How many milliliters should be given direct IV? _____

8. Order: eptoposide (VePesid) 75 mg/m²/day for 5 consecutive days q 3-4 wk. Client's weight is 134 lb and height is 66 inches.
   Use the nomogram to determine body surface areas (BSA, m²) (Figure 4E–8).
   Available:

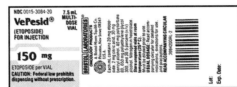

   a. What is the client's BSA? _____
   b. How many milligrams should the client receive? _____
   c. How many milliliters of drug solution should the client receive? _____
   Set and solution: Secondary set with 250 ml of D_5W to run for 60 min. Drop factor is 15 gtt/ml.
   Determine the volumetric pump for this problem in addition to the drug and IV flow calculations.

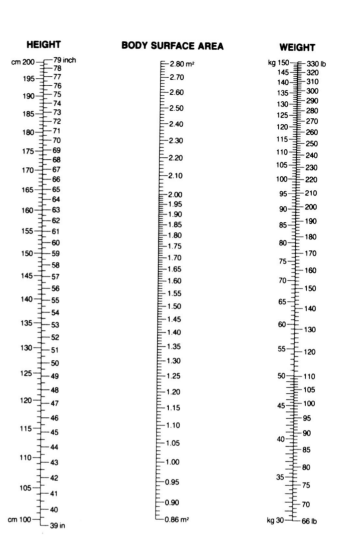

FIGURE 4E–8   Nomogram of body surface area for adults. Directions: (1) Find height. (2) Find weight. (3) Draw a straight line that connects the height and weight. (4) Where the line intersects on the body surface area column is the body surface area (m²). (Sources: Deglin, Vallerand, Russin A: *Davis's drug guide for nurses*, ed 2, Philadelphia, 1991, FA Davis; Lentner C, editor: *Geigy scientific tables*, ed 8, vol 1, Basle, Switzerland, 1981, Ciba-Geigy, pp. 226–227.)

ANSWERS TO PRACTICE PROBLEMS

1	CONTINUOUS INTRAVENOUS FLOW RATES

1. a. Microdrip set because the client is to receive 83 ml/h

b. Two-step method: for continuous IV flow rate

Step 1. $\dfrac{1000}{12} = 83$ ml/h

Step 2. $\dfrac{83 \text{ ml/h} \times \overset{1}{\cancel{60}} \text{ drops}}{\underset{1}{\cancel{60}} \text{ minutes}} = 83$ gtt/min

2. a. 1000 ml

b. 8 h

c. Step 1. $\dfrac{1000}{8} = 125$ ml/h

Step 2. $\dfrac{125 \text{ ml/h} \times \overset{1}{\cancel{15}} \text{ gtt}}{\underset{4}{\cancel{60}} \text{ minutes}} = \dfrac{125}{4} = 31$ gtt/min

3. a. Microdrip set

b. Step 1. $\dfrac{250}{24} = 10$ ml/hour

Step 2. $\dfrac{10 \text{ ml/h} \times \overset{1}{\cancel{60}} \text{ gtt}}{\underset{1}{\cancel{60}} \text{ minutes}} = 10$ gtt/min

4. a. BF: $\dfrac{D}{H} \times V = \dfrac{10}{20} \times 20 = \dfrac{200}{20} = 10$ ml KCl

b. $\dfrac{1000}{10} = 100$ ml/hour

Macrodrip set $\dfrac{100 \times \overset{1}{\cancel{15}}}{\underset{4}{\cancel{60}} \text{ min}} = 25$ gtt/min

Microdrip set $\dfrac{100 \times \overset{1}{\cancel{60}}}{\underset{1}{\cancel{60}} \text{ min}} = 100$ gtt/min

SECTION E

2 | INTERMITTENT INTRAVENOUS SET

1. Use the One-Step for Intermittent IV Flow Rate
Drug calculation:

BF: $\dfrac{D}{H} \times V = \dfrac{250 \text{ mg}}{500 \text{ mg}} \times 2 = \dfrac{500}{500}$

$= 1$ ml of kanamycin

or

RP: $\quad H \quad : \quad V \quad :: \quad D \quad : \quad x$
$500 \text{ mg} : 2 \text{ ml} :: 250 \text{ mg} : x \text{ ml}$
$500x = 500$
$x = 1$ ml of kanamycin

Flow calculation: $\dfrac{75 \text{ ml} \times 60 \text{ (set)}}{30 \text{ minutes}} = \dfrac{4500}{30}$

$= 150$ gtt/min

2. Drug calculation: Change 2 g to milligrams.

$2 \text{ g} = 2.000 \text{ mg}$

BF: $\dfrac{D}{H} \times V = \dfrac{500}{2000} \times 8 \text{ ml} = \dfrac{4000}{2000} = 2$ ml Mandol

or

DA: $\text{ml} = \dfrac{8 \text{ ml} \times \quad 1 \cancel{g} \quad \times 500 \cancel{mg}^{1}}{2 \cancel{g} \times 1000 \cancel{mg}_{2} \times \quad 1 \text{ g}} = \dfrac{8}{4}$

$= 2$ ml of Mandol

Flow calculation: $\dfrac{100 \text{ ml} \times 15 \text{ gtt (set)}^{1}}{30 \text{ minutes}_{2}}$

$= \dfrac{100}{2} = 50$ gtt/min

3. Drug calculation: BF: $\dfrac{D}{H} \times V = \dfrac{50}{80} \times 2 = \dfrac{100}{80}$

$= 1.25$ ml of tobramycin

Flow calculation: $\dfrac{100 \text{ ml} \times 60 \text{ gtt (set)}^{3}}{40 \text{ minutes}_{2}}$

$= \dfrac{300}{2} = 150$ gtt/min

Drug parameter: It is within safe parameters
($3 \text{ kg} \times 65 = 195$ mg/day).
Client is receiving $50 \text{ mg} \times 3 = 150$ mg/day.

4. Drug calculation: Convert to milligrams.

$2 \text{ g} = 2.000 \text{ mg}$

BF: $\dfrac{D}{H} \times V = \dfrac{500}{2000} \times 5 = \dfrac{5}{4} = 1.25$ ml of ampicillin

or

RP: $\quad H \quad : \quad V \quad :: \quad D \quad : \quad x$
$2000 \text{ mg} : 5 \text{ ml} :: 500 \text{ mg} : x \text{ ml}$
$2000x = 2500$
$x = 1.25$ ml of ampicillin

Flow calculation:

$\dfrac{50 \text{ ml} \times 60 \text{ gtt (set)}^{4}}{15 \text{ min}_{1}} = \dfrac{200}{1} = 200$ gtt/min

Volumetric pump rate:

$50 \text{ ml} + 1.25 \text{ ml} \div \dfrac{15}{60} = 51.25 \text{ ml} \times \dfrac{60^{4}}{15_{1}}$

$= 205$ ml/hour

5. BF: $\dfrac{D}{H} \times V = \dfrac{750 \text{ mg}}{1000 \text{ mg}} \times 4 \text{ ml} = \dfrac{3000}{1000}$

$= 3$ ml of Ticar

or

DA: $\text{ml} = \dfrac{4 \text{ ml} \times \quad 1 \cancel{g} \quad \times 750 \cancel{mg}^{3}}{1 \cancel{g} \times 1000 \cancel{mg}_{4} \times \quad 1} = \dfrac{12}{4}$

$= 3$ ml of Ticar

Flow calculation: $\dfrac{20 \text{ ml} \times 60 \text{ gtt (set)}^{2}}{30 \text{ min}_{1}} = \dfrac{40}{1}$

$= 40$ gtt/min

Volumetric pump rate:

$20 \text{ ml} + 3 \text{ ml} \div \dfrac{30}{60} = 23 \text{ ml} \times \dfrac{60^{2}}{30_{1}} = 46$ ml/h

(Increase in D_5W solution may be desired)

6. a. Drug dose is within safe drug parameters;
800 mcg/daily

$10 \text{ mcg} \times 75 \text{ kg} = 750$ mcg/day
$15 \text{ mcg} \times 75 \text{ kg} = 1125$ mcg/day

b. BF: $\dfrac{D}{H} \times V = \dfrac{400 \text{ mcg}}{500 \text{ mcg}} \times 2 \text{ ml} \times \dfrac{800}{500}$

$= 1.6$ ml of digoxin

RP: $\quad H \quad : \quad V \quad :: \quad D \quad : \quad x$
$500 \text{ mcg} : 2 \text{ ml} :: 400 \text{ mcg} : x$
$500x = 800$
$x = 1.6$ ml of digoxin per
dose

Answer: Mix 1.6 ml of digoxin with 4 ml of diluent and administer the 5.6 ml by direct IV injection over 5 or more minutes.

SECTION E

7. Client's weight: 178 lb ÷ 2.2 = 81 kg
   a. Either Cardizem vial could be used. The Cardizem 25-mg vial is preferred because the dose is less than 25 mg, and the balance of the solution would need to be discarded.
   b. 0.25 mg × 81 kg = 20.25 mg or 20 mg

   c. BF: $\dfrac{D}{H} \times V = \dfrac{20 \text{ mg}}{25 \text{ mg}} \times 5 \text{ ml} = \dfrac{100}{25}$
   $= 4 \text{ ml of Cardizem}$

8. a. Client's BSA is 1.75.
   b. 75 mg × 1.75 (BSA) = 131.25 or 131 mg

   c. $\dfrac{D}{H} \times V = \dfrac{131}{150} \times 7.5 \text{ ml} = \dfrac{982.5}{150} = 6.55 \text{ or } 6.6 \text{ ml}$

   Flow calculation with secondary set:

   $$\dfrac{250 \text{ ml} \times 15 \text{ gtt (set)}}{60 \text{ min}} = \dfrac{3750}{60} = 62.5 \text{ gtt/min}$$

   Volumetric pump rate: 250 ml + 6.6 ml

   $$(256.6 \text{ or } 257 \text{ ml}) \div \dfrac{60}{60} = 257 \text{ ml} \times \dfrac{\cancel{60}^{1}}{\cancel{60}_{1}}$$
   $$= 257 \text{ ml/hour}$$

Section 4F PEDIATRIC DRUG CALCULATIONS

OUTLINE

Objectives

Terms

Introduction

Oral

Intramuscular

Pediatric Dosage per Body Weight

Pediatric Dosage per Body Surface Area

Pediatric Dosage from Adult Dosage

Pediatric Calculations for Injectables

OBJECTIVES

- Use one of the two primary methods to determine pediatric drug dosage.
- Describe the dosage inaccuracies that may occur with pediatric drug formulas.
- Identify the steps used to determine body surface area from a pediatric nomogram.
- Calculate the drug dosages correctly in the practice problems.

TERMS

body surface area (BSA)
body weight (BW)

drug parameters

Introduction

Pediatric drug dosages differ greatly from those for adults because of the physiologic differences between the two. Neonates and infants have immature kidney and liver function, which delays metabolism and elimination of many drugs. In neonates, drug absorption is different as a result of slow gastric emptying time. Decreased gastric acid secretion in children younger than 3 years old contributes to altered drug absorption. Neonates and infants have a lower concentration of plasma proteins, which can cause toxicity with drugs that are highly bound to proteins. Young children have less total body fat and more body water; therefore lipid-soluble drugs require smaller doses when less-than-normal fat is present. Water-soluble drugs can require large doses because of a greater percentage of body water. It is the nurse's responsibility to ensure that a safe drug dosage is given and to closely monitor signs and symptoms of side effects and adverse drug reactions.

The purpose of learning how to calculate pediatric drug dosages is to ensure that children receive the correct dose within the approved therapeutic range. The two methods that are considered safe in the administration of drugs to children are the **body weight (BW)** (kg) and **body surface area (BSA, or m²)** methods. Many manufacturers supply information in their literature concerning drug doses for children according to BW. Also, manufacturers frequently give **drug parameters** for safe dose ranges. It is the nurse's responsibility to check the dose ranges given by the pharmaceutical manufacturers to be certain that the prescribed dose is within the parameters. Children's dosage can be determined from the adult dose using the BSA rule.

Oral

Oral pediatric drug delivery usually requires the use of a calibrated measuring device because most drugs for small children are in liquid form. The measuring device can be a small plastic cup, an oral dropper, a measuring spoon, or an oral syringe (Figure 4F–1). Some liquid medications come with their own calibrated droppers. The type of measuring device chosen depends on the age or the developmental level of the child. For infants and toddlers, the oral syringe and dropper can provide better drug delivery than a small cup. A young child who is cooperative is able to use a small cup or measuring spoon. The cup or spoon may be rinsed with water or juice to ensure that the child has received all of the drug. Avoid giving oral medications to a crying child or infant because the drug could be easily aspirated or the child could "spit out" the drug. For the older child, some drugs are available in chewable form. Children should be told not to chew drugs that are enteric-coated or in time-release form.

Intramuscular

Intramuscular (IM) sites for drug administration are chosen on the basis of the age and muscle development of the child (Table 4F–1). All injections should be given in a manner that minimizes physical and psychosocial trauma. Explanations of injection administration should be

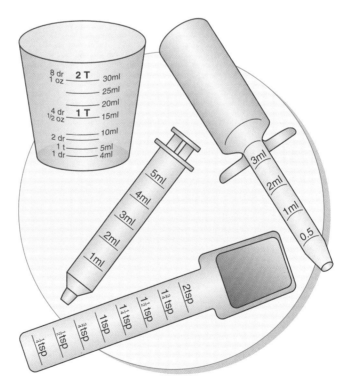

FIGURE 4F–1 Calibrated measuring devices. (From Kee JL, Marshall SM: *Clinical calculations,* ed 5, Philadelphia, 2004, Saunders, p. 232.)

Table 4F–1

Pediatric Guidelines for Intramuscular Injections According to Muscle Group*

	Amount by Muscle Group (ml)			
Age	Vastus Lateralis	Gluteus Maximus	Ventrogluteal	Deltoid
Birth to 4 months	0.5-1	Not safe	0.5-1	Not safe
Infants	0.5-1	Not safe	1	Not safe
Toddlers	0.5-2	0.5-1	0.5-1	0.5-1
Preschool and older children	2	0.5-2	2-3	0.5–1
Adolescents	2	2	2-5	1-1.5

*The safe use of all sites is based on normal muscle development and size of the child. (From Kee JL, Marshall SM: *Clinical calculations,* ed 5, Philadelphia, 2004, W.B. Saunders, p. 233.)

given to children who can comprehend. With the very young child, distraction or brief restraint may be necessary. Comfort measures should immediately follow the injection.

Pediatric Dosage per Body Weight

EXAMPLE

Order: cefaclor (Ceclor) 50 mg q.i.d. Child weighs 15 lb or 6.8 kg (15 ÷ 2.2 = 6.8)
Child's drug dosage: 20-40 mg/kg/day in three divided doses
Available:

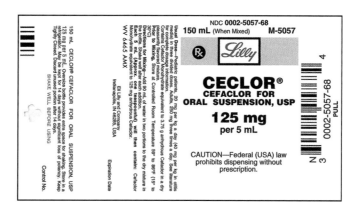

Is the prescribed dose safe? _____

Answer:

Drug parameters:	20 mg × 6.8 kg = 136 mg/day
	40 mg × 6.8 kg = 272 mg/day
Dosage order:	50 mg × 4 = 200 mg/day

Dosage is within safe drug parameters.

a. BF: $\dfrac{D}{H} \times V = \dfrac{50}{125} \times 5 = \dfrac{250}{125} = 2$ ml

b. RP:

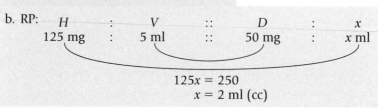

$$125x = 250$$
$$x = 2 \text{ ml (cc)}$$

Cross-multiply:

c. FE: $\dfrac{H}{V} = \dfrac{D}{X}$ $\dfrac{125 \text{ mg}}{5 \text{ ml}} = \dfrac{50 \text{ mg}}{x \text{ ml}}$

$$125x = 250$$
$$x = 2 \text{ ml}$$

d. DA: ml $= \dfrac{5 \text{ ml} \times \overset{2}{\cancel{50} \text{ mg}}}{\underset{5}{\cancel{125} \text{ mg}} \times 1} = \dfrac{10}{5} = 2 \text{ ml}$

Cefaclor 50 mg = 2 ml. Give 2 ml four times a day.

Pediatric Dosage per Body Surface Area

To calculate pediatric dose by BSA, the child's height and weight are needed. Figure 4F–2 is the nomogram used to determine the BSA for infants and children.

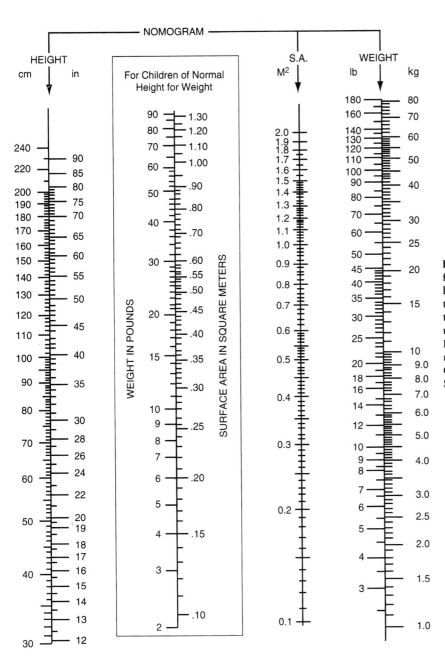

FIGURE 4F–2 Nomogram of body surface area for infants and children. Directions: (1) Find height. (2) Find weight. (3) Draw a straight line that connects the height and weight. (4) Where the line intersects on the body surface area column is the body surface area (m²). (Sources: Deglin, Vallerand, Russin A: *Davis's drug guide for nurses*, ed 2, Philadelphia, 1991, FA Davis; Lentner C, editor: *Geigy scientific tables*, ed 8, vol 1, Basle, Switzerland, 1981, Ciba-Geigy, pp. 226-227.)

SECTION F

EXAMPLE

Order: methotrexate (Mexate) 50 mg weekly. Child's height is 54 inches and weight is 90 lb (41 kg).
  Child's drug dosage: 25-75 mg/m²/week
  Child's height and weight intersect at 1.3 m² (BSA).
  Is the prescribed dose safe? _____

Answer:
Multiply the BSA, 1.3 m², by the minimum and maximum doses.

25 mg × 1.3 m² = 32.5 mg
75 mg × 1.3 m² = 97.5 mg

Dosage is considered safe within the parameters according to the child's BSA.

Pediatric Dosage From Adult Dosage

To calculate the pediatric dosage from the adult dosage, determine the child's height and weight. Where they intersect on the nomogram is the BSA in square meters. The formula for calculation is the following:

$$\frac{\text{Surface area (m}^2)}{1.73 \text{ m}^2} \times \text{Adult dose} = \text{Pediatric dose}$$

EXAMPLE

Order: erythromycin (E-Mycin) 125 mg PO q.i.d. Child's height is 42 inches and weight is 60 lb.
  Child's height and weight intersect at 0.9 m²
  The adult dose is 1000 mg/day.

$$\frac{0.9 \text{ m}^2}{1.73 \text{ m}^2} \times 1000 = \frac{900}{1.73} = 520 \text{ mg/day}$$

Drug dosage: 520 mg ÷ 4 times a day = 130 mg/dose
Dosage is within safe range.

PRACTICE
PROBLEM 1

PEDIATRIC DOSING (ORAL)

Solve the following problems using one of these three methods: BW, BSA, or pediatric dosage from adult dosage. The safe dosage is given in drug reference books.
1. Order: dicloxacillin sodium 100 mg q6h. Child weighs 55 lb (_____ kg).
   Child's drug dosage range: <40 kg, 12.5–25 mg/kg/day
   Available: dicloxacillin 62.5 mg per 5 ml
   Is the prescribed dose safe? _____ How many milliliters should be given for each dose? _____
2. Order: digoxin (Lanoxin), 35 mcg/kg/loading dose, PO.
   Child weighs 10 kg.
   Available: Lanoxin 50 mcg/ml (0.05 mg/ml)
   a. How many micrograms or milligrams should the child receive? _____
   b. How many milliliters should be given for the loading dose? _____
3 Order: amoxicillin (Amoxil) 200 mg PO q8h. Child weighs 26 lb (12 kg).
   Child's drug dosage: 20-40 mg/kg/day in three divided doses

Available:

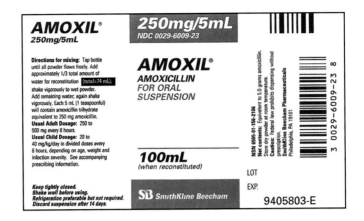

Is the prescribed dose safe? _____ How many milliliters should be given every 8 hours? _____

4. Order: azithromycin (Zithromax), PO. First day: 10 mg/kg/day; next 4 days; 5 mg/kg/day. Client weighs 44 pounds.

Available:

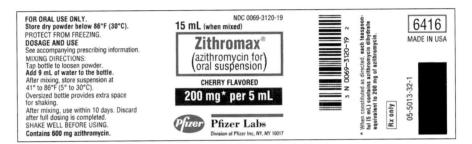

   a. How much does the child weigh in kilograms? _____
   b. How many milliliters should the child receive for the first day? _____
   c. How many milliliters should the child receive each day for the next 4 days (second to fifth days)? _____

5. Order: amoxicillin and clavulanate potassium (Augmentin) 100 mg PO q8h.
Child weighs 28 lb.
Child's drug dosage: 20-40 mg/kg/day
Available:

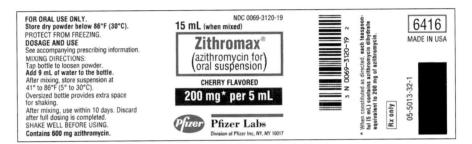

   a. Is the prescribed drug dose within safe drug parameters? _____
   b. How many milliliters should the child receive per dose? _____

6. Order: doxycycline (Vibramycin) 50 mg PO q12h.
Child is 10 years old and weighs 88 lb.
Child's drug dosage: 2.2-4.4 mg/kg/day in one to two doses

Available:

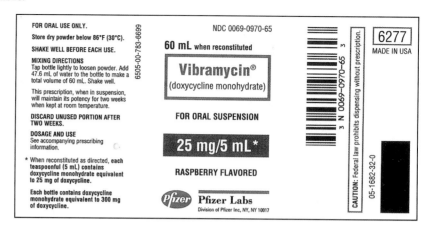

a. What would be the dosage parameter range for this child? _____
b. Is the prescribed drug dose within safe drug parameters? _____
c. How many milliliters should the child receive per dose? _____

7. Order: ampicillin 200 mg PO q6h.
   Child weighs 27 kg.
   Child's drug dosage: 25-50 mg/kg/day
   Available:

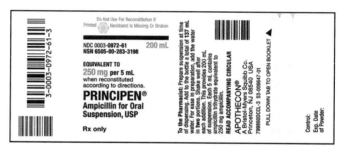

Is the prescribed dose safe? _____
How many milliliters should the child receive per dose? _____

8. Order: vinblastine (Velsar)
   Child's BSA is 1.2 m².
   Child's drug dosage: 2.5 mg/m²
   How many milligrams should the child receive? _____

Pediatric Calculations for Injectables

The same three methods used to calculate oral dosages for children are used to calculate injectable dosages. They are calculated from (1) BW (kg), (2) BSA (m²), and (3) the adult dose. Use the nomogram for BSA.

PRACTICE PROBLEM 2

PEDIATRIC INJECTABLES

Solve the following drug problems and indicate whether the drug dose is within the safe drug parameters.

1. Order: tobramycin (Nebcin) 10 mg IM q8h.
   Child weighs 10 kg.
   Child's drug dosage: 3 mg/kg/day in three divided doses

Available:

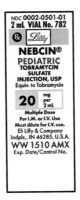

a. Is the dose within safe drug parameters? _____
b. How many milliliters should the child receive per dose? _____

2. Order: promethazine (Phenergan) 20 mg IM q6h.
   Child weighs 45 kg.
   Child's drug dosage: 0.25-0.5 mg/kg/dose; repeat every 4 to 6 h
   Available: Phenergan 25 mg/ml
   a. Is the dose within safe drug parameters? _____
   b. How many milliliters should the child receive per dose? _____

3. Order: oxacillin sodium 250 mg IM q6h.
   Child weighs 15 kg.
   Child's drug dosage: 50-100 mg/kg/day in divided doses
   Available:

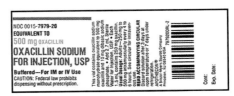

a. How many milligrams should the child receive per day? _____
b. How much diluent should be added? _____
c. How many milliliters should the child receive per dose? _____
d. Is the dose within safe drug parameters? _____

4. Order: nafcillin sodium 200 mg IM q6h.
   Child weighs 10 kg.
   Child's drug dosage: 100-300 mg/kg/day in divided doses
   Available:

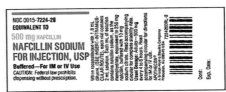

a. How many milligrams will the child receive per day? _____
b. Is the drug dosage per day within safe drug parameters? _____
c. How many milliliters should the child receive per dose? _____

5. Order: The newborn is to receive AquaMEPHYTON (vitamin K) 0.5 mg immediately after delivery.
   Available:

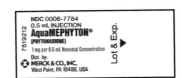   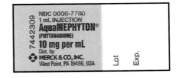

a. Which AquaMEPHYTON container should be selected? _____
b. How many milliliters should the newborn receive? _____

6. Order: cefazolin (Ancef) 125 mg IM q6h.
   Child weighs 22 kg.
   Child's drug dosage: 25-50 mg/kg/day in three to four divided doses (up to 100 mg/kg/day)
   Available:

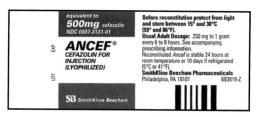

a. How many milligrams should the child receive per day? _____
b. Is the dose within safe drug parameters? _____
c. The drug label does not give the amount of diluent to add to the Ancef powder. Check the pamphlet insert. With 3.4 ml of diluent added, it is equivalent to 4 ml of drug solution.
d. How many milliliters of cefazolin should the child receive per dose? _____

7. Order: hydroxyzine (Vistaril) 50 mg IM.
   Child's height is 47 inches and weight is 45 lb.
   Child's drug dosage: 30 mg/m²
   Available: Vistaril 25 mg/ml
   Is the dose within safe drug parameters? _____

8. Order: methotrexate (Mexate) 50 mg IM weekly.
   Child's height is 56 inches and weight is 100 lb.
   Child's drug dosage: 25-75 mg/m²/week
   Available: methotrexate 2.5 mg/ml; 25 mg/ml; 100 mg/ml
   Is the dose within safe drug parameters? _____
   Which methotrexate should be selected? _____

ANSWERS TO PRACTICE PROBLEMS

1   **PEDIATRIC DOSING (ORAL) USING BASIC FORMULA, RATIO AND PROPORTION, OR DIMENSIONAL ANALYSIS**

1. a. Child weighs 25 kg (55 lb ÷ 2.2 = 25 kg)
    b. Drug parameters:
      12.5 mg × 25 kg = 312.5 mg/day
      25 mg × 25 kg = 625 mg/day

Dosage order: 100 mg × 4 times a day (q6h)
= 400 mg/day
Dosage is within safe drug parameters.

    a. BF: $\dfrac{D}{H} \times V = \dfrac{100}{62.5} \times 5 = \dfrac{500}{62.5} = 8$ ml of dicloxacillin

    b. RP:
$$H \quad : \quad V \quad :: \quad D \quad : \quad x$$
$$62.5 \text{ mg} : 5 \text{ ml} :: 100 \text{ mg} : x \text{ ml}$$
$$62.5x = 500$$
$$x = 8 \text{ ml of dicloxacillin}$$

2. Child's drug dosage:
    a. 35 mcg × 10 kg = 350 mcg, or 0.35 mg
      350 mcg = 0.350 mg

    b. $\dfrac{D}{H} \times V = \dfrac{350 \text{ mcg}}{50 \text{ mcg}} \times 1$ ml = 7 ml loading dose

    or

    $\dfrac{0.35 \text{ mg}}{0.05 \text{ mg}} \times 1$ ml = 7 ml loading dose

3. Drug parameters:
    20 mg × 12 kg = 240 mg/day
    40 mg × 12 kg = 480 mg /day

Dosage order: 200 mg × 3 (q8h) = 600 mg/day
Dosage is *not* within safe drug parameters. Dose exceeds the drug parameters.
Health care provider must be contacted.

4. a. 20 kg

b. First day: 10 mg × 20 kg = 200 mg

BF: $\dfrac{D}{H} \times V = \dfrac{\overset{1}{\cancel{200}} \text{ mg}}{\underset{1}{\cancel{200}} \text{ mg}} \times 5 \text{ ml} = 5 \text{ ml}$

or

RP: $H \quad : \quad V \quad :: \quad D \quad : x$
200 mg : 5 ml :: 200 mg : x
$200x = 1000$
$x = 5$ ml

or

DA: $\text{ml} = \dfrac{5 \text{ ml} \times \overset{1}{\cancel{200} \text{ mg}}}{\underset{1}{\cancel{200} \text{ mg}} \times 1} = 5 \text{ ml}$

First day give 5 ml.

c. Second to fifth days (next 4 days): 5 mg × 20 kg = 100 mg. Give 2.5 ml/day. Same answer worked out by BF, RP, and DA.

5. a. Drug parameters: (28 lb ÷ 2.2 = 12.7 kg)
20 mg × 12.7 kg = 254 mg/day
40 mg × 12.7 kg = 508 mg/day

Dosage order: 100 mg × 3 (q8h) = 300 mg/day
Dosage is within safe drug parameters.

b. 4 ml of Augmentin

6. a. Drug parameters: 88 mg to 176 mg per day

b. Dose is within safe drug parameters.

c. 10 ml per dose of Vibramycin

7. Drug parameters:
25 mg × 27 kg = 675 mg/day
50 mg × 27 kg = 1350 mg/day

Dosage order: 200 mg × 4 (q6h) = 800 mg/day
Dosage is within safe drug parameters.

$\dfrac{D}{H} \times V = \dfrac{200}{250} \times 5 = \dfrac{1000}{250} = 4$ ml of ampicillin

8. Drug dosage: 2.5 mg × 1.2 m² = 3 mg
Administer 3 mg vinblastine.

2 PEDIATRIC INJECTABLES

1. a. Tobramycin parameter: 3 mg/kg/day × 10 kg = 30 mg/day in three divided doses
Drug order: 10 mg × 3 (q8h) = 30 mg/day
Dosage is within safe drug parameters.

b. 10 mg = 1 ml/dose
Child should receive 1 ml per dose.

2. a. Phenergan parameters:
0.25 mg/kg/dose × 45 kg = 11.25 mg/dose
0.50 mg/kg/dose × 45 kg = 22.5 mg/dose

Drug order: Phenergan 20 mg IM per dose
Dosage is within safe drug parameters.

b. Phenergan 20 mg = 0.8 ml

3. a. 250 mg × 4 (q6h) = 1000 mg/day

b. Add 2.7 ml of diluent = 3 ml of drug solution

c. 1.5 ml

d. Dosage is within safe drug parameters.

4. a. 200 mg × 4 (q6h) = 800 mg/day

b. Dose per day is safe but not in therapeutic range. Notify health care provider.

100 mg × 10 kg = 1000 mg
300 mg × 10 kg = 3000 mg

c. Add 1.8 ml diluent = 2 ml (500 mg = 2 ml)
Nafcillin 200 mg = 0.8 ml

5. a. Preferred selection is AquaMEPHYTON
1 mg = 0.5 ml.

b. *AquaMEPHYTON 1 mg = 0.5 ml*
$\dfrac{D}{H} \times V = \dfrac{0.5 \text{ mg}}{1.0 \text{ mg}} \times 0.5 \text{ ml} = \dfrac{0.25}{1.0} = 0.25$ ml

AquaMEPHYTON 10 mg = 1 ml
$\dfrac{D}{H} \times V = \dfrac{0.5 \text{ mg}}{10 \text{ mg}} \times 1.0 \text{ ml} = \dfrac{0.5}{10} = 0.05$ ml

For AquaMEPHYTON 1 mg = 0.5 ml. Give 0.25 ml. (Use a tuberculin syringe.)
For AquaMEPHYTON 10 mg = 1 ml. Give 0.05 ml. (Use a tuberculin syringe; however, it would be difficult to give this small amount.)

6. a. 125 mg × 4 (q6h) = 500 mg

b. Drug parameters: 22 kg × 25 mg/kg/day = 550 mg
22 kg × 50 mg/kg/day = 1100 mg
22 kg × 100 mg/kg/day = 2200 mg maximum (range: 550-2200 mg)
Drug dose per day is below the suggested child's drug dose range. The nurse should contact the health care provider. The daily drug dose may need to be increased.

c. Add 3.4 ml of diluent yielding 4 ml of drug solution.

d. Give 1 ml of cefazolin (Ancef) per dose.

7. Height and weight intersect at 0.82 m².
Hydroxyzine parameter: 30 mg/m² × 0.82 m² = 24.6 mg, or 25 mg
Drug order: hydroxyzine 50 mg IM
Dosage ordered is *not* within safe parameters. Dosage exceeds the drug parameters. *Do not* give the medication. Notify the health care provider.

8. Height and weight intersect at 1.38 m².
Methotrexate parameters:
25 mg/m²/week × 1.38 m² = 34.5 mg/week
75 mg/m²/week × 1.38 m² = 103.5 mg/week

Drug order: methotrexate 50 mg/week IM
Dosage is within safe drug parameters.
(1) If methotrexate 25 mg/ml is used, give 2 ml (50 mg) or
(2) If methotrexate 100 mg/ml is used, give 0.5 ml. Because of the amount of solution, it may be more desirable to give 0.5 ml of the 100 mg/ml solution.

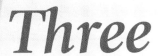

Three

Contemporary Issues in Pharmacology

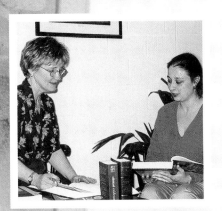

This unit comprises nine chapters that cover a range of issues affecting drug therapy and nursing. Chapter 5, The Drug Approval Process, covers drug standards and federal legislation for American and Canadian drugs that establish safety guidelines for drug use, drug names, and drug resources. Ethical considerations in the pharmacotherapeutic regimen are also addressed.

Chapter 6, Transcultural and Genetic Considerations, helps the nurse understand and respond to unique cultural and genetic factors that may influence drug therapy for a particular client. Factors such as communication styles, family organization, spirituality and religion, health beliefs and practices, and traditional and folk medicine are discussed.

Chapter 7, Drug Interaction and Over-the-Counter Drugs, and Chapter 8, Drugs of Abuse, cover drug interactions and drug abuse, two areas of special interest to nurses. Assessing drug interaction has always been and remains an ongoing function of the nurse. Because drug abuse is a national problem from which no portion of the population is immune—including health professionals—it is a topic of great concern to nurses.

Chapter 9, Herbal Therapy with Nursing Implications, explores the increasingly popular herbal-based preparations that are available over-the-counter. It covers the most commonly used herbs and discusses their indications, preparation, dosages, potential hazards, and tips for safe and effective use.

Chapter 10, Pediatric Pharmacology, and Chapter 11, Geriatric Pharmacology, cover pharmacokinetic and pharmacodynamic effects specific to these age groups. It also discusses the special attention required to administer drugs to these age groups. Specific recommendations are described.

With the increasing movement of health care into the community, nurses, above all other health care providers, are gaining more responsibilities and opportunities to guide clients in safe medication administration. Chapter 12, Medication Administration in Community Settings, focuses on aspects of drug therapy unique to the home, school, workplace, and other alternative care settings.

Chapter 13, The Role of the Nurse in Drug Research, discusses the nurse's challenges regarding drug research. In general practice the nurse identifies specific needs that may be met by medications. As part of clinical drug trials, the nurse needs to be aware of informed consent and the client's response to drugs.

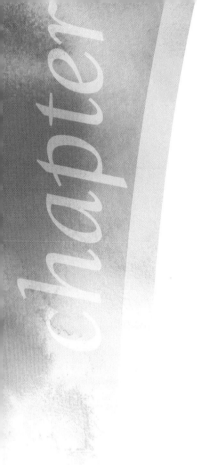

5 The Drug Approval Process

ELECTRONIC RESOURCES

Additional information can be found on the companion website at *http://evolve.elsevier.com/KeeHayes/pharmacology/* or on the companion CD-ROM, which includes:
- *NCLEX-style examination review questions*
- *Pharmacology animations*
- *Medication error and IV therapy checklists*
- *Medication calculation problems*
- *Electronic calculators*

OUTLINE

Objectives

Terms

Introduction

Drug Standards and Legislation
Drug Standards
Federal Legislation

Nurse Practice Acts

Canadian Drug Regulation

Initiatives to Combat Drug Counterfeiting

Drug Names

Drug Resources

Food and Drug Administration Pregnancy Categories

Poison Control Centers

Ethical Considerations

International Issues

Websites

Study Questions

OBJECTIVES

- Discuss the various federal legislation acts related to Food and Drug Administration drug approvals.
- Explain the three Canadian schedules for drugs sold in Canada.
- Describe the function of nurse practice acts.
- Differentiate between chemical, generic, and brand names of drugs.
- List two drug resource (reference) books.
- Explain various ethical values that the nurse should consider in relation to health care.

TERMS

American Hospital Formulary Service (AHFS) Drug Information
brand (trade) name
chemical name
controlled substances

Drug Enforcement Administration (DEA)
Drug Facts and Comparisons (F & C)
Food and Drug Administration (FDA)

generic name
malfeasance
misfeasance
nonfeasance
Physicians' Desk Reference (PDR)

pharmacology
United States Pharmacopeia —Drug Information (USP-DI)
United States Pharmacopeia National Formulary (USP-NF)

Introduction

Pharmacology is the study of the effects of chemical substances on living tissues. Early drugs were derived from plants, animals, and minerals. Records of drug use date back to 2700 BC in the Middle East and China. The drugs most commonly used then were laxatives and emetics to induce vomiting.

In 1550 BC the Egyptians wrote their empirical observations of drug therapy on what has come to be known as the Ebers Medical Papyrus. They suggested castor oil for a laxative and opium for pain. They also suggested that moldy bread be applied to wounds and bruises—3500 years before Alexander Fleming's discovery of penicillin.

The Roman physician and writer Galen (131-201 AD) was considered an authority in medicine and pharmacy for hundreds of years. He initiated the common use of prescriptions and used several ingredients to treat a specific illness.

After the fall of the Roman Empire, medicine and pharmacy returned to the realms of folklore and tradition. During this time, however, Christian monks kept information on medicine and pharmacy in their monasteries and tended the sick and needy. The medicines used by the monks were derived from plants and herbs grown in the monastery gardens.

Around 1240 AD, Arab doctors formulated the first set of drug standards and measurements (grains, drams, minims), known as the *apothecary system*. (Currently, the units of the metric system are used internationally to measure drugs; the apothecary system is being phased out.) In fifteenth-century England, apothecary shops were owned by barber-surgeons, physicians, and independent merchants dispensing herbal and chemical remedies.

In the eighteenth century, the following breakthrough drugs were introduced: the vaccine for smallpox, digitalis from the foxglove plant for strengthening and slowing the heartbeat, and vitamin C from citrus fruit. In the nineteenth century, morphine and codeine were extracted from opium; atropine, bromides, and iodine were introduced; amyl nitrite was used to relieve the pain of angina; and the anesthetics ether and nitrous oxide were discovered.

In the early twentieth century, aspirin was derived from salicylic acid, and phenobarbital, insulin, and the sulfonamides were introduced. A vast majority of modern drugs date back to the early 1940s. Antibiotics (penicillin, tetracycline, streptomycin), antihistamines, and cortisone were marketed in the 1940s. In the 1950s, antipsychotic drugs, antihypertensives, oral contraceptives, and the polio vaccine were introduced.

Drug Standards and Legislation

Drug Standards

The set of drug standards used in the United States is the *United States Pharmacopeia* of 1820. The **United States Pharmacopeia National Formulary (USP-NF)**, the current authoritative source for drug standards, is revised every 5 years by a group of experts in nursing, pharmaceutics, pharmacology, chemistry, and microbiology. Drugs included in the *USP-NF* have met high standards for therapeutic use, client safety, quality, purity, strength, packaging safety, and dosage form. Drugs that meet these standards have the initials USP following their official name.

The *International Pharmacopeia*, first published in 1951 by the World Health Organization (WHO), provides a basis for standards in strength and composition of drugs for use throughout the world. The book is published in English, Spanish, and French and, like the *USP-NF*, is revised every 5 years.

Federal Legislation

Through federal legislation, the public is protected from drugs that are impure, toxic, ineffective, or not tested before public sale. The primary purpose of this federal legislation is to ensure safety. America's first law to regulate drugs was the Federal Pure Food and Drug Act of 1906, which did not include drug effectiveness and drug safety.

1938: Food, Drug, and Cosmetic Act

The Food, Drug, and Cosmetic Act of 1938 empowered a governing body, the **Food and Drug Administration (FDA)**, to monitor and regulate the manufacture and marketing of drugs. It is the FDA's responsibility to ensure that all drugs are tested for harmful effects, have labels with accurate information, and enclose with the drug packaging detailed literature that explains adverse effects. The FDA can prevent the marketing of any drug it judges to be incompletely tested or dangerous. Only drugs considered safe by the FDA are approved for marketing.

1952: Durham-Humphrey Amendment to the 1938 Act

The Durham-Humphrey amendment to the Food, Drug, and Cosmetic Act of 1938 distinguished between drugs that can be sold with or without prescription and those that should not be refilled without a new prescription. Those drugs that should not be refilled without a new prescription, such as narcotics, hypnotics, or tranquilizers, must be so labeled.

1962: Kefauver-Harris Amendment to the 1938 Act

The Kefauver-Harris amendment to the Food, Drug, and Cosmetic Act of 1938 resulted from the widely publicized thalidomide tragedy of the 1950s in which pregnant European women who took the sedative-hypnotic thalidomide during the first trimester of pregnancy gave birth to infants with extreme limb deformities. The Kefauver-Harris amendment tightened controls on drug safety, especially experimental drugs, and required that adverse reactions and contraindications must be labeled and included in the literature. Also included in the amendment were provisions for the evaluation of testing methods used by manufacturers, the process for withdrawal of approved drugs when safety and effectiveness were in doubt, and the establishment of the effectiveness of new drugs before marketing.

1970: The Controlled Substances Act

In 1970 the Controlled Substances Act (CSA) of the Comprehensive Drug Abuse Prevention and Control Act, Title II, was passed by Congress. This act, designed to remedy the escalating problem of drug abuse, included several provisions: (1) the promotion of drug education and research into the prevention and treatment of drug dependence; (2) the strengthening of enforcement authority; (3) the establishment of treatment and rehabilitation facilities; and (4) the designation of schedules, or categories, for controlled substances according to abuse liability.

Controlled substances are described in five schedules, or categories, which are listed in Table 5-1. Schedule I drugs are *not* approved for medical use; schedule II through V drugs have accepted medical use. In addition, the abuse potential and extent of physical and psychologic dependence are greatest with schedule I drugs. This dependency decreases as one moves through the schedule, with schedule V drugs having only limited abuse potential. Some drugs might be listed in more than one schedule category. Codeine is a schedule II drug, but when it is added to acetaminophen, it becomes a schedule III drug, and when it is used in combination as a cough preparation, it becomes a schedule V drug.

Nursing Interventions: Controlled Substances

- Account for all controlled drugs.
- Keep a special controlled-substance record for required information.
- Countersign all discarded or wasted medication.
- Ensure that records and drugs on hand match.
- Keep all controlled drugs locked up; narcotics must be kept under double lock.
- Be certain that only authorized persons have access to the keys.

In 1983 the **Drug Enforcement Administration (DEA)** of the Department of Justice was charged with the role of being the nation's sole legal drug enforcement agency. The Bureau of Narcotics and Dangerous Drugs, which preceded the DEA, is defunct.

Table 5-1

Schedule Categories of Controlled Substances

Schedule	Examples of Substances	Description
I	heroin, hallucinogenics (LSD, marijuana [except when prescribed with cancer treatment], mescaline, peyote, psilocybin)	Drugs with high abuse potential. No accepted medical use. Labeled C-I.
II	meperidine (Demerol), morphine, hydrocodone, hydromorphone, methadone, oxycodone, codeine, amphetamines, secobarbital, pentobarbital	High potential for drug abuse. Accepted medical use. Can lead to strong physical and psychologic dependency. Labeled C-II.
III	codeine preparations, paregoric, nonnarcotic drugs (pentazocine, propoxyphene)	Medically accepted drugs. Potential abuse is less than that for schedules I and II. May cause dependence. Labeled C-III.
IV	phenobarbital, benzodiazepines (diazepam, oxazepam, lorazepam, chlordiazepoxide), chloral hydrate, meprobamate	Medically accepted drugs. May cause dependence. Labeled C-IV.
V	opioid-controlled substances for diarrhea and cough (e.g., codeine in cough preparations)	Medically accepted drugs. Very limited potential for dependence. Labeled C-V.

C, Control; *LSD*, lysergic acid diethylamide.

1978: Drug Regulation Reform Act

This reform act shortened the time in which new drugs could be developed and marketed.

1992: Drug Relations Act

The regulations were changed to increase the approval rate of drugs used to treat acquired immunodeficiency syndrome (AIDS) and cancer. The pharmaceutical companies pay a user fee at the time they file the application for the new drug. The fee is for the FDA drug approval process.

1997: The Food and Drug Administration Modernization Act

There are five provisions in this act, including the following: (1) review and use of new drugs is accelerated; (2) drugs can be tested in children before marketing; (3) clinical trial data are necessary for experimental drug use for serious or life-threatening health conditions; (4) drug companies are required to give information on "off-label" drugs (non-FDA approved drugs) and their uses and costs; and (5) drug companies that plan to discontinue drugs must inform health professionals and clients at least 6 months before stopping drug production.

2003: Health Insurance Portability and Accountability Act (HIPAA)

This act sets the standards for the privacy of individually identifiable health information as of 2003. This rule gives clients more control over their health information, including boundaries on the use and release of health records. See *http://hhs.Gov/admnsimp* for a summary.

Implications of HIPAA related to the individual's therapeutic regimen includes limitation on access to information from the pharmacy. For example, the client history can be released only to the client. In addition, the pharmacist must provide a private area for consultation with the client and have all clients sign a statement that they have received a copy of the privacy statement.

2003: Pediatric Research Equity Act

The FDA is authorized to require testing of drugs and biologic products for safety and effectiveness in children by drug manufacturers. One must not assume that children are small adults.

2003: Medicare Prescription Drug Improvement and Modernization Act (MMA)

The Medicare Prescription Drug Improvement and Modernization Act serves to provide financial assistance to seniors to purchase needed prescription medications. The full effect of this benefit will not be in place until January 1, 2006; however, currently pharmaceutical- and insurance-company-sponsored discount cards are available for about $30 per month and result in savings of 10% to 15%. According to the MMA, in 2006 the client is responsible for a monthly premium of $35 and a $250 annual deductible. This benefit will pay 75% of the total cost of the prescription drugs, up to a maximum of $2250. There is no drug coverage between $2250 and $5100; Medicare will pay 95% of the drug costs beyond $5100. Between $2250 and $5100, the senior will pay full price for the drugs. Medicare seniors may have supplemental insurance coverage for prescription medications; they must choose whether to continue this policy or sign up for the Medicare drug benefit. Double coverage is not an option.

Nurse Practice Acts

Every state has its own laws regarding drug administration by nurses. Generally, nurses cannot prescribe or administer drugs without a health care provider's order, but state laws vary. A practicing nurse should request a copy and be knowledgeable about the nurse practice act in the state in which she or he is licensed. In some states, a nurse who administers a drug without a physician's order is in violation of the nurse practice act and could have her or his license revoked.

In a civil court, the nurse can be prosecuted for giving the wrong drug or dosage, omitting a drug dose, or giving the drug by the wrong route. The legal terms for these offenses are the following:
- *Misfeasance.* Negligence; giving the wrong drug or drug dose that results in the client's death
- *Nonfeasance.* Omission; omitting a drug dose that results in the client's death
- *Malfeasance.* Giving the correct drug but by the wrong route that results in the client's death

Canadian Drug Regulation

In Canada the Health Protection Branch, Department of National Health and Welfare, is responsible for the administration of the two acts that are the foundation of the national drug laws. The manufacture, distribution, and sale of drugs (except narcotics) are controlled by the Canadian Food and Drug Act, amended in 1953. The manufacture, distribution, and sale of narcotic drugs are controlled by the 1961 Narcotics Control Act. Like the U.S. Controlled Substances Act, the Canadian act requires prescriptions and strict record keeping for all narcotics.

Drugs sold in Canada are assigned to one of the following schedules:
1. *Schedule F.* All prescription drugs (approximately 350) are available only with a prescription (written or verbal); thus these drugs have essentially no potential for abuse.
2. *Schedule G.* Fourteen drugs in this group require written or verbal prescription, and refills require a written prescription. These drugs have a moderate potential for abuse and must have a "G" on the label, similar to schedule III drugs in the United States.
3. *Schedule H.* These drugs have no recognized medical use and are potentially dangerous, similar to schedule I

drugs in the United States. Their use is limited primarily to specialized medical research.

4. *Narcotics.* These drugs are dispensed only with written prescription, and an "N" must appear on all advertisements and labels. Low-dose codeine (20 mg/30 ml and 8-mg tablets) is an exception and can be sold only by a pharmacist. Two additional medicinal ingredients, caffeine and acetylsalicylic acid, must be part of this codeine preparation.

Nonprescription drugs (over-the-counter [OTC] preparations) are administered by the Pharmacy Acts of the respective Canadian provinces, which identify the place and conditions of sale. These drugs are assigned to one of three categories:

1. *General proprietary.* These drugs are for treatment of self-limiting minor illness, injury, or discomfort. The packaging information is considered adequate, and the drug can be administered without consultation with a health care provider. These drugs can be purchased at any store.

2. *Availability only through pharmacies.* After consultation and approval by a health care provider, drugs designed to treat minor, self-limiting conditions are available through a pharmacy. Examples are cold remedies and laxatives that can be purchased OTC.

3. *Recommendation of a health care provider.* This category requires recommendation by a health care provider. Examples include nitroglycerin, insulin, and muscle relaxants.

To address the proliferation of a variety of provincial schedules and regulations, the Health Protection Branch has proposed to "harmonize" regulations nationwide by creating a three-schedule system:

Schedule I: All prescription drugs (schedules F and G and narcotics)
Schedule II: Nonprescription, pharmacist-monitored drugs
Schedule III: Nonprescription drugs with no restrictions placed on location of sale

The initial harmonizing work is the development of specific criteria to identify the amount of professional involvement required for the sale and use of drug preparations. The initiation of schedule II presents special challenges.

In Canada the therapeutic and toxic levels are monitored according to International System (SI) of units; this is also true in many European countries. The mole (mol) was adopted to express drug concentration in body fluid in molar units, such as millimoles per liter (mmol/L), instead of the traditional expression of mass units, milligrams per liter (mg/L). Some institutions in the United States use the SI units; however, the traditional use of mass units in the United States continues.

Initiatives to Combat Drug Counterfeiting

The numbers of counterfeit and adulterated prescription drugs are on the rise. Contributing reasons for this are that counterfeiting has features of a "perfect crime" (medicine taken and evidence is gone) and lack of mandatory reporting of counterfeit incidents. The FDA and consumer groups are working on strategies to combat this problem, including tougher oversight of distributors, a rapid alert system, and better-informed consumers. The role of the nurse is critical in consumer education. Both the nurse and the client must be ever vigilant. Strategies include being alert to slight variations in packaging or labeling (e.g., color, package seal); advising clients to report any differences in taste or in the appearance of drug or packaging; noting any unexpected side effects; buying drugs from a reputable source. Reputable on-line pharmacies have an approval seal—VIPPS—Verified Internet Pharmacy Practice Site. If any suspicion of counterfeit arises, the nurse should contact the FDA at *www.fda.gov/medwatch* or call (800) FDA-1088.

Drug Names

Each drug may have several names. The **chemical name** describes the drug's chemical structure. The **generic name** is the official or nonproprietary name for the drug. This name is not owned by any pharmaceutical (drug) company and is universally accepted. Most drugs are ordered by their generic name. The **brand (trade) name,** also known as the *proprietary name,* is chosen by the drug company and is usually a registered trademark owned by that specific manufacturer. Drug companies market a compound using their given name (brand name). For example, Narcen is the brand (proprietary) name registered with the manufacturer, and naloxone HCl is the generic name recognized by the USP.

There are pros and cons to using generic drugs (Figure 5–1). Today, generic drugs must be approved by the FDA before they can be marketed. If the generic drug is found to be bioequivalent to the brand or trade drug, then the generic drug is considered to be therapeutically equivalent and is given an "A" rating. If the peak serum concentration (C_{max}) and the plasma-concentration curve (AUC) of the generic drug fall within 80% to 125% of the brand drug, it is considered equivalent to the brand drug. Generic approved drugs can be checked on the Internet at www.fda.gov/cder/ob/default.htm. The FDA also publishes a list of approved generic drugs that are bioequiva-

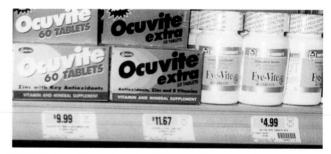

FIGURE 5–1 There is a $5 difference between the brand-name and generic-name vitamins.

lent to brand-name drugs. Generic drugs are usually cheaper and have the same active ingredients as brand-name, or trade-name, drugs. However, some generic drugs have inert fillers and binders that may result in variations of drug effectiveness. Generic drugs are less expensive because manufacturers do not have to do extensive testing because these drugs were clinically tested for safety and efficacy by the pharmaceutical company that first formulated the drug. The health care provider and client must exercise care in choosing generic drugs because there may be some variation in the action of or response to them. Brand-name drugs are preferred when ordering anticonvulsants for seizures, anticoagulants (e.g., Coumadin), medication for congestive heart failure (e.g., Lanoxin), and aspirin when giving large doses for rheumatoid arthritis. A study showed that 23 seizure-free epileptic clients who switched to the generic drug experienced renewed seizure activity. The nurse should check with the health care provider or pharmacist when generic drugs are prescribed. The health care provider must note on the prescription (computerized or paper) whether the pharmacist may substitute the generic drug when the brand name is prescribed.

Throughout this text, both generic and brand names are given for drugs. Because many brand names may exist for a single generic name, the generic name is given *first* in lower-case letters, followed by the most commonly used brand name in parentheses. With generic drugs, the name may be long and difficult to pronounce. Brand names always begin with a capital letter. An example of a generic and brand-name drug listing is "furosemide (Lasix)."

Drug Resources

There are many resource reference books on drugs, including nursing texts that identify related nursing interventions and areas for health teaching.

The *American Hospital Formulary Services (AHFS)*, *Physicians' Desk Reference (PDR)*, *Drug Facts and Comparisons (F & C)*, and the *United States Pharmacopeia—Drug Information (USP-DI)* are resources that provide valuable information for approved drugs. The method for presentation of the drugs varies.

American Hospital Formulary Service (AHFS) Drug Information is published yearly by the American Society of Health-System Pharmacists in Bethesda, Maryland. It is an excellent reference that provides accurate and complete drug information on nearly all prescription drugs marketed in the United States. This reference text contains drugs listed according to therapeutic drug classification. The information given for each drug includes chemistry and stability, pharmacologic actions, pharmacokinetics, uses, cautions per body system, precautions, contraindications, acute toxicity, drug interactions, dosage and administration, and preparations.

This reference book is updated yearly and with monthly supplements. The supplementary editions contain new marketed drugs with their dosage forms and strengths, uses, and cautions. This text is unbiased in that it does not contain information about the drug from only a pharmaceutical company. Additionally, many drug handbooks are available as quick drug references. Most of these include nursing implications. When more information is needed about a drug, the *PDR* or the *AHFS* is frequently suggested.

The *Physicians' Desk Reference (PDR)* lists several thousand drugs with complete drug information given by pharmaceutical companies. The *PDR* is published yearly. It contains seven sections, two of which are the most useful to nurses: the second (pink) section, which is the drug name index; and the sixth (white) section, which gives information about the drugs. The *PDR* is a useful drug resource, but it does not provide complete pharmacologic and therapeutic information and does not include nursing interventions. The drug information is reprinted drug package inserts supplied by pharmaceutical companies, which pay to have their drugs listed in the *PDR*.

Drug Facts and Comparisons (F & C) contains information on almost all drugs marketed in the United States. The reference consists of drug actions, indications, warnings and precautions, dosage and route for administration, adverse reactions, client information, overdosage, drug interactions, contraindications, and comparison charts and tables.

The *United States Pharmacopeia—Drug Information (USP-DI)* is a three-volume set that is available in most hospitals and pharmacies. Monthly supplements are available. Volumes IA and IB provide drug information for the health care provider. The sections in these volumes include pharmacology, precautions to consider, side and adverse effects, client consultation, general dosing information, and dosage forms. Volume II gives drug information for the client. It is a client-oriented volume that explains information in an understandable way for the client. The sections included in Volume II are administration of drug, drug effects, indications, adverse reactions, dosage guidelines, and what to do for missed doses.

The Medical Letter on drugs and therapeutics is published biweekly by the Medical Letter, Inc., in New Rochelle, New York. This is a nonprofit publication for physicians, nurse practitioners, and other health professionals. These biweekly issues cover one of two themes, such as (1) drugs for the treatment of disease entities (e.g., human immunodeficiency virus [HIV], peptic ulcers) or (2) two to four new drugs that have been approved by the FDA. The following information is included with each new drug: pharmacokinetics, clinical studies, dosage, adverse effects, interactions, and a conclusion.

Prescriber's Letter is published monthly by the Therapeutic Research Center in Stockton, California, and addresses new FDA-approved drugs, the various uses of older drugs, and FDA warnings. This is primarily a newsletter.

The *Handbook on Injectable Drugs* by Lawrence A. Trissel is published by the American Society of Hospital Pharmacists. It is an excellent reference for injectable medications and lists drug compatibility with other drugs, base fluids, and drugs available in large-volume parenterals. Also, it includes the pH of each drug and gives some dosing administration guidelines.

Numerous nursing drug reference books are updated yearly. Examples include the *Saunders' Nursing Drug Handbook* (W.B. Saunders), *Nursing Drug Guide* (Prentice Hall), and *NDR* (Delmar).

The Internet is a source for drug information. Drug-related Internet sites are listed in Appendix I. Drug information can be posted by anyone, so the information may not always be accurate and comprehensive.

Food and Drug Administration Pregnancy Categories

The FDA developed a classification system related to the effects of drugs on the unborn child (fetus). In the drug literature and drug reference books, a pregnancy category is indicated for most drugs. Categories A and B are considered to be within safe limits for drug use in pregnancy, especially in the first trimester. Table 5–2 lists the FDA pregnancy categories and describes each category's effect on the fetus.

Poison Control Centers

Poison control centers (PCCs) are present in almost all cities. The website is *www.nlu.edu/aapcc*. Telephone numbers for PCCs are listed in the front pages of most telephone books. The centers provide information about the drug or toxic chemical compounds and the immediate action that should be taken to prevent injury or death. Client education about PCCs is a function of the nurse.

Each year, PCCs respond to more than 1.5 million cases related to a possible ingested drug or chemical toxic compound. About 90% of these cases are in children younger than 3 years and occur at home. Iron tablets, chocolate-covered laxatives, flavored acetaminophen, and flavored liquid medicines are common drugs that children ingest; in large doses they can be toxic to the child. Also, the consumption of most household cleaning chemicals and insecticides is extremely toxic to children.

The mortality rate from poisoning in the United States is about 12,000 deaths per year, of which 50% are from accidental causes and 50% are from suicides. Immediate reporting of an excess drug or chemical ingestion followed by a proper action may prevent a death or more serious injury from the toxic agent.

Ethical Considerations

Ethical values related to drug administration and client care are an ongoing consideration for nurses. Nurses should be morally and ethically responsible for the client's

Table 5–2

FDA Pregnancy Categories

Pregnancy Category	Description
A	No risk to fetus. Studies have not shown evidence of fetal harm.
B	No risk in animal studies, and well-controlled studies in pregnant women are not available. It is assumed there is little to no risk in pregnant women.
C	Animal studies indicate a risk to the fetus. Controlled studies on pregnant women are not available. Risk versus benefit of the drug must be determined.
D	A risk to the human fetus has been proved. Risk versus benefit of the drug must be determined. It could be used in life-threatening conditions.
X	A risk to the human fetus has been proved. Risk outweighs the benefit, and drug should be avoided during pregnancy.

FDA, Food and Drug Administration.

BOX 5–1

American Nurses Association Code of Ethics for Nurses

1. The nurse, in all professional relationships, practices with compassion and respect for the inherent dignity, worth, and uniqueness of every individual, unrestricted by considerations of social or economic status, personal attributes, or the nature of health problems.
2. The nurse's primary commitment is to the patient, whether an individual, family, group, or community.
3. The nurse promotes, advocates for, and strives to protect the health, safety, and rights of the patient.
4. The nurse is responsible and accountable for individual nursing practice and determines the appropriate delegation of tasks consistent with the nurse's obligation to provide optimum patient care.
5. The nurse owes the same duties to self as to others, including the responsibility to preserve integrity and safety, to maintain competence, and to continue personal and professional growth.
6. The nurse participates in establishing, maintaining, and improving health care environments and conditions of employment conducive to the provision of quality health care and consistent with the values of the profession through individual and collective action.
7. The nurse participates in the advancement of the profession through contributions to practice, education, administration, and knowledge development.
8. The nurse collaborates with other health professionals and the public in promoting community, national, and international efforts to meet health needs.
9. The profession of nursing, as represented by associations and their members, is responsible for articulating nursing values, for maintaining the integrity of the profession and its practice, and for shaping social policy.

From American Nurses Association, Washington, DC (revised 2001). Available at *www.nursingworld.org/ethics/chcode.htm*.

total care. Drug administration should be correctly prepared and administered.

The American Nurses Association (ANA) and the Canadian Nurses Association (CNA) have a "Code of Ethics for Nurses." Both the ANA and CNA have developed similar standards for ethical practice in nursing. Box 5–1 lists the nine standards of the ANA Code of Ethics for Nurses.

Nurses need to respect the rights, dignity, and wishes of clients. Clients have the right to know about their drugs, drug actions, and any side effects. They have the right to refuse drugs even after a thorough explanation of the drugs and desired effects are given. According to the ANA Code of Ethics for Nurses, the nurse safeguards client's rights, safety, dignity, and health care. The nurse seeks consultation, accepts responsibility, and demonstrates competency in nursing care. The nurse's primary obligation is to the client.

International Issues

Two examples of international issues are the reduced prices of many drugs available to be bought directly from Canada and the availability of expensive drugs for AIDS sufferers in Africa. First, many drugs can be bought from Canada at a reduced rate compared with those in the United States.

There are claims that drugs available on the Canadian websites may be counterfeit drugs from unregulated sources. The second issue is that the cost of AIDS drugs is prohibitive for impoverished individuals in Africa. Recently there has been a change in the World Trade Organization (WTO) accord that now permits manufacture of the generic version of these (without regard to patents) in emergency situations, such as for people with AIDS in Africa.

WEBSITES

For further information on *The Drug Approval Process,* visit these Internet resources:

Poison Control Centers: *www.nlu.edu/aapcc*

Internet Drug Index: *www.rxlist.com*

American Nurses Association: *www.ana.org*

Food and Drug Administration: *www.fda.gov/medwatch*

Nursing Ethics Resources: *www.nursingethics.ca/*

National Council of State Boards of Nursing: *www.ncsbn.org*

Study Questions

1. What are the provisions in the Food, Drug, and Cosmetic Act of 1938? What additional safeguards are included in the Durham-Humphrey amendment of 1952 and the Kefauver-Harris amendment of 1962?

2. Which controlled substance has the higher potential for drug abuse, controlled substance schedule II or schedule IV? Explain.

3. Explain how the 1978 and 1992 drug regulation acts differ.

4. Name three of the five provisions of the Food and Drug Administration Modernization Act of 1997.

5. The Canadian Food and Drug Act of 1953 has identified three schedules for drug regulation. How does schedule F differ from schedule G?

6. Describe the implications of the Pediatric Research Equity Act of 2003.

7. List at least three factors that might alert the client or nurse that a drug is counterfeit or adulterated.

8. What are the implications of HIPAA related to drug prescriptions?

9. What are the characteristics of the chemical name, generic name, and brand or trade name of a drug?

10. What are the titles of two drug resource books that are helpful in nursing practice?

11. Your client is taking a drug that is in pregnancy category B. Would this drug be safe? Explain.

12. Ethical values toward clients is a nursing responsibility. What are some examples of nursing considerations related to ethical responsibilities of the nurse according to the ANA Code of Ethics for Nurses?

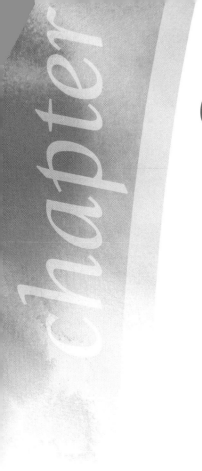

6 Transcultural and Genetic Considerations

LARRY D. PURNELL

ELECTRONIC RESOURCES

evolve

Additional information can be found on the companion website at *http://evolve.elsevier.com/KeeHayes/pharmacology/* or on the companion CD-ROM, which includes:
- *NCLEX-style examination review questions*
- *Pharmacology animations*
- *Medication error and IV therapy checklists*
- *Medication calculation problems*
- *Electronic calculators*

OUTLINE

OBJECTIVES

- Recognize verbal and nonverbal communication practices used by different ethnocultural individuals and groups.
- Assess clients in the context of biocultural ecology.
- Collaborate with traditional and folk practitioners.
- Assess clients for use of traditional and folk therapies.
- Increase the client's compliance with prescriptive therapies.

TERMS

African Americans
American Indians
Amish
Asians/Pacific Islanders
biocultural ecology

ethnocultural
European Americans
genetic
hereditary
Hispanics

Jewish Americans
racial
spatial distancing
temporality

Introduction

Racial, hereditary, and **genetic** influences have a profound effect on the way clients metabolize drugs and experience and tolerate side effects of medications (Matthews, 1995; Matthews, 1997; Soo-Jin Lee, Mountain, & Koenig, 2001; Twedell, 2003). Differences in the pharmacokinetics of drugs support processes that are biologically or chemically mediated. These processes are related to the bioavailability of drugs, protein binding, volume distribution, hepatic metabolism, and renal tubular absorption (Johnson, 1997). Factors affecting the efficacy and compliance with drug therapy include environment and culture (Finn, 1994). **Ethnocultural** perceptions and beliefs of illness and disease play an important role in the client's compliance with and understanding of medical treatment and drug therapy (Hines, 2000; Levy, 1993).

Additionally, age, diurnal rhythms, gender, dietary practices, living conditions, and high-risk behaviors affect drug metabolism, efficacy, and client compliance. To meet the needs of diverse ethnic and cultural groups, health care professionals need to have an understanding of the variables that influence compliance with medications, differences in physiologic responses to medications, and the client's beliefs regarding medication (Purnell, 2003a).

Understanding clients' beliefs related to their desire and willingness to take medications can improve the health care provider's cultural competence in designing strategies to increase compliance among diverse ethnocultural populations (Katz, 2004; Levy, 1995). This is especially important when the cultural beliefs of the nurse are different than or in conflict with the cultural beliefs of the client, family, or group.

This chapter provides a brief overview of the cultural characteristics of the following groups: **African Americans, American Indians, Amish, Asians/Pacific Islanders, Hispanics, Jewish Americans,** and **European Americans.**

The Purnell Model for Cultural Competence

This chapter uses selected domains and concepts from the Purnell Model for Cultural Competence to provide essential information in the context of ethnic, racial, and cultural responses to medication administration and compliance. The Purnell Model for Cultural Competence (Figure 6–1) is a circle with an outlying rim that represents global society, a second rim that represents community, a third rim that represents family, and an inner rim that represents the person; these are the macro aspects of the model.

The interior of the circle is divided into 12 pie-shaped wedges that depict cultural domains and their concepts. The domains have bidirectional arrows indicating that each domain relates to and is affected by all other domains; these are the micro aspects of the model.

The center of the model is empty and represents unknown aspects about the cultural group. Along the bottom of the model is an erose (jagged) line that represents the nonlinear concept of cultural competence. This nonlinear line represents the degree of cultural competence attained by the health care provider or organization. Culturally competent nursing care requires that providers understand their culture and the client's culture and negotiate and integrate folk practices with allopathic care.

The Domains of Culture

Overview/Heritage

Overview/heritage includes concepts related to origins, topography, economics, and education. Racial origin affects responses to some drugs; for example, Asian Americans have increased sensitivity to beta-blockers, whereas African Americans respond better to monotherapy for hypertension than do their European-American cohort groups (Jamerson & DeQuattro, 1996; Levy, 1993). Topography, the landscape and surface configuration of terrain, may affect clients physiologically. For example, clients coming from high-altitude mountainous climates normally have increased red blood cell counts because of the lowered oxygen tension in the high-altitude climate. Clients coming from low-lying, swampy terrain are at an increased risk for dengue fever, malaria, and sickle cell anemia. The client's socioeconomic status has an impact on his or her ability to afford expensive prescription drugs. In some cases, the nurse can recommend a generic equivalent or other acceptable drug that is more affordable. The educational status of clients may determine how the nurse provides information to the client. For clients who are unable to read or do not have English-language skills, the nurse may need to devise pictures to teach medication schedules. Directions should be provided to clients in their preferred language and at a level they can understand.

Communication

Communication includes concepts related to language, dialect, contextual use of the language, volume, and tone. **Spatial distancing,** touch, use of eye contact, preferred greetings, temporality, time, and format for names are also key concepts to understand for the nurse who wishes to be effective in the assessment and counsel of clients.

Language

Given that 16% (Minnesota) to 62.9% (California) of people speak another language besides English at home (Languages Spoken at Home, 2000), there are increased challenges for nurses to teach clients about their medication schedules and the side effects of medications. Because dialects may differ significantly, the nurse should attempt to identify a dialect-specific interpreter. Because clients may be able to read English but not speak or understand it, detailed written instructions are helpful.

The nurse needs to be aware of the contextual use of languages to better understand and communicate with culturally diverse clients. English and the Romance languages—Italian, Spanish, French, Portuguese, and Romanian—are

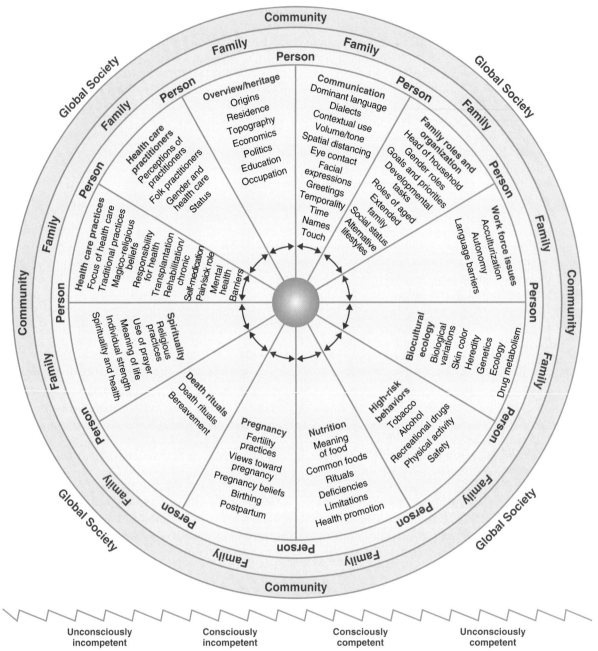

FIGURE 6–1 The Purnell Model for Cultural Competence. (Courtesy Larry Purnell, Newark, Del.)

low-contexted languages with the majority of the message in the explicit verbal mode. In low-contextual languages, many words are used to express a thought, and verbal skills are considered important. People may be uncomfortable with silence. However, in high-contexted languages, such as American Indian dialects, Chinese, and Vietnamese, the majority of the message is in the nonverbal mode. Few words are used to convey thoughts. Silence is considered important. In high-contexted languages, to interrupt someone or give a hasty response may be considered rude.

Not all languages have the numerous verb tenses that occur in the English language. For example, Finnish and Chinese only have the present tense; one must interpret the statement within its context. For example, the person may say, "I go to doctor today, I go to doctor tomorrow," or "I go to doctor yesterday." The nurse must give very precise instructions, such as "take one pill at 9 PM." Because there is no future tense, the nurse should not say, "You will/should take one pill at bedtime." Because the English language is the only language that uses contractions such as "don't" or "can't," the nurse must say "do not" or "cannot" to prevent confusion and improve understanding among culturally diverse clients.

Paralanguage

Some cultural groups, such as African Americans, European Americans, and Arabs, speak in a voice volume that may carry to those nearby. Asians and American Indians usually speak in a lower-volume voice. Because clients speak in a loud voice volume does not mean that they are angry, nor does speaking in a soft voice tone indicate that the person is reticent or not interested in the discussion. Likewise, the use of eye contact may vary among cultural groups and individuals. In general, European Americans maintain eye contact without staring when conversing, which signals that the person is listening. Arabs and Greeks usually maintain intense eye contact in conversations, which should not be interpreted as aggression. Because many Asians/Pacific Islanders do not maintain eye contact with people in a perceived higher social status, this does not mean that they are not interested or not listening to the conversation. They are demonstrating respect for the person's status.

Spatial Distancing

The physical proximity between people conversing varies between and among cultural groups. Most European Americans maintain approximately 18 to 24 inches when engaged in conversation with the health care provider. However, traditional Germans may see this as a violation of personal space, preferring to stand at a distance greater than 2 feet (Steckler, 2003). Traditional Arabs and some Hispanics may stand very close to each other with less than 18 inches between them. Although the nurse may be uncomfortable with this close personal space, he or she should not take offense but should accept it as a cultural variation.

Temporality

Temporality, whether the client stresses a past, present, or future orientation, needs to be considered when the nurse cares for clients from diverse cultures. For example, many Portuguese, Haitians, and Hispanics are primarily present oriented; whatever occurs at the moment is more important than what may occur later. With present-oriented clients, the nurse may need to take extra time and stress the importance of taking the medication. Future-oriented individuals are more likely to comply with prescription regimens.

Client orientation to clock time may also affect how the nurse perceives them. Mexican Americans (Zoucha & Purnell, 2003) and Brazilians (Purnell, 2003b) have a more relaxed perception of time than do European Americans and the dominant U.S. health care system. For Mexican Americans and American Indians (Still & Hodgins, 1998), appointments are flexible, adherence to medication schedules is more fluid, and clients expect to be seen regardless of how late they arrive. If the provider does not see them, it may be interpreted as a noncaring behavior. However, in the dominant European American health care system, a client with an appointment for 10 AM is expected to arrive before that time to ensure that he or she is ready for the appointment. For a client with a present-orientation that stresses flexibility, the nurse may need to adjust medication schedules to be congruent with the client's lifestyle.

Greetings

Culturally appropriate greetings demonstrate respect and enhance the therapeutic relationship between the nurse and client. The more informal style practiced by many Americans may not be acceptable to all cultural groups. Many traditional Asians, Hispanics, and Germans prefer to be addressed formally, using Mr., Mrs., Miss, or their title. To address them informally may be perceived as insolence or disrespectful behavior. Therefore the nurse should always greet the client formally until told otherwise.

The format for names may cause confusion for nurses unfamiliar with diverse cultures. Among Hispanics, extended family names are common and may include a woman's married name and the last names of both parents. For example, Rosa Nunez Arosemina would indicate a single woman whose father's last name is Nunez and whose mother's maiden name is Arosemina. If Rosa marries Jorge Sanchez, her complete name becomes Senora (depicting a married woman) Rosa Sanchez de Nunez Arosemina. She would be called Mrs. Sanchez in a formal setting and Rosa by her family and close friends. The traditional Korean woman does not take her husband's last name when she marries. However, because many Koreans know this causes confusion for health care providers in the United States, many are beginning to take their husband's name (Purnell & Kim, 2003). Thus the nurse needs to specifically ask the client his or her family name and given name.

Family Organization

Family organization with the concepts of head of household and gender roles must be considered when the nurse assesses and intervenes with clients. The nurse must recognize that not all individuals adhere to the U.S. value of egalitarian decision making between men and women. Among traditional Central American Indian groups, men are expected to provide for their families in terms of outside resources and protect them from harm. When a family travels from its village, the procession looks something like this: The husband (or other adult male) leads the way, followed by the children who are old enough to walk. An older child may carry a smaller child. Bringing up the rear is the wife, who may be pregnant or breastfeeding an infant. In this order, the wife can watch all of the children and the man is in a better position to protect the family from harm.

Women take care of the home and provide the majority of child care. Men work at a distance from the house or sometimes in another village, mixing more with the outside world. Therefore they have a greater sphere of knowledge from which to make decisions. In cultures in which men are expected to make most decisions, the nurse is expected to direct questions to the man, even though the woman may provide the answers with the man being the spokesperson, a culturally prescribed role. When traditional women must work outside the home, family dynamics change. Men feel guilt for being unable to provide for their families, and women feel they are abandoning their children because they are working, especially if extended family members are not available for childcare.

Biocultural Ecology

Biocultural ecology includes concepts related to biologic variations, heredity, genetics, endemics, and drug metabolism. To assess for oxygenation and cyanosis in dark-skinned people, the nurse must examine the sclera, conjunctiva, buccal mucosa, tongue, lips, nail beds, palms, and soles of the feet rather than relying on skin tone. Jaundice can be determined in dark-skinned people by examining the sclera for a yellow pigmentation.

Genetic background can affect a client's response to drugs. For example, African Americans have high rates of hypertension and respond better to monotherapy because their hypertension is usually related to volume expansion, decreased renin, and increased intracellular concentration of sodium and calcium (Levy, 1993). For people of Greek and Chinese Heritage with glucose-6-phosphate dehydrogenase deficiency, life-threatening hemolytic crises may occur if oxidating drugs such as quinine and chloramphenicol are prescribed (Purnell & Papadopoulos, 2003; Wang, 2003). Many Asians/Pacific Islanders experience increased side effects of alcohol with facial flushing, tachycardia, and palpitations (Pacquiao, 2003; Purnell & Kim, 2003; Wang, 2003).

High-Risk Behaviors

The domain *high-risk behaviors* includes the use of tobacco, alcohol, safe sex practices, and recreational drugs. Tobacco use causes more rapid elimination of medicines from the body; thus the drug does not have its full therapeutic effect. Alcohol interferes with some psychotropic medications and enhances the effects of analgesics. Recreational use of drugs such as marijuana, antihistamine combinations, and cocaine may potentiate the effects of medications, resulting in increased side effects, an enhanced therapeutic response, or an overdose.

Nutrition

The domain *nutrition* includes concepts related to common foods and food rituals, limitations in obtaining nutritious foods, enzyme deficiencies, and how foods are used for health promotion and wellness. Each ethnocultural group has preferred foods and rituals that are passed on through the generations. Traditional Appalachian people frequently use extra lard to prepare fried foods. The diets of many Asians/Pacific Islanders are high in sodium. Some African Americans use fatback to add extra flavor to vegetables. The proportion of fats, carbohydrates, and proteins may have an effect on how some drugs are absorbed or metabolized. Dietary consideration must be taken into account when prescriptions are given. Newer immigrants may have difficulty finding preferred native foods and may not be aware of which foods to substitute to provide a nutritious diet. Asians/Pacific Islanders, Hispanics, and African Americans have high incidences of lactose intolerance, resulting in maldigestion and bloating, although the condition is rare in children.

All societies have "prescriptions" for what is considered a healthy diet, although these prescriptions have great variability within each ethnocultural group. Among conservative Jews, milk and meat should not be eaten at the same meal. Among Haitians (Colin & Paperwalla, 2003), some Hispanics/Latinos (Zoucha & Purnell, 2003; Purnell, 2003c), Vietnamese (Nowak, 2003), Greeks and Greek Cypriots (Purnell & Papadopoulos, 2003), and Iranians

(Hafizi & Lipson, 2003), foods are classified as "hot" or "cold" and a balance of these foods must be consumed at each meal or illness may result. Drugs are also classified as hot or cold. Antibiotics are considered hot and therefore should not be taken with cold water because their effect would be negated; use room temperature or tap water instead. Because hot and cold foods and conditions vary within each group, the nurse must specifically ask clients their food preferences and determine whether the diet interferes with drug absorption or interactions.

Spirituality

Spirituality includes concepts related to religious preference, meaning of life, and individual sources of strength. Clients' religious practices may prescribe what is acceptable in terms of diet (e.g., Islamic and orthodox Jewish), acceptability for genetic counseling, and use and choice of contraceptive methods. Muslims who celebrate the holiday Ramadan fast from sunup to sundown. Fasting also includes not taking medications. However, in times of illness, clients are permitted to take their prescribed medications, although the more devout may be reluctant to do so. The nurse can improve medication compliance by working with the client to determine an acceptable medication schedule during religious holidays. Because clients may not eat on a normal daytime schedule, insulin administration must be adjusted accordingly.

Meaning of Life

Among people of Mexican, Guatemalan, and Panamanian ancestry, family is usually the most important aspect of their lives and gives meaning to life (Purnell, 1998; Purnell, 2000; Zoucha & Purnell, 2003). Thus it can be especially important to include the family in teaching strategies. Illness is a family affair and should be treated accordingly.

Health Care Practices

Health care practices include the focus of health care, traditional medical practices, self-medicating practices, barriers to accessing health care, the sick role, and perceptions of mental illness. The current focus of health care in the United States is undergoing a paradigm shift from acute care to one of wellness with health promotion and maintenance and disease and illness prevention. Whereas this concept is congruent with many ethnocultural groups, for some, prevention activities are unknown. For example, unacculturated Egyptian Americans may refuse to have Pap smears and mammograms because in Egypt these preventive measures are just beginning to be recognized and promoted (Purnell, 2003d).

Complementary, Alternative, and Traditional Medicine

Many people prefer their traditional medical practices either as complementary to or as an alternative to allopathic medicine (Figure 6–2; Herbal Alert 6–1). Traditional Chinese medicine, Ayurvedic medicine, herbal and naturopathic medicine, and a host of other therapies may be pre-

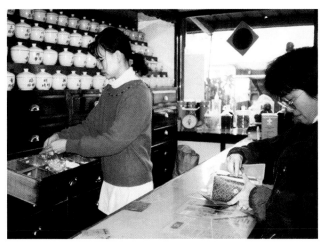

FIGURE 6–2 In some cultures, people may rely on traditional nonprescription drugs.

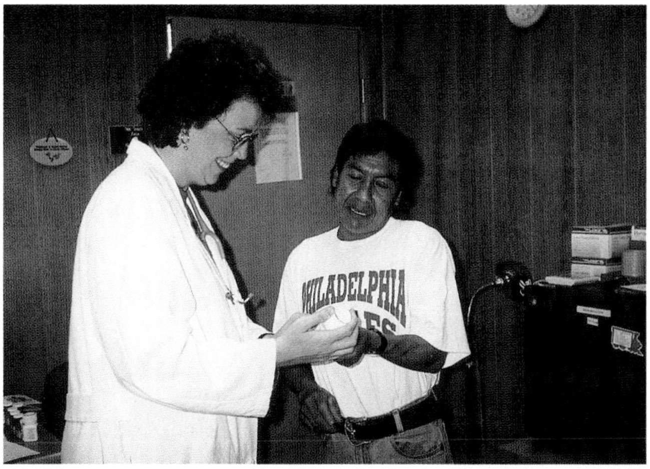

FIGURE 6–3 The nurse needs to ask the client about all medications and remedies he or she takes so that any potential interactions with the prescribed medication regimen can be identified.

HERBAL ALERT 6–1

Gender-Specific Herb Protocols

🌿 Women have traditionally sought substitutes for hormonal replacement therapy, especially if there are adverse side effects. With increased media attention given to natural hormone replacement therapies, more women are using phytoestrogens such as those found in flaxseed, licorice, black cohosh, and soybeans. Health care providers need to query their clients regarding their use of these naturally occurring phytoestrogens because they are contraindicated in women with a history or risk for hormonally mediated cancers and benign tumors.

---

ferred by some or used in conjunction with other therapies. Many ethnic people, accustomed to taking medications for only 2 or 3 days in their home countries, may believe that Western medicine is too strong, is supposed to only relieve symptoms, or has too many side effects. Thus they may stop taking the medication when symptoms disappear.

Self-Medicating Practices

All clients self-medicate to some degree. Many use over-the-counter medications or folk remedies for the initial symptoms of an illness. Additionally, some ethnic groups may have family or friends bring medication that may not be available in the United States from their home country. For example, in Panama and throughout Central America, clients can purchase a wide variety of antibiotics, injectable vitamins, and even intravenous fluids without a prescription. To prevent contraindications in medication administration, the nurse must ask clients in a nonjudgmental manner whether they take any prescription medications, nonprescription medications, or herbal therapies (Figure 6–3).

Sick Role

In some Hispanic and Arabic cultures, clients can enter the sick role without feelings of guilt or attached stigma. Any reason is acceptable for being ill, and the person is relieved of

normal responsibilities (Kulwicki, 2003; Zoucha & Purnell, 2003). However, among German and Polish people, clients may be expected to carry out their obligations unless they are severely ill (From, 2003; Steckler, 2003). This is one area in which the nurse can hasten the client's recovery with culturally appropriate counseling.

Pain

Pain—the primary reason most people see a health professional—is expressed differently among ethnocultural groups. For example, among some Asians/Pacific Islanders, clients are reluctant to express pain because they believe it is God's will or a punishment for past sins (Pacquiao, 2003; Nowak, 2003; Sharts-Hopko, 2003). Among Arabs, clients are expected to express their pain openly and expect immediate relief, preferably through injectable or intravenous medication (Purnell, 2003d).

Mental Illness

Mental illness is a culture-bound phenomenon. What is perceived as a mental illness in one culture may be seen as normal in another; for example, having visions and hallucinations about God is an expected behavior among some Hispanic groups (Dossey, 1998). Although the "evil eye" occurs in numerous cultures, someone from a culture who does not believe in the evil eye may see those who do believe in it as having a mental health problem. Thus nurses must interpret a client's behavior within cultural boundaries.

Health Care Practitioners

The domain *health care practitioners* includes concepts related to the status of health care providers, folk practitioners, and gender and health care. For Arabs and Arab Americans, the most respected health care provider is an experienced middle-aged to elderly male physician with several degrees (Hafizi & Lipson, 2003). Among Appalachian people, foreign-educated physicians may have difficulty being accepted because they are outsiders, not because of their ethnocultural background (Purnell, 2003e). In many Arab countries, nursing is not seen as a desirable profession because it requires contact between the sexes (Kulwicki, 2003).

Folk Practitioners

Many times, folk practitioners are preferred over allopathic educated physicians because treatments are less invasive. Folk practitioners are known to the client. Usually, they do not treat the symptoms of an illness; they remove the cause of the illness. Allopathic physicians can only treat the symptoms.

Gender and Health Care

Islamic women prefer health care providers of the same gender and may refuse treatment from male health care providers. However, the nurse should remind them that the *Koran* sanctions the use of male health care providers if female providers are not available. If only a male is available, physical examination should be performed through one layer of clothes or by the health care provider using gloves to prevent direct skin contact. Most European-American and African-American men and women generally accept care from either gender. More traditional and younger clients may prefer a same-gender provider for intimate care. This should be accommodated whenever possible. Table 6–1 lists characteristics of selected domains for the major cultural groups in the United States.

Nursing Process

Transcultural Considerations

ASSESSMENT

- Assess ethnocultural and racial background.
- Assess length of time away from country of origin.
- Assess travel history, both within the country and outside the country.
- Assess language ability and preferred language for instruction.
- Assess nonverbal communication practices such as spatial distancing, temporality, use of touch, and eye contact.
- Assess high-risk health behaviors.
- Assess preferred foods, preparation practices, and eating patterns.
- Assess for illness and disease patterns commonly found in client's family and cultural group.
- Assess use of traditional and folk practices.
- Assess use of traditional health care practitioners.

PLANNING

- Collaborate with client to reduce high-risk health behaviors.

- Develop a culturally congruent dietary plan that helps the client understand his or her dietary practices in relation to drug interactions.

NURSING INTERVENTIONS

- Incorporate nonharmful traditional and folk practices with biomedical prescriptions.
- Collaborate with traditional and folk practitioners.
- Maintain culturally congruent communication practices to develop a trusting relationship with the client and family.
- Conduct a nutritional assessment to determine potential for drug-food interactions.
- Incorporate cultural beliefs and practices into the plan of care.

Client Teaching

- Involve family in teaching about prescriptive therapies.
- Provide explanation for all prescriptions, treatments, and procedures.
- Provide written instruction (or videos) in the client's preferred language.

EVALUATION

- Client correctly demonstrates understanding of prescriptive therapies and treatments.
- Client is compliant with prescriptive therapies of biomedical health care practitioners.
- Family members are involved in client's overall health plan.
- Client eliminates or decreases high-risk health behaviors.
- Client selects food choices congruent with prescriptive therapies.

WEBSITES

For further information on *Transcultural and Genetic Considerations,* visit these Internet resources:

NIH Office of Dietary Supplements: *http://dietary supplements.info.nih.gov/*

Medical Herbalism: A journal for the clinical practitioner; Adverse Effects of Herbs: *http://medherb.com/ADVERSE.HTM*

Herb clinic and herb organizations: *http://www. medical.com.hk/english_site/doctor_site/herbs_clinics/ herbsclinic_m.htm*

List of herbal remedies and formulas for home remedies: *http://www.valeredenet.com*

Health Care Practices and Compliance in Various Cultural Groups

Cultural Group	Communications	Biocultural Ecology	Health Care Practices	Nutrition	Promoting Strategies for Compliance
African Americans	Dominant language is English, with dialects such as Black English, Gullah, and Pidgin. Most are dynamic and expressive with verbal and nonverbal communications. Usually comfortable with close personal space. Some older adults may avoid direct eye contact with white health care providers. Maintaining intense eye contact may be interpreted as a sign of aggression.	To assess jaundice, cyanosis, and pallor, inspect the sclera, palms of the hands, and soles of the feet. May need to feel for rashes. Less responsive than white ethnic groups to beta blockers and more responsive to monotherapy and ACE inhibitors than are white ethnic groups. Experience high rates of side effects and toxicity with psychotropic and antidepressant medications. High incidence of lactose intolerance.	Many delay seeking health care because of financial limitations and distrust in the formal medical establishment because of past inequities. Health care may be sought from family members and older community female leaders before professional health care providers.	Food, a symbol of health and wealth, is used to celebrate special events. Being overweight, compared with the dominant U.S. culture's view of what is a normal weight, usually is seen as positive. Food is also important for building blood. Diets are high in fat and low in fiber, fruits, and vegetables.	Develop a sound, trusting relationship. Identify conflicts in values and beliefs. Listen attentively. Respect cultural beliefs and values. The strengths of the family ties, church, and community organization are important resources for promoting adherence to medication regimens. Grandmothers have a significant voice in health care concerns.
Native Americans	Language and dialects vary by tribe. Most speak English, but some speak only Spanish. Talking loudly is considered rude. Silence is important, and to interrupt someone is considered rude. Touch may be unacceptable with some older adults, who are more traditional.	Increased reactions to lidocaine among the Navajo. Faster metabolism of alcohol and greater side effects than white ethnic groups. High rates of type 2 diabetes.	Spirituality is central in their health care practice. Maintaining harmony with one's environment is stressed. Health promotion and maintenance may be difficult based on past acute care survival practices.	Food has a major significance in celebrations with numerous food rituals. Corn is an important staple and is used in ceremonial dances and healing practices. Generally, food is not associated with health promotion or illness. High-fat diet predominates and a lack of fruits and vegetables exists on many reservations.	Increase access to health care. Community involvement and culturally sensitive client education are important. Do not ask questions in public. If a wrong answer is given, embarrassment may occur. Involve traditional healers and community leaders, including American Indian church, in health promotion programs.
Amish	English is used when communicating with the outside world, Deutsch at home, and High German for preaching. Conversations with outsiders are at a distance greater than 2 feet. Do not change clock settings for Day-	Incidence of dwarfism is extremely high. Incidence of hemophilia B is also high. Closed gene pools are responsible for high rates of genetic diseases, including glutaricaciduria, pyruvate kinase	Very health conscious. Obtain medical care from physicians they know in nearby communities. Traditional home remedies are commonly used. Obligation is to care for oneself first before seeing a health care provider. Most do not participate in	Food has a major nutritional and social significance. Meals are large and high in fat, carbohydrates, and calories. High incidence of obesity.	Develop a trusting relationship. Use culturally consistent communication practices. Respect their cultural beliefs and practices. Allow them time to make decisions. Must involve the family in all decisions. Incorporate traditional medicines

ACE, Angiotensin-converting enzymes

Continued

Table 6–1

Health Care Practices and Compliance in Various Cultural Groups—cont'd

Cultural Group	Communications	Biocultural Ecology	Health Care Practices	Nutrition	Promoting Strategies for Compliance
	light Savings Time.	deficiency, and maple sugar urinary disease. Twinning occurs between 15% and 21%.	immunization practices. Do not like a lot of pills and strong medicine. Health foods are increasing among denominations.		with Western practices. Expect that a telephone call from the Amish for a health-related problem is a true emergency.
Asians/Pacific Islanders: Chinese, Filipino, Japanese, Korean, Vietnamese, other Indochinese	Language varies by country of origin. Traditional maintain formal distance for conversations with outsiders. Expressing emotion is discouraged. Traditional may be uncomfortable with direct eye contact, especially with authority figures. Most are present or past oriented. Most are uncomfortable with touch but accept touch from health care providers. "Yes" does not mean I agree or understand. May mean, "I hear you." Considered rude to say "no" to questions such as, "Do you understand me?"	High degree of lactose intolerance. Determine jaundice and oxygenation by examining the sclera, palms of the hands, and soles of the feet. Skin color varies from white to light brown tones. High rates of diabetes mellitus, multiple myeloma, and cancer. More sensitive than white ethnic groups to psychotropic and antidepressant medications.	Younger generations generally practice Western medicine. Older adults try traditional methods before seeking Western medicine. Self-medication and self-diagnosis are common. Traditional therapies include the following: acupuncture, acupressure, acumassage, moxibustion therapy, coining, and Chinese herbal therapies.	Food habits are important with balancing yin and yang qualities of foods. Many rituals revolve around food. Foods at meals have a specific order. Many diets are high in sodium.	Include family members in the plan of care. Encourage client to continue treatment after the initial response; many tend to stop treatment after the initial response. Address cultural issues directly. Incorporate traditional practices into Western practices. Include physical components of mental health illnesses and concerns to improve compliance. Ask the individual what he or she thinks caused the illness/problem. Address the individual formally until requested otherwise. Confidentiality is extremely important.
Hispanics: Mexican Americans, Cuban Americans, Puerto Ricans, Latin Americans, Spanish Americans	Primary language is Spanish, with many different dialects. Many are bilingual with English as the primary or secondary language. Touch between same gender is acceptable but less so between the genders unless family or close friends. Most are modest, although physical touch is commonly accepted,	Skin color varies from white to various tones of brown, to black, depending on heritage. Being overweight is seen as positive and a sign of health. Many require lower doses of antidepressant medications than white ethnic groups. Side effects at a high rate with antituberculosis medications.	Strong valuing of the extended family. Use of home remedies, consultations with folk healers, herbalists, and masseuses influence their use of Western medicine. Fatalistic in their thinking; a higher power influences illness and health.	Many food rituals, depending on one's origin. Diet varies by country and region within the country. Hot and cold theory of balancing foods is common with most groups.	Identify conflicts in values and beliefs. Address cultural issues directly. Accommodate family values. Have instructions available in the language the client speaks or reads most easily. Demonstrate respect by addressing client formally until told otherwise. Incorporate folk and traditional practices with Western medicine. Ask about family matters first

Table 6–1

Health Care Practices and Compliance in Various Cultural Groups—cont'd

Cultural Group	Communications	Biocultural Ecology	Health Care Practices	Nutrition	Promoting Strategies for Compliance
	explain the necessity of touch during a physical examination. More traditional do not maintain eye contact with people in higher status positions.				if condition is not life-threatening. Stress individual health care provider rather than the organization.
Jewish Americans	Primary language in the United States is English. Hebrew is used for prayers. Many speak Yiddish. Orthodox men are not allowed to touch a woman other than their wives. Therapeutic touch is not recommended for this group. Most balance past, present, and future temporality.	Most have white skin, but a few from Ethiopia have black skin. Increased incidence of agranulocytosis with clozapine. High incidence of genetic diseases such as Tay-Sachs disease, familia dystonia, torsion dystonia, Gaucher's disease, mucolipidosis IV, Niemann-Pick disease, Bloom syndrome, ulcerative colitis, phenylketonuria, and familial Mediterranean fever.	Jewish Americans are health conscious and practice preventive medicine. A well-immunized population. No folk healers in this group, but there are several home remedies, chicken soup being the most known.	Meals are used to satisfy hunger and teach discipline and are the center of many religious celebrations. Food rituals are common, and the laws of kashrut dictate which foods are permissible. Among the more religious and orthodox, all meat must be Kosher, which requires a ritual slaughtering of animals wherein the animal is killed as quickly as possible and all blood is drained from the animal as quickly as possible. Avoid pork and shellfish. Religious do not mix dairy and meat at the same meal.	Health promotion and disease prevention are important. Practitioners are held in high regard.
European Americans	English is dominant language and is spoken by newer immigrants as well. Personal space is important. Maintain direct eye contact without staring during conversations. Being on time is important and majority is future oriented, although the past is well respected, especially among the English and German.	Skin color varies from white to olive. At high risk for skin cancer with exposure to the sun. Most drug testing in the United States is done on this group. High incidence of phenylketonuria among the Irish.	Most minimize or ignore symptoms until they interfere with work and activities of daily living. Sick role is not entered into easily. Use of traditional medicine varies but is common. Many are stoic with pain, but there are broad variations; Italians are more expressive than most other white ethnic groups. Expect health care providers to give explanations for all treatments and procedures.	British and French influence on U.S. diet: high in cholesterol and fat, low in fiber and complex carbohydrates. Descendants of southern Europeans have higher incidence of lactose intolerance.	Develop a sound, trusting relationship. Value the strengths of family ties and religious groups. Provide explanations for all prescriptions, treatments, and procedures.

Critical Thinking Case Study

Ana Maria de Navarro, age 63 years, picks vegetables along with several of her male relatives on a large farm. She has been recently diagnosed with hypertension and is 45 pounds overweight. She speaks minimal English, eats a traditional Mexican diet, and is the primary cook for the family. She takes furosemide, 40 mg daily. Twice within the last month, she fainted while picking vegetables. Each time, her family took her to a shaded area, where she regained consciousness within a few minutes. She admits to feeling dizzy when she awakes each morning but is glad that she no longer has headaches since she started taking her medicine. Her skin is dry and has decreased turgor. You are the public health nurse responsible for the employees in the migrant worker camp. You want her to keep a diary of her blood pressure and pulse four times a day for the next week. You speak minimal Spanish.

1. What type of medicine is furosemide?

2. Is the dose within therapeutic range?

3. Why is Ana Maria experiencing dizziness?

4. Why did Ana Maria faint twice in the last month?

5. How might you teach her family to take and record Ana Maria's blood pressure and pulse?

6. At what times each day do you recommend her vital signs be taken?

7. How will you communicate this with her and with her family?

8. What recommendation do you have for Ana Maria to combat her morning dizziness?

9. What recommendations do you have for her medication regimen?

10. If Ana Maria wanted to see a traditional healer, which one(s) might you recommend?

11. What culturally congruent goals might you collaborate on with Ana Maria?

12. What evaluation measures would you include in terms of nutrition and hydration?

Study Questions

1. How does racial origin affect metabolism of pharmacologic agents?

2. How does the topography physiologically affect clients, and what effect does it have on drug dosages?

3. What is meant by the contextual use of languages? Give an example of a high-contexted language. Give an example of a low-contexted language.

4. What are differences and similarities in nonverbal communications among Hispanics, American Indians, and European Americans?

5. What are some strategies that can be used to improve medication compliance with each of the following ethnocultural groups: African American, American Indian, Amish, Asians/Pacific Islander, Hispanic, Jewish American, and European American?

6. What is the format for names for Hispanics?

7. Why do most African Americans respond better to monotherapy than do European Americans?

8. What are several reasons why most Asians/Pacific Islanders respond differently to pharmacologic agents than European Americans and African Americans?

9. What may occur if a client with glucose-6-dehydrogenase deficiency is prescribed an oxidating agent?

10. What is meant by the "hot and cold" theory that is commonly practiced by Asian Americans, Hispanics, and Greek Americans?

11. How might you alter insulin administration for a client who celebrates Ramadan?

12. What are three reasons why some clients prefer traditional or folk practitioners instead of allopathic practitioners?

13. What are strategies that can be used to get stoic individuals to accept medication for pain?

14. With what clients may therapeutic touch not be acceptable?

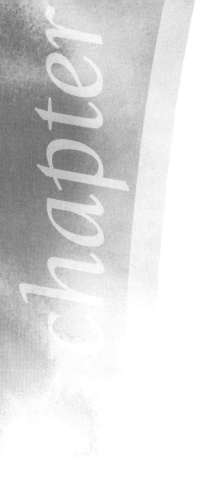

7

Drug Interaction and Over-the-Counter Drugs

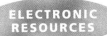

Additional information can be found on the companion website at *http://evolve.elsevier.com/KeeHayes/pharmacology/* or on the companion CD-ROM, which includes:

- *NCLEX-style examination review questions*
- *Pharmacology animations*
- *Medication error and IV therapy checklists*
- *Medication calculation problems*
- *Electronic calculators*

OUTLINE

OBJECTIVES

- Define the term *drug interaction.*
- Differentiate the four pharmacokinetic processes related to drug interaction.
- Explain the three effects associated with pharmacodynamic interactions.
- Explain the effects of drug-food interactions.
- Explain the meaning of drug-induced photosensitivity.
- Discuss the nursing implications related to clients' use of over-the-counter (OTC) drugs.

TERMS

additive effect	drug incompatibility	photosensitivity
adverse drug reaction	drug interaction	synergistic effect
antagonistic effects	over-the-counter (OTC) drugs	

Introduction

Drug therapy has become complex because of the number of drugs available. Drug-drug, drug-food, and drug-laboratory interactions have also become an increasing problem. Because of the possibility of numerous interactions, the nurse should be knowledgeable about drug interactions and should closely monitor client responses. Communication among members of the health team is essential.

Drug Interaction

A **drug interaction** is defined as an altered or modified action or effect of a drug as a result of interaction with one or more other drugs. It should not be confused with adverse drug reaction or drug incompatibility. An **adverse drug reaction** is an undesirable drug effect that ranges from mild untoward effects to severe toxic effects, including hypersensitivity reaction and anaphylaxis. **Drug incompatibility** is a chemical or physical reaction that occurs among two or more drugs in vitro (outside the body).

Drug interactions can be divided into two categories: (1) pharmacokinetic interaction and (2) pharmacodynamic interactions. These two categories of drug interaction are discussed individually.

Pharmacokinetic Interactions

Pharmacokinetic interactions are changes that occur in the absorption, distribution, metabolism or biotransformation, or excretion of one or both drugs.

Absorption

When a person takes two drugs at the same time, the rate of absorption of one or both drugs can change. One drug can block, decrease, or increase the absorption rate of another drug. It can do this in one of the three following ways:

- By decreasing or increasing gastric emptying time
- By changing the gastric pH
- By forming drug complexes

Drugs that increase the speed of gastric emptying, such as laxatives, increase gastric and intestinal motility and cause a decrease in drug absorption. Most drugs are absorbed primarily in the small intestines; exceptions include barbiturates, salicylates, and theophylline. Narcotics and anticholinergic drugs (atropinelike drugs) decrease gastric emptying time and decrease gastrointestinal (GI) motility, thus causing an increase in absorption rate. The longer the drug remains in the stomach or intestine, the greater the amount of drug absorption (only for those drugs absorbed in the stomach).

When the gastric pH is decreased, a weak acid drug, such as aspirin, is less ionized and is more rapidly absorbed. Drugs that increase the pH of gastric juices decrease absorption of weak acid drugs. Antacids, such as Maalox and Amphojel, raise the gastric pH and block or slow absorption. Some drugs may react chemically. For example, tetracycline and the heavy-metal ions (calcium, magnesium, aluminum, iron) found in antacids form a complex, and the tetracycline is not absorbed. Tetracycline also can form complexes with dairy products. Milk products and antacids should be avoided for 1 hour before and 2 hours after tetracycline consumption.

Other drugs that can cause complexes with drugs besides antacids are kaolin-pectin, certain hypocholesterol drugs such as cholestyramine and colestipol, and activated charcoal. Because of the formed complexes, the drugs are less soluble, which results in less drug absorption.

Certain broad-spectrum antibacterials (antibiotics) such as erythromycin affect the GI flora, thereby causing an increase in absorption of digoxin, which depends on the flora in the intestine to metabolize.

Distribution

A drug's distribution to tissues can be affected by its binding to plasma/serum protein. Only drugs unbound to protein are free, active agents and can enter body tissues. Two drugs that are highly protein-bound and administered simultaneously can result in drug displacements. Factors that influence displacement of drugs are (1) the drug concentration in the blood, (2) protein-binding power of the drugs, and (3) volume of distribution (Vd).

Two drugs that are highly bound to protein or albumin will compete for protein or albumin sites in the plasma. The result is a decrease in protein binding of one or both drugs; therefore more free drug circulates in the plasma and is available for drug action. This effect can lead to drug toxicity. When two highly protein-bound drugs need to be taken concurrently, drug dosage of one or both drugs may need to be decreased to avoid drug toxicity.

Examples of drugs that are highly protein bound include warfarin (anticoagulant); certain anticonvulsants, such as phenytoin and valproic acid; clofibrate; most nonsteroidal antiinflammatory drugs (NSAIDs); sulfonamides; tolbutamide; and quinidine. Warfarin is 99% protein bound, thus allowing only 1% to be free drug. If 2% to 3% of warfarin is displaced in the albumin, the amount of free warfarin would be 3% to 4% instead of 1%. This increases the anticoagulant effect, and thus excess bleeding may result.

Metabolism or Biotransformation

Many drug interactions of metabolism occur with the induction (stimulation) or inhibition of the hepatic microsomal system. A drug can increase the metabolism of another drug by stimulating (inducing) liver enzymes. Drugs that promote induction of enzymes are called *enzyme inducers*. Barbiturates (e.g., phenobarbital) are enzyme inducers. Phenobarbital increases the metabolism of beta blockers (propranolol [Inderal]), most antipsychotics, and theophylline. Increased metabolism promotes drug elimination and decreases plasma concentration of the drug. The result is a decrease in drug action. Sometimes liver enzymes convert drugs to active or passive metabolites. The drug metabolites may be excreted or may produce an active pharmacologic response. Also, some drugs are enzyme inhibitors.

The anticonvulsant drugs phenytoin and carbamazepine, alcohol, and rifampin are hepatic enzyme inducers that can increase drug metabolism, for example, for the anticoagulant drug warfarin. A larger dose of warfarin is usually needed while the client takes a hepatic inducer. The metabolism aids in decreasing the amount of drug. If the drug inducer is withdrawn, warfarin dosages need to be decreased because less drug is eliminated by hepatic metabolism. Usually interaction occurs after 1 week of drug therapy and can continue for 1 week after the drug inducer is discontinued. Drugs with narrow therapeutic ranges should be closely monitored.

Cigarette smoking increases hepatic enzyme activity and can increase theophylline clearance. For smokers who take theophylline, the theophylline dose should be increased. With chronic alcohol use, hepatic enzyme activities are increased, whereas with acute alcohol use, metabolism is inhibited.

The antiulcer drug cimetidine is an enzyme inhibitor that decreases the metabolism of certain drugs, such as theophylline (antiasthmatic). As the result of decreasing theophylline metabolism, there is an increase in the plasma concentration of theophylline. The theophylline dose needs to be decreased to avoid toxicity. If cimetidine or any enzyme drug inhibitor is discontinued, the theophylline dosage should be adjusted. Certain drugs alter hepatic blood flow, causing a decrease in liver metabolism. Table 7–1 describes the effects of drug enzyme inducers and inhibitors.

Excretion

Most drugs are excreted in the urine and filtered through the glomeruli. With some drugs, excretion occurs in the bile, which passes into the intestinal tract. Drugs can increase or decrease renal excretion and have an effect on the excretion of other drugs. Drugs that decrease cardiac output, decrease blood flow to the kidneys, and decrease glomerular filtration can also decrease or delay drug excretion. The antidysrhythmic drug quinidine decreases the excretion of digoxin (a digitalis preparation); therefore the plasma concentration of digoxin is increased and digitalis toxicity can occur.

Diuretics promote water and sodium excretion from the renal tubules. Furosemide (Lasix) acts on the loop of Henle, and hydrochlorothiazide (HydroDiuril) acts on the distal tubules. Both diuretics decrease reabsorption of water, sodium, and potassium. A loss of potassium (hypokalemia) can enhance the action of digoxin; thus digitalis toxicity could occur (see Drug-Laboratory Interactions).

Probenecid (Benemid), a drug for gout, decreases penicillin excretion by competing for tubular reabsorption of penicillin in the kidneys. In some cases, this may be desirable to increase or maintain the plasma concentration of penicillin, which has a short half-life, for a longer time.

Changing urine pH affects drug excretion. The antacid sodium bicarbonate causes the urine to be alkaline. Alkaline urine promotes the excretion of drugs that are weak acids, such as aspirin and barbiturates. Alkaline urine also promotes reabsorption of weak base drugs. Acid urine promotes the excretion of drugs that are weak bases, such as quinidine.

With clients who have decreased renal or hepatic function, there is usually an increase in free drug concentration. It is essential to closely monitor such a client for drug toxicity when he or she takes multiple drugs. Checking serum drug levels (therapeutic drug monitoring [TDM]) is especially important for drugs that have a narrow therapeutic range and are highly protein bound, such as digoxin and phenytoin. Table 7–2 summarizes the drug interactions that affect pharmacokinetics.

Pharmacodynamic Interactions

Pharmacodynamic interactions are those that result in additive, synergistic (potentiation), or antagonistic drug effects. When two drugs are given that may or may not have similar actions, the combined effect may be additive (twice the effect), synergistic (greater than twice the effect), or antagonistic (the effect of either or both drugs is decreased).

Additive Drug Effect

When two drugs with similar action are administered, the drug interaction is called an **additive effect** and is the sum of the effects of the two drugs. Additive effects can be desirable or undesirable. For example, a desirable additive drug effect occurs when a diuretic and a beta blocker are given for hypertension; used in combination, these drugs lower the blood pressure and act as antihypertensive drugs. As another example, two analgesics, aspirin and codeine, can be given together for increased pain relief.

An example of an undesirable additive effect is that from two vasodilators: hydralazine (Apresoline) prescribed for hypertension and nitroglycerin prescribed for angina. The result could be a severe hypotensive response. Another example is the interaction of aspirin and alcohol taken together, from which gastric bleeding can result. Both aspirin and alcohol can prolong bleeding time.

Table 7–1	
Drugs: Enzyme Inducer or Enzyme Inhibitor	
Drug Category	**Drug Effect**
Drug enzyme inducer	Onset and termination of drug effect is slow, approximately 1 wk. Drug dosage may need to be increased with use of drug inducer. Drug dosage should be adjusted after termination of drug inducer. Monitor serum drug levels, especially if the drug has a narrow therapeutic drug range.
Drug enzyme inhibitor	Onset of drug effect usually occurs rapidly. Half-life ($t\frac{1}{2}$) of the second drug may be increased, causing a prolonged drug effect. Interaction may occur related to the dosage prescribed. Disease entities affect drug dosing. Monitor serum drug levels, especially if the drug has a narrow therapeutic range.

wk, Week.

Table 7–2

Pharmacokinetic Interactions of Drugs

Process	Drug	Effect
Absorption	Laxatives	Speeds gastric emptying time
		Increases gastric motility
		Decreases drug absorption
	Narcotics	Slows gastric emptying time
	Anticholinergics	Decreases gastric motility
		Increases drug absorption or decreases absorption depending on where the drug is delayed (gastric vs. intestinal)
	Aspirin	Decreases gastric pH
		Increases drug absorption
	Antacids	Increases gastric pH
		Slows absorption of acid drugs
	Antacids and tetracycline	Forms drug complexes
		Blocks drug absorption
Distribution	Anticoagulant and anti-inflammatory (sulindac)	Competes for protein-binding sites
		Increases free drug (e.g., increases anticoagulant)
Metabolism or biotransformation	Barbiturates	Promotes induction of liver enzymes
		Increases drug metabolism
		Decreases drug plasma concentration of the second drug
	Antiulcer (cimetidine)	Inhibits liver enzymes release
		Decreases drug metabolism of diazepam (Valium), phenytoin (Dilantin), morphine, etc.
		Increases drug plasma concentration of the second drug
Excretion	Antidysrhythmic (quinidine)	Decreases renal excretion of second drug (e.g., digoxin)
		Increases digoxin concentration
	Antigout (probenecid)	Decreases excretion of penicillin by competing for tubular reabsorption
		Increases penicillin concentration
	Antacid (sodium bicarbonate)	Promotes excretion of weak acid drug (e.g., aspirin, barbiturates, sulfonamides)
Other: Decrease cardiac output and renal blood flow	Aspirin, ammonium chloride	Promotes excretion of weak base drugs (e.g., quinidine, theophylline)
	Most drug categories	Decreases drug excretion
		Increases drug plasma concentration

Synergistic Drug Effect or Potentiation

When two or more drugs are given together, one drug can potentiate or have a **synergistic effect** on the other drug, meaning that sometimes the effect is greater than the combined effect of two drugs from the same category. An example is the combination of meperidine (Demerol, a narcotic analgesic) and promethazine (Phenergan, an antihistamine). Promethazine enhances or potentiates the effect of meperidine. Actually, less meperidine is required when it is combined with promethazine, which can be a desirable effect. An example of an undesirable effect occurs when two drugs, alcohol and a sedative-hypnotic drug such as chlordiazepoxide (Librium) or diazepam (Valium), are combined because central nervous system (CNS) depression increases as a result.

Some antibacterials (antibiotics) have an enzyme inhibitor added to the drug to potentiate the therapeutic effect of the drug. Examples are ampicillin with sulbactam and amoxicillin with clavulanate potassium. Ampicillin and amoxicillin can be given without these inhibitors; however, the desired therapeutic effect may not occur because of the bacterial enzyme activity (e.g., beta-lactamase enzyme) that causes bacteria resistance. The combination of the antibiotic with an added enzyme inhibitor (sulbactam or clavulanate potassium) inhibits bacterial enzyme activity and thus prolongs the effect of the antibacterial agent.

The use of two prescription drugs can have an additive or synergistic effect. An example is an anticoagulant such as warfarin with another drug. The effects of the second drug can increase, decrease, or have no effects on the anticoagulant. Table 7–3 lists the drugs that may be taken with an anticoagulant and the effects that the second drug has on the anticoagulant.

Antagonistic Drug Effect

When two drugs are combined that have opposite, or **antagonistic effects,** the drugs cancel each other's drug effect. The actions of both drugs are nullified. An example of an antagonistic effect occurs when the adrenergic beta stimulant isoproterenol (Isuprel) and the adrenergic beta blocker propranolol (Inderal) are given together. The action of each drug is cancelled. Neither delivers the expected therapeutic effect.

With morphine overdose, naloxone is given as an antagonist (antidote) to block the narcotic response. This is a beneficial drug interaction of an antagonist. Table 7–4 summarizes the drug responses associated with pharmacodynamic interaction.

Table 7–3

Drug Interaction with Anticoagulants and Prescription Drugs

Prescription Drugs	Anticoagulant Effects
Selected Antilipidemics	
Fibrate group	Increased effect; may cause increase in bleeding
Statin group	
lovastatin	Increased effect
pravastatin	No known effects
Angiotensin-Converting Enzyme Inhibitors	No known effects
Aminoglycosides	No known effects
Aspirin	Strong effects; can cause bleeding
Antineoplastic Drugs	
Cytoxan, 5-fluorouracil, methotrexate, doxorubicin, vincristine	Increased effects; can cause bleeding
Cytoxan, mercaptopurine, mitotane	Decreased effects; Cytoxan may cause increased or decreased effects
Barbiturates	Reduced effect of anticoagulants
Benzodiazepines	No known effects
Beta Blockers	No known effects
Selected Cephalosporins	
Cefamandole	Increased effects; may cause bleeding
Nonsteroidal Antiinflammatory Drugs (NSAIDs)	
ibuprofen	Normal doses; no effects
diclofenac, ketoprofen, tolmetin	May increase effects
Quinolone Antibiotics	Usually no effects
ciprofloxacin, norfloxacin, ofloxacin	Increased effects in isolated cases
Sulfonamides	
Bactrim-cotrimoxazole	Increased effects in 35% of persons
Tricyclic Antidepressants	No known effects
Vitamin K	Decreased effects of anticoagulants
Food	
Aspartame (artificial sweetener)	Increased effects
Green vegetables (spinach, broccoli, Brussels sprouts)	Decreased effects; vegetables are rich in vitamin K
Alcohol	
Mild to moderate drinking	No effects unless heavy drinking
Heavy drinking	Increased effects if liver function is impaired

Drug-Food Interactions

Food is known to increase, decrease, or delay drug absorption. Food can bind with drugs, causing less or slower drug absorption. An example of food binding with a drug is the interaction of tetracycline and dairy products. The result is a decrease in the plasma concentration of tetracycline. Because of the binding effect, tetracycline should be taken 1 hour before or 2 hours after meals and *should not* be taken with dairy products. There are a few drugs in which food increases drug absorption; examples include the antiinfective agent nitrofurantoin (Macrodantin), the beta blocker metoprolol (Lopressor), and the antilipemic lovastatin (Mevacor). These drugs should be taken at mealtime or with food.

The levodopa component of Sinemet, used to treat parkinsonism, is significantly reduced when it is taken with high protein meals. A significant decrease in the serum albumin level can increase the free amount of highly protein-bound drugs such as phenytoin (Dilantin) and warfarin (Coumadin).

Table 7–4

Pharmacodynamic Interactions of Drugs

Interaction	Effect
Additive	In the same drug category, the drug effect is the sum of both drug effects.
Synergistic or potentiation	One drug potentiates or enhances the effect of the other drug (greater than effect of each alone).
Antagonistic	Two drugs in opposing drug categories cancel drug effects of both drugs.

The classic drug-food interaction occurs when an antidepressant of the monoamine oxidase (MAO) inhibitor type (e.g., Marplan) is taken with tyramine-rich foods such as cheese, wine, organ meats, beer, yogurt, sour cream, or bananas. More norepinephrine is released, and the result could be a hypertensive crisis. These foods must be avoided when taking monoamine oxidase inhibitors.

Drug-Laboratory Interactions

Abnormal plasma or serum electrolyte concentrations can affect certain drug therapies. If the client takes digoxin (a digitalis preparation) and there are decreased serum potassium and serum magnesium levels or an increased serum calcium level, digitalis toxicity may result. Certain drugs, such as those from the thiazide diuretic group, can cause abnormal electrolyte concentrations. An example is hydrochlorothiazide (HydroDiuril), which can decrease serum potassium, magnesium, and sodium levels and can increase the serum calcium level. Because HydroDiuril promotes potassium loss, the low serum potassium increases the plasma concentration of digoxin, thereby increasing the action. The result is digitalis toxicity (intoxication). When digoxin and HydroDiuril are taken together, the nurse should observe the client for digitalis toxicity (nausea, vomiting, bradycardia [pulse less than 60 beats per minute], and stated visual problems).

Drug-Induced Photosensitivity

Photosensitivity is a skin reaction caused by exposure to sunlight. It is caused by the interaction of a drug and exposure to ultraviolet A (UVA) light, which can cause cel-lular damage. Usually, the skin area that is exposed is affected.

Phototoxicity and *photoallergy* from drug-induced photosensitivity reactions are terms that are used interchangeably. Both are the result of light exposure but differ according to the wavelength of light and the photosensitive drug. Photosensitivity may be the result of the drug dose. The onset of phototoxicity with erythema can be rapid, occurring within 2 to 6 hours of sunlight exposure. Examples of drugs that can induce photosensitivity are listed in Table 7–5.

Most photosensitive reactions can be avoided by using sunscreen block (UVA protection) with a sun protection factor greater than 15 and by avoiding excessive sunlight. The higher the drug doses, the more likely that drug-induced photosensitivity will occur. Decreasing drug dose may decrease photosensitivity if treatment is necessary. It may be necessary to discontinue use of the drug.

Over-the-Counter Drugs

Multiple factors contribute to the increase in the number of and use of OTC products. Mass-media marketing surrounds us. These remedies are used by family and friends, and many people now are into "self-treatment." It is one of the nurse's responsibilities to advocate for the client making educated choices.

Over-the-counter (OTC) drugs, drugs that are available without a prescription, are found in most households (Fig-

---

Table 7–5

Drug-Induced Photosensitivity

Drug Induced	Occurrence
amantadine	Confirmed by positive photopatch testing
amiodarone	Frequency may be 10% to 75%. Sunscreen lotion with UVA can inhibit photosensitivity
benzodiazepines	Has been reported with drugs alprazolam and chlordiazepoxide
carbamazepine	Frequency is less than 1%; however, photocopy machines can trigger photosensitivity
corticosteroids	Was reported with positive photopatch testing and with use of hydrocortisone
diphenhydramine	Was reported with positive photopatch testing with topical and oral use
fluorouracil	Avoid sunlight with topical or intravenous use; erythema and hyperpigmentation could occur
NSAIDs	Aspirin, ibuprofen, and indomethacin have been reported to have low phototoxin effect; however, there is a possibility for photosensitive effect with ibuprofen (dose related)
methotrexate	Avoid sunlight to prevent severe photosensitive reaction (sunburn)
calcium blockers	diltiazem: possible phototoxic reaction nifedipine: may cause phototoxicity with high drug doses
phenothiazines	Reported cases of phototoxic reaction with chlorpromazine and other phenothiazines at high drug doses
piroxicam	Was confirmed with positive photopatch testing; photosensitive reaction occurs after a few days of piroxicam and exposure to sunlight
pyrazinamide	Skin color may change to reddish brown; usually occurrence is dose-related
quinolones (fluoroquinolones)	Phototoxicity occurs with lomefloxacin, enoxacin, ofloxacin, and nalidixic acid; ciprofloxacin causes less photosensitivity
sulfonamides	Photosensitive reaction has been reported
sulfonylureas	Photosensitive reaction has been reported
tetracyclines	Highly photosensitive; demeclocycline and doxycycline have a higher degree of photosensitive reaction than minocycline
thiazines	Thiazide-induced photosensitivity has been reported; hydrochlorothiazide has a greater photosensitivity than bendroflumethiazide
triamterene	Was confirmed by positive photopatch testing
trimethoprim	Photosensitivity has been reported
vinblastine	Photosensitivity has been reported

NSAIDs, Nonsteroidal antiinflammatory drugs; *UVA,* ultraviolet A.

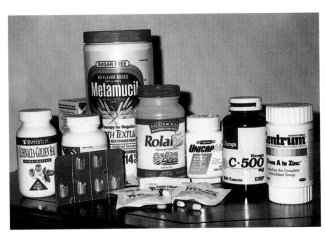

FIGURE 7–1 Commonly used over-the-counter preparations.

ure 7–1). The Food and Drug Administration (FDA) finds that OTC preparations do not require that you be in the care of a health care provider to have access to these products. More than 90% of all illnesses are initially treated with OTC drugs that are unknown to many of the health care providers. Many OTC drugs include vitamin supplements, cold and cough remedies, analgesics for pain, antacids, laxatives, antihistamines, sleep aids, nasal sprays, weight-control drugs, and herbal products. Some clients do not consider herbal products to be OTC drugs. Almost $4 billion is spent annually on herbal products, nutraceuticals, and dietary supplements; most of these products are minimally regulated by the FDA. Refer to Chapter 9, Herbal Therapy with Nursing Implications, for a detailed presentation.

Today, many of the prescriptive drugs are now available as OTC drugs, and many more are in the process of being approved as OTC drugs by the FDA (e.g., proton pump inhibitors and hyperlipidemic drugs). Because of this process, more than 700,000 OTC products have ingredients or dose strengths available only by prescription three decades ago.

The FDA has been working to standardize OTC labeling. OTC labeling should provide consumers with better information and describe the benefits and risks associated with taking the drug. New labeling for all OTC drugs is scheduled to be available by 2005.

Nurses need to be aware of OTC products and the implications of their use for their clients' drug therapy. OTC drugs provide both advantages and potential serious complications for the consumer. The nurse needs to emphasize that many of these drugs are potent medications and can cause moderate to severe side effects, especially when taken with other drugs. Self-diagnosing and self-prescribing OTC drugs may mask the seriousness of the clinical condition.

The Durham-Humphrey amendment (1952) to the Food, Drug, and Cosmetic Act of 1938 approved drugs that are safe for consumption and that could be sold as nonprescription or OTC drugs. In 1962 the Kefauver-Harris amendment required proof of efficacy and safety of the drug. OTC drugs came under the scrutiny of the FDA in 1970.

The FDA has the responsibility of monitoring the safety of drug therapy. This group of professionals is charged with (1) identifying standards for known active ingredi-

ents and (2) establishing mandatory labeling to assist the consumer in the proper use of the drug. The FDA OTC drug categories are listed in Box 7–1.

As a result of the review by the FDA panel, drugs are placed in one of three categories:

Category I: Drugs judged to be both safe and effective

Category II: Drugs judged to be either unsafe or ineffective; these drugs should not be included in nonprescription products

Category III: Drugs for which there are insufficient data to judge safety or efficacy

The FDA has recommended that drugs in category II be reformulated to be included in category I or removed from the market. (NOTE: Manufacturers can maintain the brand name after changing the components of an OTC product.) The FDA also has recommended that selected prescription drugs be reclassified so that they can be sold over the counter. As a result, it is vitally important that nurses be aware of current drug information, any changes in FDA recommendations, and the implications of this information for an informed client population. The following cautions may be of assistance when OTC preparations are considered:

- Delay in professional diagnosis and treatment of serious or potentially serious conditions may occur if the client self-prescribes OTC drugs.
- Symptoms may be masked, thereby making diagnosis more complicated.
- Labels and instructions should be followed carefully.

BOX 7–1

FDA Over-the-Counter Drug Categories

- Allergy treatment products (internal)
- Analgesics—antipyretics (internal)
- Antacids and antiflatulents
- Antidiarrheal products
- Antimicrobials
- Antiperspirants
- Antirheumatic products
- Antitussives
- Bronchodilators and antiasthmatic products
- Cold remedies and decongestants
- Contraceptive products
- Dandruff products
- Dentifrices and other dental products
- Dermatologic products
- Emetics and antiemetics
- Hematinics
- Hemorrhoidal products
- Herbal products
- Laxatives and cathartics
- Nicotine gum or transdermal patches
- Ophthalmic products
- Oral-hygiene drug products
- Sedatives and sleep aids
- Stimulants
- Sunburn prevention and treatment products
- Vitamin–mineral supplements
- Weight-loss aids
- Miscellaneous products (OTC products not covered in above categories)

FDA, Food and Drug Administration; *OTC,* over-the-counter.

- The client's health care provider or pharmacist should be consulted before OTC preparations are taken.
- Ingredients in OTC products may interact with medications that are prescribed by the health care provider or are self-prescribed by the client.
- Inactive ingredients (e.g., alcohol, dyes, preservatives) may result in adverse reactions.
- Potential for overdose exists because of the use of several preparations with similar active ingredients. A double dose does not equal quicker recovery.
- Multiple medication users, whether prescription or OTC, are at increased risk as more medications are added to a therapy regimen.
- Interactions of selected prescription medications and OTC preparations are potentially dangerous. Many individuals routinely reach for aspirin, acetaminophen, and ibuprofen to relieve a discomfort or pain without being aware of these interactions. For example, an individual taking digoxin should avoid taking ibuprofen because it may increase the serum digoxin level, thereby resulting in digoxin toxicity. Ibuprofen increases fluid retention, which could worsen the condition of a client with congestive heart failure; use of ibuprofen on a long-term basis may decrease the effectiveness of antihypertensive drugs.

Some OTC drugs were previously classified as prescription drugs, such as ibuprofen. The prescription drug Motrin became available as an OTC drug, ibuprofen, in 1984. Tagamet, another prescription drug, was also made available as the OTC drug cimetidine.

Several OTC drugs, such as cough medicines, are composed of two to four compounds. One of the compounds may interact with a prescription drug that the client takes.

Clients with asthma need to be aware that aspirin can trigger an acute asthma episode. Furthermore, aspirin is not recommended for children with flu symptoms or chickenpox because it has been associated with Reye syndrome.

Clients with impaired renal function should avoid aspirin, acetaminophen, and ibuprofen because each can further decrease renal function, especially with long-term use. Aspirin and ibuprofen increase the effects of oral anticoagulants, so clients who take these medications may be at increased risk for bleeding.

The aforementioned examples are not inclusive. Caution is advised before using any OTC preparations, including antacids, decongestants, laxatives, and cough syrup (Figure 7–2). Clients should check with their health care providers and read the drug labels before taking OTC medications so they are aware of possible contraindications and adverse reactions. Always read OTC labels and look for product name, active ingredients, purpose, uses, warnings, directions, storage information, and inactive ingredients, (e.g., color, flavors). It is a good idea to check your supply of medications at least once a year; store medications in their original container in a cool, dry place (or as directed on label); and properly dispose of expired meds. If you are pregnant or breast-feeding, consult your health care provider or pharmacist before taking any medicine.

A good source for OTC drug information is *The Handbook of Nonprescription Drugs,* published by the American Pharma-

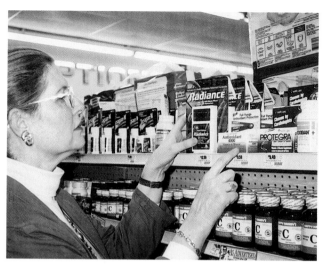

FIGURE 7–2 Consumers often have questions when choosing an over-the-counter preparation.

ceutical Association in Washington, DC ([800] 237-2742). See p. 147 for Internet resource information on OTC drugs.

Cold and Cough Remedies

Most OTC cold and cough remedies are used to relieve coughs and nasal and sinus congestion. The majority of these OTC agents are sympathomimetic (stimulating the sympathetic nervous system) and contain ingredients such as phenylpropanolamine, pseudoephedrine, analgesic, and an antihistamine. The FDA has ordered removal of phenylpropanolamine from OTC cold remedies and weight-control drugs because of the increased risk of hemorrhagic stroke in young women who take the drug. It has been reported that phenylpropanolamine may also cause psychosis, hypertension, renal failure, and cardiac dysrhythmias.

OTC cold and cough remedies are primarily safe for children older than 6 years (for children ages 2 to 6, consult with a health care provider). Clients with heart disease, hypertension, or thyroid disease should not take these OTC preparations without approval from their health care provider. Side effects of cold and cough OTC drugs that contain a sympathomimetic include headache, nervousness, increased blood pressure, and insomnia. The most common side effect of the antihistamine is drowsiness.

Health professionals should discuss the pros and cons of taking cold and cough remedies with their client and read the labels carefully. The recommended dose should not be exceeded for either adults or children.

Sleep Aids

The FDA restricts the number of OTC sleep aids. Before 1979 most of the OTC sleep aids contained bromides, scopolamine, or a combination of antihistamines. Most OTC sleep aids currently contain an antihistamine with or without an analgesic such as aspirin or acetaminophen. The side effect of an antihistamine is drowsiness, which is useful as a sleep aid. If the client has night pain that causes sleeplessness, the analgesic with the antihistamine is helpful. In small children or older adults, these sleep aids may cause CNS stimulation instead of sedation. These drugs should not be taken with a depressant because they can have an additive depressive effect on the CNS.

Weight-Control Drugs

For years, most weight-control drugs contained amphetamines. The amphetamines were prescription drugs prescribed to suppress the appetite. The effectiveness of the amphetamines was short-term because they were effective only as long as the therapeutic blood level of the drug was maintained. Drug dependence was a problem associated with amphetamines. Side effects included nervousness, heart palpitations, increased blood pressure, and insomnia.

Currently, many OTC weight-control drugs are on the market. The weight-control drugs are contraindicated for clients with heart disease, hypertension, diabetes mellitus, and thyroid disease.

Nonpharmacologic measures of consuming fewer calories and exercising more are the foundation of any weight loss program. If the client continues to eat large meals and snacks while taking weight-control drugs, little to no weight loss occurs.

Nursing Process

Drug Interactions

ASSESSMENT

■ Obtain a drug history of the OTC drugs client currently takes. There could be a drug interaction with the prescribed drug.

■ Review all literature provided by drug companies and pharmacy.

■ Assess for drug reaction when two highly protein-bound drugs are taken together daily. For example, the anticoagulant warfarin (Coumadin) and the antiinflammatory sulindac (Clinoril) have a high affinity to protein. Warfarin is displaced from the plasma protein, causing more free warfarin and a possible increase in bleeding.

■ Determine if potential for drug interaction problems related to an increased or decreased absorption rate of two drugs. Drug enzyme inducers that increase drug metabolism may result in a decrease in drug effect (increased drug metabolism leads to increased drug excretion).

■ Assess the client for drug toxicity (overdose) when a drug enzyme inducer has been discontinued or when a drug enzyme inhibitor is taken concurrently with other drugs.

■ Determine whether the client is a cigarette smoker. Tobacco is an enzyme inducer and can increase the metabolic rate of drugs. If client is taking a drug such as theophylline to control asthma and also smokes, the drug dosage needs to be increased. For nonsmokers, the theophylline dosage should be less or within the suggested drug range.

■ Determine renal function by checking for adequate urine output; it should be greater than 600 ml daily. The guideline is 25 ml/h for adults.

NURSING DIAGNOSES

■ Risk of tissue injury related to the adverse reaction to drug interaction.

PLANNING

■ Client will be aware of drug interactions and avoid drugs that may cause a severe drug reaction.

■ Client will not take any OTC drugs without consultation with health care provider.

NURSING INTERVENTIONS

■ Contact the health care provider if a drug dose adjustment has not been ordered when a drug enzyme inducer has been discontinued.

■ Recognize drugs of the same category that might have an additive effect. The additive drug effect might be undesirable and could cause a severe physiologic response.

■ Notify the health care provider of drugs ordered that have antagonistic or opposite effects, such as beta stimulants and beta blockers.

■ Consult a pharmacist about processing through a drug interaction computer program.

Client Teaching

• Advise clients not to take OTC drugs with prescribed drugs without first notifying the health care provider.

• Remind clients to be cautious about taking herbal products, especially if taking OTC or prescription medications; check with health care provider first.

EVALUATION

■ Evaluate the effectiveness of the drugs and determine that client is free of side effects.

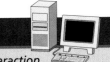

WEBSITES

For further information on *Drug Interaction and Over-the-Counter Drugs,* visit these Internet resources:

Consumer Health Products Association: *www.chpa-info.org*

Drug topics: *www.drugtopics.com*

Food and Drug Administration: *www.fda.gov*

Facts and Comparisons' Guide to Popular Natural Products: *www.drugfacts.com*

National Center for Complementary and Alternative Medicine Clearinghouse: *www.nccam.nih.gov*

National Library of Medicine fact sheets on supplements: *www.nlm.nih.gov/medlineplus/vitaminandmineralsupplements.html*

PubMed: *www.ncbi.nlm.nih.gov/PubMed*

Study Questions

1. What are the meaning and importance of drug interaction?

2. What are the four pharmacokinetic processes related to drug interaction? Describe each process.

3. What are the three main effects associated with pharmacodynamic interaction?

4. What are the effects of drugs in food interactions? What are the implications for nursing practice?

5. Define drug-induced photosensitivity. What are five drugs or drug groups that are attributed to photosensitivity?

6. What are five potential disadvantages in the use of OTC preparations?

7. Describe the three categories of OTC preparations.

8. Identify at least three chronic illnesses in which OTC weight-control drugs are contraindicated.

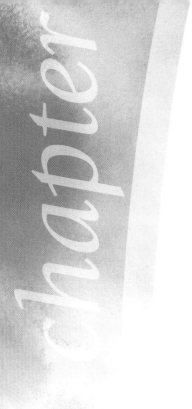

8 Drugs of Abuse

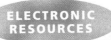

> **ELECTRONIC RESOURCES**
>
> Additional information can be found on the companion website at *http://evolve.elsevier.com/KeeHayes/pharmacology/* or on the companion CD-ROM, which includes:
> - *NCLEX-style examination review questions*
> - *Pharmacology animations*
> - *Medication error and IV therapy checklists*
> - *Medication calculation problems*
> - *Electronic calculators*

OUTLINE

OBJECTIVES

- Define the terms *drug (substance) abuse, drug (substance) misuse, addiction, dependence, tolerance, detoxification, withdrawal,* and *abstinence.*
- Describe the neurobiology of addictive drugs.
- Identify the physical and psychologic effects of commonly abused central nervous system stimulants and depressants, cannabis, psychedelic agents, and inhalants.
- Identify drugs used in the treatment of toxicity, withdrawal, and maintenance of abstinence of commonly abused drugs.
- Identify nursing interventions appropriate during management of surgical experiences and pain in clients who abuse drugs.
- Describe the nurse's role in recognizing and promoting treatment of chemical impairment among nurses.
- Describe the use of the nursing process in the care of clients who abuse drugs.

Introduction

Most drugs are used safely and within prescribed guidelines, but it is possible for all drugs to be misused or abused. Although drug abuse and **addiction** is a serious and complex social and health problem that nurses address in all areas of practice, this chapter focuses on the physiologic effects of the drugs and the pharmacologic treatment of abuse.

Terminology of Drug Abuse

Cultural Considerations

Describing what constitutes drug misuse and abuse is difficult because culture and social expectations influence the definitions and perception of drug abuse. In Moslem Middle Eastern populations, any use of alcohol or mind-altering drugs would be considered abuse. The same would be true in the United States among Mormon and some conservative Christian groups. Yet, in many European cultures, alcohol use is expected and is present in all family and social gatherings. In some subcultures in the United States, occasional use of marijuana is not considered abuse, nor is the use of psychedelic agents in some Native American religious rites. Cigarette smoking, which was glamorized in the past, is now less socially acceptable than moderate alcohol use.

Rates of drug abuse and addiction are similar among white, African American, and Hispanic populations in the United States. Native Americans, however, have much higher rates of alcoholism. White American populations tend to abuse alcohol and amphetamines, whereas African Americans and Hispanics prefer to use heroin and cocaine, respectively. The cultural influences of drug abuse are often related to other factors, such as unemployment, poverty, or adverse social conditions. A major responsibility of nurses in addressing drug abuse in ethnic and cultural groups is to assess and treat the client within his or her cultural perspective as described in Chapter 6, Transcultural and Genetic Considerations.

Definitions

Although small differences exist in their definitions, the terms *drug*, *substance*, and *chemical* are often used interchangeably within the context of drug abuse. **Drug misuse** generally refers to indiscriminate use of a chemical substance or its use for purposes other than for which it is intended. **Drug abuse** is culturally defined and may be defined as using a drug inconsistent with medical or social norms. It generally refers to an overindulgence of a chemical substance that results in a negative impact on the psychologic, physical, or social functioning of an individual. Chronic abuse of a drug may lead to addiction. **Drug addiction** should be considered a complex disease of the central nervous system (CNS) characterized by a compulsive, uncontrolled craving for and dependence on a substance to such a degree that cessation causes severe emotional, mental, or physiologic reactions. **Physical dependence** is not necessary or sufficient for addiction to occur. These and additional terms used in describing drug abuse are presented in Table 8–1.

The drugs that are abused most often are psychoactive agents that result in pleasure or modify thinking and perception. They include legal substances, such as alcohol and tobacco, and drugs with therapeutic value, such as analgesics, sedative-hypnotics, tranquilizers, and amphetamines. Common illegal substances that are abused include, in descending prevalence, marijuana and hashish, cocaine, hallucinogens, inhalants, and heroin.

Neurobiology of Addictive Drugs

Current research indicates that most addictive drugs increase the availability of dopamine and other neurotransmitters in the "pleasure" area of the mesolimbic system of the brain. This area has been identified as the **brain reward system**, an ancient system that creates the sensation of pleasure for certain behaviors necessary for survival, such as eating and sexual behavior.

Normally, dopamine is released at a slow rate in the mesolimbic system, producing a normal mood. However, certain drugs, such as opioids and cocaine, increase the release of dopamine or decrease its reuptake at the synapse. Nicotine, alcohol, marijuana, amphetamines, and caffeine are also believed to increase dopamine activity at the synapse. The resulting increase in dopamine in the system leads to mood elevation or euphoria, factors that provide strong motivation to repeat the experience. Many addictive drugs also increase the availability of other neurotransmitters, such as serotonin and gamma-aminobutyric acid (GABA), but dopamine's effect on the reward system appears to be pivotal to the addictive process.

Addiction results from the prolonged effects of addictive drugs on the brain. Repeated use of addictive drugs remodels the neural circuitry of the brain cells and reduces

Table 8–1

Terminology of Drug Abuse

Term	Definition
Abstinence	Avoidance of substance use.
Addiction	A compulsive, uncontrollable craving for and dependence on a substance to such a degree that cessation causes severe emotional, mental, or physiologic reactions.
Chemical impairment	A term used by health professionals to describe behaviors related to the effects of drugs or substances on performance
Craving	Subjective need for a substance, usually experienced after decreased use or abstinence. Cue-induced craving is stimulated in the presence of situations previously associated with drug-taking.
Dependence	Reliance on a substance that has reached the level that its absence will cause an impairment in function.
Psychologic	Compulsive need to experience pleasurable response from the substance.
Physical	Altered physiologic state from prolonged substance use; regular use is necessary to prevent withdrawal syndrome.
Drug abuse	Overindulgence in and dependence on a substance that has a negative impact on psychologic, physiologic, and social functioning of an individual; synonymous with chemical dependence.
Drug misuse	Indiscriminate use of a drug for purposes other than those for which it is intended.
Relapse	Return to substance use during abstinence.
Substance	Drug, chemical, or biologic entity.
Tolerance	Decreased effect of a substance that results from repeated exposure. It is possible to develop cross-tolerance to other substances in same category.
Withdrawal syndrome	Constellation of physiologic and psychologic responses that occur when there is abrupt cessation or reduced intake of a substance on which an individual is dependent or when the effect is counteracted by a specific antagonist.

the responsiveness of receptors. This decreased responsiveness leads to **tolerance**, the need for a larger dose of a drug to obtain the original euphoria, and also reduces the sense of pleasure from experiences that previously resulted in positive feelings. Without the drug, the individual experiences depression, anxiety, and irritability. Even to feel normal, the individual must take the drug.

Drug **craving** is another characteristic of addiction. An important type of craving experienced by addicts, **cue-induced craving**, occurs in the presence of people, places, or things that they have previously associated with drug taking. New studies indicate that these encounters produce surges in dopamine levels, and these surges push the individual toward active drug seeking and drug taking. Cue-induced craving may occur after long periods of **abstinence** and is a common cause of **relapse**.

Continued research into the biologic and genetic basis of addictions is of crucial importance in the development of drugs to treat addiction. There is increasing evidence that genetics plays a significant role in alcoholism and nicotine use and that there are significant gender differences in drug abuse risk. A natural genetic mutation that inhibits nicotine metabolism in the brain has been identified. Men with the mutation are less likely to become addicted to nicotine and find it easier to quit smoking. However, the presence or absence of the defective gene does not affect women's smoking. Initial research into the biologic and genetic basis of addictions has been used to develop drugs to treat opioid addiction, but currently no medications are approved by the Food and Drug Administration

(FDA) for treating addiction to cocaine, lysergic acid diethylamide (LSD), phencyclidine hydrochloride (PCP), marijuana, methamphetamine and other stimulants, or inhalants.

Overview of Addictive States

Intoxication

Intoxication is a state of being poisoned by a drug or other toxic substance. In the client who abuses a drug, intoxication is commonly caused by a drug overdose. The signs and symptoms that are seen are the toxic effects of the drug when taken in excessive doses.

Detoxification

Detoxification involves treating an intoxicated client to diminish or remove drugs or their effects from the body. Treatments may involve administration of antagonistic drugs, promotion of metabolism and elimination of the drug, or intensive supportive care until the drug is eliminated.

Withdrawal Syndrome

Withdrawal syndrome is a group of signs and symptoms that occur in physically dependent persons when drug use is stopped. The symptoms are often opposite the effects the drug produced before it was withdrawn. Opioids, alcohol, barbiturates, and anxiolytics cause relatively strong physical dependence and withdrawal syndrome. Cannabinoids and amphetamines cause weak physical dependence. Hallucinogens, such as LSD, do not cause physical dependence or abstinence signs. Withdrawal syndrome is treated by slow weaning of the drugs, administration of drugs to control symptoms, and supportive care.

Cessation and Maintenance of Abstinence

To promote cessation and abstinence of the abused drug, treatment with other drugs may be used to decrease craving and prevent withdrawal syndrome. Specific receptor blockers, less potent drugs of the same class, or nonaddicting substitutes are treatment options.

Stimulants

Nicotine

Nicotine is the alkaloid in tobacco that causes dependence and is the most rapidly addicting of the drugs of abuse. Smoking cigarettes is the most damaging method of nicotine use. Cigarette smoke contains more than 4000 chemicals and gases, including at least 45 cancer-causing or tumor-promoting agents and a number of hydrocarbons or solvents. Although nicotine is not believed to be carcinogenic, it is the addictive substance and has no therapeutic value.

Pharmacodynamics

In low doses, such as those obtained through cigarettes, nicotine activates nicotinic receptors. Most effects occur from activated receptors in autonomic ganglia and the adrenal medulla. In the CNS, nicotine rapidly acts on the mesolimbic reward system of the brain, promoting the release of dopamine and mimicking the effects of cocaine and other highly addictive substances.

Pharmacokinetics

Nicotine is rapidly absorbed into the blood through the lungs in smoking and more slowly through the buccal mucosa in chewing and through the nasal mucosa in snuffing. It crosses membranes easily and is widely distributed throughout the body. Nicotine passes freely into breast milk and may be toxic to the nursing infant. Plasma protein binding of nicotine is <5%. The liver is the major site of nicotine metabolism. Nicotine and its more than 20 metabolites are eliminated in the urine. The elimination half-life of nicotine is 1 to 2 hours.

Side Effects and Adverse Reactions

Stimulation of nicotinic receptors in the sympathetic ganglia and the adrenal medulla result in marked cardiovascular stimulation and increased myocardial oxygen consumption. In the brain, the action of nicotine causes general CNS stimulation. Physical effects include increased respiratory rate and tremors. Psychologic effects include increased alertness and arousal. In the gastrointestinal (GI) tract, nicotine increases GI secretions and smooth-muscle tone. Many abusers of nicotine report that nicotine has a depressant effect, promoting relaxation and relief of anxiety. However, it is thought that these effects actually occur when periodic nicotine withdrawal is relieved by further nicotine.

Nicotine causes a very strong psychologic dependence. In addition, **physiologic dependence** occurs with regular

heavy use. Withdrawal symptoms may occur within the first few hours after stopping smoking, peak in 24 to 48 hours, and last from a few weeks to several months. After withdrawal subsides, cue-induced craving may cause smoking relapse. The effects of nicotine and symptoms of withdrawal are presented in Table 8–2.

Treatment

Treatment of nicotine addiction has received considerable attention in the past few years because of its association with preventable illness and death. To help end thousands of these unnecessary health problems, nurses must be proactive, identifying and talking with tobacco users and providing them with information on ways to stop the use of tobacco. Except in special circumstances, nicotine replacement therapy or bupropion (Zyban) is recommended for all tobacco users in addition to behavioral and support therapies. Nicotine-replacement systems in the form of gum, lozenges, transdermal patches, nasal spray, and inhalers have been approved by the FDA to reduce the craving and withdrawal symptoms associated with tobacco cessation. These agents enable a smoker to reduce nicotine previously obtained from cigarettes with a system that provides slower delivery of the drug and eliminates the carcinogens and gases associated with tobacco smoke. Table 8–3 describes the various nicotine replacement products.

Bupropion is an atypical (heterocyclic) antidepressant that is unrelated to nicotine; it has also been approved by the FDA for smoking cessation. The mechanism of action of bupropion is unknown. It is a relative weak inhibitor of neuronal uptake of norepinephrine, serotonin, and dopamine that reduces the urge to smoke and reduces some symptoms of nicotine withdrawal (see Chapter 26, Antidepressants and Mood Stabilizers).

Nortriptyline (Aventyl, Pamelor), clonidine (Catapres), and mecamylamine (Inversine) are used as second-line drugs to reduce withdrawal symptoms and promote cessation. These drugs are not approved by the FDA for this purpose, and their action in nicotine addiction is not clearly understood. Nortriptyline is a tricyclic antidepressant (see Chapter 26, Antidepressants and Mood Stabilizers). Clonidine is a centrally acting alpha$_2$-agonist, and mecamylamine is a ganglionic blocker. Both drugs are used to treat hypertension (see Chapter 42, Antihypertensive Drugs).

Research related to the development of new agents and new uses of approved drugs in smoking cessation is a priority of the National Institute for Drug Abuse. Clinical trials are currently in progress that are examining the effects of various combinations of nicotine-replacement agents, combinations of nicotine-replacement agents with antidepressants, neurotransmitter modulators, nicotine vaccines that produce antibodies that bind in the blood with nicotine, and nicotine receptor-blocking agents. (See Chapter 39, Drugs for Acute and Chronic

Table 8–2

Effects of Frequently Abused Drugs

Substance	Physiologic and Psychologic Effects	Toxicity	Withdrawal Syndrome
Stimulants			
Nicotine	Increased arousal and alertness; performance enhancement; increased heart rate, cardiac output, and blood pressure; cutaneous vasoconstriction; fine tremor, decreased appetite; antidiuretic effect; increased gastric motility	Rare: Nausea, abdominal pain, diarrhea, vomiting, dizziness, weakness, confusion, decreased respirations, seizures, death from respiratory failure	Craving, restlessness, depression, hyperirritability, headache, insomnia, decreased blood pressure and heart rate, increased appetite
Cocaine/amphetamines amphetamine (Benzedrine) benzphetamine (Didrex) dextroamphetamine (Dexedrine) methamphetamine (Desoxyn) methylphenidate (Ritalin) pemoline (Cylert) phenmetrazine (Preludin)	Euphoria, grandiosity, mood swings, hyperactivity, hyperalertness, restlessness, anorexia, insomnia, hypertension, tachycardia, marked vasoconstriction, tremor, dysrhythmias, seizures, sexual arousal, dilated pupils, diaphoresis	Agitation; increased temperature, pulse, respiratory rate, blood pressure; cardiac dysrhythmias, myocardial infarction, hallucinations, seizures, possible death	Severe craving, severely depressed mood, exhaustion, prolonged sleep, apathy, irritability, disorientation
Caffeine	Mood elevation, increased alertness, nervousness, jitteriness, irritability, insomnia, increased respirations, increased heart rate and force of myocardial contraction, relaxation of smooth muscle, diuresis	Rare: Nervousness, confusion, psychomotor agitation, anxiety, dizziness, tinnitus, muscle twitching elevated blood pressure, tachycardia, extrasystoles, increased respiratory rate	Headache, irritability, drowsiness, fatigue
Depressants			
Alcohol Sedative-hypnotics Barbiturates secobarbital (Seconal) pentobarbital (Nembutal) amobarbital (Amytal) Benzodiazepines diazepam (Valium) chlordiazepoxide (Librium) alprazolam (Xanax) Nonbarbiturates nonbenzodiazepines methaqualone (Quaalude) chloral hydrate (Noctec)	Initial relaxation, emotional lability, decreased inhibitions, drowsiness, lack of coordination, impaired judgment, slurred speech, hypotension, bradycardia, bradypnea, constricted pupils	Shallow respirations; cold, clammy skin; weak, rapid pulse; hyporeflexia, coma, possible death	Anxiety, agitation, insomnia, diaphoresis, tremors, delirium, seizures, possible death
Opioids heroin morphine opium codeine fentanyl (Sublimaze) meperidine (Demerol) hydromorphone (Dilaudid) propoxyphene (Darvon) oxycodone (OxyContin, Percocet) methadone (Dolophine)	Analgesia, euphoria, drowsiness, detachment from environment, relaxation, constricted pupils, constipation, nausea, decreased respiratory rate, slurred speech, impaired judgment, decreased sexual and aggressive drives	Slow, shallow respirations; clammy skin; constricted pupils; coma; possible death	Watery eyes, dilated pupils, runny nose, yawning, tremors, pain, chills, fever, diaphoresis, nausea, vomiting, diarrhea, abdominal cramps

Continued

Table 8–2

Effects of Frequently Abused Drugs—cont'd

Substance	Physiologic and Psychologic Effects	Toxicity	Withdrawal Syndrome
Cannabis			
Marijuana Hashish	Relaxation, euphoria, amotivation, slowed time sensation, sexual arousal, abrupt mood changes, impaired memory and attention, impaired judgment, reddened eyes, dry mouth, lack of coordination, tachycardia, increased appetite	Fatigue, paranoia, panic reactions, hallucinogen-like psychotic states	Rare: insomnia, hyperactivity
Psychedelics			
lysergic acid diethylamide (LSD) psilocybin (mushrooms) dimethyltryptamine (DMT) diethyltryptamine (DET) 3,4-methylendioxy-amphetamine (MDMA, Ecstasy) mescaline (peyote) phencyclidine (PCP)	Perceptual distortions, hallucinations, delusions (PCP), depersonalization, heightened sensory perception, euphoria, mood swings, suspiciousness, panic, impaired judgment, increased body temperature, hypertension, flushed face, tremor, dilated pupils, constricted pupils (PCP), nystagmus (PCP), violence (PCP)	Prolonged effects and episodes, anxiety, panic, confusion, blurred vision, increases in blood pressure and temperature	No physical withdrawal, but psychologic desire may occur
Inhalants			

Aerosol propellants
  fluorinated hydrocarbons
Nitrous oxide (in deodorants, hair spray, pesticide, whipped cream spray, spray paint, cookware coating products)
Solvents
  Gasoline, kerosene, nail polish remover, typewriter correction fluid, cleaning solutions, lighter fluid, paint, paint thinner, glue
Anesthetic agents
  Nitrous oxide, chloroform
Nitrites
  Amyl nitrite, butyl nitrite
	Euphoria, decreased inhibitions, giddiness, slurred speech, illusions, drowsiness, clouded sensorium, tinnitus, nystagmus, dysrhythmias, cough, nausea, vomiting, diarrhea, irritation to eyes, nose, mouth	Anxiety, respiratory depression, cardiac dysrhythmias, loss of consciousness, sudden death	None

Lower Respiratory Disorders, for more information on nicotine abuse and its effects.)

Cocaine

Cocaine is the most potent of the abused stimulants. It is an alkaloid that was originally obtained from the leaves of the coca plant, but today it can be prepared synthetically. Historically it was used as a local anesthetic, but it has been largely replaced by synthetic agents with no abuse potential. Cocaine is a Schedule II drug under the Controlled Substances Act. Ilicit cocaine is available as a white powder (cocaine hydrochloride) and as cocaine base (alkaloidal cocaine, freebase), a crystalline substance. "Crack," a cocaine base that gets its name from the popping sound the crystals make when heated, is popular because it is less expensive, readily available, easy to use, and has increased purity over cocaine hydrochloride.

Pharmacodynamics

Cocaine inhibits the neuronal uptake of dopamine in the brain and increases the activation of dopamine receptors in the brain reward system. This action magnifies pleasures and leads to rapid dependence. Cocaine also increases norepinephrine at postsynaptic receptor sites, producing intense vasoconstriction and cardiovascular stimulation. Drug interactions with cocaine are identified in Table 8–8.

Table 8-3

Nicotine-Replacement Agents

General Considerations for Nicotine Replacement Therapy (NRT):
- NRT should not be used by pregnant or nursing women.
- Smoking while using NRT may cause nicotine overdose.
- Tapering of all agents except transdermal patches is required.
- Replacement agents used are usually a matter of personal preference.
- The stronger doses of agents should be used by heavy smokers.
- Using more than one agent at the same time should be discussed with the health care provider.
- Generic preparations are available for some of the agents.

Agents	Absorption	Side Effects	Considerations
Gum (OTC) Nicorette 2, 4 mg	Buccal mucosa	Hiccoughs, mouth ulcers, indigestion, jaw pain	Specific 30-min chewing regimen with periods of holding the gum between cheek and teeth; food and drink should be avoided 15 min before, or during use.
Lozenge (OTC) Commit 2, 4 mg	Buccal mucosa	Nausea and indigestion, hiccoughs, headache, cough, mouth soreness, flatulence	Dissolves in the mouth in 20-30 min; chewing and swallowing the lozenge increases GI side effects.

Patch (OTC)
  NicoDerm CQ
  Nicotine
  Transdermal system
  18-, 24-hr doses
	Skin	Skin rash at patch site, headache, dizziness, weakness, indigestion, diarrhea, sleep disturbances with 24-hr patch	Differs from other agents in that it helps prevent craving; cannot be used by those with adhesive allergies.

Nasal Spray Nicotrol NS	Nasal mucosa	Nose and throat irritation, sneezing, rhinitis, watery eyes, cough	Requires a prescription; nasal irritation may limit use; affects airways and not a good choice for those with asthma, allergies, or sinus problems.

Inhaler
  Nicotrol nicotine
  inhalation system,
  delivers 4 mg
	Oral mucosa	Cough; nose, mouth, and throat irritation; heartburn and nausea	Requires a prescription; simulates smoking with mouthpiece and nicotine cartridge; may not be advisable for those with asthma or pulmonary disease.

GI, Gastrointestinal; *OTC*, over the counter.
Additional information and client instructions are available from the American Lung Association at *http://www.lungusa.org*.

Pharmacokinetics

Absorption rates of cocaine depend on the route of administration. Cocaine hydrochloride is usually "snorted" intranasally. Cocaine can also be smoked as "crack" cocaine or in "freebase" form, injected intravenously (IV), taken orally, or absorbed through mucous membranes. Smoking and IV methods result in the fastest absorption and the highest rush. Peak blood levels develop within 5 to 30 minutes with most methods of administration. The longest effects occur following intranasal use because absorption is delayed by vasoconstriction of the nasal vessels. Cocaine is rapidly metabolized by the liver. Elimination half-lives by oral, intranasal, and IV routes are 50, 80, and 60 minutes, respectively. Cocaine readily crosses the placenta in pregnant women and accumulates in the fetal circulation. Conflicting research exists about the effect of prenatal cocaine exposure on the development of the child.

Side Effects and Adverse Reactions

At usual doses cocaine produces euphoria and increased energy and alertness. In addition to stimulation of the CNS, effects include peripheral adrenaline-like actions (see Table 8–2). Chronic use may lead to impairment of concentration and memory, irritability and mood swings, paranoia, and depression.

A stimulant psychosis may occur with the chronic use of any stimulant. A cocaine psychosis usually progresses from paranoid delusions to visual hallucinations of "snow lights," (colored lights when cocaine is administered) and tactile hallucinations of bugs crawling under the skin. Skin excoriations from scratching; needle marks; and elevated blood pressure, heart rate, and temperature are findings that help differentiate a stimulant psychosis from schizophrenia.

Acute cocaine toxicity may be manifested by cardiac palpitations, tachycardia, increased respiratory rate, and fever. At high levels of overdose, grand mal seizures, hypertension, and dysrhythmias or myocardial ischemia can occur. The client experiences restlessness, paranoia, agitated delirium, confusion, and repetitive stereotyped behaviors. Death is often related to a cerebrovascular accident, fatal dysrhythmias, or myocardial infarction.

Although cocaine withdrawal is not usually accompanied with obvious physical signs, an intense psychologic response occurs (see Table 8–2). In the first 9 hours to 14 days, withdrawal is characterized by intense craving and cocaine-seeking behavior. Some individuals experience marked agitation, feelings of depression, exhaustion, and a need to sleep. Eventually, mood becomes more normal, but a desire to return to the drug, especially prompted by cue-induced craving, remains for an indefinite period. In rare instances withdrawal can be prolonged and difficult.

Treatment

Emergency management of cocaine toxicity depends on the client findings at the time of treatment. Treatment may be complicated by the possibility that the client has combined the use of cocaine with heroin, alcohol, or PCP. There is no specific antidote for cocaine toxicity, but during an overdose most symptoms can be controlled with a variety of drugs. Emergency interventions for assessment findings in cocaine toxicity are presented in Table 8–4.

Cessation of cocaine abuse and maintenance of abstinence with behavioral therapies have been difficult to achieve in most users. No drugs are currently approved to promote cocaine abstinence, and most that have been tried have had little effect. Current studies are investigating the effects of propranolol (Inderal), amantadine (Symmetrel), mecamylamine (Inversine), and selegiline (Eldepryl) in cocaine abstinence. In addition, a medication used to treat epilepsy outside the United States, vigabatrin (GVG), has been found to block the biochemical effects of addictive drugs such as nicotine, morphine, psychostimulants, ecstasy, and alcohol. Initial clinical trials are being conducted in the United States to evaluate GVG's effectiveness in treating cocaine addiction.

Amphetamines

Amphetamine is a synthetic drug and, with its derivatives and similar stimulants, is strictly regulated today as a Schedule II drug of the Controlled Substance Act. Specific drugs classified as amphetamines are identified in Table 8–2 and Chapter 19, Central Nervous System Stimulants. Because amphetamines may be used therapeutically as CNS stimulants, abuse may rise out of slow escalation of a prescribed dose. However, they are more often initially used as the "poor man's cocaine." Methamphetamine (crank) and methamphetamine crystals (crystal meth, ice) are produced illegally in clandestine laboratories and are in great demand on the black market.

Pharmacodynamics

Amphetamines act similarly to cocaine, stimulating the release of dopamine and norepinephrine in the brain and the sympathetic nervous system. The dopamine release in the brain reward system produces euphoria and an increase in self-confidence. Drug interactions with amphetamines are identified in Table 8–8 on p. 163.

Pharmacokinetics

Amphetamines are usually taken orally with peak effects occurring within 60 to 90 minutes and may last 2 to 4 hours. More rapid effects are obtained by smoking, snorting, or by IV injection. Amphetamines have a longer half-life than cocaine and, because they are more often taken

---

Table 8–4

Drug Therapy for Cocaine and Amphetamine Toxicity

Assessment Findings	Drug Therapy
Cardiovascular	
Palpitations	Establish IV access and initiate fluid replacement as appropriate.
Tachycardia	Anticipate the need for propranolol (Inderal) or labetalol (Normodyne) for hypertension
Hypertension	and tachycardia.
Dysrhythmias	Severe hypertension may require administration of nitroprusside (Nipride) or phentolamine
Myocardial ischemia or infarction	(Regitine).
	Treat ventricular dysrhythmias as appropriate with lidocaine, bretylium (Bretylol), or procainamide (Pronestyl).
	Aspirin may be administered to lower the risk of myocardial infarction.
Central Nervous System (CNS)	
Feeling of impending doom	Naloxone (Narcan) IV should be given if CNS depression is present and concurrent opiate
Euphoria	use is suspected.
Agitation	Administer diazepam (Valium) or lorazepam (Ativan) IV for agitation and seizures.
Combativeness	Administer chlorpromazine (Thorazine) or haloperidol (Haldol) IV for psychosis and
Seizures	hallucinations.
Hallucinations	
Confusion	
Paranoia	
Fever	

IV, Intravenous.

orally, have a longer effect. See Chapter 19, Central Nervous System Stimulants, for additional information regarding the pharmacodynamics and pharmacokinetics of amphetamines.

Side Effects and Adverse Reactions

Initial use of amphetamines results in increased alertness, improved performance, relief of fatigue, and anorexia. Stimulation of the sympathetic nervous system leads to cardiovascular stimulation with increased heart rate and blood pressure. Amphetamines used over time may lead to irritability, anxiety, paranoia, and hostile and violent behaviors.

Toxic reactions to amphetamines are also similar to those of cocaine. Increased levels of stimulation, sometimes described as "overamping," may result in amphetamine psychosis, paranoia, seizures, and death (see Table 8–2). Without medical intervention, death may occur as a result of dysrhythmias, myocardial infarction, hyperthermia, and cerebral hemorrhage.

Withdrawal symptoms of amphetamines are similar to those of cocaine use and are presented in Table 8–2. Amphetamines usually cause only mild physical dependence, but craving can be intense during abstinence. IV use will cause the onset of withdrawal symptoms in approximately 2 hours, whereas oral use results in withdrawal symptoms in 8 to 10 hours.

Treatment

Clients often seek treatment for complications of amphetamine abuse, such as panic reactions or temporary psychosis related to intoxication, overdose, or withdrawal. Emergency management of amphetamine toxicity is the same as that for cocaine. Elevated blood pressure and tachycardia can be controlled with vasodilators and adrenergic beta-blockers. Drug elimination can be enhanced by administering agents that acidify the urine, such as ammonium chloride. Emergency treatment of amphetamine toxicity is presented in Table 8–4.

Cessation of sex and maintenance of abstinence are difficult in amphetamine abuse. Like cocaine, withdrawal causes more psychologic symptoms than physical symptoms. Depression can last for months and is a common cause of relapse. No specific drug therapy is recommended to help maintain abstinence. It is possible that agents being tested to promote cocaine abstinence may also be effective for amphetamine abuse.

Caffeine

Caffeine is the most widely used psychoactive substance in the world. Its use to promote alertness and to alleviate fatigue is safe in most people. Although weaker than other stimulant drugs, caffeine shares characteristics of intoxication, tolerance, and withdrawal symptoms in some individuals.

Pharmacodynamics

Caffeine is a methylxanthine that stimulates the CNS, especially the medullary respiratory center. It also is a diuretic and myocardial stimulant. It relaxes smooth muscles and promotes peripheral vasodilation and cerebral vasoconstriction.

Pharmacokinetics

Caffeine is readily absorbed from the GI tract and reaches peak plasma levels in about 1 hour. See Chapter 19, Central Nervous System Stimulants, for additional information regarding the pharmacodynamics and pharmacokinetics of caffeine.

Side Effects and Adverse Reactions

Oral doses of 200 mg (two cups of coffee) can elevate mood, produce insomnia, increase irritability, cause anxiety, and offset fatigue. Heavy intake of 500 mg or more per day is known to cause intoxication manifested by nervousness, insomnia, gastric hyperacidity, muscle twitching, confusion, and tachycardia or cardiac dysrhythmias. Ingestion of a lethal dose is extremely rare but could occur with caffeine-containing drugs or the oral ingestion of 10 g (70 to 100 cups of coffee). In toxic doses, caffeine influences behavior patterns and may precipitate panic states.

Physical and psychologic dependence on caffeine have been found with chronic use of more than 500 mg daily. However, dependence may occur in some individuals at lower doses. The most commonly reported withdrawal symptoms are headache, irritability, drowsiness, and fatigue occurring within 12 to 24 hours following abstinence. Caffeine withdrawal may be responsible for some cases of headache that occur after general anesthesia. It is also thought that weekend headaches may also be related to caffeine withdrawal because caffeine consumption in many individuals is higher at work than at home. The effects of caffeine are presented in Table 8–2.

Treatment

Toxic reactions to caffeine and lethal doses of caffeine are managed symptomatically. Attention is given to controlling hypertension, dysrhythmias, and seizures as with other CNS stimulants. Management of the client with symptoms of caffeine dependence includes assisting the client to reduce gradually or to stop the intake of caffeine. A list of caffeinated products with their dosages may be helpful to the client. Substituting decaffeinated beverages may also help. Decaffeinated coffee and tea contain 2 to 4 mg of caffeine per cup.

Depressants

Drugs classified as depressants have common physiologic and psychologic effects. Drugs in this category include alcohol, sedative-hypnotics, anxiolytics, and opioid narcotics. With the exception of alcohol and some federally regulated drugs, most CNS depressants are medically useful. These drugs are also widely recognized for their abuse potential, which leads to rapid tolerance, dependence, and medical emergencies involving overdose and withdrawal.

Alcohol

Alcohol is the most widely consumed substance of abuse in the United States. Most people use alcohol in moderation, with some positive cardiovascular benefits. Abuse of alcohol, however, can lead to dependence and significant health, social, legal, and interpersonal problems. Alcoholism, or alcohol dependency, is currently viewed as a chronic, progressive, potentially fatal disease if left untreated.

Pharmacodynamics

Alcohol affects almost all cells of the body and has complex effects on the neurons in the CNS. Alcohol is a general CNS depressant. In addition, alcohol binds with receptors in the brain reward system, promoting the release of dopamine and the addictive process.

Pharmacokinetics

Alcohol is absorbed directly from the stomach and small intestine. Absorption from the stomach is slower in the presence of water or food, especially proteins and fats. Faster absorption occurs when alcohol is mixed with carbonated liquids. Alcohol is distributed to all body tissues and fluids. It crosses the placenta and can affect fetal development. Alcohol is primarily metabolized in the liver, although a small amount is metabolized in the stomach. Unlike most other drugs in which the metabolic rate increases as plasma drug levels rise, alcohol is usually metabolized at a relatively constant rate. In an occasional or moderate drinker, that metabolic rate is approximately one drink (7 g of alcohol) per hour. One drink is equal to 12 ounces beer, 5 ounces wine, or 1 ounce of distilled spirits. However, regular or heavy use of alcohol induces liver metabolism of itself and other drugs, resulting in more rapid metabolism. Because women have significantly lower rates of stomach metabolism, they have higher blood alcohol levels than men after the same amount of alcohol intake.

The concentration of alcohol in the body can be determined by assessing the blood alcohol concentration (BAC). For the nondependent drinker, the BAC is fairly predictable of alcohol's effects and is presented in Table 8–5. The relationship between BAC and behavior is different in a person who has developed tolerance to alcohol and its effects. This individual is commonly able to drink large amounts without obvious impairment at BAC levels several times higher than levels that would produce obvious impairment in the nontolerant drinker. However, little tolerance develops to respiratory depression. Chronic heavy alcohol users reach the lethal BAC at almost the same level as nonusers.

Alcohol interacts with many commonly prescribed or over-the-counter medications (see Table 8–8). Potentiation and cross-tolerance with other CNS depressants also may occur. **Potentiation** occurs when an additional CNS depressant is taken with alcohol, increasing the effect. **Cross-tolerance**, the need for an increased dose of other drugs, also develops to general anesthetics, barbiturates, and other general CNS depressants. No cross-tolerance develops to opioids.

Side Effects and Adverse Reactions

Alcohol intoxication is evidenced with an increasing BAC and results in behavioral and physical changes described in Tables 8–2 and 8–5. Acute overdose produces vomiting, coma, and respiratory depression. Alcohol-induced hypotension may lead to renal failure and cardiogenic shock, common causes of alcohol-related death.

The effects of chronic alcohol use are numerous. One condition that can be prevented is **Wernicke's encephalopathy**, an inflammatory, hemorrhagic, degenerative condition of the brain resulting from a deficiency of thiamine. Untreated or progressive Wernicke's encephalopathy may lead to **Korsakoff's psychosis**, a form of amnesia characterized by loss of short-term memory and an inability to learn.

Table 8–5

Blood Alcohol Concentration and Related Effects

BAC* (mg%)	Physical and Psychologic Effects
20 (0.02)	Light and moderate drinkers begin to feel some effects after one drink.
40 (0.04)	Most people begin to feel relaxed.
60 (0.06)	Judgment is mildly impaired. People are less able to make rational decisions about their capabilities (e.g., driving skills).
80 (0.08)	Definite impairment of muscle coordination and driving skills occurs. Person is legally intoxicated in some states.
100 (0.10)	Clear deterioration of reaction time and control is observed. Person is legally intoxicated in most states.
120 (0.12)	Vomiting occurs unless this level is reached slowly.
150 (0.15)	Balance and movement are impaired. Equivalent of one half pint of whiskey is circulating in the bloodstream.
300 (0.30)	Many people lose consciousness.
400 (0.40)	Most people lose consciousness, and some die.
450 (0.45)	Breathing stops; person eventually dies.

*Blood alcohol concentration (BAC) is generally recorded in milligrams of alcohol per deciliter (mg/dl) of blood or milligrams percent (mg%). Percentage is used for legal definitions of intoxication. BAC is dependent on how much alcohol is consumed, how fast it is consumed, and the individual's weight.

After excessive drinking, nondependent individuals experience hangovers manifested by malaise, nausea, headache, thirst, and a general feeling of fatigue. In alcoholics, sudden withdrawal may have life-threatening effects. Withdrawal syndrome should be anticipated if the individual reports consumption of more than 10 drinks every day for a period of 2 weeks. Four characteristic signs of withdrawal are gross tremors, seizures, hallucinations, and alcohol withdrawal delirium.

The onset of withdrawal symptoms is variable, depending on the person's drinking pattern. Symptoms may occur the first 4 to 6 hours after the last drink, peak at 24 to 28 hours, and last up to 5 days. Anticipation of withdrawal syndrome should always include assessment of the time of the last alcohol intake. Characteristic symptoms are presented in Table 8–2. Seizures are most likely to occur 7 to 48 hours after the last drink. Alcohol withdrawal delirium is a serious complication that may occur from 30 to 120 hours after the last drink. Delirium components include disorientation, visual or auditory hallucinations, and increased hyperactivity without seizures. Death may be caused by hyperthermia, peripheral vascular collapse, or cardiac failure.

Treatment

Initial treatment of acute alcohol intoxication or overdose requires implementation of the basic principles of airway, breathing, and circulation (ABCs). No antidote for alcohol is available, and stimulants should not be given. Alcohol-induced hypotension cannot be corrected with vasoconstrictors. Alcohol may be removed from the body by gastric lavage and dialysis. Because symptoms of Wernicke's encephalopathy may be difficult to distinguish from those of intoxication, and because it is potentially reversible, IV thiamine at a dose of 300 mg daily is often administered to intoxicated clients. Clients with alcohol intoxication may also be hypoglycemic because of a lack of food intake. Glucose solutions may precipitate Wernicke's encephalopathy in a previously unaffected client. For this reason, thiamine should be started before treatment with IV glucose solution in all clients with alcoholism and continued until the client resumes a normal diet.

Although specific drugs are not indicated for acute alcohol toxicity, drugs are available to facilitate alcohol withdrawal and help maintain abstinence. Management of alcohol withdrawal frequently includes the use of a variety of drugs. Anticipating withdrawal syndrome in clients is important because alcohol withdrawal delirium can usually be prevented by administration of benzodiazepines, such as lorazepam (Ativan). Benzodiazepines (see Chapter 20, Central Nervous System Depressants) with long half-lives are the most effective drugs in alcohol withdrawal to stabilize vital signs, reduce symptoms, and decrease the risk of seizures and delirium. Additional drugs used as adjuncts to benzodiazepines are included in Table 8–6.

Rehabilitation and sustained abstinence are the primary long-term goals of alcohol treatment. Drugs approved to maintain abstinence may be used in addition to behavioral therapy for long-term therapy. These include disulfiram (Antabuse), which prevents drinking by causing an unpleasant reaction if alcohol is consumed, and naltrexone (ReVia), which blocks the desired effects of alcohol. Disulfiram disrupts alcohol metabolism, causing accumulation of acetaldehyde when alcohol is ingested. An adverse reaction to the accumulated acetaldehyde begins with flushing in the face and develops into intense vasodilation of the face, neck, and upper part of the body. Hyperventilation and palpitations may occur. Nausea occurs in 30 to 60 minutes with copious vomiting. Headache, sweating, thirst, chest pain, weakness, blurred vision, and hypotension follow. Blood pressure may decline to shock levels. The reaction lasts from 30 minutes to several hours and can be brought on by ingesting as little as 7 ml of alcohol. In its most severe form, it can be life threatening. In the absence of alcohol, disulfiram may cause drowsiness and skin eruptions that diminish over time.

Disulfiram is metabolized by the liver, and excretion of metabolites occurs through the kidneys and lungs. Up to 20% of the drug is excreted unchanged in the feces. Effects may persist for up to 2 weeks after the last dose is taken. Client education regarding disulfiram therapy is extremely important. Clients must be made aware that consumption of any alcohol while taking disulfiram can cause a severe, potentially fatal reaction. All food and liquid medication labels must be checked for the presence of alcohol, and alcohol must not be used on the skin. Because disulfiram is self-administered, clients must be highly motivated to abstain from alcohol for it to be effective.

Naltrexone is a pure opioid antagonist that decreases craving for alcohol and blocks the "high" of alcohol use. It was originally approved for treatment of opioid addiction but was approved for alcohol dependency when clinical trials found that it reduced alcohol relapse rates by 50% when combined with extensive counseling. Naltrexone is discussed with opioid abuse later in this chapter and in Chapter 21, Drugs for Pain Management: Nonnarcotic and Narcotic Analgesics.

Acamprosate (Campral) was recently approved to decrease craving and distress during abstinence from alcohol. It is thought to act on the brain pathways related to alcohol abuse. Acamprosate is not addicting, and the most common adverse events reported include headache, diarrhea, flatulence, and nausea.

Table 8–6

Drug Therapy for Alcohol Withdrawal

Clinical Manifestations	Medications
Minor Withdrawal Syndrome	
Tremulousness, anxiety	Long-acting benzodiazepines (e.g., lorazepam [Ativan], chlordiazepoxide
Insomnia	[Librium]) to stabilize vital signs, reduce anxiety, and prevent seizures and delirium
Increased heart rate	Thiamine to prevent Wernicke's encephalopathy
Increased blood pressure	Multivitamins (folic acid, B vitamins) for nutritional support
Sweating	Magnesium sulfate if serum magnesium is low
Nausea	Glucose solutions IV if hypoglycemia present (after thiamine)
Hyperreflexia	
Major Withdrawal Syndrome	
Disorientation	Continue use of benzodiazepines and add:
Visual/auditory hallucinations	Antipsychotic drugs (e.g., haloperidol [Haldol]) for hallucinations and delirium
Increased hyperactivity without seizures	Carbamazepine (Tegretol) or phenytoin (Dilantin) to prevent or treat seizures
Gross tremors	
Seizures	
Alcohol withdrawal delirium	

IV, Intravenous.

Ondansetron (Zofran) is an antagonist of receptors in the brain reward system that decreases motivation for drinking in early onset alcoholism and is currently in clinical trials.

Sedative-Hypnotics

Commonly abused sedative-hypnotic agents include barbiturates, benzodiazepines, and barbiturate-like drugs. Benzodiazepines have largely replaced barbiturates as therapeutic agents for anxiety and insomnia because they have less risk of toxicity, tolerance, and dependence. The short-acting barbiturates are preferred as recreational drugs because they more frequently produce euphoric effects (see Chapter 20, Central Nervous System Depressants).

Pharmacodynamics and Pharmacokinetics

Sedative-hypnotic drugs act primarily on the CNS. Benzodiazepines enhance the effects of gamma-aminobutyric acid (GABA), an inhibitory neurotransmitter in the brain. Barbiturates not only enhance the inhibitory effect of GABA, but they can directly mimic the actions of GABA. Barbiturates are powerful respiratory depressants and can readily cause death by overdose. See Chapter 20, Central Nervous System Depressants, for a description of the pharmacodynamics and pharmacokinetics of these drugs.

Side Effects and Adverse Reactions

The abuse potential is much greater for barbiturates than benzodiazepines. The drugs are usually taken orally, but both may be injected intravenously. Excessive doses produce an initial euphoria and intoxication similar to that of alcohol. The effects of sedative-hypnotics are presented in Table 8-2.

Tolerance develops rapidly to the sedative effects of barbiturates, requiring higher doses to achieve euphoria. Little tolerance develops to respiratory depression, however, and increasing doses may trigger hypotension and respiratory depression, resulting in death. Cross-tolerance also develops between barbiturates and other CNS depressants such as alcohol, benzodiazepines, and general anesthetics. Little cross-tolerance occurs with opioids, however. In addition, many drug interactions are associated with barbiturates and benzodiazepines (see Table 8-8).

An overdose of a sedative-hypnotic produces respiratory depression and coma. Other symptoms of overdose are listed in Table 8-2.

Withdrawal from sedative-hypnotics can be very serious. In the first 12 to 16 hours following the last dose, the client may develop anxiety, tremors, weakness, nausea or vomiting, muscle cramps, and increased reflexes. After 24 hours the client is craving the drug and may experience delirium, grand mal seizures, and respiratory and cardiac arrest (see Table 8-2). Symptoms of withdrawal peak on the second or third day for short-acting drugs (e.g., alprazolam, secobarbital, pentobarbital) and on the seventh or eighth day for long-acting drugs (e.g., diazepam, chlordiazepoxide, phenobarbital).

Treatment

Overdoses of benzodiazepines are treated with flumazenil (Romazicon), a specific benzodiazepine antagonist. No antagonists are known to counteract the effects of barbiturates or other sedative-hypnotic drugs. Emergency life support measures must be taken in cases of overdose. Gastric lavage may be used if the drug was taken orally within 4 to 6 hours. Dialysis may be required to decrease the drug level. Gradual withdrawal of the drug is required during withdrawal syndrome. Phenobarbital, a long-acting barbiturate, may be used to control withdrawal symptoms in a client dependent on barbiturates. Phenobarbital is then gradually withdrawn when the client is stable. Hospitalization is recommended during drug withdrawal for individuals who have been abusing large amounts of barbiturates to manage their symptoms safely.

Opioids

Opioids include the naturally occurring opiates derived from opium in addition to the many semisynthetic and synthetic narcotic agents used as analgesics (see Table 8-2). Individuals who abuse opioids include those who use illegal drugs sold on the street and individuals who misuse opioids in a medical setting. Those who begin drug use illegally constitute the largest group of abusers. Street use usually involves the use of heroin. In a medical setting, some people misuse prescribed analgesics. A significant group in the medical setting includes health care professionals, who may have the highest rate of opioid abuse and dependence of any middle-class population. Ready access to drugs, stresses of the workplace environment, and long hours that interfere with family life are considered contributing factors in health care professionals. Drug abuse and chemical dependency in nurses are discussed later in this chapter.

Pharmacodynamics and Pharmacokinetics

The pharmacodynamics and pharmacokinetics of opioids are presented in Chapter 21, Drugs for Pain Management: Narcotic and Nonnarcotic Analgesics. Important to the abuse potential of opioids is their ability to activate the brain reward system, reinforcing their addictive effect. As drugs of abuse, opioids are taken orally, sniffed, smoked, or injected subcutaneously ("skin-popping") or intravenously ("mainlining"). IV use will produce effects in seconds. Smoking or sniffing produces a longer onset and effect. Drug interactions with opioids are identified in Table 8-8.

Side Effects and Adverse Reactions

The primary effects of opioids include analgesia, drowsiness, slurred speech, and detachment from the environment. IV use usually causes a "rush" of feelings in the lower abdomen, along with warm skin flushing and a strong sense of euphoria (see Table 8-2). Opioid use leads to rapid tolerance and physical dependence after short-term use. Cross-tolerance among the opioids is common, but cross-tolerance to other CNS depressants does not occur. However, additive effects of other CNS depressants may lead to increased CNS depression.

Signs of overdose of opioids include pinpoint pupils, clammy skin, depressed respiration, coma, and death, if not treated. Unintentional overdose frequently occurs with recreational use of the drugs because of the unpredictability in potency and purity. Signs of toxicity are presented in Table 8–2.

Withdrawal symptoms occur with decreased amounts or cessation of the drug after prolonged moderate to heavy use. The administration of a narcotic antagonist, such as naloxone (Narcan), will cause withdrawal symptoms in dependent individuals. Symptoms may include craving, abdominal cramps, diarrhea, nausea, and vomiting. Additional symptoms are presented in Table 8–2. Symptoms appear about 8 to 10 hours after the last dose, peak within 36 to 48 hours, and usually subside in 96 hours. Although opioid withdrawal is acutely uncomfortable, it is not usually life threatening, as is withdrawal from other CNS depressants.

Treatment

Overdose of opioids can precipitate a medical emergency. A narcotic antagonist such as naloxone (Narcan) should be given as soon as life support is instituted. The use of naloxone and other narcotic antagonists is discussed in Chapter 21, Drugs for Pain Management: Narcotic and Nonnarcotic Analgesics.

Treatment of withdrawal syndrome is symptom based and does not always require the use of medication. Methadone (Dolophine) in decreasing doses over 10 to 14 days is the drug most often used during opioid detoxification to decrease symptoms. Some clients obtain relief from withdrawal symptoms with the use of clonidine (Catapres), a centrally acting alpha$_2$-adrenergic agonist that may also be used for nicotine addiction (see Chapter 42, Antihypertensive Drugs). It is most effective against GI hyperactivity, but it does not decrease craving. The action of clonidine in nicotine and opioid addiction is not fully understood.

Long-term management of opioid addiction involves the use of opioid agonists, opioid antagonists, and mixed opioid agonist-antagonists (see Table 8–7 and Chapter 21, Drugs for Pain Management: Narcotic and Nonnarcotic Analgesics). Methadone is the most commonly used opioid agonist. By substituting oral methadone for the abused opioid, withdrawal syndrome can be avoided and the euphoria that leads to craving can be prevented. Levomethadyl (Orlaam) is a long-acting analog of methadone that has been used to maintain abstinence. However, it was withdrawn from the market by the manufacturer in 2004 because of continuing reports of serious cardiac adverse effects. Methadone is an addictive drug, but its use in maintenance programs alters the drug-using lifestyle, reduces exposure to infectious disease, and controls drug use. To

prevent methadone abuse, it is available for addiction treatment only through agencies approved by the FDA and state authorities.

Naltrexone (Trexan, ReVia) is an opioid antagonist that blocks euphoria and all other opioid effects. Like naloxone, it will precipitate withdrawal symptoms when administered to opioid-dependent individuals. When naltrexone is used, administration of an opioid produces no effect, eliminating the reinforcing properties of drug use. It does not prevent craving, however. Naltrexone is used for long-term abstinence maintenance because it can be taken orally and has a long half-life.

Buprenorphine is an agonist-antagonist opioid that may be used for detoxification and maintenance therapy. Because of its action on specific opiate receptors, it can decrease the symptoms of withdrawal and suppress drug craving, yet it has a low potential for abuse. For treatment of withdrawal symptoms, it is available in a sublingual tablet marketed as Subutex. For long-term maintenance it is combined with naltrexone in a sublingual tablet marketed as Suboxone. In this preparation, naltrexone is added to the buprenorphine to prevent addicts from injecting the tablets intravenously, which has happened with tablets containing only buprenorphine. Because it contains naloxone, Suboxone can produce intense withdrawal symptoms if it is used intravenously by opioid-addicted individuals. Buprenorphine in other forms (e.g., Buprenex) is not approved for treatment of opioid addiction and is used only as a Schedule III analgesic.

Other Drugs of Abuse

Cannabis

In North America, cannabis is usually sold as marijuana or hashish. Tetrahydrocannabinol (THC) is the active ingredient in cannabis that is responsible for most of the psychoactive effects. Although a number of potential benefits of THC have been reported, the only approved THC preparation is dronabinol (Marinol). It is used to control nausea and vomiting resulting from cancer chemotherapy and to simulate the appetite in clients with acquired immunodeficiency syndrome (AIDS).

Pharmacodynamics

At low to moderate doses, THC produces fewer physiologic and psychologic alterations than do other classes of psychoactive drugs, including alcohol. Although its mechanism of action is uncertain, THC affects cannabinoid receptors in the brain and may act in part through the same reward system as opioids and cocaine.

Pharmacokinetics

When marijuana is smoked, effects usually occur in about 20 to 30 minutes and may last up to 7 hours. Because it is stored in body fat, it is eliminated slowly, resulting in a half-life of 2 to 7 days. When taken orally, it is almost completely absorbed but undergoes extensive first-pass metabolism.

Table 8–7

Drugs Used in Opioid Addiction

State with Signs and Symptoms	Drugs
Toxicity 　Respiratory depression 　Coma	Opioid antagonists: 　naloxone (Narcan): Short acting and may need to be repeated until opioid levels decrease; too much will cause withdrawal symptoms. 　Nalmefene (Revex): Long acting; may cause prolonged withdrawal if dose is excessive
Detoxification/withdrawal 　Nausea, vomiting, diarrhea 　Abdominal cramping 　Bone and muscle pain 　Muscle spasms 　Tremor, chills, diaphoresis	Opioid substitution: 　methadone (Dolophine): An opioid agonist that may be used to prevent withdrawal syndrome; when used for withdrawal, it is given in decreasing oral doses over 10 to 14 days after the client is stabilized. 　buprenorphine (Subutex): an opioid agonist-antagonist that can be substituted for abused opioids to prevent withdrawal syndrome but can cause withdrawal if an opioid agonist is in the bloodstream; for treatment of withdrawal, it must be given after withdrawal symptoms begin. Centrally acting alpha$_2$-adrenergic agonist: 　clonidine (Catapres): effective in decreasing GI hyperactivity and some other symptoms of withdrawal but does not reduce craving for the drug.
Maintenance of abstinence 　Craving, cue-induced craving	Opioid agonists: 　methadone (Dolophine): substitution for abused opioids may be used for long-term treatment of dependency. Addiction is maintained with this method and withdrawal occurs if methadone is stopped, but drug use can be controlled and drug-using lifestyles changed with methadone maintenance. Opioid antagonists: 　naltrexone (ReVia, Trexan): blocks opioid receptors, preventing the desired effects if opioids are used; is a long-acting oral preparation that must be used voluntarily. Mixed opioid agonist/antagonists: 　buprenorphine (Subutex), a sublingual tablet, can be used instead of methadone for maintenance therapy. To prevent abuse of buprenorphine itself, it is also marketed in combination with naltrexone as Suboxone. If this preparation is crushed and injected, opioid withdrawal will occur in an opioid-addicted individual. When Suboxone is used sublingually, the opioid agonist effect predominates.

Side Effects and Adverse Reactions

Marijuana and hashish are usually smoked as a cigarette. Usual effects include euphoria, sedation, and hallucinations. Responses are varied and depend on dose, expectations of the user, and the setting of drug use. The most commonly affected organs are the brain and the cardiovascular and respiratory systems. Decreased sperm production and decreased reproductive hormones in both men and women may occur. Signs of intoxication are presented in Table 8–2. Problems of chronic heavy use include impaired short-term memory, decreased motor coordination, tremors, and increased heart and respiratory rates. A condition known as amotivational syndrome, characterized by apathy, dullness, and disinterest, may also occur.

Acute reactions, including intoxication and withdrawal, are usually mild and time limited. Complications may result when marijuana is used with other drugs, such as heroin and cocaine (see Table 8–8). Tolerance to many of its effects occurs, but physical dependence does not usually develop, even with long-term heavy use. Marijuana has low toxicity, and there is no known level of lethal dose. In rare instances withdrawal can be prolonged and difficult.

Treatment

Individuals using marijuana may seek treatment for panic reactions or may be treated for toxic reactions to a combination of drugs that includes marijuana. Treatment is directed toward relief of symptoms, and the administration of drugs is avoided if possible. There is no antidote or substitution therapy for cannabis.

Psychedelic Agents

Psychedelic drugs are often referred to as hallucinogens. These drugs produce a change in level of consciousness and induce hallucinations and mental states that resemble psychosis. Primarily they bring about alterations in thoughts, perceptions, and feelings that only occur in dreams. Common agents and their effects are identified in Table 8–2. Although LSD originally was thought to provide a model for study of psychosis, this idea was found to be incorrect. As a result, the drugs have no recognized medical use. Currently Ecstasy (3,4-methylenediosymethamphetamine or MDMA) is the most commonly used psychedelic. It is a popular drug among adolescents and young adults at nightclubs and all-night dance parties known as "raves." It also may be used as a date-rape drug.

Table 8–8

Drug Interactions: Drugs of Abuse

Drug of Abuse	Interacting Drugs	Effects
Nicotine/smoking*	isoproterenol (Isuprel) phenylephrine (Neo-Synephrine)	Increased effects with use of nicotine/smoking (After smoking cessation, dosages may need to be increased.)
	pentazocine (Talwin) propoxyphene (Darvon) Benzodiazepines (e.g., diazepam [Valium]) Tricyclic antidepressants propranolol (Inderal) theophylline heparin insulin	Decreased effects with use of nicotine/smoking (After smoking cessation, dosages may need to be reduced.)
Cocaine	Sympathomimetics/adrenomimetics CNS stimulants Cholinesterase inhibitors (e.g., neostigmine)	May increase CNS and cardiac effects of cocaine.
	Tricyclic antidepressants, digoxin, methyldopa	May increase cocaine-induced dysrhythmias.
	Adrenergic beta-blockers	Cocaine may decrease effects.
Amphetamines	Tricyclic antidepressants Sympathomimetics/adrenomimetics CNS stimulants	Increased effect of tricyclics and sympathomimetics; increased effect of amphetamines
	GI antacids/urinary alkalinizing agents MAO inhibitors	Increased amphetamine effect
	meperidine (Demerol)	Amphetamines increase analgesic effect; meperidine increases risk of seizures and vascular collapse.
	thyroid hormone	Reciprocal increase in effects
	Adrenergic blockers Antihistamines Antihypertensives	Amphetamines may decrease effects.

Alcohol	Other CNS depressants:
	  Sedative-hypnotics
	  Opioids
	  General anesthetics
		Increased CNS depression with increased risk of death from respiratory depression

	Nonsteroidal antiinflammatory drugs	Combined effect increases risk of gastric bleeding.
	acetaminophen (e.g., Tylenol)	Increased risk of liver injury
	Antihypertensives	Decreased effect of antihypertensives

Barbiturates	Other CNS depressants:
	  alcohol
	  Opioids
	  General anesthetics
	  Other sedative/hypnotics
	  MAO inhibitors
	  valproic acid (Depakene)
		Increased CNS depression

	Oral anticoagulants Cortico- and other steroid hormones griseofulvin doxycycline	Effect decreased by barbiturates

Benzodiazepines	Other CNS depressants:
	  alcohol
	  Opioids
	  General anesthetics
	  Other sedative/hypnotics
	Herbs:
	  kava kava
	  valerian
		Increased CNS depression

Opioids	Other CNS depressants:
	  alcohol
	  General anesthetics
	  Sedative/hypnotics
	  Phenothiazines
	  Antiemetics
		Increased CNS depression

CNS, Central nervous system; *GI*, gastrointestinal; *MAO*, monoamine oxidase.
*Interactions may be due to nicotine or the effect on the liver by hydrocarbons found in cigarette smoke.

Continued

Table 8–8

Drug Interactions: Drugs of Abuse—cont'd

Drug of Abuse	Interacting Drugs	Effects
Opioids—cont'd	Mixed agonist/antagonist opioids	Reduces the effect of pure opioid agonists and may precipitate withdrawal syndrome
	MAO inhibitors	May cause severe, fatal reaction.
	Diuretics	Opioids may decrease effect.
Marijuana/hashish	CNS stimulants/sympathomimetics	Additive hypertension, tachycardia, drowsiness
	Anticholinergic agents	
	Tricyclic antidepressants	
	CNS depressants	Additive drowsiness and CNS depression
	theophylline	Decreased effect of theophylline

The effects of psychedelic use are primarily psychologic, but cardiovascular and neurologic toxicity may occur. Little or no physical dependence develops, but acute panic reactions are common with toxicity. Panic attacks may be treated with an antianxiety agent such as diazepam (Valium) and by providing a nonthreatening environment. Although a toxic reaction may mimic a psychosis, the use of antipsychotic agents such as phenothiazines (e.g., haloperidol, chlorpromazine) can intensify the experience.

Inhalants

Inhalation is the major route of ingestion for a number of common household and industrial volatile substances. Forms of use include sniffing, huffing, bagging, or spraying. Because inhalants are readily accessible, inexpensive, and produce a rapid high, their use among preadolescents and adolescents is high.

The four main classes of inhalants are volatile solvents, aerosols, anesthetic agents, and nitrites. They act as CNS depressants but are also extremely damaging to the cardiovascular and respiratory systems. Common agents and their effects are presented in Table 8–2. Users may develop peripheral neuropathies and exhibit tremors and weakness. Sudden death may occur from direct toxic effects, aspiration of gastric contents, trauma, and suffocation. No antidotes are available for these substances, and treatment of toxicity is symptomatic.

Special Needs of Drug-Abusing Clients

Surgical Clients

An individual who abuses dugs is at high risk for drug interactions, complications, and death when surgery is required. Preoperative assessment of all clients must include an assessment of drug use. Respiratory changes in smokers make introduction of endotracheal and suction tubes more difficult and increase the risk for postoperative respiratory problems. Postoperative headaches may be caused by caffeine withdrawal in heavy users. During the client's

postoperative period, the nurse should be alert for signs and symptoms of drug interactions with pain medications or anesthesia and for signs of drug withdrawal. Reactions that should be considered in surgical clients who abuse drugs are presented in Box 8–1.

Special precautions must be taken for the client who is intoxicated or alcohol dependent and requires surgery. Alcohol use may be overlooked in an accident victim if there are injuries that cause CNS depression. In addition, many persons are undiagnosed as alcoholics at the time of admission for elective surgery. The client who is alcohol dependent but is not currently drinking usually requires an increased level of anesthesia because of cross-tolerance. The intoxicated individual needs a decreased level of anesthesia because of the synergistic effect of alcohol. Whenever possible, surgery is postponed in alcohol-intoxicated individuals until the BAC is less than 200 mg%. Synergistic effects occur with anesthesia when the BAC is >150 mg%, and a client with a BAC >250 mg% has a significantly increased surgical risk and mortality rate. Alcohol-withdrawal delirium may be triggered by surgery and the cessation of alcohol consumption. Anesthetics and pain

BOX 8–1

Surgical Considerations: Clients with Drug Abuse

Standard amounts of anesthetic and analgesic medication may not be sufficient because of cross-tolerance.

Anesthetic agents may have a prolonged sedative effect if the client has liver dysfunction.

Increased doses of pain medication may be required if the client is dependent on opioids.

Dosage of pain medications must be reduced gradually.

Clients have an increased susceptibility to cardiac and respiratory depression.

Clients have an increased risk for bleeding, postoperative complications, and infection.

Withdrawal symptoms from central nervous system (CNS) depressants may be delayed for up to 5 days because of effects of anesthetics and pain medications.

medications used in the acute period can delay withdrawal syndrome for up to 5 days postoperatively.

Pain Management

Although nurses and physicians may be reluctant to administer opioids to drug-dependent clients for fear of promoting or enhancing addictions, there is no evidence that providing opioid analgesia to these clients in any way worsens their addictive disease. When addicted clients experience any type of acute pain, the goal is to treat the pain. Addiction treatment is not the priority while the client is in pain.

If the client acknowledges opioid use, it is important to determine the types and amounts of drugs used. It is best to avoid exposing the client to the drug of abuse, and effective equianalgesic doses of other opioids can be determined if daily drug doses are known. If a history of drug abuse is unknown, or if the client does not acknowledge drug abuse, the nurse should suspect abuse when normal doses of analgesics do not relieve the client's pain or signs of withdrawal occur. Withdrawal symptoms can exacerbate pain and lead to drug-seeking behavior or illicit drug use. Toxicology screens may be helpful in determining recently used drugs.

Severe pain should be treated with opioids but at much higher doses than those used with drug-naïve clients. The use of one opioid is preferred. Mixed opioid angonist-antagonists, such as butorphanol (Stadol) or buprenorphine (Buprenex), should be avoided because these may precipitate withdrawal symptoms. Nonopioid and adjuvant analgesics and nonpharmacologic pain relief measures may also be used. To maintain opioid blood levels and prevent withdrawal symptoms, analgesics should be provided around the clock. Supplemental doses should be used to treat breakthrough pain. Although patient-controlled analgesia (PCA) is controversial for treating addicted clients, its use may improve pain control and reduce drug-seeking behavior.

A written agreement or treatment plan that describes the pain management should be developed with the client. The plan should assure that pain will be treated based on the client's perception and report of pain but also clearly outline the gradual tapering of the analgesic dose and eventual substitution of long-acting oral preparations for parenteral analgesics.

Chemical Impairment in Nurses

Drug abuse is a serious concern in the nursing profession. It is estimated that 10% to 20% of nurses (i.e., 300,000 to 600,000) have substance-abuse problems and that 3% to 6% (i.e., 90,000 to 180,000) demonstrate impaired practice resulting from the use of drugs (chemicals). Alcohol is the most commonly abused drug among nurses. Other drugs include meperidine (Demerol), oxycodone (Percodan), diazepam (Valium), and alprazolam (Xanax).

Contributing Factors

A number of contributing factors to drug abuse among nurses have been identified. Specific stressors that are commonly thought to contribute to this problem include chronic fatigue, illness, responsibility for clients' responses to illness and dying, professional dissatisfaction, access to drugs, marital and child care problems, and downsizing. Other factors include nurses' false beliefs that drugs can relieve problems or that knowledge of drugs provides immunity to drug problems. The issue has become less of a priority within the nursing community over the past several years, partly because the nursing shortage and workplace hazards have received more attention. Yet these current trends lead to increasing stressful working conditions that put nurses at even greater risk for substance-related disorders.

Characteristics

Evidence of chemical dependence may be seen by changes in personality and behavior, job performance, and attendance. Behaviors related to the influence of the drug or signs of withdrawal may also be present. Poor judgement, errors, inappropriate behavior, and illogical documentation are common in the chemically impaired nurse. Discrepancies in controlled-drug handling and records may indicate drug diversion, the deliberate redirecting of a drug from a client or facility to the employee for his or her own or others use. Nurses often enable substance abuse to continue among co-workers by covering their mistakes or tardiness, excusing their behavior, or simply ignoring obvious signs and symptoms. When it is recognized that a nurse is impaired, help for the nurse requires sharing observations and concerns with the nurse and supervisor to provide the means for rehabilitation.

Management

Management of drug abuse in nurses largely depends on the state in which the nurse practices and the policies of the employing facility. Sometimes the nurse is simply terminated, allowing the nurse to work elsewhere with no resolution of the problem. Some states or facilities require that management report the nurse to regulatory agencies that will revoke the nurse's license or result in referral to the criminal justice system. These approaches are disciplinary and contribute to the reluctance by nurses to report impaired co-workers.

The tragedy of allowing a treatable disease to go untreated is costly in both human and economic terms. In an effort to help impaired nurses, the American Nurses Association, the National Student Nurse Organization, and other nursing organizations and nurse substance-abuse experts strongly advocate rehabilitation for nurses who are chemically dependent. Alternatives to discipline have developed in most states. Alternatives include diversion programs associated with the state board of nursing that allow nurses to maintain their licenses while being monitored through recovery; state nurses' association peer assistance programs; and employee assistance programs. The goals of these programs are to protect the safety of the public, to maintain the integrity of the profession, and to ensure that the nurse is offered the possibility of treatment and rehabilitation before the license to practice is revoked or the job is terminated. Other efforts are under way to prevent chemical dependency in nurses through substance abuse educational programs, both for nursing students and nurse employees.

Summary

All nurses care for clients dependent on drugs, whether they are identified as dependent or not, simply because of the prevalence of drug abuse. It is important for nurses to suspect, identify, and intervene with clients who are abusing drugs. Knowledge of the commonly abused drugs and their treatment during intoxication, overdose, withdrawal, and cessation is critical to maintaining life and promoting healthy, drug-free lifestyles.

Nursing Process

Smoking (Nicotine) Cessation

ASSESSMENT

- Assess current smoking status and smoking history.
- Identify the cultural context of client's smoking pattern.
- Determine the willingness of client to attempt to quit.
- Have client identify negative consequences of smoking and the potential benefits of quitting.
- Ask client to identify any barriers or impediments to quitting.
- Identify what rewards for quitting are most important to client.

NURSING DIAGNOSES

- Health-seeking behavior

PLANNING

- Client will eliminate tobacco use.

NURSING INTERVENTIONS

- Set a quit date with client, ideally within 2 weeks.

- Teach client about the nicotine-replacement systems and other agents available to assist in smoking cessation.
- Help client choose the best method to quit smoking based on his or her preferences and anticipated benefits.
- Refer client to support groups or quit-tobacco programs available in the community.
- Teach client to anticipate withdrawal symptoms and challenges of quitting.
- Teach client to keep a list of "slips" and near-slips to learn to avoid their causes.
- Teach client to avoid environments and activities previously associated with smoking.
- Schedule frequent follow-up contacts with client to offer encouragement, and help the client deal with lapses.

EVALUATION

- Evaluate the effectiveness of the cessation plan, including the use of drugs and support systems to avoid relapses.
- Determine the smoking status of client.

WEBSITES

For further information on *Drugs of Abuse,* visit these Internet resources:

American Cancer Society: Complete Guide to Quitting: *www.cancer.org*

American Heart Association: How Can I Quit Smoking?: *http://americanheart.org*

American Lung Association: *www.lungusa.org*

American Society of Addiction Medicine: *www.asan.org*

National Clearinghouse for Alcohol and Drug Information: *www.health.org/about/*

National Institute on Drug Abuse: *www.drugabuse.gov*

Tobacco Information and Prevention Source (TIPS): *www.cdc.gov/tobacco*

International Nurses Society on Addictions: *www.intnsa.org*

Critical Thinking Case Study

L.M., a 57-year-old farmer, is admitted to the surgical unit in preparation for back surgery after conservative treatment for a recent back injury has not relieved his pain. His wife tells the nurse she hopes the surgery will be successful because her husband has just been sitting around the house drinking more beer than usual because he has not been able to work. Mr. M. appears relaxed and unconcerned about his anticipated surgery. He jokes with the nurse, telling her that his back would be cured if "a cute, young thing like her would only rub his back."

1. What assessments of L.M.'s alcohol use should the nurse make and communicate to the surgeon and anesthesiologist before he is further prepared for surgery?

2. How would the nurse's approximation of L.M.'s BAC affect his surgical experience?

3. During L.M.'s postoperative period, when would the nurse expect signs of withdrawal syndrome to occur and why?

4. What early signs and symptoms would alert the nurse to the development of withdrawal syndrome?

5. What drug regimens might be used during L.M.'s postoperative period to manage problems associated with his alcohol use?

Study Questions

1. What is the difference between drug misuse and drug abuse? Between physical dependency and psychologic dependency?

2. Describe the brain reward system and how it contributes to addiction.

3. What drugs commonly cause withdrawal syndrome, and which ones cause little or no withdrawal symptoms?

4. What approach should be used by the nurse when a client tells the nurse that he has tried to quit smoking several times unsuccessfully but wants to quit permanently?

5. A client admitted to the emergency department has chest pain and palpitations. What assessment findings by the nurse would indicate acute cocaine toxicity in the client?

6. What teaching would the client who is to use disulfiram (Antabuse) for alcohol treatment need from the nurse?

7. What is the safest and most effective method to withdraw the drug in a client dependent on barbiturates?

8. What is the rationale for the use of long-term methadone (Dolophine) treatment of opioid addiction?

9. Identify the drugs of abuse that have specific antidotes approved for overdose.

10. What problems occur with long-term heavy marijuana use?

11. What approach should the nurse take in providing analgesics to a client addicted to opioids?

12. What factors contribute to chemical impairment in nurses? How is chemical impairment identified?

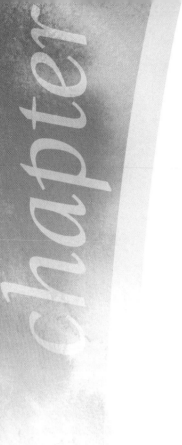

9

Herbal Therapy with Nursing Implications

ELECTRONIC RESOURCES

Additional information can be found on the companion website at *http://evolve.elsevier.com/KeeHayes/pharmacology/* or on the companion CD-ROM, which includes:
- *NCLEX-style examination review questions*
- *Pharmacology animations*
- *Medication error and IV therapy checklists*
- *Medication calculation problems*
- *Electronic calculators*

OUTLINE

OBJECTIVES

- Discuss at least four important points associated with consumer and health care provider education.
- Compare at least four common herbs and their associated toxicity.
- Differentiate at least eight of the most common herbal therapies and at least one situation in which they seem to be helpful.
- Describe the recommendations for labels on herbal therapy.
- Discuss the nursing implications, including client teaching, related to herbal products.

TERMS

Current Good Manufactur-
  ing Practices (CGMPs)
Dietary Supplement
  Health and Education
  Act of 1994 (DSHEA)

dried herbs
extracts
fresh herbs
herb

herbal monographs
oils
phytomedicine
salves

syrups
teas
tinctures

Introduction

The purpose of this chapter is to inform nurses about herbal therapy and the herbal products that clients may use. It is critical for nurses to know about herbs and include herbal preparations as part of their assessment. Herbal products can have both positive and negative effects and important interactions with medications. Nurses are in an excellent position to foster clients' sharing of such information.

An **herb**, according to *Webster's New Collegiate Dictionary*, is a "plant or plant part valued for its medicinal, savory, or aromatic qualities." Herbs have strong roots in Judeo-Christianity (e.g., the tree of life). Also, herbs have long been and continue to be sources of old and new drugs, such as foxglove (source of digitalis), snakeroot (source of reserpine), willow bark (source of aspirin), and Pacific yew tree (source of Taxol). The therapeutic value of **phytomedicine** relates to several factors including dosage, potency, and purity. Research into the effects of herbal medicine is increasing. Although much of this research is conducted in the Orient, more is being done in the West.

Many Americans are using herbal products for therapeutic or preventive reasons. Herbs are the earliest form of medicine, and many cultural groups continue to routinely use herbs as medicine. Herbal therapy has surged in popularity in recent years. Marketing and the media have fueled the hype. Magazines, newspapers, billboards, and displays in grocery and drug stores are ablaze with products and advertisements. Herbal therapy has grown into a multimillion-dollar business as a result of the "back to nature" movement of the 1970s and the more health-conscious modern citizenry. In addition, herbal therapy is now being addressed in the professional literature with increasing frequency and seriousness. Health care providers and consumers are asking questions about herbal therapy, such as, "How effective is it?," "Are herbs toxic?," and "In what ways do herbs mix with current medications?" What do these questions mean for consumers and their health? Consumers should be skeptical of potentially dangerous TV, radio, and other advertisements that infer that herbs will cure anything. Herbs *can* be useful, but they can also be useless or even dangerous (see Herbal Alert 9–1).

Herbs were the original medicines and are still in wide use throughout the world. It is estimated that phytomedicines are prescribed by the majority of physicians in Germany. This practice is promoted because the government's health insurance pays for botanical remedies. Americans have long used botanicals—but outside the mainstream. The United States exports significant quantities of herbs to Europe. Few pharmacy schools in the United States offer courses in botanical remedies.

In 1992, Congress instructed the National Institutes of Health to develop an Office of Alternative Medicine to support studies of alternative therapies. This office is now called the National Center for Complementary and Alternative Medicine (NCCAM).

It is reasonable to expect an associated expense of $350 million to bring a new drug to market. A botanical remedy cannot be patented; thus manufacturers generally cannot justify this expense in an already booming conventional medicine economy.

This chapter describes selected aspects of herbal therapy including (1) herbal monographs, (2) the Dietary Supplement Health and Education Act of 1994, (3) varieties of herbal preparations, (4) the most commonly used herbs, (5) herbs used to treat selected common ailments, (6) potential hazards of herbs, (7) tips for consumers and health care providers, and (8) herbal resources.

Herbal Monographs

The two primary types of **herbal monographs** are therapeutic and qualitative. Therapeutic monographs contain information on use, dosage, side effects, and contraindications. Qualitative monographs have information on areas such as compliance with compounding guidelines and standards of purity. Integrating herbs into the American health care system requires both types of monographs, which the United States currently does not have.

Work to develop these monographs is in progress by several organizations including the United States Pharmacopeia (USP), World Health Organization (WHO), American Herbal Pharmacopeia (AHP), European Scientific Cooperative of Phytomedicines (ESCOP), and German Commission E.

> ### HERBAL ALERT 9-1
> **Client Responsibility**
> To optimize the therapeutic regimen, the client has the responsibility to (1) consult with the health care provider before taking any herbal preparation, (2) report all herbal preparations taken to all health care providers, and (3) inform health care providers of any allergic or sensitivity to any herbal products.

Table 9–1	
Selected Herbal Products with Standardized Concentrations	
Herb	**Standardized Concentration of Active Ingredient**
Bilberry	25% anthanocyanosides
Feverfew	0.2% parthenolide
Ginkgo biloba	24% flavone glycosides; 6% terpene lactones
Goldenseal	8%-12% alkaloid
Hawthorn	20% procyanidins
St. John's wort	0.13%-0.30% hypericin
Saw palmetto	85%-95% fatty acids

The American Botanical Council has translated the German Commission E monographs into English as an effort to bring more information to the American public. Much work remains to be done related to effects of preparations and the improvement of manufacturing and marketing processes.

The German Commission E (in Germany), an oversight commission, works to determine the safety of an herbal product with "reasonable certainty." In addition, "standardized" is an important feature within herbal products. "Standardization" is movement toward consistency and comparison. A standardized herbal extract has one or multiple ingredients whose levels are guaranteed in the sold product. Examples of standardized herbal products are presented in Table 9–1.

Dietary Supplement Health and Education Act of 1994

The **Dietary Supplement Health and Education Act of 1994 (DSHEA)** clarified marketing regulations for herbal remedies. Furthermore, it reclassified them as "dietary supplements," distinct from food or drugs. Herbal supplements can be marketed with suggested dosages. Consumers are reminded that premarket testing for safety and efficacy is not required, and manufacturing is not standardized. The physiologic effects of the product can be noted, but no claims can be made about preventing or curing specific conditions. For example, a claim cannot say the agent "prevents heart disease," but it can say that the agent "helps to increase blood flow to the heart." In addition, there is need for a disclaimer that indicates that the herb is not approved by the Food and Drug Administration (FDA) and that it is not meant to be used as a drug.

In January 2000 the FDA finalized rules for claims on dietary supplements noting that supplements may make structure and function claims without FDA approval. However, it may not be claimed that the supplement can prevent, treat, cure, mitigate, or diagnose diseases. This ruling may cause label changes on products but is not expected to affect product availability or consumer access. Health maintenance claims (e.g., "maintain a healthy immune system") and claims for minor symptoms related to life stages (e.g., "alleviates hot flashes") are acceptable because they do not relate to disease. Dietary supplement manufacturers are still required to substantiate any claims they make.

Proposed Standards

The FDA proposed standards for marketing and labeling for dietary supplements in 2003. Known as the **Current Good Manufacturing Practices (CGMPs)**, these standards are multifaceted and require that package labels give quality and strength of all contents and that product be free of contaminants and impurities. Manufacturing quality control procedures are part of the CGMPs.

Herbal Preparations

Herbal remedies are available in a variety of preparations and form. Examples include fresh aloe, dried ginger, peppermint oil, elderberry syrup, and chamomile tea. Following is a description of selected preparations and forms of herbs including dried kelp extracts, fresh oils, salves, teas, tinctures, syrups, capsules, and tablets. The consumer and health care provider also need to be knowledgeable about the differences in dosages between extracts and powders as well as issues associated with standardization.

Dried herbs are fresh herbs that have had the moisture removed by sun or heat. They can be stored for about 6 months. **Extracts** are made by isolating certain components, resulting in more reliable dosing. Dissolving the herb in a solvent such as alcohol or water is a common way to prepare an extract, which may or may not be standardized. **Fresh herbs** may decay after a few days because of enzyme activity; hence, they have a short life. Drying is a means of preservation. **Oils** are made by soaking dried herb in olive or vegetable oil and then heating for an extended time. The vegetable oil promotes the concentration of some of the active components, and it may last for months if stored correctly. These infused oils are *not* essential oils. **Salves**, semisolid fatty preparations, are made by melting a wax in oil and allowing it to cool and harden. If stored correctly, they last for several months as balms, creams, and ointments. **Teas** are made by steeping fresh or dried herbs in boiling water. Tea made from bark and roots is often simmered. It is recommended that only a 2- to 3-day supply be prepared at one time and that it be stored in the refrigerator. Teas may be used as a drink, added to baths, and applied topically in a compress. **Tinctures** are commonly made by soaking fresh or dried herbs in solvent such as water or alcohol. Both water- and fat-soluble components are concentrated in the final form. Alcohol promotes preservation, yielding a shelf life of 1 year. Alcohol-free, glycerin-based tinctures are available for people who do not consume alcohol. **Syrups** are made by adding a sweetener, usually honey or sugar, to the herb and then cooking it. Syrups are used to treat colds, coughs, and sore throats.

Capsules are commonly a powdered form of dried supplement, but they may hold juices or oils. They have a slower effect than liquids because of decreased absorption. They store and travel well. *Tablets* are similar to capsules; they are a powder compressed with stabilizers and binders.

Commonly Used Herbal Remedies

Most herbal therapies are used for chronic conditions, are unlikely to cause harm, and may provide some relief in selected situations (Figure 9–1). This section discusses some of the more commonly used herbs.

Aloe Vera *(Aloe barbadensis)*

The juice is used externally for treatment of minor burns, insect bites, and sunburn. There has been some success with the treatment of dandruff, oily skin, and psoriasis. Taken internally, aloe vera is a powerful laxative. Menstrual flow is increased with small doses.

Chamomile *(Matricaria recutita)*

Dried flower heads of *Matricaria recutita* are ingredients of a popular tea for relief of digestive and gastrointestinal (GI) complaints. The tea is used for relief of irritable bowel syndrome and infant colic through antispasmodic and antiinflammatory effects on the GI tract. In addition, chamomile may have sedative effects.

Chamomile tea is prepared by steeping one teaspoon of flower heads for 10 to 15 minutes in boiling water and drinking three to four times per day. An extremely rare allergic reaction of urticaria and bronchoconstriction may occur in an individual allergic to daisy or ragweed-type

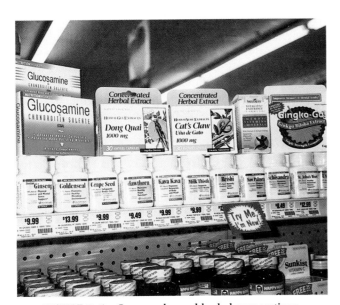

FIGURE 9–1 Commonly used herbal preparations.

plants. Pharmacokinetics and pharmacodynamics are not known.

Dong Quai *(Angelica sinensis)*

Dong quai, an all-purpose woman's tonic herb, has long been popular in China and Japan for the treatment of menstrual cramps and to regulate the menstrual cycle. This herb has not been well studied, and preparations are frequently mixed with fillers. It contains vitamin B_{12}, which may promote manufacture of blood cells. Rare side effects include fever and excessive menstrual bleeding. Pharmacokinetics and pharmacodynamics are not known.

Echinacea *(Echinacea angustifolia)*

Echinacea, a popular supplement, is used as an immune enhancer; it acts by furthering phagocytosis by means of increasing leukocytes and spleen cells and activating granulocytes. In addition, echinacea inhibits hyaluronidase activity and increases the release of tumor necrosis factor. The leaf preparation is given for respiratory and urinary tract infections. The root extract is used to treat flulike symptoms. German Commission E recommends that echinacea preparations be avoided by persons with autoimmune diseases and those with abnormal T-cell functioning (e.g., human immunodeficiency virus [HIV], acquired immunodeficiency syndrome [AIDS], tuberculosis). Echinacea is used by Native Americans to treat snakebites and has many other uses.

Echinacea should be purchased only from reliable sources; there are many reports of fraudulent substitution with other plants and varying potency. There is inconsistent recommendation of duration of treatment. German Commission E recommends use of up to 8 weeks; others recommend a week's "drug holiday" (i.e., not taking the preparation for a specific time period) before continuing therapy. Pharmacokinetics is unknown. Immunosuppression may occur after extended therapy.

Feverfew *(Chrysanthemum parthenium)*

The plant compound parthenolide is believed to act as a serotonin antagonist, a mediator of vascular headaches from platelets. Feverfew is popular for the relief of migraine headaches and their accompanying nausea and vomiting.

Only standardized extracts should be used. Wide variation in the amount of active compound in plants and commercial capsules is a potential dosing problem. Pharmacokinetics and pharmacodynamics are not known.

Garlic *(Allium sativum)*

Garlic, frequently called the "herb of endurance," is reported to lower cholesterol and triglyceride levels, decrease blood pressure, and reduce the clotting capability of blood. It also acts as an antibiotic to treat infections and wounds both internally and externally. Warm garlic oil is used in the ear for treatment of earache. Garlic may be used for some types of heavy-metal poisoning. Pharmacokinetics and pharmacodynamics are not known.

Ginger (Zingiber officinale)

Ginger boosts the immune system. It is used to treat migraine headache, stomach problems, and digestive disorders, including motion sickness. Long-time use as relief from nausea is validated by modern research. In addition, it may provide relief from pain, swelling, and stiffness of both osteoarthritis and rheumatoid arthritis (dosage is 500 to 4000 mg daily). Pharmacokinetics and pharmacodynamics are limited. Metabolites are excreted via urine within 24 hours, and it is 90% protein bound.

Ginkgo (Ginkgo biloba)

Ginkgo biloba, extract of one of the oldest plant species, is the most commonly prescribed herbal remedy worldwide. When it crosses the blood–brain barrier, ginkgo has central nervous system (CNS) effects, increasing both cerebral arterial dilation and uptake of oxygen and glucose. It assists cells during periods of hypoxia (e.g., during transient ischemic attacks) and decreases free-radical damage to neurons. In addition, there is inhibition of platelet adhesion and degranulation. German Commission E monograph #55 lists the use of ginkgo for dementia syndromes, intermittent claudication, vertigo, and tinnitus when these symptoms are secondary to diminished blood flow. In addition, there is some evidence that it improves cognition and may be helpful in Alzheimer's disease, early stroke, and Raynaud's phenomenon.

Ginkgo biloba is generally given as 120 to 240 mg daily in two to three divided doses for up to 90 days. Rare side effects include headache and GI disturbances. Limited information is available on pharmacokinetics and pharmacodynamics. Bioavailability not affected by food; excretion <30% metabolites.

Ginseng (Panax ginseng)

Preparations of ginseng are taken for short-term relief of stress, to boost energy, and to give digestive support. Ginseng tends to support the immune system and assist in the prevention of chronic infections. Red Korean or Chinese ginseng may be overstimulating in chronic inflammatory conditions such as arthritis. Pharmacokinetics and pharmacodynamics are not known.

Goldenseal (Hydrastis canadensis)

Goldenseal is frequently used with echinacea to ward off infection and promote wound healing. Common uses include treatment of GI ulcers, mouth ulcers, bladder infection, and postpartum hemorrhage. It is used to treat congestion associated with the common cold. In addition, it is used as a tonic and astringent. Active ingredients are deactivated in the stomach. Goldenseal is expensive and scarce; thus it is frequently adulterated with fillers. Its ability to stimulate the immune system has been questioned, and it can be toxic if overused. Pharmacokinetics and pharmacodynamics are not known.

Kava (Piper methysticum)

Kava has practical and ceremonial roles in the Pacific Island cultures. The root promotes sleep and muscle relaxation and is an antiepileptic, antidepressant, and antipsychotic; it also promotes wound healing. Tea can help with urinary tract infections. Kava may be used in combination with other herbs, such as valerian and St. John's wort, for relaxation. Little is known about its pharmacokinetics and pharmacodynamics. Kava may cross the placenta and be in breast milk.

Licorice (Glycyrrhiza glabra)

Licorice may have physiologic effects similar to aldosterone and corticosteroids related to glycyrrhizin, a major ingredient. Licorice may help with chronic fatigue syndrome. The deglycyrrhizinated form is used to treat ulcers. It relieves heartburn and indigestion by decreasing stomach acid; it also has a laxative effect. Side effects from excessive use of licorice include increased blood pressure, headache, lethargy, water retention, increased potassium excretion, and, rarely, heart failure. Licorice root is considered safe in dosages of 5 to 15 mg when taken as tea. Its recommended use is limited to 6 weeks. Pharmacokinetics and pharmacodynamics are not known.

Milk Thistle (Silybum marianum)

This herbal extract has the remarkable ability to prevent damage to liver cells and stimulate regeneration of liver cells. These findings have been validated by research. Milk thistle is widely used in Europe to treat hepatitis, cirrhosis, and fatty liver associated with drugs and alcohol. Pharmacokinetics and pharmacodynamics are not known.

Peppermint (Mentha piperita)

Peppermint stimulates appetite and aids in digestion when taken internally. The digestive tract is protected by the tannins, and peppermint is used in treatment of bowel disorders. Hot peppermint tea stimulates circulation, reduces fever, clears congestion, and helps restore energy. Peppermint oil is an effective treatment for tension headache when rubbed on the forehead. In research in Germany, peppermint has been shown to be comparable with acetaminophen (extra-strength Tylenol) in relieving headache. Pharmacokinetics and pharmacodynamics are not known.

St. John's Wort (Hypericum perforatum)

Current research suggests St. John's wort is not effective when used by individuals with moderate to severe depression. Botanical experts indicate it is to be used for mild depression. St. John's wort has at least 10 pharmacologically active components. The compound used for standardization is hypericin. Researchers recommend that prospective trials be conducted to compare St. John's wort with standard antidepressant medication and to identify dosages, effectiveness in different stages of depression, and implications of long-term use. St. John's wort has been nicknamed "herbal Prozac" because of its great popularity in the

United States and its use as a "tonic" for the nervous system. St. John's wort is used in combination with yarrow to treat enuresis. When taken with a prescription antidepressant, suicidal ideations is an adverse effect. It is considered a dietary supplement in the United States and has not been FDA approved; it is licensed in Germany for relief of anxiety, depression, and insomnia.

The 1984 German Commission E monograph on hypericin indicated the agent was an experimental monoamine oxidase (MAO) inhibitor for use in depression, anxiety, and psychogenic disturbances. The mechanism of action is unknown.

The usual dose of St. John's wort is 300 mg t.i.d. of extract (standardized to 0.3% hypericin). A tea can be prepared from 1 to 2 teaspoonful of herb steeped for 10 minutes. One to two cups of tea per day for 4 to 6 weeks is recommended. Users need to apply sunscreen freely when outdoors, although phototoxicity has not been reported in humans. Users of St. John's wort do not need to avoid tyramine-rich foods. Minimal information is known about the pharmacokinetics and pharmacodynamics. St. John's wort crosses blood-brain and placental barriers and may enter breast milk.

Saw Palmetto (Serenoa repens)

Double-blind studies indicate that the herb saw palmetto relieves symptoms of benign prostatic hypertrophy and urinary conditions. Saw palmetto has earned the name "plant catheter." Other indications for this herb include use as an expectorant and treatment for colds, asthma, bronchitis, and thyroid deficiency. The recommended dose is 160 mg of standardized extract twice a day. Pharmacokinetics and pharmacodynamics are not known.

Valerian (Valeriana officinalis)

Valerian, a mild sedative and sleep-inducing agent, has an effect similar to benzodiazepines. It is popularly known as "herbal Valium." Most researchers report no hangover effect. A "dirty socks" odor is related to the dried plant, resulting in no risk of overdose. Preparations from fresh root are reported to be better relaxants and have a sweet aroma. There have been no reports of habituation and addiction. Drowsiness may occur, as with any relaxant. The dosage depends on the symptoms, such as insomnia and anxiety. To treat insomnia, 400 mg of tincture extract is recommended: 2.5 to 5 mg of solid extract at bedtime. For anxiety, a tea steeped with 1 teaspoonful of dried herb is taken several times a day. About 5% to 10% of users report a stimulant effect. Pharmacokinetics and pharmacodynamics are not known.

Summary of Commonly Used Herbal Remedies

A summary of selected herbs' actions/uses, dosage, interactions, and side/adverse effects is given in Table 9–2. Vitamins and elements commonly used in conjunction with herbal therapy are vitamins B_6, A, C, E, selenium, and zinc. The American Herbal Products Association has categorized herbal products based on "reasonable use" of the herb into four classes. Refer to the note at the end of Table 9–2 (p. 180) for a description of the classes.

Using Herbs to Treat Selected Common Ailments

Herbs also seem helpful for conditions such as cough, sore throat, cuts, and as "cholesterol chaser." For example, oil of eucalyptus is found in many cough medicines. Breathing and respiratory ailments are frequently eased with eucalyptus tea. The effectiveness of the aloe vera plant is known to many; gel from a broken leaf of the aloe potted houseplant is spread directly on minor cuts and burns. The fresh plant, which is easily grown in pots or a garden, is superior to commercial preparations. Lowering cholesterol levels may be the most documented values of garlic and onions.

Potential Hazards of Herbs

Both consumers and health care providers need to remember that although herbs are natural substances, they are not necessarily safe. No preparations are safe in all situations, and herbs are no exception. Consumers and health care providers need to be alert to potential hazards with herbal therapy. It is essential that the health care provider get a complete list of *all* the herbal preparations the client takes, the reason they are taken, and their perceived effectiveness. This assessment needs to be updated regularly along with information on clients' prescription and over-the-counter (OTC) drug use.

Contamination is one area of concern, most likely resulting from lack of standards in manufacture and regulation of herbs. It is the responsibility of consumers to educate themselves about herbs before use and to purchase products only from reputable dealers. Determination of the purity and concentration of a particular product can be done only through assays, a costly process; thus most products have not had appropriate human toxicologic analysis.

Interaction with conventional drugs is another area in which health care providers should be alert. For example, an additive effect of digoxin can result from the use of the laxative herbs cascara and senna. Also, elevation of lithium in the blood level may result from juniper, dandelion, and other herbs with diuretic properties.

Refer to Appendix D for a table on herbal ingredients and drug interactions.

All compounds are not safe via all routes. For example, comfrey (*Symphytum officinale*) has both internal and external preparations. Internal use is discouraged because hepatic damage may be fatal. For external use, comfrey is used as an ointment for relief of swelling associated with abrasions and sprains.

In 1997 the FDA proposed controls on dietary supplements containing ephedra, also known as *ma huang*, which is used for weight loss and to boost energy. Use of this supplement has markedly declined since reports of adverse

Text continued on p. 180

Table 9–2

Summary Table of Selected Herbs

Herb	Actions and Uses	Dosage	Interactions/Precautions	Side/Adverse Effects
Common and *botanical* names Class and part used				

Aloe/aloe Vera
Aloe barbadenis
Class 1
  Leaf gel
Class 2b/2d
  Dried, juice
Class 2d
  Topical
  Bladelike leaf
	Uses: Internal for constipation; externally to relieve pain and promote healing of burns, wounds, sunburn, psoriasis	Internal:
		Tincture/extract: 50-300 mg
		External: t.i.d. or PRN
			Internal use contraindicated if pregnant, lactating, children <12 y
			Consult with HCP before taking if have ulcerative colitis or Crohn's disease, taking cardiac glycosides, artiarrythmics, thiazide diuretics, licorice, or corticosteroids
			Monitoring of electrolytes
				Internal: Overdose/long-term may cause arrhythmias, neuropathies, edemas, albuminuria, hematuria (side effects are rare)

Bilberry *Vaccinium myrtillus L.* Class 4 Extract of dried fruit and leaf	Uses: Fruit may promote healthy vision, increase visual pigment regeneration; decrease diarrhea in children Leaf used for diabetes, arthritis, dermatitis, gout	Fruit extract: 80-160 mg t.i.d. (St: 25% anthocyanosides) Leaf: no information	Avoid with pregnancy, lactation, children No reported significant interaction with fruit Leaf: May decrease blood sugar and triglyceride levels; may increase action of anticoagulants and NSAIDs; monitor for dose adjustments	Leaf: Long-term higher doses (in animals) anemia, icterus, excitation, death

Black cohosh (bugwort, snakeroot, squaw root)
Cimicifuga racemosa
Class 2b/2c
  Root
	Suppresses luteinizing hormone, optimizes estrogen levels
	Uses: Antispasmodic, astringent, diuretic, vasodilator, PMS, dysmenorrhea, infertility, menopausal symptoms
		Cap/tab: 20 mg b.i.d.
		Tincture:
		  2-5 mg b.i.d
			Avoid with pregnancy, lactation, children
			Limit use to 6 mo; no data on long-term use
			Under supervision of qualified herbalist, increases action of antihypertensives; may alter effects of HRT
			May decrease iron absorption
				Higher doses: dizziness, headache, nausea, change in heart rate

Chamomile (green chamomile) *Matricaria recutita* Class 2b Dried flower tops	Stimulates normal digestion, antiinflammatory, antispasmodic, mild sedative, mild diuretic, mild antibacterial with topic use Uses: Anxiety, insomnia, indigestion, inflammatory skin conditions	Between meals: Cap/tab: 2-3 g t.i.d., Tea: 1-4 c/d Tincture: max: 1 tsp t.i.d.	Avoid if allergic to daisy family (e.g., ragweed, asters, chrysanthemums) May increase effects of sedatives and interfere with action of anticoagulants. H/F, H/H: None known.	None known
Cranberry *Vaccinium macrocarpon Ait.* Class 4 Berries	Prophylaxis (not treatment) of urinary tract infections; to treat kidney stones	Extract: 300-400 mg concentrated juice b.i.d. Cocktail: 300 ml/d commercial cranberry juice	Caution: avoid use with oliguria and anuria. Clients with DM should use sugar-free cranberry juice; lactating clients, children <12 y, and clients with history of oxalate kidney stones limit to 1 L/day. H/D, H/K, H/H: None known	Doses of >3 L/day may produce diarrhea

b.i.d., Twice a day; *c,* cup; *cap,* capsule; *DM,* diabetes mellitus; *HCP,* health care provider; *H/D,* herb-drug interaction; *H/F,* herb-food interaction; *H/H,* herb-herb interaction; *HRT,* hormone replacement therapy; *max,* maximum; *NSAIDs,* nonsteroidal antiinflammatory drugs; *PMS,* premenstrual syndrome; *PRN,* as needed; *St,* standarized to; *tab,* tablet; *t.i.d.,* three times a day; *y,* year.

Table 9–2

Summary Table of Selected Herbs—cont'd

Herb	Actions and Uses	Dosage	Interactions/Precautions	Side/Adverse Effects
Dong Quai *Angelica Sinensis* Class 2b (root) Roots, rhizomes	Phytoestrogen activity; vasodilation, small muscle relaxation Decreased IgE antibody production Uses: PMS, menopausal symptoms, cardiovascular support	Tea: 1-4 c/d (equivalent 1-2 g dried herb) Tincuture: $^1/_2$-4 ml, Max: 6×/d	AVOID USE OF THIS HERB Avoid use with prescription anticoagulants, history of bleeding disorders, pregnancy, if at risk for breast cancer Herb-Drug Interaction: additive bleeding effect with anticoagulants, aspirin, NSAIDs	Rash and photosensitivity; fever, bleeding
Echinacea (purple cornflower) *E. purpura; E. angustifolia, E. pallida* Class 1 (root/seed) Aerial parts of *E. pallida*; root of *E. pallida* and angustifolia	Stimulates immune system; antibacterial, antiviral, antipyretic Antifungal as topical Uses: Prevention and early treatment of colds and flu; recurrent respiratory, ear, and urinary tract infections Topical: Canker sores, fungal infections Investigational use: Stimulate immune system of HIV/AIDS clients.	Tab: 500 mg-1 g t.i.d. Tea: 1-5 c/d Tincture: max: 2 tsp t.i.d.	Short-term use: 2 wk; 8 wk if low dose; may be hepatotoxic if taken continuously Avoid use with immunosuppressants such as corticosteroids (may counteract); persons with chronic systemic disease of immune system (e.g., SLE, HIV, TB, MS) Safety not determined in pregnancy lactation, and in children under 2 y	Lozenge/tincture: Temporary numbness or tingling of tongue Cross-sensitivity in clients allergic to daisy family, GI upset, diarrhea
Evening primrose *Oenothera biennis* Class 4 Oil of seed	Natural estrogen promoter Uses: PMS, problems with synthesis of fatty acids, abnormal prostaglandin production, diabetic neuropathies, chronic inflammatory conditions (eczema), overactive immune systems	Take with meals (increases absorption): Oil: PMS: 3-6 g/d for 6 mo, 14 days before menses Inflammatory conditions: 4-8 g/d for 3-4 mo MS: 500 mg/d for 3 wk with exacerbation	Avoid use during pregnancy and lactation May lower seizure threshold if taken with anticonvulsants; anticonvulsant dose may need modification or do not use concurrently. H/F, H/H: None known	GI upset, nausea, headache, rash. Immunosuppression with long-term use
Feverfew *Tanacetum parthenium; chrysanthemum parthenium* Class 2b (whole herb) Leaves, flowering tops	Interferes with platelet aggregation, inhibits release of serotonin from platelets, blocks proinflammatory mediators, digestive relaxant Uses: Prevention and long-term management of migraine headaches; rheumatoid arthritis; menstrual problems; allergies	Cap/tab (at least 2% parthenolide) 125 mg/d; increase to 1-2 g with acute attack	May be 4-6 wk before effect; continuous use for best outcome Cross sensitivity to plants in daisy family Avoid with pregnancy, lactation, with prescription anticoagulants, and in children <2 y Consult HCP before using herb if taking prescription NSAIDs (decreases effectiveness) May interfere with SSRI antidepressants (e.g., Prozac)	Possible gastric distress or mouth sores if using raw leaves; muscle stiffness; may have rebound headache if discontinued abruptly

AIDS, acquired immunodeficiency syndrome; *c*, cup; *d*, day; *GI*, gastrointestinal; *HIV*, human immunodeficiency virus; *mo*, month; *MS*, multiple sclerosis; *SLE*, systemic lupus erythematosus; *SSRI*, selective serotonin reuptake inhibition; *TB*, tuberculosis; *wk*, week.

Continued

Table 9–2

Summary Table of Selected Herbs—cont'd

Herb	Actions and Uses	Dosage	Interactions/Precautions	Side/Adverse Effects
Garlic *Allium sativum* Class 2c Bulb	Detoxifies body and increases immune function; decreases platelet aggregation; increases HDL and decreases cholesterol and triglycerides, broad antimicrobial activity, mild antihypertensive; hypoglycemia Uses: Hypercholesterolemia, mild HTN, colds and flu	Caps (enteric coated): (ED of 5000 mcg of allicin/d in divided doses) Raw garlic clove is best source; minimum: 1/d	Avoid use during pregnancy and lactation (may stimulate labor or cause infant colic) and hypothyroidism Blood pressure may decrease in 30 min and return to baseline in about 2 hr Caution: Use with anticoagulants because of increased fibrinolysis and decreased platelet aggregation; modify antidiabetic doses. H/F: None; H/H: Acidophilus deceases absorption of garlic	Heartburn, flatulence, gastric irritation, decreased RBCs; dizziness diaphoresis

Ginger
Zingiber officinale
Class 1 (fresh root)
  Class 2b/2d
  Dried root
  Rhizome
	Stimulates digestion, increases bile and motility; antispasmodic; decreased platelet aggregation; decreases absorption and increases excretion of cholesterol; antioxidant
	
	Uses: Nausea, pregnancy morning sickness (short term, low dose ONLY); motion sickness; gastric protection with NSAIDs
		Take with food
		Cap/tab/tea: 2-4 g in 2-3 divided doses
		For motion sickness start 2 d to 2 hr before travel
		Inflammatory joint disease: 4 g in 2-3 divided doses
		Nausea-pregnancy related: 1 g in divided doses for 1-4 d
		Tincture: 1.5-3 ml in 8 oz juice q.i.d., PRN
			Avoid long-term use with pregnancy, thrombocytopenia (abortificiant in large amounts)
			Caution: With prescription anticoagulants (additive effect)
			Consult with HCP before use if have gallstones
			May increase absorption of all PO medications H/F, H/H: None known
				May cause gastric discomfort if not taken with food; anorexia

Ginkgo biloba *Gingko folium* Class 1 (leaf) Leaves	Antioxidant; peripheral vasodilation and increased blood flow to CNS, reduces platelet aggregation Uses: Allergic rhinitis, Alzheimer's disease, anxiety/stress, dementia, Raynaud's disease, tinnitus, vertigo, impotence, poor circulation; altitude sickness	Cap/tab: 120-240 mg/d in 2-3 divided doses (standardized to at least 24% ginkgo flavone glycosides and 6% Terpene lactones) Tincture: 5-10 ml b.i.d., t.i.d. Circulation/memory: 120 mg/d in 2-3 divided doses Alzheimer's dementia, tinnitus: up to 240 mg/d in 2-3 divided doses	Effects seen in 2-3 wk; 12-wk course recommended Avoid use in pregnancy, lactation, children, and with MAOIs Caution: With prescription anticoagulants monitor bleeding and prothrombin times. Extra caution if using ginger, garlic, or feverfew May increase BP if used with thiazide diuretics Discontinue 2 wk before surgery Ginkgo fruit may result in severe rash; seeds are toxic. H/F, H/H: None known	Initially, mild transient headache that usually stops in 2 d; mild gastric distress Toxicity: vomiting, diarrhea, dermitis, irritability

BP, Blood pressure; *ED*, effective dose; *HCP*, health care provider; *HDL*, high density lipoprotein; *HTN*, hypertension; *MAOIs*, monoamine oxidase inhibitors; *PO*, orally; *PMS*, premenstrual syndrome; *RBCs*, red blood cells.

Table 9–2

Summary Table of Selected Herbs—cont'd

Herb	Actions and Uses	Dosage	Interactions/Precautions	Side/Adverse Effects
Ginseng, eleuthera or siberian *Eleutheroccus senticosus, Acanthopanax senticosus* Class 2b/2c/2d Root	Supports adrenal glands, enhances energy levels by inhibiting alarm phase SNS response, stimulates RBC production, decreases blood sugar levels, protects from cellular mutation from carcinogens Uses: Cold and flu prevention, adaptation to stress, chronic fatigue syndrome, SLE, HIV, mental fatigue and physical exhaustion, following chemotherapy or radiation treatments, recovery from chronic or long-term illness	Cap/tab: 2-3 g/d in 3-4 divided doses Tea: 1-4 c/d Tincture: 5-20 ml/d in 3-4 divided doses	Take for 6-8 wk; then 1 wk drug holiday, and resume for total of 3 mo Avoid with BP >170/90; pregnancy, lactation, children, bipolar or psychic disorders, DM, may increase or decrease anticoagulants, dependent on species; anticoagulants May increase effects of caffeine and HRT; falsely elevate digoxin levels, and interact with antipsychotic drugs. H/F: Overstimulation may be with caffeinated coffee, cola, and tea. H/H: None	Hypertension, palpitations, occasional diarrhea; possible insomnia if taken at bedtime Ginseng abuse syndrome: Edema, insomnia, and hypertonia, may be life threatening
Goldenseal *Hydrastis canadensis* Class 2b Root, rhizome	Stimulates immune system and bile secretion, antipyretic, broad spectrum antibiotic activity Uses: For infection: respiratory, digestive, urinary tract, mucous membranes; cholecystitis, cirrhosis	Cap/tab: 2-4 g/d in divided doses (standardized to 8%-12% alkaloid content)	Avoid with pregnancy, lactation, children, HTN Dosing >5-7 d of higher doses may increase liver enzymes or malabsorption of B vitamins May decrease effect of heparin, anticoagulants, cardiac glycosides; increased effect of antiarrhythmics, antihypertensives, beta-blockers, and CNS depressants Caution: In clients with cardiovascular disease, DM, or glaucoma	In higher doses may be hepatotoxic Toxicity: CNS depression, restlessness, seizures, cardiovascular collapse Endangered plant species
Hawthorn *Crataegus laevigata, C. oxycantha, C. monogyna* Class 1 Ripe fruit, leaves, flowers	Peripheral dilation and increased coronary circulation, improves cardiac oxygenation, antioxidants, mild diuretic, decreases proinflammatory substances Uses: Mild HTN, early CHF, stable angina	Cap/tab: 100-900 mg/d in divided doses (standardized to 20% procyanidins) Average/dose: 100-250 mg t.i.d. Tea: 2.5–5 ml t.i.d. Tea: 1 c t.i.d. (4-5 g dried/day)	May need to modify doses of beta blockers, digitalis, and ACE inhibitors Increased effects of digitalis, beta blockage, ACE inhibitors, CNS depressants High doses contraindicated with chronic atrial fibrillation and hypotension from dysfunction of valve: IH/F None known; H/H increases action of Lily of the Valley	Hypotension, fatigue Sedation, nausea, vomiting, anorexia

ACE, angiotensin-converting enzyme; *CHF,* congestive heart failure; *CNS,* central nervous system; *SNS,* sympathetic nervous system.   *Continued*

Table 9–2

Summary Table of Selected Herbs—cont'd

Herb	Actions and Uses	Dosage	Interactions/Precautions	Side/Adverse Effects
Kava *Piper methysticum* Class 2b/2c/2d Dried rhizome, roots	CNS sedation without loss of mental acuity or memory Uses: Anxiety, insomnia, skeletal muscle spasm Good with psychotic disorders, no risk of tolerance	Cap/tab: Anxiety: 50-100 mg up to t.i.d. Insomnia: 180-210 mg at bedtime (standardized to 70% kavalactones) Max: 300 g/wk	Avoid with pregnancy, lactation, parkinsonism, and if taking levodopa; not for young children Avoid alcohol use and if need to be alert or operate machinery Increases CNS sedating drugs, especially benzodiazipines Fat soluble so may have delayed effects. H/F increased absorption when taken with food; H/H: None known	Unstable gait, numb tongue, mild GI upset High doses may cause loss of balance, pulmonary hypertension May cause liver toxicity. Banned in several European countries. Use >3 mo may turn skin yellow: discontinue drug HTN, headache, weakness.
Licorice *Glycyrrhiza glabra* Class 2b/2c/2d (root) Root, leaf	Antiinflammatory, antibacterial, antiviral, hepato and gastric protective, antidepressant, estrogenic, laxative Uses: Viral infection, upper respiratory infection, inflammation, Addison's disease, depression, ulcers Topically: Herpes, psoriasis, eczema DCL: IBS, mouth ulcers	Cap/tab: 200-600 mg glycyrrhizen in 3 divided doses; max: 4-6 wk Tea: 3 c/d (equivalent to 1-2 g/d) Tincture: 2.5-5 ml t.i.d. DGL: 300-380 mg; max: 1200 mg/d in chewable form 20 min before meals for 8-16 wk	Avoid with pregnancy, lactation, children, HTN, kidney or liver disorders, or if at risk for hypokalemia Caution with DM Increased aldosterone effect with increasing dose and duration Antagonizes antihypertensive meds and spirolactone Potentiates corticosteroids and digitalis. H/F none known; H/H may cause hypokalemia with aloe	Doses >5000 mg/d results in aldosterone-like syndrome that reverses when herb discontinued
Milk thistle (Mary thistle wild artichoke) *Silybum manarum* Class 1 Seeds of dried flowers	Increased regeneration of liver cells; increases antioxidant activity Uses: Liver disease (hepatitis), cholecystitis, psoriasis	Cap/tab: Initially: 500 mg/d in 3 divided doses for 6-8 wk With improvement: 120-240 mg/d in divided doses; may take 7-10 d for effect; 4-8 wk if liver diseased with alcohol Tincture: 1 ml t.i.d. (avoid ETOH-based tinctures)	Avoid use in pregnancy, lactation, in children, with drugs metabolized by P-450 enzyme Herb does not reverse cirrhotic liver changes but disease may be slowed with increased quality of life. H/F, H/H: None known	Diarrhea first days of therapy, nausea, vomiting; menstrual changes
Peppermint *Mentha piperita, var. officinalis or vulgaris* Class 4 Aerial parts	Antispasmodic; increase bile flow; carminative, external analgesic Uses: IBS, indigestion, cholecystitis, infant colic, nasal decongestant Topically: Musculo-skeletal pain, itching, colds	Cap/tab: enteric coated: 1-2 t.i.d. between meals Tea: 2-3 c/d (equivalent 3-6 g dried herb) Tincture/oil: 6-12 gtts/d diluted in divided doses	Consult HCP before taking if have cholecystitis or obstructed bile duct No known drug interactions; may interfere with iron absorption	None known

DCL, Deglycyrrhizinated licorice; *Eq,* equivalent to; *ETOH,* alcohol; *IBS,* irritable bowel syndrome.

Table 9–2

Summary Table of Selected Herbs—cont'd

Herb	Actions and Uses	Dosage	Interactions/Precautions	Side/Adverse Effects
Psyllium *Plantago psyllium* Class 4	Uses: Laxative, treatment of hemorrhoids, colitis, Crohn's disease, IBS	$\frac{1}{2}$ t soaked in water for 15-60 min at bedtime with at least 8 oz water	Major ingredient in Metamucil May decrease lithium absorption	None known
Sage *Salvia officinalis* Class 2b/2d (leaf) Whole plant	Herb of longevity, poultice: wound healing effects Gargle tea for sore throat, dries up mother's milk, decreases hot flashes	PO extract: 1-4 ml t.i.d.	Avoid use during pregnancy, lactation, in children Limit use to 2 wk to avoid toxic effects of tannins Caution clients with DM and seizure disorders	Nausea, vomiting, anorexia, oral irritation
St. John's wort *Hypercium perforatum* Class 2d Flowers	Antidepressant and antiviral activity Uses: Mood swings, mild to moderate depression, anxiety, sleep disorders Topically: Burns/wounds	Take with food Cap/tab: (standardized to at least 0.1% hypericin) 300 mg t.i.d. Tea: 1-2 c/d for 4-6 wk Tincture: 1-2 ml t.i.d.	Long-term use recommended; effects seen in 4-8 wk Avoid with pregnancy, lactation, prescription antidepressants, MAOIs, children <2 y indinavir May decrease effect of digoxin related to bioavailability Monitor serum digoxin levels Use with amphetamines, tiazodone; tricyclics may cause serotonin syndrome Interferes with absorption of iron and other minerals; high doses may increase liver enzymes	Skin photosensitivity, headache, occasional GI upset, dry mouth, dizziness, confusion
Saw palmetto *Serenoa repens,* *Sabazi serrulata* Class 4 Berries	Decreases size of prostate; increases breakdown of estrogen, progesterone, and prolactin: antiandrogenic Diuretic Uses: BPH, chronic cystitis; sexual potency	Cap/tab: 230 mg/d in 1-2 doses (standardized to 85%-95% fatty acids) Tea: 1 c t.i.d. (equivalent dose 1-2 g/d) Liquid extract: 5-6 ml daily	Recommend 45-90 d of treatment; effects seen after 30 d. If effective, may take long term Avoid in pregnancy, lactation, in children, in clients with breast cancer Effectiveness of prophylactic treatment not shown May interfere with PSA test; discontinue herb 1-2 wk before test May increase or decrease effects of antiinflammatories and immunostimulants; may antagonize hormone therapy	Headache, dysuria, back pain Gastric disturbance (rare)

BPH, Benign prostatic hypertrophy.

Continued

Table 9-2

Summary Table of Selected Herbs—cont'd

Herb	Actions and Uses	Dosage	Interactions/Precautions	Side/Adverse Effects
Valerian *Valeriana officinalis* Class 1 Root	Sedative/hypnotic, antispasmodic, increases deep sleep Uses: Insomnia, stress headaches, mild anxiety, muscle cramps, and spasms	Cap/tab: (standardized to 0.5% essential oils, equivalent to 2-3 g up to b.i.d.) Tea: 1-3 c/d or at bedtime Tincture: 1-3 ml; may repeat 2 × over 6 h	Effects may take several doses For long-term use; monitor liver function if elevated, discontinue herb Avoid in pregnancy, lactation, children, with prescription sedative/ hypnotics, MAOIs, anticoagulants Increased sedative effect with barbiturates; negates effects of phenytoin Foul smell; no dependence or tolerance	Anxiety, headache, occasional GI upset and hang-over effect with high doses, CNS depression

MAOIs, Monoamine oxidase inhibitors.

Note: The American Herbal Products Association (described in the Botanical Safety Handbook) has categorized herbal products based on "reasonable use" of the herb into the following four classes:

Class 1   Herbs that can be safely consumed when used appropriately

Class 2   Herbs for which the following use restrictions apply, unless otherwise directed by an expert qualified in the use of the described substance:
    2a: For external use only
    2b: Not to be used during pregnancy
    2c: Not to be used while nursing
    2d: Other specific use restrictions as noted

Class 3   Herbs for which significant data exist to recommend the following labeling: "To be used only under the supervision of an expert qualified in the appropriate use of this substance." Labeling must include proper use information as follows: Dosage, contraindications, potential adverse effects and drug interactions, and any other relevant information related to safe use of the substance

Class 4   Herbs for which insufficient data are available for classification

effects came to light (e.g., palpitations, stroke). Ephedrine and pseudoephedrine, components of ephedra, have stimulant and bronchodilation effects. The FDA proposed that the dosage not exceed 24 mg ephedrine per day as a dietary supplement.

Currently ephedra is banned from the market. See Herbal Alert 9-2.

All the herbal products listed in Herbal Alert 9-3 have significance for clients going to have surgery. Other products may interfere with the absorption, breakdown, and excretion of anesthetics, anticoagulants, and other surgery related medications. For example, valerian may increase or prolong the sedative effects of anesthetic agents. Echinacea and St. John's wort have the potential of immunosupopression required for transplant surgeries. Consult the health care provider about the length of herb free "washout" before surgery.

Herbal-product advocates have petitioned the FDA to reconsider herbal dietary supplement classification and change to a drug model consistent with European herbal regulation. The FDA is currently formulating rules that set standards for preparing and labeling dietary supplements to enable the consumer to make more informed choices; for example, the appropriate dosage.

Tips for Consumers and Health Care Providers

The following are guidelines about prudent use of herbs:
• Do not take herbs if pregnant or attempting to become pregnant.
• Do not take herbs if nursing.
• Do not give herbs to infants or young children.

HERBAL ALERT 9-2

Ephedra

🐾 On December 31, 2003, the FDA banned ephedra based on links to heart problems, strokes, and death.

HERBAL ALERT 9-3

Anticoagulants

🐾 The following commonly used herbal products have been reported to interfere with anticoagulants: Bilberry, Cat's claw, chamomile (German), dong quai, feverfew, garlic, ginger, ginkgo, and licorice.

- Do not take a large quantity of any one herbal preparation.
- Buy only preparations that have the plant and their quantities listed on the packet; there is no guarantee of safety.
- Contact a health care provider *before* stopping use of a prescription medication.
- Store herbal remedy in a cool, dry, dark place; dark glass containers are preferred.
- Use only herbs that are bought currently and are fresh.
- Do *not* delay in seeking care from the health care provider for persisting or severe symptoms.
- Advise against belief in unsubstantiated claims of "miracle cures."

It is essential that both consumers and health care providers become aware of several crucial factors before trying the herbal therapy approach. Alschuler et al. (1997) identified these as the following:

- Consumers need to think of herbs as medicines; more is not necessarily better.
- Herbs are not placebos.
- Most herbal remedies are less potent than conventional drugs. However, when prescription and OTC drugs and herbs with similar actions are combined, there is an increased risk of adverse reactions.
- Results from conventional medicine may come faster.
- Safety, efficacy, and dosage are important; thus multiple reliable sources should be consulted.

Labeling of herbal products is an important aspect. The following recommended information should be on the label of herbal products:

- Scientific name of the product and the parts of the plant used in the preparation
- Manufacturer's name and address
- Batch and lot number
- Dates of manufacture and expiration; many products have a short shelf life

Nursing Process

Herbal Preparations

ASSESSMENT

- Obtain baseline information about the client's use of nonconventional therapeutic agents.
- Determine product name, brand, dosage, frequency, side effects, and client's perception of effectiveness.
- Identify all prescription and over-the-counter (OTC) medications taken by client; include dosage, frequency, side effects, and perceived effectiveness.

NURSING DIAGNOSES

- Deficient knowledge about therapeutic regimen
- Imbalanced nutrition: less than body requirement
- Fatigue

PLANNING

- Client/family will verbalize understanding of herbal therapy.
- Client/family will verbalize understanding of prescription and OTC medications.
- Client/family will verbalize understanding of interaction between herbal therapy and prescription and OTC medications.
- Client/family will identify strategies for optimal participation in their therapeutic regimen.

NURSING INTERVENTIONS

- Check client's response to herbal therapy.
- Monitor client's response to prescription and OTC medications.
- Consult dietitian and other specialists as necessary.
- Continue with same brand of herbal therapy; notify health care provider if considering changing brands/preparations.

Client Teaching

General
- Explain rationale for herbal therapy (see Herbal Alert 9–1).
- Instruct client to first notify health care provider before substituting herbal product for prescription or OTC medication.
- Encourage client to read labels and heed the recommended information displayed on the label.
- Advise client of portion of plant used in preparation (e.g., flower or root).
- Inform client about optimal storage conditions of the herbal remedy.

Diet
- Teach client about foods that enhance or diminish the action of the specific herbs.
- Advise client about foods to avoid, if any, while taking herbs.

Side Effects
- Advise client of potential side effects of herbal therapy.
- Instruct client of symptoms that require prompt reporting to the health care provider.

Self-Administration
- Instruct client about preparation of special remedies (e.g., steeping of specific teas).

Cultural Considerations
- Assess personal beliefs of clients from different cultures.
- Modify communication to meet client/family cultural needs.
- Communicate respect for client/family culture.
- Evaluate effectiveness of cultural competence in interactions.

- Do not criticize folk practices; it deters clients from seeking follow-up care and decreases trust and confidence.
- Inquire about nutritional practices and incorporate harmless or nonconflicting practices into diet.
- Refrain from making prejudicial comments that may inhibit collaboration with folk healers.
- Obtain an interpreter when necessary; try not to rely on family members, who may not fully disclose because of honor or guilt.

EVALUATION

- Evaluate the effectiveness of herbal remedies for alleviating symptoms.
- Evaluate client's use of resources.

Herbal Resources

Multiple herbal resources are available on the Web. Of course, the reader needs to evaluate the website and decide if the information is appropriate. Following are a few examples of the many Internet resources that provide herbal information. Also see the Websites box.

Organizations

American Botanical Council
P.O. Box 201660
Austin, TX 78720
amebotcncl@aol.com
www.herbalgram.org

United States Pharmacopeia
12601 Twinbrook Parkway
Rockville, MD 20852
(301) 816-8250

Research Databases

Herbnet: *www.herbnet.com*
Herb Research Foundation: *www.herbs.org*

Summary

Herbal medicine is the most widely used and oldest form of medicine in the world. Currently, there is no pressure from the U.S. government to enforce quality control of herbal products. Hence, the buyer needs to be informed before purchasing the products and should deal only with reputable dealers. It is important for clients to share with the health care provider use and anticipated use of herbal products so an optimal therapeutic plan can be implemented.

WEBSITES

For further information on *Herbal Therapy with Nursing Implications*, visit these Internet resources:

Herb Research Foundation: *www.herbs.or*
Medical Herbalism: *www.medherb.com*
American Herbalists Guild: *www.healthy.net/herbalists*
U.S. Office of Dietary Supplement: *http://ods.od.nih.gov*
National Cancer Institute: *www.cancer.gov*
Department of Health and Human Services: *www.healthfinder.gov*

Info on consistency, potency, & purity: *www.ConsumerLab.com*
The Mayo Clinic: *http://mayoclinic.com*
HerbMed: *http://www.herbmed.org*
About herbs and botanicals: *www.mskcc.org/mskcc/html/11570.cfm*
American Herbal Pharmacopoeia: *www.herbal-ahp.org*
Focus on Alternative and Complementary Therapies (FACT): *www.exeter.ac.uk/FACT/*
National Center for Complementary and Alternative Medicine: *www.nccam.nih.gov*
Natural Health Village (legislative issues): *www.netvillage.com*
The Alternative Medicine Home Page: *www.pitt.edu/~cbw/atlm.html*
The Review of Natural Products: *www.drugfacts.com*
The U.S. Department of Agriculture Agricultural Genome Information System: *probe.nalusda.gov*

 Critical Thinking Case Study

A.B., a 49-year-old female accountant, reports periods of feeling tired that are increasing in frequency and intensity. On her health history she lists "no medications on a regular basis." During the nursing history, you learn that she has been taking ginseng, ginkgo biloba 300 mg b.i.d., and licorice root 2 mg b.i.d. for the past 6 months. Occasionally she takes 300 mg t.i.d. of St. John's wort extract.

1. Is A.B. taking the recommended dose of ginseng and ginkgo biloba? If not, what modifications would you suggest that she consider?

2. A.B. tells you that she has arthritis. What modifications would be appropriate based on this new information?

3. What specific client teaching is appropriate for A.B. at this time?

Study Questions

1. What is the most authoritative source for therapeutic substances?

2. What information is recommended to be placed on labels of herbal products?

3. What are the stipulations of the Dietary Supplement Health and Education Act of 1994?

4. What claims can be made about herbal remedies relative to preventing or curing specific conditions?

For questions 5 through 7, identify a common herb that best matches each of the following descriptions:

5. Serotonin antagonist for relief of migraine headache; requires refrigeration.

6. Most commonly prescribed herbal remedy used in the treatment of dementia syndromes, vertigo, and tinnitus for up to 90 days.

7. Has at least 10 pharmacologically active components for the relief of depression and anxiety. Should users avoid tyramine-rich foods?

8. List at least three recommended pieces of information that should be on labels of herbal products.

9. What are five important areas of client teaching related to herbal therapy? Describe at least one specific suggestion for each area.

10 Pediatric Pharmacology

JUDITH W. HERRMAN

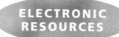

Additional information can be found on the companion website at *http://evolve.elsevier.com/KeeHayes/pharmacology/* or on the companion CD-ROM, which includes:
- *NCLEX-style examination review questions*
- *Pharmacology animations*
- *Medication error and IV therapy checklists*
- *Medication calculation problems*
- *Electronic calculators*

OUTLINE

OBJECTIVES

- Apply the principles of pharmacokinetics and pharmacodynamics to pediatric medication administration.
- Differentiate components of pharmacology unique to pediatric clients.
- Discuss key nursing implications as they relate to pediatric medications and administration.

TERMS

chronologic age
developmental age

pharmacodynamics

pharmacokinetics

Introduction

A nurse who provides care to children must make certain adaptations in assessments, treatments, and evaluations of nursing care because of physiologic, psychologic, and developmental differences inherent in this population. This is especially true in the science of pharmacology—both in the administration of medications to children and in the evaluation of the therapeutic and adverse effects of a medication. This chapter addresses these adaptations and discusses the impact that growth and development have on the many aspects of pharmacology, such as pharmacokinetics, pharmacodynamics, dosing and monitoring, methods of medication administration, and nursing implications.

Pharmacology as it relates to the nursing of infants, children, and adolescents is limited by the research available in providing protocols of recommend dosages, safe practices, key assessments, and important nursing implications. Most information available about medications is concluded from studies that use adult samples, small sample sizes, or samples with healthy children. Few studies have been conducted with children diagnosed as having applicable illnesses to determine the effectiveness of medication for the target population. Generalizing results of these studies to pediatric populations, as in applying principles of adult pharmacology to dictate pediatric nursing practice, may result in serious errors and negate the impact of growth and development on pharmacology.

Research related to pediatric clients is limited as a result of several factors. It is difficult to obtain a pediatric sample because of informed consent and research risks. Parents and guardians are reluctant to provide consent for children to participate in research studies because of the risk involved and the potentially invasive nature of the studies. Pharmaceutical companies tend to put fewer resources toward pediatric drug research because of the smaller market share afforded to pediatric medications. Many perceive pediatric pharmacologic research as unethical because of these factors. In contrast, others contend that this lack of pediatric data reflects a lack of ethics, especially when medications are administered to pediatric clients without supporting research data on which to base safe practices. As a result, less is known about the effects, uses, and dosages of pediatric medications. Nurses need to investigate pediatric medications carefully to provide knowledgeable nursing care for children.

Closely aligned with the conflicts that impact pediatric pharmacologic research are those associated with medication labels and dosing instructions. Because many drugs have not undergone the clinical trials required for federal approval, many drugs have not been approved for pediatric use. Indications of safe use for children may be guided by small studies or the judgment of the clinician and may be based on anecdotal rather than scientific study. These conflicts generated new legislation designed to protect the client and provide health care professionals with the optimal information and resources.

Approximately one quarter of all medications carry federally approved indications for use in children, but almost 75% of all drugs marketed for adults in the United States are also prescribed for children. As a result of legislation presented in 1992 and 1994, the Food and Drug Administration (FDA) now requires many medications to include known dosages, adverse effects, precautions, and effectiveness, which allows health care professionals and the public some level of security when using medications. A law known as the Pediatric Research Equity Act in 2003, along with the Best Pharmaceuticals Act of 2002, requires drug manufacturers to study pediatric medication use and offers incentives for pediatric pharmacology research. Even with increasing data, many drugs are prescribed via off-label instructions based on expert opinions, small clinical trials, or practitioners' personal experiences with the medication.

Pharmacokinetics

Significant differences exist in the pharmacokinetics when implicating the pediatric population. These differences stem from differences in body composition and organ maturity and appear to be more pronounced in neonates and younger infants and less significant in older school-age and adolescent children. **Pharmacokinetics** may be defined as the study of the time course of drug absorption, distribution, metabolism, and excretion.

Absorption

The degree and rate of absorption are based on many factors, such as age, the child's health status, and the route of administration. As children grow and develop, the absorption of medications generally becomes more effective; therefore absorption in infants and neonates must be considered in dosing and administration. A contradiction to this occurs during the adolescent years, during which poor nutritional habits, changes in physical maturity, and hormonal differences may provide for poorer medication absorption. The presence of underlying disease, hydration status, and gastrointestinal (GI) disorders in the child may be a significant factor in the absorption of medications.

Absorption is initially impacted by the route of administration. For oral medication, conditions in the stomach and intestine affect the absorption of the drug. Such conditions include gastric acidity, gastric emptying, gastric motility, GI surface area, enzyme levels, and intestinal flora. The lack of maturation of the GI tract is most pronounced in infancy, making the neonatal and infancy periods those most affected by changes in physiology. Gastric pH is alkaline at birth, and acid production begins in the neonatal period. Gastric pH may reach adult acidity between 1 and 3 years of age. A low pH or acidic environment favors acidic drug absorption, whereas a high pH or alkaline environment favors basic drug formulations; therefore differences in pH may hinder or enhance the absorption of medications. Gastric emptying is generally prolonged in neonates and infants but increases as the child grows. Nurses should be aware that delayed emptying in children reduces the peak concentrations of medications.

Varying transit times throughout the GI system may also hinder or enhance absorption, depending on the usual site of chemical absorption. In line with this issue, the feeding method may impact infant absorption; for example, breast-fed infants have longer GI transit times than formula-fed infants. Frequent infant feedings also affect GI transit times. The more frequent the feedings, the less time the food is in contact with the gastric or intestinal lining.

Irregular peristalsis, associated with immaturity or with symptoms of vomiting or diarrhea, decreases the absorption time available for medications. In contrast, many pediatric medications actually cause diarrhea, which again bears impact on absorption rates. In younger infants and children, the GI surface area is greater than in adults. This allows for more absorptive area in the stomach and intestines and may affect the speed and effectiveness of absorption, especially in the small intestine. Immature enzyme function may impact drug absorption; for example, low lipase levels deter the absorption of lipid-soluble medications. The colonization of the intestine, as it changes with pH and flora, creates different environments that are available to change medication absorption. All these factors should be considered when assessing the effectiveness of medications administered by the oral route (Figure 10–1).

For medications administered via the subcutaneous or intramuscular (IM) routes, absorption occurs at the tissue level. Intravenous (IV) medications are administered directly into the bloodstream. The level of peripheral perfusion and effectiveness of circulation has an effect on the ability of medications to be absorbed. Conditions that alter perfusion, such as dehydration, cold temperatures, and alterations in cardiac status, may impede absorption of medications at the tissue level.

Topical medications, or those absorbed through the skin, may be altered by the condition of the skin tissue. Because the skin of children is thinner and more porous, absorption may be enhanced. Because the skin surface area for children is proportionately higher than for adults, many medications are more readily absorbed, and there-fore the child may not only have the expected topical effect but also unwanted systemic effects.

Distribution

The distribution of a medication throughout the body of a child is impacted by factors such as body-fluid composition, body-tissue composition, protein-binding capability, and effectiveness of various barriers to medication transport. In neonates and young infants, the human body is about 70% water. As the child grows, this percentage decreases to 50% to 60%. This increased body-fluid proportion for weight allows for a greater volume of fluid in which to distribute the medication and a decreasing concentration of the drug. Younger pediatric clients, until about 2 years of age, therefore require higher doses of water-soluble medications to achieve therapeutic levels. Younger clients also have higher levels of extracellular fluids, which increases the tendency for children to become dehydrated and changes the distribution of water-soluble medications.

Neonates and young infants tend to have less body fat than older children. This difference causes young clients to require less fat-soluble medications relative to adult populations because fat-soluble drugs saturate fat tissue before acting on body tissues. Less fat available for saturation creates a need for less medication.

Drugs become bound to circulating plasma proteins in the body. Only drugs that are free, or unbound, are available to cross the cell membrane and exert an effect. Infants and neonates have less albumin than older clients and less protein receptor sites available for binding with medication. This allows medication to be more available for use and dictates a decrease in the dosage needed in young clients to produce the same therapeutic effect. Greater quantities of circulating drugs caused by reduced plasma proteins increase the propensity for adverse or toxic reactions in infants less than 1 year of age. In neonates, high bilirubin levels may pose a health risk with regard to the administration of medications. These bilirubin molecules may bind with plasma protein sites, making them unavailable to medications. This allows large amounts of medication to be available for effect. If neonatal medications are needed, the dose needs to be decreased and closely monitored to ensure therapeutic effectiveness and avoid adverse effects.

The barriers to medication distribution, such as the skin or the blood-brain barrier, must be considered. Infants' blood-brain barriers are relatively immature, allowing medications to pass easily into nervous system tissue. This increases the likelihood for toxicity in young infants. The skin is also more absorptive in young children, as described, and provides for rapid distribution of medication. As the child matures, both of these barriers become more impervious to medication, and dosages need to be titrated accordingly.

Metabolism

The metabolism of medications is impacted by the maturation level of the child, and this process varies greatly from child to child. Metabolism is carried out primarily in the liver, with the kidneys and lungs playing a small part in

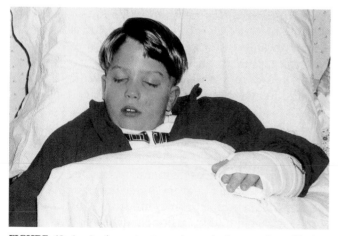

FIGURE 10–1 An important nursing role is assessing effectiveness of medication on each child.

the metabolic stage. For most infants, until about 2 years of age, sustained decreases in levels of hepatic enzymes result in a slower metabolism of medications. Hepatic metabolic activity is lower in neonates; infant hepatic function matures at 1 to 2 months of age. This issue, as with other pharmacokinetic factors, reinforces the importance for the nurse to evaluate therapeutic effects and monitor adverse effects of medications.

Children inherently have a higher metabolic rate than adults, causing metabolism to occur more rapidly. This may necessitate a higher medication requirement than for adults. For example, pain medication for children may require increased dosages or decreased durations between medications. Oral medications absorbed are then subject to metabolism in the liver. This phenomenon, called the *first-pass effect*, provides that drugs administered through the oral route and absorbed via the GI tract undergo some metabolism in the hepatocytes in the liver before they are made available to the body tissues. For select medications, when the oral route is ordered, the first-pass effect must be considered in the calculation of dosages. Some medications are administered via the rectal route to avoid the hepatic first-pass effect.

Excretion

The excretion of medications occurs in the kidneys, intestines, lungs, sweat glands, salivary glands, and mammary glands, with the kidneys providing the most elimination. Before about 9 months of age, infants experience a reduction in the elimination capacity of the kidneys because of decreases in renal blood flow, decreases in glomerular filtration rate, and reductions in renal tubular function. Because medications are excreted more slowly as a result of this decreased renal function, medications accumulate and may reach toxic levels. At the onset of adolescence, renal tubular function is again decreased. Water is needed for the effective excretion of medication; therefore clients need to be evaluated for dehydration, which could lead to toxic drug levels. Nurses need to carefully monitor renal function, urine flow, and medication effectiveness to evaluate the impact of medication excretion for clients.

Pharmacodynamics

Pharmacodynamics have also been used to describe differences in pediatric pharmacology. **Pharmacodynamics** refers to the mechanisms of action and effect of a drug on the body and includes the onset, peak, and duration of effect of a medication. It can also be described as the intensity and time course of therapeutic and adverse effects of medications. The variables of pharmacokinetics—absorption, distribution, metabolism, and excretion—all impact the parameters of

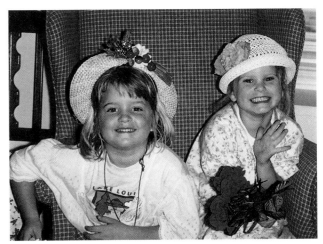

FIGURE 10–2 What special concerns related to medications should a caregiver of these two 7-year-olds playing "dress up" need to consider?

pharmacodynamics. These processes affect the time a medication begins to function, reaches its peak, and sustains its length of action. The half-life of a medication may be different in children than in adults. Pediatric variables, such as organ function, developmental implications, and administration issues, impact the pharmacodynamics and require nurses to knowledgeably evaluate the action and effectiveness of pediatric medications (Figure 10–2).

Nursing Implications

Pediatric Medication Dosing and Monitoring

Because of the changes in pharmacokinetics and pharmacodynamics inherent of pediatric clients, a key nursing role is to monitor the client for therapeutic effect and adverse reactions. The processes described earlier may be measured using plasma or serum drug levels, which indicate the amount of medication in a client's body. The monitoring of serum drug levels can assist in the establishment of appropriate dosages, schedules, and routes of medications for a client. It can also assist in indicating when the dose is too high (toxic) or too low (not therapeutic). The ranges established for many drug levels are based on studies on adults, which indicates the importance for the nurse to assess pediatric clients in conjunction with monitoring blood levels. Serum blood levels are not available for all medications because of the lack of methods available to measure medications. As a result, client clinical responses to medication is especially important in the monitoring of medications.

The calculation of pediatric dosages, as discussed earlier, is based in part on FDA recommendations, approved protocols, research studies, and provider experience. Most medications are ordered based on the child's weight in kilograms; therefore a dose per unit of weight calculation is required. However, some medications, such as chemotherapies, are prescribed based on body surface area (BSA) (e.g., mg/m^2). BSA provides a good indication of the distribution, metabolism, and excretion of medications.

When the pediatric dosages are not available, the dose may be extrapolated based on the adult dose. Using a nomogram (see Chapter 4, Medications and Calculations, Section F), the BSA for the child is determined (Figure 10–3). The following equation then may be used to find the pediatric dosage for the child:

$$\text{child's dose} = \frac{\text{m}^2 \text{ (body surface area)}}{1.73 \text{ m}^2} \times \text{adult dose}$$

Although this is not the recommended method to calculate pediatric medication dosages, it can be used when medication ranges based on the child's weight are not easily accessible. BSA calculators have been developed to reduce errors that may occur when using the nomogram, and it may be easier to use. Other rules that have been used in the past to calculate pediatric dosages are no longer considered safe or accurate. Dosing must also consider the individual child's status, including age, organ function, health, and the route of administration.

Pediatric Medication Administration

A key issue with pediatric medication administration is the identification of the client who is to receive the dose. Using the client's identification wristband in inpatient settings is the most effective method to ensure client identity; outpatient and other settings pose a greater challenge in establishing client identity. Children may not know or want to divulge their name. A safe method to identify clients for each setting must be created to ensure safe medication administration.

Developmental and cognitive differences must always be considered when administering medication to children. It is important for the nurse to differentiate the child's **developmental age** from the **chronologic age** because this has an impact on the child's response and responsiveness to medication. The child's ability to understand the process and reasons for medication and the capacity to cooperate with the procedure must always figure clearly into the pediatric nurses' plan of care. The child's temperament may influence this understanding and level of cooperation. When possible, family members or caregivers should be solicited to assist in medication administration, taught how to administer the medications, and instructed on methods to evaluate effectiveness. In addition, these significant persons in the child's life, who know the child on a day-to-day basis, are usually in the best position to evaluate the effectiveness of a medication and observe for adverse reactions. Some of the adverse reactions of medications, such as ringing in the ears or nausea, may be difficult to evaluate in a child, and those closest to the child may be in the best position to assess for these responses. In contrast, parents or other family members may request not to participate in invasive procedures but can be encouraged to provide comfort to the child after the medication is administered. This request should be respected and caregivers should be supported in their caring function so that the child feels safe and secure.

Cognitive issues, such as the ability to understand (1) the reason for the medication, (2) the need for the medication despite unpleasant taste or method of administration, and (3) the need to complete all doses and courses of medication, must be addressed. When the family is taught about pediatric drug administration, education for the child—at a developmentally appropriate level—must also be included. Communication with the child and family must always consider the level of knowledge, developmental age, cultural factors, and levels of anxiety. The nurse should use optimal interpersonal skills to ensure the safe administration of medications.

The primary concerns in administering medications to infants are maintaining safety with the minimum restraint necessary, administering the correct dosage, and providing care with as much comforting as possible. Toddlers may react violently and negatively to medication administration. Simple explanations, a firm approach, and enlisting the imagination of a toddler through play may enhance success with medication administration. Preschoolers are fairly cooperative and respond well to age-appropriate explanations. Allowing some level of choice and control may enlist success with preschool children. School-age children, though cooperative, may fear bodily injury and need even more control, involvement in the process, and information. Age-appropriate fears related to pain, changes in body image, and injury are prevalent among older school-

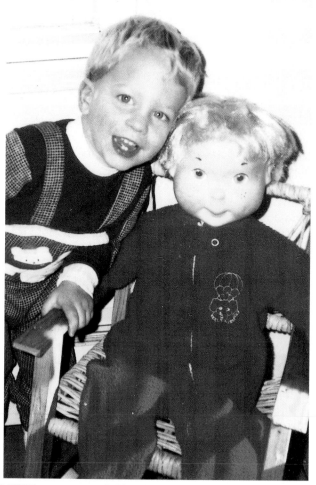

FIGURE 10–3 Many children's medication dosages are calculated based on a child's weight.

age and adolescent clients. The nurse should establish a positive rapport with the client, contract with the adolescent related to the plan of care, and ensure privacy in all aspects of medication administration.

Most pediatric medications are administered via the oral route. This route is the least invasive, is the easiest to use, and can be used by family and home caregivers. Nonetheless, the subcutaneous (subQ), IM, topical, rectal, and IV routes are also used to deliver medications to clients for whom the oral route is contraindicated. Because of tissue differences among children, the IV route is more predictable than other routes.

Most oral medications are administered to a child using an oral syringe. Oral syringes ensure more exact dosing of medication and are relatively easy to use. Syringes may be marked to ensure correct dosages. The syringe is inserted into the mouth and pointed toward the buccal mucosa on either side of the mouth. Allowing the medication to fall too close to the front of the mouth increases the likelihood that medication will be spit out. Pointing the syringe directly toward the back of the mouth may increase the risk for gagging or choking. Younger infants may suck medication from a bottle nipple in which medication has been "squirted" from the oral syringe. At times, blowing in the face of the infant will stimulate the swallow reflex and facilitate medication administration. Preschool and school-age children are usually able to inject the medication themselves into their mouth, enhancing their level of control of the situation.

Nurses may need to crush pills or dissolve capsules in fluid for administration to pediatric clients. It is the nurse's responsibility to access information on the ability to crush or dissolve a medication before administration; some medications, such as time-release and enteric-coated medications, should not be crushed or dissolved before administration. Some medications may be made more palatable by adding jelly, syrup, or honey (infants less than 1 year old should not be given honey because of the risk of botulism). Small volumes should be used to dilute medications so that the client is ensured the entire dose. As pediatric medication research increases, more medication will be available in stable, liquid pediatric forms. Until then, the nurse should work closely with the pharmacist and hospital policies to ensure safe administration of oral medications to children. Medications should not be added to formula so that future food aversions are avoided. For children who refuse to take medication by mouth or for children who have intestinal tubes, medications can be administered via nasogastric, orogastric, or gastrostomy tubes. Precautions required when giving medications via this route are similar to those implemented when administering feedings.

The administration of subcutaneous, IM, and IV medications to children includes many of the same principles as adults, with some additional considerations. Safe restraint and atraumatic care principles should be used when possible. Wong (2003) defines *atraumatic care* as the delivery of therapeutic care through the implementation of interventions that "eliminate or minimize the psychologic and physical distress experienced by children and their families in the health care system" (p. 15). Depending on developmental age, the child may have incorrect interpretations about the need for medication, believing that the medication is a punishment or a result of wrongdoing. The nurse should provide preparation for the procedure at the appropriate level for the child and involve caregivers in all aspects of care. One method to ensure atraumatic care is through the use of topical analgesics on the site before IM, subQ, or IV injections. Eutectic mixture of local anesthetics (EMLA) a topical cream, anesthetizes the site of injection if applied 1 to 2.5 hours before injection (Wong, 2003). After EMLA is applied to the injection site, the site is covered with a transparent dressing for containment. Also available are iontophoresis (Numby Stuff), a vasocoolant spray, or buffered lidocaine injections (Wong, 2003). Distraction and other nonpharmacologic methods of pain and anxiety control can also be used, based on the cognitive level of the child, to decrease the perception of pain. The use of creative imagery with toddlers and preschool children has been explored as a pain-management strategy (Ott, 1996). Injections should never be given to a sleeping child with the intent to surprise the child with a quick procedure. As a result, the child may experience a lack of trust and be reluctant to sleep in the future.

IV infusion sites must also be protected, especially in infants and toddlers, who do not understand the rationale or importance of maintaining the IV site. The patency of an IV site should be checked before each medication administration to avoid infiltration and extravasation. Any injection site on a preschooler should be covered with a bandage, preferably a decorated one, so that the young child does not fear "leakage" from the area. Selection of injection and IV sites are made based on developmental variables, site of preference, and access to administration sites. IM injections should not be given in the gluteal muscle until children have been ambulating for a full year. The ventrogluteal or the vastus lateralis are the preferable sites for pediatric IM injections (Wong, 2003). The length of the needle depends on the child's muscle mass, subQ tissue, and the site of injection. The child may prefer subQ injections in the leg or upper arm, rather than in the abdomen. IV sites may be difficult to find in children based on amount of fat tissue, the hydration status of the child, and the ability to isolate and immobilize veins.

Some key aspects of pediatric medication administration identified by Miller and Fiorvanti (1997) include the following: (1) honesty is a priority; (2) careful attention to vocabulary should be maintained; (3) forceful restraint should never be used; (4) praise should be given to the child after successful administration of the medication; and (5) the child should not be threatened or shamed into taking a medication. These principles may be used throughout the pediatric life span and highlight the need for nursing intervention that is sensitive, individualized, and caring.

Nursing Process

When working with pediatric clients, key developmental differences need to be considered when administering and monitoring medications. The nursing process provides the framework to guide nursing practice in administering medications, planning and evaluating nursing care, providing client and family teaching, and incorporating the family into all aspects of care.

Teaching is a key component for the family and client. Much of the information the nurse has knowledge of should be passed on to the client and family as well. Issues such as the indications for the medication, the side effects, the dose, how to measure the dose, how to administer the dose, the therapeutic effect of the medication, any adverse effects to be monitored, the duration, and the frequency are all important information needed by the family or caregiver. Specifics such as the need for refrigeration, the need to shake the medicine, the difference between household and prescriptive teaspoons, and other issues should be addressed to ensure client safety. Adherence to the medication regimen is of paramount importance with children and families; providing written instructions or a medication calendar may facilitate this through concrete reminders.

Considerations for the Adolescent

Nursing care of the adolescent client warrants individualized care specific for this developmental stage. These age-oriented developmental considerations include physical changes, cognitive level and abilities, emotional factors, and the impact of chronic illness.

Physically, adolescence is a highly diverse period of growth and development. Growth rates during the teen years may be impacted by nutrition, factors within the environment, genetics and heredity, and gender. A group of adolescents of similar ages may manifest very different sizes, height-to-weight proportions, secondary sex characteristics, and other indicators of physical maturity. These differences may warrant individualization of dosages based on weight or body surface area, even when the adolescent meets or exceeds the size of standard adults. For example, an adjustment may be required in the dosage of a lipid-soluble medication because changes in lean-to-fat body mass, especially in young adolescent males, coincide with physical maturation. Hormonal changes and growth spurts may necessitate changes in medication dosages; many children with chronic illness require dosage adjustments in the early teen years as a result of these transitions. Teens' sleep requirements and metabolic rates may greatly increase during the teen years, along with appetites and food consumption, which may affect their scheduling of and response to medications. Although adolescents resemble the physical appearance and organ structure and function of adults, their body continues to grow and change, requiring increased vigilance in monitoring therapeutic and toxic drug levels.

The cognitive level and abilities of the adolescent may pose even greater challenges to the pediatric nurse. As dictated by cognitive theorists, adolescents progress from concrete to abstract reasoning (Wong, 2003). Individuals who are still in the concrete operational stage may have difficulty comprehending how a medication exerts its effects on the body and the importance of meticulous dosing and admin-

istration. Teens may also have difficulty understanding such concepts as drug interactions, side effects, adverse reactions, and therapeutic levels. For example, the client taking birth control pills may or may not be able to comprehend the potential implications and extra precautions necessary when taking an antagonistic antibiotic during an acute infection. Client teaching must consider the cognitive level of the individual; as adolescents learn to reason in an abstract manner, teaching may be based on more complex information.

Teens' difficulty in relating future consequences to current actions and their commonly perceived invulnerability may dictate that the nurse adapt teaching to address specific adolescent thought processes. The adolescent who is told that an insulin injection schedule must be adhered to in order to avoid long-term complications may not understand the rationales for treatment if only substantiated by abstract, future-oriented risks. That same teen may find the relationship between insulin to maintain normoglycemia and the ability to participate in sports more immediate and relevant. Although teens may physically resemble soon-to-be adults, the nurse must continue to assess clients' cognitive levels as they relate to medications.

The emotional development of the teen also occurs on an individual basis. The teen years are characterized by sensation seeking, risk taking, questioning, formation of identity, and increasing influences exerted by peer groups. The nurse should assess for high-risk behaviors, including use of alcohol, tobacco, and recreational drugs, to avoid potential drug interactions. Other issues, including sexual practices, stressful family and social situations, and lifestyle behaviors may impact the client's response to medications. Nurses must be respectful of the emotional needs of adolescence while attending to the mental health issues that may surface during the teen years. A comprehensive history must be solicited from the teen client to ensure appropriate medication administration.

The nurse is often in a key role to establish a working relationship with the client and to provide the client with appropriate levels of privacy. Allowing the adolescent to verbalize concerns about the medication and the regimen may offer the opportunity for clarification of misconceptions and learning of new concepts. The nurse must also be conscious of the need to exercise care in offering confidentiality in the event that information needs to be divulged to other health care providers, parents, or caregivers to ensure client safety.

As adolescents attain greater levels of independence from their parents, self-care can be increased. The nurse should assess the teen's abilities to self-administer medication and self-monitoring of therapeutic and adverse reactions. Teens who spend less time with parents and caregivers may need increased instruction about their medication regimen and the key observations that are needed. Although during the teen years young people frequently display this "breaking away" from parental bonds, teens continue to role model adult parent or caregiver medication habits. These may have a bearing on the teen's medication behaviors.

For the child with chronic illness, issues may change throughout the teen years. Engaging peers in the medication plan of care, allowing the teen safe choices and flexibility within that plan, setting up mutual medication contracts with adolescent clients, and permitting the teen to design his or her own adult-monitored medication regimen may facilitate compliance. For many children with chronic illness, the family's key role in disease management changes during adolescence. Such issues as rebellion from rules, refusal to take medications, and participation in high-risk behaviors may ensue. The nurse can facilitate required adaptations and support the client and family during these trying times.

Teens needing to receive medications may require assistance with decision making; organization of a medication schedule; and understanding of the key physical, cognitive, and emotional changes characteristic of this stage. Nurses' levels of knowledge and caring support may offer a great contribution to adolescent clients and their families.

Nursing Process

Pediatrics

ASSESSMENT

■ Record the age, weight, and height of the child. Drug calculations are based on these three factors.
■ Assess developmental age, health status, and nutritional and hydration statuses.
■ Assess history of drug use (prescriptions, over-the-counter (OTC), herbal).
■ Assess family understanding and child cognitive level.

NURSING DIAGNOSES

■ Delayed growth and development
■ Ineffective tissue perfusion
■ Impaired urinary elimination
■ Knowledge deficit
■ Risk for injury

PLANNING

■ The child receives drug dosage based on age, weight, and height. Most drug calculations for children are related to weight in kilograms or body surface area (BSA) (see Chapter 4, Medications and Calculations, Section F).

NURSING INTERVENTIONS

■ Use appropriate drug references to obtain the drug parameters or ranges, side effects, and contraindications for use of the drug when administering drugs to children.
■ Monitor infants closely for side effects of drugs because of their immature liver and kidneys. Because infants and young children have limited communication skills, changes in their usual behavior pattern may be indicative of side effects.

■ Communicate with the health care provider about drug dosages that are questionable for infants because of the drug's prolonged half-life and the infant's decreased drug excretion.
■ Calculate the child's drug dose according to weight in kilograms or BSA.

Client Teaching

• Instruct the responsible family member not to give OTC drugs to children without asking the health care provider.
• Instruct the family member to report side effects of the medication immediately to the health care provider.
• Advise mothers who are breastfeeding their newborn or infant to avoid taking OTC drugs or another person's medication because a portion of most drugs is excreted in breast milk.
• Advise the family member to keep medications out of reach of children.
• Instruct the family member to use child-resistant medication containers.

Cultural Considerations

• Consider parenting, caregiving, and cultural differences when providing care and teaching to children and families about medications.
• When soliciting adolescent health histories, consider issues related to sexual practices, risk behaviors, recreational drug use, and other lifestyles may impact medication administration and safety.

EVALUATION

■ Evaluate the family member's knowledge concerning the drug, drug dosage, schedule for drug administration, and side effects.
■ Evaluate the child's physiologic and psychologic response to the drug regimen.
■ Evaluate the therapeutic and adverse effects of the medication(s).

WEBSITES

For further information on *Pediatric Pharmacology,* visit these Internet resources:

General information for parents, teens, and children: *www.kidshealth.org*

Society of Pediatric Nursing: *www.pedsnurses.org*

General information about medications: *http://pediatrics.about.com/ce/childhoodmedications*

American Academy of Pediatrics: *www.aap.org*

General pediatric information: *www.keepkidshealthy.com*

Critical Thinking Case Studies

A.J. is a 9-month-old infant admitted for congestive heart failure secondary to an unrepaired congenital heart defect. The infant is ordered to receive several medications by mouth. You are providing discharge teaching to the family.

1. How does a nurse adapt teaching methods when the client is an infant?

2. A.J. does not readily take the medications by mouth. What suggestions could you offer this family to enhance medication administration?

3. The mother is concerned with the child's current diarrhea. With your knowledge of absorption, distribution, metabolism, and excretion, what impact may this symptom have on the effectiveness of the medications?

C.C. is a 12-year-old boy receiving daily injections of growth hormone. He is extremely afraid of injections.

4. What advice could you offer his caregivers to facilitate injection technique?

5. The family is considering using topical anesthetic to ease the administration of injections. Why may this be an effective strategy?

6. Based on C.C.'s developmental level, how could the nurse facilitate cooperation in C.C.?

Study Questions

1. What are the dangers of focusing on infants and children as small adults?

2. If a water-soluble drug is to be administered to an infant, what adjustments should be made? If a fat-soluble medication is to be administered to an infant, what adjustments should be made?

3. A child is to receive a medication with a dosage of 30 mg/kg. What is the appropriate dosage for a child who weighs 15 kg?

4. A child is to receive a chemotherapy in which the dose is based on body surface area. The dosage recommendation is 4.5 g/m^2/24 hours in three divided doses. The child's body surface area has been calculated as 1.7 m^2. What is the total daily dose and each t.i.d. dose of the medication?

5. What are the following pharmacokinetics related to children and drug therapy?
   • Gastric emptying time
   • Protein-binding sites
   • Liver function
   • Kidney function

6. What are some methods that enhance cooperation during medication administration in toddlers, preschool, school-age, and adolescent children?

7. What are two key developmental considerations for each childhood stage that impacts medication administration?

8. What are methods that provide restraint when an infant is to receive an intramuscular medication in the right thigh?

9. What are major aspects to be included when teaching a family about medications for its child?

10. What is the nurse's role in pharmacology research when applied to pediatric clients?

11. Discuss two developmental characteristics specific to adolescence that impact medication administration and monitoring.

11 Geriatric Pharmacology

OUTLINE

OBJECTIVES

- Explain the physiologic changes of the aging process that have a major effect on drug therapy.
- Explain the pharmacokinetics and pharmacodynamics of the older adult that relate to drug dosing.
- Differentiate the effects of two drug categories on the older adult.
- Discuss reasons for noncompliance to drug regimen by the older adult.
- Give nursing implications related to drug therapy in the older adult.

compliance	noncompliance	pharmacodynamics	polypharmacy
nonadherence	older adult	pharmacokinetics	

Introduction

Older Americans constitute almost 20% of the population; thus all nurses will care for increasing numbers of elders representing the "core business" of health care. Geriatric pharmacology for the **older adult** (elderly client) requires increased attention to the age-related factors of drug absorption, distribution, metabolism, and excretion. Drug dosages are adjusted according to the older adult's weight, adipose tissue, laboratory results (e.g., serum protein, electrolytes, liver enzymes, blood urea nitrogen [BUN], creatinine), and current health problems. Modifications in drug therapy for the older adult are frequently required. Because of the declining organ functions in the older adult, the effect of drug therapy should be closely monitored to prevent the risk of adverse reactions to drugs and possible drug toxicity.

About 13% of the U.S. population are persons older than 65 years of age; this age group consumes approximately 30% of all prescribed medications and 40% of over-the-counter (OTC) drugs. By 2030 it is expected that the number of older adults will be nearly twice the number in 2000. It is predicted that in the older population there will be a greater increase in the number of Hispanics, Asians, and African Americans than in whites. Women 65 years of age outnumber 65-year-old men by 134 to 100; in the 75-year-old age group, there are 100 women to 55 men. A fast-growing population is those 85 years and older; their use of drug therapy will continue to grow. The cost of drugs in the United States reached more than $160 billion annually, much of it spent by elderly. However, medications save money spent on hospitalizations and surgeries.

Approximately 70% of clients older than 65 years of age take at least one or two prescribed drugs daily, and the other 30% of older adults take five or more prescribed drugs daily. Older adults take pain, sleep, and laxative OTC drugs more frequently than does the general population. At the time of hospital admission, about 15% of clients older than 65 years are not taking any medications. During hospitalization, older adults take an average of three to five drugs. One third of clients in nursing homes receive 6 to 12 drugs daily. Figure 11–1 shows a client with a "handful" of drugs.

The adverse reactions and drug interactions that occur in the older adult are three to seven times greater than those for middle-aged and young adults. Older adults consume numerous drugs because of chronic and multiple illnesses; therefore they are susceptible to adverse reactions and interactions. Additional problems that can cause adverse reactions from drugs include self-medicating with

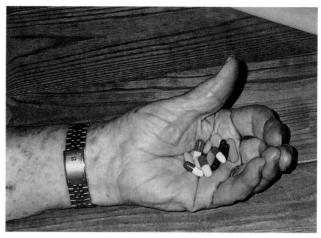

FIGURE 11–1 Does the client know what the medications are for and whether they are all necessary?

OTC drugs, taking drugs that were prescribed for other health problems, consuming drugs ordered by several different health care providers, overdosing when symptoms do not subside, using drugs that were prescribed for another person, and, of course, the ongoing physiologic aging process.

Drug toxicity may develop in the older adult for drug doses that are within therapeutic range for the average adult. These therapeutic drug ranges are usually safe for young and middle-aged adults but are not always within safe range for older adults. It has been suggested that the drug dose for older adults should initially be at a low to low-average therapeutic range and then gradually increased according to tolerance and lack of adverse reactions; start low and go slow. This prevents a toxic reaction to the drug in older adults.

Physiologic Changes

The physiologic changes associated with the aging process have a major effect on drug therapy. Table 11–1 describes the physiologic changes that occur in the gastrointestinal (GI), cardiac and circulatory, hepatic (liver), and renal (kidney) systems of the older adult and how these changes can affect pharmacologic response to drug therapy.

Polypharmacy

Polypharmacy (administration of many drugs together) is more common in older adults because of the use of (1) multiple health care providers, (2) herbal therapy, (3) OTC drugs, and (4) discontinued prescription drugs. Polypharmacy can cause confusion, falls, malnutrition,

Table 11–1

Physiologic Changes in the Older Adult

System	Physiologic Change	Effect on Drug Administration
Gastrointestinal	↑ pH (alkaline) gastric secretions ↓ peristalsis with delayed intestinal emptying time ↓ motility ↓ first-pass effect	Slower absorption of oral drugs
Cardiac and circulatory	↓ cardiac output ↓ blood flow	Impaired circulation can delay transportation of drugs to the tissues
Hepatic	↓ enzyme function ↓ blood flow	Drugs metabolized more slowly and less completely
Renal	↓ blood flow ↓ functioning nephrons (kidney cells) ↓ glomerular filtration rate	Drugs excreted less completely

↓: Decrease; ↑: increase.

renal and liver dysfunction, and nonadherence. The nurse needs to coordinate the health care, including drug therapy, for older adults to avoid duplication of drugs from various health care providers and misuse of OTC and herbal drugs. For example, an older client may take a prescribed drug, ranitidine (Zantac), with an OTC drug, famotidine (Pepcid AC), for GI discomfort; this drug combination causes duplication to occur. Some older adults do not think herbal drugs are actually drugs that could cause adverse reactions when taken with other prescription or OTC drugs. Older adults should be encouraged to use the same pharmacy and give the pharmacist a list of all drugs they take, both prescribed and OTC drugs. Pharmacists conduct clinical reviews of medications that focus primarily on drug interactions.

Pharmacokinetics

Parameters of **pharmacokinetics** for the older adult are described in Table 11–2.

Absorption

Drug absorption from the GI tract is slowed in the older adult because of decreases in both blood flow and GI motility. In the older adult, acidic drugs are poorly absorbed because of their increased alkaline gastric secretions. Drugs remain in the GI tract because there is a

Table 11–2

Pharmacokinetics in Geriatric Pharmacology

Phases	Body Effects and Possible Drug Responses
Absorption	A decrease in gastric acidity (increased gastric pH) alters absorption of weak acid drugs, such as aspirin. A decrease in blood flow to the GI tract (40%-50% less) is caused by a decrease in cardiac output. Because of the reduction of blood flow, absorption is slowed but not decreased. A reduction in GI motility rate (peristalsis) may delay onset of action. A reduction in gastric emptying time occurs.
Distribution	Because of a decrease in body water in the older adult, water-soluble drugs are more concentrated. There is an increase in fat-to-water ratio in the older adult; fat-soluble drugs are stored and are likely to accumulate. Older adults have a decrease in circulating serum protein. The two most common proteins are albumin and alpha$_1$ acid glycoprotein. Acidic drugs (e.g., nonsteroidal antiinflammatory drugs [NSAIDs] including aspirin, benzodiazepines, phenytoin, and warfarin) bind to albumin, and the basic drugs (e.g., beta-adrenergic blockers, tricyclic antidepressants, lidocaine) bind to alpha$_1$ acid glycoprotein. With fewer protein-binding sites, there is more free drug. It is the free, unbound drug that is available to body tissue at receptor sites. Drugs with a high affinity for protein (>90%) compete for protein-binding sites with other drugs. Drug interactions result because of a lack of protein sites and an increase in free drugs.
Metabolism	In the older adult, there is a decrease in hepatic enzyme production, hepatic blood flow, and total liver function. These decreases cause a reduction in drug metabolism. With a reduction in metabolic rate, the $t^1/_2$ of drugs increases, and drug accumulation can result. Metabolism of a drug inactivates the drug and drug metabolite and prepares it for elimination via the kidneys. When drug clearance by the liver is decreased, the drug $t^1/_2$ is prolonged, and when drug clearance is increased, the drug $t^1/_2$ is shortened. With prolonged $t^1/_2$, drug accumulation can result and drug toxicity could occur.
Excretion	The older adult has a decrease in renal blood flow and a decrease in glomerular filtration rate of 40% to 50%. With a decrease in renal function, there is a decrease in drug excretion, and drug accumulation results. Drug toxicity should be assessed continually while the client takes the drug.

GI, Gastrointestinal; $t^1/_2$, half-life.

decrease in gastric motility. However, the absorption amount of an oral dose is not affected by age. Enteric-coated tablets dissolved in alkaline fluid can break down more rapidly. Iron and calcium tablets may not be absorbed as readily. Generally, the amount of an oral dose that is absorbed is not affected by age.

Distribution

Older adults have a loss of protein-binding sites for drugs, which causes increased circulation of free drug and increased chance for adverse drug reaction. During the aging process, there is a loss of body water; thus water-soluble drugs become more concentrated in the body. Because of an increase in body fat in the older adult, the lipid-soluble drugs are absorbed into the fat, which causes a decrease in desired drug effects.

Metabolism or Biotransformation

Hepatic blood flow in the older adult may be decreased by 40% to 45%. Also, aging causes a decrease in liver size. Drug clearance by hepatic metabolism is affected more in older male adults than in female adults.

Liver dysfunction caused by the aging process decreases enzyme function, which decreases the liver's ability to metabolize and detoxify drugs, thereby increasing the risk of drug toxicity.

The liver, as well as the kidneys, is a major organ responsible for drug clearance from the body. *Biotransformation* refers to drug metabolism that occurs in the liver (hepatic cells) and contributes to the clearance of drugs. Biotransformation can occur either in phase I by oxidation reaction or in phase II by conjugation reaction. The hepatic microsomal enzymes are responsible for phase I, oxidation reaction. The hepatic microsomal oxidation can be impaired by the aging process, liver diseases (e.g., cirrhosis, hepatitis), and drugs that reduce oxidation capability. Drug clearance by the liver is then reduced. An example of a drug that undergoes a phase I biotransformation oxidation reaction is diazepam (Valium). Diazepam is biotransformed to its active metabolites, desmethyldiazepam. In the older adult, the plasma-serum diazepam level would remain high because of an impaired phase I oxidation reaction. Other drugs that are biotransformed by phase I include barbiturates, codeine, ibuprofen, phenytoin, meperidine, lidocaine, certain benzodiazepines (alprazolam, flurazepam, midazolam, prazepam), and warfarin (Coumadin).

Phase II of biotransformation involves the conjugation or attachment of the drug to an inactive state. The hepatic conjugation is usually not influenced by older age, liver diseases, or drug interaction, so the drug is inactivated and excreted in the urine. Examples of drugs that are biotransformed or metabolized by phase II are aspirin, acetaminophen, certain benzodiazepines (lorazepam, oxazepam, temazepam), procainamide, and sulfanilamide. The benzodiazepines lorazepam, oxazepam, and temazepam that undergo conjugation reaction do not have active metabolites. The drug metabolic process, phase I or II, for drug clearance for the older adult client is an important consideration with drug selection.

To assess liver function, the liver enzymes need to be checked. Elevated levels indicate possible liver dysfunction. However, normal liver enzyme results may not indicate normal drug metabolism. The older adult could have normal liver function test results and still have impaired hepatic microsomal enzyme–drug oxidation reactions.

Excretion

Cardiac output and blood flow throughout the circulatory system are decreased in older adults, which affects blood flow to the liver and kidneys. After 65 years of age, nephron function may be decreased by 35%, and after 70 years of age, blood flow to the kidneys may be decreased by 40%.

Kidney function is assessed by monitoring urine output, laboratory values of BUN and serum creatinine (Cr), and the creatinine clearance (Cl_{cr} or CrCl) test (estimated). Creatinine clearance is an indicator of glomerular filtration rate (GFR). To evaluate renal function based on serum creatinine alone may not be accurate for the older adult because of the decrease in muscle mass. Creatinine is a byproduct of muscle catabolism; however, creatinine is primarily excreted by the kidneys. A decrease in muscle mass can cause a decrease in serum creatinine. With older clients, serum creatinine may be within normal values because of a lack of muscle mass, but there still could be a decrease in renal function. With the young or middle-aged adult, serum creatinine would be increased with a decrease in renal function.

The 24-hour creatinine clearance test and the serum creatinine level should be used to evaluate renal function. If a 24-hour creatinine clearance test is not feasible, the following formulas can be used to estimate creatinine clearance:

$$Cl_{cr}(\text{males}) = \frac{(140 - \text{age}) \times \text{kg}}{72 \times \text{serum Cr level}} = \text{ml/min}$$

$$Cl_{cr}(\text{females}) = \text{value of males} \times 0.85 = \text{ml/min}$$

The normal creatinine clearance value for an adult is 80 to 130 ml/min.

With liver and kidney dysfunction, the efficacy of a drug dose is usually reduced. Multiple drug use may intensify drug effect in the older adult. When the efficiency of the hepatic and renal systems is reduced, the half-life of the drug is prolonged and drug toxicity is probable.

Factors contributing to adverse reactions in the older adult include a loss of protein-binding sites, which increases the amount of free circulating drug; a decline in hepatic first-pass metabolism; and a prolonged half-life of the drug because of decreased liver and kidney function. As a result of this, the time interval between doses of a drug may need to be increased for the older client.

Pharmacodynamics

Pharmacodynamics refers to how a drug interacts at the receptor site or at the target organ. Because there is a lack of affinity to receptor sites throughout the body in the older adult, the pharmacodynamic response may be altered. The older adult could be more or less sensitive to drug action because of age-related changes in the central nervous system (CNS), changes in the number of drug receptors, and changes in the affinity of receptors to drugs. Frequently, the drug dose needs to be lowered. Changes in organ functions are important to consider in drug dosing.

With the older adult, the compensatory response to physiologic changes is decreased. When a drug with vasodilator properties is administered and the sympathetic feedback does not occur quickly, orthostatic hypotension (i.e., rapid decrease in blood pressure when standing up quickly) could result. In the younger adult, the sympathetic response of vasoconstriction works to avert a severe hypotensive effect.

Effects of Selected Drug Groups on Older Adults

Hypnotics, diuretics and antihypertensives, cardiac glycosides, anticoagulants, antibacterials (antibiotics), GI drugs (antiulcer, laxatives), antidepressants, and narcotic analgesics are drug categories for which drug effects on the older adult are possible. The number of drugs taken, drug interactions (see Chapter 7, Drug Interaction and Over-the-Counter Drugs), and physical health of the older adult (cardiac, renal, and hepatic function) are factors associated with drug effects in the older adult population. Drug selection is extremely important. Drugs with a shorter half-life are less likely to cause problems as a result of drug accumulation than drugs with a long half-life. If severe side effects occur, the drug with a shorter half-life is eliminated more quickly than the drug with a longer half-life.

Drugs that are classified as phase II (biotransformation) are tolerated and eliminated more quickly than are those from phase I (oxidation). If phase I drugs are used, drug selection should be from those agents that have fewer active metabolites. Evaluation of hepatic and renal functions is imperative, especially if the older adult takes multiple drugs. When side effects and adverse reactions occur, prescription and nonprescription drugs should be assessed (Herbal Alert 11–1).

Hypnotics

Insomnia is a frequent problem for older adults. Sedatives and hypnotics are the second most common group of drugs prescribed or taken OTC. Insomnia may be described as having difficulty in falling asleep, frequently awakening during the night, or awakening early in the morning with difficulty falling back to sleep. Types of

hypnotics differ according to the cause of insomnia. Five benzodiazepine hypnotics (flurazepam, quazepam, temazepam, triazolam, and estazolam) have been approved by the U.S. Food and Drug Administration (FDA) as hypnotics to control insomnia. For the older client, low doses of benzodiazepines with short or intermediate half-lives usually are prescribed. Short-term therapy is suggested. Usually, benzodiazepines are prescribed at higher doses for sedative and hypnotic effects and at lower doses for antianxiety effects. About 35% of the older adult population takes a hypnotic.

Flurazepam HCl (Dalmane), the first benzodiazepine hypnotic, was introduced in 1970. It has three metabolites; thus it is considered to be a short- and long-acting hypnotic. Its principal metabolite is desalkylflurazepam, which is long-acting, has a long half-life, and is slowly eliminated. This drug is not suggested for persons older than age 65. Drug hangover is a problem. Quazepam (Doral) has effects similar to flurazepam. It is a precursor of desalkylflurazepam and has a prolonged half-life.

Temazepam (Restoril) was introduced in 1981. It is biotransformed in the liver by conjugation and not by oxidation; thus it is prescribed frequently for the older adult client. Its principal metabolite, glucuronide, is conjugated with no pharmacologic effects and is excreted in the urine. Temazepam is slowly absorbed, so it should be taken 1 to 2 hours before bedtime. It is classified as an intermediate-acting benzodiazepine. Food delays its action. Temazepam is more effective for frequent awakenings during the night than for problems falling asleep.

Triazolam (Halcion) is an intermediate-acting benzodiazepine. It has a short half-life and at low doses (0.0625 to 0.125 mg) is considered safe for the older adult. It is metabolized by hepatic microsomal oxidation, although the drug doses differ from oxidized benzodiazepines. Triazolam helps with falling asleep, and it also decreases frequent awakenings during the night. When stopping the drug, doses should be tapered rather than abruptly discontinued to avoid rebound insomnia.

Estazolam, a new benzodiazepine, is an intermediate- to long-acting drug. It is metabolized in the liver to two metabolites that are not highly potent.

Other benzodiazepines, lorazepam and oxazepam, can be used for insomnia. These agents have an intermediate half-life and should be taken 1 hour before bedtime. Other benzodiazepines are more effective as anxiolytics (antianxiety drugs) than as hypnotics.

Diuretics and Antihypertensives

Diuretics are frequently prescribed for treatment of hypertension or congestive heart failure (CHF). For the older adult, the dose is usually reduced because of dose-related side effects. Hydrochlorothiazide (HydroDiuril) is prescribed in low doses of 12.5 mg. Doses of 25 to 50 mg daily with chron-ic use can cause electrolyte imbalances (e.g., hypokalemia, hyponatremia, hypomagnesemia, hypercalcemia), hyperglycemia, hyperuricemia, and hypercholesterolemia.

HERBAL ALERT 11–1

Older Adults

✎ Advise clients to consult with health care provider before starting herbal products. Common herbal preparations interact with many drugs (e.g., anticoagulants) that elderly clients take to treat chronic health disorders.

Many older adults are hypertensive (blood pressure >140/90 mmHg). Nonpharmacologic methods such as exercise, weight reduction if obese, reduction of salt and alcohol intake, and adequate rest are suggested to reduce blood pressure. (See Chapter 42, Antihypertensive Drugs, for a detailed discussion of these medications.) These actions can reduce the systolic and diastolic pressure by 8 to 10 mmHg. Drugs such as diuretics, beta-adrenergic blockers or antagonists, calcium channel blockers, angiotensin-converting (ACE) inhibitors, angiotensin II receptor antagonists (A-II blockers), and centrally acting alpha$_2$-agonists are used as antihypertensive drugs. Calcium blockers, angiotension-converting inhibitors, and A-II blockers are frequently the agents of choice because of their low incidence of electrolyte imbalance and CNS side effects. Usually, antihypertensive dosing for older adults begins with reduced doses that are gradually increased according to need, tolerance, and adverse reactions. Alpha$_1$-blockers or antagonists (prazosin, terzosin) and centrally acting alpha$_2$-agonists (methyldopa, clonidine, guanabenz, guanfacine) infrequently are prescribed for older adult clients because of their adverse reactions, such as orthostatic hypotension.

Cardiac Glycosides

Digoxin is commonly prescribed for older adults; however, long-term use of the drug should be carefully monitored because of its narrow therapeutic range (0.5 to 2 ng/ml) and the possibility of digitalis toxicity occurring. It is given for left ventricular heart failure, chronic atrial fibrillation, and atrial tachycardia. Its half-life is doubled (70 hours) in clients who are older than 80 years of age. Most of the digoxin is eliminated by the kidneys, so a decline in kidney function (decreased GFR) could cause digoxin accumulation. With close monitoring of serum digoxin levels, creatinine clearance test, and vital signs (pulse should not be <60 beats per minute), digoxin is considered safe for the older adult.

Anticoagulants

Bleeding may occur with chronic use of anticoagulants in older adult clients. Warfarin (Coumadin) is 99% protein bound; with a decrease in serum albumin, which is common among older adults, there is an increase in free, unbound circulating warfarin. There is a potential risk for bleeding. Older adult clients should have their prothrombin time (PT) or international normalized ratio (INR) checked periodically, and the nurse should check for signs of bleeding.

Antibacterials

Penicillins, cephalosporins, tetracyclines, and sulfonamides are considered safe for the older adult. If the older adult client has a decrease in renal drug clearance and the drug has a prolonged half-life, the drug dose should be reduced. Aminoglycosides, fluoroquinolones (quinolones), and vancomycin are excreted in the urine. These drug agents are not frequently prescribed for clients older than 75 years, and if they are prescribed, the drug dose is usually reduced.

Gastrointestinal Drugs

Histamine (H$_2$) blockers and sucralfate are safer drugs than other antiulcer agents for the treatment of peptic ulcers. Cimetidine (Tagamet) was the first histamine blocker or antagonist and is not suggested for the older adult because of its side effects and multiple potential drug interactions. Ranitidine, famotidine, and nizatidine may be prescribed for the older adult client instead of cimetidine.

Laxatives are frequently taken by the older adult. In long-term facilities such as nursing homes, 75% of older adult clients take laxatives on a daily basis. Fluid and electrolyte imbalances may occur with excessive use. Increased GI motility with laxative use could decrease other drug absorptions. Nonpharmacologic measures should be encouraged, such as increasing fluid intake, consuming high-fiber foods such as prunes, and exercising.

Antidepressants

The antidepressant drug dose for the older adult is normally 30% to 50% of the dose for young and middle-aged adults. Drug dose should be gradually increased according to the client's tolerance and the desired therapeutic effect. Close monitoring for possible adverse reactions is important.

The tricyclic antidepressants are effective for the older adult client. However, they do have anticholinergic properties that can cause the following side effects: dry mouth, tachycardia, constipation, and urinary retention; they also can contribute to narrow-angle glaucoma. Fluoxetine (Prozac), a bicyclic antidepressant, has fewer side effects than the tricyclics; the side effects are mostly dose related. The monoamine oxidase (MAO) inhibitors are not often prescribed for older adults because of their adverse reactions, such as drug-food interactions, which could result in hypertensive crisis and severe orthostatic hypotension. (See Chapter 26, Antidepressants and Mood Stabilizers, for a detailed description of these medications.)

Narcotic Analgesics

Narcotics can cause dose-related adverse reactions when taken by the older adult. Hypotension and respiratory depression may result from narcotic use. Close monitoring of vital signs is important while the older adult takes narcotic analgesics.

Noncompliance/Nonadherence

Nonadherence with a drug regimen can be a problem in all client age groups, but it is especially troublesome with older adults. Frequently, the older adult fails to ask questions during interactions with health care providers; therefore the drug regimen may not be fully understood or pre-

Table 11–3

Barriers to Effective Medication Use by Older Adults

Causes	Nursing Actions
Taking too many medications at different times (see Figure 11–2)	Develop a chart indicating times to take drugs. Provide space to place a mark for each drug taken. Use an organizer device to mark with days and weeks.
Failure to understand the purpose or reason for drug	Explain the purpose, drug action, and importance of the medications. Provide time for questions and reinforcement. Reinforce with written information.
Impaired memory	Encourage family members or friends to monitor drug regimen.
Decreased mobility and dexterity	Advise family members or friends to have drugs and water or other fluid accessible. Assist older adult as needed.
Visual and hearing disturbances	Suggest eye and ear examinations (glasses or hearing aids).
High cost of prescriptions	Contact the social services department of your institution; contact "compassionate care programs" as appropriate.
Childproof drug bottles	Suggest that the client request non-childproof bottle caps.
Side effects or adverse reactions from the drug	Educate client and family about side effects to report to health care provider.

cisely followed. Nonadherence can cause underdosing or overdosing that could be harmful to the older adult client's health. Some barriers to effective medication use by older adult are listed in Table 11–3.

Working with the older adult is an ongoing nursing responsibility. The nurse should plan strategies with the older adult and family or friends to encourage **compliance**. Daily contact with the client may be necessary at first. Mere ordering of medication does not mean that the client is able to get the drugs or is taking them correctly. Figure 11–2 shows the different medications to be taken by a client at different times; this complicated array of drugs can result in confusion and **noncompliance.** Older adults often do not have insurance that pays for medications, and instead they choose to buy food rather than medications. Some older adults delay purchasing or never purchase the drugs. The older adult is more apt to experience serious side effects from drug administration than the young or middle-aged adult. If a drug such

as ibuprofen (Motrin) irritates the GI tract, the older adult frequently will *not* take the drug. However, another drug, such as magnesium hydroxide (Maalox), may be given before the ibuprofen dose to decrease the side effects. Food can also decrease gastric irritation from ibuprofen.

Health Teaching with the Older Adult

A comprehensive discussion of health teaching is presented in Chapter 2, Nursing Process and Client Teaching. Guidelines for health teaching with the older client include:

- Be sure that the client is wearing clear eyeglasses and has working hearing aids in place, if needed.
- Speak in tone of voice that client can hear; sit facing the client.
- Treat the client with respect; expect that he or she can learn.
- Use large print and bright colors in teaching aids.
- Review all medications at each client visit.
- Encourage a simple dosing schedule when possible.
- With onset of new confusion or disorientation, suspect recently prescribed medication(s).
- Encourage the client to report that a drug is not improving the condition for which it was prescribed.

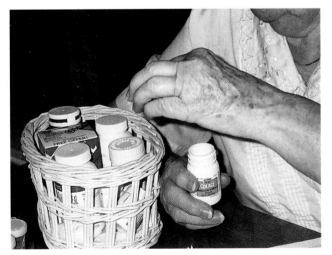

FIGURE 11–2 A possible cause of noncompliance in an older adult client is the need to take many different medications at different times.

Nursing Process

Geriatrics

ASSESSMENT

■ Assess the older adult's sensorium, mental awareness, and visual and auditory acuity. Is the person confused or disoriented? Is this state transitory? Does the older adult live alone with or without social support?

■ Obtain a history of kidney, liver, or GI disorder, and determine whether eyesight is failing. Kidney or liver disorders can cause a decrease in the function of these organs and can increase the half-life of drugs. Longer drug half-life and frequent drug dosing can result in drug toxicity. Assess the older adult's use of eyeglasses, and check the date of the last eye examination.

■ Determine whether the older adult takes OTC drugs, including herbal preparations, how often, and for what length of time. Specifically ask about laxatives and antacids, which can affect gastric pH, electrolyte balance, and GI motility; many people do not think of these agents as drugs. Remind the older adult or the family to tell the pharmacist about prescribed drugs when contemplating the purchase of OTC preparations.

■ Assess for compliance of taking drugs correctly and reasons for noncompliance. Does the older adult have problems opening drug containers?

NURSING DIAGNOSES

■ Perceived constipation
■ Urinary retention related to drug therapy
■ Imbalanced nutrition: less than body requirements
■ Ineffective health maintenance
■ Deficient knowledge
■ Noncompliance
■ Wandering

PLANNING

■ The older adult will take the prescribed medications as ordered.
■ The drug therapy will be effective with no or few side effects.

NURSING INTERVENTIONS

■ Monitor the older adult's laboratory results in relation to kidney and liver function. Are the blood urea nitrogen (BUN), serum creatinine, and creatinine clearance levels within normal range (reference values)? Are the liver enzymes within normal range? Discuss the findings with the health care provider.

■ Check the older adult's serum drug level as ordered, and report abnormal findings to the charge nurse or health care provider. Because of their reduced body water, older adults who take water-soluble drugs such as digoxin are likely to have higher blood levels.

■ Communicate with the pharmacist or health care provider when the drug dose is in question. Check drug reference books for recommended drug doses for older adults.

■ Observe the client for adverse reactions when multiple drugs are being taken. An older adult with hypertension and a failing heart (e.g., congestive heart failure) might take a diuretic (e.g., hydrochlorothiazide [HydroDiuril]) and digoxin. The diuretic may cause potassium loss and, if potassium replacement is not ordered, digitalis toxicity may occur. Hypokalemia (low serum potassium) enhances the action of digoxin, causing the toxicity. The symptoms of digitalis toxicity may be a slow or irregular pulse rate (bradycardia, <60 beats/min), nausea and vomiting, and blurred vision.

■ Recognize a change in usual behavior or an increase in confusion. One of the first signs of drug toxicity is confusion. Report these changes to the health care provider.

■ Ascertain whether the older adult has a financial problem in purchasing prescribed drugs.

Client Teaching

General

• Review the medications with the older adult and the family, including the reason for the medication, its route of administration, how often it is to be taken, common side effects, and when to notify the health care provider.

• Explain to the older adult or the family the importance of adherence with the drug regimen. Emphasize taking the drug as prescribed, discarding unused or old drugs, and keeping a record of medication taken for reference. REMEMBER: The drugs are the property of client and may not be disposed of without his or her permission.

• Be available to answer client's questions. Be supportive of the older adult and the family. Discuss problems related to the medications.

• Instruct the older adult not to share prescribed medications with others or to take medications prescribed for another person.

• Inform the older adult to use one pharmacy to fill prescribed drug orders. Tell client to inform the pharmacist of all OTC and herbal drugs that are taken.

• If the older adult has arthritis in the hand joint or has difficulty opening childproof bottle caps, inform the client to request a non-childproof cap from the pharmacy. Most likely, the client will need to sign permission at the pharmacy.

Self-Administration

• Instruct the older adult to keep a medication record of drugs and when they are to be taken. This removes barriers and increases drug adherence and avoids drug errors.

Diet

• Instruct the older adult who is taking a potassium-wasting diuretic (e.g., hydrochlorothiazide [HydroDiuril]) to control hypertension to eat foods rich in potassium, such as fruits and vegetables, and to take potassium supplements if indicated by the health care provider.

• Inform the older adult about how to maintain a well-balanced diet and give examples.

Side Effects

- Advise the older adult and family to report mental and physiologic changes, such as confusion and GI bleeding, immediately to the health care provider.

Cultural Considerations ⊕

- Recognize that older adults in various cultural groups may have language difficulty in understanding the drug regimen. Many of these older adults do not speak English.
- Provide additional time for verbal and written explanation to ensure that the older adult will take the drugs as prescribed.
- The more traditional and older individuals in some cultures do not maintain eye contact. Do not assume that lack of eye contact means the client is not listening or does not care; it might indicate respect.

EVALUATION

- Evaluate the older adult's compliance to the drug regimen, and answer any questions the older adult may have.
- Evaluate the drug effect and the lack of side effects or adverse reactions.

WEBSITES

For further information on *Geriatric Pharmacology*, visit these Internet resources:

Beers' Criteria for Potentially Inappropriate Medication Use in the Elderly: *www.hartfordign.org*

American Society of Consultant Pharmacists: *www.ascp.com*

Senior Care Pharmacist: *www.Seniorcarepharmacist.com*

Peter Lamy Center for Drug Management and Aging: *lamycenter@rx.umaryland.edu*

Critical Thinking Case Study

R.T., a 72-year-old woman, has osteoarthritis. She had taken aspirin and later was prescribed naproxen (Naprosyn). Both drugs caused her GI distress. The health care provider discontinued the naproxen and prescribed celecoxib (Celebrex), 100 mg twice a day. Celecoxib is a nonnarcotic, cyclooxygenase-2 (COX-2) inhibitor.

1. How does celecoxib differ from naproxen? NOTE: Refer to Chapter 21, Drugs for Pain Management, and Chapter 27, Antiinflammatory Drugs.

2. Describe the advantages and disadvantages of R.T. taking celecoxib.

3. What is the rationale for checking R.T.'s renal and liver function before prescribing celecoxib? Explain.

4. What should be included in the nursing assessment in regard to her physical and drug histories?

R.T. states that her arthritic pain is not relieved with this new drug. She wants to take naproxen with the celecoxib.

5. Explain the effects of these two medications when taken together.

6. What is the most appropriate response by the nurse to R.T.'s request? Explain.

7. Develop a teaching plan for R.T. that includes medication use and nursing measures to relieve pain.

Study Questions

1. What are the following pharmacokinetics related to drug therapy and older adults?
   a. GI absorption
   b. Body water and water-soluble drugs
   c. Fat-soluble drugs
   d. Effect of liver function and metabolism on half-life
   e. Renal function

2. What is polypharmacy? How does polypharmacy affect the older adult?

3. What are the possible effects that may occur when combining prescribed drugs with OTC and herbal drugs? Explain.

4. What are major factors in each bodily system that influence the effect of drugs on older adults?

5. List at least three reasons for nonadherence to the drug regimen that are common in the older adult.

6. What nursing measures remove barriers and help to improve drug regimen adherence?

12 Medication Administration in Community Settings

 ELECTRONIC RESOURCES

 evolve

Additional information can be found on the companion website at *http://evolve.elsevier.com/KeeHayes/pharmacology/* or on the companion CD-ROM, which includes:
- *NCLEX-style examination review questions*
- *Pharmacology animations*
- *Medication error and IV therapy checklists, and*
- *Medication calculation problems*
- *Electronic calculators*

OUTLINE

OBJECTIVES

- Describe common elements of client teaching about medication administration in community settings.
- Explain specific points related to administration of medications in the home.
- Discuss specific points related to administration of medications in the school.
- Describe specific points related to administration of medications in the work site.
- Explain the application of the nursing process to medication administration in community settings.

Introduction

Health and illness care has shifted from traditional institutions to community settings. The faces of a community are many, varied, and ever changing (Figure 12–1). With the movement of health care into the community, nurses—more than any other health care provider—have the opportunity to shape the health care of society. This chapter describes selected aspects of medication administration of prescription, over-the-counter (OTC), and herbal preparations within each of the major community settings: home, school, and work. In all settings, client safety is the primary concern. (See Chapter 3, Principles of Drug Administration, for a detailed presentation on medication administration.)

The process of medication administration in the home, school, and work site must be consistent with professional, legal, and regulatory requirements. In each setting, it must first be determined what the nursing personnel will teach clients about medications and then the routes by which the medications can be administered. Once these

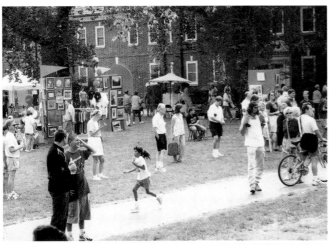

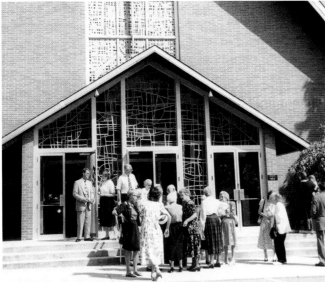

FIGURE 12–1 A community has many different faces.

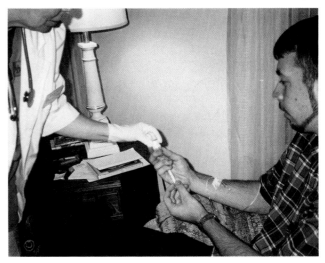

FIGURE 12–2 Effective client teaching is based on the individual client's learning needs.

decisions have been made, criteria for administration, instruction and client teaching, and ongoing supervision need to be developed, implemented, and evaluated. Mechanisms for communication and paper tracking must be in place to promote efficacy of the medication and avoidance of untoward responses and medication errors.

With the sky-rocketing costs of medications, the nurse in any community setting is likely to become aware of clients who need assistance with paying for prescription medications. Ready resources for the nurse and client are pharmaceutical companies' assistance programs. See the selected websites at the end of this chapter.

The backbone of health promotion and disease prevention is the client knowledge base. The role of the nurse in establishing this base is critical. (See Chapter 2, Nursing Process and Client Teaching, for a comprehensive discussion of client teaching.) Assessment of learning needs and styles is another essential component to achieve the identified teaching goal (Figure 12–2).

Client Teaching

Regardless of the state and agency regulations related to medication administration in community settings, the following hints for client teaching are associated with medication administration. These hints are grouped into five categories: (1) general, (2) diet, (3) self-administration, (4) side effects, and (5) cultural considerations.

General

Within the general area, client safety is of primary concern. Thus a client's physical abilities require ongoing assessment. Capabilities of the client may be temporarily impaired with the use of certain drugs (e.g., narcotics, selected eye medications, psychotropics). It is essential that clients be advised not to operate hazardous machinery during such times and to use caution at all other times. It is appropriate to discuss with clients and families what

PREVENTING MEDICATION ERRORS

Safety alert:

- Do not give (or take) medications in the dark; proper lighting is important to avoid errors.

HERBAL ALERT 12–1

Community

Encourage client/family to consult the health care provider before taking herbal preparations; some products may interact with prescription or other over-the-counter (OTC) medications they are taking.

situations in the daily routine require full alertness and cannot be influenced by medication for the sake of safety.

Numerous safety concerns are associated with the storage of medications. Medications should be kept in their original labeled containers, with childproof caps when needed.

The client or family should be provided with written instructions (audio instructions if client is sight impaired) about the drug regimen. Large print may be helpful or necessary. Another part of the teaching plan is to advise the client or family about any necessary laboratory tests to monitor the blood level of the medication and any possible drug-laboratory test interactions. This information should be included in the written instructions as well.

An important yet frequently misunderstood component of the written instructions is the expected therapeutic effect and the length of time required to achieve a therapeutic response from the medication. These vary widely among different medications (e.g., most narcotics act within 30 minutes; many antibiotics act within 24 hours; some psychotropics act within 6 weeks). Having clients understand the expected time frame for results can markedly diminish their concerns and promote adherence to the therapeutic plan.

The client or family must also be aware of the need to have an adequate supply of necessary medications available at all times—at home, school, work, and while traveling. It is best to order prescription refills in advance. If the pharmacy is local, at least 1 week should be allowed; several weeks should be allowed if drugs are ordered through the mail. It is a good idea to pack extra medication when going on trips, both short and extended. This is preferred at all times and is essential for foreign travel.

Impress on the client or family to *first* contact the health care provider *before* using OTC preparations. Common OTC preparations that may cause problems are laxatives, diet aids, cold and cough preparations, and overdose of fat-soluble vitamins. Reinforce with the client or family the importance of follow-up appointments with health care providers. Encourage wellness checkups, including preventive and restorative dental care, because the presence of other conditions may impact on the current therapeutic regimen. In addition, advise clients of the need to complete laboratory studies in a timely manner. Encourage clients to wear Medic-alert bands that indicate medications taken and any allergies. (See Herbal Alert 12–1.)

Reinforcement of the availability of community resources is important. Availability does not always equate with accessibility, so the client or family needs to know how to mobilize them according to individual needs.

Matching community resources and client needs is a prerequisite. While acknowledging the variability of each, the following are offered as examples:

- The telephone book is a frequently overlooked resource that can direct clients and families to contacts and addresses of associations of relevant health conditions (e.g., American Heart Association, American Cancer Society). Most agencies and associations have or can direct the caller to a wealth of health education resources available in a variety of media (e.g., written, audiocassettes, videotapes, occasionally braille).
- Churches may have outreach groups in which volunteers pick up prescriptions and deliver them to homebound clients.
- Pharmacists can frequently clarify a client's or family's concern over the telephone.
- Meals on Wheels enables clients to remain at home and adhere to taking medications with food.
- In a college town, students of the health professions may be motivated caregivers to assist clients or families in the community.

Clients or families need to be encouraged to have a contact person for their concerns and questions, frequently a nurse. Use of appropriate resources is likely to increase compliance with and effectiveness of the therapeutic regimen.

Diet

Diet is the second area that requires the nurse's attention. There is an overall need to advise clients or families about possible drug-food interactions, detailing which foods are to be avoided and which foods are encouraged for specific nutrient value. For example, tyramine-rich foods are contraindicated with monoamine oxidase (MAO) inhibitors, and potassium-rich foods are recommended for clients taking potassium-wasting diuretics. Alcohol may be contraindicated with selected medications. Lists of foods—and pictures when appropriate—may be helpful to clients and others involved with their diet.

Self-Administration

The third area of concern is self-administration of medications. Based on the level of the client's or family's knowledge, instructions should be given on all skills related to the drug regimen, for example, how to take the pulse for clients who take digitalis preparations, correct use and cleaning of inhalers, techniques for successful administration of parenteral medications, and how to decrease risks of infection for clients taking immunosuppressants.

The nurse should allow time for instruction and questions, including demonstration of the skill and return demonstration. Clients should be given graphic illustrations for future reference as appropriate. It is essential that the nurse provide the client or family with the name of a contact person and telephone number for questions and concerns. It is not uncommon for a client or family member to return-demonstrate a skill (e.g. administration of insulin, use of inhaler) with relative ease and then forget information or become confused when trying self-administration of the drug when alone.

Side Effects

Side effects are the fourth area for client teaching. The client or family should be advised about general side effects of the medications. This is not done to scare clients but rather to inform them about the more commonly occurring side effects. Clients need to know when to notify their health care provider if they experience an adverse reaction.

Cultural Considerations

Cultural considerations are the fifth general area of concern. Initially the nurse assesses the client's personal beliefs (Figure 12–3). Based on these beliefs, the nurse then modifies communications to meet client or family cultural practices. The nurse needs to communicate respect for the client or family culture at all times. It is incumbent on the nurse to assess his or her own beliefs and biases related to cultural competence and diversity. Then one needs to evaluate the effectiveness of interactions and their acceptability within the cultural realm. (See Chapter 6, Transcultural Considerations, for a comprehensive presentation of cultural considerations.)

Culturally sensitive and competent health care promotes client or family compliance with the therapeutic regimen. Respect for cultural diversity may be demonstrated by inclusion of traditional and folk practices into the plans for improved communication, health promotion, and disease prevention. Although applicable to multiple settings, the following are some common cultural concerns presented as examples for illustrative purposes (Purnell, 1998):

Home Care

Hispanics and Asians/Pacific Islanders frequently say they agree with the plan out of respect for health care providers, although they may not intend to follow the plan. This practice may have dangerous or life-threatening outcomes. Egyptians are accustomed to the oral tradition of communication and thus may not keep reliable written records for medication schedules and glucose monitoring results. A call from an Amish family is probably a true emergency because of their religious and cultural obligations to care for themselves first before seeking outside resources. Food rituals are important to the Appalachian, Jewish, Muslim, and Asian/Pacific Island people and must be incorporated into the plan of care if a prescription is to be followed. Self-medication and self-diagnosis are common among Asians.

School

African-American grandmothers play a significant role in dealing with health care concerns and must be included in the plans for care. Because being overweight is seen as positive to many African Americans, the health care provider may need to reeducate clients (children and families) in this cultural group frequently and carefully explain the health risks associated with obesity.

Work Site

African Americans have increased risk for development of hypertension. They prefer to be addressed formally. For Asians/Pacific Islanders, confidentiality is especially important, and they may not provide needed information if they perceive that the information might be shared and other community members may obtain knowledge about their health problems. It may be difficult for outsiders to develop rapport with Appalachian people because of past inequities from government agencies.

A summary of these guidelines is presented in Box 12–1.

Community-Based Settings

Home Setting

The home setting provides nurses with many challenges related to medication administration. A major question that quickly arises is, "Who can administer medications in the home setting?" The response does not develop so quickly.

In general, medications are administered by licensed nurses in the home setting according to the order of the health care provider. Drugs that are administered by nursing personnel in the home must be approved by the Food and Drug Administration (FDA). The nurse also initiates instructions about the medication to the client or family (Figure 12–4). The licensed nurse may also administer the medication on a short-term basis for a disease-related con-

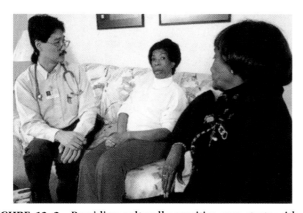

FIGURE 12–3 Providing culturally sensitive care starts with an assessment of the client's and family's particular beliefs, customs, and preferences. (From Swanson JM, Nies MA: *Community health nursing: promoting the health of aggregates,* ed 2, Philadelphia, 1997, Saunders.)

Summary of Client Teaching Hints About Medication Use and Administration in the Community

General

- Client safety is of primary concern.
- Client's physical abilities require ongoing assessment.
- Keep or store medications in original labeled containers with childproof caps when needed.
- Provide client or family with written instructions (audio instructions if sight impaired) about the drug regimen.
- Advise client or family about the expected therapeutic effect and length of time to achieve a therapeutic response from the medication; also inform clients of the expected duration of treatment.
- Advise client or family about possible drug-laboratory test interaction.
- Advise client of nonpharmacologic measures to promote therapeutic response.
- Advise client or family to have adequate supply of necessary medications available.
- Caution against the use of over-the-counter (OTC) preparations without *first* contacting the health care provider.
- Reinforce the importance of follow-up appointments with health care providers.
- Encourage clients to wear Medic-alert band that indicates medications and allergies.
- Reinforce that community resources are available and need to be mobilized according to the client or family needs.

Diet

- Advise client/family/student/employee about possible drug-food interactions.
- Advise client/family/student/employee what foods are contraindicated.
- Advise client/family/student/employee regarding alcohol use.

Self-Administration

- Instruct client/family/student/employee regarding drug dose and dosing schedule.
- Instruct client/family/student/employee on all psychomotor skills related to the drug regimen.
- Provide client/family/student/employee with contact person and telephone number for questions and concerns.

Side Effects

- Advise client/family/student/employee about general side effects and adverse reactions of the medications.
- Advise client/family/student/employee when to notify health care provider.

Cultural Considerations

- Assess personal beliefs of client/family/student/employee.
- Modify communications to meet cultural needs of client/family/student/employee.
- Communicate respect for client/family/student/employee culture.

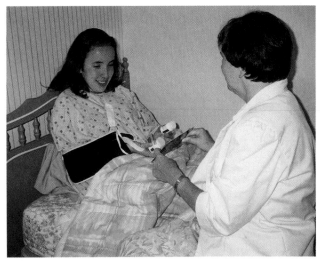

FIGURE 12–4 A vital aspect of home care is teaching clients about medications.

dition if a caregiver with an order from the health care provider is unable to do so.

The order from the health care provider must be current and complete (drug, dosage, frequency, route of administration, and signature). The medication must be labeled by the pharmacist or health care provider. The nurse should not administer any medication that is not properly labeled. It is the nurse's responsibility to contact the health care provider, pharmacist, or other group identified by the agency with any concerns about the medication for a specific client. The expiration date must be checked at the time of each administration. Storage and deterioration of the medication are also evaluated. Significant side effects, allergies, and adverse reactions are reported promptly to the health care provider; each client is assessed for allergies *before* administering the drug.

The establishment of policy and procedures for medication administration promotes safety and consistency; however, errors do occur. When a medication error occurs, it is reported to the health care provider and nursing supervisor. The client and family are instructed when to notify the nurse or health care provider about adverse drug reactions; the health care provider is notified of all adverse drug reactions.

An agency policy for medication administration generally addresses guidelines for specific medications. Examples of these specific agents include allergy vaccines, chemotherapy, gamma globulin, gold, experimental drugs, and narcotics. The guidelines are agency specific and may include that the first dose of allergy vaccine be given by the health care provider in a controlled environment or that family members be taught how to administer narcotics to the client by the parenteral route if the order is so written by the health care provider. When the order is discontinued, the health care provider needs to be notified if any unused narcotics are in the home. Licensed practical nurses may not administer gamma globulin intravenously, and family members may not be taught to administer selected drugs (e.g., iron dextran [Imferon]). Chemotherapy for cancer commonly presents a special challenge. The client's blood work must be current before the administration of the chemotherapeutic drugs, the client must be under regular and ongoing care of a physician, and safety requirements may be identified (e.g., gloves and goggles may be used).

Certified home health aides work under the supervision of the registered nurse. Home health aides are commonly asked to administer medications to the clients by the client, family, or friends. In the current health care environment, the home health aide may receive pressure to administer medications. However, the home health aide may only *assist* a client with medications that the client customarily *self-administers.*

Additional challenges related to medication administration in the home setting include adherence to the therapeutic regimen, especially the right drug, right dose, and right time. Some clients need but do not have a primary caregiver to oversee follow-up with medications and other aspects of care. The quality and preparation of meals may also be a factor related to medication administration, such as what foods to avoid with certain medications and what foods complement a medication. In addition, it may be difficult for clients to get their medications and to get them in a timely manner. Furthermore, coordinated skill may be required by the client or family, for example, with the use of an inhaler or administration of insulin. In all these situations, the nurse is frequently the person who coordinates the resources.

School Setting

Health and education are natural partners. The ability to learn is influenced by health factors.

Administration of medications in the school setting is of special concern. School health services are not immune from the phenomenon of downsizing personnel. Thus many school systems are dealing with questions such as "Where are the nurses?" and "Who is responsible for the administration of medication?"

In the absence of federal and state law, some school districts have elected not to employ school nurses. The average national caseload for a school nurse is an alarming 3098 students. This is a reality despite the long-standing recommendation of having one registered nurse for every 750 students. Coupled with this is the impact of a federal law that entitles children with handicaps to attend public schools in their residential areas. Hence it is reasonable to assume that these children have special needs that require professional nursing services (Figure 12–5).

In 1990 the Office of School Health Policy of the University of Colorado Health Sciences Center recognized that medication administration was a serious policy issue. Massachusetts developed its model with a goal "to develop regulations that provided minimum standards for the safe and proper administration of prescription med-

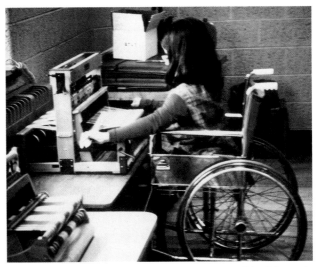

FIGURE 12–5 Many schoolchildren have special health needs.

ications in the Commonwealth schools" (Sheetz & Blum, 1998). The development of this model has many strengths, including representation of professional associations, community groups, and regulatory bodies. Consistent consent forms were designed and adopted, and orientation and training programs were instituted for all personnel in school health positions. The established regulations apply to both public and nonpublic schools. This model appears to have applicability to other states that are grappling with the important child health issue of medication administration in the schools.

It is essential that the nurse be aware of the policies and procedures for medication administration in the specific state, county, and schools. The policy for medication administration is necessary and should promote self-management programs of students with chronic conditions such as asthma and diabetes. Nurses must be actively involved in developing this policy and in ensuring that the needs of the individual students are met.

In some states or school systems, persons who are not nurses may be responsible for medication administration. This presents additional concerns that need to be addressed, such as adherence to instructions and to the principle that medication administration is a process, more than merely "giving the student a pill." A major component of medication administration is assessment of the need for the medication and its effectiveness of action. The effectiveness of action includes being alert to side effects and adverse reactions that the client may experience.

While recognizing the variability among policies on medication administration, Igoe and Speer (1996) identified the following basic requirements for administration of medications in schools:

1. Medications are given only with parents' written permission.

2. Medications requiring a prescription are given only on the written authorization of a health care provider.

3. For medications requiring a prescription, there must be an individual pharmacy-labeled bottle for each student.

4. Medications must be recorded by the school personnel who administer them. This record states the student's name, medication, dosage, time, and the name of the person administering the medication.

5. Medications must be stored in a secure, locked, clean container or cabinet.

Child care and adult day care services have similar rules for the administration of medications. In general, these facilities administer medications or supervise self-administration within the Nurse Practice Act of the specific state. In addition, most facilities require labeling of medications in accordance with the Pharmacy Rules and Regulations of the specific state. Guidelines for safe storage of medications must be followed, including being only accessible to personnel responsible for distribution of self-administration or administration of medications. Some states require that internal and external medications be stored separately. Care must be taken to ensure that prescription medications be used only for whom the medication was prescribed.

The National Association of School Nurses *(www.nasn.org)* is a good resource for information on the many faceted aspects of school nursing.

Work Setting

Most adult Americans and many youth are employed and spend a significant amount of time at the work site on a regular basis. Thus the work site is an ideal setting to promote personal health behaviors and decrease environmental hazards.

Healthy employees are more productive than unhealthy employees. This fact, coupled with the escalating costs of health care and insurance, has inspired many businesses to offer some type of health care at the work site. This care ranges from emergency first aid and work-related health and safety problems to the provision of primary care and referral services.

Occupational and environmental health nursing is the specialty practice that provides for and delivers health care services to workers and worker populations. The practice is autonomous and focuses on the promotion, protection, and restoration of workers' health within the context of a safe and healthy work environment. According to the American Association of Occupational Health Nurses (AAOHN), occupational and environmental health nurses may function in a variety of roles, including (but not limited to) solo practitioner, manager, educator, consultant, nurse practitioner, case manager, and corporate director, and they often work with the other members of an occupational health and safety team (e.g., medicine, safety, industrial hygiene) (AAOHN, 2001).

The nurse needs to be aware of the policies and procedures for administration of medication at the specific work site. There is great diversity in policy and procedure among settings. For example, the following are two of the many current practices at work sites:

• At one setting the registered nurse essentially follows protocols for selected employee complaints (e.g., back injuries: acute and chronic; burns: thermal, chemical, and electrical; eye emergencies; herpes; adult immunizations). Each protocol includes the following areas with relevant information for the specific complaint: assessment, treatment/medications, client education, referral, and follow-up. Medications are identified as appropriate and noted under the treatment/medications section with the stated drug, dosage, frequency, and route.

• Another work site has established self-care stations for minor illnesses and injuries. Each station has designated criteria for use. Examples of stations include colds, superficial cuts, and menstrual cramps. Employees are oriented to this service as part of the orientation process. Upon arrival at the stations, employees note date, time, and signature on the sign-in sheet posted at each station. Employees indicate the chief complaint or reason for seeking medication and the specific OTC medications they have taken from the OTC preparations supplied at each station.

An excellent resource for care of clients in the work setting is the AAOHN *(www.aaohn.org)*.

Summary

This chapter discusses only a minute, but significant, portion of the nurse's role in a variety of community settings. Specifically, the focus is on selected concerns associated with the administration of medications and the need to practice in accordance with the Nurse Practice Act of a specific state. The role of the nurse in drug administration is growing in complexity. The nurse in the twenty-first century must have a strong knowledge base.

Nursing Process

Overview of Medication Administration

ASSESSMENT

■ Obtain appropriate vital signs and relevant laboratory test results for future comparisons and evaluation of the therapeutic response.

■ Obtain drug history (prescription, over-the-counter, and herbal preparations), including drug allergies.

■ Identify high-risk clients/students/employees for reactions.

■ Assess client's/student's/employee's capability to follow therapeutic regimen.

■ Determine client/student/employee learning needs.

NURSING DIAGNOSES

- Risk for injury related to possible adverse reaction
- Risk for ineffective therapeutic regimen management
- Deficient knowledge related to therapeutic regimen

PLANNING

- Identify goals.
- Promote therapeutic response and prevent or minimize adverse reactions.
- Identify strategies to promote adherence.
- Identify interventions.

NURSING INTERVENTIONS

- Prepare equipment and environment; wash hands.
- Determine allergies and other assessment data.
- Check drug label three times; check expiration date.
- Be certain of drug calculation; verify dose with another registered nurse as necessary.
- Pour liquids at eye level.
- Keep all drugs stored properly, especially related to temperature, light, and moisture.
- Avoid contact with topical and inhalation preparations.
- Verify client/student/employee identification.
- Administer only drugs you have prepared.
- Assist the client to desired position.
- Discard needles and syringes in "sharps" container.
- Follow policy related to discarding drugs and controlled substances.
- Report drug errors immediately.
- Document all appropriate information in a timely manner.
- Record effectiveness of drugs administered and reason for any drugs refused.

Cultural Considerations ⊕

- When language barriers are present, use literature and videos in client's preferred language and with pictures of that group to promote compliance with health interventions.
- Obtain an interpreter when necessary; do not rely on family members, who may not fully disclose because of honor and shame. Provide interpreter with the same ethnic background and gender if possible, especially with sensitive topics.
- When offering a prescription, instructions, or pamphlets to Asians and Pacific Islanders, use both hands to show respect.
- Include grandmothers when providing support and health teaching in the African American population.
- Encourage clients to disclose the use of folk healers and treatments prescribed. Incorporate harmless and nonconflicting practices into the therapeutic plan.

EVALUATION

- Evaluate effectiveness of medication(s) administered.
- Identify expected time frame of desired drug response; consider need for modification of therapy.
- Determine client/student/employee satisfaction with regimen.
- Determine client/student/employee knowledge of medication regimen.

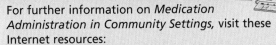

WEBSITES

For further information on *Medication Administration in Community Settings*, visit these Internet resources:

AstraZeneca Foundation Patient Assistance Program: *www.astrazeneca-us.com/pap/pap.asp*; (800) 424-3727

GlaxoWellcome Patient Assistance Program: *www.ipp.gsk.com*; (800) 722-9294

Novartis: *www.novartis.com*; (800) 277-2254

Smith Kline Beecham Foundation: *www.ipp.gsk.com*; (800) 546-0420

Directory of Prescription Drug Patient Assistance Programs: *www.phrma.org*

American Association of Occupational Health Nurses (AAOHN): *www.aaohn.org*

National Association of School Nurses (NASN): *www.nasn.org*

Critical Thinking Case Study

The Rivera family (José, age 30; wife, Maria, age 29, 7 months pregnant; children José Jr., age 11; Angel, age 8; Tony, age 7) recently moved into a new community. José is employed full time by a large credit card corporation, and Maria handles the child care and works part time as a cashier.

1. Give examples of culturally sensitive and competent care for the Rivera children in the school setting.
2. Identify culturally sensitive and competent care for the parents at the work sites.
3. What modifications would you suggest for a family of African-American heritage?

Study Questions

1. When teaching a client, student, or employee about OTC preparations, what information does the nurse need to include?

2. What is the role of the certified home health aide in the administration of medications in the home?

3. Why is it important to advise the client, student, or employee of the expected length of time for therapeutic effects of the medication?

4. What are the cultural considerations applicable to administration of medication in general? List at least four examples related to specific cultures.

5. What are the five basic requirements for administration of medication in the school according to Igoe and Speer?

6. What are the major points in the application of the nursing process to the administration of medications?

13 The Role of the Nurse in Drug Research

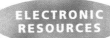

Additional information can be found on the companion website at *http://evolve.elsevier.com/KeeHayes/pharmacology/* or on the companion CD-ROM, which includes:

- *NCLEX-style examination review questions*
- *Pharmacology animations*
- *Medication error and IV therapy checklists*
- *Medication calculation problems*
- *Electronic calculators*

OUTLINE

OBJECTIVES

- Identify basic ethical principles.
- Relate three basic ethical principles governing informed consent and risk-to-benefit ratio.
- Describe the objectives of each phase of human clinical experimentation.
- Describe the role of the nurse in clinical drug trials using the nursing process.

TERMS

active control
autonomy
beneficence
control group
Declaration of Helsinki
double-blind

experimental group
FDA Modernization Act
Good Clinical Practice (GCP)
informed consent
open-label study

placebo
Prescription Drug User Fee Act
single-blind
triple-blind

Introduction

News broadcasts or headlines often announce the release of a new drug for the treatment of acquired immunodeficiency syndrome (AIDS) or multiple sclerosis, an increase in a drug company's research and development budget, Food and Drug Administration (FDA) approval for promising drugs, or similar pharmacology-related news. Such news items signal increasing awareness of the importance of drug research. Drug research involves risk and is also a "high-cost item," with the estimated average cost to develop each new drug being more than $800 million.

Drug research and development are complex processes that are of interest and importance to professional nursing practice. The nursing process facilitates the integration of cutting-edge research.

This chapter is devoted to a description of basic ethical principles governing informed consent and risk-to-benefit ratio, preclinical testing and human clinical experimentation, and the role of the nurse in clinical drug trials using the nursing process.

Basic Ethical Principles

Four basic ethical principles are relevant to research involving human subjects: (1) respect for persons, (2) beneficence, (3) justice, and (4) truth telling.

Respect for Person

Individuals undergoing treatment in any health care system should be treated as independent persons who are capable of making decisions in their own interest. Individuals whose decision-making capability is diminished are entitled to protection. The nurse can determine this with consistent reassessment of the client's cognitive state. Clients should be made aware of the alternatives available to them in their health care, as well as the consequences that stem from those alternatives. Furthermore, the client's choice should be honored whenever possible. It is imperative that the nurse recognize when the client is not capable of rational decision making and is therefore entitled to protection.

Autonomy is an integral component of respect for person. **Autonomy** is the right of self-determination. In health care settings, health care personnel must respect the clients' right to make decisions about themselves, even if the decision is not what the personnel wanted or thought was best for the client. Generally clients can refuse any and all treatments *(right of autonomy)* except when the decision poses a threat to others, such as with tuberculosis, when taking medications is legally mandated. Clients have the right to refuse to participate in a research study and may withdraw from the study at any time without penalty of any kind.

Beneficence

Beneficence is the duty to not harm others, to maximize possible benefits, and to minimize possible harm that might occur in research. It is often not possible to know whether something is beneficial unless it is tested and individuals have been exposed to the risks. A central question to this issue is, Who makes this decision—the client or those caring for the client?

Justice

Justice requires that all people be treated fairly. Expansion of justice includes equal access to health care for all. Justice can be limited when it interferes with the rights of others. The principle of justice in the context of clinical drug trials means that social benefits and burdens can be allocated objectively and that those with equivalent circumstances should be treated equally. A challenge to the nurse is the allocation of scarce resources.

Truth telling (veracity) is a principle that requires health care personnel to tell the truth and the whole truth. When there is "bad news" to tell the client, the health care provider may be reluctant to tell the truth and answer questions honestly. The client has the right to know the truth, including "the bad news."

The principles of respect for person, beneficence, justice and truth telling are integral to the issues of informed consent and risk-to-benefit ratio in research involving human subjects.

Informed Consent

Informed consent has its roots in the Nuremberg Code, the two most relevant aspects being the participant's right to be informed and that participation is voluntary, without coercion. If the nurse suspects that a client is being coerced to participate in the study, the nurse is obligated to report this promptly to the party named on the informed consent (the client should have copy of consent for reference). **Informed consent** has dimensions beyond protection of the individual client's choice and includes the following:

1. Promotion of individual autonomy
2. Protection of clients and subjects from harm
3. Avoidance of fraud and duress in health care
4. Encouragement for professionals to be thorough and clear in communicating information
5. Promotion of educated decision making among clients
6. Promotion of self-determination of the client

It is the role of the health care providers, *not* the nurse, to explain the study to the client, including the expectations of the client, and to respond to questions. During this time of giving written consent, the client must be alert and able to comprehend.

It is the nurse's role to protect clients from any anticipated harm. The nurse, in collaboration with the health care provider and pharmacist, must be knowledgeable about all aspects of the drug study, including all inclusion and exclusion criteria for participants (see Box 13–3 on p. 216).

See Figure 13–1 for an example of Permission for Clinical Investigation and Box 13–1 for an Informed Consent Checklist form.

Memorial Hospital

PERMISSION FOR CLINICAL INVESTIGATION

Completed by Client:

1. I hereby authorize Dr. _____ and/or such assistants as may be selected by him/her to conduct studies upon _____ for the following: _____ _____ _____

2. I further authorize Dr. _____ and/or such assistants as may be selected by him/her, to prescribe drugs or to perform certain procedures in connection with the diagnosis and treatment of my condition including the following drugs and/or extraordinary procedures: _____ _____ _____ _____

3. I have (have not) been made aware of certain risks, possible consequences and discomfort associated with these drugs or extraordinary procedures which are: _____ _____ _____

4. I understand that no guarantee or assurance has been made as to the results that may be obtained although I have (have not) been advised of the possibility that certain benefits may be expected such as: _____ _____

5. I have (have not) had explained to me alternative procedures/treatments/drugs that may be advantageous and they include the following: _____ _____

6. I have (have not) received an offer to answer any inquiries concerning the procedures involved _____

7. I have (have not) had explained to me all medical terminology in connection with this study _____

8. I understand that it is in the intent of the principal investigator to maintain the confidentiality of records identifying subjects in this study. The Food and Drug Administration, however, may possibly inspect the records to monitor compliance with published federal regulations.

9. I understand that I may withdraw this consent and discontinue participation in this study at any time, without prejudice to my care, by informing Dr. _____ of my desire to withdraw. _____ Yes, I understand   _____ No, I do not understand

10. I understand that Department of Health and Human Services regulations require the Memorial Hospital to inform me of any provisions to provide for medical treatment for any physical injury which may occur as a result of this study. In this connection, I understand that the Memorial Hospital does not have a formal plan or program to provide for the cost of medical treatment or compensation for any physical injury which occurs as a result of this study and for which they do not have legal liability. However, in the unlikely event that I am injured as a result of my participation, I understand that I should promptly inform Dr. _____

    SIGNED _____

    RELATIONSHIP _____

    ADDRESS _____ _____

    DATED _____

Completed by witness:

I, the undersigned, hereby acknowledge that I was present during the explanation of the above consent for clinical investigation given by Dr. _____ to _____ during which the nature, purpose, risks, complications and consequences thereof were fully set forth and all questions answered and I was present while _____ signed the above consent.

Dated _____

_____
(witness)

_____
(address)

FIGURE 13–1   Example of informed consent.

Informed Consent Checklist

- Participates voluntarily
- Identifies related drugs, treatments, and techniques
- Describes benefits and risks
- Describes other forms of treatment available
- Describes laboratory tests to monitor client's reactions
- Identifies extent of confidentiality of results
- Describes availability of emergency treatment for illness/injury, if any
- States compensation for study-related injury, if any
- States compensation for participation, if any
- Writes consent clearly and understands easily at the 10th-grade reading level
- Provides name and telephone number of contact person for client questions and concerns

Risk-to-Benefit Ratio

The risk-to-benefit ratio is one of the most complex problems faced by the researcher. All possible consequences of a clinical study must be analyzed and balanced with the inherent risks and the anticipated benefits. Physical, psychological, and social risks must be identified and weighed against the benefits. A requirement of the Department of Health and Human Services (DHHS) is that institutional review boards (IRBs) determine that "risks to subjects are reasonable in relation to anticipated benefits, if any, to subjects" (DHHS, 1981). No matter how noble the intentions, the calculation of risks and benefits by the researcher cannot be totally accurate or comprehensive.

Varying amounts of time are required for the process of identifying a potentially useful chemical and having it become available to the general population; in many cases, 10 years may elapse. Only 1 in 10,000 potential drugs endures the research and development process and is used in a clinical situation. Box 13–2 lists the basic sequence of the development of a new drug.

Objectives and Phases of Human Clinical Experimentation

Good Clinical Practice (GCP), a standard for the design, conduct, performance, monitoring, auditing, recording, analysis, and reporting, is the foundation of clinical trials. Guidance and information sheets are available from the

Basic Sequence of New Drug Development

1. Identification of potentially clinically useful chemical entity
2. Preclinical testing
3. Study designs
4. Human clinical experimentation
   - Phase I
   - Phase II
   - Phases III and IV

FDA on multiple topics related to clinical trials. Examples include information sheets for IRBs and Clinical Investigators and Choice of Control Groups and Related Issues in Clinical Trials. See the websites at the end of the chapter for detailed information on GCP. In addition, the World Medical Association **Declaration of Helsinki** has crafted ethical principles for medical research involving human subjects. Please see websites at the end of the chapter for information on the Declaration of Helsinki.

Preclinical Testing

Preclinical testing consists of in vitro and in vivo systems. In vitro experimentation is generally conducted in a test tube or other laboratory equipment, and in vivo testing is conducted with living organisms. This testing is followed by toxicity screening for the purposes of identifying (1) abnormal changes in animal organs related to drug administration and (2) the parameters of the safe therapeutic dose. Control and experimental groups of animals are compared. Participants in the **experimental group** receive the experimental intervention or treatment. Those in the **control group** do not receive the experimental intervention or treatment and provide a baseline against which to measure the effects of the treatment. Before initiating human studies, an assessment is made of the seriousness of the disease to be treated using this drug in relation to the drug's toxicity.

Human Clinical Experimentation

For every 5000 to 10,000 compounds screened as potential new medications, only five are entered into clinical trials. To bring a new drug to market takes an average of 9 to 12 years, and costs continue to rise. The cost is currently at $1.1 billion per drug. The **FDA Modernization Act** of 1997 increases the minimum age for subjects of human clinical experimentations. The Act has five provisions, one of which requires pediatric evaluation of new products intended for use by children. The Act advocates for children and appropriate testing for drugs to be used by the pediatric population. Refer to Chapter 5, The Drug Approval Process, for a listing of all of the provisions of this act.

Clinical experimentation in drug research and development encompasses four phases, each with its own objectives. A multidisciplinary team approach (nurses, physicians, pharmacologists, statisticians, and research associates) is required to ensure throughout the phases that the data collected will answer the clinical questions. A brief description of each phase follows.

Phase I

Phase I trials are primarily designed to assess safety. The objectives of phase I are to determine the human dosage range based on response in healthy human subjects and to identify the pharmacokinetics (i.e., absorption, distribution, metabolism/biotransformation, excretion/elimination) of the drug. Progression to the next phase occurs if no serious adverse effects are demonstrated, the drug is eliminated in a reasonable amount of time, and the dose range is below that known to induce pathology in animals.

Phase II

The objective of phase II is to demonstrate the safety and efficacy of the drug in subjects ($n = 100$) who have the disease the drug is designed to treat. Phase III is initiated only when acceptable efficacy and safety data are generated and clearly documented.

Phases III and IV

Phase III studies involve large numbers of subjects with the disease intended for treatment. The objectives of phases III and IV are to demonstrate the safety and efficacy of the drug for a wide client population and to include long-term data if a chronic regimen is under consideration. Phase IV studies may also examine potential new indications for approved drugs. The sponsor submits all relevant and analyzed data in a new drug application (NDA) to the FDA. In time, the FDA decides to approve, reject, or recommend withdrawal or resubmission. After the NDA research has been approved, phase IV addresses the long-term use of the drug.

The pharmaceutical industry is eager to get new drugs to market. Delays in the FDA approval process were decreasing the valuable life of a drug's patent; therefore in 1992 Congress passed the **Prescription Drug User Fee Act,** which provided the FDA with funds to expedite the review process. As a result, the average drug approval time has decreased from 30 to 12 months.

Study Designs

An appropriate experimental design is important in being able to answer questions about drug safety and efficacy. The experimental design uses different groups of subjects (i.e., some experimental groups who receive treatment and control groups who receive no treatment or an alternative method of treatment or a combination of both), and assigns subjects randomly to treatment or control groups. Treatment groups and control groups do not differ in terms of baseline characteristics or demographics. If the subjects are different, variability is introduced and it becomes more difficult to determine a treatment effect.

The following examples illustrate selected research designs:

A *quasi-experimental* design is a comparison of intermittent intravenous (IV) device patency of those hospitalized clients who received heparin flushes and those who received saline flushes. This study has a nonmatched comparison group but had no random assignment to a treatment group. Such quasi-experimental designs may contribute valuable information but lack the power to ascribe cause because the variables are uncontrolled and potentially influential. Ethical decisions do not permit the use of the experimental design in all situations. For example, an experimental study to determine whether nicotine causes cancer would be unethical because individuals would have to be exposed to a carcino-

genic substance. However, in this example it is possible to use an already exposed group (smokers) as comparator.

The researcher designs the study to show the effect of the independent variable (the drug) on the dependent variables (clinical responses or reactions). Intervening variables are specific to the research question and may include age, sex, weight, disease and its state of severity, diet, and the subject's social environment. It is important to control for as many of the intervening variables as possible to make it easier to determine whether there is a drug effect. Controlled treatment groups in drug research trials can receive no drug, a different drug, a **placebo** (pharmacologically inert substance), or the same drug with a different dose, route, or frequency of administration. A control group receiving a different drug is called an **active control.** In some cases, such as cancer treatment, it would not be ethical to use a placebo as a control.

A *crossover* design uses each subject in several different situations. In the first instance, the experimental group receives the drug and the control group receives an alternative form of treatment or no treatment. Then both groups receive no therapy. Finally, the experimental group receives the control form of therapy and the control group receives the drug. In this design, the subject serves as his or her own control.

The researcher wants to generalize the findings from the sample of subjects to the larger target population, such as all women with breast cancer. A statistical method called *probability sampling* (subjects are randomly selected from the entire population) is typically used to provide relative confidence in the generalization of findings.

Various designs and techniques assist the researcher to reach valid, generalizable conclusions. In a *matched-pair* design, the researcher identifies several variables that may influence the outcome, such as age, weight, or family history; then the subjects are matched for these variables. One of the pair is randomly assigned to the experimental group and the other to the control group. A less effective technique is nonrandom assignment to treatment group.

The **double-blind** technique is a powerful tool wherein neither the health care provider nor the subject knows whether the subject is receiving the experimental or control form of therapy. In **triple-blind** studies, a researcher other than the prescribing health care provider collects data and is also unaware of the subject's treatment group. In a **single-blind** study, only the subject is unaware of which group to which he or she is assigned. An **open-label study** indicates that all parties—data collectors, prescribing health care provider, and subject—know the treatment group assignment. The double-blind and triple-blind techniques are preferred for drug research because those involved in the study are not aware of the subject's treatment group, thereby removing a source of bias.

Nurse's Role

The nurse has a pivotal role in drug clinical trials. The research and development process for drug research requires the multifaceted roles of professional nursing practice. The nurse must first consider her or his own thoughts, feelings, and beliefs about clinical trials. The nurse is both the client and family advocate and the liaison between the client, health care provider, and research nurse responsible for the specific protocol. Communication that is both thorough and timely is essential in all aspects of the nurse's role. Nursing involvement is essential to the successful completion of clinical trials.

Asking relevant questions about informed consent and risk-to-benefit ratio is a major role of the nurse. Refer to the website for the Health Insurance Portability and Accountability Act (HIPAA) implications for clinical trials (e.g., consent and privacy issues). Awareness of initial indicators of change in the client and prediction of increased risk for adverse drug reaction are also dimensions of professional nursing practice.

Nursing responsibilities related to the specific research or clinical trial span the nursing process. Critical to the assessment phase are the recruitment and assessment of study subjects; a thorough understanding of the protocol, including inclusion and exclusion criteria for subjects; validity and reliability of measurement instruments; ongoing teamwork; and communication with the health care providers and sponsors.

Nursing input is important in the budget negotiations of the clinical trial as well as staff education on protocol requirements. Protocol guidelines are an essential component of staff education with special attention to ensuring that the subject's consent is "informed consent" obtained by the health care provider. The nurse is an ongoing resource for the subject and family questions.

Protocol-based nursing implementations include comprehensive screening of subjects and monitoring parameters per protocol with relevant and timely communication with the entire health care team. Documentation on all predetermined components throughout the clinical trial is mandatory, including input from study subjects.

During the evaluation phase, the nurse's role involves examining the research statement or question. In addition, it considers elements such as, are the conclusions valid and data based? Are the findings clinically significant?

Recent Developments and What Is on the Horizon

Tomorrow's anti-human immunodeficiency virus (HIV) drugs will block HIV from entering the cell; other compounds will promote plaque regression in individuals with Alzheimer's disease; and there is the expectation of more powerful drugs to supplement—and possibly replace—selected cardiac surgery. Anticancer drugs will attack only cells with abnormal growth (not healthy cells). In addition, there is major vaccine research for AIDS, Alzheimer's disease, and cancer. Highly lucrative drugs go "off patent." When a drug goes "off patent," other companies are free to make their own form of the same drug, thus increasing competition among the pharmaceutical companies and resulting in a lower cost of the drug.

BOX 13-3

Inclusion/Exclusion Criteria for a Hypothetic Protocol for an Experimental Diuretic Medication

Inclusion

• Men and women between the ages of 18 and 65 years
• Weight between 50 and 100 kg
• Subjects receive cardiac medications only if dose has been stable for past 3 months
• Subjects on sodium-restricted diet

Exclusion

• Pregnant or nursing women
• All women of childbearing age who do not responsibly use oral contraceptives
• Persons with severe damage or disease of cardiac, hepatic, renal, neurologic, or musculoskeletal system
• Clinically significant laboratory values

Synthetic antibiotics, such as linezolid (Zyvox), are one of the first new class of antibiotics in 30 years. Objective, reliable data are needed about which drugs are most effective. Currently there is public outcry for these data because Medicare is about to spend $400 billion over the next decade on new drug benefits. The FDA approves drugs based on safety and efficacy but does not address whether the drug is safer or more effective than other drugs.

Nursing Process

Clinical Drug Trials

ASSESSMENT

■ Explore own beliefs about clinical trials.
■ Recruit subjects.
■ Assess subjects.
■ Assess protocol.
■ Demonstrate thorough knowledge of all inclusion/exclusion criteria for subjects (Box 13-3).
■ Articulate observations and concerns to health care providers and sponsors/pharmaceutical company.
■ Communicate need for drug to address a specific need with the appropriate individuals.

PLANNING

■ Develop fact sheet of protocol guidelines.
■ Educate involved staff about protocol requirements.
■ Provide input into budget negotiations.
■ Coordinate personnel and budget, including office visits, special tests, and laboratory work.
■ Ensure that subject consent is informed (see Box 13-1 and Figure 13-1).
■ Respond to subject's questions.

NURSING INTERVENTIONS

■ Screen subjects accurately and thoroughly based on established protocol.

■ Adhere to protocol guidelines, including administration of drug.

■ Monitor selected parameters. Observe and report toxicities promptly.

■ Collect all data required by the sponsor (e.g., drug company).

■ Communicate information in a complete, concise, accurate, and timely manner to the principal investigator and sponsor.

■ Document data in a clear and timely manner.

■ Record subjects' own evaluation; *seemingly unrelated responses may be significant.* At times, a drug is actually marketed for a different indication than the original testing.

■ Report *all* deaths to physician, sponsor, Institutional Review Board, and FDA, whether or not the cause of death is drug related.

Cultural Considerations

• Be alert to specific side effects in selected drug groups from clients of different ethnic backgrounds (e.g., African Americans and tricyclics and other psychotropic medications).

• Use an interpreter when necessary, preferably from the same ethnicity and gender, especially for sensitive and anxiety-raising topics.

• Depending on client's background, include the extended family in the teaching and support system.

EVALUATION

■ Was the research design appropriate and maintained?

■ Are the conclusions valid and based on data?

■ Are the clinical findings significant?

WEBSITES

For further information on *The Role of the Nurse in Drug Research,* visit these Internet resources:

Good Practices: *http://www.fda.gov/oc/gcp/default.htm*

Good Practices: *http://www.allconferences.com/conferences/20030114093418/*

Biotech Media: The Good Clinical Practice Journal: *http://www.biotechmedia.com/y2001-ed-gcpj.html*

Declaration of Helsinki: Recommendation for Conduct of Clinical Research: *http://www.bioscience.org/guides/declhels.htm*

Declaration of Helsinki: Ethical Principles for Medical Research Involving Human Subjects: *http://www.med.or.jp/wma/helsinki02_e.html*

Health Insurance Portability and Accountability Act: (HIPAA): *http://www.cms.hhs.gov/hipaa/*

Study Questions

1. What are the four basic ethical principles? Discuss the meaning of each.

2. What document is the root of informed consent? What are the two most relevant aspects to clinical trials and the nurse's role?

3. In what ways are informed consent and risk-to-benefit ratio related to drug research?

4. What are the objectives of the four phases of human experimentation?

5. What are the advantages and disadvantages of the various research designs?

6. What are the implications of the Declaration of Helsinki for clinical trials?

7. Identify at least two cautions related to drug development. What are the implications for your nursing practice?

8. What are the implications of clinical drug research for your nursing practice? Apply the nursing process.

Four

Nutrition and Electrolytes

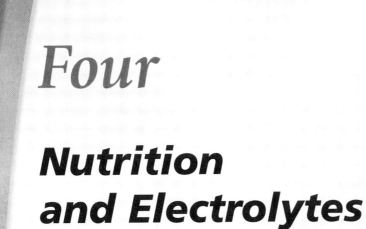

The body requires vitamins, minerals, and electrolytes for cellular function. When there is a lack of these chemical components, replacement drug therapy is necessary. With regular nutritional dietary intake, vitamin, mineral, and electrolyte replacements are not needed.

Multiple vitamins have the highest sales volume of any over-the-counter (OTC) drugs. Usually, vitamin replacements are not necessary, especially for those who maintain a nutritionally balanced daily diet.

The vitamins discussed in Chapter 14, Vitamin and Mineral Replacement, include the fat-soluble vitamins (vitamins A, D, E, and K) and the water-soluble vitamins (vitamin B complex [B_1, B_2, B_3, B_6, and B_{12}] and C). Iron is the primary mineral described. Other minerals discussed are copper, zinc, chromium, and selenium.

Body electrolytes are plentiful in extracellular and intracellular fluids and in the gastrointestinal mucosa. The cations (positively charged ions or electrolytes)—potassium (K), sodium (Na), calcium (Ca), and magnesium (Mg)—promote transmission and conduction of nerve impulses and contractibility of muscles. Inadequate dietary intake and many disease entities contribute to electrolyte imbalances. Electrolyte replacements are discussed in Chapter 15, Fluid and Electrolyte Replacement, and nutritional support is discussed in Chapter 16, Nutritional Support.

14 Vitamin and Mineral Replacement

ELECTRONIC RESOURCES

Additional information can be found on the companion website at *http://evolve.elsevier.com/KeeHayes/pharmacology/* or on the companion CD-ROM, which includes:
- *NCLEX-style examination review questions*
- *Pharmacology animations*
- *Medication error and IV therapy checklists*
- *Medication calculation problems*
- *Electronic calculators*

OUTLINE

OBJECTIVES

- List the four justifications for the use of vitamin supplements.
- Differentiate between water- and fat-soluble vitamins.
- Relate food sources and deficiency conditions associated with each vitamin.
- Define the term *recommended dietary allowance (RDA)*.
- Explain the need for iron and foods that are high in iron content.
- Explain the uses for iron, copper, zinc, chromium, and selenium.
- Describe the nursing interventions, including client teaching, related to vitamin and mineral uses.

TERMS

fat-soluble vitamins
free radicals
iron

megavitamin therapy
minerals

recommended dietary allowance (RDA)
water-soluble vitamins

Introduction

This chapter discusses two topics: vitamins and minerals. These substances are needed in correct portions for normal body function. Overuse of vitamins and minerals, particularly fat-soluble vitamins and iron, may lead to vitamin or iron toxicity.

Vitamins

Vitamins are organic chemicals that are necessary for normal metabolic functions and for tissue growth and healing. The body needs only a small amount of vitamins daily, which can be easily obtained through one's diet. A well-balanced diet has all the vitamins and minerals needed for body functioning. The intake of vitamins should be increased by those experiencing periods of rapid body growth, by those who are pregnant or are breastfeeding, by those with a debilitating illness, and by those with inadequate diets (e.g., alcoholics, some geriatric clients). Children who have poor nutrient intake or are malnourished may need vitamin replacement. Persons on fad or restrictive diets frequently have vitamin deficiencies.

The sale of vitamins in the United States is a multibillion-dollar business (Figure 14–1). Some people take vitamins to relieve tiredness or to improve general overall health, both of which are inappropriate indications for vitamin therapy. Today numerous vitamins and herbal medications are available for various specialized needs, such as cholesterol, memory, menopause, prostate, and others (Figure 14–2). Before purchasing these agents, the client should discuss with the health care provider the health value and use of multiple vitamins and herbal medications. Vitamins are *not* necessary if the individual is well and consumes a well-balanced daily diet on a regular basis.

Vitamin deficiencies can cause cellular and organ dysfunction that may result in a slow recovery from illness. Vitamin supplements are necessary for the vitamin deficiencies described in Table 14–1, but vitamins frequently are taken prophylactically rather than therapeutically.

The United States Department of Agriculture (USDA) provides *MyPyramid: Steps to a Healthier You* as a guide to

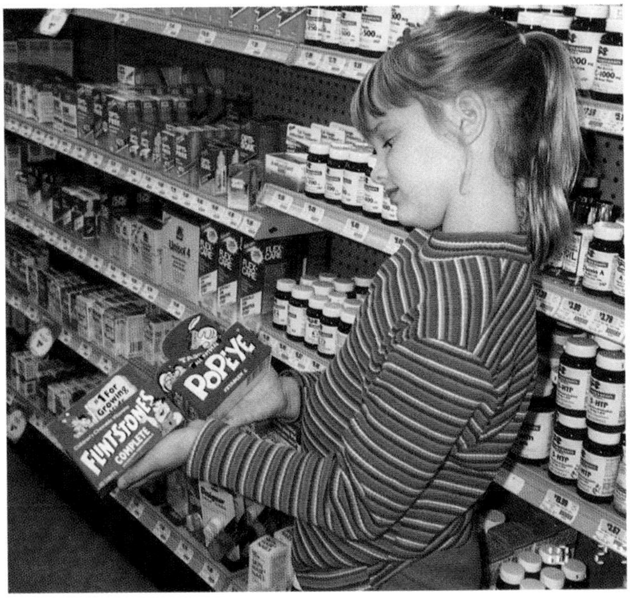

FIGURE 14–1 Would a less-expensive generic children's vitamin be just as good?

Table 14–1

Justification for Vitamin Supplements

Categories	Deficiencies
Inadequate absorption	Malabsorption, diarrhea, infectious and inflammatory diseases
Inability to use vitamins	Liver disease (cirrhosis, hepatitis), renal disease, certain hereditary deficiencies
Increased vitamin losses	Fever from infectious process, hyperthyroidism, hemodialysis, cancer, starvation, crash diets
Increased vitamin requirements	Early childhood, pregnancy, debilitating disease (cancer, alcoholism), gastrointestinal surgery, special diets

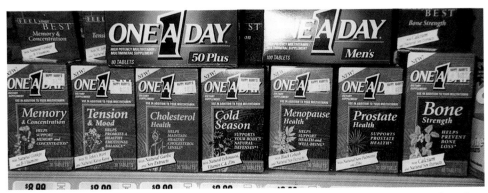

FIGURE 14–2 Drug companies offer vitamin and herbal supplements for specialized needs. Some of these agents have a combination of vitamins, minerals, and herbs.

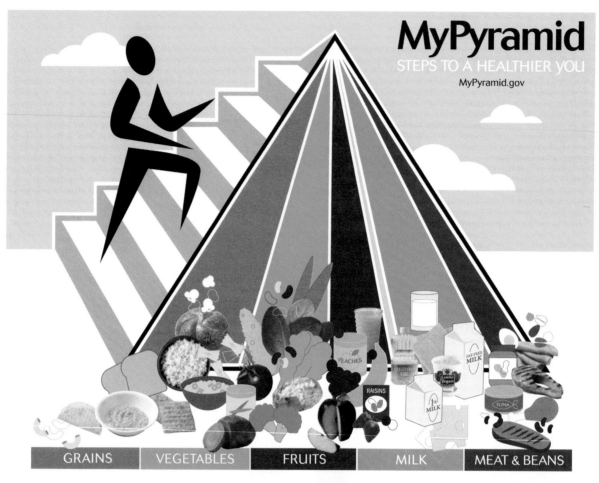

MyPyramid
STEPS TO A HEALTHIER YOU
MyPyramid.gov

| GRAINS | VEGETABLES | FRUITS | MILK | MEAT & BEANS |

GRAINS Make half your grains whole	VEGETABLES Vary your veggies	FRUITS Focus on fruits	MILK Get your calcium-rich foods	MEAT & BEANS Go lean with protein
Eat at least 3 oz. of whole-grain cereals, breads, crackers, rice, or pasta every day 1 oz. is about 1 slice of bread, about 1 cup of breakfast cereal, or ½ cup of cooked rice, cereal, or pasta	Eat more dark-green veggies like broccoli, spinach, and other dark leafy greens Eat more orange vegetables like carrots and sweetpotatoes Eat more dry beans and peas like pinto beans, kidney beans, and lentils	Eat a variety of fruit Choose fresh, frozen, canned, or dried fruit Go easy on fruit juices	Go low-fat or fat-free when you choose milk, yogurt, and other milk products If you don't or can't consume milk, choose lactose-free products or other calcium sources such as fortified foods and beverages	Choose low-fat or lean meats and poultry Bake it, broil it, or grill it Vary your protein routine — choose more fish, beans, peas, nuts, and seeds

For a 2,000-calorie diet, you need the amounts below from each food group. To find the amounts that are right for you, go to MyPyramid.gov.

| Eat 6 oz. every day | Eat 2½ cups every day | Eat 2 cups every day | Get 3 cups every day; for kids aged 2 to 8, it's 2 | Eat 5½ oz. every day |

Find your balance between food and physical activity
- Be sure to stay within your daily calorie needs.
- Be physically active for at least 30 minutes most days of the week.
- About 60 minutes a day of physical activity may be needed to prevent weight gain.
- For sustaining weight loss, at least 60 to 90 minutes a day of physical activity may be required.
- Children and teenagers should be physically active for 60 minutes every day, or most days.

Know the limits on fats, sugars, and salt (sodium)
- Make most of your fat sources from fish, nuts, and vegetable oils.
- Limit solid fats like butter, stick margarine, shortening, and lard, as well as foods that contain these.
- Check the Nutrition Facts label to keep saturated fats, *trans* fats, and sodium low.
- Choose food and beverages low in added sugars. Added sugars contribute calories with few, if any, nutrients.

MyPyramid.gov
STEPS TO A HEALTHIER YOU

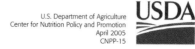

U.S. Department of Agriculture
Center for Nutrition Policy and Promotion
April 2005
CNPP-15

USDA

FIGURE 14–3   The U.S. Department of Agriculture food guide pyramid, showing the MyPyramid Plan.

daily food choices (Figure 14–3). Eating a variety of foods and getting the appropriate number of calories and grams of fat for a healthy weight are recommended. Visit the interactive website at *http://mypyramid.gov* to develop an individualized plan based on your needs.

The National Academy of Sciences Food and Nutrition Board publishes the U.S. **recommended dietary allowance (RDA)** for daily dose requirements of each vitamin. The Food and Drug Administration (FDA) requires that all vitamin products be labeled according to the amount of vitamin content and the proportion of the RDA provided by the vitamin product. Individuals should be encouraged to check the RDA listed on a vitamin container to determine whether the product provides the RDA dose requirements. The RDA may need to be modified for clients who are ill.

Fat-Soluble Vitamins

Vitamins fall into two general categories: fat-soluble and water-soluble. The **fat-soluble vitamins** are A, D, E, and K. They are metabolized slowly; can be stored in fatty tissue,

liver, and muscle in significant amounts; and are excreted in the urine at a slow rate. Vitamins A and D are toxic if taken in excessive amounts over time. Vitamin A can be stored in the liver for up to 2 years. Vitamins E and K are less toxic than vitamins A and D. Foods rich in vitamin A are fruits, yellow and green vegetables, fish, and dairy products; foods rich in vitamin D are dairy products and margarine; foods rich in vitamin E are oils, margarine, milk, grains, and meats; and foods rich in vitamin K are green leafy vegetables, meats, eggs, and dairy products.

Vitamin A

Vitamin A is essential for the maintenance of epithelial tissues, skin, eyes, hair, and bone growth. It has been used for the treatment of skin disorders such as acne; however, excess doses can be toxic. During pregnancy, excess amounts of vitamin A (>6000 international units) might have a teratogenic effect (birth defect) on the fetus. Prototype Drug Chart 14–1 describes the effects of vitamin A. The nursing process is applied as the drug data are obtained and

---

PROTOTYPE DRUG CHART 14–1

VITAMIN A

Drug Class

Fat-soluble vitamin
Trade names: Acon, Aquasol A
Pregnancy Category: A (X if doses are above RDA)

Dosage

Severe deficiency:
A & C >8 y: PO: 100,000-500,000 international units daily × 3 d; then 50,000 daily × 14 d
Maintenance:
10,000-20,000 international units daily × 60 d
1-8 y: PO/IM: 17,000-35,000 international units daily × 10 d
Dietary supplement:
4-8 y: PO: 15,000 international units daily
1 < 4 y: PO: 10,000 international units daily

Contraindications

Hypervitaminosis A, pregnancy (massive doses)

Drug-Lab-Food Interactions

Drug: May decrease absorption of mineral oil, cholestyramine
Lab: May increase BUN, calcium, cholesterol triglycerides; may lower erythrocyte, leukocyte counts
Food: None known

Pharmacokinetics

Absorption: PO: 1 h
Distribution: PB: UK
Metabolism: t½: weeks-months
Excretion: Urine

Pharmacodynamics

PO: Onset: 1-2 h
Peak: 4-5 h
Duration: UK

Therapeutic Effects/Uses

To treat vitamin A deficiency (biliary tract or pancreatic disease, colitis, cirrhosis, celiac disease, sprue), prevent night blindness, treat skin disorders, promote bone development
Mode of Action: Essential for growth, bone and teeth development, vision, integrity of skin and mucous membranes, and reproduction

Side Effects

Headache, fatigue, drowsiness, irritability, anorexia, vomiting, diarrhea, dry skin, visual changes

Adverse Reactions

Evident only with toxicity: leukopenia, aplastic anemia, papilledema, increased intracranial pressure, hypervitaminosis A, bulging fontanelles in infants

---

A, Adult; *C,* child; *d,* day; *h,* hour; *IM,* intramuscular; *PB,* protein-binding; *PO,* by mouth; *RDA,* recommended daily allowance; *t½,* half-life; *UK,* unknown; *y,* year; <, less than; > greater than.

the drug is administered. IM administration is only in acutely ill or clients refractory to the oral route, such as those with gastrointestinal (GI) malabsorption syndrome.

Pharmacokinetics

When a person is deficient in vitamin A, the vitamin is absorbed faster than if there is no deficiency or intestinal obstruction. A portion of vitamin A is stored in the liver, and this function can be inhibited with liver disease. Massive doses of vitamin A may cause hypervitaminosis A, symptoms of which are hair loss and peeling skin.

The RDA for vitamin A supplement is 5000 international units. Excess use of vitamin A should be avoided unless warranted because this vitamin is stored in the liver, kidneys, and fat and is slowly excreted from the body. Excess vitamin A is stored in the liver for up to 2 years. Vitamin A toxicity affects multiple organs, especially the liver. The dose for healthy clients should not be greater than 7500 international units to prevent the occurrence of vitamin A toxicity.

Mineral oil, cholestyramine, alcohol, and antilipemic drugs decrease the absorption of vitamin A. Vitamin A is excreted through the kidneys and feces.

Pharmacodynamics

Vitamin A is necessary for many biochemical processes. It aids in the formation of the visual pigment needed for night vision, it is needed in bone growth and development, and it promotes the integrity of the mucosal and epithelial tissues. An early sign of vitamin A deficiency (hypovitaminosis A) is night blindness. This may progress to dryness and ulceration of the cornea and to blindness.

Vitamin A taken orally begins to take effect in 1 to 2 hours and peaks in 4 to 5 hours. Its duration of action is unknown. Because vitamin A is stored in the liver, the vitamin may be available to the body for days, weeks, or months.

Vitamin D

Vitamin D has a major role in regulating calcium and phosphorus metabolism and is needed for calcium absorption from the intestines. Dietary vitamin D is absorbed in the small intestine and requires bile salts for absorption. There are two compounds of vitamin D: vitamin D_2, ergocalciferol (a synthetic fortified vitamin D), and vitamin D_3, cholecalciferol (a natural form of vitamin D influenced by ultraviolet sunlight through the skin). Once absorbed, vitamin D is converted to calcifediol in the liver. Calcifediol is then converted to an active form, calcitriol, in the kidneys.

Calcitriol, the active form of vitamin D, functions as a hormone and, with parathyroid hormone (PTH) and calcitonin, regulates calcium and phosphorus metabolism. Calcitriol and PTH stimulate bone reabsorption of calcium and phosphorus. Excretion of vitamin D is primarily in bile; only a small amount is excreted in the urine. If serum calcium levels are low, more vitamin D is activated; when serum calcium levels are normal, activation of vitamin D is decreased.

Excess vitamin D ingestion (>40,000 international units) results in hypervitaminosis D and may cause hypercalcemia (an elevated serum calcium level). Anorexia, nausea, and vomiting are early symptoms of vitamin D toxicity.

Vitamin E

Vitamin E has antioxidant properties that protect cellular components from being oxidized and red blood cells from hemolysis. Vitamin E depends on bile salts, pancreatic secretion, and fat for its absorption. Vitamin E is stored in all tissues, especially the liver, muscle, and fatty tissue. About 75% is excreted in bile.

It has been reported that taking 400 to 800 international units of vitamin E per day reduces the number of nonfatal myocardial infarctions (MIs). Also, it has been stated that taking 200 international units a day for several years can reduce the risk of coronary artery disease (CAD). Today the use of vitamin E for CAD is being questioned. However, many still state that this vitamin protects the heart and arteries and aids in the prevention of macular degeneration because of its antioxidant effects (i.e., it inhibits the oxidation of other compounds by blocking a group of harmful chemicals called **free radicals**).

Side effects of large doses of vitamin E may include fatigue, weakness, nausea, GI upset, headache, and breast tenderness. Vitamin E may prolong the prothrombin time (PT). Persons taking warfarin should have their PT monitored closely. Iron and vitamin E should not be taken together because iron can interfere with the body's absorption and use of vitamin E.

Vitamin K

Vitamin K occurs in four forms: vitamin K_1 (phytonadione) is the most active form; vitamin K_2 (menaquinone) is synthesized by intestinal flora; and vitamin K_3 (menadione) and vitamin K_4 (menadiol) have been produced synthetically. Vitamin K_2 is not commercially available. Vitamin K_1 and K_2 are absorbed in the presence of bile salts. Vitamin K_3 and K_4 do not need bile salts for absorption. After vitamin K is absorbed, it is stored primarily in the liver and in other tissues. Half of vitamin K comes from the intestinal flora, and the remaining portion comes from one's diet.

Vitamin K is needed for synthesis of prothrombin and the clotting factors VII, IX, and X. For oral anticoagulant overdose, vitamin K_1 (phytonadione) is the vitamin that is most effective in preventing hemorrhage. The commercial drugs for vitamin K_1 are Mephyton, AquaMEPHYTON, and Konakion, and the commercial drug for vitamin K_4 is Synkayvite.

Water-Soluble Vitamins

Water-soluble vitamins are the B-complex vitamins and vitamin C. This group of vitamins is not usually toxic unless taken in extremely excessive amounts. Water-soluble vitamins are not stored by the body and are readily excreted in the urine. Protein binding of water-soluble vitamins is min-

PREVENTING MEDICATION ERRORS

Do not confuse...

- **Aquasol A** or **Aqusol E** with **Anusol**, an anti-inflammatory generally used to treat hemorrhoids

imal. Foods that are high in vitamin B are grains, cereal, bread, and meats. Citrus fruits and green vegetables are high in vitamin C. If the fruits and vegetables are cut, washed, or cooked, a large amount of vitamin C is lost.

Vitamin B Complex

Vitamin B_1 (thiamine), vitamin B_2 (riboflavin), vitamin B_3 (nicotinic acid, or niacin), and vitamin B_6 (pyridoxine) are four of the vitamin B–complex members. This B-complex group is water soluble. Thiamine is used to treat peripheral neuritis, which may occur from alcoholism or beriberi. Riboflavin may be given to manage dermatologic problems, such as scaly dermatitis, cracked corners of the mouth, and inflammation of the skin and tongue. Niacin is given to alleviate pellagra and hyperlipidemia, for which large doses are required. See Chapter 44, Antilipids and Peripheral Vasodilators, for a discussion of niacin used to reduce cholesterol levels. However, large doses may cause GI irritation and vasodilation, resulting in a flushing sensation. Pyridoxine is administered to correct vitamin B_6 deficiency. It may also help alleviate the symptoms of neuritis caused by isoniazid (INH) therapy for tuberculosis.

Vitamin B_6 (pyridoxine) is an essential building block of nucleic acids, red blood cell formation, and synthesis of hemoglobin. Pyridoxine is readily absorbed in the jejunum and stored in the liver, muscle, and brain. It is metabolized in the liver and excreted in the urine. This vitamin is used to treat vitamin B_6 deficiency caused by lack of adequate diet, inborn error of metabolism or drug induced by INH, penicillamine, or cyclosporine. It is also used to treat neonates with seizures refractive to traditional therapy.

Vitamin C

Vitamin C (ascorbic acid) is absorbed from the small intestine. Vitamin C aids in the absorption of iron and in the conversion of folic acid. Vitamin C is not stored in the body and is excreted readily in the urine. A high serum vitamin C level that results from excessive dosing of vitamin C is excreted by the kidneys unchanged.

The average dose of vitamin C for an adult per day is 50 to 100 mg. Some individuals take as much as 500 to 6000 mg a day to treat upper respiratory infections, cancer, or hypercholesterolemia. Massive doses of vitamin C can cause diarrhea and GI upset. Reduce vitamin C dose gradually; abrupt withdrawal can result in rebound defi-

ciency. Prototype Drug Chart 14–2 gives drug information on vitamin C.

Pharmacokinetics

Vitamin C is absorbed readily through the GI tract and is distributed throughout the body fluids. The kidneys completely excrete vitamin C, mostly unchanged.

Pharmacodynamics

Vitamin C is needed for carbohydrate metabolism and protein and lipid synthesis. Collagen synthesis also requires vitamin C for capillary endothelium, connective tissue and tissue repair, and osteoid tissue of the bone.

Large doses of vitamin C may decrease the effect of oral anticoagulants. Oral contraceptives can decrease vitamin C concentration in the body. Smoking decreases serum vitamin C levels.

The use of **megavitamin therapy**, massive doses of vitamins, is questionable at best. Megadoses of vitamins can cause toxicity and might result in minimal desired effect. Most authorities believe that vitamin C does not cure or prevent the common cold; rather, they believe that vitamin C has a placebo effect. Moreover, megadoses of vitamin C taken with aspirin or sulfonamides may cause crystal formation in the urine (crystalluria). Excessive doses of vitamin C can cause a false-negative occult (blood) stool result and false-positive sugar result in the urine when tested by the Clinitest method. If large doses of megavitamins are to be discontinued, a gradual reduction of dosage is necessary to avoid vitamin deficiency.

Folic Acid (Folate)

Folic acid is absorbed from the small intestine, and the active form of folic acid (folate) is circulated to all tissues. One third of folate is stored in the liver, and the rest is stored in tissues. Four fifths of folate is excreted in bile and one fifth in urine.

Folic acid is essential for body growth. It is needed for deoxyribonucleic acid (DNA) synthesis, and without folic acid there is a disruption in cellular division. Chronic alcoholism, poor nutritional intake, malabsorption syndromes, pregnancy, and drugs that cause inadequate absorption (phenytoin, barbiturates) or folic acid antagonists (methotrexate, triamterene, trimethoprim) are causes of folic acid deficiencies. Symptoms of folic acid deficiencies include anorexia, nausea, stomatitis, diarrhea, fatigue, alopecia, and blood dyscrasias (megaloblastic anemia, leukopenia, thrombocytopenia). These symptoms are usually not noted until 2 to 4 months after folic acid storage is depleted.

Folic acid deficiency during the first trimester of pregnancy can affect the development of the central nervous system (CNS) of the fetus. This may cause neural tube defects (NTDs) such as spina bifida (defective closure of the bony structure of the spinal cord) or anencephaly (lack of brain mass formation). It is imperative that pregnant women take adequate folic acid supplements, 400 mcg daily, starting with the first trimester of pregnancy to prevent the development of CNS anomalies.

There is some evidence that 400 to 800 mcg (0.4 to 0.8 mg) of folic acid per day can decrease the incidence of CAD. It is thought that folic acid decreases the amino acid homocysteine in the blood, which may contribute to heart disease.

Excessive doses of folic acid may mask signs of vitamin B_{12} deficiency, which is a risk in older adults. Clients taking phenytoin (Dilantin) to control seizures should be cautious about taking folic acid. This vitamin can lower the

PREVENTING MEDICATION ERRORS

Do not confuse...

- **Pyridoxine** with **paroxetine (Paxil),** an antidepressant

- **Pralidoxine,** an antidote used to treat poisoning with organophosphate pesticides and chemicals that have antocholinesterase activity

- **Phenazopyridine (Pyridium),** a urinary analgesic

PROTOTYPE DRUG CHART 14–2

VITAMIN C

Drug Class	Dosage
Water-soluble vitamin Trade names: Ascorbicap, Cecon, Cevalin, Solucap C, ♦ Apo-C, Ce-Vi-Sol, Redoxon *Pregnancy Category:* A (C if used in doses above RDA)	*Prophylactic:* **A: PO:** 45-60 mg/d **C: PO:** 20-50 mg/d *Severe deficit:* Scurvy **A: PO: IM: IV:** 150-500 mg/d in 1 to 2 divided doses **C: PO: IM: IV:** 100-300 mg/d in 1 to 2 divided doses *Pregnancy and lactation:* **A: PO:** 60-80 mg/d
Contraindications	**Drug-Lab-Food Interactions**
Caution: Renal calculi, gout, anemia: sickle cell, sideroblastic, thalassemia	*Decrease* ascorbic acid uptake taken with salicylates; may decrease effect of oral anticoagulants; may decrease elimination of aspirins **Lab:** May decrease bilirubin, urinary pH; may increase uric acid, uric oxalate **Food:** None known
Pharmacokinetics	**Pharmacodynamics**
Absorption: PO: quickly **Distribution:** PB: 25% **Metabolism:** t½: UK **Excretion:** In the urine; unchanged with high doses	**PO:** Onset: >2 d Peak: UK Duration: UK

Therapeutic Effects/Uses

To prevent and treat vitamin C deficiency (scurvy); increase wound healing; for burns. Preserves integrity of blood vessels.
Mode of Action: A water-soluble vitamin, essential for collagen formation and tissue repair (bones, skin, blood vessels). Synthesis of lipids, protein, carnitine.

Side Effects	Adverse Reactions
Nausea, vomiting, diarrhea; increase urination with dose >19. Parenteral: flushing, headache, dizziness, soreness at injection site	Kidney stones, crystalluria, hyperuricemia **Life-threatening:** Sickle cell crisis, deep vein thrombosis

A, Adult; *C,* child; *d,* day; *IM,* intramuscular; *IV,* intravenous; *PB,* protein-binding; *PO,* by mouth; *t½,* half-life; *UK,* unknown; >, greater than; ♦, Canadian drug names.

PREVENTING MEDICATION ERRORS

Do not confuse...

- **Folvite** with **florvite**, a fluoride supplement put in the water

serum phenytoin level, which could increase the risk of seizures. The phenytoin dose would need to be adjusted in such clients.

Vitamin B₁₂

Vitamin B₁₂, like folic acid, is essential for DNA synthesis. Vitamin B₁₂ aids in the conversion of folic acid to its active form. With active folic acid, vitamin B₁₂ promotes cellular division. It is also needed for normal hematopoiesis (de-

velopment of red blood cells in bone marrow) and to maintain nervous system integrity, especially the myelin.

The gastric parietal cells produce an intrinsic factor that is necessary for the absorption of vitamin B₁₂ through the intestinal wall. Without the intrinsic factor, little or no vitamin B₁₂ is absorbed. After absorption, vitamin B₁₂ binds to the protein transcobalamin II and is transferred to the tissues. Most vitamin B₁₂ is stored in the liver. Vitamin B₁₂ is slowly excreted, and it can take 2 to 3 years for stored vitamin B₁₂ to be depleted and a deficit noticed.

Vitamin B₁₂ deficiency is uncommon unless there is a disturbance of the intrinsic factor and intestinal absorption. Pernicious anemia (lack of the intrinsic factor) is the major cause of vitamin B₁₂ deficiency. Vitamin B₁₂ deficiency can develop in strict vegetarians who do not consume meat, fish, or dairy products. Other possible causes of vitamin B_{12} deficiency include malabsorption syndromes (cancer, celiac disease, certain drugs), gastrectomy, Crohn's disease, and liver and kidney diseases. Symptoms may include numbness and tingling in the lower extremities, weakness, fatigue, anorexia, loss of taste, diarrhea, memory loss, mood changes, dementia, psychosis, megaloblastic anemia with macrocytes (over enlarged erythrocytes [red blood cells]) in blood, and megaloblasts (over enlarged erythroblasts) in the bone marrow.

To correct vitamin B_{12} deficiency, cyanocobalamin in crystalline form can be given for severe deficits intramuscularly. It cannot be given intravenously because of possible hypersensitive reactions. It also can be given orally and is found in multiple vitamin preparations.

Table 14–2 lists both the fat- and water-soluble vitamins with their functions, suggested food sources, and selected deficiency conditions. Table 14–3 lists fat- and water-soluble vitamins, their RDA values, dosages for vitamin deficiencies, and therapeutic serum blood or urine ranges.

Table 14–2

Vitamins: Functions, Suggested Food Sources, and Selected Deficiency Conditions

Vitamin	Function	Food Sources	Deficiency Conditions
A	Required for development and maintenance of healthy eyes, gums, teeth, skin, hair, and selected glands. Needed for fat metabolism.	Whole milk, butter, eggs, leafy green and yellow vegetables and fruits* Natural vitamin A, found only in animal sources: cod, halibut, shark, tuna	Dry skin, poor tooth development, night blindness
B_1 (thiamine)	Promotes use of sugars (energy). Required for good function of nervous system and heart.	Enriched breads and cereals, yeast, liver, pork, fish, milk	Sensory disturbances, retarded growth, fatigue, anorexia
B_2 (riboflavin)	Promotes body's use of carbohydrates, proteins, and fats by releasing energy to cells. Required for tissue integrity.	Milk, enriched breads and cereals, liver, lean meat, eggs, leafy green vegetables†	Visual defects, such as blurred vision and photophobia; cheilosis; rash on nose; numbness of extremities
B_6 (pyridoxine)	Important in metabolism, synthesis of proteins, and formation of red blood cells.	Lean meat, leafy green vegetables, whole-grain cereals, yeast, bananas	Neuritis, convulsions, dermatitis, anemia, lymphopenia
B_{12} (cobalamin)	Functions as a building block of nucleic acids and to form red blood cells. Facilitates functioning of nervous system.	Liver, kidney, fish, milk	Gastrointestinal disorders, poor growth, anemias
folic acid (folvite)	Helps in formation of genetic materials and proteins for the cell nucleus. Assists with intestinal functioning and prevents selected anemias.	Leafy green vegetables, yellow fruits and vegetables, yeast, organ meats	Decreased white blood cell count and clotting factors, anemias, intestinal disturbances, depression
pantothenic acid	Promotes body's use of carbohydrates, fats, and proteins. Essential for formation of specific hormones and nerve-regulating substances.	Eggs, leafy green vegetables, nuts, liver, kidney, skim milk	Natural deficiency unknown in man
niacin	In all body tissues. Necessary for energy-producing reactions. Assists nervous system.	Eggs, meat, liver, beans, peas, enriched bread, and cereals	Retarded growth, pellegra, headache, memory loss, anorexia, insomnia
biotin	Synthesis of fatty acids and energy production from glucose. Required by body chemical systems.	Eggs, milk, leafy green vegetables, liver, kidney	Natural deficiency unknown in man
C (ascorbic acid)	Helps tissue repair and growth. Required in formation of collagen.	Citrus fruits, tomatoes, leafy green vegetables, potatoes, strawberries	Poor wound healing, bleeding gums, scurvy, predisposition to infection
D (calciferol)	Promotes use of phosphorus and calcium. Important for strong teeth and bones.	Vitamin D–fortified milk, egg yolk, tuna, salmon	Rickets, deficit of phosphorus and calcium in blood
E	Protects fatty acids and promotes the formation and functioning of red blood cells, muscle, and other tissues.	Whole-grain cereals, wheat germ, vegetable oils, lettuce, sunflower seeds, milk, eggs, meat	Breakdown of red blood cells
K	Essential for blood clotting.	Leafy green vegetables, liver, cheese, egg yolk, vegetable oil, tomatoes	Increased clotting time, leading to increased bleeding and hemorrhage

*Yellow fruits and vegetables include apricots, cantaloupe, carrots, rutabaga, pumpkin, squash, and sweet potatoes.
†Leafy green vegetables include Brussels sprouts, chard, broccoli, kale, spinach, and turnip and mustard greens.

Table 14–3

Fat- and Water-Soluble Vitamins

Vitamin	RDA	Dosages for Vitamin Deficiencies	Therapeutic Ranges
Fat-Soluble			
A	Men: 1000 mcg or 5000 international units Women: 800 mcg or 4000 international units Preg: 1000 mcg, 5000 international units Lact: 1200 mcg, 6000 international units	10,000-20,000 international units or 3000-6000 mcg/dl	30-70 mcg/dl Deficit: <20 mcg/dl
D	Men and women: 40-80 mcg; 200-400 international units	Mild: 50-125 mcg/dl Moderate to severe: 2.5-7.5 mg/d; 2500-7500 mcg	Unknown
E	Men: 10 mg/d; 15 international units Women: 8 mg/d; 12 international units Preg: 10-12 mg/d	Malabsorption: 30-100 mg/d Severe deficit: 1-2 mg/kg/d or 50-200 international units/kg/d	0.5-0.7 mg/dl Deficit: <0.5 mg/dl
K	Men: 70-80 mcg/d Women: 60-65 mcg/d Taking broad-spectrum antibiotic: 140 mcg/d Preg: 65 mcg/d	5-15 mg/d	Based on prothrombin time (PT) results
Water-Soluble			
C	Men and Women: 60 mg/d Preg: 70 mg/dl Lact: 95 mg/dl	150-300 mg *Burns:* 500-2000 mg/d	Serum: >1.30 mg/dl WBC: >15 mg/dl *Deficit:* Serum <0.2 mg/dl WBC: <7 mg/dl
B$_1$ (thiamine)	Men: 1.5 mg Women: 1.1 mg Preg: 1.5 mg Lact: 1.6 mg	30-60 mg/d	Urine: <50 mcg/d
B$_2$ (riboflavin)	Men: 1.4-1.7 mg Women: 1.2-1.3 mg Preg: 1.6 mg Lact: 1.8 mg	5-25 mg/d Prophylactic: 3 mg/d	Urine: <50 mcg/d
B$_3$ (nicotinic acid or niacin)	Men: 15-19 mg/d Women: 13-15 mg/d Preg: 18 mg/d Lact: 20 mg/d	Prevention: 5-20 mg/d Deficit: 50-100 mg/d *Pellagra:* 300-500 mg in 3 divided doses *Hyperlipidemia:* 1-2 g/d in 3 divided doses	Unknown
B$_6$ (pyridoxine)	Men: 2.0 mg/d Women: 1.6 mg/d Preg: 2.1 mg/d Lact: 2.2 mg/d	25-100 mg/d *Isoniazid therapy prophylaxis:* 25-50 mg/d *Peripheral neuritis:* 50-200 mg/d	Serum: >50 ng/ml Urine: <1 mg/d
Folic acid (folate)	Men and Women: 400 mcg/d Preg: 600-800 mcg/d Lact: 600-800 mcg/d	1-2 mg/d	Serum folate: 6-20 ng/ml RBC: 160-600 ng/ml *Deficit:* Serum: <3-4 ng/ml RBC: <140 ng/ml
B$_{12}$	Men and Women: 3 mcg/d Preg: 4 mcg/d	100 mg/dl 14 d *Pernicious anemia:* 50-100 mcg /d or 1000 mcg/wk × 3 wk	150-900 pg/ml *Deficit:* <100 pg/ml *Schilling test* >30% normal

d, Day; *lact,* lactation; *preg,* pregnancy; *RBC,* red blood cell; *WBC,* white blood cell; *wk,* week; >, greater than; <, less than.

Nursing Process

Vitamins

ASSESSMENT

▪ Check client for vitamin deficiency before start of therapy and regularly thereafter. Explore such areas as inadequate nutrient intake, debilitating disease, and GI disorders.
▪ Obtain 24- and 48-hour diet history analysis.

NURSING DIAGNOSES

▪ Imbalanced nutrition; less than body requirements
▪ Deficient knowledge

PLANNING

▪ Client will eat a well-balanced diet that includes the foods and servings recommended in the food pyramid.
▪ Client with vitamin deficiency will take vitamin supplements as prescribed.

NURSING INTERVENTIONS

▪ Administer vitamins with food to promote absorption.
▪ Store drug in light-resistant container.
▪ When administering vitamins in drop form, use the supplied calibrated dropper for accurate dosing. Solution may be administered mixed with food or dropped into the mouth.
▪ Administer IM primarily for clients unable to take by PO route (e.g., GI malabsorption syndrome).
▪ Recognize need for vitamin E supplements for infants receiving vitamin A to avoid hemolytic anemia.
▪ Monitor for vitamin A therapeutic serum levels (80-300 international units/ml).

Client Teaching

General
• Instruct client to take the prescribed amount of drug.
• Inform clients (adults and children) to read vitamin labels to determine which vitamin is most appropriate for them (Figure 14–4).
• Instruct client to consult with health care provider/ pharmacist regarding interactions with prescription and OTC medications (e.g., vitamin B_6 interferes with action of levodopa).
• Discourage client from taking megavitamins over a long period unless these are prescribed for a specific purpose by the health care provider. To discontinue long-term megavitamin therapy, a gradual decrease in vitamin intake is advised to avoid a vitamin deficiency. Megadoses of vitamins can be toxic.
• Inform client that missing vitamins for 1 or 2 days is not a cause for concern because deficiencies do not occur for some time.

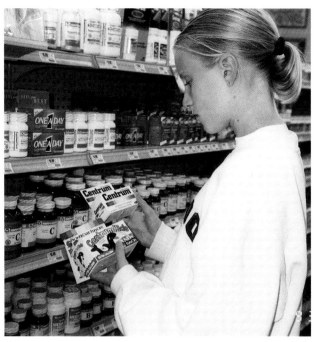

FIGURE 14–4   This 12-year-old is trying to decide whether an adult's or a children's vitamin is more appropriate for her needs.

• Advise client to check the expiration dates on vitamin containers before purchasing and taking them. Potency of the vitamin is reduced after the expiration date.
• Instruct client to avoid taking mineral oil with vitamin A on a regular basis because it interferes with the absorption of the vitamin. If needed, take mineral oil at bedtime.
• Explain to client that there is no scientific evidence that megadoses of vitamin C (ascorbic acid) will cure a cold.
• Alert client not to take megadoses of vitamin C with aspirin or sulfonamides because crystals may form in the kidneys and urine.
• Instruct client to avoid excessive intake of alcoholic beverages. Alcohol can cause vitamin B-complex deficiencies.

Diet
• Advise client to eat a well-balanced diet that includes the recommended amounts and types of food detailed in the food pyramid. Vitamin supplements are not necessary if the person is healthy and receives proper nutrition on a regular basis.
• Instruct client about foods rich in vitamin A, including whole milk, butter, eggs, leafy green and yellow vegetables, fruits, and liver. Foods rich in other vitamins are listed in Table 14–2.

Side Effects
• Instruct client that nausea, vomiting, headache, loss of hair, and cracked lips (symptoms of hypervitaminosis A) should be reported to the health care provider. Early symptoms of hypervitaminosis D are anorexia, nausea, and vomiting.

Cultural Considerations

- Food and food choices have strong cultural roots. Determine the client's preferred and culturally meaningful foods, and incorporate them into food and supplement plan.
- Ask about folk practices and incorporate as appropriate.
- Use interpreters as appropriate.

EVALUATION

■ Evaluate the effectiveness of client's diet for the inclusion of the appropriate amounts and types of food from the food pyramid. Have client keep a periodic diet chart for a complete week.

■ Determine whether client with malnutrition is receiving appropriate vitamin therapy.

Minerals

Various **minerals,** such as iron, copper, zinc, chromium, and selenium, are needed for body function.

Iron

Iron (ferrous sulfate, gluconate, or fumarate) is vital for hemoglobin regeneration. Sixty percent of the iron in the body is found in hemoglobin. One of the causes of anemia is iron deficiency. A normal diet contains 5 to 20 mg of iron per day. Foods rich in iron include liver, lean meats, egg yolks, dried beans, green vegetables (e.g., spinach), and fruit. Food and antacids slow the absorption of iron, and vitamin C increases iron absorption.

During pregnancy, an increased amount of iron is needed, but during the first trimester of pregnancy, megadoses of iron are contraindicated because of its possible teratogenic effect on the fetus. Larger doses of iron are required during the second and third trimesters of pregnancy.

The dose of iron for infants and children, 6 months to 2 years of age, is 1.5 per kilogram of body weight. For the adult, 50 mg daily is needed for hemoglobin regeneration. The ferrous sulfate tablet is 325 mg, of which 65 mg is elemental iron. Therefore one tablet of ferrous sulfate is sufficient as a daily iron dose when indicated. Prototype Drug Chart 14-3 describes the effects of iron preparations.

Pharmacokinetics

Iron is absorbed by the intestines and goes into the plasma as heme, or it may be stored as ferritin. Although food decreases absorption by 25% to 50%, it may be necessary to take iron preparations with food to avoid GI discomfort. Vitamin C may slightly increase iron absorption, whereas tetracycline and antacids can decrease absorption. See Herbal Alert 14-1.

HERBAL ALERT 14-1

Iron

🌿 Chamomile, feverfew, peppermint, and St. John's wort interfere with the absorption of iron and other minerals.

Pharmacodynamics

Iron replacement is given primarily to correct or control iron-deficiency anemia, which is diagnosed by a laboratory blood smear. Positive findings for this anemia are microcytic (small), hypochromic (pale) erythrocytes (red blood cells [RBCs]). Clinical signs and symptoms include fatigue, weakness, shortness of breath, pallor, and, in cases of severe anemia, increased GI bleeding. The dosage of ferrous sulfate for prophylactic use is 300 to 325 mg daily; for therapeutic use, the dosage is 600 to 1200 mg daily in divided doses.

The onset of action for iron therapy takes days, and its peak action does not occur for days or weeks; therefore the client's symptoms are slow to improve. Increased hemoglobin and hematocrit levels occur within 3 to 7 days.

Iron toxicity is a serious cause of poisoning in children. As few as 10 tablets of ferrous sulfate (3 g) taken at one time can be fatal within 12 to 48 hours. The child can hemorrhage because of the ulcerogenic effects of unbound iron, causing shock. Parents should be cautioned against leaving iron tablets that look like candy (e.g., M&M's) within a child's reach; most iron products are distributed in bubble packs.

Copper

Copper is needed for the formation of RBCs and connective tissues. Copper is a cofactor of many enzymes, and its function is in the production of norepinephrine and dopamine (neurotransmitters). Excess serum copper levels may be associated with Wilson's disease, which is an inborn error of metabolism that allows for large amounts of copper to accumulate in the liver, brain, cornea (brown or green Kayser-Fleischer rings), or kidneys.

A prolonged copper deficiency may result in anemia, which is not corrected by taking iron supplements. Abnormal blood and skin changes caused by a copper deficiency include a decrease in white blood cell count, glucose intolerance, and a decrease in skin and hair pigmentation. Mental retardation might also occur in the young.

The RDA for copper is 1.5 to 3 mg per day. Most adults consume about 1 mg per day. Foods rich in copper are shellfish (crab, oysters), liver, nuts, seeds (sunflower, sesame), legumes, and cocoa.

Zinc

The use of zinc has greatly increased in the past few years (Figure 14-5). Some believe zinc can alleviate the common cold. Some individuals take as much as 200 mg daily. The adult RDA is 12 to 19 mg. Foods rich in zinc include beef, lamb, eggs, and leafy and root vegetables.

Large doses, more than 150 mg, may cause a copper deficiency, a decrease in high-density lipoprotein (HDL) cholesterol ("good" cholesterol), and a weakened immune response. Zinc can inhibit tetracycline absorption. Clients taking zinc and an antibiotic should not take them together; zinc should be taken at least 2 hours after taking an antibiotic.

Chromium

Chromium is said to be helpful in the control of type 2 diabetes (non–insulin-dependent diabetes). It is thought that this mineral helps to normalize blood glucose by increasing the effects of insulin on the cells. If a client is taking large doses of chromium and an oral hypoglycemic agent

PROTOTYPE DRUG CHART 14–3

IRON

Drug Class	**Dosage**
Mineral for antianemia Trade names: *ferrous sulfate* (Feosol, Fer-Iron) *ferrous gluconate* (Fergon, Fertinic) *ferrous fumarate* (Feostat, Fumerin) *Pregnancy Category:* A	A: PO: 300-325 mg q.i.d.: increase to 650 mg q.i.d. as needed or tolerated *Pregnancy:* PO: 300-600 mg/d C ≥2 y: PO 8 mg/kg daily in divided doses
Contraindications	**Drug-Lab-Food Interactions**
Hemolytic anemia, hemosiderosis, peptic ulcer, ulcerative colitis *Caution:* Bronchial asthma, iron hypersensitivity	*Increased* effect of iron with vitamin C; *decreased* effect of tetracycline, antacids, penicillamine **Lab:** May increase bilirubin, may decrease calcium **Food:** None known
Pharmacokinetics	**Pharmacodynamics**
Absorption: PO: 10%-30% intestines **Distribution:** PB: UK **Metabolism:** t½: 6 h **Excretion:** Urine, feces, sweat	PO: Onset: 4 d Peak: 7-14 d Duration: 3-4 mo

Therapeutic Effects/Uses

To prevent and treat iron deficiency anemia
Mode of Action: Enables RBC development and oxygen transport via hemoglobin

Side Effects	**Adverse Reactions**
Nausea, vomiting, diarrhea, constipation, epigastric pain; elixir may stain teeth	Existing GI conditions may be aggravated Pallor, drowsiness **Life-threatening:** Iron poisoning (mostly in children) and may result in cardiovascular collapse, metabolic acidosis

A, Adult; *C,* child; *d,* day; *GI,* gastrointestinal; *h,* hour; *mo,* month; *PB,* protein-binding; *PO,* by mouth; *q.i.d.,* four times a day; *RBC,* red blood cell; *t½,* half-life; *UK,* unknown; ≥, greater than or equal to.

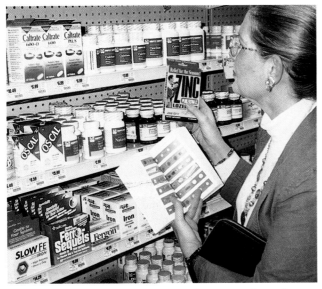

FIGURE 14–5 The use of zinc and other mineral supplements, such as iron and selenium, is on the rise.

or insulin, the glucose level should be monitored closely for a hypoglycemic reaction. The dose of an oral hypoglycemic drug or insulin may need to be decreased. Some clients with an impaired glucose tolerance or clients who do not have diabetes may benefit by taking chromium.

There is no RDA for chromium; however, 50 to 200 mcg per day is considered within the normal range for children older than 6 years old and adults. Foods rich in chromium include meats, whole-grain cereals, and brewer's yeast.

Selenium

Selenium acts as a cofactor for an antioxidant enzyme that protects protein and nucleic acids from oxidative damage. Selenium works with vitamin E. It is thought that selenium has an anticarcinogenic effect, and doses greater than 200 mcg may reduce the risk of lung, prostate, and colorectal cancer. Excess doses of more than 200 mcg might cause weakness, a loss of hair, dermatitis, nausea, diarrhea, and abdominal pain. Also, there may be a garlic-like odor from the skin and breath.

The RDA for selenium is 40 to 75 mcg (higher dose for men and a lower dose for women). Foods rich in selenium include meats (especially liver), seafood, eggs, and dairy products.

Nursing Process

Antianemia, Mineral: Iron

ASSESSMENT

■ Obtain a drug history of current drugs and herbs client is taking.

■ Obtain a history of anemia or health problems that may lead to anemia.

■ Assess client for signs and symptoms of iron deficiency anemia, such as fatigue, malaise, pallor, shortness of breath, tachycardia, and cardiac dysrhythmia.

■ Assess client's RBC count, hemoglobin, hematocrit, iron level, and reticulocyte count before start of therapy and throughout thereafter.

NURSING DIAGNOSES

■ Fatigue

■ Imbalanced nutrition; less than body requirements

■ Knowledge deficit of foods high in iron

PLANNING

■ Client will name six foods high in iron content.

■ Client will consume foods rich in iron.

■ Client with iron deficiency anemia or with low hemoglobin will take iron replacement as recommended by the health care provider, resulting in laboratory results within the desired range.

NURSING INTERVENTIONS

■ Encourage client to eat a nutritious diet to obtain sufficient iron. Iron supplements are not needed unless the person is malnourished, pregnant, or has abnormal menses.

■ Store drug in light-resistant container.

■ Administer IM injection of iron by the Z-track method to avoid leakage of iron into the subQ tissue and skin, because it irritates and stains the skin.

Client Teaching

General

• Instruct client to take the tablet or capsule between meals with at least 8 ounces of juice or water to promote absorption. If gastric irritation occurs, instruct the client to take with food.

• Advise client to swallow the tablet or capsule whole.

• Instruct client to maintain sitting upright position for 30 minutes to prevent esophageal corrosion from reflux.

• Do not administer the iron tablet within 1 hour of ingesting antacid, milk, ice cream, or other milk products such as pudding.

• Inform client that certain herbal drugs can decrease absorption of iron and other minerals. See Herbal Alert 14–1.

• Advise client to increase fluids, activity, and dietary bulk to avoid or relieve constipation. Slow-release iron capsules decrease constipation and gastric irritation.

• Instruct adults not to leave iron tablets within reach of children. If a child swallows many tablets, induce vomiting and immediately call the local poison control center; the telephone number is in the front of most telephone books (include this number on emergency reference list). Keep ipecac available; it is an OTC drug.

• Encourage client to take prescribed amount of drug to avoid iron poisoning.

• Be alert that iron content varies among iron salts; therefore do not substitute one for another.

• Advise client that drug treatment for anemia is generally less than 6 months.

Diet

• Counsel client to include iron-rich foods in diet, such as liver, lean meats, egg yolk, dried beans, green vegetables, and fruit.

Side Effects

• Advise client taking the liquid iron preparation to use a straw to prevent discoloration of teeth enamel.

• Alert client that the drug turns stools a harmless black or dark green.

• Instruct client about signs and symptoms of toxicity, including nausea, vomiting, diarrhea, pallor, hematemesis, shock, and coma, and report occurrence to health care provider.

Cultural Considerations

• Ask about folk practices, and incorporate as appropriate.

• Use interpreter as needed.

EVALUATION

■ Evaluate the effectiveness of the drug therapy by determining that client is not fatigued or short of breath and that the hemoglobin is within the desired range.

WEBSITES

For further information on *Vitamin and Mineral Replacement,* visit these Internet resources:

Center for Food Safety and Applied Nutrition: *http://vm.cfaan.fda.gov*

Drug Topics: *http://www.drugtopics.com*

MyPyramid Plan: *http://www.mypyramid.gov*

National Library of Medicine: *http://www.nlm.nih.giv*

Critical Thinking Case Study

A.P. is pregnant and is taking two tablets of 325 mg of ferrous sulfate. She has a 2-year-old daughter.

1. What precautions should A.P. take in regard to the container of ferrous sulfate? Explain.

2. If A.P. asks whether she should take more than two tablets of iron a day, how should you respond?

3. A.P. states that she is constipated and wonders if the iron is the cause. How can this problem be alleviated? What would be an appropriate response?

4. Develop a safety plan with A.P. related to medication safety in the home with children.

Study Questions

1. Vitamin A is classified in what vitamin category? What foods are high in vitamin A? How does vitamin A differ from vitamin C?

2. What are the nursing interventions when megadoses of vitamins are discontinued?

3. Why is vitamin D important?

4. Which is the most active form of vitamin K? Where is this vitamin stored in the body?

5. What is the approved use of vitamin C (ascorbic acid)? What is the nonapproved use of the drug?

6. What are the common names of vitamins B_1, B_2, B_3, and B_6? What are the uses of these vitamin B-complex drugs?

7. How are folic acid and vitamin B_{12} similar? Why is folic acid important during the first trimester of pregnancy?

8. What is the most common cause of vitamin B_{12} deficiency? Explain.

9. List three nursing interventions and client teaching guides for clients receiving iron preparations. High doses of ferrous sulfate can result in what condition?

10. List at least six client teaching interventions related to vitamins.

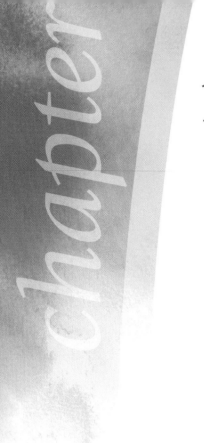

15 Fluid and Electrolyte Replacement

ELECTRONIC RESOURCES

Additional information can be found on the companion website at *http://evolve.elsevier.com/KeeHayes/pharmacology/* or on the companion CD-ROM, which includes:
- *NCLEX-style examination review questions*
- *Pharmacology animations*
- *Medication error and IV therapy checklists*
- *Medication calculation problems*
- *Electronic calculators*

OBJECTIVES

- Define *osmolality* and *tonicity.*
- Give the iso-osmolality range for serum and isotonicity of intravenous solutions.
- Describe the four classifications of intravenous fluids.
- Differentiate between cations and anions of electrolytes.
- List the major functions of cations.
- List examples of potassium, calcium, and magnesium supplements.
- Explain the methods used to correct potassium, calcium, and magnesium excess.
- Describe several signs and symptoms of hypokalemia, hyperkalemia, hyponatremia, hypernatremia, hypocalcemia, and hypercalcemia.
- Explain the pharmacokinetics and pharmacodynamics of oral and intravenous potassium chloride and calcium salts.
- Describe the assessments, nursing interventions, and client teaching for fluid, potassium, sodium, calcium, and magnesium imbalances.

TERMS

anion

cation

electrolytes

hypercalcemia

hyperkalemia

hypermagnesemia

hypernatremia

hyperosmolar

hypocalcemia

hypokalemia

hypomagnesemia

hyponatremia

hypo-osmolar

iso-osmolar

osmolality

tonicity

Introduction

Fluid replacement is based on body fluid needs. The adult body is approximately 60% water, the human embryo is 97% water, and the newborn infant is 77% water. Of the 60% adult body water (fluid), 40% is intracellular fluid (ICF; cells), and 20% is extracellular fluid (ECF), of which 15% is interstitial (tissue) fluid and 5% is intravascular or vascular fluid (Table 15–1).

Electrolytes in the body are substances that carry either a positive charge **(cation)** or a negative charge **(anion)**. Cations and anions are described in Table 15–2. The functions of cations are to transmit nerve impulses to muscles and to contract skeletal and smooth muscles.

The cations of the electrolytes are most plentiful in the cells (potassium, magnesium, and some calcium), in the ECF that is within the blood vessels and tissue spaces (sodium and some calcium), and in the gastrointestinal (GI) tract. Anions are attached to cations. Figure 15–1 illustrates those electrolytes that are plentiful in the stomach and in the intestines.

This chapter describes fluid and electrolyte replacements based on fluid and specific electrolyte deficits and excesses.

Body Fluids

The concentration of body fluid is described as **osmolality** and osmolarity; these terms are frequently used interchangeably. Osmolality is the osmotic pull exerted by all particles (solutes) per unit of water, expressed as osmoles or milliosmoles per kilogram (mOsm/kg) of water. Three types of fluid concentration are based on the osmolality of body fluids:

1. **Iso-osmolar** fluid, which has the same proportion of weight of particles (e.g., sodium, glucose, urea, protein) and water
2. **Hypo-osmolar** fluid, which has fewer particles than water
3. **Hyperosmolar** fluid, which has more particles than water. The plasma/serum osmolality (concentration of circulating body fluids) can be calculated if the serum

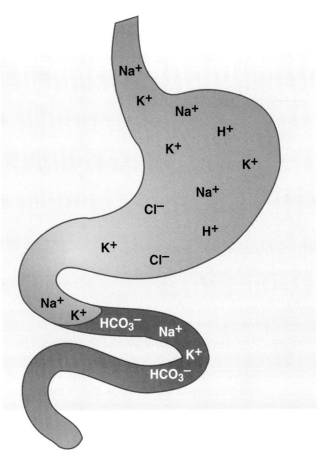

FIGURE 15–1 Plentiful electrolytes in the gastrointestinal tract include potassium (K^+), sodium (Na^+), hydrogen (H^+), bicarbonate (HCO_3^-), and chloride (Cl^-).

Table 15–1

Adult Body Fluid Volume

Fluid Compartment		Percentage
Intracellular (cellular) fluid (ICF)		40%
Extracellular fluid (ECF)		20%
Interstitial fluid (tissue spaces)	15%	
Intravascular fluid (vascular fluid)	5%	
Total body fluid		60%

Table 15–2

Cations and Anions

Cations	Anions
Potassium (K^+)	Chloride (Cl^-)
Sodium (Na^+)	Bicarbonate (HCO_3^-)
Calcium (Ca^{2+})	Phosphate (PO_4^-)
Magnesium (Mg^{2+})	Sulfate (SO_4^-)

sodium level is known or the sodium, glucose, and blood urea nitrogen (BUN) levels are known. Sodium is the main extracellular electrolyte, and its major function is to regulate body fluids. The two formulas used to estimate serum osmolality are the following:

a. Double the serum sodium (Na) = serum osmolality

b. $2 \times \text{serum Na} + \dfrac{\text{BUN}}{3} + \dfrac{\text{Glucose}}{18} = \text{serum osmolality}$

The second formula is more accurate in estimating the correct serum osmolality.

Normal serum osmolality is 275 to 295 mOsm/kg. If the serum osmolality is less than 275 mOsm/kg, the body fluid is hypo-osmolar (fewer particles than water); if the serum osmolality is greater than 295 mOsm/kg, the body fluid is hyperosmolar (more particles, less water). Hypo-osmolality of body fluid may be the result of excess water intake or fluid overload (edema) caused by an inability to excrete excess water. Hyperosmolality of body fluid could be caused by severe diarrhea, increased salt and solutes (protein) intake, inadequate water intake, diabetes, ketoacidosis, or sweating.

Osmolality and Tonicity

The terms osmolality and **tonicity** have been used interchangeably, and although they are similar, they are different. Osmolality is the concentration of body fluids, and tonicity is the effect of fluid on cellular volume. Increased osmolality (hyperosmolality) can result from impermeable solutes such as sodium and permeable solutes such as urea (BUN). Hypertonicity results from an increase of impermeable solutes such as sodium but *not* of permeable solutes such as BUN. Hyperosmolality of body fluid occurs with increased serum sodium and BUN levels; however, it may also cause isotonicity because BUN does not affect tonicity. Serum osmolality is a better indicator of the concentration of solutes in body fluids than tonicity. Tonicity is used primarily as a measurement of the concentration of intravenous (IV) solutions.

Fluid Replacement

Intravenous Solutions

With fluid volume deficit from the extracellular body compartment, there is a loss of fluid from the interstitial (tissue) spaces and from the vascular (blood vessel) spaces. IV fluids in various concentrations are available to replace body fluid loss. The tonicities of many IV fluids are similar to serum osmolality, with the exception that the tonicity of solutions is wider. The average serum osmolality is 290 mOsm/kg water. For an IV solution, the isotonicity range is 240 to 340 mOsm/L. This is determined by using a factor of 50: subtract 50 from 290 mOsm to equal 240, and add 50 to 290 to equal 340. If the tonicity of the IV solution is less than 240 mOsm, it is a hypotonic solution; if it is greater than 340 mOsm, it is a hypertonic solution. Isotonic solutions include dextrose 5% in water (D_5W), which has 250 mOsm;

normal saline solution or 0.9% sodium chloride (NaCl), which has 310 mOsm; lactated Ringer's solution, which has 275 mOsm; and Ringer's solution, which has 310 mOsm. These isotonic solutions have osmolalities similar to the ECFs and intracellular fluids. With fluid volume loss, isotonic IV solutions are usually indicated.

Dextrose in water, when used continuously or administered rapidly, becomes a hypotonic solution instead of an isotonic solution. The dextrose is rapidly metabolized to water and carbon dioxide (CO_2). Five percent dextrose in water (D_5W) should only be given IV and never subcutaneously (subQ). Normal saline solution or an isotonic solution of dextrose and saline may be administered subcutaneously.

The following are the four classifications of IV solutions used for fluid replacements:
- Crystalloids
- Colloids
- Blood and blood products
- Lipids

Crystalloids include dextrose, saline, and lactated Ringer's solutions. This group of solutions is used for replacement and maintenance fluid therapy.

Colloids are volume expanders that include dextran solutions, amino acids, hetastarch, and Plasmanate. Dextran is not a substitute for whole blood because it does not have any products that can carry oxygen. Dextran 40 tends to interfere with platelet function and can prolong bleeding time. Hetastarch is a nonantigenic volume expander and lasts for more than 24 hours, but it may persist for weeks in the body. Hetastarch is an isotonic solution (310 mOsm/L) that can decrease platelet and hematocrit counts and is contraindicated for clients with bleeding disorders, congestive heart failure (CHF), and renal dysfunction. Plasmanate is a commercially prepared protein product that is used instead of plasma or albumin to replace body protein.

Blood and blood products are whole blood, packed red blood cells (RBCs), plasma, and albumin. A unit of packed RBCs contains whole blood without plasma. The advantages for using packed cells instead of whole blood are that there is a decreased chance for causing circulatory overload, a smaller risk of a reaction to plasma antigens, and a possible reduction in the risk of transmitting serum hepatitis. Whole blood should not be used to correct anemia unless the anemia is severe. A unit of whole blood elevates the hemoglobin by 0.5 to 1 g, and a unit of packed RBCs elevates the hematocrit by three points.

Lipids are administered as fat emulsion solution and are usually indicated when IV therapy lasts longer than 5 days. Lipids add to balancing the client's nutritional needs. Total parenteral nutrition (TPN) or hyperalimentation (HA) is normally implemented for clients who require long-term IV therapy. TPN is discussed in Chapter 16, Nutritional Support.

See **evolve**, the online resource, for a table of various IV solutions in the four classifications, listed according to their tonicity, caloric and electrolyte compositions, and general comments.

Daily water requirements differ according to age and medical problems. The approximate daily water need for a client weighing 70 kg is 30 ml per kg of body weight, or 2000 ml per day. In pounds, the calculation is 15 ml per pound. A client weighing 150 pounds should receive 2250 ml of water daily. If the client has a fever, water needs increase by 15%. A client loses water daily: 400 to 500 ml through skin by normal evaporation, 400 to 500 ml from breathing, 100 to 200 ml in feces, and 1000 to 1200 ml in urine.

When IV fluids are prescribed for 24 hours, the total amount ordered is usually 2000 to 3000 ml. Normally, there is more than one type of solution used. Three liters of D_5W per day causes a hypo-osmolar body fluid state, and water intoxication (intracellular fluid volume excess) can occur. If hypertonic IV solutions such as dextrose in normal saline solution only are used, dehydration can occur as a result of hyperosmolality, which pulls fluid from the cells and promotes fluid excretion. Usually one or two isotonic solutions (this could include D_5W) and one or two hypertonic solutions are administered per day.

Nursing Process

Fluid Replacement

ASSESSMENT

- Assess vital signs and use for future baseline values. Report abnormal findings.
- Check client's laboratory findings, especially the hematocrit and blood urea nitrogen (BUN). If both values are elevated, this may be because of fluid volume deficit (dehydration). If the BUN is >60 mg/dl, renal impairment is most likely the cause.
- Determine urine output. Report if the urine output is <25 ml/h or 600 ml/day. Normal urine output should be >35 ml/hr or 1000 to 1200 ml/day.
- Obtain urine specific gravity (SG). Normal range is 1.005 to 1.030. If the urine specific gravity is >1.030, hypovolemia or dehydration may be the cause.
- Check the types of IV fluid ordered per day. Report to the health care provider if there is continuous use of one type of IV fluid such as 5% dextrose in water (D_5W). This could cause hypo-osmolality of body fluid.
- Record client's weight for a baseline level.

NURSING DIAGNOSES

- Risk for fluid volume excess related to excess volume infused, rapidly infused IV fluids, or volume infused too great for client's physical size or condition
- Risk for deficient fluid volume related to inadequate fluid intake
- Ineffective tissue perfusion (vascular) related to decreased blood circulation or inadequate fluid replacement
- Deficient knowledge

PLANNING

- Client will not develop fluid volume deficit or excess as the result of IV fluid replacement.
- Client will be hydrated; vital signs and urine output will be within the normal ranges.

NURSING INTERVENTIONS

- Monitor vital signs and report abnormal findings. Rapid pulse rate could be indicative of hypovolemia (decrease in body fluids). Blood pressure changes should be reported. Decrease in blood pressure occurs when hypovolemia is severe and shock is occurring.
- Monitor urine output. Report if the urine output is less than 600 ml/day. This could be caused by fluid volume deficit or congestive heart failure from fluid overload.
- Measure weight daily. A gain of 2.2 to 2.5 pounds is equivalent to 1 L of fluid. If the client gained 5 pounds in one day, it may indicate that client is retaining 2 L of fluid. This could be a sign of fluid overload.
- Check for signs and symptoms of fluid volume deficit (dehydration) such as excess thirst (mild dehydration). Marked thirst, dry mucous membranes, poor skin turgor, decrease in urine output, tachycardia, and slight decrease in systolic blood pressure are indicators of marked dehydration.
- Observe for signs and symptoms of fluid volume excess (fluid overload) such as constant, irritated cough; dyspnea; neck vein engorgement; hand vein engorgement; and moist rales in the lung.
- Monitor laboratory results daily, especially BUN, hemoglobin, and hematocrit. Elevated values can indicate dehydration.
- Monitor the types of fluids client is receiving. Report if only one type of IV fluid is being prescribed daily. This can cause fluid imbalance (hypo-osmolality or hyperosmolality).
- Check IV injection site for infiltration or phlebitis.

Client Teaching

- Instruct client that thirst means there is a mild fluid deficit. Increasing fluid intake is important. Older clients' thirst mechanisms are frequently decreased. The nurse should offer fluids as needed to older adults.
- Advise client to report frequent vomiting or diarrhea. When vomiting and diarrhea occur constantly or over several days, severe fluid volume imbalance can result.
- Encourage client to monitor fluid intake and output. Inform client to report abnormal findings such as diuresis, weight gain or loss, peripheral edema, or tight shoes and rings to the health care provider.

- Use an interpreter as appropriate.
- Involve the extended family in health teaching and support.
- Incorporate wise food choices that are culturally acceptable.

EVALUATION

■ Evaluate that the IV therapy has replaced client's body fluids.

■ Evaluate that the IV therapy has not caused a deficit or an excess of client's body fluids.

Electrolytes

Potassium

Potassium (K⁺), an important cellular cation, is 20 times more prevalent in the cells (ICF) than in the vessels (intravascular fluid, or plasma). The normal plasma or serum level (these terms are frequently used interchangeably) for potassium is 3.5 to 5.3 milliequivalents per liter (mEq/L). A serum potassium level less than 3.5 mEq/L is called **hypokalemia,** and a serum potassium level greater than 5.3 mEq/L is called **hyperkalemia.** Potassium has a narrow normal range. Too little potassium (hypokalemia), less than 2.5 mEq/L, or too much potassium (hyperkalemia), more than 7.0 mEq/L, may lead to cardiac arrest.

Potassium is poorly stored in the body, so daily potassium intake is necessary. The recommended potassium intake is approximately 40 to 60 mEq daily, consumed in such foods as fruits, fruit juices, and vegetables, or in the form of potassium supplements. Bananas and dried fruits are higher in potassium content than oranges and fruit juices.

Functions

Potassium is necessary for the transmission and conduction of nerve impulses and for the contraction of skeletal, cardiac, and smooth muscles. It is also needed for the enzyme action used to change carbohydrates to energy (glycolysis) and amino acids to protein. Potassium promotes glycogen (energy) storage in hepatic (liver) cells. It also helps in the regulation of osmolality (solute concentration) of cellular fluids.

Hypokalemia

Whenever cells are damaged from trauma, injury, surgery, or shock, potassium leaks from the cells into the intravascular fluid and is excreted by the kidneys. With cellular loss of potassium, potassium shifts from the blood plasma into the cell to restore the cellular potassium balance; thus hypokalemia usually results. Vomiting and diarrhea also decrease serum potassium levels. Between 80% and 90% of potassium in the body is excreted in the urine; 8% is excreted in the feces. If the kidneys shut down or are dis-

eased, potassium accumulates in the intravascular fluid and hyperkalemia results.

When the serum potassium level is between 3.0 and 3.5 mEq/L, 100 to 200 mEq of potassium chloride (KCl) is needed to increase the serum potassium level 1 mEq (e.g., 3.0 to 4.0 mEq). If the serum potassium level is less than 3.0 mEq/L, then 200 to 400 mEq of KCl is needed to increase the serum potassium level 1 mEq. Administering potassium chloride cannot rapidly correct a severe potassium deficit.

Potassium can be given orally or IV and is combined with an anion, such as chloride or bicarbonate. Oral potassium can be given as a liquid, powder, or tablet. Potassium is extremely irritating to the gastric and intestinal mucosa, so *it must be given with at least a half glass of fluid* (juice or water) or, preferably, a full glass of fluid. Because cardiac arrest (standstill) results from excessive potassium, IV potassium *must be diluted* in IV fluids—it cannot be given as an IV push or IV bolus. Nurses must remember that, when administering any type of potassium, *it must be diluted.* Table 15–3 lists the potassium preparations used to treat hypokalemia.

Signs and symptoms of hypokalemia include nausea and vomiting, dysrhythmias, abdominal distention, and soft, flabby muscles. If the serum potassium level is a low normal, foods high in potassium should be suggested, such as fruit juices, citrus fruits, dried fruits, bananas, nuts (peanut butter), some sodas and tea, and vegetables such as potatoes, broccoli, and green leafy vegetables.

Certain drugs promote potassium loss, such as potassium-wasting diuretics (hydrochlorothiazide [HydroDiuril], furosemide [Lasix], ethacrynic acid [Edecrin]) and

Table 15–3

Potassium Supplements

Preparation	Drug
Oral liquid	potassium chloride: 10% = 20 mEq/15 ml, 20% = 40 mEq/15 ml
	Kay Ciel (potassium chloride)
	Kaochlor 10% (potassium chloride)
	Kaon-Cl 20% (potassium chloride)
	potassium triplex: potassium acetate, bicarbonate, citrate. Rarely used.
Oral tablet or capsule	potassium chloride (enteric-coated tablet)
	Kaon (potassium gluconate)
	Kaon-Cl (potassium chloride)
	Slow-K (potassium chloride), 8 mEq
	Kaochlor (potassium chloride)
	K-Lyte (potassium bicarbonate), effervescent tablet
	K-Lyte/Cl (potassium chloride)
	K-Dur (potassium chloride)
	Micro-K (potassium chloride)
	Ten-K (potassium chloride)
	K-Tab (potassium chloride)
Intravenous potassium	potassium chloride in clear liquid in multidose vial or ampule (2 mEq/ml)

cortisone preparations. Clients receiving these drugs should increase their potassium intake by consuming foods rich in potassium or by taking potassium supplements. Their serum potassium levels should be monitored for abnormal serum potassium levels. Potassium must be used cautiously in clients with renal insufficiency. If the urine output is less than 600 ml per day, the health care provider should be notified, especially if a potassium supplement is ordered.

Prototype Drug Chart 15–1 compares the pharmacokinetics and pharmacodynamics of oral and IV potassium preparations. The nursing process is based on the drug data.

Pharmacokinetics

Oral liquid potassium is absorbed faster than tablets or capsules; the pharmaceutic phase is decreased. Sustained-release capsules such as Micro-K, Slow-K, and K-tab release the potassium over a period of time. Plenty of water—no less than 4 ounces—must be taken with oral potassium prepara-

tions. The capsule may be taken with a meal or immediately after eating. IV potassium is immediately absorbed in the vascular fluids. IV potassium must be diluted in IV solutions and *never* given as a bolus or an IV push. REMEMBER: 80% to 90% of the potassium in body fluids is excreted in the urine; 8% is excreted in feces. Renal function should be monitored.

Pharmacodynamics

Potassium maintains neuromuscular activity. Onset of action of oral potassium may be within 30 minutes; for IV potassium, it is immediate. Duration of action of potassium is not known; however, it may vary according to the dose taken. An electrocardiogram (ECG) and serum potassium levels should be closely monitored when large doses are administered.

Hyperkalemia

Hyperkalemia usually results from renal insufficiency or from the administration of large doses of potassium over time. For a mildly elevated serum potassium level, such as

---

PROTOTYPE DRUG CHART 15–1

POTASSIUM

Drug Class	**Dosage**
Electrolyte Trade names: Kaochlor, Kaon-Cl, Kay Ciel, Micro-K, K-Dur *Pregnancy Category:* A	*Hypokalemia (maintenance):* A: PO: 20 mEq in 1 or 2 divided doses *Hypokalemia (correction):* PO: 40-80 mEq in 3 or 4 divided doses A: IV: 20-40 mEq diluted in 1 L of IV solution
Contraindications	**Drug-Lab-Food Interactions**
Renal insufficiency or failure, Addison's disease, hyperkalemia, severe dehydration, acidosis, potassium-sparing diuretics *Caution:* Cardiac disorders, burns	**Drug:** *Increase* serum potassium level with ACE inhibitors, potassium-sparing diuretics, NSAIDs, potassium-sparing diuretics, beta adrenergic blockers, heparin, salt substitutes. **Lab:** May *increase* serum potassium level (>5.5 mEq/L) **Food:** None known
Pharmacokinetics	**Pharmacodynamics**
Absorption: PO: rapidly absorbed, 95% in body fluids **Distribution:** PB: UK **Metabolism:** t½: UK **Excretion:** 80%-90% in urine; 10% in feces	**PO:** Onset: 30 min Peak: 1-2 h Duration: UK **IV:** Onset: Rapid Peak: 1-1.5 h Duration: UK

Therapeutic Effects/Uses

To correct potassium deficit; strengthen cardiac and muscular activities; prevent hypokalemia in at-risk clients.
Mode of Action: Transmits and conducts nerve impulses; contracts skeletal, smooth, and cardiac muscles.

Side Effects	**Adverse Reactions**
Nausea, vomiting, diarrhea, abdominal cramps, irritability, rash (rare); phlebitis with IV administration	Hyperkalemia (elders with renal impairment); oliguria, ECG changes (peaked T waves, widened QRS complex, prolonged PR interval), GI ulceration **Life-threatening:** Cardiac dysrhythmias, respiratory distress, cardiac arrest

A, Adult; *ACE,* angiotensin-converting enzyme; *ECG,* electrocardiogram; *GI,* gastrointestinal; *h,* hour; *IV,* intravenous; *PB,* protein-binding; *PO,* by mouth; *t½,* half-life; *UK,* unknown; >, greater than.

5.3 to 5.5 mEq/L, restricting foods rich in potassium may correct the excess potassium level. If renal insufficiency or failure is present, additional measures must be taken.

Drugs that might be ordered for hyperkalemia (serum potassium >5.3 mEq/L) are listed in Table 15–4. To decrease immediately a temporary potassium excess in the serum potassium level, sodium bicarbonate, calcium gluconate, or insulin and glucose may be prescribed. Sodium polystyrene sulfonate (Kayexalate) with sorbitol is ordered for severe hyperkalemia. This drug therapy exchanges a sodium ion for a potassium ion in the body and is a more permanent means of correcting hyperkalemia.

Signs and symptoms of hyperkalemia include nausea, abdominal cramps, oliguria (decreased urine output), tachycardia and later bradycardia, weakness, and numb-ness or tingling in the extremities. For mild hyperkalemia, foods rich in potassium are usually restricted.

Effect of Drugs on Potassium Balance

Potassium-wasting diuretics are a major cause of hypokalemia. Diuretics are divided into two categories: potassium-wasting and potassium-sparing drugs. Potassium-wasting diuretics excrete potassium and other electrolytes such as sodium and chloride in the urine. Potassium-sparing diuretics retain potassium but excrete sodium and chloride in the urine. Table 15–5 lists the trade and generic names of potassium-wasting and potassium-sparing diuretics and combined potassium-wasting/potassium-sparing diuretics.

Table 15–4

Correction of Potassium Excess (Hyperkalemia)

Treatment Methods	Rationale
Potassium restriction	Restriction of potassium intake will slowly lower the serum level. For mild hyperkalemia (slightly elevated K levels) (i.e., 5.4-5.6 mEq/L, potassium restriction is normally effective).
Intravenous sodium bicarbonate (NaHCO$_3$)	By elevating the pH level, potassium moves back into the cells, thus lowering the serum level. This is a temporary treatment.
10% calcium gluconate	Calcium decreases the irritability of the myocardium resulting from hyperkalemia. It is a temporary treatment and does not promote K loss. *Caution:* Administering calcium to a client on digitalis can cause digitalis toxicity.
Insulin and glucose (10%-50%)	The combination of insulin and glucose moves potassium back into the cells. It is a temporary treatment, effective for approximately 6 h and is not always as effective when repeated.
Kayexalate (sodium polystyrene) and sorbitol 70%	Kayexalate is used as a cation exchange for severe hyperkalemia and can be administered orally or rectally. Approximate dosages are as follows: *Orally:* Kayexalate—10-20 g 3 to 4 times daily Sorbitol 70%—20 ml with each dose *Rectally:* Kayexalate—30-50 g Sorbitol 70%—50 ml; mix with 100-150 ml water (Retention enema—20-30 min)

From Kee JL, Paulanka BJ, Purnell LD: *Fluids and electrolytes with clinical applications,* ed 7, New York, 2004, Delmar.
h, Hour; *min,* minute.

Table 15–5

Potassium-Wasting and Potassium-Sparing Diuretics

Potassium-Wasting Diuretics	Potassium-Sparing Diuretics
Thiazides	Aldosterone antagonist
Chlorothiazide/Diuril	Spironolactone/Aldactone
Hydrochlorothiazide/	Triamterene/Dyrenium
HydroDIURIL	Amiloride/Midamor
Loop diuretics	
Furosemide/Lasix	**Combination: K-Wasting**
Ethacrynic acid/Edecrin	**and K-Sparing Diuretics**
Carbonic anhydrase	Aldactazide
inhibitors	Spironazide
Acetazolamide/Diamox	Dyazide
Osmotic diuretic	Moduretic
Mannitol	

From Kee JL, Paulanka BJ, Purnell LD: *Fluids and electrolytes with clinical applications,* ed 7, New York, 2004, Delmar.

Nursing Process

Electrolyte: Potassium

ASSESSMENT

■ Assess for signs and symptoms of hypokalemia (decreased serum potassium) and hyperkalemia (elevated serum potassium). Symptoms of hypokalemia include nausea, vomiting, cardiac dysrhythmias, abdominal distention, and soft flabby muscles. Symptoms of hyperkalemia include oliguria, nausea, abdominal cramps, and tachycardia and, later, bradycardia, weakness, and numbness or tingling in the extremities.

■ Assess serum potassium level; normal serum potassium level is 3.5 to 5.3 mEq/L. Report serum potassium deficit or excess to the health care provider.

■ Obtain baseline vital sign (VS) and electrocardiograph (ECG) readings. Report abnormal findings. The VS and ECG results can be compared with future VS and ECG readings.

■ Check client for signs and symptoms of digitalis toxicity when receiving a digitalis preparation (digoxin) and a potassium-wasting diuretic (hydrochlorothiazide, furosemide) or a cortisone preparation (prednisone). A decreased serum potassium level enhances the action of digitalis. Signs and symptoms of digitalis toxicity are nausea, vomiting, anorexia, bradycardia (pulse rate <60 or markedly decreased), cardiac dysrhythmias, and visual disturbances.

NURSING DIAGNOSES

■ Imbalanced nutrition, less than body requirements
■ Impaired tissue integrity
■ Deficient knowledge

PLANNING

■ Client's serum potassium level will be within normal range in 2 to 4 days.
■ Client with hypokalemia will eat foods rich in potassium, such as fruits, fruit juices, and vegetables. Client with hyperkalemia will avoid potassium-rich foods.

NURSING INTERVENTIONS

■ Give oral potassium with a sufficient amount of water or juice (at least 6 to 8 ounces) or at mealtime. Potassium is extremely irritating to the gastric mucosa.

■ Dilute IV potassium chloride in the IV bag and invert the bag several times to promote thorough mixing of potassium with IV fluids. Potassium *cannot* be given IM. *Potassium should never be given as an IV bolus or push.* Giving IV potassium directly into the vein causes cardiac dysrhythmias and cardiac arrest.

■ Check the amount of urine output. If client is receiving potassium and the urine output is <25 ml/h or <600 ml/d, potassium accumulation occurs. REMEMBER: 80% to 90% of potassium is excreted in the urine. Report results to the health care provider.

■ Determine the serum potassium level. Hypokalemia occurs if the serum potassium value is <3.5 mEq/L; hyperkalemia occurs when the serum potassium value is >5.3 mEq/L.

■ Monitor the ECG. With hypokalemia, the T wave is flat or inverted, the ST segment is depressed, and the QT interval is prolonged. With hyperkalemia, the T wave is narrow and peaked, the QRS complex is spread, and the PR interval is prolonged.

■ Check the IV site for infiltration if client is receiving potassium in the IV fluids. Potassium can cause tissue necrosis if it infiltrates into the fatty tissue (subcutaneous tissue). The IV fluid with potassium should be discontinued when infiltration occurs.

■ Monitor clients receiving various medications for hyperkalemia (e.g., sodium bicarbonate, calcium gluconate, insulin and glucose, sodium polystyrene sulfonate [Kayexalate], sorbitol) for signs and symptoms of continuing hyperkalemia or of developing hypokalemia.

■ Prepare and administer sodium polystyrene sulfonate (Kayexalate) orally or by retention enema, according to the drug circular. Client should have a cleansing enema before the retention enema. A suggested method for preparation and administration of sodium polystyrene sulfonate (Kayexalate) retention enema is as follows:

1. Use warm fluid to prepare (do not heat).
2. Mix with 20% dextrose in water or sorbitol.
3. Keep particles in suspension by stirring periodically and administer at body temperature by gravity.
4. Encourage client to retain the enema for a minimum of 30 to 60 minutes.
5. Flush tubing with 50 to 100 ml of fluid before clamping for retention.
6. After completion, irrigate the colon with 2 quarts of flushing liquid and drain the fluid contents.

Client Teaching

General

• Advise client to have the serum potassium level checked at regular intervals when taking drugs that are potassium supplements or that decrease potassium levels.
• Instruct client to drink a full glass of water or juice when taking oral potassium supplements. Potassium preparations can be taken during or after a meal. Explain to client that potassium is very irritating to the stomach.
• Encourage client to comply with the prescribed potassium dose, regular laboratory tests, and medical follow-up related to the health problem and drug regimen.

Diet

• Instruct client who is taking a potassium-wasting diuretic or a cortisone preparation to eat potassium-rich foods, including citrus fruit juice, fruits (bananas, plums, oranges, cantaloupes, raisins), vegetables, and nuts.

Side Effects

• Instruct client to report signs and symptoms of hypokalemia and hyperkalemia (see Assessment for the list). When taking large amounts of potassium supplements, hyperkalemia could result.

Cultural Considerations ⊕

• Use an interpreter as appropriate.
• Involve the extended family in health teaching and support.
• Incorporate wise food choices that are culturally acceptable.

EVALUATION

■ Evaluate client's serum potassium level and ECG. Report to the health care provider if the level remains abnormal. Potassium replacements and diet may need modification.

Laxatives, corticosteroids, antibiotics, and potassium-wasting diuretics are the major drug groups that can cause hypokalemia. The drug groups that may cause hyperkalemia include oral and IV potassium salts, central nervous system (CNS) agents, and potassium-sparing diuretics. Table 15–6 lists the drugs that affect potassium balance.

Sodium

Sodium is the major cation in the ECF (vessels and tissue spaces). The normal serum or plasma sodium level is 135 to 145 mEq/L. A serum sodium level less than 135 mEq/L

is called **hyponatremia**, and a serum sodium level greater than 145 mEq/L is called **hypernatremia**.

Functions

Sodium is the major electrolyte that regulates body fluids. It promotes the transmission and conduction of nerve impulses. It is part of the sodium/potassium pump that causes cellular activity. Sodium shifts into cells as potassium shifts out of the cells, repeatedly, to maintain water balance and neuromuscular activity. When sodium shifts into the cell, depolarization occurs; when sodium shifts out of the cell, potassium shifts back into the cell and repolarization occurs. Sodium combines readily with chloride (Cl^-) or bicarbonate (HCO_3^-) to promote acid-base balance.

Hyponatremia

Sodium loss can result from vomiting, diarrhea, surgery, and potent diuretics. Signs and symptoms of hyponatremia include muscular weakness, headaches, abdominal

Table 15–6

Drugs Affecting Potassium Balance

Potassium Imbalance	Substances	Rationale
Hypokalemia (serum potassium deficit)	Laxatives	Laxative abuse can cause potassium depletion.
	Enemas (hyperosmolar)	
	Corticosteroids	
	Cortisone	Ion-exchange agent.
	Prednisone	Steroids promote potassium loss and sodium retention.
	Kayexalate	Exchange potassium ion for a sodium ion.
	Licorice	Licorice action is similar to aldosterone, promoting K loss and Na retention.
	Levodopa/L-dopa	Increases potassium loss via urine.
	Lithium	
	Antibiotic I	
	Amphotericin B	Toxic effect on renal tubules, thus decreasing potassium reabsorption.
	Polymyxin B	
	Tetracycline (outdated)	
	Gentamicin	
	Neomycin	
	Amikacin	
	Tobramycin	
	Cisplatin	
	Antibiotic II	
	Penicillin	Potassium excretion is enhanced by the presence of non-reabsorbable anions.
	Ampicillin	
	Carbenicillin	
	Ticarcillin	
	Nafcillin	
	Piperacillin	
	Azlocillin	
	Alpha-adrenergic blockers	These agents promote movement of potassium into cells, thus lowering the serum potassium level.
	Insulin and glucose	
	Beta$_2$-agonists	Beta$_2$ agonists promote potassium loss.
	Terbutaline	
	Albuterol	
	Estrogen	
	Potassium-wasting diuretics	See Table 15–5

From Kee JL, Paulanka BJ, Purnell LD: *Fluids and electrolytes with clinical applications*, ed 7, New York, 2004, Delmar.

cramps, nausea, and vomiting. The serum sodium level should be monitored as necessary.

For a serum sodium level between 125 and 135 mEq/L, normal saline (0.9% sodium chloride) may increase the sodium content in the vascular fluid. If the serum sodium level is 115 mEq/L, a hypertonic, 3% saline solution may be necessary.

Hypernatremia

When the serum sodium level is elevated above 145 mEq/L, sodium restriction is indicated. Signs and symptoms of hypernatremia are flushed skin, elevated body temperature and blood pressure, and rough, dry tongue. An increase in serum sodium can result from consuming certain drugs, such as cortisone preparations, cough medications, and selected antibiotics.

Nursing Process

Electrolyte: Sodium

ASSESSMENT

■ Assess client for signs and symptoms of hyponatremia and hypernatremia. See signs and symptoms in this chapter.
■ Check the serum sodium level. Report abnormally low sodium levels (<125 mEq/L), because prompt medical care is required.
■ Obtain history of health problems that may lead to sodium loss or excess.

Table 15–6

Drugs Affecting Potassium Balance—cont'd

Potassium Imbalance	Substances	Rationale
Hyperkalemia (serum potassium excess)	Potassium chloride (oral or IV) Potassium salt substitutes K penicillin KPO₄ enema	Excess ingestion or infusion of these agents can cause a potassium excess.
	Angiotensin-converting enzyme (ACE) inhibitors Captopril (Capoten) Quinapril HCl (Accupril) Ramipril (Altace) and others	Increase the state of hypoaldosteronism (decrease sodium and increase potassium) and impair renal potassium excretion.
	Angiotensin II receptor antagonists Losartan potassium (Cozaar)	Decrease adrenal synthesis of aldosterone; potassium is retained and sodium excreted.
	Beta-adrenergic blockers Propranolol (Inderal) Nadolol (Corgard) and others	Decrease cellular uptake of potassium and decrease Na-K-ATPase function.
	Digoxin	Therapeutic dose is not affected; however, with overdose, potassium excess may occur.
	Heparin (>10,000 units/d) Low-molecular-weight heparin (LMWH)	Inhibits adrenal aldosterone production. Decreases potassium homeostasis; renal excretion of potassium is reduced.
	Immunosuppressive drugs Cyclosporine Tacrolimus Cyclophosphamide	Reduce potassium excretion by induction of hypoaldosteronism; loss of potassium from cells.
	Nonsteroidal anti-inflammatory drugs (NSAIDs) Ibuprofens and others Indomethacin	Impair potassium homeostasis and block cellular potassium uptake.
	Succinylcholine: intravenous	Allows for leakage of potassium out of cells.
	CNS agents Barbiturates Sedatives Narcotics Heroin Amphetamines	These CNS agents are usually characterized by muscle necrosis and cellular shift of potassium from cells to serum.
	Potassium-sparing diuretics	See Table 15–5.

ATPase, Adenosine triphosphate; *CNS,* central nervous system; *d,* day; *IV,* intravenous.

NURSING DIAGNOSES

■ Risk for imbalanced (excess) fluid volume related to water retention
■ Deficient knowledge

PLANNING

■ Client's serum sodium level will be within normal range in 3 to 5 days.
■ Edema will be decreased in client with sodium retention.

NURSING INTERVENTIONS

■ Monitor the medical regimen for correction of hyponatremia, such as water restriction, IV normal saline (0.9% sodium chloride), and 3% saline solution to correct a serum sodium level of <115 mEq/L.
■ Monitor serum sodium levels. Report abnormal level.

Client Teaching

• Instruct client with hypernatremia to avoid foods rich in sodium, such as canned foods, lunch meats, ham, pork, pickles, potato chips, and pretzels. Instruct the client to avoid using salt when cooking or adding salt to food at the table.
• Emphasize the importance of reading labels on food products.

Cultural Considerations (⊕)

• Use an interpreter as appropriate.
• Involve the extended family in health teaching and support.
• Incorporate wise food choices that are culturally acceptable.

EVALUATION

■ Evaluate client's serum sodium level. Report if sodium imbalance continues.

Calcium

Calcium is found in approximately equal proportion in the ICF and ECF. The serum calcium range is 4.5 to 5.5 mEq/L, or 8.5 to 10.5 (9 to 11) mg/dl. A calcium deficit, less than 4.5 mEq/L, is called **hypocalcemia,** and a calcium excess, greater than 5.5 mEq/L, is called **hypercalcemia.** About half of the calcium in the body fluid is bound to protein. Calcium that is unbound to protein is free, ionized calcium and can cause a physiologic response. If the serum protein (albumin) levels are decreased, there is more free circulating calcium even when the serum calcium level is decreased.

Modern blood analyzers allow the ionized calcium (iCa) level to be measured. The normal serum iCa range is

2.2 to 2.5 mEq/L, or 4.25 to 5.25 mg/dl. Certain changes in the blood composition can either increase or decrease the serum iCa level. When an individual is acidotic, calcium is released from the serum protein and increases the serum iCa level. During alkalosis, calcium is bound to protein and there is less iCa.

Functions

Calcium promotes normal nerve and muscle activity. It increases contraction of the heart muscle (myocardium). This cation also maintains normal cellular permeability and promotes blood clotting by converting prothrombin into thrombin. In addition, calcium is needed for the formation of bone and teeth.

Vitamin D is needed for calcium absorption from the GI tract. Aspirin and anticonvulsants can alter vitamin D, affecting calcium absorption. Loop or high-ceiling diuretics (furosemide [Lasix]; see Chapter 41, Diuretics), steroids (cortisone), magnesium preparations, and phosphate preparations promote calcium loss. Conversely, thiazide diuretics (hydrochlorothiazide [HydroDiuril]) increase the serum calcium level.

Hypocalcemia

Inadequate calcium intake causes calcium to leave the bone to maintain a normal serum calcium level. Fractures may occur if calcium deficit persists because of calcium loss from the bones (bone demineralization). Hypoparathyroidism, vitamin D deficiency, and multiple blood transfusions are causes of hypocalcemia.

Signs and symptoms of hypocalcemia include anxiety, irritability, and tetany (twitching around the mouth, tingling and numbness of fingers, carpopedal spasm, spasmodic contractions, laryngeal spasm, and convulsions). If metabolic acidosis is present with hypocalcemia, tetany symptoms are absent because calcium leaves protein sites during an acidotic state; thus more ionized calcium is available. During an alkalotic state, more calcium binds with protein. There is less ionized calcium, and tetany symptoms usually occur.

Many calcium preparations can be administered orally or IV. For treatment of calcium deficit, oral calcium tablets, capsules, or powder and IV calcium solutions may be given. Calcium preparations are combined with various salts, such as chloride, carbonate, gluconate, gluceptate, and lactate. Calcium for IV use should be mixed with D_5W and *not mixed* in a saline solution. Sodium encourages calcium loss. Prototype Drug Chart 15–2 compares the pharmacokinetics and pharmacodynamics of calcium preparations.

Pharmacokinetics

Vitamin D promotes calcium absorption from the GI tract; phosphorus inhibits calcium absorption. The pH affects the amount of circulating, free ionized calcium. When pH is decreased (acidic), there is more free calcium because it has been released from protein-binding sites. With an increased pH (alkalosis) more calcium is bound to protein.

PROTOTYPE DRUG CHART 15–2

CALCIUM

Drug Class

Electrolyte
Trade names:
calcium carbonate (Os-cal, Tums, Caltrate, Megacal)
calcium gluconate (Kalcinate)
Pregnancy Category: C
Drug Forms: Tablet, capsule, liquid, injection

Dosage

Antacid use:
A: PO: 0.5-1 g q4-6h (dose varies according to the
  calcium salt)
Osteoporosis:
A: PO: 1200 mg/d
Tetany:
A: IV: 4-16 mEq
C: IV: 0.5-0.7 mEq/kg t.i.d., q.i.d.
Hypocalcemia:
A: PO: 500 mg/d in divided doses

Contraindications

Hypercalcemia, renal calculi, digitalis toxicity,
  ventricular fibrillation
Caution: Renal or respiratory disorders, GI hypomotility

Drug-Lab-Food Interactions

Drug: *Increase* digitalis toxicity: digoxin; *decrease* calcium
  effect: saline solution; *decrease* effect of calcium channel blockers, verapamil; *decrease* absorption of tetracycline; *increase* serum calcium level: thiazide diuretics
Lab: May increase calcium gastrin, pH; may decrease
  phosphate, potassium
Food: None known

Pharmacokinetics

Absorption: PO: 35% absorbed, requires vitamin D
Distribution: PB: UK
Metabolism: t½: UK
Excretion: 20% in urine, 70% in feces, some in saliva

Pharmacodynamics

PO: Onset: UK
  Peak: UK
  Duration: 2-4 h
IV: Onset: Rapid
  Peak: UK
  Duration: 2-3 h

Therapeutic Effects/Uses

To correct calcium deficit or tetany symptoms, prevent osteoporosis
Mode of Action: Transmits nerve impulses, contracts skeletal and cardiac muscles, maintains cellular permeability; promotes strong bone and teeth growth

Side Effects

PO: Nausea, vomiting, constipation, pain, drowsiness,
  headache, muscle weakness

Adverse Reactions

Hypercalcemia, ECG changes (shortened QT interval),
  metabolic alkalosis, heart block, rebound hyperacidity
Life-threatening: Renal failure, cardiac dysrhythmias,
  cardiac arrest

A, Adult; *C,* child; *d,* day; *ECG,* electrocardiogram; *GI,* gastrointestinal; *h,* hour; *IV,* intravenous; *PB,* protein-binding; *PO,* by mouth;
q.i.d., four times a day; *t½,* half-life; *t.i.d.,* three times a day; *UK,* unknown.

Pharmacodynamics

A calcium deficit causes tetany symptoms and, if severe, can be life-threatening. Rapid administration of IV calcium may cause tingling, warm sensations, and a metallic taste. Calcium needs to be administered at a moderate rate, and infiltration should be avoided. Calcium can be given
undiluted IV in emergency situations.

Hypercalcemia

Elevated serum calcium may be a result of hyperparathyroidism, hypophosphatemia, tumors of the bone, prolonged immobilization, multiple fractures, and drugs such
as the thiazide diuretics. Pathologic fractures might occur

because of thinning of the bone resulting from calcium
loss from the bony structure. Calcium leaves the bone and
accumulates in the vascular fluid. Signs and symptoms of
hypercalcemia are flabby muscles, pain over bony areas,
and kidney stones of calcium composition.

Effect of Drugs on Calcium Balance

Phosphate preparations, corticosteroids, loop diuretics, aspirin, anticonvulsants, magnesium sulfate, and mithramycin
are some of the groups of drugs that can lower the serum calcium level. Excess calcium salt ingestion and infusion and

Table 15–7

Drugs Affecting Calcium Balance

Calcium Imbalance	Drugs	Rationale
Hypocalcemia (serum calcium deficit)	Magnesium sulfate Propylthiouracil/Propacil Colchicine Plicamycin/Mithracin Neomycin Excessive sodium citrate	These agents inhibit parathyroid hormone/PTH secretion and decrease the serum calcium level.

	Acetazolamide
	Aspirin
	Anticonvulsants
	Glutethimide/Doriden
	Estrogens
	Aminoglycosides
	  Gentamicin
	  Amikacin
	  Tobramycin
		These agents can alter the vitamin D metabolism that is needed for calcium absorption.

	Phosphate preparations:
	Oral, enema, and intravenous
	  Sodium phosphate
	  Potassium phosphate
		Phosphates can increase the serum phosphorus level and decrease the serum calcium level.

	Corticosteroids
	  Cortisone
	  Prednisone
		Steroids decrease calcium mobilization and inhibit the absorption of calcium.

	Loop diuretics Furosemide/Lasix	Loop diuretics reduce calcium absorption from the renal tubules.
Hypercalcemia (serum calcium excess)	Calcium salts Vitamin D	Excess ingestion of calcium and vitamin D and infusion of calcium can increase the serum Ca level.
	IV lipids	Lipids can increase the calcium level.

	Kayexalate, androgens
	Diuretics
	  Thiazides
	  Chlorthalidone/Hygroton
		These agents can induce hypercalcemia.

From Kee JL, Paulanka BJ, Purnell LD: *Fluids and electrolytes with clinical applications*, ed 7, New York, 2004, Delmar.
IV, Intravenous; *PTH*, parathyroid hormone.

thiazide and chlorthalidone diuretics are conditions that can increase the serum calcium level. Table 15–7 lists the drugs that affect calcium balance.

Clinical Management of Calcium Imbalance

Clinical management of hypocalcemia consists of oral supplements and IV calcium diluted in D_5W. Calcium should *not* be diluted in a normal saline solution (0.9% NaCl) because the sodium promotes calcium loss. Table 15–8 lists the oral and IV preparations of calcium salts, their dosages, and drug form. Calcium carbonate can cause GI upset because it produces carbon dioxide. For better calcium absorption, calcium supplements should contain vitamin D and oral calcium should be taken 30 minutes before meals. Table 15–9 gives guidelines for the suggested clinical management for hypocalcemia.

The goal for managing hypercalcemia is to correct the underlying cause of the serum calcium excess. Drugs such as calcitonin or IV saline solution administered rapidly and followed by a loop diuretic can be used to promote rapid urinary excretion of calcium.

Table 15–8

Calcium Preparations

Calcium Name	Drug Form	Drug Dose
Orals		
Calcium carbonate	650- to 1500-mg tablets	400 mg/g*
Calcium citrate	950-mg tablet	211 mg/g*
Calcium lactate	325- to 650-mg tablets	130 mg/g*
Calcium gluconate	500- to 1000-mg tablets	90 mg/g*
Intravenous		
Calcium chloride	10-ml size	272 mg/g*; 13.5 mEq
Calcium glucaptate	5-ml size	90 mg/g*; 4.5 mEq
Calcium gluconate	10-ml size	90 mg/g*; 4.5 mEq

From Kee JL, Paulanka BJ, Purnell LD: *Fluids and electrolytes with clinical applications*, ed 7, New York, 2004, Delmar.
*Elemental calcium is 1 g.

Table 15–9

Suggested Clinical Management for Hypocalcemia

Calcium Deficit	Suggested Clinical Management
Mild	Oral calcium salts with vitamin D, take twice a day.
	10% IV calcium gluconate (10 ml) in D_5W solution. Administer slowly, 1-3 ml/min.
Moderate	10% IV calcium gluconate (10-20 ml) in D_5W solution. Administer slowly, 1-3 ml/min.
Severe	10% IV calcium gluconate (100 ml) in 1 L of D_5W. Administer over 4 h.

From Kee JL, Paulanka BJ, Purnell LD: *Fluids and electrolytes with clinical applications*, ed 7, New York, 2004, Delmar.
D_5W, Dextrose 5% in water; *h*, hour; *IV*, intravenous.

Nursing Process

Electrolyte: Calcium

ASSESSMENT

■ Assess client for signs and symptoms of hypocalcemia (decreased serum calcium), such as tetany (twitching of the mouth, tingling and numbness of the fingers, facial spasms, spasms of the larynx, and carpopedal spasm), muscle cramps, bleeding tendencies, and weak cardiac contractions.

■ Check the serum calcium levels (normal, 4.5-5.5 mEq/L, or 8.5-10.5 mg/dl) for hypocalcemia and hypercalcemia. Report abnormal test results. Serum ionized calcium (iCa) (normal, 2.2-2.5 mEq/L, or 4.25-5.25 mg/dl) indicates free circulating calcium and is more accurate for determining calcium imbalance.

■ Obtain vital signs (VS) and electrocardiograph (ECG) readings. Report abnormal findings. VS and ECG results can be compared with future VS and ECG readings.

■ Gather current drug history for client. Calcium enhances the effect of digoxin. An elevated serum calcium level, when taken with digoxin, can cause digitalis toxicity. Signs and symptoms of digitalis toxicity include nausea, vomiting, anorexia, bradycardia (pulse rate <60 or markedly decreased), cardiac dysrhythmias, and visual disturbances. Thiazide diuretics can increase the serum calcium level. Drugs that decrease the effect of calcium are calcium channel blockers, tetracycline, and sodium chloride.

NURSING DIAGNOSES

■ Imbalanced nutrition, less than body requirements
■ Impaired tissue integrity
■ Deficient knowledge

PLANNING

■ Client's serum calcium level will be within normal range by 3 to 7 days.
■ Tetany symptoms will cease. Client will eat foods rich in calcium or take calcium supplements as ordered.
■ Client with hypercalcemia will avoid foods rich in calcium, such as milk products.

NURSING INTERVENTIONS

■ Monitor VS. Report abnormal findings. Compare with baseline VS. Monitor pulse rate if client is taking digoxin. Bradycardia is a sign of digitalis toxicity.

■ Administer IV fluids slowly with 10% calcium gluconate or chloride. Calcium should be administered with D_5W and not saline solution because sodium promotes calcium loss. Calcium should not be added to solutions containing bicarbonate because rapid precipitation occurs.

■ Check IV site for infiltration if client is receiving calcium in IV fluids. Calcium can cause tissue necrosis (sloughing of the tissue) if it infiltrates into the subcutaneous tissue. Calcium gluceptate is the only calcium preparation that can be given IM.

■ Monitor the serum calcium and iCa levels. Hypocalcemia occurs if the serum calcium value is <4.5 mEq/L, or <8.5 mg/dl, or if iCa is <2.2 mEq/L. Hypercalcemia occurs if the serum calcium value is >5.5 mEq/L, or >10.5 mg/dl, or if iCa is >2.5 mEq/L.

■ Monitor ECGs. With hypocalcemia, the ST segment is lengthened and the QT interval is prolonged. With hypercalcemia, the ST segment is decreased and the QT interval is shortened.

Client Teaching

General

• Instruct client to avoid overuse of antacids and to prevent the habit of chronic use of laxatives. Excessive use of certain antacids may cause alkalosis, decreasing calcium ionization. Chronic use of laxatives decreases calcium absorption from the GI tract. Suggest fruits and foods rich in fiber for improving bowel elimination.

• Encourage client taking calcium supplements to check that the calcium tablet is absorbable. To do this, put 1 tablet into 1 ounce of white vinegar. Stir every 3 minutes. The tablet should break up or dissolve within 30 minutes.

• Advise clients to take oral calcium supplements with meals or after meals to increase absorption.

Diet

• Suggest that client consume foods high in calcium, such as milk, milk products, and protein-rich foods. Protein and vitamin D are needed to enhance calcium absorption.

Side Effects
- Instruct client to report symptoms related to calcium excess or hypercalcemia, including flabby muscles, pain over bony areas, ECG changes, and kidney (calcium form) stones.

Cultural Considerations
- Use an interpreter as appropriate.
- Involve the extended family in health teaching and support.
- Incorporate wise food choices that are culturally acceptable.

EVALUATION

- Evaluate client's serum calcium level. Report if calcium imbalance continues.
- Determine whether side effects caused by previous untreated hypocalcemia are absent.

Magnesium

Magnesium, a sister cation to potassium, is most plentiful in the ICF. When there is a loss of potassium, there is also a loss of magnesium. The normal serum magnesium level is 1.5 to 2.5 mEq/L or 1.8 to 3 mg/dl. A magnesium deficit is called **hypomagnesemia,** and a magnesium excess is called **hypermagnesemia.** Daily magnesium requirement is 8 to 20 mEq.

Functions

Magnesium promotes the transmission of neuromuscular activity; it is an important mediator of neural transmission in the CNS. Like potassium, it promotes contraction of the myocardium. It activates many enzymes for the metabolism of carbohydrates and protein. It is responsible for the transportation of sodium and potassium across cell membranes.

When there is a magnesium deficit, there frequently is a potassium or calcium deficit. A serum magnesium deficit increases the release of acetylcholine from the presynaptic membrane of the nerve fiber. This increases neuromuscular excitability. A serum magnesium excess has a sedative effect on the neuromuscular system, which can result in a loss of deep tendon reflexes. Cardiac (ventricular) dysrhythmias can occur as a result of hypomagnesemia. Hypotension and heart block may result from hypermagnesemia.

Hypomagnesemia is probably the most undiagnosed electrolyte deficiency. This is most likely because hypomagnesemia is asymptomatic until the serum magnesium level approaches 1 mEq/L. The total serum magnesium concentration is not representative of the cellular magnesium levels.

To correct severe hypomagnesemia, IV magnesium sulfate may be given. For hypermagnesemia, calcium gluconate may be given to decrease the serum magnesium level.

Effect of Drugs on Magnesium Balance

Sodium inhibits tubular absorption of magnesium and calcium. Long-term administration of saline infusions may result in losses of magnesium and calcium. Diuretics, certain antibiotics, laxatives, and steroids are drug groups that promote magnesium loss. Hypomagnesemia, like hypokalemia, enhances the action of digitalis and causes digitalis toxicity. Magnesium sulfate corrects hypomagnesemia and symptoms of digitalis toxicity.

An excess intake of magnesium salts is the major cause of serum magnesium excess. Two drug groups that contain magnesium and could cause hypermagnesemia are laxatives (e.g., magnesium sulfate, milk of magnesia, magnesium citrate) and antacids (e.g., Maalox, Mylanta, Di-Gel). Table 15–10 lists the drugs that affect magnesium balance.

Nursing Process

Electrolyte: Magnesium

ASSESSMENT

- Assess client for signs and symptoms of magnesium deficit or excess. Hypomagnesemia includes tetany-like symptoms caused by hyperexcitability (tremors, twitching of the face) and ventricular tachycardia that leads to ventricular fibrillation and hypertension. Hypermagnesemia includes lethargy, drowsiness, weakness, paralysis, loss of deep tendon reflexes, hypotension, and heart block.
- Check serum magnesium levels for magnesium imbalance. Symptoms of magnesium deficit may or may not be seen until the serum level is below 1 mEq/L.
- Observe clients receiving digitalis preparations for digitalis toxicity. A magnesium deficit, as with a potassium deficit, enhances the action of digitalis, causing digitalis toxicity.

NURSING DIAGNOSES

- Imbalanced nutrition: less than body requirements related to insufficient intake of foods that are rich in magnesium
- Decreased cardiac output related to hypomagnesemia or hypermagnesemia
- Deficient knowledge

PLANNING

- Client's serum magnesium level will be within normal range in 2 to 5 days.

NURSING INTERVENTIONS

- Report to the health care provider if client is NPO (nothing by mouth) and receiving IV fluids without magnesium salts for weeks. Administer IV magnesium sulfate in solution slowly to prevent a hot or flushed feeling. Monitor vital signs.
- Monitor urinary output. Most of the body's magnesium is excreted by the kidneys. Report if the urine output is <600 ml/day.
- Check hypomagnesemia clients who are taking digoxin for digitalis toxicity (e.g., nausea and vomiting,

bradycardia). Magnesium deficit enhances the action of digoxin (digitalis preparations).

■ Monitor vital signs. Report abnormal findings to the health care provider.

■ Monitor serum electrolyte results. Report a low serum potassium or calcium level. Low serum magnesium levels may be attributed to hypokalemia or hypocalcemia. When correcting a potassium deficit, potassium is not replaced in the cells until magnesium is replaced. A serum magnesium level of 1 mEq/L or less can cause cardiac arrest.

■ Check for Trousseau's and Chvostek's signs of severe hypomagnesemia. Tetany symptoms occur in both magnesium and calcium deficits.

■ Have IV calcium gluconate available for emergency reversal of hypermagnesemia from overcorrection of a magnesium deficit.

Client Teaching

• Advise client to eat foods rich in magnesium (green vegetables, fruits, fish and seafood, grains, nuts, and peanut butter).

• Instruct client with hypermagnesemia to avoid routine use of laxatives and antacids that contain magnesium. Suggest that client check drug labels.

Cultural Considerations

• Use an interpreter as appropriate.
• Involve the extended family in health teaching and support.
• Incorporate wise food choices that are culturally acceptable.

EVALUATION

■ Evaluate client's serum magnesium level. Report if the serum level remains abnormal.

■ Observe for signs and symptoms of hypomagnesemia and hypermagnesemia.

WEBSITES

For further information on *The Role of the Nurse in Drug Research,* visit these Internet resources:

Medicine books: *www.Medicine-book.com/*

Nutritional supplements: *http://www.e-caps.com/*

Table 15–10

Drugs Affecting Magnesium Balance

Magnesium Imbalance	Drugs	Rationale

Hypomagnesemia (serum magnesium deficit)	Diuretics
	    furosemide (Lasix)
	    ethacrynic acid (Edecrin)
	    mannitol
		Diuretics promote urinary loss of magnesium.

	Antibiotics
	    gentamicin
	    tobramycin
	    carbenicillin
	    capreomycin
	    neomycin
	    polymyxin B
	    amphotericin B
	Digitalis
	Calcium gluconate
	Insulin
		These agents can cause magnesium loss via kidney.

	Laxatives cisplatin	Laxative abuse causes magnesium loss via the gastrointestinal tract.

	Corticosteroids
	    cortisone
	    prednisone
		Steroids can decrease serum magnesium level.

Hypermagnesemia (serum magnesium excess)	Magnesium salts
	Oral and enema
	    magnesium hydroxide (MOM)
	    magnesium sulfate (Epsom) salt
	    magnesium citrate
	    magnesium sulfate (maternity)
		Excess use of magnesium salts could increase serum magnesium level.

		Use of excess $MgSO_4$ in treatment of toxemia could cause hypermagnesemia.
	lithium	Hypermagnesemia is associated with lithium.

From Kee JL, Paulanka BJ: *Fluids and electrolytes with clinical applications,* ed 7, New York, 2004, Delmar.

Critical Thinking Case Study

J.S., 72 years old, has been vomiting and has had diarrhea for 2 days. J.S. takes digoxin 0.25 mg/day and hydrochlorothiazide (HydroDiuril) 50 mg/day. His serum potassium level is 3.2 mEq/L. He complains of being dizzy. His blood pressure is slightly lower than usual. The nurse assesses his physiologic status and notes that his muscles are weak and flabby, his abdomen is distended, and peristalsis is diminished.

1. What contributing factors causes J.S.'s potassium imbalance?

2. What signs and symptoms indicate that J.S. is in potassium imbalance?

3. What interventions should be taken for alleviating this potassium imbalance?

4. How much potassium chloride would be needed to elevate J.S.'s serum potassium by 1 mEq?

J.S. was ordered intravenously 1 L of 5% dextrose in water (D$_5$W) with 30 mEq of potassium chloride (KCl), and 1 L of 5% dextrose in 0.45% NaCl ($^1/_2$ of normal saline). He was also prescribed oral KCl 15 mEq, three times a day for 2 days. Oral KCl is available in 15 mEq/10 ml.

5. Explain the method for diluting KCl in IV fluids. Can KCl be given intramuscularly, subcutaneously or as an IV bolus (push)? Explain.

6. What instructions would you give J.S. for taking oral potassium supplements?

7. What happens if J.S.'s urine output decreases while he is receiving IV and oral potassium? What would be your responsibility?

8. Because J.S. is taking a diuretic and digoxin, what should the nurse include with client teaching? Give examples.

Study Questions

1. What is the average range of the osmolality of body fluids? If your client's serum sodium is 140 mEq/L, BUN is 12 mg/dl, and glucose is 100 mg/dl, what is your client's serum osmolality?

2. The client is receiving 1000 ml of D$_5$/0.9% NaCl (5% dextrose in normal saline solution). What is the osmolality of this IV solution? Explain.

3. What is the difference between crystalloids and colloids? Give examples of each.

4. Your client gained 15 pounds in 2 days. It is determined that the weight gain is caused by body-fluid retention. The weight gain could be equivalent to how many liters of fluid (water)?

5. Describe at least eight nursing interventions (with rationale) for clients receiving fluid replacement.

6. What is the normal serum potassium range? Your client has been vomiting and has weak, flabby muscles. The client's pulse is irregular. What type of potassium imbalance would you suspect?

7. What are the nursing implications of giving oral potassium supplements and for giving IV potassium chloride? Name the groups of foods that are rich in potassium.

8. What are the drugs used to correct severe hyperkalemia? How are they administered?

9. What drugs may cause an elevated serum sodium level? What health problem may result?

10. In hypocalcemia, the serum calcium level is less than what level? What are the symptoms of hypocalcemia?

11. Why are clients with hypocalcemia and hypercalcemia at high risk of having fractures?

12. What are the functions of magnesium? Describe specific client teaching for clients with hypomagnesemia or hypermagnesemia.

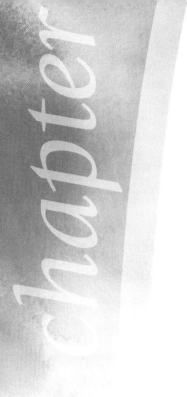

16 Nutritional Support

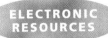

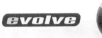
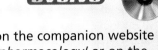

Additional information can be found on the companion website at *http://evolve.elsevier.com/KeeHayes/pharmacology/* or on the companion CD-ROM, which includes:

- *NCLEX-style examination review questions*
- *Pharmacology animations*
- *Medication error and IV therapy checklists*
- *Medication calculation problems*
- *Electronic calculators*

OUTLINE

Objectives

Terms

Introduction

Enteral Nutrition
Routes for Enteral Feedings
Enteral Solutions
Methods for Delivery
Complications
Enteral Medications

Nursing Process: Enteral Nutrition

Parenteral Nutrition
Total Parenteral Nutrition
Complications
Nursing Process: Total Parenteral Nutrition

Websites

Critical Thinking Case Study

Study Questions

OBJECTIVES

- Explain the differences between enteral nutrition and parenteral nutrition.
- Describe the routes for enteral feedings.
- Give examples of enteral solutions and explain the differences.
- Explain the advantages and differences of the methods used to deliver enteral nutrition.
- Describe the complications that may occur with use of enteral nutrition and parenteral nutrition.
- List the nursing interventions for clients receiving enteral nutrition and parenteral nutrition.

TERMS

bolus
continuous feedings
cyclic method
enteral nutrition
hyperalimentation (HA)

intermittent enteral feedings
intermittent infusion
nasogastric tube
nutritional support
parenteral nutrition

total parenteral nutrition
  (TPN)
Valsalva maneuver

Introduction

Nutrients are needed for cell growth, cellular function, enzyme activity, carbohydrate-fat-protein synthesis, muscular contraction, wound healing, immune competence, and gastrointestinal (GI) integrity. Inadequate nutrient intake can result from surgery, trauma, malignancy, and other catabolic illnesses. Without adequate nutritional support, protein catabolism (breakdown), malnutrition, and diminished organ functioning affect the GI, liver, renal, cardiac, and respiratory systems. The functioning of the immune system also is decreased.

Clients who are well nourished can usually tolerate a lack of nutrients for 14 days without major health problems. However, clients who are critically ill may only tolerate a lack of nutrient support for a short period (a few days to a week) before signs of impaired organ function, infection, or morbidity result. If nutritional support is started within hours of an injury, as in the cases of severe trauma or burns, recovery is more rapid. When the injury is a result of minor surgery, no severe bodily harm results from lack of nutritional support for days. Early nutritional support improves intestinal and liver blood flow and function, enhances wound healing, decreases the occurrence of infection, and improves the general outcome of the health situation for the critically ill and for clients with minor injuries. "Early fed" injured clients have a positive nitrogen balance and less chance for bacterial infections; thus they also have a decrease in institutional length of stay.

Dextrose 5% in water (D_5W), normal saline, and lactated Ringer's solution are not forms of nutritional support, although these solutions do provide fluids and some electrolytes. A client requires 2000 calories per day; critically ill clients may require 3000 to 5000 calories per day. In cases of burns, the caloric need could be greater. Clients who receive nothing by mouth (NPO) for an extended period become malnourished. Delayed nutritional support by even 5 days for a client experiencing trauma or neurologic damage (e.g., cervical fracture) could hamper wound healing and increase the risk of developing an infection.

There are two routes for administering **nutritional support:** enteral and parenteral. **Enteral nutrition,** which involves the GI tract, can be given orally or by feeding tubes (tube feeding). If the client can swallow, the nutrient preparations can be taken by mouth; if the client is unable to swallow, a tube is inserted into the stomach or small intestine. **Parenteral nutrition** involves administering high-caloric nutrients through large veins, for example, the subclavian vein. This method is called **total parenteral nutrition (TPN)** or **hyperalimentation (HA).** Parenteral nutrition is more costly (approximately three times more expensive) than enteral nutrition, and the benefits are not significant. In fact, with TPN there is a higher infection rate. The use of TPN does not promote effective GI integrity, liver function, or body weight gain, as does enteral nutrition. Enteral feedings require a functioning small intestine. TPN is necessary when the GI tract is incapacitated; if there is intestinal obstruction, uncontrolled vomiting, or high risk for aspiration; or to supplement inadequate oral intake.

This chapter is divided into enteral nutrition and parenteral nutrition. Routes for nutritional administration, nutritional preparations, methods for delivery, complications, and the nursing process are discussed for each.

Enteral Nutrition

When enteral nutrition is prescribed, there should be adequate small bowel function with digestion, absorption, and GI motility. To determine whether there is a lack of GI motility, the nurse assesses for abdominal distention and a decrease or absence of bowel sounds. In critically ill clients, frequently there is a decrease or absence in gastric emptying time; then TPN may be necessary. The preferred method for nutritional support is enteral feedings for clients with intact gastric emptying and with a decreased risk of aspiration.

Routes for Enteral Feedings

Oral, gastric by **nasogastric tube** or gastrostomy, and small intestinal by nasoduodenal/nasojejunal or jejunostomy tube are the routes used for enteral feedings. Use of nasogastric tube through oral (mouth) or nasal cavities is the most common route for short-term enteral feedings. The gastrostomy, nasoduodenal/nasojejunal, and jejunostomy tubes are used for long-term enteral feedings. Figure 16–1 displays the four types of GI tubes used for enteral feedings. If aspiration is a concern, the small intestinal route is suggested.

Enteral Solutions

Several types of liquid formulas are commercially available for enteral feedings. These solutions differ according to their various nutrients, caloric values, and osmolality. There are three groups of solutions for enteral nutrition: blenderized; polymeric, which includes milk-based and lactose-free; and elemental or monomeric. Examples of commercial preparations are listed according to their groups in Table 16–1. Components of the enteral solutions include (1) carbohydrates in the form of dextrose, sucrose, lactose, starch or dextrin (the first three are simple sugars that can be absorbed quickly); (2) protein in the form of intact proteins, hydrolyzed proteins, or free amino acids; and (3) fat in the form of corn oil, soybean oil, or safflower oil (some have a higher oil content than others). With all enteral nutrition, sufficient water to maintain hydration is essential.

Blended formulas for enteral solutions are liquid in consistency so they are able to pass through the tube. These are individually prepared based on the client's nutritional need. Frequently, baby food is used with liquid added. If the food particles are too large, the tube can become clogged.

The two groups of polymeric solutions are milk-based and lactose-free. Most of the milk-based polymeric preparations come in powdered form to be mixed with milk or

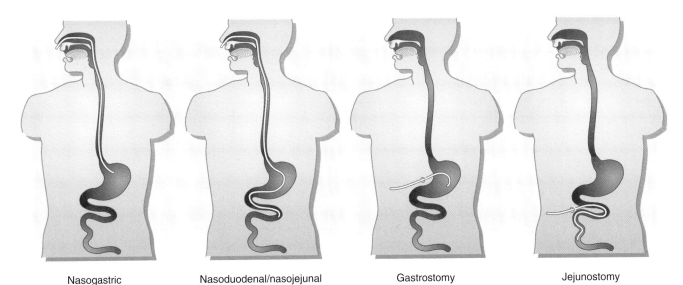

Nasogastric Nasoduodenal/nasojejunal Gastrostomy Jejunostomy

FIGURE 16–1 Types of gastrointestinal tubes used for enteral feedings. A nasogastric tube is passed from the nose into the stomach. A weighted nasoduodenal/nasojejunal tube is passed through the nose into the duodenum/jejunum. A gastrostomy tube is introduced through a temporary or permanent opening on the abdominal wall (stoma) into the stomach. A jejunostomy tube is passed through a stoma directly into the jejunum.

Table 16–1

Commercial Preparations for Enteral Feeding

Type	Commercial Preparations (Manufacturer)	Comments
Blenderized	Compleat B (Sandoz) Formula 2 (Cutter) Vitaneed (Sherwood)	Blended natural foods; ready to use
Polymeric *Milk-based*	Meritene (Sandoz) Instant Breakfast (Carnation) Sustacal Powder (Mead Johnson)	Pleasant tasting oral supplements; provide intact nutrients
Lactose-free	Ensure, Jevity, Osmolite (Ross) Sustacal Liquid, Isocal, Ultracal (Mead Johnson) Fibersource, Resource (Sandoz) Entrition, Nutren (Clintec) Attain, Comply (Sherwood)	May be used as tube feeding, meal replacement, or oral supplement; made with intact protein isolates, oligosaccharides and starches, and fats; provide 1 kcal/ml (others available providing up to 2 kcal). Adequate quantities meet reference daily intakes for vitamins and minerals; ready to use; isotonic (except Ensure and Sustacal)
Elemental or monomeric formulas	Vital HN (Ross) Vivonex T.E.N. (Sandoz) Criticare HN (Mead Johnson) Travasorb (Clintec) Peptamen (Clintec) Reabilan (O'Brian)	Partially digested nutrients for feeding; hypertonic (except for Reabilan and Peptamen); require reconstitution (except for Peptamen, Reabilan, and Criticare)

From Davis JR, Sherer K: *Applied nutrition and diet therapy for nurses,* ed 2, Philadelphia, 1994, Saunders, p. 349.

water. Many of these milk-based polymeric solutions do not provide complete nutritional requirements unless given in large amounts. Frequently, they are used as a supplement to meet nutritional needs. The lactose-free polymeric solutions are commercially prepared in liquid form for replacement feedings. Many of these solutions are isotonic (300 to 340 mOsm/kg water), and the breakdown of nutrients includes 50% carbohydrates, 15% protein, 15% fat, and 20% other nutrients. Examples of polymeric solutions include Ensure, Isocal, and Osmolite (Figure 16–2). These solutions provide 1 calorie per milliliter of feeding.

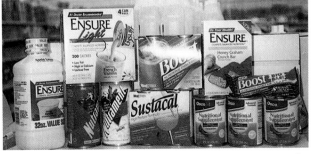

FIGURE 16–2 A typical selection of over-the-counter supplemental feeding products.

Characteristics of the formula may be targeted to treat a specific group of disorders. For those with diabetes mellitus, Glucerna and Diabetic Resource (low-carbohydrate, high-fat, lactose-free products), are most helpful. Nutri-Hep (low-fat, lactose-free product) is recommended to treat hepatic disorders. For individuals with pulmonary disorders, Pulmocare or Respalor (low-carbohydrate, high-fat products) are commonly prescribed. Nepro and Novasource Renal (low-fat amino acids, water-soluble vitamins) are used to treat those with renal disorders.

The elemental or monomeric solutions are useful for partial GI tract dysfunction. They are available in powdered and liquid forms. The nutrients from these solutions are rapidly absorbed in the small intestine. They are more expensive than the other enteral solutions.

Methods for Delivery

Enteral feedings may be given by bolus, intermittent drip or infusion, continuous drip, or cyclic infusion. The bolus method was the first method used to deliver enteral feedings. With the **bolus** method, 250 to 400 ml of solution is rapidly administered through a syringe or funnel into the tube four to six times a day. This method takes about 10 minutes each feeding, and many times is not tolerated well because a massive volume of solution is given in a short period. This method can cause nausea, vomiting, aspiration, abdominal cramping, and diarrhea. A healthy client can tolerate the rapidly infused solution. This method is seldom used unless the client is ambulatory.

Intermittent enteral feedings are administered every 3 to 6 hours over 30 to 60 minutes by gravity drip or pump infusion. At each feeding, 300 to 400 ml of solution is usually given. A feeding bag is commonly used. **Intermittent infusion** is considered an inexpensive method for administering enteral nutrition.

Continuous feedings are prescribed for the critically ill or for those who receive feedings into the small intestine. The enteral feedings are given by an infusion pump, such as the Kangaroo set, at a slow rate over 24 hours. Approximately 50 to 125 ml of solution is infused per hour (Figure 16–3).

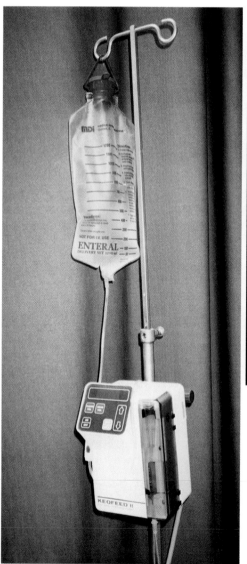
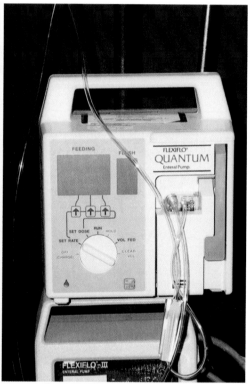

FIGURE 16–3 Examples of enteral infusion pumps for intermittent, continuous, and cyclic enteral feedings.

The **cyclic method** is another type of continuous feeding that is infused over 8 to 16 hours daily (day or night). Administration during daytime hours is suggested for clients who are restless or for those who have a greater risk for aspiration. The nighttime schedule allows more freedom during the day for the clients who are ambulatory.

Complications

Dehydration can occur if an insufficient amount of water is given with the feedings or between feedings. Some of the enteral solutions are hyperosmolar and can draw water out of the cells to maintain serum iso-osmolality.

Aspiration may occur if the client is fed while lying down or unconscious. The head of the bed should be elevated at least 30 degrees. The nurse should check for gastric residual by gently aspirating the stomach contents before administering the next enteral feeding.

One of the major problems of enteral feeding is diarrhea. This could be caused by rapid administration of feeding, high caloric solutions, malnutrition, GI bacteria (*Clostridium difficile*), and drugs. Antibacterials (antibiotics) and drugs that contain magnesium, such as antacids (Maalox) and sorbitol (used as a filler for certain drugs), are associated with the occurrence of diarrhea. Many oral liquid drugs are hyperosmolar, which tends to pull water into the GI tract and cause diarrhea.

Diarrhea usually can be managed or corrected by decreasing the rate of infusion of the solution, diluting the solution, changing the enteral solution, discontinuing the drug, or increasing the client's daily water intake.

Enteral Medications

Pancreatic enzymes such as precreatin (Creon) and pancrelipase (Viokase) are products used by individuals with a pancreatic enzyme deficiency as a result of conditions such as pancreatectomy, pancreatic obstruction, and cystic fibrosis. Both these preparations promote digestion and absorption of foods normally accomplished by natural amylase, lipase, and protease. Best given before meals, these artificial enzymes promote digestion and absorption of food.

Most drugs that can be administered orally can also be given via enteral tube. The drug must be in liquid form or dissolved into a liquid. Drugs that cannot be dissolved are time-release forms, enteric-coated forms, sublingual forms, and bulk-forming laxatives.

The liquid medication must be properly diluted when administered through the feeding tube. The drug dose is usually given as a bolus and then followed with water. Most liquid medications are hyperosmolar (>1000 mOsm/kg water) compared with the osmolality of the secretions of the GI tract (130 to 350 mOsm/kg water). Although the hyperosmolality of liquid medication was once thought to be well tolerated by the GI tract, abdominal distention and cramping, vomiting, and diarrhea can result from the administration of undiluted hyperosmolar liquid medications and electrolyte solutions. Liquid medication should be diluted with water to reduce the osmolality to 500 mOsm/kg H_2O (mildly hypertonic) to decrease GI intolerance. Table 16–2 lists the osmolalities of various commercial drug suspensions and solutions.

Calculation for Dilution of Enteral Medications

The following three steps should be followed to determine the amount of water needed for diluting liquid medications:

Step 1. Calculate the drug order to find the volume of the drug:

$$\frac{D}{H} \times V \text{ or } H:V::D:x$$

D: Desired dose: drug dose ordered by health care provider

H: On-hand dose: drug dose on label of container (e.g., bottle, vial, or ampule)

V: Vehicle: form and amount in which the drug is available (e.g., tablet, capsule, liquid)

Step 2. Find the osmolality of the drug (check drug literature or with pharmacist) and liquid dilution. Use 500 mOsm as a constant for the desired osmolality.

$$\frac{\text{know mOsm}}{\text{desired mOsm}} \times \text{volume of drug} = \text{total volume of liquid}$$

Step 3. Determine the volume of water for dilution:

total volume of liquid − volume of drug =
volume of water for dilution

Order: acetaminophen 650 mg, q6h PRN for pain
Available: Acetaminophen elixir 65 mg/ml
Average mOsm/kg = 5400 (see Table 16–2)

Table 16–2

Osmolality of Selected Drugs

Drug	Average mOsm
acetaminophen elixir, 65 mg/ml	5400
amoxicillin suspension, 50 mg/ml	2250
cephalexin (Keflex) suspension, 50 mg/ml	1950
cimetidine (Tagamet) solution, 60 mg/ml	5500
digoxin elixir, 50 mcg/ml	1350
docusate sodium (Colace) syrup, 3.3 mg/ml	3900
furosemide (Lasix) solution, 10 mg/ml	2050
lithium citrate syrup, 1.6 mEq/ml	6850
milk of magnesia suspension	1250
potassium chloride liquid, 10%	3550
prochlorperazine syrup, 1 mg/ml	3250
theophylline solution, 5.33 mg/ml	800

Step 1. Calculate the volume of drug:

$$\frac{D}{H} \times V = \frac{650 \text{ mg}}{65 \text{ mg}} \times 1 \text{ ml} = 10 \text{ ml}$$

or

$$H : V \qquad D : x$$
$$65 \text{ mg} : 1 \text{ ml} :: 650 \text{ mg} : x \text{ ml}$$
$$65x = 650$$
$$x = 10 \text{ ml of drug}$$

Step 2. Find the osmolality of drug and total liquid dilution:

$$\frac{\text{know mOsm (5400)}}{\text{desired mOsm (500)}} \times \text{volume of drug (10)} =$$

$$\frac{5400}{500} \times 10 = 108 \text{ ml of liquid}$$

Step 3. Determine the volume of water for dilution:

$$\text{total volume of liquid (108 ml)} - \text{volume of drug (10 ml)}$$
$$= 98 \text{ ml of water for dilution}$$

Nursing Process

Enteral Nutrition

ASSESSMENT

■ Confirm that the tape around the tube is secured.
■ Assess client's tolerance to the enteral feeding, including possible GI disturbance (nausea, cramping, diarrhea). These are common complications of enteral feeding.
■ Determine urine output. Record result for future comparison.
■ Obtain client's weight, which can be used for future comparisons.
■ Listen for bowel sounds. Diminished or absent bowel sounds should be reported immediately to the health care provider.
■ Assess baseline laboratory values. Compare with future laboratory results.

NURSING DIAGNOSES

■ Risk for fluid volume deficit related to inadequate fluid intake or excess fluid loss
■ Risk for diarrhea related to enteral feedings
■ Risk for aspiration related to enteral feedings via nasogastric tube

PLANNING

■ Client will receive adequate nutritional support through enteral feedings.

■ The complication of diarrhea related to enteral feedings will be managed.

NURSING INTERVENTIONS

■ Check tube placement by aspirating gastric secretion or injecting air into the tube to listen by stethoscope for air movement in the stomach. However, injecting air to check for placement may be misleading because the tube may be in the base of the lung and air flow there produces similar sounds as when the tube is placed in the stomach. For placement of the tube for small intestine route, confirmation by radiograph may be needed.
■ Determine the gastric residual before enteral feeding. A residual of more than 50% of previous feeding indicates delayed gastric emptying. Notify the health care provider. Usually the residual is 0 to 100 ml.
■ Check continuous route for gastric residual every 2 to 4 hours. If residual is more than 50 ml, stop infusion for 30 minutes to 1 hour and then recheck.
■ Before feeding, raise the head of the bed to a 30-degree angle. If elevating the head of the bed is not advisable, then position client on his/her right side.
■ Deliver the enteral feeding according to the method ordered: bolus, gastric, or small intestine.
■ Flush feeding tube accordingly: intermittent feeding, 30 ml before and after; continuous feeding, every 4 hours; medications, 30 ml before and after. If tube obstruction occurs, flush with warm water or cola.
■ Monitor adverse effects of enteral feedings such as diarrhea. To manage or correct diarrhea, decrease flow rate for the enteral feedings and, as diarrhea lessens, gradually increase the feeding rate. Enteral solution may be diluted and then gradually increased to full strength. However, diluted solution can decrease the nutrient intake. Determine whether the drugs could be causing the diarrhea.
■ Dilute the drug solution's osmolality to 500 mOsm when giving liquid medication through the tube. Use the formula in the text. Consult with the health care provider.
■ Monitor vital signs. Report abnormal findings.
■ Give additional water during the day to prevent dehydration. Consult with the health care provider.
■ Weigh client to determine weight gain or loss. Compare with the baseline weight. Client should be weighed at the same time each day, with the same scale and the same amount of clothing.
■ Change feeding bag daily. Do not add new solution to old solution in the feeding bag. The nutritional solution should not be ice cold but at room temperature.

Client Teaching

• Instruct client to report any problems related to enteral feedings such as diarrhea, sore throat, and abdominal cramping.

Cultural Considerations ⊕

- Respect cultural beliefs concerning refusal to receive enteral or TPN. Explain the need for adequate nutrition, and find ways that nutritional needs can be met.
- Communicate, verbally or in writing, how enteral nutrition is used by various cultural groups such as those in third-world countries.
- Use an interpreter as appropriate.

EVALUATION

■ Determine that client is receiving prescribed nutrients daily and is free of complications associated with enteral feedings.

Parenteral Nutrition

Total Parenteral Nutrition

Total parenteral nutrition (TPN), also called hyperalimentation (HA) or IV hyperalimentation (IVH), is the primary method for providing complete nutrients by the parenteral or IV route. TPN is an infusion of hyperosmolar glucose, amino acids, vitamins, electrolytes, minerals, and trace elements; it can meet a client's total nutritional needs. TPN is indicated for clients with severe burns who are in negative nitrogen balance; clients with GI disorders, when the GI tract needs a complete rest; and clients with debilitating diseases such as metastatic cancer or acquired immunodeficiency syndrome (AIDS).

The average percent of dextrose in TPN is 25%. This high glucose concentration is mixed with commercially prepared protein and lipid sources. Fat emulsion supplement therapy provides an increased number of calories and is a carrier of fat-soluble vitamins. Vitamins and electrolytes are added before administration. Electrolytes are frequently added immediately before the infusion according to the client's serum electrolyte levels. High glucose concentrations are irritating to peripheral veins, so TPN is administered through central venous lines such as the subclavian or internal jugular.

Enteral feedings should be considered before TPN. Enteral feeding poses less risk of sepsis, maintains GI integrity, and is less costly. When enteral nutrition cannot be used because of severe GI disorders, TPN should be prescribed. TPN does enhance wound healing and provides the necessary nutrients to prevent cellular catabolism.

To avoid exogenous contamination during enteral feeding, the following guidelines are suggested. Wash hands before handling the feeding system; use a system with medication ports, and wipe with alcohol before and after administering drugs; wear nonsterile disposable gloves; wear a mask if you have a cold; discard the feeding system every 24 hours (48 hours in a closed system). Do not touch any part of system in contact with formula, and do not use feeding system after the expiration date on label.

Complications

Complications associated with TPN can result from catheter insertion and TPN infusion. Table 16–3 lists the complications associated with TPN.

Table 16–3

Complications of Total Parenteral Nutrition

Complication	Causes	Symptoms
Catheter Insertion		
Pneumothorax	Accidental puncture of the pleural cavity.	Sharp chest pain; decreased breath sounds
Hemothorax	Catheter damages the large vein.	Same as pneumothorax
Hydrothorax	Catheter perforates the vein, releasing solution into the chest.	Same as pneumothorax
Total Parenteral Nutrition Infusion		
Air embolism	Intravenous (IV) tubing disconnected. Catheter not clamped. Injection port fell off. Improper changing of IV tubing (no Valsalva maneuver).	Coughing, shortness of breath, chest pain, cyanosis
Infection	Poor aseptic technique when catheter inserted. Contamination when changing tubing, mixing solution, or changing dressing.	Temperature >100° F (37.7° C). Tachycardia; chills; sweating; redness; swelling; drainage at insertion site; pain in the neck, arm, or shoulder; lethargy
Hyperglycemia	Fluid infused too rapidly. Insufficient insulin coverage. Infection.	Nausea, headache, weakness, thirst, elevated blood glucose
Hypoglycemia	Fluids stopped abruptly. Too much insulin infused.	Pallor, cold, clammy skin. Increased pulse rate, "shaky feeling," headache, blurred vision
Fluid overload hypervolemia	Increased IV rate. Fluids shift from cellular to vascular spaces because of hypertonic solutions.	Cough, dyspnea, neck vein engorgement, chest rales, weight gain

Complications include pneumothorax, hemothorax, hydrothorax, air embolism, infection, hyperglycemia, hypoglycemia, and fluid overload (hypervolemia). To prevent an air embolism, the client should be taught the **Valsalva maneuver,** which is to take a breath, hold it, and bear down while the nurse is changing infusion bags or bottles and changing tubing. Strict asepsis is necessary when changing IV tubing and dressings at the insertion site. Gloves, masks, and antibacterial ointment usually are necessary. TPN solution is an excellent medium for organism growth. Hypertonic dextrose in a protein hydrolysate solution promotes yeast and bacteria growth. It has been reported that these organisms do not grow as rapidly in the preferred crystalline amino acid solution as they do in a protein hydrolysate solution. Most TPN solutions are prepared by the pharmacist with the use of a laminar airflow hood.

Hyperglycemia occurs primarily as the result of the hypertonic dextrose solution when TPN is initiated. This occurs until the pancreas adjusts to the hyperglycemic load and therefore may be transient. It also occurs when the infusion rate for TPN is too rapid. In some cases, insulin is added to the TPN solution, which tends to be more effective than administering the insulin subcutaneously. Usually 1 L of solution is ordered for the first 24 hours when initiating TPN therapy. This allows the pancreas to accommodate to the increased glucose concentration of the solution. Additional daily increases of 500 to 1000 ml are ordered until the desired daily volume of 2.5 to 3 L is reached.

Sudden interruption of TPN therapy can cause hypoglycemia. After the glucose level is decreased, the insulin level remains, causing a hypoglycemic state. It is suggested that an isotonic dextrose solution be administered for 12 to 24 hours after TPN therapy is discontinued. A gradual decrease in the hourly infusion rate of TPN may also be used to discontinue TPN therapy. This process decreases the possibility of a hypoglycemic reaction.

TPN solutions and tubing should be changed every 24 hours. Dressing changes are required every 48 to 72 hours, according to the hospital policy. In some institutions, the dressing is changed every 24 hours for the first 7 to 10 days.

Nursing Process

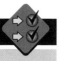

Total Parenteral Nutrition

ASSESSMENT

■ Obtain baseline vital signs for future comparison.
■ Confirm baseline weight.
■ Determine laboratory results. Electrolytes, glucose, and protein levels frequently change during TPN therapy. Early laboratory results are useful for future comparison.

■ Check urine output. Report abnormal findings.
■ Read the label on the TPN solution. Compare the solution with the order.

NURSING DIAGNOSES

■ Risk for fluid volume excess related to excess fluid infusion or renal dysfunction
■ Risk for fluid volume deficit related to osmotic diuresis resulting from hyperosmolar TPN solution
■ Risk for infection related to TPN solution that has a high glucose concentration
■ Ineffective breathing pattern related to complication from the insertion of subclavian line

PLANNING

■ Client's nutrient needs will be met via TPN.
■ The common complication from TPN therapy—infection—will be avoided.

NURSING INTERVENTIONS

■ Check vital signs. Report changes.
■ Determine body weight and compare with baseline weight.
■ Monitor laboratory results and report abnormal findings, especially electrolytes, protein, glucose. Compare laboratory changes with the baseline findings.
■ Measure intake and output. Fluid volume deficit or excess could occur. Because the TPN solution is hyperosmolar, fluid shift occurs, which can cause osmotic diuresis.
■ Monitor temperature changes for possible infection or febrile state. Use aseptic technique when changing dressings and solution bottles or bags.
■ Check blood glucose level periodically. When TPN therapy is started, there may be a transient elevated glucose level until the beta cells adjust to the secretion of insulin. If this occurs, the flow rate for TPN should be started slowly and gradually increased as the blood glucose level decreases. Regular insulin may be added to the TPN fluids to correct elevated glucose levels.
■ Refrigerate TPN solution that is not in use. High glucose concentration is an excellent medium for bacterial growth.
■ Monitor the flow rate of TPN. Start with 60 to 80 ml/hour and increase the rate slowly to the ordered level to avoid hyperglycemia.
■ Have client perform the Valsalva maneuver to avoid air embolism by taking a breath, holding it, and bearing down. If the line is opened to air when changing the solution bag or bottle and IV tubing, an air embolus could occur.

■ Observe cardiac status because the Valsalva's maneuver can cause cardiac dysrhythmias.

■ Check for signs and symptoms of overhydration, including coughing, dyspnea, neck vein engorgement, or chest rales. Report findings.

■ Follow the institution's procedure for changing dressing and tubing. Usually, the tubing is changed daily and the dressing is changed every 24 hours for the first 10 days and then every 48 hours thereafter.

■ Do not draw blood, give medications, or check central venous pressure via the TPN line. Results could be invalid.

Client Teaching

• Provide emotional support to client and family before and during TPN therapy.

• Be available to discuss client's concerns or refer client to the appropriate health care provider.

• Instruct client to notify the health care provider immediately with any discomforts or reactions.

• Keep client informed of progress and effectiveness of TPN.

Cultural Considerations

• Respect client's cultural beliefs about refusing TPN.

• Explain reasons for adequate nutrition and find ways to meet nutritional needs.

• Use an interpreter as appropriate.

EVALUATION

■ Evaluate client's positive and negative response to the TPN therapy.

■ Determine periodically whether client's serum electrolytes, protein, and glucose levels are within desired ranges.

■ Evaluate nutritional status by weight changes, energy level, feeling of well-being, symptom control, or healing.

WEBSITES

For further information on *The Role of the Nurse in Drug Research*, visit these Internet resources:

Medical source: *www.nutritionalsupport.org*

Nutritional support at home: *http://www.rxkinetics.com/tpntutorial/4_1.html*

Enteral nutritional support: *http://rnbob.tripod.com/enteralnutritionalsupport.htm*

Nutritional support and adult access devices: *http://main.uab.edu/ipnec/show.asp?durki=35535*

Critical Thinking Case Study

M.M. had abdominal surgery and received D$_5$W and D$_5$ 0.45% NaCl for 4 days. A nasogastric tube was inserted for enteral nutrition. It was determined that the function of M.M.'s GI tract was intact.

1. Why would M.M. receive enteral nutrition? Is it needed for short-term or long-term therapy?

2. Differentiate between the Ensure solution that M.M. is receiving and other forms of enteral solutions.

3. M.M. is at risk for complications related to enteral nutrition. Discuss each potential complication and give specific nursing interventions for each.

4. Differentiate methods of delivery of enteral nutrition. Describe nursing interventions related to each method.

5. Give the rationale for changing M.M.'s enteral nutrition from bolus method to intermittent method.

M.M. was ordered amoxicillin suspension 250 mg, q.i.d., and potassium chloride solution 10% (15 mEq/10 ml), every 12 hours. These medications are to be given through the enteral tubing.

6. How many milliliters of amoxicillin should M.M. receive per dose? How much water dilution is needed to reduce the drug osmolality to 500 mOsm?

7. How many milliliters of potassium chloride should M.M. receive per dose? How much water dilution is needed to reduce the drug osmolality to 500 mOsm?

Study Questions

1. What are the differences between enteral nutrition and parenteral nutrition? Would D_5W, normal saline solution (0.9% NaCl), and lactated Ringer's solution be a form of nutritional support? Explain.

2. What are the four methods of delivery for enteral nutrition? How do these four methods differ from each other?

3. What are the three groups of solution used for enteral nutrition? Give an example from each group.

4. What complications can occur with the use of enteral feedings? Explain.

5. Your client is receiving cimetidine (Tagamet) solution 200 mg, t.i.d. How many milliliters should your client receive? How much water is needed to reduce the osmolality to 500 mOsm?

6. When is TPN therapy preferred over enteral therapy for nutritional support?

7. What is the composition of TPN solution? What is the normal dextrose percent?

8. What is the osmolality of TPN solution?

9. What are the major complications associated with TPN? Explain.

10. How is the Valsalva maneuver performed? What is its purpose?

11. If the blood glucose level is elevated, what are some interventions to reduce the glucose level?

12. Discuss at least eight nursing interventions related to the care of the client receiving enterable nutrition? TPN?

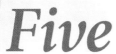

Five

Autonomic Nervous System Agents

The *central nervous system (CNS)*, the body's primary nervous system that consists of the brain and spinal cord, was previously discussed in the Unit IV introduction. The *peripheral nervous system (PNS)*, located outside the brain and spinal cord, is made up of two divisions: the autonomic and the somatic. After interpretation by the CNS, the PNS receives stimuli and initiates responses to those stimuli.

The *autonomic nervous system (ANS)*, also called the *visceral system*, innervates (acts on) smooth muscles and glands. Its functions include control and regulation of the heart, respiratory system, gastrointestinal (GI) tract, bladder, eyes, and glands. The ANS is an involuntary nervous system over which a person has little or no control. We breathe, our hearts beat, and peristalsis occurs without our realizing it. However, unlike the ANS, the somatic nervous system is a voluntary system that innervates skeletal muscles over which there is control.

The two sets of neurons in the autonomic component of the PNS are the (1) afferent (sensory) neurons and the (2) efferent (motor) neurons. The *afferent neurons* send impulses to the CNS, where they are interpreted. The *efferent neurons* receive the impulses (information) from the brain and transmit those impulses through the spinal cord to the effector organ cells. The efferent pathways in the ANS are divided into two branches: the sympathetic and the parasympathetic nerves, which are collectively called the *sympathetic nervous system* and the *parasympathetic nervous system* (Figure V–1).

The sympathetic and parasympathetic nervous systems act on the same organs but produce opposite responses to provide homeostasis (balance) (Figure V–2). Drugs act on the sympathetic and parasympathetic nervous systems by either stimulating or depressing responses.

Sympathetic Nervous System

The *sympathetic nervous system* is also called the *adrenergic system* because, at one time, it was believed that *adrenaline* was the *neurotransmitter* that innervated the smooth muscle. The neurotransmitter is, however, *norepinephrine*.

The adrenergic receptor organ cells are of four types: alpha$_1$, alpha$_2$, beta$_1$, and beta$_2$ (Figure V–3). Norepinephrine is released from the terminal nerve ending and stimulates the cell receptors to produce a response.

Parasympathetic Nervous System

The **parasympathetic nervous system** is called the **cholinergic** system because the neurotransmitter at the end of the neuron that innervates the muscle is **acetylcholine.**

The cholinergic receptors at organ cells are either nicotinic or muscarinic, meaning that they are stimulated by the alkaloids nicotine and muscarine, respectively (see Figure V–3). Acetyl-

FIGURE V–1 Subdivisions of the peripheral nervous system.

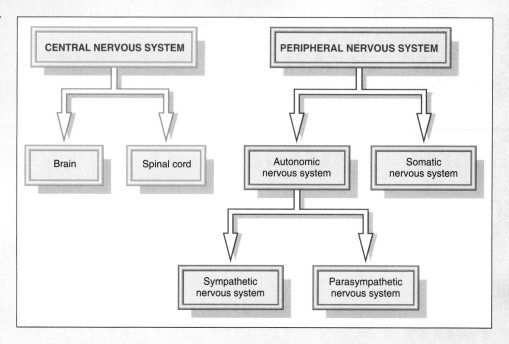

FIGURE V–2 Sympathetic and parasympathetic effects on body tissues.

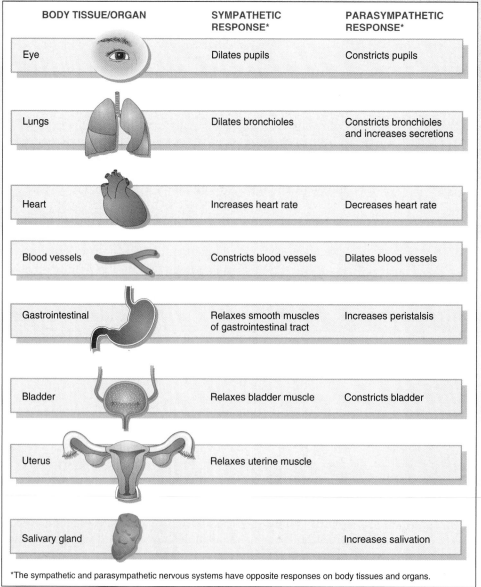

BODY TISSUE/ORGAN	SYMPATHETIC RESPONSE*	PARASYMPATHETIC RESPONSE*
Eye	Dilates pupils	Constricts pupils
Lungs	Dilates bronchioles	Constricts bronchioles and increases secretions
Heart	Increases heart rate	Decreases heart rate
Blood vessels	Constricts blood vessels	Dilates blood vessels
Gastrointestinal	Relaxes smooth muscles of gastrointestinal tract	Increases peristalsis
Bladder	Relaxes bladder muscle	Constricts bladder
Uterus	Relaxes uterine muscle	
Salivary gland		Increases salivation

*The sympathetic and parasympathetic nervous systems have opposite responses on body tissues and organs.

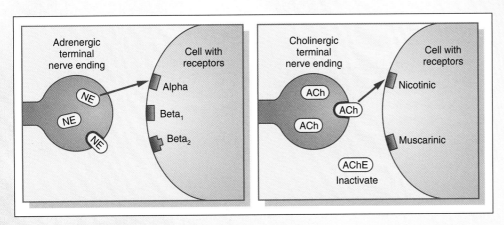

FIGURE V–3 Sympathetic and parasympathetic transmitters and receptors. *ACh,* Acetylcholine; *AChE,* acetylcholinesterase; *NE,* norepinephrine.

choline stimulates the receptor cells to produce a response, but the enzyme, acetylcholinesterase, may inactivate acetylcholine before it reaches the receptor cell.

Drugs that mimic the neurotransmitters norepinephrine and acetylcholine produce responses opposite to each other in the same organ. For example, an adrenergic drug (sympathomimetic) increases the heart rate, whereas a cholinergic drug (parasympathomimetic) decreases the heart rate (see Figure V–2). However, a drug that mimics the sympathetic nervous system and a drug that blocks the parasympathetic nervous system can cause similar responses in the organ. For instance, the sympathomimetic and the parasympatholytic drugs both increase the heart rate; the adrenergic blocker and the cholinergic drug both decrease heart rate.

Many name classifications are given to drugs that mimic or block both the sympathetic nervous system and the parasympathetic nervous system (Table V–1). The nurse needs to become familiar with these names. Drug names and specific actions are discussed in Chapters 17, Adrenergics and Adrenergic Blockers, and 18, Cholinergics and Anticholinergics.

Table V–1

Autonomic Nervous Systems: Sympathetic and Parasympathetic

Sympathetic Stimulants	Parasympathetic Stimulants
	Direct-Acting
Sympathomimetics (adrenergics, adrenomimetics, or adrenergic agonists)	**Parasympathomimetics (cholinergics or cholinergic agonists)**
Action:	*Action:*
Increase blood pressure	Decrease blood pressure
Increase pulse rate	Decrease pulse rate
Relax bronchioles	Constrict bronchioles
Dilate pupils of eyes	Constrict pupils of eyes
Relax uterine muscles	Increase urinary contraction
Increase blood sugar	Increase peristalsis
	Indirect-Acting
	Cholinesterase inhibitors (anticholinesterase)
	Action:
	Increase muscle tone
Sympathetic Depressants	**Parasympathetic Depressants**
Sympatholytics (adrenergic blockers, adrenolytics, or adrenergic antagonists)	**Parasympatholytics (anticholinergics, cholinergic antagonists, or antispasmodics)**
Action:	*Action:*
Decrease pulse rate	Increase pulse rate
Decrease blood pressure	Decrease mucous secretions
Constrict bronchioles	Decrease gastrointestinal motility
	Increase urinary retention
	Dilate pupils of eyes

Opposite responses on organ tissue are caused by sympathomimetics and parasympathomimetics and by sympatholytics and parasympatholytics. Sympathomimetics and parasympatholytics cause similar organ responses as do sympatholytics and parasympathomimetics.

Summary

There are two subdivisions of the autonomic nervous system: the sympathetic and the parasympathetic nervous systems. These nervous systems have opposite effects on organ tissues. Drugs can either stimulate or block both of these nervous systems through their receptors. Table V–2 lists the organ responses from drugs that act on these systems.

Table V–2

Sympathetic and Parasympathetic Responses to Drugs

Sympathetic	Parasympathetic	Response
Sympathomimetic	Parasympathomimetic	Opposite response
Sympatholytic	Parasympatholytic	Opposite response
Sympathomimetic	Parasympatholytic	Similar response
Sympatholytic	Parasympathomimetic	Similar response

17 Adrenergics and Adrenergic Blockers

ELECTRONIC RESOURCES

Additional information can be found on the companion website at *http://evolve.elsevier.com/KeeHayes/pharmacology/* or on the companion CD-ROM, which includes:
- *NCLEX-style examination review questions*
- *Pharmacology animations*
- *Medication error and IV therapy checklists*
- *Medication calculation problems*
- *Electronic calculators*

OUTLINE

Objectives

Terms

Introduction

Adrenergics
Inactivation of Neurotransmitters
Classification of Sympathomimetics/
  Adrenomimetics
Epinephrine
Albuterol
Isoproterenol Hydrochloride

Clonidine and Methyldopa
Nursing Process: Adrenergic Agonist

Adrenergic Blockers (Antagonists)
Alpha-Adrenergic Blockers
Beta-Adrenergic Blockers
Nursing Process: Adrenergic Neuron Blockers
Adrenergic Neuron Blockers

Websites

Critical Thinking Case Studies

Study Questions

OBJECTIVES

- Name the adrenergic receptors and give examples of their major responses.
- Describe the difference between selective and nonselective adrenergic drugs.
- Give drug names of selective and nonselective adrenergic drugs.
- List the major side effects of adrenergic drugs.
- Explain nursing interventions, including client teaching, associated with adrenergic drugs.
- List examples of drugs that are selective and nonselective adrenergic blockers.
- Describe the uses of alpha-blockers and beta-blockers.
- List the general side effects of adrenergic blockers.
- Describe nursing interventions, including client teaching, associated with adrenergic blockers.

TERMS

adrenergic blockers
adrenergic neuron blockers
adrenergic receptor
alpha-blockers

beta-blockers
catecholamines
nonselective
selective

sympatholytics
sympathomimetics

Introduction

This chapter discusses two groups of drugs that affect the sympathetic nervous system: the *adrenergics* (**sympathomimetics** or *adrenomimetics*) and the *adrenergic blockers* (**sympatholytics** or *adrenolytics*). Adrenergic drugs and adrenergic blockers are listed here along with their dosages and uses.

Adrenergics

Drugs that stimulate the sympathetic nervous system are called adrenergics, adrenergic agonists, sympathomimetics, or adrenomimetics because they mimic the sympathetic neurotransmitters (i.e., norepinephrine, epinephrine). They act on one or more **adrenergic receptor** sites located on the cells of smooth muscles, such as the heart, bronchiole walls, gastrointestinal (GI) tract, urinary bladder, and ciliary muscle of the eye. There are many adrenergic receptors; the four main receptors are alpha$_1$, alpha$_2$, beta$_1$, and beta$_2$, which mediate the major responses described in Table 17–1 and illustrated in Figure 17–1.

Table 17–1

Effects of Adrenergics at Receptors

Receptor	Physiologic Responses
Alpha$_1$	Increases force of heart contraction; vasoconstriction increases blood pressure; mydriasis (dilation of pupils) occurs; salivary glands decrease secretion; bladder and prostate capsule increases contraction and ejaculation
Alpha$_2$	Inhibits the release of norepinephrine; dilates blood vessels; produces hypotension; decreases gastrointestinal motility and tone
Beta$_1$	Increases heart rate and force of contraction; increases renin secretion, which increases blood pressure
Beta$_2$	Dilates the bronchioles; promotes gastrointestinal and uterine relaxation; promotes increase in blood sugar through glycogenolysis in the liver; increases blood flow in the skeletal muscles

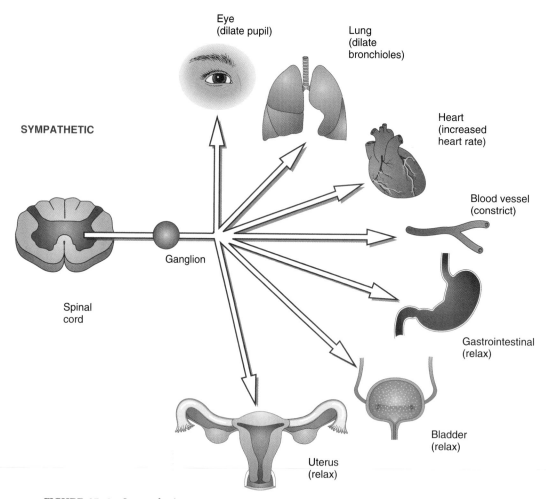

FIGURE 17–1   Sympathetic responses. Stimulation of the sympathetic nervous system or use of sympathomimetic (adrenergic) drugs can cause the pupils and bronchioles to dilate; the heart rate to increase; blood vessels to constrict; and the muscles of the gastrointestinal tract, bladder, and uterus to relax, thereby decreasing contractions.

The alpha-adrenergic receptors are located in the vascular tissues (vessels) of smooth muscles. When the *alpha$_1$*-receptor is stimulated, the arterioles and venules constrict, thereby increasing peripheral resistance and blood return to the heart. Circulation is improved and blood pressure is increased. When there is too much stimulation, the blood flow is decreased to the vital organs. The *alpha$_2$*-receptor is located in the postganglionic sympathetic nerve endings. When stimulated, it inhibits the release of norepinephrine thus leading to a decrease in vasoconstriction. This results in a decrease in blood pressure.

The *beta$_1$*-receptors are located primarily in the heart. Stimulation of the beta$_1$-receptor increases myocardial contractility and heart rate. The *beta$_2$*-receptors are found mostly in the smooth muscles of the lung, the arterioles of skeletal muscles, and the uterine muscle. Stimulation of the beta$_2$-receptor causes (1) relaxation of the smooth muscles of the lungs, resulting in bronchodilation; (2) an increase in blood flow to the skeletal muscles; and (3) relaxation of the uterine muscle, resulting in a decrease in uterine contraction (see Table 17–1 and Figure 17–2).

Another adrenergic receptor is dopaminergic and is located in the renal, mesenteric, coronary, and cerebral arteries. When this receptor is stimulated, the vessels dilate and blood flow increases. Only dopamine can activate this receptor.

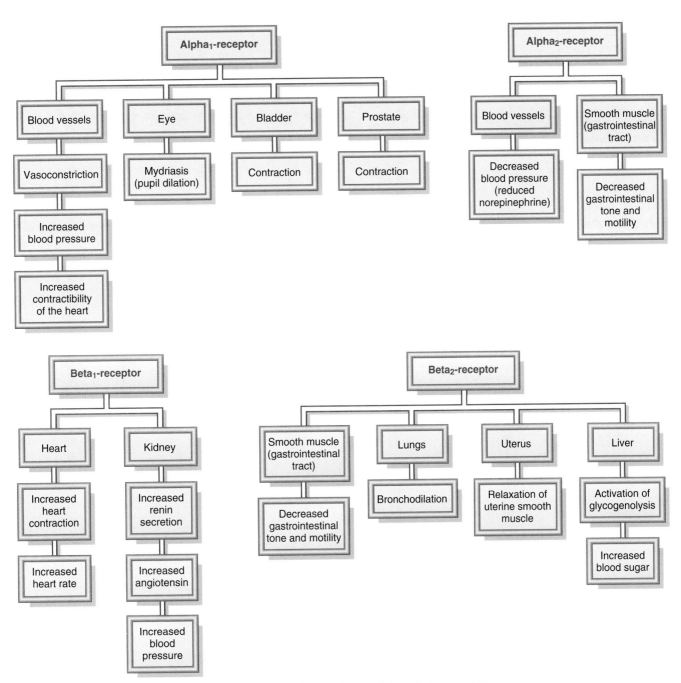

FIGURE 17–2   Effects of activation of alpha$_1$-, alpha$_2$-, beta$_1$-, and beta$_2$- receptors.

Inactivation of Neurotransmitters

After the transmitter (e.g., norepinephrine) has performed its function, the action must be stopped to prevent prolonging the effect. Transmitters are inactivated by (1) reuptake of the transmitter back into the neuron (nerve cell terminal), (2) enzymatic transformation or degradation, and (3) diffusion away from the receptor. The mechanism of norepinephrine reuptake plays a more important role in inactivation than the enzymatic action. Following the reuptake of the transmitter in the neuron, the transmitter may be degraded or reused. The two enzymes that inactivate the metabolism of norepinephrine are (1) monoamine oxidase (MAO), which is inside the neuron; and (2) catechol-O-methyltransferase (COMT), which is outside the neuron.

Drugs can stop the termination of the neurotransmitter (e.g., norepinephrine) by either (1) inhibiting the norepinephrine reuptake, which prolongs the action of the transmitter; or by (2) inhibiting the degradation of norepinephrine by enzyme action.

Classification of Sympathomimetics/ Adrenomimetics

The sympathomimetic drugs that stimulate adrenergic receptors are classified into three categories according to their effects on organ cells: (1) *direct-acting sympathomimetics,* which directly stimulate the adrenergic receptor (e.g., epinephrine or norepinephrine); (2) *indirect-acting sympathomimetics,* which stimulate the release of norepinephrine from the terminal nerve endings (e.g., amphetamine); and (3) *mixed-acting sympathomimetics* (both direct and indirect acting), which stimulate the adrenergic receptor sites and stimulate the release of norepinephrine from the terminal nerve endings (Figure 17–3).

Ephedrine is an example of a mixed-acting sympathomimetic. This drug acts *indirectly* by stimulating the release of norepinephrine from the nerve terminals and acts *directly* on the alpha$_1$-, beta$_1$-, and beta$_2$-receptors. Ephedrine-like epinephrine increases heart rate and blood pressure, but it is not as potent a vasoconstrictor as epinephrine. Ephedrine is helpful to treat idiopathic orthostatic hypotension and hypotension that results from spinal anesthesia. It also stimulates beta$_2$-receptors, which dilate bronchial tubes, and is useful to treat mild forms of bronchial asthma.

Catecholamines are the chemical structures of a substance (either endogenous or synthetic) that can produce a sympathomimetic response. Examples of endogenous catecholamines are epinephrine, norepinephrine, and dopamine. The synthetic catecholamines are isoproterenol and dobutamine. *Noncatecholamines* (e.g., phenylephrine, metaproterenol, albuterol) stimulate the adrenergic receptors. Most noncatecholamines have a longer duration of action than the endogenous or synthetic catecholamines.

Many of the adrenergic drugs stimulate more than one of the adrenergic receptor sites. An example is epinephrine (Adrenalin), which acts on alpha$_1$-, beta$_1$-, and beta$_2$-adrenergic receptor sites. The responses from these receptor sites include an increase in blood pressure, pupil dilation, increase in heart rate (tachycardia), and bronchodilation. In certain types of shock (i.e., cardiogenic, anaphylactic), epinephrine is useful because it increases blood pressure, heart rate, and airflow through the lungs through bronchodilation. Because epinephrine affects three different adrenergic receptors, it is not **selective;** in other words, it is considered **nonselective** to one receptor. Side effects result when more responses occur than are desired. Prototype Drug Chart 17–1 lists the pharmacologic behavior of epinephrine.

Epinephrine

Pharmacokinetics

Epinephrine can be administered subcutaneously, intravenously, topically, or by inhalation. It should not be given orally because it is rapidly metabolized in the GI tract and liver; thus inadequate serum levels occur.

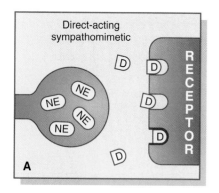
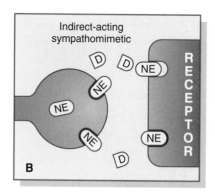
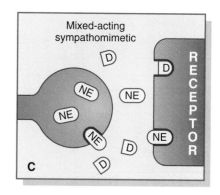

> [D] = Sympathomimetic drug
> (NE) = Norepinephrine

FIGURE 17–3 A, Direct-acting sympathomimetics; **B,** indirect-acting sympathomimetics; and **C,** mixed-acting sympathomimetics.

PROTOTYPE DRUG CHART 17–1

EPINEPHRINE

Drug Class

Sympathomimetic
Trade Name: Adrenalin
Pregnancy Category: C

Dosage

Severe anaphylactic shock:
A: **subQ:** 0.1-0.5 ml of 1:1000 PRN
IV: 0.1-0.25 ml of 1:1000 with additional dilution
IV: 1-2.5 ml of 1:10,000 infused over 5-10 min
C: **subQ:** 0.01 ml/kg of 1:1000
IV: 0.01 ml/kg of 1:1000 with additional dilution
IV: 0.1 mg or 10 ml of 1:100,000

Contraindications

Cardiac dysrhythmias, cerebral arteriosclerosis,
  pregnancy, narrow-angle glaucoma, cardiogenic shock
Caution: Hypertension, prostatic hypertrophy,
  hyperthyroidism, pregnancy, diabetes mellitus
  (hyperglycemia could result)

Drug-Lab-Food Interactions

Drug: Decrease epinephrine effect with methyldopa,
  beta blockers, and alpha-adrenergic blockers (e.g.,
  phentolamine)
Lab: Increase blood glucose, serum lactic acid

Pharmacokinetics

Absorption: subQ/IM/IV: Rapidly
Distribution: PB: UK; in breast milk
Metabolism: t½: UK
Excretion: In urine unchanged

Pharmacodynamics

subQ/IM: Onset: 3-10 min
  Peak: 20 min
  Duration: 20-30 min
IV: Onset: Immediate
  Peak: 2-5 min
  Duration: 5-10 min
Inhal: Onset: 1 min
  Peak: 3-5 min
  Duration: 1-3 min

Therapeutic Effects/Uses

To treat allergic reaction, anaphylaxis, bronchospasm, cardiac arrest

Mode of Action: Action on one or more adrenergic sites; promotion of CNS and cardiac stimulation
  and bronchodilation

Side Effects

Anorexia, nausea, vomiting, nervousness, tremors, agitation, headache, pallor, insomnia, syncope, dizziness

Adverse Reactions

Palpitations, tachycardia, dyspnea
Life-threatening: Ventricular fibrillation, pulmonary
  edema

A, Adult; *C,* child; *CNS,* central nervous system; *IM,* intramuscular; *Inhal,* inhalation; *IV,* intravenous; *min,* minute; *PB,* protein-
binding; *PRN,* as needed; *subQ,* subcutaneous; *t¹/₂,* half-life; *UK,* unknown.

The percentage by which the drug is protein bound and its half-life are unknown. Epinephrine is metabolized by the liver and excreted in the urine.

Pharmacodynamics

Epinephrine is frequently used in emergencies to combat anaphylaxis, which is a life-threatening allergic response. It is a potent inotropic (force of muscular contraction) drug that causes the blood vessels to constrict; thus the blood pressure increases, the heart rate increases, and the bronchial tubes dilate. High doses can result in cardiac dysrhythmias; therefore the electrocardiogram (ECG) should be monitored. Epinephrine can also cause renal vasoconstriction, thereby decreasing renal perfusion and urinary output.

The onset of action and peak concentration times are rapid. The use of decongestants with epinephrine has an additive effect. When epinephrine is administered with digoxin, cardiac dysrhythmias may oc-cur. Beta-blockers can cause a decrease in action of epinephrine. Epinephrine is also discussed in Chapter 57, Adult and Pediatric Emergency Drugs, with the drugs used during emergencies.

Albuterol

Albuterol sulfate (Proventil) is selective for beta₂-adrenergic receptors, so the response is purely bronchodilation. An asthmatic client may therefore respond better by taking albuterol than isoproterenol because its primary action is on the beta₂-receptor. By using selective sympathomimetics, fewer undesired responses (i.e., side effects) will occur. However, high dosages of albuterol may affect the beta₁ receptors, causing an increase in heart rate. Prototype Drug Chart 17–2 lists the drug data related to albuterol.

Pharmacokinetics

Albuterol sulfate (Proventil, Ventolin) is well absorbed from the GI tract and is extensively metabolized by the liver. The half-life of the drug differs slightly according to the route of administration (oral route is 2.5 hours; inhalation route is 3.5 hours).

Pharmacodynamics

The primary use of albuterol is to prevent and treat bronchospasms. With inhalation, the onset of action of albuterol is faster than with oral administration, although the duration of action is the same for both oral and inhalation preparations.

Tremors, restlessness, and nervousness may occur when high doses of albuterol are taken—side effects that are most likely caused by the reflex effect of beta$_1$-receptors. If albuterol is taken with an MAO inhibitor, a hy-

pertensive crisis can result. Beta-blockers may inhibit the action of albuterol. Albuterol and the beta$_2$ drugs are also discussed in Chapter 39, Drugs for Acute and Chronic Lower Respiratory Disorders.

Isoproterenol Hydrochloride

Isoproterenol hydrochloride (Isuprel), an adrenergic drug, activates beta$_1$- and beta$_2$-receptors. It is more specific than epinephrine because it acts on two different adrenergic receptors but is not completely selective. The response to beta$_1$ and beta$_2$ stimulation is bronchodilation and an increase in heart rate. For example, when a client takes isoproterenol to control asthma for dilating the bronchi, an increase in heart rate also occurs as a result of beta$_1$

PROTOTYPE DRUG CHART 17–2

ALBUTEROL

Drug Class	**Dosage**
Beta$_2$-adrenergic agonist Trade Name: Proventil, Salbutamol, Ventolin, ✤ Novo-Salmol *Pregnancy Category:* C	A: PO: 2-4 mg, t.i.d., q.i.d.; *max:* 32 mg/d in 4 divided doses SR: 4-8 mg, q12h Inhal: 1-2 puffs q4-6h PRN Nebulizer: 0.5 ml of 0.5% sol in 3 ml of 0.9% NaCl in 5-15 min C 2-6 y: PO: 0.1 mg/kg/t.i.d. 6-12 y: PO: 2 mg, t.i.d., q.i.d. 6-12 y: Inhal: Same as adult
Contraindications	**Drug-Lab-Food Interactions**
Caution: Severe cardiac disease, hypertension, hyperthyroidism, diabetes mellitus, pregnancy	*Drug: Increase* effect with other sympathomimetics; may *increase* effect with MAO inhibitors and tricyclic antidepressants *Antagonize* effect with beta-adrenergic blockers (beta-blockers) *Lab:* May *increase* glucose level slightly; may *decrease* serum potassium level
Pharmacokinetics	**Pharmacodynamics**

Absorption: Well absorbed from the GI tract
Distribution: PB: UK
Metabolism: t½: PO: 2.5–6 h; Inhal: 3.5–5 h
Excretion: 75% excreted in the urine
	PO: Onset: 30 min
	   Peak: 2-3 h
	   Duration: 4-6 h
	Inhal: Onset: 5-15 min
	   Peak: 0.5-2 h
	   Duration: 3-6 h

Therapeutic Effects/Uses

To treat bronchospasm, asthma, bronchitis, and other COPD
Mode of Action: Stimulates the beta$_2$-adrenergic receptors in the lungs, which relaxes the bronchial smooth muscles

Side Effects	**Adverse Reactions**
Tremor, dizziness, nervousness, restlessness	Palpitations, reflex tachycardia, hallucinations **Life-threatening:** Cardiac dysrhythmias

A, Adult; *C,* child; *COPD,* chronic obstructive pulmonary disease; *d,* day; *GI,* gastrointestinal; *h,* hour; *Inhal,* inhalation; *MAO,* monoamine oxidase; *min,* minute; *PB,* protein-binding; *PO,* by mouth; *PRN,* as needed; *q.i.d.,* four times a day; *SR,* sustained release; *t½,* half-life; *t.i.d.,* three times a day; *UK,* unknown; *y,* year; ✤, Canadian drug name.

stimulation. When isoproterenol is used excessively, severe tachycardia can result.

Clonidine and Methyldopa

Clonidine (Catapres) and methyldopa (Aldomet) are selective alpha$_2$-adrenergic drugs that are used primarily to treat hypertension. The accepted theory for the action of alpha$_2$ drugs is that they regulate the release of norepinephrine by inhibiting its release. Alpha$_2$ drugs are also believed to produce a cardiovascular depression by stimulating alpha$_2$ receptors in the central nervous system (CNS), leading to a decrease in blood pressure (see Chapter 42, Antihypertensive Drugs).

Side Effects and Adverse Reactions

Side effects frequently result when the drug dosage is increased or the drug is nonselective (i.e., it acts on several receptors). Side effects commonly associated with adrenergic drugs include hypertension, tachycardia, palpitations, dysrhythmias, tremors, dizziness, urinary difficulty, nausea, and vomiting.

Names of adrenergic drugs, the receptors they activate, dosage information, and common uses are listed in Table 17–2.

Nursing Process

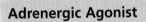

Adrenergic Agonist

ASSESSMENT

■ Record vital signs for future comparison. Epinephrine stimulates the alpha$_1$ (increases blood pressure), beta$_1$ (increases heart rate), and beta$_2$ (dilates bronchial tubes) receptors. Isoproterenol (Isuprel) stimulates the beta$_1$ and beta$_2$ receptors. Albuterol (Proventil) stimulates the beta$_2$-receptor.

■ Assess the drugs client takes and report possible drug-drug interactions. Beta-blockers decrease the effect of epinephrine.

■ Determine client's health history. Most adrenergic drugs are contraindicated if the client has cardiac dysrhythmias, narrow-angle glaucoma, or cardiogenic shock.

■ Evaluate the results of laboratory values and compare with future laboratory findings.

NURSING DIAGNOSES

■ Risk for impaired tissue integrity
■ Decreased cardiac output

PLANNING

■ Client's vital signs will be closely monitored and will be within normal or acceptable ranges.

NURSING INTERVENTIONS

■ Record client's vital signs. Report signs of increasing blood pressure and increasing pulse rate. If client receives an alpha-adrenergic drug intravenously for shock, the blood pressure should be checked every 3 to 5 minutes or as indicated to avoid severe hypertension.

■ Report side effects of adrenergic drugs, such as tachycardia, palpitations, tremors, dizziness, and increased blood pressure.

■ Check client's urinary output and assess for bladder distention. Urinary retention can result from high drug dose or continuous use of adrenergic drugs.

■ For cardiac resuscitation, administer epinephrine 1:1000 IV (1 mg/ml), which may be diluted in 10 ml of saline solution (as prescribed).

■ Monitor IV site frequently when administering norepinephrine bitartrate (Levarterenol) or dopamine (Intropin) because infiltration of these drugs causes tissue necrosis. These drugs should be diluted sufficiently in IV fluids. An antidote for norepinephrine (Levophed) and dopamine is phentolamine mesylate (Regitine) 5 to 10 mg, diluted in 10 to 15 ml of saline infiltrated into the area.

■ Offer food to client when giving adrenergic drugs to avoid nausea and vomiting.

■ Evaluate laboratory test results. Blood glucose levels may be increased.

Client Teaching

General

• Instruct client to read labels on all over-the-counter (OTC) drugs for cold symptoms and diet pills. Many of these have properties of sympathetic (adrenergic, sympathomimetics) drugs and should not be taken if client is hypertensive or has diabetes mellitus, cardiac dysrhythmias, or coronary artery disease.

• Advise mothers not to take drugs that contain sympathetic drugs while nursing infants. These drugs pass into the breast milk.

• Explain to client that continuous use of nasal sprays or drops that contain adrenergics may result in nasal congestion rebound (inflamed and congested nasal tissue).

Self-Administration

• Inform client and family how to administer cold medications by spray or drops in the nostrils. Spray should be used with the head in an upright position. The use of nasal spray while lying down can cause systemic absorption. Coloration of nasal spray or drops might indicate deterioration.

Table 17–2

Adrenergic Drugs (Alpha₁, Beta₁, and Beta₂)

Generic (Brand)	Route and Dosage	Uses and Considerations
epinephrine (Adrenalin) Alpha₁, beta₁, and beta₂	See Prototype Drug Chart 17–1.	
ephedrine HCl, ephedrine sulfate (Ephedsol, Ectasule) Alpha₁, beta₁, and beta₂	A: PO: 25-50 mg t.i.d./q.i.d. subQ/IM: 12.5-50 mg; IV: 10-25 mg PRN; *max:* 150 mg/24 h C: >2 y: PO: 2-3 mg/kg/d in 4-6 divided doses; *max:* 75 mg/24 h	To treat hypotensive states, bronchospasm, nasal congestion, and orthostatic hypotension. Effective for relief of symptoms of hay fever, sinusitis, and allergic rhinitis. Also may be used to treat mild cases of asthma. Drug resistance may occur with prolonged use of ephedrine. If this occurs, stop drug for 3-5 d and then resume. *Pregnancy category:* C; PB: UK; t½: 3-6 h
norepinephrine bitartrate (Levarterenol, Levophed) Alpha₁ and beta₁	A: IV: 4 mg in 250-500 ml of D₅W or NSS infused initially 8-12 mcg/min, then 4 mcg/min; monitor blood pressure	For shock. It is a potent vasoconstrictor. It increases blood pressure and cardiac output. The blood pressure should be closely monitored every 2-5 min during infusion. IV flow is titrated according to blood pressure. *Pregnancy category:* D; PB: UK; t½: UK
metaraminol bitartrate (Aramine) Alpha₁ and beta₁	A: IV/Inf: 15-100 mg in 500 ml of D₅W C: IV/Inf: 0.04 mg/kg (each 1 mg diluted in 25 ml of D₅W)	Treatment of acute hypotension. Infusion rate should be adjusted according to blood pressure. *Pregnancy category:* C; PB: UK; t½: UK
dopamine HCl (Intropin) Alpha₁ and beta₁	A: IV/INF: 1-5 mcg/kg/min initially; gradually increase 5-10 mcg/kg/min; *max:* 50 mcg/kg/min C: IV: Usually the same	To correct hypotension. It does not decrease renal function in doses <5 mcg/kg/min. *Pregnancy category:* C; PB: UK; t½: 2 min
midodrine (ProAmatine) Alpha₁	A: PO: 10 mg t.i.d.	To treat symptomatic orthostatic hypotension. Blood pressure may increase by 15 to 30 mm Hg in 1 h with one 10-mg dose. *Pregnancy category:* C; PB: UK; t½: 3-4 h
phenylephrine HCl 12-hour spray/ oxymetazoline HCl (Neo-Synephrine) Alpha	*Nasal decongestant:* A: Instill: 2-3 sprays or gtt of 0.25%-0.5% sol C: <6 y: Instill: 2-3 gtt of 0.125% sol C: 6-12 y: Instill: 2-3 gtt of 0.25% sol Also available IM, IV	To treat nasal congestion; acts as a decongestant. Used for clients with common cold, sinusitis, and with allergic rhinitis. Have client blow nose before drug is administered. *Pregnancy category:* C; PB: UK; t½: 2.5 h
pseudoephedrine HCl (Sudafed, Actifed, Co-Tylenol, PediaCare) Alpha and beta₁	*Nasal decongestant:* A: PO: 60 mg q.i.d./q6h PO/SR: 120 mg q12h; *max:* 240 mg/d C: 2-6 y: PO: 15 mg q6h; *max:* 60 mg/d C: 6-12 y: PO: 30 mg q6h; *max:* 120 mg/d	To treat nasal congestion. OTC drug. Check label for contraindications. Avoid taking with a history of hypertension, cardiac disease, diabetes mellitus. *Pregnancy category:* C; PB: UK; t½: 9-16 h
phenylpropanolamine HCl (Dimetapp, Dristan, Contac 12 Hour, Triaminicol, Triaminic)	*Nasal decongestant:* A: PO: 25 mg q4h PRN PO/SR: 75 mg q12h PRN C: 2-6 y: PO: 6.25 mg q4h PRN C: 6-12 y: 12.5 mg q4h PRN	To treat nasal congestion; acts as OTC drugs. FDA has required that phenylpropanolamine be withdrawn from OTC weight-control products and other OTC drugs. In some cases, pseudoephedrine has been used in place of phenylpropanolamine.

A, Adult; *C,* child; *d,* day; *FDA,* Food and Drug Administration; *gtt,* drops; *h,* hour; *IM,* intramuscular; *inf,* infusion; *inhal,* inhalation; *IPPD,* intermittent positive pressure breathing; *IV,* intravenous; *min,* minute; *NSS,* normal saline solution; *OTC,* over-the-counter; *PB,* protein-binding; *PO,* by mouth; *PRN,* as needed; *q.i.d.,* four times a day; *SL,* sublingual; *SR,* sustained release; *subQ,* subcutaneous; *t½,* half-life; *t.i.d.,* three times a day; *UK,* unknown; *y,* year; >, greater than; <, less than.

Table 17–2

Adrenergic Drugs (Alpha₁, Beta₁, and Beta₂)—cont'd

Generic (Brand)	Route and Dosage	Uses and Considerations
Dexatrim, Dietac, Control Alpha and beta₁	*Appetite suppressant:* A: PO/SR: 75 mg daily (before breakfast); PO: 25 mg t.i.d. a.c.	OTC drug used to control weight gain. Client should check with health care provider before taking an appetite suppressant. *Pregnancy category:* C; PB: UK; t½: 3-4 h
albuterol (Proventil, Ventolin) Beta₂	See Prototype Drug Chart 17–2.	To relieve bronchospasm caused by acute and chronic obstructive airway disease (e.g., asthma, bronchitis, emphysema). It stimulates the beta₂-receptors of the bronchi thus promoting bronchodilation. *Pregnancy category:* C; PB: UK; t½: 2.5-5 h
metaproterenol sulfate (Alupent, Metaprel) Beta₁ (some) and beta₂	A & C: >9 y: PO: 10-20 mg t.i.d./q.i.d. C: <6 y: PO: 1-2.6 mg/kg/d in 3-4 divided doses C: 6-9 y: PO: 10 mg t.i.d./q.i.d. A & C: >12 yr: Inhal: 2-3 puffs q3-4h; *max:* 12 puffs/d	Treatment for bronchospasm, acute heart block (only used in atropine-refractory bradycardia). By stimulating beta₁, the heart rate is increased but not as strongly as with isoproterenol HCl. The drug dilates the bronchial tubes. *Pregnancy category:* C; PB: UK; t½: UK
isoproterenol HCl (Isuprel) Beta₁ and beta₂	A: SL: 10-20 mg t.i.d.; *max:* 60 mg/d; Inhal: 1-2 puffs q4-6h PRN; IV: 0.01-0.02 mg OR 2-20 mcg/min via infusion C: SL: 5-10 mg t.i.d.; Inhal: same as adult; IV: 2.5 mcg/min OR 0.1 mcg/kg/min via infusion	To treat cardiac decompensation, congestive heart failure (increases myocardial blood flow and cardiac output), and asthmatic attack. This drug increases heart rate and dilates bronchial tubes. *Pregnancy category:* C; PB: UK; t½: 2.5-5 min
dobutamine HCl (Dobutrex) Beta₁	A & C: IV: 2.5-10 mcg/kg/min initially; increase dose gradually; *max:* 40 mcg/kg/min	To treat cardiac decompensation by enhancing myocardial contractility, stroke volume, and cardiac output, which may result from cardiogenic shock or cardiac surgery. *Pregnancy category:* C; PB: UK; t½: 2 min
isoetharine HCl (Bronkosol) Beta₂	A: IPPB: 0.5-1.0 ml of 0.5% sol OR 0.5 ml of 1% sol diluted in 3 ml of NSS A: Inhal: 1-2 puffs	To control asthma and chronic obstructive pulmonary disease by dilating the bronchial tubes. *Pregnancy category:* C; PB: UK; t½: UK
terbutaline sulfate (Brethine, Brethaire, Bricanyl) Beta₂	*Bronchodilator:* A: PO: 2.5-5 mg t.i.d. OR q8h; SC: 0.25 mg initially; no more than 0.5 mg in 4 h Inhal: 2 puffs q4-6h C: >12 y: PO: 2.5 mg t.i.d. OR q8h *Premature labor:* A: PO: 2.5 mg q4-6h; IV: 10 mcg/min, gradually increase; *max:* 80 mcg/min	Primary use is to correct bronchospasm. Unofficial use is during premature labor to prevent premature-term birth. *Pregnancy category:* B; PB: 25%; t½: 3-11 h
ritodrine HCl (Yutopar) Beta₂ and some beta₁	A: PO: Initially 10 mg q2h for first 24 h; maint: 10-20 mg q4-6h; *max:* 120 mg/d IV: 50-100 mcg/min; dose may gradually increase to 300 mcg/min	Used to decrease and/or stop uterine contraction. To be effective, the heart rate must be more than 100 beats per minute. Because there are many side effects, the drug is not used as frequently to control premature labor as it once was. *Pregnancy category:* C; PB: UK; t½: 1.6-2.6 h

- Direct client not to excessively use bronchodilator sprays. If client uses a nonselective adrenergic drug that affects beta$_1$- and beta$_2$-receptors, tachycardia may occur.

Side Effects

- Encourage client to report side effects (e.g., rapid heart rate, palpitations, dizziness) to a health care provider.

Cultural Considerations (⊕)

- Decrease language barriers by decoding the jargon of the health care environment for clients with language difficulties and for those who do not work in the health care field.

EVALUATION

■ Evaluate client's response to the adrenergic drug. Continue monitoring client's vital signs and report abnormal findings.

Adrenergic Blockers (Antagonists)

Drugs that block the effects of the adrenergic neurotransmitter are called **adrenergic blockers,** adrenergic antagonists, or sympatholytics. They act as antagonists to the adrenergic agonists by blocking the alpha- and beta-receptor sites. Most adrenergic blockers block either the alpha- or the beta-receptor. They block the effects of the neurotransmitter either *directly* by occupying the alpha- or the beta-receptors or *indirectly* by inhibiting the release of the neurotransmitters norepinephrine and epinephrine. The three sympatholytic receptors are alpha$_1$, beta$_1$, and beta$_2$. Table 17–3 lists the effects of alpha- and beta-blockers.

Alpha-Adrenergic Blockers

Drugs that block or inhibit a response at the alpha-adrenergic receptor site are called *alpha-adrenergic blockers,* or more commonly, **alpha-blockers.** Alpha-blocking agents are divided into two groups: *selective alpha-blockers* that block alpha$_1$ and *nonselective alpha-blockers* that block alpha$_1$ and alpha$_2$. Because alpha-adrenergic blockers can cause orthostatic hypotension and reflex tachycardia,

Table 17–3

Effects of Adrenergic Blockers at Receptors

Receptor	Responses
Alpha$_1$	Vasodilation: decreases blood pressure; reflex tachycardia might result; miosis (constriction of pupil) occurs; suppresses ejaculation; reduces contraction of the smooth muscles in the bladder neck and prostate gland
Beta$_1$	Decreases heart rate; reduces force of contractions
Beta$_2$	Constricts bronchioles; contracts uterus; inhibits glycogenolysis, which can decrease blood sugar

many of these drugs are not as frequently prescribed as the beta-blockers. The alpha-blockers are helpful in decreasing symptoms of benign prostatic hypertrophy (BPH).

The alpha-blockers promote vasodilation, thus causing a decrease in blood pressure. If the vasodilation is long-standing, orthostatic hypotension can result. Dizziness may also be a symptom of a drop in blood pressure. As the blood pressure decreases, pulse rate usually increases to compensate for the low blood pressure and inadequate blood flow. The alpha-blockers can be used to treat peripheral vascular disease (e.g., Raynaud's disease). Vasodilation occurs, permitting more blood flow to the extremities. The alpha blockers are also discussed in Chapter 42, Antihypertensive Drugs.

Beta-Adrenergic Blockers

Beta-adrenergic blockers, commonly called **beta-blockers,** decrease heart rate; a decrease in blood pressure usually follows. Some of the beta-blockers are nonselective, blocking both beta$_1$- and beta$_2$-receptors. Not only does the pulse rate decrease because of beta$_1$-blocking, but bronchoconstriction also occurs. Nonselective beta-blockers (beta$_1$ and beta$_2$) should be used with extreme caution in any client who has chronic obstructive pulmonary disease (COPD) or asthma. If the desired effect is to decrease pulse rate and blood pressure, then a selective beta$_1$-blocker, such as metoprolol tartrate (Lopressor), may be ordered.

An intrinsic sympathomimetic activity (ISA) causes partial stimulation of beta receptors. Certain nonselective beta blockers (block both beta$_1$ and beta$_2$) that have ISA are carteolol, carvedilol, penbutolol, and pindolol. The selective blocker (blocks beta$_1$ only) that has ISA is acebutolol. These agents reportedly cause fewer serious side effects and are helpful to clients experiencing severe bradycardia.

Propranolol hydrochloride (Inderal) was the first beta-blocker prescribed to treat angina, cardiac dysrhythmias, and hypertension. Although it is still prescribed today, it has many side effects, partly because of its nonselective response in blocking both beta$_1$- and beta$_2$-receptors. It is contraindicated for clients with asthma or second- or third-degree heart block. Propranolol is extensively metabolized by the liver (hepatic first-pass); thus only a small amount of the drug reaches the systemic circulation. Prototype Drug Chart 17–3 describes the pharmacologic behavior of propranolol.

Pharmacokinetics

Propranolol is well absorbed from the GI tract. It crosses the blood-brain barrier and the placenta and is found in breast milk. It is metabolized by the liver and has a short half-life of 3 to 6 hours.

Pharmacodynamics

By blocking both types of beta-receptors, propranolol decreases the heart rate and, secondarily, the blood pressure. It also causes the bronchial tubes to constrict and the uterus to contract. It is available

PROTOTYPE DRUG CHART 17–3

ATENOLOL

Drug Class

Beta$_1$-adrenergic blocker
Trade Name: Tenormin, Apo-Atenolol
Pregnancy Category: C

Dosage

Hypertension
A: PO: 50-100 mg/d
Elderly: PO: 25-50 mg/d
Myocardial Infarction
A: IV: 5 mg q5min × 2, then 10 min after second dose 50 mg PO, then 50 mg PO 12 h later, then 50 mg bid for 6-9 d

Contraindications

Sinus bradycardia, heart block > first degree, cardiogenic shock, overt cardiac failure
Caution: Renal dysfunction, peripheral arterial circulatory disorders, asthma, COPD, hyperthyroidism, concurrent use of diuretics and digitalis

Drug-Lab-Food Interactions

Drug: Increased absorption with atropine and other anticholinergics, decreased effects with NSAIDs, increased risk of hypoglycemia with insulin and sulfonylureas, increased hypotension with prazosin and terazosin, increased lidocaine and verapamil levels with toxicity

Pharmacokinetics

Absorption: Well-absorbed
Distribution: PB: 6-16%
Metabolism: t½: 6-7 h
Excretion: Urine

Pharmacodynamics

PO: Onset: 2.7-7.7 h
Peak: 2-4 h
Duration: 24 h
IV: Onset: UK
Peak: 5 min
Duration 24 h

Therapeutic Effects/Uses

To treat hypertension, angina pectoris, and myocardial infarction
Mode of Action: Selectively blocks beta$_1$-adrenergic receptor sites, decreases sympathetic outflow to the periphery, suppresses renin-angiotensin-aldosterone system

Side Effects

Drowsiness, dizziness, fainting, weakness, nausea, vomiting, diarrhea, cool extremities, leg pain

Adverse Effects

Bradycardia, hypotension, heart failure, masking of hypoglycemia
Life-threatening: Agranulocytosis, laryngospasm, respiratory distress, pulmonary edema, dysrhythmias

A, Adult; *COPD,* chronic obstructive pulmonary disease; *h,* hour; *IV,* intravenously; *min,* minute; *NSAID,* nonsteroidal antiinflammatory drug; *PB,* protein-binding; *PO,* by mouth; *t½,* half-life; *UK,* unknown.

orally in tablets and sustained-release capsules and intravenously. The onset of action of the sustained-release preparation is longer than that of the tablet; peak time and duration of action are also longer for the sustained-release formulation. This form is effective for dosing once a day, especially for clients who do not comply with drug doses of several times a day.

Drug Interactions

Many drugs interact with propranolol. Phenytoin, isoproterenol, nonsteroidal antiinflammatory drugs (NSAIDs), barbiturates, and xanthines (caffeine, theophylline) decrease the drug effect of propranolol. When propranolol is taken with digoxin or a calcium blocker, atrioventricular (AV) heart block may occur. The blood pressure can be decreased if propranolol is taken with another antihypertensive, although this may be the desired result.

Beta-blockers are useful in treating cardiac dysrhythmias, mild hypertension, mild tachycardia, and angina pectoris. The use of beta-blockers as antihypertensives, antidysrhythmics, and drugs for angina is discussed in Chapter 40, Cardiac Glycosides, Antianginals, and Antidysrhythmics, and Chapter 42, Antihypertensive Drugs. Table 17–4 lists the alpha- and beta-blockers and their dosages, uses, and considerations.

Side Effects and Adverse Reactions

General side effects of alpha-adrenergic blockers include cardiac dysrhythmias, flush, hypotension, and reflex tachycardia. The side effects commonly associated with beta-blockers are bradycardia, dizziness, hypotension, headache, hyperglycemia, intensified hypoglycemia, and agranulocytosis. Usually the side effects are dose related.

Table 17–4

Adrenergic Blockers

Generic (Brand)	Route and Dosage	Uses and Considerations
tolazoline (Priscoline HCl) Alpha$_1$	A: subQ/IM/IV: 10-50 mg q.i.d. *Pulmonary hypertension:* NB: IV: 1-2 mg/kg infused over 10 min, followed by 1-2 mg/kg/h for 24–48 h	For peripheral vascular disorder and for persistent pulmonary hypertension in the newborn. Also for emergency hypertension. *Pregnancy category:* C; PB: UK; t^1/$_2$: 3-10 h
phentolamine mesylate (Regitine) Alpha$_1$	A: IM/IV: 2.5-5 mg, repeat q5min until controlled, then q2-3h PRN C: IM/IV: 0.05-0.1 mg/kg, repeat PRN	Management of peripheral vascular disorder and hypertensive emergency. Antidote for dopamine infiltration. *Pregnancy category:* C; PB: UK; t^1/$_2$: 20 min
doxazosin mesylate (Cardura) Alpha$_1$	A: PO: 1 mg/d, titrate dose up to *max:* 16 mg/d; *maint:* 4-8 mg/d Elderly: PO: 0.5 mg/d initially; may increase dose	For mild to moderate hypertension and BPH. Check for orthostatic hypotension. Dizziness, headache, syncope may occur. *Pregnancy category:* C; PB: 98%; t^1/$_2$: 9-12 h
prazosin HCl (Minipress) Alpha$_1$	A: PO: 1 mg b.i.d./t.i.d.; *maint:* 3-15 mg/d; *max:* 20 mg/d in divided doses	Management of mild to moderate hypertension. May be used in combination with other antihypertensive drugs. *Pregnancy category:* C; PB: 95%; t^1/$_2$: 3 h
terazosin HCl (Hytrin) Alpha$_1$	A: PO: 1 mg at bedtime, *maint:* 1-5 mg in 1-2 divided doses; *max:* 20 mg/d	For hypertension. May be used in combination with diuretic or other antihypertensive drugs. May also be used for BPH. May cause dizziness, headache, edema, orthostatic hypotension. *Pregnancy category:* C; PB: UK; t^1/$_2$: 9-12 h
carvedilol (Coreg) Alpha$_1$, beta$_1$, and beta$_2$	A: PO: 6.25 mg b.i.d.; may increase to 12.5 mg b.i.d.; *max:* 50 mg/d	For treatment of hypertension. Can be used alone or with a thiazide diuretic. Used also for mild to moderate heart failure. *Pregnancy category:* C; PB: UK; t^1/$_2$: 7-10 h
labetalol (Normodyne, Trandate) Alpha$_1$, beta$_1$, and beta$_2$	A: PO: 100 mg b.i.d.; dose may be increased; *max:* 2.4 g/d; IV: 20 mg OR 1-2 mg/kg; repeat 20-80 mg at 10-min interval; *max:* 300 mg/d	To treat mild to severe hypertension; angina pectoris; used during surgery to manage blood pressure. *Pregnancy category:* C; PB: 50%; t^1/$_2$: 6-8 h
carteolol HCl (Cartrol) Beta$_1$ and beta$_2$	A: PO: 2.5-5.0 mg/d	For hypertension and glaucoma. Primarily blocks beta$_1$ adrenergic receptor; however, in large doses it blocks beta$_2$. *Pregnancy category:* C; PB: 23%-30%; t^1/$_2$: 4-6 h
penbutolol (Levatol) Beta$_1$ and beta$_2$	A: PO: 10-20 mg/d; *max:* 80 mg/d	To treat mild to moderate hypertension. Clients with asthma should avoid taking the drug. *Pregnancy category:* C; PB: 80%-98%; t^1/$_2$: 5 h
propranolol HCl (Inderal)	A: PO: Initially: 10-20 mg tid-qid; *maint:* 20-60 mg tid-qid; *max:* 320 mg/day; SR: 80-160 mg/day	Management of angina pectoris, myocardial infarction, hypertension, dysrhythmias, thyrotoxicosis. *Pregnancy category:* C; PB: 93%; t^1/$_2$: 2-4 h
nadolol (Corgard) Beta$_1$ and beta$_2$	A: PO: 40-80 mg/d; *max:* 320 mg/d	Management of hypertension and angina pectoris. Contraindicated in bronchial asthma and severe COPD because it blocks beta$_2$. *Pregnancy category:* C; PB: 30%; t^1/$_2$: 10-24 h
pindolol (Visken) Beta$_1$ and beta$_2$	A: PO: 5 mg b.i.d./t.i.d.; *maint:* 10-30 mg in divided doses; *max:* 60 mg/d in divided doses	Management of hypertension and angina pectoris. Contraindicated in asthma, COPD, and second- and third-degree heart block. *Pregnancy category:* B; PB: 40%; t^1/$_2$: 3-4 h
sotalol (Betapace) Beta$_1$ and beta$_2$	A: PO: 80 mg b.i.d.; may increase gradually. Average: 240-320 mg/d	To treat life-threatening ventricular arrhythmias and chronic angina pectoris. *Pregnancy category:* B; PB: 0; t^1/$_2$: 12 h
timolol maleate (Blocadren) Beta$_1$ and beta$_2$	A: PO: Initially 10 mg b.i.d.; *maint:* 20-40 mg/d in 2 divided doses; *max:* 60 mg/d	Management of mild to moderate hypertension, dysrhythmias, and postmyocardial infarction. Also may be used as prophylaxis of migraine headache. For ophthalmic use to treat IOP. Use with caution for clients with asthma or COPD. *Pregnancy category:* C; PB: <10%; t^1/$_2$: 3-4 h

A, Adult; *b.i.d.,* two times a day; *BPH,* benign prostatic hypertrophy; *bpm,* beats per minute; *C,* child; *COPD,* chronic obstructive pulmonary disease; *d,* day; *h,* hour; *IM,* intramuscular; *IOP,* intraocular pressure; *IV,* intravenous; *NB,* newborn; *PB,* protein-binding; *PO,* by mouth; *PRN,* as necessary; *q.i.d.,* four times a day; *subQ,* subcutaneous; *t^1/$_2$,* half-life; *t.i.d.,* three times a day; *UK,* unknown; >, greater than; <, less than.

Table 17–4

Adrenergic Blockers—cont'd

Generic (Brand)	Route and Dosage	Uses and Considerations
Selective Beta-Adrenergic Blockers		
metoprolol tartrate (Lopressor) Beta$_1$	*Hypertension:* A: PO: 50-100 mg/d in 1-2 divided doses; *maint:* 100-450 mg/d in divided doses; *max:* 450 mg/d in divided doses *Myocardial infarction:* A: IV: 5 mg q2min 3 doses, then PO: 100 mg b.i.d.	Management of hypertension, angina pectoris, postmyocardial infarction. Bradycardia, dizziness, and gastrointestinal distress may occur. *Pregnancy category:* C; PB: 12%; t$^1/_2$: 3-4 h
atenolol (Tenormin) Beta$_1$	See Prototype Drug Chart 17–3.	
acebutolol HCl (Sectral) Beta$_1$	A: PO: Initially: 200-400 mg/d A: PO: maint; 200-800 mg/d in 1-2 divided doses; *max:* 1200 mg/d	Treatment for mild to moderate hypertension, angina pectoris, and supraventricular dysrhythmias. Check apical pulse; do not give if <60 bpm. *Pregnancy category:* B; PB: 26%; t$^1/_2$: 3-13 h
betaxolol (Kerlone) Beta$_1$	A: PO: 10-20 mg/d. Also for ophthalmic use: glaucoma	For hypertension and glaucoma. Ophthalmic preparation is used to decrease IOP. *Pregnancy category:* C; PB: UK; t$^1/_2$: 14-22 h
bisoprolol fumarate (Zebeta) Beta$_1$	A: PO: Initially: 5 mg/d; maint: 2.5-20 mg/d	For hypertension and angina pectoris. Long-acting beta blocker. Heart rate and blood pressure may be decreased. *Pregnancy category:* C; PB: <30%; t$^1/_2$: 9-12 h
esmolol HCl (Brevibloc) Beta$_1$	A: IV: Loading dose: 500 mcg/kg/min for 1 min; then 50 mcg/kg/min for 4 min	For treatment of supraventricular tachycardia, atrial fibrillation/flutter, and hypertension *Contraindications:* heart block, bradycardia, cardiogenic shock, uncompensated congestive heart failure. *Pregnancy category:* C; PB: UK; t$^1/_2$: 9 min

Adrenergic Neuron Blockers

Drugs that block the release of norepinephrine from the sympathetic terminal neurons are called **adrenergic neuron blockers,** which are classified as a subdivision of the adrenergic blockers. The clinical use of neuron blockers is to decrease blood pressure. Guanethidine monosulfate (Ismelin) and guanadrel sulfate (Hylorel), examples of adrenergic neuron blockers, are potent antihypertensive agents.

Nursing Process

Adrenergic Neuron Blockers*

ASSESSMENT

■ Obtain baseline vital signs and electrocardiogram for future comparison. Bradycardia and decrease in blood pressure are common cardiac effects of beta-adrenergic blockers. Beta-adrenergic blockers are frequently called beta-blockers because they block beta$_1$ and beta$_2$ (nonselective) or beta$_1$ (cardiac selective) receptors.

■ Assess whether client has respiratory problems by listening for signs of wheezing or noting dyspnea (difficulty in breathing). If the beta-blocker is nonselective, not only does the pulse rate decrease but also bronchoconstriction can result. Clients with asthma should take a beta$_1$ blocker such as metoprolol (Lopressor) and avoid nonselective beta-blockers.

■ Determine the drugs client currently takes. Report if any are phenothiazines, digoxin, calcium channel blockers, or other antihypertensives.

■ Record client's urine output and use for future comparison.

NURSING DIAGNOSES

■ Decreased cardiac output
■ Impaired tissue integrity

PLANNING

■ Client will comply with the drug regimen.
■ Client's vital signs will be within the desired range.

---

*Alpha- and beta-adrenergic blockers are also presented within the antidysrhythmic (Chapter 40), antianginal (Chapter 40), and antihypertensive (Chapter 42) sections.

NURSING INTERVENTIONS

■ Monitor client's vital signs. Report marked changes such as marked decrease in blood pressure and pulse rate.

■ Administer IV propranolol undiluted or diluted in D₅W.

■ Note any complaints of excessive dizziness or light-headedness.

■ Report any complaint of a stuffy nose. Vasodilation results from the use of alpha-adrenergic blockers, and nasal congestion can occur.

■ Determine whether client has diabetes and receives a beta-adrenergic blocker; the insulin dose or oral hypoglycemic may need to be adjusted.

■ Clients who take beta-blockers do not have normal compensatory mechanisms while in states of shock. To resuscitate such clients, glucagon must be given in high doses to counteract the sympatholytic effects of beta-blockers.

Client Teaching

General

• Advise client to avoid abruptly stopping a beta-blocker; rebound hypertension, rebound tachycardia, or an angina attack could result.

• Instruct client to comply with the drug regimen.

• Educate clients about insulin therapy that early warning signs of hypoglycemia (e.g., tachycardia, nervousness) may be masked by the beta-blocker.

• Direct clients on insulin therapy to monitor their blood sugar carefully and to follow diet orders.

Self-Administration

• Teach client and family how to take the pulse and blood pressure.

Side Effects

• Encourage client to avoid orthostatic (postural) hypotension by slowly rising from supine or sitting positions to standing.

• Inform client and family of possible mood changes when taking beta blockers. Mood changes can include depression, nightmares, and suicidal tendencies.

• Warn male client that certain beta blockers (e.g., propranolol, metoprolol, pindolol) and alpha blockers (e.g., prazosin) may cause impotence or a decrease in libido. Usually the problem is dose related.

Cultural Considerations ⊕

• Obtain an interpreter when necessary; do not rely on family members, who may not fully disclose because of honor or shame.

• When translation is needed, discuss the ethnicity of the interpreter as well as the language desired. Provide an interpreter with the same ethnic background and gender if possible, especially when sensitive topics are being addressed.

EVALUATION

■ Evaluate the effectiveness of the adrenergic blocker. Vital signs must be stable within the desired range.

Critical Thinking Case Studies

V.T., age 79, has asthma. An adrenergic drug is selected.

1. What are the drug advantages and disadvantages associated with the use of ephedrine, isoproterenol, metaproterenol, albuterol, and terbutaline for V.T.? Explain.

2. Is age a factor in drug selection? Explain.

H.P., age 69, has hypertension and asthma. An adrenergic blocker is selected.

1. What are the drug advantages and disadvantages associated with the use of doxazosin, prazosin, propranolol, metoprolol, atenolol, and acebutolol for H.P.? Explain.

2. What needs to be included when teaching H.P. about the use of an adrenergic blocker?

Study Questions

1. What are the divisions of the central nervous system and the peripheral nervous system? What is their interrelationship?

2. What does the autonomic nervous system control and regulate? What does the somatic nervous system control and regulate?

3. Drugs that mimic and block the sympathetic and parasympathetic nervous systems have opposite and similar effects on organ tissue. What is the explanation for this phenomenon?

4. What terms are used to classify sympathetic stimulants and depressants? What are their actions on the body?

5. What terms are used to classify parasympathetic stimulants and depressants? What are their actions on the body?

6. What are the adrenergic receptors? What are the major physiologic responses of each?

7. What is the difference between selective and nonselective adrenergic drugs? Give examples of each.

8. What are the major side effects of adrenergic drugs? What are the implications for client teaching?

9. What drugs are selective and nonselective adrenergic blockers? What are the uses of alpha-blockers and beta-blockers?

10. What are the side effects of adrenergic blockers?

11. What are the nursing interventions associated with the use of adrenergic drugs?

18 Cholinergics and Anticholinergics

OUTLINE

OBJECTIVES

- Compare the two cholinergic receptors.
- Describe the responses of cholinergic drugs and anticholinergic drugs.
- Differentiate between direct-acting and indirect-acting cholinergic drugs.
- Compare the major side effects of cholinergic and anticholinergic drugs.
- Differentiate the uses of cholinergics and anticholinergics.
- Explain the nursing process, including client teaching, associated with cholinergics and anticholinergics.

TERMS

acetylcholine (ACh)
anticholinergics
anticholinesterases
cholinergics
cholinergic blocking agents
cholinesterase (ChE)
direct-acting cholinergics
indirect-acting cholinergics
miosis
muscarinic receptors
mydriasis
nicotinic receptors
parasympatholytics
parasympathomimetics

Introduction

The two groups of drugs that affect the parasympathetic nervous system are the (1) *cholinergics* (parasympathomimetics) and the (2) *anticholinergics* (parasympatholytics). See the Unit V opener for a discussion and comparison of the parasympathetic nervous system (parasympathomimetics and parasympatholytics) and the sympathetic nervous system.

Cholinergics

Drugs that stimulate the parasympathetic nervous system are called **cholinergics**, or **parasympathomimetics**, because they mimic the parasympathetic neurotransmitter acetylcholine. Cholinergic drugs are also called *cholinomimetics, cholinergic stimulants,* or *cholinergic agonists.* **Acetylcholine (ACh)** is the neurotransmitter located at the ganglions and the parasympathetic terminal nerve endings that innervates the receptors in organs, tissues, and glands. The two types of cholinergic receptors are (1) **muscarinic receptors,** which stimulate smooth mus-

cle and slow the heart rate; and (2) **nicotinic receptors** (neuromuscular), which affect the skeletal muscles. Many cholinergic drugs are nonselective because they can affect both the muscarinic and the nicotinic receptors. However, there are selective cholinergic drugs for the muscarinic receptors that do *not* affect the nicotinic receptors. Figure 18–1 illustrates the effects of parasympathetic or cholinergic stimulation.

There are direct-acting cholinergic drugs and indirect-acting cholinergic drugs. *Direct-acting cholinergic drugs* act on the receptors to activate a tissue response (Figure 18–2, *A*). *Indirect-acting cholinergic drugs* inhibit the action of the enzyme **cholinesterase (ChE)** (acetylcholinesterase) by forming a chemical complex, thus permitting acetylcholine to persist and attach to the receptor (Figure 18–2, *B*). Drugs that inhibit cholinesterase are called *cholinesterase inhibitors, acetylcholinesterase (AChE) inhibitors,* or **anticholinesterases.** Cholinesterase may destroy acetylcholine before it reaches the receptor or after it has attached to the site. By inhibiting or destroying the enzyme cholinesterase, more acetylcholine is available to stimulate the receptor and remain in contact with it longer.

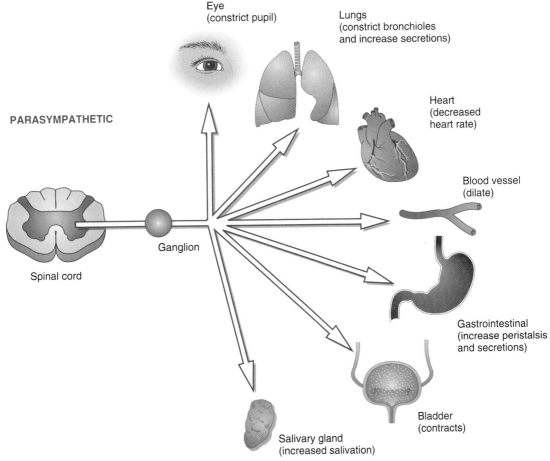

FIGURE 18–1 **Parasympathetic responses. Stimulation of the parasympathetic nervous system or use of parasympathomimetic drugs will cause the pupils to constrict, the bronchioles to constrict and increase bronchial secretions, the heart rate to decrease, the blood vessels to dilate, peristalsis and gastric secretions to increase, the bladder muscle to contract, and the salivary glands to increase salivation.**

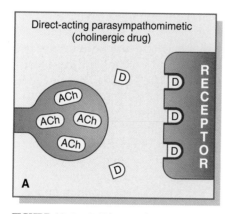
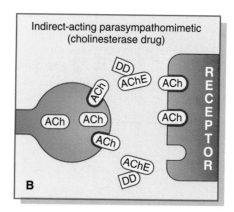

FIGURE 18–2 A, Direct-acting parasympathomimetic (cholinergic drugs). Cholinergic drugs resemble acetylcholine and act directly on the receptor. **B,** Indirect-acting parasympathomimetic (cholinesterase inhibitors). Cholinesterase inhibitors inactivate the enzyme acetylcholinesterase (cholinesterase) thus permitting acetylcholine to react to the receptor. *ACh,* Acetylcholine; *AChE,* acetylcholinesterase or cholinesterase; *D,* cholinergic drug; *DD,* cholinesterase inhibitor (anticholinesterase).

The cholinesterase inhibitors (anticholinesterases) can be separated into reversible inhibitors and irreversible inhibitors. The reversible inhibitors bind the enzyme, cholinesterase, for several minutes to hours, and the irreversible inhibitors bind the enzyme permanently. The resulting effects vary with how long the cholinesterase is bound.

The major responses of cholinergic drugs are to stimulate bladder and gastrointestinal (GI) tone, constrict pupils of the eyes **(miosis)**, and increase neuromuscular transmission. Other effects of cholinergic drugs include decreased heart rate and blood pressure and increased salivary, GI, and bronchial glandular secretions. Table 18–1 lists the functions of direct- and indirect-acting cholinergic drugs.

Direct-Acting Cholinergics

Many drugs classified as **direct-acting cholinergics** are primarily selective to the muscarinic receptors but are nonspecific because the muscarinic receptors are located in the smooth muscles of the GI and genitourinary tracts, glands, and heart. Bethanechol chloride (Urecholine), a direct-acting cholinergic drug, acts on the muscarinic (cholinergic) receptor and is used primarily to increase urination. Metoclopramide HCl (Reglan) is a direct-acting cholinergic drug that is usually prescribed to treat gastroesophageal reflux disease (GERD). Metoclopramide increases gastric emptying time. Prototype Drug Chart 18–1 details the pharmacologic behavior of bethanechol.

Direct-Acting Cholinergics: Eye

Pilocarpine is a direct-acting cholinergic drug that constricts the pupils of the eyes thus opening the canal of Schlemm to promote drainage of aqueous humor (fluid). This drug is used to treat glaucoma by relieving fluid (intraocular) pressure in the eye. Pilocarpine also acts on the nicotinic receptor, as does carbachol. Both agents are dis-

Table 18–1
Effects of Cholinergic Drugs

Body Tissue	Response
Cardiovascular*	Decreases heart rate, lowers blood pressure because of vasodilation, and slows conduction of atrioventricular node.
Gastrointestinal†	Increases the tone and motility of the smooth muscles of the stomach and intestine. Peristalsis is increased, and the sphincter muscles are relaxed.
Genitourinary	Contracts the muscles of the urinary bladder, increases tone of the ureters, and relaxes the bladder's sphincter muscles. Stimulates urination.
Ocular†	Increases pupillary constriction, or miosis (pupil becomes smaller), and increases accommodation (flattening or thickening of eye lens for distant or near vision).
Glandular*	Increases salivation, perspiration, and tears.
Bronchial (lung)*	Stimulates bronchial smooth muscle contraction and increases bronchial secretions.
Striated muscle†	Increases neuromuscular transmission and maintains muscle strength and tone.

*Tissue responses to large doses of cholinergic drugs.
†Major tissue responses to normal doses of cholinergic drugs.

cussed in more detail in Chapter 47, Drugs for Disorders of the Eye and the Ear.

Pharmacokinetics

Bethanechol chloride (Urecholine) is poorly absorbed from the GI tract. The percentage of protein-binding and the half-life are unknown. The drug is most likely excreted in the urine.

PROTOTYPE DRUG CHART 18–1

BETHANECHOL CHLORIDE

Drug Class Cholinergic/parasympathomimetic Trade Name: Urecholine, 🍁 Duvoid, Urecholine *Pregnancy Category:* C	**Dosage** A: PO: 10-50 mg b.i.d./ t.i.d./q.i.d.; *max:* 120 mg/d subQ: 2.5-5 mg, repeat at 15-30 min intervals; PRN Do *NOT* give IM or IV. C: PO: 0.5 mg/kg/d in 3-4 divided doses

Contraindications
Severe bradycardia or hypotension, chronic obstructive
  pulmonary disease, asthma, peptic ulcer, parkinsonism,
  hyperthyroidism
	Drug-Lab-Food Interactions
	Drug: Decrease bethanechol effect with anti-
	  dysrhythmics
	Lab: Increase AST, bilirubin, amylase, lipase

Pharmacokinetics
Absorption: PO: Poorly absorbed
Distribution: PB: UK
Metabolism: t½: UK
Excretion: In urine
	Pharmacodynamics
	PO: Onset: 0.5-1.5 h
	  Peak: 1-2 h
	  Duration: 4-6 h
	subQ: Onset: 5-15 min
	  Peak: 0.5 h
	  Duration: 2 h

Therapeutic Effects/Uses

To treat urinary retention, abdominal distention
Mode of Action: Stimulate the cholinergic (muscarinic) receptor; promote contraction of the bladder; increase GI
  peristalsis, GI secretion, pupillary constriction, and bronchoconstriction

Side Effects
Nausea, vomiting, diarrhea, salivation, sweating,
  flushing, frequent urination, rash, miosis, blurred vision,
  abdominal discomfort
	Adverse Reactions
	Orthostatic hypotension, bradycardia, muscle weakness
	Life-threatening: Acute asthmatic attack, heart block,
	  circulatory collapse, cardiac arrest

A, Adult; *AST,* aspartate aminotransferase; *b.i.d.,* two times a day; *d,* day; *GI,* gastrointestinal; *h,* hour; *IM,* intramuscular; *IV,* intravenous; *min,* minute; *PB,* protein-binding; *PO,* by mouth; *PRN,* as needed; *q.i.d.,* four times a day; *subQ,* subcutaneous; *t½,* half-life;
t.i.d., three times a day; *UK,* unknown; 🍁, Canadian drug names.

Pharmacodynamics

The principal use of bethanechol is to promote micturition (urination)
by stimulating the muscarinic cholinergic receptors to increase urine output. The client voids approximately 30 minutes to 1.5 hours after taking
an oral dose of bethanechol because of the increased tone of the detrusor
urinae muscle. Bethanechol also increases peristalsis in the GI tract. The
drug should be taken on an empty stomach. It should not be administered intramuscularly (IM) or intravenously (IV), but it can be given subcutaneously (subQ). Micturition usually occurs within 15 minutes via the
subQ route. The duration of action is 4 to 6 hours for oral administration
and 2 hours for the subQ route.

Side Effects and Adverse Reactions

Mild to severe side effects of most muscarinic agonists such
as bethanechol include hypotension, bradycardia, excessive salivation, increased gastric acid secretion, abdominal
cramps, diarrhea, bronchoconstriction, and, in some cases,
cardiac dysrhythmias. This group of agents should be prescribed cautiously for clients with low blood pressure and
heart rates. Muscarinic agonists are contraindicated for
clients with intestinal or urinary tract obstruction and for
those with active asthma.

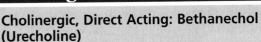

Nursing Process

Cholinergic, Direct Acting: Bethanechol (Urecholine)

ASSESSMENT

- Note baseline vital signs for future comparison.
- Assess urine output (should be >600 ml/d). Report
decrease in urine output.
- Obtain a history from client of health problems,
such as peptic ulcer, urinary obstruction, or asthma.
Cholinergics can aggravate symptoms of these
conditions.

NURSING DIAGNOSES

- Urinary retention
- Anxiety

PLANNING

- Client will have increased bladder and GI tone after taking cholinergics.
- Client will have increased neuromuscular strength.

NURSING INTERVENTIONS

Direct Acting

- Monitor client's vital signs. Pulse rate and blood pressure decrease when large doses of cholinergics are taken. Orthostatic hypotension is a side effect of a cholinergic such as bethanechol.
- Record fluid intake and output. Decreased urinary output should be reported because it may be related to urinary obstruction.
- Give cholinergics 1 hour before or 2 hours after meals. If client complains of gastric pain, the drug may be given with meals.
- Check serum enzyme values for amylase and lipase, as well as aspartate aminotransferase and bilirubin levels. These laboratory values may increase slightly when taking cholinergics.
- Observe client for side effects, such as gastric pain or cramping, diarrhea, increased salivary or bronchial secretions, bradycardia, and orthostatic hypotension.
- Auscultate for bowel sounds. Report decreased or hyperactive bowel sounds.
- Auscultate breath sounds for rales (cracking sounds from fluid congestion in lung tissue) or rhonchi (rough sounds resulting from mucous secretions in lung tissue). Cholinergic drugs can increase bronchial secretions.
- Have IV atropine sulfate (0.6 mg) available as an antidote for cholinergic overdose. Early signs of overdosing include salivation, sweating, abdominal cramps, and flush.
- Note that diaphoresis (excessive perspiration) may occur; linens should be changed as needed.

Indirect Acting

- Beware of the possibility of cholinergic crisis (overdose); symptoms include muscular weakness and increased salivation.

Client Teaching

Direct Acting
General

- Instruct client to take the cholinergic as prescribed. Compliance with the drug regimen is essential.

Side Effects

- Direct client to report severe side effects, such as profound dizziness or a decrease in pulse rate below 60 beats/min.
- Teach client to arise from a lying position slowly to avoid dizziness; this is most likely a result of orthostatic hypotension.
- Encourage client to maintain effective oral hygiene if excess salivation occurs.

- Advise client to report any difficulty in breathing as a result of respiratory distress.

Indirect Acting (see drugs for myasthenia gravis)

- Direct client to take the drug on time to avoid respiratory muscle weakness.
- Instruct client to assess changes in muscle strength. Cholinesterase inhibitors (anticholinesterases) increase muscle strength.

Cultural Considerations ⊕

- When offering a prescription, instructions, or pamphlets to Asians and Pacific Islanders, use both hands to show respect.
- The extended-family structure is important for teaching health strategies and providing support. Recognize the importance in including women in decision making and disseminating health information.

EVALUATION

- Determine the effectiveness of the cholinergic or anticholinesterase drug.
- Evaluate the stability of client's vital signs and note the presence of side effects or adverse reactions.

Indirect-Acting Cholinergics

The **indirect-acting cholinergics** do not act on receptors; instead they inhibit or inactivate the enzyme cholinesterase, thus permitting acetylcholine to accumulate at the receptor sites (see Figure 18–2, *B*). This action gives them the name *cholinesterase (ChE) inhibitors, acetylcholinesterase (AChE) inhibitors,* or *anticholinesterases,* of which there are two types: reversible and irreversible.

The function of the enzyme cholinesterase is to break down into choline and acetic acid. A small amount of cholinesterase can break down a large amount of acetylcholine in a short period. A cholinesterase inhibitor drug binds with cholinesterase thus allowing the acetylcholine to activate the muscarinic and nicotinic cholinergic receptors. This action permits skeletal muscle stimulation, which increases the force of muscular contraction. Because of this action, the cholinesterase inhibitors are useful to increase muscle tone for clients with myasthenia gravis (a neuromuscular disorder). By increasing acetylcholine, additional effects occur, such as increase in GI motility, bradycardia, miosis, bronchial constriction, and increased micturition.

The primary use of cholinesterase inhibitors is to treat myasthenia gravis. Other uses are to treat glaucoma, Alzheimer's disease, and muscarinic antagonist poisoning.

Reversible Cholinesterase Inhibitors

Reversible cholinesterase inhibitors are used (1) to produce pupillary constriction in the treatment of glaucoma and (2) to increase muscle strength in clients with myasthenia gravis. Drug effects persist for several hours. Drugs used to increase muscular strength in myasthenia gravis include neostigmine (Prostigmin [short-acting]), pyridostigmine bromide (Mestinon [moderate-acting]), ambenonium chloride (Mytelase [long-acting]), and edrophonium chloride (Tensilon [short-acting for diagnostic purposes]). These drugs are discussed in more detail in Chapter 24, Drugs for Neuromuscular Disorders: Myasthenia Gravis, Multiple Sclerosis, and Muscle Spasms. A reversible ophthalmic anticholinesterase drug is physostigmine (Eserine). Ophthalmic agents are further discussed in Chapter 47, Drugs for Disorders of the Eye and the Ear.

Side Effects

Caution in taking reversible cholinesterase inhibitors is required for clients who have bradycardia, asthma, peptic ulcers, or hyperthyroidism. Cholinesterase inhibitors are contraindicated for clients with intestinal or urinary obstruction.

Irreversible Cholinesterase Inhibitors

Irreversible cholinesterase inhibitors are potent agents because of their long-lasting effect. The enzyme cholinesterase must be regenerated before the drug effect diminishes, a process that may take days or weeks. These drugs are used to produce pupillary constriction and to manufacture organophosphate insecticides.

With irreversible cholinesterase inhibitors, the bond between the irreversible cholinesterase inhibitor and cholinesterase is considered permanent; however, this bond can be broken with the use of the drug pralidoxime (Protopam). Pralidoxime is an antidote to reverse the irreversible organophosphate. The effect is at the neuromuscular junction. See Table 18–2 for examples of cholinergic drugs and their standard dosages and common uses.

Anticholinergics

Drugs that inhibit the actions of acetylcholine by occupying the acetylcholine receptors are called **anticholinergics** or **parasympatholytics**. Other names for anticholinergics are **cholinergic blocking agents**, *cholinergic* or *muscarinic antagonists, antiparasympathetic agents, antimuscarinic agents,* or *an-*

Table 18–2

Cholinergics

Generic (Brand)	Route and Dosage	Uses and Considerations
Direct-Acting Cholinergics		
bethanechol Cl (Urecholine)	See Prototype Drug Chart 18–1.	
metoclopramine HCl (Reglan, Maxolon)	A: PO: 10-15 mg t.i.d. a.c. C: PO/IM/IV: 0.4-0.8 mg/kg/d in 4 divided doses	For GERD and gastroparesis. It is a central dopamine receptor antagonist. It increases gastric emptying time. *Pregnancy category:* B; PB: UK; t^1/$_2$: 2.5-6 h
carbachol (Miostat)	Ophthalmic: 0.75%-3%, 1-2 gtt, 3 × daily	To reduce IOP, miosis. See Chapter 47.
pilocarpine HCl (Pilocar)	Ophthalmic: 0.5%-4%, 1 gt	To reduce IOP, miosis. See Chapter 47.
Cholinesterase Inhibitor		
tacrine HCl (Cognex)	*Alzheimer's disease:* A: PO: 10 mg, q.i.d., increase dose at 6-wk intervals A: PO: 40-160 mg/d p.c.; *max:* 160 mg/d	To improve memory in mild to moderate Alzheimer's dementia. Drug enhances cholinergic function. *Pregnancy category:* C; PB: 55%; t^1/$_2$: 1.5-3.5 h
donepezil HCl (Aricept); rivastigmine (Exelon)	See Chapter 23, Table 23-8.	
Indirect-Acting Cholinergics or Cholinesterase Inhibitors for the Eye		
demecarium bromide (Humorsol)	0.125%-0.25%, 1 gt q12-48 h	To reduce IOP in glaucoma; long-acting miotic. See Chapter 47.
echothiophate iodide (Phospholine Iodide)	0.03%-0.25%, 1 gt daily or b.i.d.	To reduce IOP; long-acting miotic. See Chapter 47.
isoflurophate (Floropryl)	0.25%, ointment q8-72 h	To treat glaucoma. Apply to the conjunctival sac. See Chapter 47.
Reversible Cholinesterase Inhibitors: Myasthenia Gravis		
ambenonium Cl (Mytelase)	A: PO: 2.5-5.0 mg t.i.d./q.i.d.; dose may be increased; *maint:* 5-25 mg t.i.d./q.i.d.	To increase muscle strength in myasthenia gravis; long-acting. May be used with glucocorticoids. *Pregnancy category:* C; PB: UK; t^1/$_2$: UK
edrophonium Cl (Tensilon)	A: IV: 2 mg; then 8 mg if no response IM: 10 mg; may repeat with 2 mg in 30 min C: <34 kg: IV: 1 mg; repeat in 30-45 sec if no response; *max:* 5 mg C: >34 kg: IV: 2 mg; repeat with 1 mg if no response; *max:* 10 mg	To diagnose myasthenia gravis; very short-acting. *Pregnancy category:* C; PB: UK; t^1/$_2$: 1.2-2 h

A, Adult; *a.c.,* before meals; *b.i.d.,* two times a day; *C,* child; *d,* day; *GERD,* gastroesophageal reflux disease; *GI,* gastrointestinal; *gt,* drop; *gtt,* drops; *h,* hour; *IM,* intramuscular; *IOP,* intraocular pressure; *IV,* intravenous; *maint,* maintenance; *PB,* protein-binding; *p.c.,* after meals; *PO,* by mouth; *PRN,* as needed; *q.i.d.,* four times a day; *sec,* second; *SR,* sustained-release; *t^1/$_2$,* half-life; *t.i.d.,* three times a day; *UK,* unknown; >, greater than; <, less than.

Continued

Table 18-2

Cholinergics—cont'd

Generic (Brand)	Route and Dosage	Uses and Considerations
Reversible Cholinesterase Inhibitors: Myasthenia Gravis—cont'd		
neostigmine (Prostigmin); neostigmine methylsulfate (injectable form)	A: PO: Initially 15 mg t.i.d.; *maint:* 150 mg/d in divided doses; range: 15-375 mg/d IM/IV: 0.5-2.5 mg PRN C: PO: 2 mg/kg/d in 6 divided doses	To increase muscle strength in myasthenia gravis; short-acting. Used also to prevent or treat postoperative urinary retention. *Pregnancy category:* C; PB: 15%-25%; $t^1/_2$: 1-1.5 h
physostigmine salicylate (Eserine Salicylate)	0.25%-0.5%, 1 gt daily or q.i.d.	To reduce IOP, miosis; short-acting
pyridostigmine bromide (Mestinon)	A: PO: 60-120 mg t.i.d./q.i.d.; *maint:* 600 mg/d in 3-4 divided doses; *max:* 1.5 g/d SR: 180-540 mg daily or b.i.d. IM/IV: 2 mg q2-3h C: PO: 7 mg/kg/d in 5-6 divided doses	To increase muscle strength in myasthenia gravis; moderate-acting. Prevents the destruction of the neurotransmitter acetylcholine. *Pregnancy category:* C; PB: <10%; $t^1/_2$: 3-4 h
Antidote for Irreversible and Reversible Cholinesterase Inhibitors		
pralidoxime Cl (Protopam)	A: IM: 1-2 g, repeat in 1-2 h, then 10 to 12 h intervals A: IV: 1-2 g in 100 ml of saline solution infused over 15-30 min A: PO: 1-3 g, repeat in 5 h PRN C: IV: 20-40 mg/kg/dose; repeat in 1-2 h; 10- to 12-h intervals PRN	To treat overdose of organophosphate pesticides that cause muscle paralysis and to treat an overdose of a cholinesterase inhibitor for myasthenia gravis. *Pregnancy category:* C; PB: UK; $t^1/_2$: 1-2.7 h

tispasmodics. The major body tissues and organs affected by the anticholinergic group of drugs are the heart, respiratory tract, GI tract, urinary bladder, eyes, and exocrine glands. By blocking the parasympathetic nerves, the sympathetic (adrenergic) nervous system dominates. Anticholinergic and adrenergic drugs produce many of the same responses.

Anticholinergic and cholinergic drugs have opposite effects. The major responses to anticholinergics are a decrease in GI motility, a decrease in salivation, dilation of pupils **(mydriasis)**, and an increase in pulse rate. Other effects of anticholinergics include decreased bladder contraction, which can result in urinary retention, and decreased rigidity and tremors related to neuromuscular excitement. Anticholinergics can act as an antidote to the toxicity caused by cholinesterase inhibitors and organophosphate ingestion. The various effects of anticholinergics are described in Table 18–3.

Muscarinic receptors, also called *cholinergic receptors*, are involved in tissue and organ responses to anticholinergics, because anticholinergics inhibit the actions of acetylcholine by occupying these receptor sites. Figure 18–3 illustrates this action of anticholinergic drugs. Anticholinergic drugs may block the effect of direct-acting parasympathomimetics, such as bethanechol and pilocarpine, and of indirect-acting parasympathomimetics, such as physostigmine and neostigmine.

Atropine

Atropine sulfate, first derived from the belladonna plant *(Atropa belladonna)* and purified in 1831, is a classic anticholinergic, or muscarinic antagonist drug. Scopolamine was the second belladonna alkaloid produced. Atropine and scopo-

Table 18-3

Effects of Anticholinergic Drugs

Body Tissues	Responses
Cardiovascular	Increases heart rate with large doses. Small doses can decrease heart rate.
Gastrointestinal (GI)	Relaxes smooth muscle tone of GI tract, decreasing GI motility and peristalsis. Decreases gastric and intestinal secretions.
Urinary tract	Relaxes the bladder detrusor muscle and increases constriction of the internal sphincter. Urinary retention can result.
Ocular	Dilates pupils (mydriasis) and paralyzes ciliary muscle (cycloplegia), causing a decrease in accommodation.
Glandular	Decreases salivation, perspiration, and bronchial secretions.
Bronchial	Dilates the bronchi and decreases bronchial secretions.
Central nervous system	Decreases tremors and rigidity of muscles. Drowsiness, disorientation, and hallucination can result from large doses.

lamine act on the muscarinic receptor, but they have little effect on the nicotinic receptor. Atropine is useful (1) as a preoperative medication to decrease salivary secretions, (2) as an antispasmodic drug to treat peptic ulcers because it relaxes the smooth muscles of the GI tract and decreases peristalsis, and (3) as an agent to increase the heart rate when

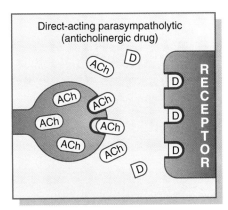

FIGURE 18–3 Anticholinergic response. The anticholinergic drug occupies the receptor sites, thus blocking acetylcholine. *ACh*, Acetylcholine; *D*, anticholinergic drug.

bradycardia is present. Atropine can also be used as an antidote for muscarinic agonist poisoning caused by an overdose of a muscarinic drug such as bethanechol or of a cholinesterase inhibitor. However, if a client takes atropine or an atropine-like drug (antihistamine) for a long period, side effects can occur. Prototype Drug Chart 18–2 details the pharmacologic behavior of atropine.

Synthetic anticholinergic drugs are also used as antispasmodics to treat peptic ulcers and intestinal spasticity. One example is propantheline bromide (Pro-Banthine), which has been available for several decades. It decreases gastric secretions and GI spasms. Since the introduction of the histamine (H_2) blockers, anticholinergic agents such as propantheline are not used as frequently to decrease gastric secretions.

PROTOTYPE DRUG CHART 18–2

ATROPINE

Drug Class

Anticholinergic/parasympatholytic
Trade Name: Atropine, Atropisol (Optic), ✦ Atropair
Pregnancy Category: C

Dosage

A: PO/IM/IV: 0.4–0.6 mg q4-6h PRN
C: PO/IM/IV: 0.01 mg/kg/dose; *max:* 0.4 mg/dose, q4-6h, PRN

Contraindications

Narrow-angle glaucoma, obstructive GI disorders, paralytic ileus, ulcerative colitis, tachycardia, benign prostatic hypertrophy, myasthenia gravis, myocardial ischemia
Caution: Renal or hepatic disorders, COPD, congestive heart failure

Drug-Lab-Food Interactions

Drug: Increase anticholinergic effect with phenothiazines, antidepressants, MAOIs, amantadine; may *increase* effects of atenolol

Pharmacokinetics

Absorption: PO/IM: Well absorbed
Distribution: PB: UK; crosses the placenta
Metabolism: t½: 2-3 h
Excretion: 75% excreted in urine

Pharmacodynamics

PO: Onset: 0.5-1 h
 Peak: 1-2 h
 Duration: 4 h
IM: Onset: 10-30 min
 Peak: 0.5 h
 Duration: 4 h
IV: Onset: Immediate
 Peak: 5 min
 Duration: UK
Instill: Onset: 20-30 min
 Peak: 30-40 min
 Duration: days

Therapeutic Effects/Uses

Preoperative medication to reduce salivation, increase heart rate, dilate pupils
Mode of Action: Inhibition of acetylcholine by occupying the receptors; increase heart rate by blocking vagus stimulation; promote dilation of the pupils by blocking iris sphincter muscle

Side Effects

Dry mouth, nausea, headache, constipation, rash, dry skin, flush, blurred vision, photophobia

Adverse Reactions

Tachycardia, hypotension, pupillary dilation, abdominal distention, palpitations, nasal congestion
Life-threatening: Paralytic ileus, coma

A, Adult; *C,* child; *COPD,* chronic obstructive pulmonary disease; *GI,* gastrointestinal; *h,* hour; *IM,* intramuscular; *instill,* instillation; *IV,* intravenous; *MAOI,* monoamine oxidase inhibitor; *min,* minute; *PB,* protein-binding; *PO,* by mouth; *PRN,* as needed; *t½,* half-life; *UK,* unknown; >, greater than; ✦, Canadian drug names.

Pharmacokinetics

Atropine sulfate is well absorbed orally and parenterally. It crosses the blood-brain barrier and exerts its effect on the central nervous system (CNS). The protein binding is unknown. It crosses the placenta. Atropine has a short half-life; therefore there is little cumulative effect. Most of the absorbed atropine is excreted in the urine (75% to 95%).

Pharmacodynamics

Atropine sulfate blocks acetylcholine by occupying the muscarinic receptor. It increases the heart rate by blocking vagus stimulation and promotes dilation of the pupils by paralyzing the iris sphincter. The two most frequent uses of atropine are to decrease salivation and respiratory secretions preoperatively and to treat sinus bradycardia by increasing the heart rate. Atropine also is used ophthalmically for mydriasis and cycloplegia before eye refraction and to treat inflammation of the iris (iritis) and uveal tract.

Its onset of action orally is between 0.5 to 1 hour and peaks at 2 to 4 hours. For the IM route, the onset of action is 10 to 30 minutes and peaks at 30 minutes. The duration for oral and IM routes is 4 hours; via the IV route, the onset of action is immediate and peak action is at 5 minutes.

Side Effects and Adverse Reactions

The common side effects of atropine and atropine-like drugs include dry mouth, decreased perspiration, blurred vision, tachycardia, constipation, and urinary retention. Other side effects and adverse reactions are nausea, headache, dry skin, abdominal distention, hypotension or hypertension, impotence, photophobia, and coma.

Nursing Process

Anticholinergic Drugs: Atropine

ASSESSMENT

■ Obtain baseline vital signs for future comparison. Tachycardia is a side effect that occurs with large doses of anticholinergics such as atropine sulfate.
■ Assess urine output. Urinary retention may occur.
■ Check client's medical history. Atropine and atropine-like drugs are contraindicated if client has narrow-angle glaucoma, obstructive gastrointestinal (GI) disorder, paralytic ileus, ulcerative colitis, benign prostatic hypertrophy, or myasthenia gravis.
■ Determine a history of the drugs client takes. Phenothiazines and antidepressants increase the effect of anticholinergics.

NURSING DIAGNOSES

■ Urinary retention
■ Impaired oral mucous membrane
■ Constipation

PLANNING

■ Client's secretions will be decreased before surgery.

■ Client will not have side effects that may become a health problem.

NURSING INTERVENTIONS

■ Monitor client's vital signs. Report if tachycardia occurs.
■ Determine fluid intake and output. Encourage client to void before taking the medication. Report decreased urine output. Anticholinergics can cause urinary retention. Maintain adequate fluid intake.
■ Record bowel sounds. Absence of bowel sounds may indicate paralytic ileus resulting from a decrease in GI motility (peristalsis).
■ Check for constipation caused by the decrease in GI motility. Encourage the client to ingest foods that are high in fiber, to drink adequate amounts of fluids, and to exercise if able.
■ Raise bedside rails for clients who are confused and debilitated. Atropine could cause central nervous system stimulation (excitement, confusion) or drowsiness.
■ Provide mouth care. Atropine decreases oral secretions and can cause dryness of the mouth.
■ Administer IV atropine undiluted or diluted in 10 ml of sterile water. Rate of administration is 0.6 mg/min.

Client Teaching

General

• Direct client to avoid hot environments and excess physical exertion. Elevations in body temperature can result from diminished sweat gland activity.
• Teach client with glaucoma to avoid atropine-like drugs. Anticholinergics cause mydriasis and increase the intraocular pressure. Clients should be alerted to check labels on over-the-counter drugs to determine whether they are contraindicated for glaucoma.
• Instruct client not to drive a motor vehicle or participate in activities that require alertness. Drowsiness is common.
• Advise client to avoid alcohol, cigarettes, caffeine, and aspirin at bedtime to decrease gastric acidity.
• Tell client with mydriasis from an eye examination to use sunglasses in bright light because of photophobia (intolerance of bright light).

Side Effects

• Advise client of common side effects, such as dry mouth, decrease in urination, and constipation, that occur as a result of long-term use of anticholinergics.
• Direct client to increase fluid intake to prevent constipation when taking anticholinergics for a prolonged period.
• Instruct client to urinate before taking the anticholinergic. Urinary retention can be a problem. Client should report a marked decrease in urine output.

- Suggest that client use hard candy, ice chips, or chewing gum. Maintain effective oral hygiene if client's mouth is dry. Anticholinergics decrease salivation.
- Encourage client to use eye drops to moisten dry eyes that result from decreased lacrimation (tearing).

Diet
- Suggest that client's diet include foods high in fiber and increased water intake to prevent constipation.

Cultural Considerations ⊕
- Obtain an interpreter when necessary; do not rely on family members, who may not fully disclose because of honor and shame.
- Ask open-ended questions and have clients demonstrate, rather than verbalize, their understanding of treatments. Because politeness and "saving face" prevail, do not assume that a positive response means a definite *yes*.

EVALUATION
- Evaluate client's response to the anticholinergic.
- Determine whether constipation, urine retention, or increased pulse rate is or remains a problem.

Antiparkinson–Anticholinergic Drugs

At one time, atropine was given to clients with Parkinson's disease to decrease salivation and drooling. It was also found to have some effect on the motor manifestation of this disease by decreasing tremors and rigidity. Additional studies indicate that anticholinergic (antimuscarinic) agents affect the CNS as well as the parasympathetic nervous system. These anticholinergic drugs affect the CNS by suppressing the tremors and muscular rigidity of parkinsonism, but they have little effect on mobility and muscle weakness. As a result of these findings, several anticholinergic drugs were developed, such as trihexyphenidyl hydrochloride (Artane), procyclidine (Kemadrin), biperiden (Akineton), and benztropine (Cogentin), for the treatment of Parkinson's disease. These drugs can be used alone in early stages of parkinsonism. They may be used in combination with levodopa to control parkinsonism or used alone to treat pseudoparkinsonism, which results from the side effects of the phenothiazines in antipsychotic drugs. Drugs used to treat parkinsonism are described in more detail in Chapter 23, Drugs for Neurological Disorders: Parkinsonism and Alzheimer's Disease. Prototype Drug Chart 18–3 lists the drug data related to trihexyphenidyl, which is used for pseudoparkinsonism.

Pharmacokinetics

Trihexyphenidyl is well absorbed from the GI tract. Its protein-binding percentage and half-life are unknown. It is excreted in the urine.

Pharmacodynamics

Trihexyphenidyl decreases involuntary movement and diminishes the signs and symptoms of tremors and muscle rigidity that occur with Parkinson's disease and pseudoparkinsonism. It is available as a tablet, elixir, and sustained-release capsule. The duration of action of the sustained-release preparation is twice as long as that for the oral and elixir forms. Alcohol, narcotics, amantadine, phenothiazines, and antihistamines may increase the effect of trihexyphenidyl. The side effects are similar to other anticholinergic drugs.

Antihistamines for Treating Motion Sickness

The effects of anticholinergics on the CNS benefit clients prone to motion sickness. An example of such an anticholinergic, classified as an antihistamine for motion sickness, is scopolamine. It is available topically as a skin patch (Transderm Scōp) that is placed behind the ear. The transdermal scopolamine is delivered over 3 days and is frequently prescribed for activities such as flying, cruising on the water, and bus or automobile trips. Other drugs classified as antihistamines for motion sickness are dimenhydrinate (Dramamine), cyclizine (Marezine), and meclizine hydrochloride (Bonine). Most of these drugs can be purchased over-the-counter (OTC), with the exception of Transderm Scōp.

Examples of anticholinergic drugs and their dosages and common uses are found in Table 18–4. Dosages may vary according to age, sex, and weight. Because anticholinergic drugs can increase intraocular pressure, they should *not* be administered to clients diagnosed with glaucoma.

Side Effects and Adverse Reactions

Side effects of antihistamines used as anticholinergics include dry mouth, visual disturbances (especially blurred vision resulting from pupillary dilation), constipation secondary to decreased GI peristalsis, urinary retention related to decreased bladder tone, tachycardia (when taken in large doses), hypotension, skin rash, muscle weakness, and flush.

WEBSITES

For further information on *Cholinergics and Anticholinergics*, visit these Internet resources:

Information on bethanechol:
www.healthdigest.org/drugs/bethanechol-chloride.html

Information on atropine:
www.nurse-anesthesia.com/tdm%2Catropine.htm

PROTOTYPE DRUG CHART 18–3

TRIHEXYPHENIDYL HCl

Drug Class

Antiparkinson: anticholinergic agent
Trade Name: Artane, Trihexane, Trihexy, 🍁 Aparkane,
 Apo-Trihex, Novohexidyl
Pregnancy Category: C

Dosage

Parkinsonism:
A: PO: Initially 1-2 mg/d; increase to 6-10 mg/d in
 3 divided doses; *max:* 15 mg/dl
Extrapyramidal symptoms (drug induced):
A: PO: 1 mg/d; increase to 5-15 mg/d in divided doses

Contraindications

Narrow-angle glaucoma, GI obstruction, urinary retention,
 severe angina pectoris, myasthenia gravis
Caution: Tachycardia, benign prostatic hypertrophy,
 children, elderly, nursing mothers

Drug-Lab-Food Interactions

Drug: Increase anticholinergic effect with phenothiazines, antihistamines, tricyclic antidepressants,
 amantadine, quinidine
Decrease trihexyphenidyl absorption with antacids

Pharmacokinetics

Absorption: PO: Well absorbed
Distribution: PB: UK
Metabolism: t½: 5-10 h
Excretion: In urine

Pharmacodynamics

PO: Onset: 1 h
 Peak: 2-3 h
 Duration: 6-12 h
SR/PO: Onset: UK
 Peak: UK
 Duration: 12-24 h

Therapeutic Effects/Uses

To decrease involuntary symptoms of parkinsonism or drug-induced parkinsonism by inhibiting acetylcholine
Mode of Action: Blocks cholinergic (muscarinic) receptors thus decreases involuntary movements

Side Effects

Nausea, vomiting, dry mouth, constipation, anxiety,
 restlessness, headache, dizziness, blurred vision,
 photophobia, pupil dilation, dysphagia

Adverse Reactions

Tachycardia, palpitations, urticaria, postural hypotension, urinary retention
Life-threatening: Paralytic ileus

A, Adult; *d,* day; *GI,* gastrointestinal; *h,* hour; *IV,* intravenous; *PB,* protein-binding; *PO,* by mouth; *SR,* sustained-release; *t½,* half-life;
UK, unknown; 🍁, Canadian drug names.

Table 18-4

Anticholinergics

Generic (Brand)	Route and Dosage	Uses and Considerations
Anticholinergics: Gastrointestinal or Cholinergic Blockers		
atropine sulfate	See Prototype Drug Chart 18–2.	
dicyclomine HCl (Bentyl, Antispas, Di-Spaz)	A: PO: 10-20 mg t.i.d./q.i.d. IM: 20 mg q6h C: >2 y: PO: 10 mg t.i.d./q.i.d.	For IBS. Avoid use in clients with narrow-angle glaucoma, severe ulcerative colitis, paralytic ileus. *Pregnancy category:* B; PB: UK; $t^1/_2$: 9-10 h
glycopyrrolate (Robinul)	*GI disorders:* A: PO: 1-2 mg b.i.d./t.i.d. IM/IV: 0.1-0.2 mg t.i.d./q.i.d. *Preoperative:* A: IM: 4.4 mcg/kg 30 min-1 h before surgery	Presurgery to reduce secretions and for peptic ulcer. Contraindicated in clients with narrow-angle glaucoma, obstructive GI tract, ulcerative colitis. *Pregnancy category:* B; PB: UK; $t^1/_2$: 1-4.5 h
hyoscyamine SO₄ (Cystospaz, Anaspaz, Levsin)	A: PO/SL: 0.125-0.25 mg t.i.d./q.i.d. a.c. and at bedtime SR: 0.375-0.75 mg/q12h subQ/IM/IV: 0.25-0.5 mg b.i.d./q.i.d., PRN C: 2-10 y: half of the adult dose or individualized	Treatment of peptic ulcer and IBS. Controls gastric secretion and spastic bladder. Contraindicated in clients with narrow-angle glaucoma and severe ulcerative colitis. *Pregnancy category:* C; PB: 50%-60%; $t^1/_2$: 3.5 h
isopropamide iodide (Darbid)	A: PO: 5 mg b.i.d. or q12h; may increase to 10 mg b.i.d.	To treat peptic ulcer and IBS. Not for use in children under 12 y. *Pregnancy category:* C; PB: UK; $t^1/_2$: UK
methscopolamine bromide (Pamine)	A: PO: 2.5 mg a.c. and 2.5-5.0 mg at bedtime	Treatment of peptic ulcer, IBS. Avoid use in clients with prostatic hypertrophy and intestinal atony. *Pregnancy category:* C; PB: UK; $t^1/_2$: UK
oxyphencyclimine HCl (Daricon)	A: PO: 5-10 mg b.i.d., t.i.d.	For peptic ulcer, IBS. Not for use in children under 12 y. *Pregnancy category:* C; PB: UK; $t^1/_2$: UK
propantheline bromide (Pro-Banthine)	A: PO: 15 mg a.c. t.i.d.; 30 mg at bedtime; *max:* 120 mg/d Elderly: 7.5 mg a.c. t.i.d.; *max:* 90 mg/d	Antispasmodic for peptic ulcer, IBS. Also used for pancreatitis and urinary bladder spasm. *Pregnancy category:* C; PB: UK; $t^1/_2$: 9 h
scopolamine hydrobromide (also hyoscine hydrobromide)	*Preoperative:* A: PO: 0.5-1 mg subQ/IM/IV: 0.3-0.6 mg C: subQ: 0.006 mg/kg or 0.2 mg/m²; *max:* 0.3 mg *Motion sickness:* A: PO: 0.3-0.6 mg; transderm patch: 1 patch behind ear q72h	For preanesthetic drug, IBS, motion sickness, and delirium. Contraindicated in clients with narrow-angle glaucoma, obstructive GI disease, severe ulcerative colitis, and paralytic ileus. *Pregnancy category:* C; PB: <30%; $t^1/_2$: 8 h
Cholinergic Antagonists: Eye		
cyclopentolate HCl (Cyclogyl)	0.5%-2%, sol, 1-2 gtt	For mydriasis and cycloplegia for eye examination. See Chapter 47.
homatropine (Isopto Homatropine)	2%-5% sol, 1-2 gtt	For mydriasis and cycloplegia (paralysis of ciliary muscle resulting in loss of accommodation) for eye examination. See Chapter 47.
tropicamide (Mydriacyl Ophthalmic)	0.5%-1% sol, 1-2 gtt	For mydriasis and cycloplegia for eye examination. See Chapter 47.
Anticholinergic–Antiparkinson Drugs		
benztropine mesylate (Cogentin)	*Parkinsonism:* A: PO: IV: Initially 0.5-1.0 mg/d in 1-2 divided doses (larger dose at bedtime); maint: 0.5-6 mg/d in 1-2 divided doses EPR: A: PO: 1-2 mg, b.i.d.	Treatment of parkinsonism and drug-induced extrapyramidal syndrome. See Chapter 23.
biperiden lactate (Akineton)	*Parkinsonism:* A: PO: 2 mg t.i.d./q.i.d. IM/IV: 2 mg q30min for 4 doses Elderly: PO: 2 mg in 1 or 2 divided doses	Same as benztropine mesylate. See Chapter 23.
procyclidine HCl (Kemadrin)	*Parkinsonism:* A: PO: 2.5-5 mg p.c. t.i.d.; *maint:* 10-20 mg/d	Same as benztropine mesylate. See Chapter 23.
trihexyphenidyl HCl (Artane, Trihexy)	See Prototype Drug Chart 18–3.	

A, Adult; *a.c.*, before meals; *b.i.d.*, two times a day; *C*, child; *d*, day; *EPR*, extrapyramidal reaction; *GI*, gastrointestinal; *gtt*, drops; *h*, hour; *IBS*, irritable bowel syndrome; *IM*, intramuscular; *inhal*, inhalation; *IV*, intravenous; *maint*, maintenance; *min*, minute; *PB*, protein-binding; *p.c.*, after meals; *PO*, by mouth; *PRN*, as needed; *q.i.d.*, four times a day; *subQ*, subcutaneous; *SL*, sublingual; *sol*, solution; *SR*, sustained-release; $t^1/_2$, half-life; *t.i.d.*, three times a day; *UK*, unknown; >, greater than; <, less than. *Continued*

Table 18–4

Anticholinergics—cont'd

Generic (Brand)	Route and Dosage	Uses and Considerations
Anticholinergic–Antimuscarinic Drugs		
tolterodine tartrate (Detrol, Detrol LA)	See Prototype Drug Chart 18–4.	
Others		
ipratropium bromide (Atrovent)	A: Inhal: 2 inhal q.i.d. C: >3 y: Inhal: 1 or 2 inhal t.i.d.	An anticholinergic bronchodilator to treat chronic obstructive pulmonary disease by blocking the action of acetylcholine at the bronchial smooth muscle sites thus promoting bronchodilation. *Pregnancy category:* B; PB: UK; $t^1/_2$: UK. See Chapter 39.

PROTOTYPE DRUG CHART 18–4

TOLTERODINE TARTRATE

Drug Class

Antimuscarinic agent: Anticholinergic
Trade name: Detrol, Detrol LA
Pregnancy Category: C

Dosage

A: PO: 2 mg b.i.d. or 4 mg SR daily

Contraindications

Hypersensitivity, urinary retention, gastric retention, uncontrolled narrow-angle glaucoma
Caution: Controlled narrow-angle glaucoma, cardiovascular disease, urinary bladder outflow obstruction, pyloric stenosis or other GI obstructive disorders, paralytic ileus, ulcerative colitis, renal or hepatic dysfunction, lactation

Drug-Lab-Food Interactions

Drug: Increased effects with amantadine, amoxapine, bupropion, clozapine, cyclobenzaprine, disopyramide, maprotiline, olanzapine, orphenadrine, H_1 blockers, phenothiazines, and tricyclic antidepressants; decreased effects with azole antifungals (e.g., ketoconazole) or macrolide antibiotics (e.g., erythromycin), cyclosporine, and fluoxetine

Pharmacokinetics

Absorption: GI absorption decreased with food
Distribution: PB: 96%
Metabolism: $t^1/_2$: 2-4 h
Excretion: urine and feces

Pharmacodynamics

PO: Onset: UK
Peak: 1-2 h
Duration: UK

Therapeutic Effects/Uses

To decrease urinary frequency, urgency, and incontinence.
Mode of Action: Blocks cholinergic (muscarinic) receptors selectively in urinary bladder

Side Effects

Dry mouth and eyes, headache, dizziness, fainting, nervousness, nausea, vomiting, diarrhea, abdominal pain, dyspepsia, flatulence, dysuria, weight gain, arthralgia, urinary retention, UTI, URI, rash, pruritis, dry skin

Adverse Reactions

Bronchitis, visual abnormalities, chest pain, hypertension

A, Adult; *b.i.d.,* two times a day; *GI,* gastrointestinal; H_1, histamine 1, *h,* hour; *PB,* protein-binding; *PO,* by mouth; *SR,* sustained-release; $t^1/_2$, half-life; *UK,* unknown; *URI,* upper respiratory tract infection; *UTI,* urinary tract infection.

Critical Thinking Case Study

J.S., age 56, is scheduled for surgery to remove gallstones. He has been in good health, and his only other clinical problem is glaucoma. Preoperative medications, meperidine 75 mg and atropine sulfate 0.4 mg, were given intramuscularly 1 hour before surgery.

1. What are the advantages of giving atropine sulfate before surgery?

2. If J.S. received an atropine-like drug for several months, what assessments should be made related to the effects of the atropine-like drug?

3. How does atropine sulfate differ from bethanechol chloride?

J.S. receives ophthalmic pilocarpine drops to control glaucoma.

4. How does pilocarpine differ from physostigmine? Explain.

5. What client teaching should the nurse include related to the use of pilocarpine?

Study Questions

1. What are the actions of cholinergic and anticholinergic drugs? Differentiate between direct-acting and indirect-acting cholinergic drugs.

2. What are the major side effects of cholinergic and anticholinergic drugs? What are the implications for client teaching for each of these classes of drugs?

3. What are the general uses and indications for cholinergic and anticholinergic drugs?

4. What are the nursing implications associated with the use of cholinergic and anticholinergic drugs?

5. Your client has glaucoma. What should you instruct the client regarding OTC drugs? The same client is scheduled for surgery and atropine has been ordered. What are your nursing responsibilities?

Six

Neurologic and Neuromuscular Agents

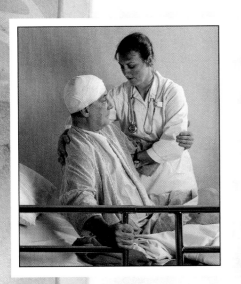

The nervous system is composed of all nerve tissues: brain, spinal cord, nerves, and ganglia. The purpose of the nervous system is to receive stimuli and transmit information to nerve centers for an appropriate response. There are two types of nervous systems: the central nervous system and the peripheral nervous system.

The *central nervous system (CNS)*, composed of the brain and spinal cord, regulates body functions (Figure VI–1). The CNS interprets information sent by impulses from the *peripheral nervous system (PNS)* and returns the instruction through the PNS for appropriate cellular actions. Stimulation of the CNS may either increase nerve cell *(neuron)* activity or block nerve cell activity.

The PNS consists of two divisions: the *somatic nervous system (SNS)* and the *autonomic nervous system (ANS)*. The SNS is voluntary and acts on skeletal muscles to produce locomotion and respiration. The ANS, also called the *visceral system,* is involuntary and controls and regulates the functioning of the heart, respiratory system, gastrointestinal system, and glands. The ANS, a large nervous system that functions without our conscious control, has two subdivisions: the sympathetic and the parasympathetic nervous systems.

The sympathetic nervous system of the ANS is called the *adrenergic system* because its neurotransmitter is norepinephrine. The parasympathetic nervous system is called the *cholinergic system* because its neurotransmitter is acetylcholine. Because organs are innervated by both the sympathetic and the parasympathetic systems, they can produce opposite responses. The sympathetic response is excitability, and the parasympathetic response is inhibition.

The sympathetic and the parasympathetic nerve pathways originate from different locations in the spinal cord. These nervous systems send information by two types of nerve fibers, the preganglionic and the postganglionic, and by the ganglion between these fibers (Figure VI–2). The preganglionic nerve fiber carries messages from the CNS to the ganglion, and the postganglionic fiber transmits impulses from the ganglion to body tissues and organs.

The sympathetic nervous system is also called the *thoracolumbar division* of the ANS because the preganglionic fibers originate from the thoracic (T1 to T12) and the upper lumbar segments (L1 and L2) of the spinal cord. The sympathetic preganglionic fibers are short from the spinal cord to the ganglion, and the sympathetic postganglionic fibers are long from the ganglion to the body cells. Figure VI–3 illustrates the sympathetic preganglionic fibers from the spinal cord.

The parasympathetic nervous system is called the *craniosacral division* of the ANS because the preganglionic fibers originate with the cranial nerves III, VII, IX, and X from the brainstem and the sacral segments S2, S3, and S4 from the spinal cord. The parasympathetic preganglionic fibers are long from the spinal cord to the ganglion, and the parasympathetic postganglionic fibers are short from the ganglion to the body cells. Figure VI–4 illustrates the parasympathetic preganglionic fibers from the spinal cord.

Drugs that stimulate and depress the CNS are discussed in Chapters 19, Central Nervous System Stimulants; 20, Central Nervous System Depressants, and 21, Drugs for Pain Management:

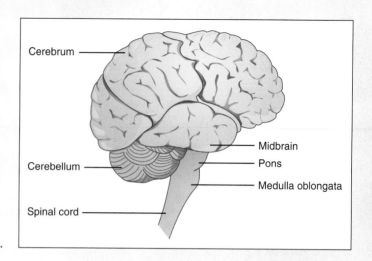

FIGURE VI–1   Brain and spinal cord.

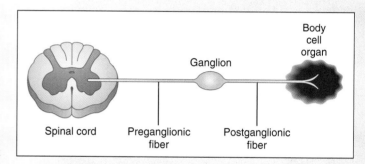

FIGURE VI–2   Preganglionic and postganglionic nerve fibers.

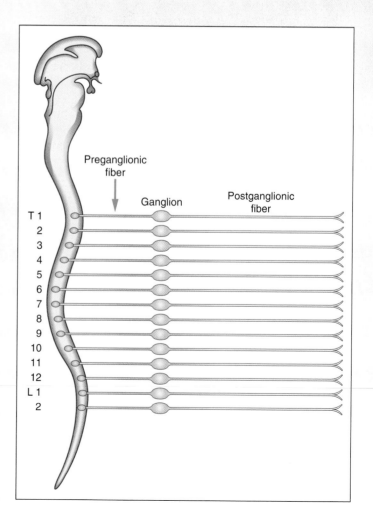

FIGURE VI–3   Sympathetic nerve fibers.

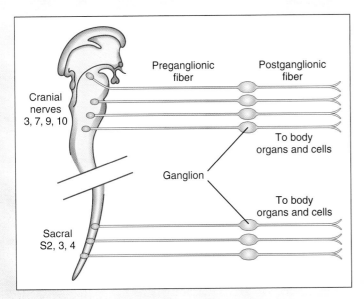

FIGURE VI–4   Parasympathetic nerve fibers.

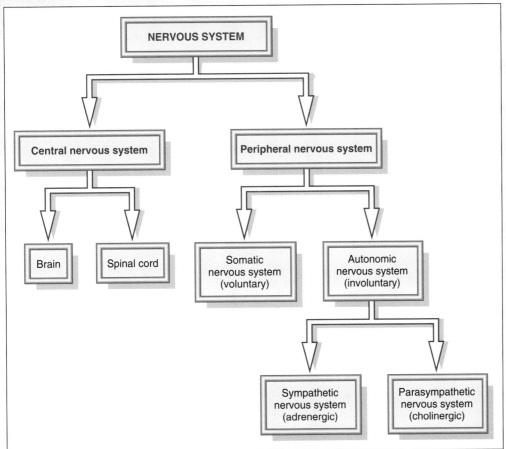

FIGURE VI–5   The body's nervous system.

Nonnarcotic and Narcotic Analgesics. Amphetamines, amphetamine-like drugs, anorexiants, analeptics, and xanthines (caffeine) stimulate the CNS. Some of these drugs are used therapeutically for attention deficit/hyperactivity disorder (ADHD) and narcolepsy. The groups of drugs that depress the CNS are sedative-hypnotics, anesthetics, narcotics, and nonnarcotic agents. Drugs used to control convulsions (see Chapter 22, Anticonvulsants) are considered CNS depressants. The drug groups used to control psychiatric and depressive disorders (see Chapters 25, Antipsychotics and Anxiolytics, and 26, Antidepressants and Mood Stabilizers) also affect CNS response. Drugs that affect the sympathetic and the parasympathetic nervous systems are discussed in Chapters 17, Adrenergics and Adrenergic Blockers, and 18, Cholinergics and Anticholinergics. The drugs used to treat neuromuscular disorders, such as parkinsonism, myasthenia gravis, multiple sclerosis, and Alzheimer's disease, have varying effects on the nervous system and muscles (see Chapters 23, Drugs for Neurologic Disorders: Parkinsonism and Alzheimer's Disease, and 24, Drugs for Neuromuscular Disorders: Myasthenia Gravis, Multiple Sclerosis, and Muscle Spasms).

Figure VI–5 is a schematic breakdown of the nervous systems in the body.

19 Central Nervous System Stimulants

ELECTRONIC RESOURCES

Additional information can be found on the companion website at *http://evolve.elsevier.com/KeeHayes/pharmacology/* or on the companion CD-ROM, which includes:
- *NCLEX-style examination review questions*
- *Pharmacology animations*
- *Medication error and IV therapy checklists*
- *Medication calculation problems*
- *Electronic calculators*

OBJECTIVES

- Explain the effects of stimulants on the central nervous system (CNS).
- Define attention deficit/hyperactivity disorder and narcolepsy.
- List the drugs that are used for attention deficit/hyperactivity disorder and narcolepsy.
- Identify the common side effects of amphetamines, anorexiants, analeptics, doxapram, and caffeine.
- List the drug categories along with the drug names for the treatment of migraine headaches.
- Identify at least four nursing interventions when administering CNS stimulants.

TERMS

amphetamines
analeptics
anorexiants
attention deficit/hyperactivity disorder (ADHD)

central nervous system (CNS)
cluster headaches
dependence
hyperkinesis

migraine headaches
narcolepsy
neurotransmitters
tolerance

Introduction

Numerous drugs can stimulate the **central nervous system (CNS)**, but the medically approved use of these drugs is limited to the treatment of attention deficit/hyperactivity disorder (ADHD) in children, narcolepsy, obesity, and the reversal of respiratory distress. The major group of CNS stimulants includes amphetamines and caffeine, which stimulate the cerebral cortex of the brain; analeptics and caffeine, which act on the brainstem and medulla to stimulate respiration; and anorexiants, which act to some degree on the cerebral cortex and on the hypothalamus to suppress appetite. The amphetamines and related anorexiants are greatly abused. Long-term use of amphetamines can produce psychologic **dependence** and **tolerance,** a condition in which larger and larger doses of a drug are needed to reproduce the initial response. Gradually increasing a drug dose and then abruptly stopping the drug may result in depression and withdrawal symptoms.

Drugs used to treat migraine and cluster headaches include analgesics, ergot alkaloids, and selective serotinin$_1$ receptor agonists (triptans). The triptan group, which is frequently prescribed, causes vasoconstriction to the blood vessels in the cortex.

Pathophysiology

Attention deficit/hyperactivity disorder (ADHD), formerly called *attention deficit disorder (ADD)*, might be caused by a disregulation of the transmitters—serotonin, norepinephrine, and dopamine. ADHD occurs primarily in children, usually before the age of 7, but may continue through the teenage years. However, it may not be first identified until early adulthood. The incidence of ADHD is three to seven times more common in boys than in girls. Characteristic behaviors include inattentiveness, inability to concentrate, restlessness (fidgety), hyperactivity (excessive and purposeless activity), inability to complete tasks, and impulsivity.

The child with ADHD may display poor coordination, and there may be abnormal electroencephalographic (EEG) findings. Intelligence is usually not affected. This disorder has also been called *minimal brain dysfunction, hyperactivity* in children, **hyperkinesis,** and *hyperkinetic syndrome with learning disorder.* Some professionals state that ADHD is often incorrectly diagnosed, which results in many children receiving unnecessary treatment for months or years.

Narcolepsy is characterized by falling asleep during normal waking activities, such as driving a car or talking with someone. Sleep paralysis, the condition of muscle paralysis that is normal during sleep, usually accompanies narcolepsy and affects the voluntary muscles. The person is unable to move and may collapse.

Amphetamines

Amphetamines stimulate the release of the **neurotransmitters**—norepinephrine and dopamine—from the brain and the sympathetic nervous system (peripheral nerve terminals). The amphetamines cause euphoria and alertness; however, they can also cause sleeplessness, restlessness, tremors, and irritability. Cardiovascular problems, such as increased heart rate, palpitations, cardiac dysrhythmias, and increased blood pressure, can result from continuous use of amphetamines.

The half-life of amphetamines varies from 4 to 30 hours. Acidic urine excretes amphetamines faster than it excretes alkaline urine. When CNS toxicity or cardiac toxicity is suspected, decreasing the urine pH (acidity) aids in the excretion of the drug. Acidic urine decreases the half-life of the amphetamine. Amphetamines are prescribed for narcolepsy, and in some cases for ADHD, when amphetamine-like drugs are ineffective. Amphetamine (Adderall) has been effective for controlling ADHD. Dextroamphetamine (Dexedrine) and methamphetamine (Desoxyn) may also be prescribed for some ADHD clients.

Side Effects and Adverse Reactions

Amphetamines can cause adverse effects in the central nervous, cardiovascular, gastrointestinal (GI), and endocrine systems. The side effects and adverse reactions include restlessness, insomnia, tachycardia, hypertension, heart palpitations, dry mouth, anorexia, weight loss, diarrhea or constipation, and impotence.

Amphetamine-Like Drugs for ADHD and Narcolepsy

Methylphenidate (Ritalin), dexmethylphendate (Focalin), and pemoline (Cylert), amphetamine-like drugs, are given to increase the child's attention span and cognitive performance (e.g., memory, reading) and to decrease impulsiveness, hyperactivity, and restlessness. Methylphenidate and pemoline are also used to treat narcolepsy. Pemoline should *not* be considered a first-line drug for ADHD because it can cause hepatic failure. There is less potential abuse of pemoline than methylphenidate; thus it is classified as a controlled-substance schedule (CSS) IV drug. Prototype Drug Chart 19–1 illustrates the pharmacokinetics, pharmacodynamics, and therapeutic effects of methylphenidate in the treatment of ADHD and narcolepsy. Amphetamine and amphetamine-like drugs should not be taken in the evening or before bedtime because insomnia may result.

Modafinil (Provigil) is another drug prescribed for narcolepsy. It increases the amount of time that clients with narcolepsy feel awake. Its mechanism of action is not fully known.

Methylphenidate is the most frequently prescribed drug to treat ADHD. Table 19–1 lists the amphetamines and amphetamine-like drugs and their dosages, uses, and considerations.

Pharmacokinetics

Methylphenidate and pemoline are well absorbed from the GI mucosa. Although pemoline has a longer half-life than methylphenidate, the drugs are usually administered to children once a day before breakfast. However, methylphenidate may be given twice a day, before breakfast and lunch. Be-

PROTOTYPE DRUG CHART 19–1

METHYLPHENIDATE

Drug Class

Amphetamine-like drug (CNS stimulant)
Trade Names:
methylphenidate HCl: Ritalin, Ritalin SR, Metadate CD, Concerta SR
CSS II
Pregnancy Category: C

Dosage

Attention deficit/hyperactivity disorder (ADHD):
C >6 y: PO: 5 mg before breakfast and lunch; if necessary increase dosage weekly by 5-10 mg; *max:* 60 mg/d
SR: Not recommended for initial treatment
Narcolepsy:
A: PO: 10 mg, 2-3 times/day 30 min before meals

Contraindications

Hypersensitivity, hyperthyroidism, anxiety, history of seizures, motor tics, Tourette's syndrome, glaucoma
Caution: Not to be used for children <6 y
Hypertension, depression, alcoholism, pregnancy

Drug-Lab-Food Interactions

Drug: May *decrease* effects of decongestants, antihypertensives, barbiturates; may alter effects of insulin therapy
Increases hypertensive crisis with MAOIs; *increases* effects of oral anticoagulants, anticonvulsants, tricyclic antidepressants
Food: Caffeine (coffee, tea, colas, chocolate) may *increase* effects

Pharmacokinetics

Absorption: Well absorbed from GI tract
Distribution: PB: UK
Metabolism: t½: 1-3 h
Excretion: 40% excreted unchanged in urine

Pharmacodynamics

PO: Onset: 0.5-1 h
  Peak: 1-3 h
  Duration: 4-6 h
  SR: 4-8 h

Therapeutic Effects/Uses:

To correct hyperactivity caused by ADHD, increase attention span, treat fatigue, and control narcolepsy
Mode of action: Acts primarily on the cerebral cortex, reticular activatory system

Side Effects

Anorexia, vomiting, diarrhea, insomnia, dizziness, nervousness, restlessness, irritability

Adverse Reactions

Tachycardia, growth suppression
Palpitations, transient loss of weight in children, increased hyperactivity
Life-threatening: Exfoliative dermatitis, uremia, thrombocytopenia

A, Adult; *ADHD,* attention deficit/hyperactivity disorder; *C,* child; *CD,* controlled dose; *CNS,* central nervous system; *CSS,* Controlled Substances Schedule; *d,* day; *GI,* gastrointestinal; *h,* hour; *MAOI,* monoamine oxidase inhibitor; *min,* minute; *PB,* protein-binding; *PO,* by mouth; *SR,* sustained release; *t½,* half-life; *UK,* unknown; *y,* year.

---

cause food affects the absorption rate, the drugs should be given 30 to 45 minutes before meals. These drugs should not be given within 6 hours before sleep because they may cause insomnia. Both drugs are excreted in the urine; 40% of methylphenidate is excreted unchanged.

Pharmacodynamics

Methylphenidate and pemoline help to correct ADHD by decreasing hyperactivity and improving attention span. These drugs may also be prescribed for treating narcolepsy. These amphetamine-like drugs are considered more effective in treating ADHD than amphetamines, except for Adderall. Amphetamines are generally avoided because they have a higher potential for abuse, habituation, and tolerance. Methylphenidate is slightly more effective than pemoline for ADHD. Sympathomimetic drugs, such as decongestants, enhance the actions of methylphenidate and pemoline. Antihypertensives and barbiturates can decrease the action

of these drugs. Foods that contain caffeine should be avoided because they increase drug action.

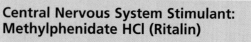

Nursing Process

Central Nervous System Stimulant: Methylphenidate HCl (Ritalin)

ASSESSMENT

■ Determine whether there is a history of heart disease, hypertension, hyperthyroidism, parkinsonism, or glaucoma; in such cases, drug is usually contraindicated.

■ Record vital signs to be used for future comparisons. Pay close attention to clients with cardiac disease because drug may reverse effects of antihypertensives.
■ Ascertain client's mental status (e.g., mood, affect, aggressiveness).
■ Evaluate height, growth, weight of children.
■ Assess complete blood count (CBC), differential white blood cells (WBCs), and platelets before and during therapy.

NURSING DIAGNOSES

■ Disorganized behavior (e.g., impulsiveness, short attention span, distractibility) related to interference with peer relationships, learning, and discipline
■ Interrupted family processes related to dysfunctional behavior

PLANNING

■ Client will be free of hyperactivity.
■ Client will increase attention span.
■ Client will not experience side effects or adverse reactions to therapy.

NURSING INTERVENTIONS

■ Monitor vital signs. Report irregularities.
■ Record height, weight, and growth of children.
■ Observe client for withdrawal symptoms (e.g., nausea, vomiting, weakness, headache).
■ Monitor client for side effects (e.g., insomnia, restlessness, nervousness, tremors, irritability, tachycardia, elevated blood pressure). Report findings.

Table 19–1

Amphetamines and Amphetamine-Like Drugs

Generic (Brand Name)	Route and Dosage	Uses and Considerations
Amphetamines		
amphetamine sulfate (Adderall) CSS II	*Narcolepsy:* A: PO: 5-20 mg, daily-t.i.d.; *max:* 60 mg/d C >6-12 y: PO: 5 mg/d *ADHD:* C: 3-5 y: PO: 2.5 mg/d C: 6-12 y: PO: 5 mg/d, *max:* 40 mg/d	For narcolepsy, ADHD. Dosage should be minimal to control symptoms in ADHD. CNS and cardiac toxicity could occur. *Pregnancy category:* C; PB: UK; t½: 10-30 h
dextroamphetamine sulfate (Dexedrine) CSS II	*ADHD:* C: 3-5 y: PO: 2.5 mg/d C: 6-12 y: PO: 5 mg/d, *max:* 40 mg/d	Uses similar to those of amphetamines. Drug has been used for obesity and narcolepsy. *Pregnancy category:* C; PB: UK; t½: UK
methamphetamine HCl (Desoxyn) CSS II	C: PO: 2.5-5 mg daily; increase to 20 mg as needed in two divided doses	For ADHD. Could cause CNS and cardiac toxicity. *Pregnancy category:* C; PB: UK; t½: UK
Amphetamine-Like Drugs		
methylphenidate HCl (Ritalin) CSS II	See Prototype Drug Chart 19–1.	
pemoline (Cylert) CSS IV	C: >6 y: PO: 37.5 mg/d; may increase weekly; *max:* 112.5 mg/d	For narcolepsy, ADHD, increasing attention span, and treating fatigue; *Pregnancy category:* B; PB: 50%; t½: 10-14 h
modafinil (Provigil) CSS IV	A: PO: 200 mg/d. With hepatic dysfunction: 100 mg/d Elderly: Reduce dose	For narcolepsy. It does not disrupt nighttime sleep. Common side effects include headaches, nausea, diarrhea, and nervousness. *Pregnancy category:* C; PB: UK; t½: 15 h.
dexmethylphenidate (Focalin)	A & C: PO: >6 y 2.5 mg twice daily; may increase 2.5 mg/d at weekly intervals; *max:* 20 mg/d	For ADHD. *Pregnancy category:* C; PB: UK; t½: 2.2 h
atomoxetine (Strattera)	A: PO: 40 mg/d; may increase after 3 d; *max:* 100 mg/d; C: PO: 0.5 mg/kg/d; may increase after 3 d; *max:* 1.4 mg/kg/d or 100 mg, whichever is less	For ADHD. *Pregnancy category:* C; PB: 98%; t½: 2.2 h

A, Adult; *ADHD,* attention deficit/hyperactivity disorder; *C,* child; *CNS,* central nervous system; *CSS,* controlled substance schedule; *d,* day; *h,* hour; *PB,* protein-binding; *PO,* by mouth; *t½,* half-life; *UK,* unknown; *y,* year; *>,* greater than.

Client Teaching

General
- Instruct client to take drug before meals.
- Direct client to avoid alcohol consumption.
- Encourage the use of sugarless gum to relieve dry mouth.
- Teach client to monitor weight twice a week and to report weight loss.
- Advise client to avoid driving and using hazardous equipment when experiencing tremors, nervousness, or increased heart rate.
- Instruct client not to abruptly discontinue the drug; the dose must be tapered off to avoid withdrawal symptoms. Consult health care provider before modifying the dose.
- Encourage client to read the labels on OTC products because many contain caffeine. A high caffeine plasma level could be fatal.
- Teach nursing mother to avoid taking all CNS stimulants. These drugs pass into the breast milk and can cause the infant to be hyperactive or restless.
- Direct family to seek counseling for children with attention deficit/hyperactivity disorder. Drug therapy alone is not an appropriate therapy program. Notify school nurse of drug therapy regimen.
- Explain to client or family that long-term use may lead to drug abuse.

Diet
- Advise client to avoid foods that contain caffeine.
- Instruct parents to provide children with a nutritional breakfast because drug may have anorexic effects.

Side Effects
- Teach client about drug side effects and the need to report tachycardia and palpitations. Monitor children for onset of Tourette's syndrome.

Cultural Considerations ⊕
- Decrease language barriers by decoding the jargon of the health care environment for those with language difficulties and for those who are not in the health care field.

EVALUATION

- Evaluate the effectiveness of drug therapy, level of hyperactivity and the presence of adverse effects.
- Monitor weight, sleep patterns, and mental status.

Anorexiants

Obesity has been treated with prescribed amphetamines or over-the-counter (OTC) amphetamine-like drugs. Amphetamines have been recommended as **anorexiants** (appetite suppressants) for short-term use (4 to 12 weeks). Because of tolerance, psychologic dependence, and abuse, amphet-amines currently are *not* recommended for use as appetite suppressants. The Food and Drug Administration (FDA) has ordered the removal of phenylpropanolamine from OTC weight loss drugs and cold remedies. A study has shown that there is an increased risk of hemorrhagic stroke in young women who take drugs containing phenyl-propanolamine and a 16 times greater risk in women who take the drugs as appetite suppressants. However, this drug was not associated with an increased risk of stroke in men. It also has been suggested that phenylpropanolamine might cause renal failure, psychosis, hypertension, and cardiac dysrhythmias. Topical use of the drug has not been associated with systemic effects. Most of the anorexiants used to suppress appetite (Table 19–2) do not have the serious side effects associated with amphetamines. To lose weight, emphasis should be placed on proper diet, exercise, and behavioral modifications. Reliance on appetite suppressants should be discouraged. Individuals who take anorexiants should be under the care of a health care provider.

Side Effects and Adverse Reactions

Children younger than 12 years old should *not* take anorexiants, and self-medication with anorexiants should be discouraged. Long-term use of these drugs frequently results in such severe side effects as nervousness, restlessness, irritability, insomnia, heart palpitations, and hypertension.

Analeptics

Analeptics, which are CNS stimulants, mostly affect the brainstem and spinal cord but also affect the cerebral cortex. The primary use of an analeptic is to stimulate respiration. One subgroup of analeptics is the xanthines (methylxanthines), of which caffeine and theophylline are the main drugs. Depending on the dose, caffeine stimulates the CNS, and large doses stimulate respiration. The concentration of caffeine in various beverages is listed on the Evolve website. Newborns with respiratory distress might be given caffeine to increase respiration. Theophylline is used mostly to relax the bronchioles; however, it has also been used to increase respiration in newborns. See Chapter 39, Drugs for Acute and Chronic Lower Respiratory Disorders, for further explanation of theophylline. Table 19–2 lists the analeptics and their dosages, uses, and considerations.

Side Effects and Adverse Reactions

The side effects from caffeine are similar to those from anorexiants: nervousness, restlessness, tremors, twitchings, palpitations, and insomnia. Other side effects include diuresis (increased urination), GI irritation (e.g., nausea, diarrhea), and, rarely, tinnitus (ringing in the ear). More than 500 mg of caffeine affects the CNS and heart. High doses of caffeine in coffee, chocolate, and cold-relief medications can cause psychologic dependence. The half-life of caffeine is 3.5 hours; however, metabolism is slowed and the half-life is prolonged in clients with liver disease and

Table 19–2

Anorexiants and Analeptics

Drug	Route and Dosage	Uses and Considerations
Anorexiants		
benzphetamine HCl (Didrex) CSS III	A: PO: 25-50 mg daily-t.i.d.	Similar to amphetamines. Potential for abuse. Avoid taking drug during pregnancy. *Pregnancy category:* X; PB: UK, t^1/$_2$: 6-12 h
dextroamphetamine sulfate (Dexedrine) CSS II	A: PO: 5-10 mg 1 to 3 × 3 d 30-60 min a.c.	To treat obesity. Can cause restlessness and insomnia. For short-term use. *Pregnancy category:* C; PB: UK; t^1/$_2$: 30-35 h
diethylpropion HCl (Dospan, Tenuate, Tepanil, ♣ Nobesine) CSS IV	A: PO: 25 mg t.i.d.; SR: 75 mg daily	For appetite suppression by stimulating the appetite control center in the hypothalamus. Take 1 h before meals. For short-term use. *Pregnancy category:* B; PB: UK; t^1/$_2$: 2-3 h
phentermine HCl (Fastin, Ionamin, Zantryl, Adipex-P, Obe-Nix-30) CSS IV	A: PO: 8 mg 3 × daily or 15-37.5 mg daily	For appetite suppression *Pregnancy category:* C; PB: UK; t^1/$_2$: 19-24 h
Without phenylpropanolamine HCl: Acutrim, Control, Dexatrim, Dexatrim Natural, Prolamine	A: PO: 1 tablet in morning	To control weight gain. FDA has ordered removal of drugs containing phenylpropanolamine HCl because it may cause stroke, hypertension, or cardiac dysrhythmias.
Analeptics		
Methylxanthines		
caffeine	*Neonatal apnea:* Infant and C: PO-IM-IV: 5-10 mg/kg on day 1; then 2.5-5 mg/d *Therapeutic range:* 5-20 mg/ml	Used for newborns with apnea to stimulate respiration; increases heart rate and blood pressure. Given through an NGT, IM, or IV. *Pregnancy category:* C; PB: 25%-35%; t^1/$_2$: A: 3-5 h, neonate: 40-144 h
OTC drugs (NōDōz, Tirend), coffee	A: 100-200 mg q3-4h as needed	Restores mental alertness. Contains citrated caffeine. Brewed coffee contains 60-180 mg of caffeine per cup.
theophylline	Infants: NGT: 5 mg/kg on day 1; then 2 mg in divided doses	Used for newborns with apnea to stimulate respiration. Given through an NGT.
Respiratory Stimulant		
doxapram HCl (Dopram)	A: IV: 0.5-1 mg/kg; infusion: 1-2 mg/min; *max:* 3 g/d *Neonatal apnea:* Initially: 0.5 mg/kg/h; *maint:* 0.5-2.5 mg/kg/h titrated to lowest effective rate	Used for respiratory depression. It can increase blood pressure. *Pregnancy category:* B; PB: UK; t^1/$_2$: A: 2.5-4 h, neonate: 7-10 h

A, Adult; *a.c.*, before meals; *C*, child; *CSS*, Controlled Substances Schedule; *d*, day; *FDA*, Food and Drug Administration; *h*, hour; *IM*, intramuscular; *IV*, intravenous; *MAOI*, monoamine oxidase inhibitor; *max*, maximum; *min*, minute; *NGT*, nasogastric tube; *PB*, protein-binding; *PO*, by mouth; *subQ*, subcutaneous; *SR*, sustained-release; *t^1/$_2$*, half-life; *t.i.d.*, three times a day; *UK*, unknown; ♣, Canadian.

who are pregnant. Caffeine is contraindicated during pregnancy because its effect on the fetus is unknown.

Respiratory Central Nervous System Stimulant

Doxapram (Dopram), a CNS and respiratory stimulant, is used to treat respiratory depression caused by drug overdose, pre- and postanesthetic respiratory depression, and chronic obstructive pulmonary disease (COPD). It should be used with caution for the treatment of neonatal apnea. It is administered intravenously, and its onset of action is within 20 to 40 seconds with a peak action within 2 minutes. Side effects are infrequent; however, with an overdose, hypertension, tachycardia, trembling, and convulsions may occur. Mechanical ventilation is more effective than doxapram for treating clients who experience respiratory distress as a result of using certain drugs.

Headaches: Migraine And Cluster

Migraine headaches are characterized by a unilateral throbbing head pain, accompanied by nausea, vomiting, and photophobia. These symptoms frequently persist for

4 to 24 hours and for several days in some cases. Two thirds of migraine headaches are experienced by women in their 20s and 30s. Symptoms usually decrease or are absent during pregnancy and menopause. The intensity of the pain can disrupt the client's daily activities.

Pathophysiology

Migraine headaches are caused by inflammation and dilation of the blood vessels in the cranium. The etiology is unknown; however, some theories suggest an imbalance in the neurotransmitter serotonin (5-hydroxytryptamine [5-HT]) that causes vasoconstriction and suppresses migraine headaches. The tendency of calcitonin gene-related peptide (CGRP) is to promote a migraine attack. The serum CGRP levels are elevated during a migraine attack. Foods such as cheese, chocolate, and red wine can trigger an attack.

The two types of migraine are (1) *classic migraines*, which are associated with an aura that occurs minutes to 1 hour before onset, and (2) *common migraines*, which are not associated with an aura.

Cluster headaches are characterized by a severe unilateral nonthrobbing pain usually located around the eye. They occur in a series of cluster attacks—one or more attacks every day for several weeks. They are not associated with an aura and do not cause nausea and vomiting. Men are more commonly affected by cluster headaches than women.

Treatment of Migraine Headaches

Preventive treatment for migraines includes (1) beta-adrenergic blockers such as propranolol (Inderal) and atenolol (Tenormin); (2) anticonvulsants, such as valproic

---

Table 19–3

Drugs to Treat Severe Migraine Headaches

Drug	Route and Dosage	Uses and Considerations
Ergot Alkaloids		
ergotamine tartrate	A: SL: 2 mg, may repeat in 30 min; *max:* 6 mg/24 h A: Inhal: 1 inhal; may repeat in 5 min A: Intranasal: 1 spray (0.5 mg) in each nostril; repeat in 15 min A: IM/IV: 1 mg at start of headache; repeat 1 h later	An antimigraine drug. To prevent or abort migraine attack. Not for prolonged use. *Pregnancy category:* D; PB: UK; $t^1/_2$: varies
dihydroergotamine meslyate (Migranal)	A: Intranasal: 1 spray in each nostril; may repeat in 15 min A: IM/IV: 1 mg; may repeat in 1 h; *max:* 3 mg IM and 2 mg IV	To prevent or abort migraine attack. *Pregnancy category:* X; PB: UK; $t^1/_2$: 21-32 h
Selective Serotinin₁ Receptor Agonists (Triptans)		
sumatriptan succinate (Imitrex)	A: PO: 25 mg; may repeat in 2 h; *max:* 100 mg A: subQ: 6 mg, may repeat in 1 h A: Intranasal: 5-10-20 mg in nostril; repeat once in 2 h	To treat acute migraine attacks and cluster headaches. Promotes vasoconstriction *Pregnancy category:* C; PB: 10%-20%; $t^1/_2$: 2 h
naratriptan (Amerge)	A: PO: 1-2.5 mg; may repeat in 4 h; *max:* 5 mg/24 h	For acute migraines. It has a longer half-life; thus duration of action is longer. Causes vasoconstriction of cranial carotid arteries. Avoid if client has severe hypertension, IHD, MI. *Pregnancy category:* C; PB: 28%-31%; $t^1/_2$: 6 h
rizatriptan benzoate (Maxalt, Maxalt MLT)	A: PO: 5-10 mg; may repeat in 2 h; *max:* 30 mg/24 h	For acute migraines. Two types of tablets: regular and melt-in mouth. Second tablet does not need to be taken by water. Avoid if client has uncontrolled hypertension, IHD, previous MI. *Pregnancy category:* C; PB: UK; $t^1/_2$: 2-3 h
zolmitriptan (Zomig)	A: PO: 2.5-5 mg; may repeat in 2 h; *max:* 10 mg/24 h	For acute migraines. 65% of clients respond in 2 h. Avoid if client has uncontrolled hypertension, IHD, previous MI. *Pregnancy category:* C; PB: 25%; $t^1/_2$: 3 h
almotriptan (Axert)	A: PO: 6.25-12.5 mg; may repeat in 2 h; *max:* 25 mg/24 h	To treat acute migraines. *Pregnancy category:* C; PB: 35%; $t^1/_2$: 3-4 h
frovatriptan (Frova)	A: PO: 2.5 mg; may repeat in 2 h; *max:* 7.5 mg/24 h	To treat acute migraines. *Pregnancy category:* C; PB: 15%; $t^1/_2$: 26 h
eletriptan (Relpax)	A: PO: 20-40 mg; may repeat in 2 h; *max:* 80 mg/24 h	To treat acute migraines. *Pregnancy category:* C; PB: 85%; $t^1/_2$: 4 h

A, Adult; *h,* hour; *IHD,* ischemic heart disease; *IM,* intramuscular; *IV,* intravenous; *max,* maximum; *MI,* myocardial infarction; *min,* minute; *PB,* protein-binding; *PO,* by mouth; *SL,* sublingual; *subQ,* subcutaneous; *t¹/₂,* half-life; *UK,* unknown.

acid (Depakote) and gabapentin (Neurontin); and (3) tricyclic antidepressants, such as amitriptyline (Elavil) and imipramine (Tofranil).

Treatment or cessation of a migraine attack depends on the intensity of pain. Drugs used to treat migraines include analgesics, opioid analgesics, ergot alkaloids, and selective serotinin₁ (5-HT) receptor agonists, also known as *triptans*. For mild migraine attacks, aspirin, acetaminophen, or nonsteroidal antiinflammatory drugs (NSAIDs), such as ibuprofen or naproxen (Aleve), may be prescribed. Aspirin may be used in combination with caffeine. Meperidine (Demerol) and butorphanol nasal spray (Stadol NS) are opioid analgesics that are occasionally used.

Ergotamine tartrate, a nonspecific serotonin agonist and vasoconstrictor, has been prescribed for years to treat moderate to severe migraine headaches. It should be taken early during a migraine attack. Nausea and vomiting might occur; antiemetics decrease these symptoms. Ergotamine is available in sublingual tablets or with caffeine in oral tablets and suppositories. Dihydroergotamine, an ergot alkaloid, can be administered subcutaneously, intramuscularly, intravenously, and by means of a nasal spray.

The triptans (5-HT₁ receptor agonists) are the most recently developed group of drugs for the treatment of migraine headaches. Sumatriptan (Imitrex), a selective serotonin receptor agonist with a short duration of action, was the first triptan drug. It is considered more effective than ergotamine in treating acute migraine attacks. Table 19–3 lists the ergot alkaloids and the selective serotinin₁ (5-HT) receptor agonists and their dosages, uses, and considerations. Do not confuse sumatriptan with zolmitriptan. Both drugs are triptans but have different dosages. Also, do not confuse Amerge (triptan used for migraines) with Amaryl (sulfonylurea used for diabetes mellitus) or Altace (angiotensin-converting enzyme inhibitor) used for hypertension and heart failure. See Prototype Drug Chart 19–2 for further pharmacology of sumatriptan.

PROTOTYPE DRUG CHART 19–2

SUMATRIPTAN

Drug Class
5-HT₁ receptor antagonist (antimigraine)
Trade Name: Imitrex
Pregnancy Category: C

Dosage
A: PO: 25-50 mg for 1 dose, may repeat once after 2 h, *max:* 200 mg/24 h
A: subQ: 6 mg, may repeat with 6 mg at least 1 h after first injection, *max:* 12 mg/24 h
A: Intranasal: 5-20 mg in one nostril, may repeat after 2 h, *max:* 40 mg/24 h

Contraindications
Hypersensitivity, coronary artery disease, hypertension, obesity, diabetes mellitus, smoking
Caution: Liver or renal dysfunction

Drug-Lab-Food Interactions
Drug: Risk of vasospasm and blood pressure elevation with dihydroergotamine and other ergo alkaloids; Increased levels and toxicity within 2 wk of MAO inhibitors

Pharmacokinetics
Absorption: Rapidly absorbed following subQ injection
Distribution: PB: 10%-20%
Metabolism: t½: 2 h
Excretion: Urine and feces

Pharmacodynamics
PO: Onset: 1-1½ h
subQ: 10 min
Peak: PO: 2-4 h
subQ: 2 h
Duration: UK

Therapeutic Effects/Uses:
To treat migraine and cluster headaches
Mode of action: Causes vasoconstriction of cranial carotid arteries to relieve migraine attacks

Side Effects
Dizziness, fainting, tingling, numbness, warm sensation, drowsiness, muscle cramps, nausea, vomiting, diarrhea, abdominal cramping

Adverse Reactions
Hypotension, hypertension, heart block, angina, dysrhythmias, thromboembolism, seizures, central nervous system hemorrhage, stroke
Life-threatening: Coronary artery vasospasm, myocardial infarction, cardiac arrest

A, Adult; *h,* hour; *MAO,* monoamine inhibitor; *max,* maximum; *min,* minute; *PB,* protein-binding; *PO,* by mouth; *subQ,* subcutaneous; *t½,* half-life; *uk,* unknown; *wk,* week.

WEBSITES

For further information on *Central Nervous System Stimulants,* visit these Internet resources:

Information on methylphenidate:
www.nida.nih.gov/Infofax/ritalin.html

Information on zolmitriptan: *www.zomig.com*

More information on zolmitriptan:
www.centerwatch.com/patient/drugs/dru681.html

Information on sumatriptan:
www.fda.govmedwatch/SAFETY/2003/03Jul_PI/ Imitrex_PI.pdf

Critical Thinking Case Study

M.P., 67 years old, wants to lose 30 pounds. She wants to take an OTC diet pill but does not want to exercise or be on a diet.

1. Would you suggest a diet pill? Why or why not?

2. What does the nurse need to assess concerning this client's physical status before suggesting a diet pill or weight loss program?

3. What behavior modification may you suggest related to losing weight?

4. In what ways could diet control and exercise help this client? Explain.

5. Would you suggest a weight-loss program such as Weight Watchers or Jenny Craig? How do these programs differ? Would one program benefit her more than the other? Explain.

Study Questions

1. A 5-year-old boy is diagnosed with attention deficit/hyperactivity disorder (ADHD). What is ADHD? What drugs effectively control this disorder?

2. What is the pharmacologic name for appetite suppressants? Why are amphetamines not recommended for the treatment of obesity?

3. The client has hypertension. Why are amphetamines not recommended for hypertensive clients? What are the side effects of amphetamines?

4. Why were products containing phenylpropanolamine removed from the market by FDA?

5. A mother is breastfeeding her infant daughter. She wants to lose 30 pounds and plans to take an OTC anorexiant. What would your response be? Explain.

6. What drug groups are used for preventive treatment of migraine headaches and for aborting or treating migraine attacks? Differentiate between the ergot alkaloids and the triptans.

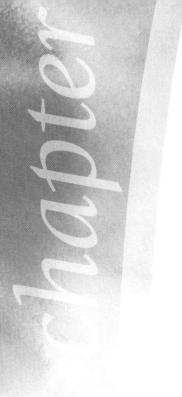

20 Central Nervous System Depressants

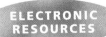

Additional information can be found on the companion website at *http://evolve.elsevier.com/KeeHayes/pharmacology/* or on the companion CD-ROM, which includes:
- *NCLEX-style examination review questions*
- *Pharmacology animations*
- *Medication error and IV therapy checklists*
- *Medication calculation problems*
- *Electronic calculators*

OBJECTIVES

- Identify the types and stages of sleep.
- Identify several nonpharmacologic ways to induce sleep.
- Define these adverse effects: *hangover, dependence, tolerance, withdrawal symptoms,* and *rapid eye movement (REM) rebound.*
- List drugs that might cause the preceding adverse effects.
- List examples of short-acting and intermediate-acting barbiturates that are used as sedative hypnotics.
- List three benzodiazepines developed for hypnotic use.
- Differentiate nursing interventions related to barbiturates and benzodiazepine hypnotics.

● Describe the stages of anesthesia.

● Explain the uses for topical anesthetics.

● Identify examples of general and local anesthetics and their major side effects.

TERMS

anesthetics	hangover	rapid eye movement	spinal block
balanced anesthesia	hypnotic effect	(REM) sleep	tolerance
barbiturates	insomnia	saddle block	withdrawal symptoms
caudal block	nerve block	sedation	
dependence	nonrapid eye movement	spinal anesthesia	
epidural block	(NREM) sleep		

Introduction

Drugs that are central nervous system (CNS) depressants cause varying degrees of depression (reduction in functional activity) within the CNS. The degree of depression depends primarily on the drug and the amount of drug taken. The broad classification of CNS depressants includes sedative-hypnotics, general and local anesthetics, analgesics, narcotic and nonnarcotic analgesics, anticonvulsants, antipsychotics, and antidepressants. The last five groups of depressant drugs are presented in separate chapters. Sedative-hypnotics and general and local anesthetics are discussed in this chapter.

Types and Stages of Sleep

Sleep disorders, such as **insomnia** (inability to fall asleep), occur in 5% to 10% of healthy adults, 20% to 25% of hospitalized clients, and approximately 75% of psychiatric clients. Insomnia occurs more frequently in women and increases with age. Sedative-hypnotics are frequently ordered for treatment of sleep disorders.

People spend approximately one third of their lives, or as much as 25 years, sleeping. Normal sleep is composed of two definite phases: **rapid eye movement (REM) sleep** and **nonrapid eye movement (NREM) sleep**. Both REM and NREM occur cyclically during sleep at about 90-minute intervals (Figure 20–1). The four succeedingly deeper stages of NREM sleep end with an episode of REM sleep, and the cycle begins again. If sleep is interrupted, the cycle begins again with stage 1 of NREM sleep.

It is during the REM sleep phase that individuals experience most of their recallable dreams. Individuals perform better during their waking hours if they experience all types and stages of sleep. Children have few REM sleep periods and have longer periods of stage 3 and 4 NREM sleep. Older adults experience a decrease in stages 3 and 4 of NREM sleep and have frequent waking periods.

It is difficult to rouse a person during REM sleep. The period of REM sleep episodes becomes longer during the sleep process. Frequently, if the person is roused from REM sleep, he or she may recall a vivid, bizarre dream. If these

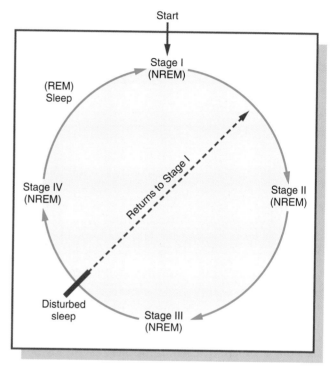

FIGURE 20–1   Types and stages of sleep. *NREM,* Nonrapid eye movement (four stages); *REM,* rapid eye movement (dreaming).

dreams are unpleasant, they may be called *nightmares.* Sleep-walking or nightmares that occur in children take place during NREM sleep.

Nonpharmacologic Methods

Various nonpharmacologic methods should be used to promote sleep before using sedative-hypnotics or over-the-counter (OTC) sleep aids. Once the nurse discovers why the client cannot sleep, the following ways to promote sleep may be suggested:

1. Arise at a specific hour in the morning.
2. Take few or no daytime naps.
3. Avoid drinks that contain caffeine 6 hours before bedtime.
4. Avoid heavy meals or strenuous exercise before bedtime.
5. Take a warm bath, read, or listen to music before bedtime.

6. Decrease exposure to loud noises.
7. Avoid drinking copious amounts of fluids before sleep.
8. Drink warm milk before bedtime.

Sedative-Hypnotics

The mildest form of CNS depression is **sedation,** which diminishes physical and mental responses at lower dosages of certain CNS depressants but does not affect consciousness. Sedatives are used mostly during the daytime. Increasing the drug dose can produce a **hypnotic effect**—not hypnosis but a form of "natural" sleep. Sedative-hypnotic drugs are sometimes the same drug; however, certain drugs are used more often for their hypnotic effect. With very high doses of sedative-hypnotic drugs, anesthesia may be achieved. An example of an ultrashort-acting barbiturate used to produce anesthesia is thiopental sodium (Pentothal).

Sedatives were first prescribed to reduce tension and anxiety. Barbiturates were initially used for their antianxiety effect, until the early 1960s when benzodiazepines were introduced. Because of the many side effects of barbiturates and their potential for physical and mental dependency, they are now less frequently prescribed. Similarly, the chronic use of any sedative-hypnotic should be avoided.

Because of the high incidence of sleep disorders, hypnotic drugs are one of the most frequently prescribed drugs. More than $35 million is spent each year on OTC sleep aids such as Nytol, Sominex, Sleep-Eze, and Tylenol PM. The primary ingredient in OTC sleep aids is an antihistamine, such as diphenhydramine, and not barbiturates or benzodiazepines.

There are short-acting hypnotics and intermediate-acting hypnotics. Short-acting hypnotics are useful in achieving sleep because they allow the client to awaken early in the morning without experiencing lingering side effects. Intermediate-acting hypnotics are useful for sustaining sleep; however, after using one the client may experience residual drowsiness, or **hangover,** in the morning. This may be undesirable if the client is active and requires mental alertness. The ideal hypnotic promotes natural sleep without disrupting normal patterns of sleep and produces no hangover or undesirable effect. Table 20–1 lists the common side effects and adverse reactions associated with sedative-hypnotic use and abuse.

Hypnotic drug therapy should be short term to prevent drug **dependence** and drug **tolerance.** Interrupting hypnotic therapy can decrease drug tolerance. However, abruptly discontinuing a high dose of hypnotic that has been taken over a long period could cause **withdrawal symptoms.** At high doses, the dose should be tapered to avoid withdrawal symptoms. The lowest dose should be taken to obtain sleep. Clients with severe respiratory disorders should avoid hypnotics, which could cause an increase in respiratory distress. Normally, hypnotics are contraindicated during pregnancy.

The category of sedative-hypnotics includes barbiturates, benzodiazepines, nonbenzodiazepines, and piperidinediones, among others. Each of these is discussed separately. Prototype drug charts are included for barbiturates and benzodiazepines.

Table 20–1	
Common Side Effects and Adverse Reactions of Sedative-Hypnotics	
Side Effects and Adverse Reactions	**Explanation of the Effects**
Hangover	A hangover is residual drowsiness resulting in impaired reaction time. The intermediate- and long-acting hypnotics are frequently the cause of drug hangover. The liver biotransforms these drugs into active metabolites that persist in the body, causing drowsiness.
REM rebound	REM rebound, which results in vivid dreams and nightmares, frequently occurs after taking a hypnotic for a prolonged period and then abruptly stopping. However, it may occur after taking only one hypnotic dose.
Dependence	Dependence is the result of chronic hypnotic use. Physical and psychologic dependence can result. Physical dependence results in the appearance of specific withdrawal symptoms when a drug is discontinued after prolonged use. The severity of withdrawal symptoms depends on the drug and the dosage. Symptoms may include muscular twitching and tremors, dizziness, orthostatic hypotension, delusions, hallucinations, delirium, and seizures. The withdrawal symptoms start within 24 hours and can last for several days.
Tolerance	Tolerance results when there is a need to increase the dosage over time to obtain the desired effect. It is mostly caused by an increase in drug metabolism by liver enzymes. The barbiturate drug category can cause tolerance after prolonged use. Tolerance is reversible when the drug is discontinued.
Excessive depression	Long-term use of a hypnotic may result in depression, which is characterized by lethargy, sleepiness, lack of concentration, confusion, and psychologic depression.
Respiratory depression	High doses of sedative-hypnotics can suppress the respiratory center in the medulla.
Hypersensitivity	Skin rashes and urticaria can result when taking barbiturates. Such reactions are rare.

REM, Rapid eye movement.

Table 20–2

Sedative-Hypnotics: Barbiturates and Others

Generic (Brand)	Route and Dosage	Uses and Considerations
Barbiturates: Short-Acting		
pentobarbital sodium (Nembutal Sodium) CSS II	*Sedative:* A: PO: 20-30 mg t.i.d. C: PO: 2-6 mg/kg/d in 3 divided doses. *max:* 100 mg/d *Hypnotic:* A: PO: 100-200 mg at bedtime; IM: 150-200 mg C: PO: 30-100 mg at bedtime; IM 2-6 mg/kg; max: 100 mg/d *Preoperative:* A: PO/IM/IV: 100-200 mg in 2 divided doses See Prototype Drug Chart 20–1.	For sedation, sleep, or preanesthetic. *Pregnancy category:* D; PB: 35%-45%; t^1/$_2$: 4-50 h
secobarbital sodium (Seconal Sodium) CSS II		
Barbiturates: Intermediate-Acting		
amobarbital sodium (Amytal Sodium) CSS II	*Sedative:* A: PO: 30-50 mg b.i.d., t.i.d. C: PO: 2 mg/kg/d in 3-4 divided doses *Hypnotic:* A: PO/IM: 65-200 mg at bedtime C: IM: 2-3 mg/kg A and C: IV: 65-200 mg	As a sedative and short-term hypnotic, to control acute convulsive episodes, and for insomnia. Take 0.5-1 h before bedtime. *Pregnancy category:* D; PB: 50%-60%; t^1/$_2$: 20-40 h
aprobarbital (Alurate) CSS III	*Sedative:* A: PO: 40 mg t.i.d. *Hypnotic:* A: PO: 40-160 mg at bedtime	As a sedative and short-term hypnotic; use no longer than 2 wk. *Pregnancy category:* D, PB: <50%; t^1/$_2$: 15-40 h
butabarbital sodium (Butisol Sodium) CSS III	*Sedative:* A: PO: 15-30 mg t.i.d., q.i.d. *Hypnotic:* A: PO: 50-100 mg at bedtime *Preoperative sedative:* A: PO: 50-100 mg, 1-1.5 h before surgery	To relieve anxiety and as short-term hypnotic for insomnia. Avoid alcohol with all barbiturates. *Pregnancy category:* D; PB: <50%; t^1/$_2$: 60-120 h
Other Sedative-Hypnotics		
chloral hydrate CSS IV	*Sedative:* A: PO: 250 mg t.i.d. p.c. C: PO: 8.3 mg/kg t.i.d. p.c.; *max:* 1000 mg/d or 500 mg/dose *Hypnotic:* A: PO: 500 mg-1g at bedtime C: PO: 50 mg/kg at bedtime; *max:* 1000 mg	For sedative or sleep. Used in mid-1800s. No hangover and less respiratory depression. Give with meals or fluids to prevent gastric irritation. Give 15-30 min before sleep. *Pregnancy category:* C; PB: 70%-80%; t^1/$_2$: 8-10 h
ethchlorvynol (Placidyl) CSS IV	*Sedative:* A: PO: 100-200 mg, b.i.d., t.i.d. *Hypnotic:* A: PO: 0.5-1 g, at bedtime for 1 wk only	A barbiturate-like drug. For sedation and sleep. Use no longer than 1 wk. Caution: renal or liver disease and drug abuse. Give with food or fluid to decrease nausea and vomiting. It has a short duration of action. *Pregnancy category:* C; PB: UK; t^1/$_2$: 20-100 h
paraldehyde (Paral) CSS IV	*Sedative:* A: PO: 5-0 ml q4-6h PRN in water or juice; *max:* 30 ml C: PO: 0.3 ml/kg *Hypnotic:* A: PO: 10-30 ml at bedtime	Exhaled via the lungs. Strong odor and disagreeable taste. Seldom used today; has been used to control delirium tremens (DTs) in alcoholics. Can be used for drug poisoning, status epilepticus, and tetanus to control convulsions. *Pregnancy category:* C; PB: UK; t^1/$_2$: 7.5 h

A, Adult; *b.i.d.,* two times a day; *C,* child; *CSS,* Controlled Substances Schedule; *d,* day; *h,* hour; *IM,* intramuscular; *IV,* intravenous; *max,* maximum; *PB,* protein-binding; *p.c.,* after meals; *PO,* by mouth; *PRN,* as needed; *q.i.d.,* four times a day; t^1/$_2$, half-life; *t.i.d.,* three times a day; *UK,* unknown; *wk,* week; <, less than.

PROTOTYPE DRUG CHART 20–1

SECOBARBITAL SODIUM

Drug Class	**Dosage**
Sedative-Hypnotic: Barbiturate Trade Names: Seconal Sodium, CSS II *Pregnancy Category:* D	*Sedative:* **A: PO:** 100-300 mg/d **C: PO:** 4-6 mg/kg/d in 3 divided doses *Hypnotic:* **A: PO:** 100-200 mg at bedtime *Preoperative:* **A: PO:** 100-300 mg 1-2 h before surgery
Contraindications	**Drug-Lab-Food Interactions**
Respiratory depression, severe hepatic disease, pregnancy (fetal immaturity), nephrosis, hypersensitivity *Caution:* liver or kidney dysfunction; elderly, children, and debilitated individuals	*Drug:* *Decrease* respiration with alcohol, CNS depres- sants, and MAOIs
Pharmacokinetics	**Pharmacodynamics**

Absorption: PO: 90% absorbed from GI tract
Distribution: PB: UK
Metabolism: t½: 15-40 h
Excretion: In urine as metabolites
	PO: Onset: 15-30 min
	    Peak: 0.5-1 h
	    Duration: 3-4 h

Therapeutic Effects/Uses

To treat insomnia; used for sedation, preoperative medication
Mode of Action: Depression of the CNS, including the motor and sensory activities

Side Effects	**Adverse Reactions**
Lethargy, drowsiness, hangover, dizziness, paradoxical excitement in the elderly	Drug dependence or tolerance **Life threatening:** Respiratory distress, laryngospasm

A, Adult; *C,* child; *CNS,* central nervous system; *CSS,* Controlled Substances Schedule; *d,* day; *GI,* gastrointestinal; *h,* hour; *MAOIs,*
monoamine oxidase inhibitors; *min,* minute; *PB,* protein-binding; *PO,* by mouth; *t½,* half-life, *UK,* unknown.

Barbiturates

Barbiturates were introduced as a sedative in the early 1900s. More than 2000 barbiturates have been developed, but only 12 are currently marketed. Barbiturates are classified as long-acting, intermediate-acting, short-acting, and ultrashort-acting.

- The *long-acting* group includes phenobarbital and mephobarbital and is used to control seizures in epilepsy. Phenobarbital, introduced in 1912, is still in use.
- The *intermediate-acting* barbiturates amobarbital (Amytal), aprobarbital (Alurate), and butabarbital (Butisol) are useful as sleep sustainers for maintaining long periods of sleep. Because these drugs take approximately 1 hour for the onset of sleep, they are not prescribed for those who have trouble getting to sleep. Vital signs should be closely monitored in persons who take intermediate-acting barbiturates.
- The *short-acting* barbiturates secobarbital (Seconal) and pentobarbital (Nembutal) are used to induce sleep for those who have difficulty falling asleep. These drugs may cause the person to awaken early in the morning. Vital signs should be closely monitored in persons who take short-acting barbiturates.
- The *ultrashort-acting* barbiturate, thiopental sodium (Pentothal), is used as a general anesthetic.

Barbiturates should be restricted to short-term use (2 weeks or less) because of their numerous side effects, including tolerance to the drug. In the United States barbiturates are classified as class II in the schedule of the Controlled Substances Act. In Canada, barbiturates are classified as schedule G. Barbiturates are listed in Table 20–2 and described in more detail in Prototype Drug Chart 20–1, with a focus on the short-acting barbiturate secobarbital (Seconal). The nursing process is based on the drug data.

Pharmacokinetics

Pentobarbital (Nembutal) has been available for nearly half a century and was the hypnotic of choice until the introduction of benzodiazepines in the 1960s. It has a slow absorption rate and is moderately protein-bound. The long half-life is mainly because of the formation of active metabolites resulting from liver metabolism.

HERBAL ALERT 20-1

Sedatives

Kava kava should not be taken in combination with CNS depressants, such as barbiturates and opioids. This herb may increase the sedative effect.

Valerian, when taken with alcohol and other CNS depressants, such as barbiturates, may increase the sedative effects of the prescribed drug.

Pharmacodynamics

Pentobarbital and secobarbital are used primarily for sleep induction and for sedation needs. They have a rapid onset with a short duration of action; thus they are considered short-acting barbiturates. The onset of action of pentobarbital is slower when administered intramuscularly (IM) than when administered orally (PO). Do not confuse pentobarbital with phenobarbital. See Herbal Alert 20-1.

Many drug interactions are associated with barbiturates. Alcohol, narcotics, and other sedative-hypnotics used in combination with barbiturates may further depress the CNS. Pentobarbital increases hepatic enzyme action, thus causing an increased metabolism and decreased effect of drugs such as oral anticoagulants, glucocorticoids, tricyclic antidepressants, and quinidine. Pentobarbital may cause hepatotoxicity if taken with large doses of acetaminophen.

Nursing Process

Sedative-Hypnotic: Barbiturate

ASSESSMENT

■ Obtain a drug history of the current drugs and herbs the client is taking.
■ Record baseline vital signs for future comparison.
■ Determine whether there is a history of insomnia or sleep disorder.
■ Assess renal function. Urine output should be >600 ml/day. Renal impairment could prolong drug action by increasing the half-life of the drug.
■ Assess potential for fluid volume deficit, which would potentiate hypotensive effects.

NURSING DIAGNOSIS

■ Disturbed sleep pattern

PLANNING

■ Client will receive adequate sleep without hangover when taking the hypnotic.

NURSING INTERVENTIONS

■ Recognize that continuous use of a barbiturate might result in drug abuse.
■ Monitor vital signs, especially respirations and blood pressure.

■ Raise bedside rails of older adults and clients who are receiving a hypnotic for the first time. Confusion may occur, and injury may result.
■ Observe client, especially an older adult or a debilitated client, for adverse reactions to the secobarbital; see Prototype Drug Chart 20-1.
■ Check client's skin for rashes. Skin eruptions may occur in clients taking barbiturates.
■ Assess client for withdrawal symptoms when barbiturates have been taken over a prolonged period of time and then discontinued.
■ Administer IV pentobarbital at a rate of less than 50 mg/min. Do *not* mix pentobarbital with other medications. IM injection should be given deep in a large muscle such as the gluteus medius.

Client Teaching

General

• Teach client to use nonpharmacologic ways to induce sleep, such as enjoying a warm bath, listening to music, drinking warm fluids, and avoiding drinks with caffeine for 6 hours before bedtime.
• Instruct client to avoid alcohol and antidepressant, antipsychotic, and narcotic drugs while taking the barbiturate. Respiratory distress may occur when these drugs are combined.
• Inform client that certain herbs (see Herbal Alert 20-1) may interact with CNS depressants such as barbiturates. The herb may need to be discontinued or the drug dose may need to be modified.
• Advise client not to drive a motor vehicle or operate machinery. Caution is always encouraged.
• Instruct client to take the hypnotic 30 minutes before bedtime. Short-acting hypnotics take effect within 15 to 30 minutes.
• Encourage client to check with the health care provider about OTC sleeping aids. Drowsiness may result from taking these drugs; therefore caution while driving is advised.

Side Effects

• Advise client to report adverse reactions, such as hangover, to the health care provider. Drug selection or dosage might need to be changed.
• Instruct client that hypnotics such as secobarbital should be gradually withdrawn, especially if it has been taken for several weeks. Abrupt cessation of the hypnotic may result in withdrawal symptoms (e.g., tremors, muscle twitching).

Cultural Considerations

• Explain and reexplain relevant points to compensate for client's knowledge deficit or language limitations.

Benzodiazepines

Selected benzodiazepines (minor tranquilizer or anxiolytic), introduced with chlordiazepoxide (Librium) in the 1960s as antianxiety agents, are ordered as sedative-hypnotics for inducing sleep. Several benzodiazepines marketed as hypnotics include flurazepam (Dalmane), temazepam (Restoril), triazolam (Halcion), estazolam (ProSom), and quazepam (Doral) (see Table 20–2). Increased anxiety might be the cause of insomnia for some clients, so lorazepam (Ativan) and diazepam (Valium) can be used to alleviate the anxiety. These drugs are classified as schedule IV according to the Controlled Substances Act. The benzodiazepines increase the action of the inhibitory neurotransmitter gamma-aminobutyric acid (GABA) to the GABA receptors. The neuron excitability is reduced. Do not confuse lorazepam with alprazolam.

Benzodiazepines (except for temazepam) can suppress stage 4 of NREM sleep, which may result in vivid dreams or nightmares and can delay REM sleep. Benzodiazepines are effective for sleep disorders for several weeks longer than other sedative-hypnotics; however, they should not be used for longer than 3 to 4 weeks as a hypnotic to prevent *REM rebound.*

Flurazepam (Dalmane) was the first benzodiazepine hypnotic introduced. Triazolam (Halcion) is a short-acting hypnotic with a half-life of 2 to 5 hours. It does not produce any active metabolites. Complaints of adverse reactions to prolonged use of triazolam, such as loss of memory, led to its removal from the market in Great Britain. The advisory group in Great Britain is recommending that the legislative body reinstate triazolam. Its use is under review by the Food and Drug Administration (FDA). Currently, it is seldom prescribed.

Small doses of benzodiazepine are recommended for clients with renal or hepatic dysfunction. For benzodiazepine overdose, the benzodiazepine antagonist flumazenil may be prescribed. Benzodiazepines prescribed as antianxiety drugs are discussed in Chapter 25, Antipsychotics and Anxiolytics.

Pharmacokinetics

Benzodiazepines are well absorbed through the gastrointestinal (GI) mucosa. Flurazepam is rapidly metabolized in the liver to active metabolites, and it has a long half-life of 45 to 100 hours. Flurazepam is highly protein bound, and if it is taken with other highly protein bound drugs, more free drug is available, which increases the risk of adverse effects.

Pharmacodynamics

Benzodiazepines are used to treat insomnia by inducing and sustaining sleep. They have a rapid onset of action and intermediate- to long-acting effects. The normal recommended dose of a benzodiazepine may be too much for the older adult, so half of the dose is recommended initially to prevent overdosing.

Alcohol or narcotics taken with a benzodiazepine may cause an additive depressive CNS response. Triazolam (Halcion) may cause rebound insomnia and temazepam (Restoril) may cause euphoria and palpitations.

Nonbenzodiazepines

Zolpidem (Ambien) is a nonbenzodiazepine that differs in its structure from benzodiazepines; however, it is used for short-term treatment (<10 days) of insomnia. Its duration of action is 6 to 8 hours with a short half-life of 2 to 2.5 hours. Zolpidem is metabolized in the liver to three inactive metabolites and is excreted in bile, urine, and feces. When zolpidem is prescribed for older adults, the dose should be decreased. Table 20–3 lists the benzodiazepines and nonbenzodiazepines that are used as sedative-hypnotics and their dosages, uses, and considerations. Zolpidem is described in Prototype Drug Chart 20–2.

Piperidinediones

The piperidinediones resemble barbiturates. These sedative-hypnotics were introduced in the mid-1950s and include glutethimide, which has effects similar to the short-acting barbiturates. These drugs were marketed to be nonaddictive; however, they can be addictive and can cause severe adverse reactions, such as vasomotor collapse, serious blood dyscrasias (aplastic anemia), and allergic reactions. Gastric irritation rarely occurs. Over the past decade, the use of the piperidinedione group has declined.

Chloral Hydrate

Chloral hydrate was first introduced in the 1860s. It is used to induce sleep and to decrease nocturnal awakenings; it does not suppress REM sleep. There is less occurrence of hangover, respiratory depression, and tolerance with chloral hydrate than with other sedative-hypnotics. Its use is effective in older adults. Chloral hydrate can be given to clients with mild liver dysfunction, but it should be avoided if severe liver or renal disorder is present. Gastric irritation is a common complaint, so the drug should be taken with sufficient water. Drugs that interact with chloral hydrate include other CNS depressants, furosemide, and oral anticoagulants.

Sedatives and Hypnotics for Older Adults

Identifying the cause of insomnia in an older adult should be the first consideration, and nonpharmacologic methods should be used before sleep medications are prescribed. The use of hypnotics can cause various side effects, especially in older adults because of their physiologic changes.

Barbiturates increase CNS depression and confusion in older adults and should not be taken for sleep. The short-

Table 20–3

Sedative-Hypnotics: Benzodiazepines and Nonbenzodiazepines

Generic (Brand)	Route and Dosage	Uses and Considerations
Benzodiazepines		
alprazolam (Xanax) CSS IV	A: PO: 0.25-0.5 mg at bedtime	For alleviating anxiety that may cause sleeplessness. *Pregnancy category:* D; PB: UK; t¹/₂: 12-15 h
estazolam (ProSom) CSS IV	A: PO: 1-2 mg at bedtime Elderly: PO: 0.5 mg at bedtime	New benzodiazepine hypnotic for treatment of insomnia. Should not be used for longer than 6 wk. Decreases the frequency of nocturnal awakeness. *Pregnancy category:* X; PB: 93%; t¹/₂: 10-24 h
flurazepam HCl (Dalmane) CSS IV	A: PO: 15-30 mg at bedtime Elderly: PO: 15 mg at bedtime	For insomnia. *Pregnancy category:* X; PB: 97%; t¹/₂: 2-3 h
lorazepam (Ativan) CSS IV	*Insomnia:* A: PO: 2-4 mg at bedtime	Used as a preoperative sedative and to reduce anxiety. *Pregnancy category:* D; PB: 85%; t¹/₂: 12-14 h
quazepam (Doral) CSS IV	A: PO: 7.5-15 mg at bedtime	To treat insomnia and to decrease nocturnal awakenings. Avoid alcohol with this drug and all benzodiazepines. *Pregnancy category:* X; PB: >95%; t¹/₂: 39 h
temazepam (Restoril) CSS IV	*Hypnotic:* A: PO: 15-30 mg at bedtime	To treat insomnia and to decrease nocturnal awakenings. Also has sedative effects. *Pregnancy category:* X; PB: 96%; t¹/₂: 10-20 h
triazolam (Halcion) CSS IV	*Hypnotic:* A: PO: 0.125-0.5 mg at bedtime (0.5 mg with caution) Elderly: PO: 0.125-0.25 mg at bedtime	For management of insomnia. Should not be used for longer than 7-10 d at a time to avoid tolerance. Avoid alcohol and smoking when taking triazolam. *Pregnancy category:* X; PB: 89%; t¹/₂: 2-4 h
Benzodiazepine Antagonist		
flumazenil (Romazicon)	A: IV: 0.2 mg over 30 sec; may repeat with 0.3 mg in 30 sec; *max:* 3 mg total dose	Management of benzodiazepine overdose or reversal of sedative effects of benzodiazepine with general anesthesia. *Pregnancy category:* UK; PB: UK; t¹/₂: UK.
Nonbenzodiazepine		
zolpidem tartrate (Ambien) CSS IV	See Prototype Drug Chart 20–2.	
Piperidinedione		
Glutethimide (Doriden) CSS III	*Hypnotic:* A: PO: 250-500 mg at bedtime; repeat in 4 h if necessary	For insomnia. Resembles barbiturates. *Caution in use:* renal disease and mental depression. Withdraw drug gradually to prevent withdrawal symptoms (rebound insomnia). *Pregnancy category:* C; PB: 50%; t¹/₂: 10-20 h

A, Adult; *CSS,* Controlled Substances Schedule; *d,* day; *h,* hour; *IV,* intravenous; *max,* maximum; *PB,* protein-binding; *PO,* by mouth; *sec,* second; *t¹/₂,* half-life; *UK,* unknown; *wk,* week.

to intermediate-acting benzodiazepines, such as estazolam (ProSom), temazepam (Restoril), and triazolam (Halcion), are considered safer than barbiturates. In addition, the long-acting hypnotic benzodiazepines, such as flurazepam (Dalmane), quazepam (Doral), and diazepam (Valium), should be avoided. In many cases, older adults should be instructed to take the benzodiazepine no more than four times a week to avoid side effects and drug dependency. They can choose selected nights to take the benzodiazepine.

The main sleep problem experienced by older adults is more frequent awakenings. Reports have shown that older women experience more difficult sleep patterns than men. Sleep disturbance may be caused by discomfort and pain. To alleviate pain and aid in sleep, the OTC drug Tylenol PM, which contains acetaminophen and diphenhydramine (an antihistamine), may be taken. Occasionally, a non-steroidal antiinflammatory drug (NSAID), such as ibuprofen, may alleviate the discomfort that prevents sleep.

Nursing Process

Sedative-Hypnotic: Benzodiazepine

ASSESSMENT

■ Record baseline vital signs and laboratory tests (e.g., AST, ALT, bilirubin) for future comparisons.

- Obtain drug history. Taking CNS depressants with benzodiazepine hypnotics can depress respirations.
- Ascertain client's problem with sleep disturbance.

NURSING DIAGNOSIS

- Disturbed sleep pattern

PLANNING

- Client will remain asleep for 6 to 8 hours.

NURSING INTERVENTIONS

- Monitor vital signs. Check for signs of respiratory distress, such as slow, irregular breathing patterns.
- Raise bedside rails of older adults or clients receiving sedative-hypnotics for the first time. Confusion may occur, and injury may result.
- Observe client for side effects of sedative-hypnotics, such as hangover (residual sedation), light-headedness, dizziness, or confusion.

Client Teaching

General

- Teach client to use nonpharmacologic ways to induce sleep, such as enjoying a warm bath, listening to music, drinking warm fluids such as milk, and avoiding drinks with caffeine after dinner.
- Instruct client to avoid alcohol and antidepressant, antipsychotic, and narcotic drugs while taking sedative-hypnotics. Severe respiratory distress may occur when these drugs are combined.
- Advise client to take sedative-hypnotic before bedtime. Flurazepam takes effect within 15 to 45 minutes.
- Suggest that client urinate before taking sedative-hypnotic to prevent sleep disruption.
- Encourage client to check with the health care provider about OTC sleeping aids. Drowsiness may result from taking these drugs; therefore caution while driving is advised.

Side Effects

- Instruct client to report adverse reactions, such as hangover, to the health care provider. Drug selection or dosage may need to be changed if hangover occurs.

PROTOTYPE DRUG CHART 20–2

ZOLPIDEM TARTRATE

Drug Class
Sedative-Hypnotic: non-benzodiazepine
Trade Name: Ambien
CSS IV
Pregnancy Category: B

Dosage
A: PO: 5-10 mg at bedtime; *max:* 7-10 mg/d
Elderly: PO: 5 mg at bedtime; *max:* 7-10 mg/d

Contraindications
Hypersensitivity to benzodiazepine, lactation
Caution: Renal or liver dysfunction; pregnancy; children, elderly, and debilitated individuals

Drug-Lab-Food Interactions
Drug: Decrease CNS function with alcohol, CNS depressants, anticonvulsants, and phenothiazines
Food: Decreases absorption

Pharmacokinetics
Absorption: PO: well absorbed
Distribution: PB: 79%-96%
Metabolism: t½: 2-2.5 h
Excretion: In bile, urine, and feces

Pharmacodynamics
PO: Onset: 7-27 min
Peak: 0.5-2.3 h
Duration: 6-8 h

Therapeutic Effects/Uses
To treat insomnia
Mode of Action: Depression of the CNS, neurotransmitter inhibition

Side Effects
Drowsiness, lethargy, hangover (residual sedation), irritability, dizziness, anxiety, nausea, vomiting, confusion, disorientation

Adverse Reactions
Tolerance, psychologic or physical dependence

A, Adult; *CNS,* central nervous system; *CSS,* Controlled Substances Schedule; *d,* day; *h,* hour; *min,* minute; *PB,* protein-binding; *PO,* by mouth; *t½,* half-life.

Cultural Considerations ⊕

- Ask the transcultural person about methods that family members have used to promote sleep.
- Suggest nonpharmacologic alternatives that may be effective to induce sleep for the person.

EVALUATION

■ Evaluate the effectiveness of sedative-hypnotic in promoting sleep.

■ Determine whether side effects such as hangover occur after several days of taking sedative-hypnotic. Another hypnotic may be prescribed if side effects remain.

Anesthetics

Anesthetics are classified as general and local. General anesthetics depress the CNS, alleviate pain, and cause a loss of consciousness. The first anesthetic, nitrous oxide ("laughing gas"), was used for surgery in the early 1800s. It is still an effective anesthetic and is frequently used in dental surgery. In the mid-1800s, ether and chloroform were introduced. Ether, a highly flammable volatile liquid, has a pungent odor and can cause nausea and vomiting after it has been administered. It is seldom used, probably because of the hazard of possible explosion and its noxious odor. Chloroform is toxic to liver cells and is no longer used.

Pathophysiology

Several theories exist regarding how inhalation anesthetics cause CNS depression and a loss of consciousness. The differing theories suggest the following about inhalation anesthetics:

1. The lipid structure of cell membranes is altered, resulting in impaired physiologic functions.
2. The inhibitory neurotransmitter gamma-aminobutyric acid (GABA) is activated to the GABA receptor that pushes chloride ions into the neurons. This greatly decreases the fire action potentials of the neurons.

3. The ascending reticular activating system is altered; thus the neurons cease to transmit information (stimuli) to the brain.

Balanced Anesthesia

Balanced anesthesia, a combination of drugs, is frequently used in general anesthesia. Balanced anesthesia generally includes the following:

1. A hypnotic given the night before;
2. Premedication, such as a narcotic analgesic or a benzodiazepine (e.g., midazolam [Versed]) and an anticholinergic (e.g., atropine), given about 1 hour before surgery to decrease secretions;
3. A short-acting barbiturate, such as thiopental sodium (Pentothal), given;
4. An inhaled gas, such as nitrous oxide and oxygen, administered;
5. A muscle relaxant given as needed.

Balanced anesthesia minimizes cardiovascular problems, decreases the amount of general anesthetic needed, reduces possible postanesthetic nausea and vomiting, minimizes the disturbance of organ function, and increases recovery from anesthesia. Because the client does not receive large doses of general anesthetics, fewer adverse reactions occur.

Stages of General Anesthesia

General anesthesia proceeds through four stages (Table 20–4). The surgical procedure is usually performed during the third stage. If an anesthetic agent is given immediately before the inhalation anesthesia, the third stage can occur without the early stages of anesthesia being observed. However, if the drug is given slowly, all stages of anesthesia are usually observed.

Assessment Before Surgery

The client's response to anesthesia may differ according to variables related to the health status of the individual. These variables include age (young and elderly), a current health disorder (e.g., renal or liver), pregnancy, history of heavy smoking, obesity, and frequent use of alcohol and drugs. These problems must be identified *before* surgery be-

Table 20–4

Stages of Anesthesia

Stage	Name	Description
1	Analgesia	Begins with consciousness and ends with loss of consciousness. Speech is difficult; sensations of smell and pain are lost. Dreams and auditory and visual hallucinations may occur. This stage may be called the *induction stage.*
2	Excitement or delirium	Produces a loss of consciousness caused by depression of the cerebral cortex. Confusion, excitement, or delirium occur. Short induction time.
3	Surgical	Surgical procedure is performed during this stage. There are four phases. The surgery is usually performed in phase 2 and upper phase 3. As anesthesia deepens, respirations become more shallow and respiratory rate is increased.
4	Medullary paralysis	Toxic stage of anesthesia. Respirations are lost and circulatory collapse occurs. Ventilatory assistance is necessary.

cause the type and amount of anesthetic required might need adjustment.

Inhalation Anesthetics

During the third stage of anesthesia, inhalation anesthetics (i.e., gas or volatile liquids administered as gas) are used to deliver general anesthesia. Certain gases, such as nitrous oxide and cyclopropane, are absorbed quickly, have a rapid action, and are eliminated rapidly. Cyclopropane was a popular inhalation anesthetic from 1930 to 1960, but because of its highly flammable state as ether, it is no longer used. In the late 1950s, halothane was introduced as a nonflammable alternative. Other inhalation drugs introduced as anesthetics include methoxyflurane in the 1960s, enflurane in the 1970s, isoflurane in the 1980s, desflurane in 1992, and the newest, seroflurane, in 1995.

Inhalation anesthetics typically provide smooth induction. Upon discontinuing administration of halothane (Fluothane), isoflurane (Forane), and enflurane (Ethrane), recovery of consciousness usually occurs in approximately 1 hour. Recovery from desflurane (Suprane) and sevoflurane (Ultane) is within minutes. Inhalation anesthetics are usually combined with a barbiturate (e.g., thiopental), a strong analgesic (e.g., morphine), and a muscle relaxant (e.g., pancuronium) for surgical procedures.

Adverse effects from inhalation anesthetics include respiratory depression, hypotension, dysrhythmias, and hepatic dysfunction. In clients at risk, these drugs may trigger malignant hyperthermia. The newer drugs primarily cause less nausea and vomiting than the older anesthetics.

Intravenous Anesthetics

Intravenous (IV) anesthetics may be used for general anesthesia or for the induction stage of anesthesia. For outpatient surgery of short duration, an intravenous anesthetic might be the preferred form of anesthesia. Previously, thiopental sodium (Pentothal), an ultrashort-acting barbiturate, was the general anesthetic used for short-term surgery. It is still used for the rapid induction stage of anesthesia and in dental procedures. Presently, droperidol (Innovar), etomidate (Amidate), and ketamine hydrochloride (Ketalar) are also used intravenously as general anesthetics. IV anesthetics have rapid onsets and short durations of action. Table 20–5 describes the inhalation and intravenous anesthetics used for general anesthesia.

Midazolam (Versed) and propofol (Diprivan) are commonly administered for the induction and maintenance of anesthesia or conscious sedation for minor surgery or procedures, such as mechanical ventilation or intubation. Clients are sedated and relaxed but responsive to commands.

Adverse effects from IV anesthetics include respiratory and cardiovascular depression. Also, propofol supports microbial growth and may increase the risk of bacterial infection. Precautions, such as discarding opened vials within 6 hours, are necessary to prevent sepsis.

Topical Anesthetics

Use of topical anesthetic agents is limited to mucous membranes, broken or unbroken skin surfaces, and burns. Topical anesthetics come in different forms, such as solution, liquid spray, ointment, cream, and gel. Topical anesthetics decrease the sensitive nerve endings of the affected area.

Local Anesthetics

Local anesthetics block pain at the site where the drug is administered, allowing consciousness to be maintained. Uses for local anesthetics include performing dental procedures, suturing skin lacerations, performing short-term (minor) surgery at a localized area, blocking nerve impulses (nerve block) below the insertion of a spinal anesthetic, and performing diagnostic procedures such as lumbar puncture and thoracentesis.

Most local anesthetics are divided into two groups, the esters and the amides, according to their basic structures. The amides have a very low incidence of causing an allergic reaction.

The first local anesthetic used was cocaine hydrochloride in the late 1800s. Procaine hydrochloride (Novocain), a synthetic of cocaine, was discovered in the early 1900s. Lidocaine hydrochloride (Xylocaine) was developed in the mid-1950s to replace procaine, except in dental procedures. Lidocaine has a rapid onset and a long duration of action, is more stable in solution, and causes fewer hypersensitivity reactions than procaine. Since the introduction of lidocaine, many local anesthetics have been marketed. Table 20–6 describes the various types of local anesthetics according to short-, moderate-, and long-acting effects.

The PainFree pump system, developed by Sgarlato Labs, controls discomfort in the first 24 to 96 hours postoperatively. This spring loaded pump administers a local anesthetic by continuous infusion to surgical wound sites. The pump is portable and can be worn in the accompanying carrying case.

Benefits of the pain pump include increased mobility as well as reduced narcotic use, drowsiness, nausea, and hospital stay. The pain pump method also provides compliance with Joint Commission on Accreditation of Health-Care Organizations (JCAHO) recommendations for pain management. This pain control method may be used in many types of surgeries, such as orthopedic joint surgeries, mastectomy, cesarean section, hysterectomy, hernia repair, and cholecystectomy. For example, the client who has a bilateral hernia repair has a catheter inserted into deep fascia of the lower abdominal area. A continuous flow of bupivacaine (Marcaine), a local anesthetic, is delivered via a Y-connector to both sides at a flow rate of approximately 2 ml per hour.

Spinal Anesthesia

Spinal anesthesia requires that a local anesthetic be injected in the subarachnoid space at the third or fourth lumbar space. If the local anesthetic is given too high in the spinal column, the respiratory muscles could be af-

Table 20–5

Inhalation and Intravenous Anesthetics

Drug	Induction Time	Considerations
Inhalation: Volatile Liquids		
ether	Slow	Highly flammable. Has no severe effect on the cardiovascular system or liver.
halothane (Fluothane)	Rapid	Introduced in the 1950s. Highly potent anesthetic. Rapid recovery. Could decrease blood pressure. Has a bronchodilator effect. Contraindicated in obstetrics.
methoxyflurane (Penthrane)	Slow	Introduced in the 1960s. Used during labor. Drug dose is usually less than other anesthetics and it does not suppress uterine contraction. Could cause hypotension. Contraindicated in renal disorders.
enflurane (Ethrane)	Rapid	Introduced in 1970s. Similar to halothane. Can depress respiratory function; thus ventilatory support may be necessary. Not to be used during labor because uterine contractions could be suppressed. Avoid with clients with seizure disorders.
isoflurane (Forane)	Rapid	Introduced in 1980s. Frequently used in inhalation therapy. Has a smooth and rapid induction of anesthesia and rapid recovery. Could cause hypotension and respiratory depression. Not to be used during labor because it suppresses uterine contractions. Has minimal cardiovascular effect.
desflurane (Suprane)	Rapid	Introduced in 1992 as a volatile liquid anesthetic. Similar to isoflurane. Rapid recovery after anesthetic administration has ceased. Could cause hypotension and respiratory depression.
sevoflurane (Ultane)	Rapid	For induction and maintenance during surgery. It may be given alone or combined with nitrous oxide. Rate of elimination is similar to desflurane.
Inhalation: Gas		
nitrous oxide (laughing gas)	Very rapid	Rapid recovery. Has minimal cardiovascular effect. Should be given with oxygen. Low potency.
cyclopropane	Very rapid	Highly flammable and explosive. Seldom used.
Intravenous (Ultra-Short Barbiturates)		
thiopental sodium (Pentothal)	Rapid	Has short duration of action. Used for rapid induction of general surgery. Keep client warm; shivering and tremors may occur. Can depress respiratory center, and ventilatory assistance might be necessary.
methohexital sodium (Brevital sodium)	Rapid	Has a short duration. Frequently used for induction and with other drugs as part of balanced anesthesia. An inhalation anesthesia usually follows.
thiamylal sodium (Surital)	Rapid	Used for induction of anesthesia and anesthesia for electroshock therapy.
Benzodiazepines		
diazepam (Valium)	Moderate to rapid	For induction of anesthesia. No analgesic effect.
midazolam (Versed)	Rapid	For induction of anesthesia and for endoscopic procedures. IV drug can cause conscious sedation. Avoid if a cardiopulmonary disorder is present.
Others		
droperidol and fentanyl (Innovar)	Moderate to rapid	A neuroleptic analgesic when combined with fentanyl (potent opiate narcotic). Frequently used with a general anesthetic. Can also be used as a preanesthetic drug. Also used for diagnostic procedures. May cause hypotension and respiratory depression.
etomidate (Amidate)	Rapid	Used for short-term surgery, or as induction of anesthesia, or with a general anesthetic to maintain the anesthetic state.
ketamine hydrochloride (Ketalar)	Rapid	Used for short-term surgery or for induction of anesthesia. It increases salivation, blood pressure, and heart rate. May be used for diagnostic procedures. Avoid with history of psychiatric disorders.
propofol (Diprivan)	Rapid	For induction of anesthesia and may be used with general anesthesia. Short duration of action. May cause hypotension and respiratory depression. Pain can occur at the injection site; thus may be mixed with a local anesthetic such as lidocaine to decrease pain.

h, Hour; *IV,* intravenous; *min,* minute.

Table 20-6

Local Anesthetics

Anesthetics	Type	Uses and Considerations
Short-Acting ($\frac{1}{2}$-1 h)		
chloroprocaine (Nesacaine)	Ester	For infiltration, caudal and epidural anesthesia. Onset of action is 6-12 min.
procaine HCl (Novocain)	Ester	Introduced in 1905. For nerve block, infiltration, epidural, and spinal anesthesias. Useful in dentistry. Caution in use for clients allergic to ester-type anesthetics.
Moderate-Acting (1-3 h)		
lidocaine (Xylocaine)	Amide	Introduced in 1948. For nerve block, infiltration, epidural, and spinal anesthesias. Allergic reaction is rare. Used to treat cardiac dysrhythmias (see Chapter 39).
mepivacaine HCl (Carbocaine HCl; Isocaine; Polocaine)	Amide	For nerve block, infiltration, caudal, and epidural anesthesias. May be used in dentistry.
prilocaine HCl (Citanest)	Amide	For peripheral nerve block, infiltration, caudal, and epidural anesthesias. May be used in dentistry.
Long-Acting (3-10 h)		
bupivacaine (Marcaine, Sensorcaine)	Amide	For peripheral nerve block, infiltration, caudal, and epidural anesthesias.
dibucaine HCl (Nupercainal)	Amide	For topical use (creams and ointment) to affected areas.
etidocaine (Duranest)	Amide	For peripheral nerve block, infiltration, caudal, and epidural anesthesias.
tetracaine HCl (Pontocaine)	Ester	For spinal anesthesia (high and low saddle block). Also for topical use to affected areas such as to the eye to anesthetize the cornea, to the nose and throat for bronchoscopy, to the skin for relief of pain and pruritus (itching).

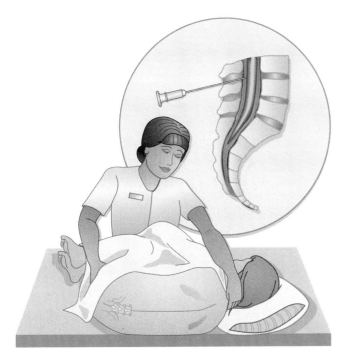

FIGURE 20-2 Positioning a client for spinal anesthetic.

fected, and respiratory distress or failure could result. Headaches might result following spinal anesthesia (a "spinal"), possibly because of a decrease in cerebrospinal fluid pressure caused by a leak of fluid at the needle insertion. Encouraging the client to remain flat following surgery with spinal anesthesia and to take increased fluids usually decreases the likelihood of leaking spinal fluid. Hypotension also can result following spinal anesthesia.

Various sites of the spinal column can be used for a **nerve block** with a local anesthetic (Figure 20-2). A **spinal block** is the penetration of the anesthetic into the subarachnoid membrane, the second layer of the spinal cord. An **epidural block** is the placement of the local anesthetic in the outer covering of the spinal cord, or the dura mater. A **caudal block** is placed near the sacrum. A **saddle block** is given at the lower end of the spinal column to block the perineal area. Blood pressure should be monitored during administration of these types of anesthesia because a decrease in blood pressure resulting from the drug and procedure might occur. A saddle block is frequently used for women in labor during childbirth (see Chapter 52, Drugs Associated with the Female Reproductive Cycle II: Labor, Delivery, and the Preterm Neonate).

Nurses play an important role in client assessment before and after general and local anesthesia is administered. Preparing the client for surgery by explaining the preparations and completing the preoperative orders, including premedications, are necessary to enhance the safety and effectiveness of the anesthesia and surgery.

Nursing Process

Anesthetics

ASSESSMENT

- Record baseline vital signs.
- Obtain a drug history, noting drugs that affect the cardiopulmonary systems.

NURSING DIAGNOSIS

■ Pain

PLANNING

■ Client will participate in preoperative preparation and understand postoperative care.
■ Client's vital signs will remain stable following surgery.

NURSING INTERVENTIONS

■ Monitor client's postoperative state of sensorium. Report if client remains nonresponsive or confused for a time.
■ Check preoperative and postoperative urine output. Report deficit of hourly or 8-hour urine output.
■ Record vital signs following general and local anesthesia; hypotension and respiratory distress may result.
■ Administer an analgesic or a narcotic-analgesic with caution until client fully recovers from the anesthetic. To prevent adverse reactions, dosage might need to be adjusted if client is under the influence of the anesthetic.

Client Teaching

• Explain to client the preoperative preparation and postoperative nursing assessment and interventions.

Cultural Considerations ⊕

• Failing to allow adequate time for information processing may result in an inaccurate response or no response. Allow time for people to respond to questions, especially for those who have language barriers. Speak clearly and slowly, giving time for translation. Obtain an interpreter if necessary.

EVALUATION

■ Evaluate client's response to the anesthetics. Continue to monitor client for adverse reactions.

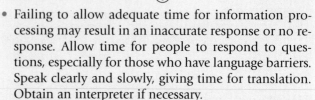

WEBSITES

For further information on *Central Nervous System Depressants*, visit these Internet resources:

Information on zolpidem:
www.nlm.nih.gov/medlineplus/druginfo/medmaster/a693025.html

More information on zolpidem:
www.sanofi-synthelabous.com/products/pi_ambien/pi_ambien.html

---

Critical Thinking Case Study

J.Z., a 72-year-old woman, has difficulty staying asleep. She asks the nurse whether she should take Nytol or Sominex before bedtime.

1. Before J.Z. takes any sleep aid or hypnotic, what nursing assessments should be made?

2. Describe the nursing plan that should be presented to J.Z. that might help her sleep disturbance.

3. Would J.Z. be a candidate for taking a barbiturate or a benzodiazepine? Explain.

4. What follow-up plan should the nurse have related to J.Z.'s sleep problem?

Study Questions

1. What are the advantages of using benzodiazepine hypnotics instead of barbiturates for sleep disorders?

2. Why should renal function be assessed by the nurse? What minimal daily urine output is considered adequate?

3. What is a hangover resulting from a hypnotic? What are the nursing interventions?

4. What is the meaning of *withdrawal symptoms* from hypnotic use? How can they be prevented? What

are the symptoms and the nursing interventions for each?

5. Why should vital signs be closely monitored following general and local anesthesia?

6. What is balanced anesthesia? Give the rationale for its use.

7. What are the nursing interventions, including client teaching, of a client who receives spinal anesthesia?

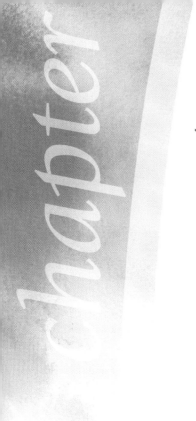

21 Drugs for Pain Management: Nonnarcotic and Narcotic Analgesics

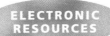
ELECTRONIC RESOURCES

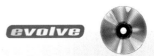
evolve

Additional information can be found on the companion website at *http://evolve.elsevier.com/KeeHayes/pharmacology/* or on the companion CD-ROM, which includes:
- *NCLEX-style examination review questions*
- *Pharmacology animations*
- *Medication error and IV therapy checklists*
- *Medication calculation problems*
- *Electronic calculators*

OBJECTIVES

- Define the following types of pain: acute, chronic, superficial, visceral, and somatic.
- Differentiate between nonnarcotic and narcotic analgesics and include an explanation of when these drug groups are indicated.
- Compare the serum therapeutic ranges of acetaminophen and aspirin.
- Contrast the side effects of aspirin and narcotics.
- Explain the methadone treatment program.
- Give the nursing interventions, including client teaching, related to nonnarcotic and narcotic analgesics.

TERMS

abstinence syndrome
analgesics
methadone treatment
  program
mixed narcotic agonist-
  antagonist

narcotic
narcotic agonist
narcotic antagonist
nociceptors
nonnarcotic

nonsteroidal antiinflam-
  matory drugs (NSAIDs)
orthostatic hypotension
patient-controlled analgesia (PCA)

prostaglandins
somatic
visceral

Introduction

Analgesics, both **nonnarcotic** and **narcotic,** are prescribed for the relief of pain; the choice of drug depends on the severity of the pain. Mild to moderate pain of the skeletal muscles and joints frequently is relieved with the use of nonnarcotic analgesics. Moderate to severe pain in the smooth muscles, organs, and bones usually requires a narcotic analgesic.

Pain management is regarded as such a significant component of nursing care that pain has recently become known as the "fifth vital sign". The Joint Commission on the Accreditation of Healthcare Organizations (JCAHO) has incorporated the assessment, documentation, and management of pain into its standards (JCAHO, 2003), which reflects the importance of this vital sign. The nurse's role is to assess the client's pain level, alleviate the client's pain through nonpharmacologic and pharmacologic treatments, thoroughly document the client's response to treatment, and teach the client and their significant others to manage pain control themselves when appropriate.

Drugs used for pain relief are presented in this chapter. Many of the same nonnarcotic analgesics, such as the nonsteroidal antiinflammatory drugs (NSAIDs), that are taken for pain are also taken for antiinflammatory purposes. These drugs are also covered in Chapter 27, Antiinflammatory Agents.

Pathophysiology

When tissue damage occurs, injured cells release chemical mediators, such as bradykinin, serotonin, and **prostaglandins,** that affect the exposed nerve endings of the **nociceptors** (pain receptors). Nociceptors are found in all types of tissue, such as the skin, muscles, and organs. Although there are few nociceptors in body organs, the **visceral** (organ) nociceptors located here are more sensitive to stretching, inflammation, and ischemia than are nociceptors located elsewhere in the body.

The seven classifications and types of pain are (1) *acute pain,* which can be mild, moderate, or severe and usually lasts for the duration of tissue injury; (2) *cancer pain* caused by pressure or blockage to body tissues and cells; (3) *chronic pain* that is persistent; (4) *somatic pain* from the bones, skeletal muscles, and joints; (5) *superficial pain* that results from skin and mucous membrane injury; (6) *vascular pain* caused by vascular and perivascular conditions; and (7) *visceral pain,* or body-organ pain.

To ascertain the individual's severity of pain, the health care provider should ask the client to rate the degree of pain on a scale of 1 to 10, with 10 being the worst or most severe pain. The client's comfort level should also be determined. A client who indicates a pain level of 9 may verbalize a decrease in pain to a level of 3 within 30 to 45 minutes after receiving pain medication. Table 21–1 lists the types of pain and the drug groups that may be effective in relieving each type of pain.

Nonnarcotic Analgesics

The nonnarcotic analgesics of aspirin, acetaminophen, ibuprofen, and naproxen are not addictive and are less potent than narcotic analgesics. They are used to treat mild to moderate pain and may be purchased over-the-counter (OTC). These drugs are effective for the dull, throbbing pain of headaches, dysmenorrhea (menstrual pain), inflammation, minor abrasions, muscular aches and pain, and mild to moderate arthritis. Most analgesics will lower an elevated body temperature, thus having an antipyretic effect. Some analgesics, such as aspirin, have antiinflammatory and antiplatelet effects as well.

Salicylates and Nonsteroidal Antiinflammatory Drugs

All **nonsteroidal antiinflammatory drugs (NSAIDs)** have an analgesic effect as well as an antipyretic and antiinflammatory action. Aspirin (ASA), ibuprofens (Motrin IB, Nuprin, Advil, Medipren), and naproxen (Aleve) can be purchased as OTC drugs. Aspirin, a salicylate, is an NSAID and is the oldest nonnarcotic analgesic drug still in use. Adolf Bayer marketed the original formulation in 1899, and currently aspirin can be purchased under many names and with added ingredients. Examples are Bufferin, Ecotrin (enteric-coated tablet), Anacin (containing caffeine), and Alka-Seltzer. Aspirin's primary effect is as an analgesic for pain, but it also has an antipyretic effect.

In children younger than 12 years of age, aspirin should not be used and is contraindicated for any elevated temperature, regardless of the cause, because of the danger of Reye syndrome (neurologic problems associated with viral infection and treated with salicylates). In these circumstances, acetaminophen (Tylenol) is used instead of aspirin.

In addition to its analgesic, antipyretic, and antiinflammatory properties, aspirin decreases platelet aggregation

Table 21-1

Types of Pain

Type of Pain	Definition	Drug Treatment
Acute	Pain occurs suddenly and responds to treatment. It can result from trauma, tissue injury, inflammation, or surgery	Mild pain: Nonnarcotic (acetaminophen, NSAIDs [aspirin, Motrin, Advil]) Moderate pain: Combination of nonnarcotic and narcotic (codeine and acetaminophen) Severe pain: Narcotic
Cancer	Pain from pressure on nerves and organs, blockage to blood supply, or metastasis to bone	NSAIDs and narcotic drugs administered PO, transdermal, IM, IV, or PCA
Chronic	Pain persists for greater than 6 mo and is difficult to treat or control	Nonnarcotic drugs are suggested. Narcotics if used should meet these criteria: • Be by oral route or transdermal • Have a long duration of action • Include adjunct therapy • Cause minimal respiratory depression
Somatic	Pain of the skeletal muscle, ligaments, and joints	Nonnarcotics: NSAIDs (aspirin, Motrin, Advil). Also act as an antiinflammatory drug and muscle relaxant
Superficial	Pain from surface areas such as the skin and mucous membrane	Mild pain: Nonnarcotic Moderate pain: Combination of narcotic and nonnarcotic analgesic drug
Vascular	Pain from vascular or perivascular tissues contributing to headaches or migraines	Nonnarcotic drugs
Visceral	Pain from smooth muscles and organs	Narcotic drugs

IM, Intramuscular; *IV*, intravenous; *NSAIDs*, nonsteroidal antiinflammatory drugs; *PCA*, patient-controlled analgesia; *PO*, by mouth.

(clotting). Some health care providers may therefore prescribe one 81-mg, 162-mg, or 325-mg aspirin tablet every day or one 325-mg tablet every other day as a preventive measure against transient ischemic attacks (TIAs, or "small strokes"), heart attacks, or any thromboembolic episode.

Aspirin is also classified as an antiinflammatory drug and is discussed in depth in Chapter 27, Antiinflammatory Agents, along with the NSAIDs.

Aspirin and other NSAIDs relieve pain by inhibiting the enzyme *cyclooxygenase,* which is needed for the biosynthesis of prostaglandins. There are two enzyme forms of cyclooxygenase, symbolized as COX-1 and COX-2. COX-1 protects the stomach lining and regulates blood platelets, thus promoting blood clotting. COX-2 triggers pain and inflammation at the injured site. Two groups of analgesics, salicylates (aspirin) and NSAIDs, inhibit or block both COX-1 and COX-2. By inhibition of COX-1, protection to the stomach lining is markedly decreased, fever and pain are reduced, and blood clotting is decreased. Stomach bleeding and ulcers may occur when COX-1 is blocked; thus aspirin and NSAID agents can cause gastric discomfort and bleeding. When COX-2 is inhibited, pain is reduced and inflammation is suppressed.

Pharmaceutical companies have developed new analgesics especially for arthritic clients that would block only COX-2 for decreasing pain and inflammation and would not block COX-1 (Figure 21–1). Therefore the stomach lining would still be intact (i.e., no gastric bleeding and ulcers), and the pain and inflammation would be decreased.

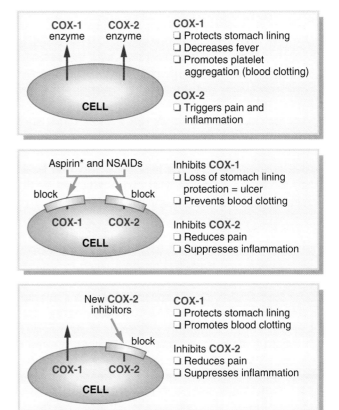

*Aspirin is only one of the NSAIDs.

FIGURE 21–1 Uses of COX-1 and COX-2 inhibitors.

PREVENTING MEDICATION ERRORS

Do not confuse...

- **Celebrex** with **Celexa** or **Celebyx**. These drug names look alike, but the drugs are different.

A COX-2 inhibitor that is approved by the Food and Drug Administration (FDA) is celecoxib (Celebrex, manufactured by Monsanto). Similar types of COX-2 inhibitor are meloxicam (Mobic) and nabumetone (Relafen, manufactured by SmithKline Beecham). Clients at risk for stroke or heart attack who take aspirin to prevent blood clotting by decreasing platelet aggregation would not benefit from COX-2 inhibitors. If COX-1 enzyme were not blocked, increased blood clotting would remain even though the stomach lining is protected.

Many researchers believe that COX-2 inhibitors may prevent some types of cancer (e.g., colon cancer). Fruits and vegetables block COX-2 enzyme naturally, protecting the colon from malignant growths.

Side Effects and Adverse Reactions

A common side effect of aspirin and NSAIDs is gastric irritation. These drugs should be taken with food, at mealtime, or with a full glass of fluid to help reduce this problem.

If aspirin or an NSAID is taken for dysmenorrhea during the first two days of menstruation, excess bleeding might occur (more so with aspirin than with ibuprofen).

Some clients are hypersensitive to aspirin. Tinnitus, vertigo, bronchospasm, and urticaria are some of the symptoms that indicate hypersensitivity or overdose of the salicylate product. Certain foods contain salicylates, such as prunes, raisins, paprika, and licorice. Those who have a hypersensitivity to aspirin and salicylate products may be sensitive to other NSAIDs. This hypersensitivity may be related to inhibition of the enzyme cyclo-oxygenase by the salicylate product.

Acetaminophen

The analgesic acetaminophen (paraaminophenol derivative) is a popular nonprescription drug taken by infants, children, adults, and older adults to relieve pain, discomfort, and fever (Figure 21–2). Acetaminophen is a nonnarcotic drug, but it is not an NSAID. Acetaminophen does not have the antiinflammatory properties of aspirin, so it is not the drug of choice for any inflammatory process. It constitutes 25% of all OTC drugs sold. Examples of OTC products that contain acetaminophen include Actifed: Cold & Allergy, Sinus; Anacin; Excedrin; Goody's Powders; Midol: Maximum Strength Menstrual Formula; Percogesic; and Vicks: Cold & Flu Relief. Examples of prescription products on the market that contain acetaminophen include Darvocet-N 100, Lortab, Percocet, and Vicodin.

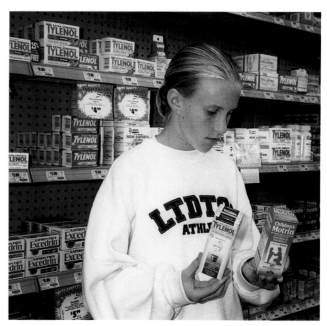

FIGURE 21–2   This 12-year-old girl injured her foot playing soccer. Which of these analgesics—acetaminophen (Tylenol) or ibuprofen (Motrin)—should she choose to relieve her pain and inflammation?

Acetaminophen (Tylenol, Panadol, Tempra), first marketed in the mid-1950s, is a safe, effective analgesic and antipyretic drug used for muscular aches and pains and for fever caused by viral infections. It causes little to no gastric distress and does not interfere with platelet aggregation. There is no link between acetaminophen and Reye syndrome, and it does not increase the potential for excessive bleeding if taken for dysmenorrhea, as do aspirin and NSAIDs. See Prototype Drug Chart 21–1.

Pharmacokinetics

Acetaminophen is well absorbed from the gastrointestinal (GI) tract. Rectal absorption may be erratic because of the presence of fecal material or a decrease in blood flow to the colon. Because of acetaminophen's short half-life, it can be administered every 4 hours as needed with a maximum dose of 4 g/day. However, it is suggested that a client who frequently takes acetaminophen limit the dose to 2000 mg/day (2 g/d) to avoid the possibility of hepatic or renal dysfunction. More than 85% of acetaminophen is metabolized to drug metabolites by the liver.

Large doses or overdoses can be toxic to the hepatic cells; therefore when large doses are administered over a long period, the level of acetaminophen in serum should be monitored. The therapeutic serum range is 5 to 20 mcg/ml. Liver enzyme levels (aspartate aminotransferase [AST], alanine aminotransferase [ALT], alkaline phosphatase [ALP]), and serum bilirubin should be monitored.

Pharmacodynamics

Acetaminophen weakly inhibits the prostaglandin synthesis, which decreases pain sensation. It is effective in eliminating mild to moderate pain and headaches and is useful for its antipyretic effect. It does not possess antiinflammatory action. Its onset of action is rapid, and the duration of action is 5 hours or less. Severe adverse reactions may occur with an overdose, so acetaminophen in liquid or chewable form should be kept out of a child's reach.

PROTOTYPE DRUG CHART 21–1

ACETAMINOPHEN

Drug Class	**Dosage**
Analgesic Trade Names: Tylenol, Tempra, Panadol, 🍁 Robigesic, Atasol *Pregnancy Category:* B	**A: PO:** 325-650 mg q4-6h PRN; *max:* 4000 mg/d; rectal supp: 650 mg q.i.d. **C: 0-3 mo: PO:** 40 mg 4-5×/d **4 mo-1 y: PO:** 80 mg 4-5×/d **1-2 y: PO:** 120 mg 4-5×/d **2-3 y: PO:** 160 mg 4-5×/d **4-5 y: PO:** 240 mg 4-5×/d **6-8 y: PO:** 320 mg 4-5×/d **9-10 y: PO:** 400 mg 4-5×/d **>11 y: PO:** 480 mg 4-5×/d **C: 2-5 y: Rectal:** 120 mg 4-5×/d **6-12 y: Rectal:** 325 mg 4-5×/d

Contraindications	**Drug-Lab-Food Interactions**
Severe hepatic or renal disease, alcoholism; hypersensitivity	*Increase* effect with caffeine, diflunisal *Decrease* effect with oral contraceptives, anticholinergics, cholestyramine, charcoal

Pharmacokinetics	**Pharmacodynamics**

Absorption: PO: rapidly absorbed; rectal: erratic
Distribution: PB: 20%-50%; crosses the placenta, in breast milk
Metabolism: t½: 1-3.5 h
Excretion: In urine as metabolites
	PO: Onset: 10-30 min
	  Peak: 1-2 h
	  Duration: 3-5 h
	Rectal: Onset: UK
	  Peak: UK
	  Duration: 4-6 h

Therapeutic Effects/Uses

To decrease pain and fever
Mode of Action: Inhibition (weakly) or prostaglandin synthesis, inhibition of hypothalamic heat-regulator center

Side Effects	**Adverse Reactions**
Anorexia, nausea, vomiting, rash	Severe hypoglycemia, oliguria, urticaria **Life-threatening:** Hemorrhage, hepatotoxicity, hemolytic anemia, leukopenia, thrombocytopenia

A, Adult; *C,* child; *d,* day; *h,* hour; *min,* minute; *PB,* protein-binding; *PO,* by mouth; *q.i.d.,* four times a day; *t½,* half-life; *UK,* unknown; *y,* year; *>,* greater than; 🍁, Canadian drug names.

Side Effects and Adverse Reactions

An overdose of acetaminophen can be extremely toxic to the liver cells, causing hepatotoxicity. Death could occur in 1 to 4 days from hepatic necrosis. If a child or adult ingests excessive amounts of acetaminophen tablets or liquid, a poison control center should be contacted *immediately* and the child or adult should be taken to the emergency department. Early symptoms of hepatic damage include nausea, vomiting, diarrhea, and abdominal pain.

Table 21–2 lists the commonly used nonnarcotic analgesics, their dosage, uses, and considerations.

Nursing Process

Analgesic: Acetaminophen

ASSESSMENT

■ Obtain a medical history of liver dysfunction. Overdosing or extremely high doses of acetaminophen can cause hepatotoxicity.

■ Ascertain the severity of the pain. Nonnarcotic NSAIDs such as ibuprofen or a narcotic may be necessary to relieve pain.

NURSING DIAGNOSES

■ Risk for injury
■ Pain

PLANNING

■ Client's pain will be relieved or controlled.

NURSING INTERVENTIONS

■ Check liver enzyme tests such as alanine aminotransferase, alkaline phosphatase, gamma-glutamyl transferase, 5′ nucleotidase, and bilirubin for elevations in clients taking high doses or overdoses of acetaminophen.

Client Teaching

General

• Instruct client to keep acetaminophen out of children's reach. Acetaminophen for children is available in flavored tablets and liquid. High doses can cause hepatotoxicity. Self-medication of acetaminophen should not be longer than 10 days for adults and 5 days for children without the health care provider's approval.
• Direct the parent to call the poison control center immediately if a child has taken a large or unknown amount of acetaminophen.
• Check acetaminophen dosage on package level. Do *not* exceed the recommended dosage. It is suggested that

---

Table 21–2

Analgesics

Generic (Brand)	Route and Dosage	Uses and Considerations
Salicylates		
aspirin (Bayer, Ecotrin, Astrin)	*Analgesic:* A: PO: 325-650 mg, q4h, *max:* 4 g/d C: PO: 40-65 mg/kg/d in 4-6 divided doses; *max:* 3.6 g/d	Effective in relieving headaches, muscle pain, inflammation and pain from arthritis, and as mild anticoagulant. Serum therapeutic range: *headache:* 5 mg/dl; *inflammation:* 15-30 mg/dl. Can displace other highly protein-bound drugs. If taken with acetaminophen, GI bleeding could result. Side effects: gastric discomfort, tinnitus, vertigo, deafness (reversible), increased bleeding. Should be taken with foods or at mealtime. It should *not* be taken with alcohol. *Pregnancy category:* D; PB: 55%-90%; $t^1/_2$: 2-20 h (high doses)
diflunisal (Dolobid)	A: PO: Initially 1000 mg; *maint:* 500 mg q8-12h	Used for mild to moderate pain. Considered to be less toxic than aspirin. *Pregnancy category:* C; PB: 99%, $t^1/_2$: 8-12 h
COX-2 Inhibitors		
celecoxib (Celebrex)	A: PO: 200 mg/d or 100 mg, b.i.d. Elderly: Same as adult dose	Treatment of osteoarthritis and rheumatoid arthritis. Not indicated for clients <18 y old. Use caution for clients with severe renal or liver disorders and for those allergic to sulfonamides. *Pregnancy category:* C; PB: UK; $t^1/_2$: 11.2 h
meloxicam (Mobic)	A: PO: Initially 7.5 mg/d; *max:* 15 mg/d	Treatment of pain from osteoarthritis. *Pregnancy category:* C (first and second trimester), D (third trimester); PB: 99%; $t^1/_2$: 15-20 h
nabumetone (Relafen)	A: PO: 1000 mg/d; *max:* 2000 mg/d	Treatment of pain from osteoarthritis, rheumatoid arthritis. *Pregnancy category:* C; PB: 99%; $t^1/_2$: 24 h
Paraaminophenol		
acetaminophen (Tylenol, Panadol, Tempra)	See Prototype Drug Chart 21–1.	
NSAIDs: Propionic Acid		
ibuprofen (Motrin, Advil, Nuprin, Medipren)	*Pain:* A: PO 200-800 mg q4-6h; *max:* 3200 mg/d	For mild to moderate muscle aches and pains. Causes some gastric distress but less than aspirin. Should be taken with food, at mealtime, or with plenty of fluids. *Pregnancy category:* B; PB: 98%; $t^1/_2$: 2-4 h

A, Adult; *b.i.d.,* twice a day; *C,* child; *d,* day; *GI,* gastrointestinal; *h,* hour; *IM,* intramuscular; *IV,* intravenous; *maint,* maintenance; *max,* maximum; *min,* minute; *NSAIDs,* nonsteroidal antiinflammatory drugs; *PB,* protein-binding; *PO,* by mouth; *PRN,* as needed; *$t^1/_2$,* half-life; *UK,* unknown; *y,* year; >, greater than; <, less than.

the safe acetaminophen dose is 2000 mg/d (2 g/day), not to exceed 4 g/day to avoid liver damage.

Side Effects

- Teach client to report side effects. Overdosing can cause severe liver damage and death.
- Inform the parent that liver damage may occur with continuous use of acetaminophen.
- Check the serum acetaminophen level when toxicity is suspected. The normal serum level is 5 to 20 mcg/ml; the toxic level is >50 mcg/ml. Levels of >200 mcg/ml could indicate hepatotoxicity. The antidote for acetaminophen is acetylcysteine (Mucomyst). The dosage is based on the serum acetaminophen level.

Cultural Considerations ⊕

- The extended family structure is important for teaching health strategies and providing support. Recognize the importance of including women in decision making and disseminating health information.

EVALUATION

- Evaluate the effectiveness of acetaminophen in relieving pain. If pain persists, another analgesic may be needed.
- Determine whether client is taking the dose as recommended. Observe and report any side effects.

Narcotic Analgesics

Narcotic analgesics, called **narcotic agonists**, are prescribed for moderate and severe pain. In the United States the Harrison Narcotic Act of 1914 required that all forms of opium be sold with a prescription and that it no longer be used as a nonprescription drug. The Controlled Substances Act of 1970 classified addicting drugs, such as narcotics, in five schedule categories according to their potential for drug abuse (see Chapter 8, Drugs of Abuse).

Opium was used as early as 350 BC to relieve pain. In 1803 a German pharmacist isolated morphine from opium. Morphine, a prototype opioid, is obtained from

Table 21–2

Analgesics—cont'd

Generic (Brand)	Route and Dosage	Uses and Considerations
NSAIDs: Propionic Acid—cont'd		
naproxen (Naprosyn, Naprelan, EC-Naprosyn, Aleve, Anaprox, Anaprox-DS)	*Mild to moderate pain:* A: PO: initially 500 mg, then 200-250 mg q6-8h; *max:* 1250 mg/d C: PO: >2 y: 5-7 mg/kg q8-12h *Inflammatory disease:* A: PO: 250-500 mg b.i.d.; *max:* 1000 mg/d; C: PO: >2 y: 10-15 mg/kg q8-12h; *max:* 1000 mg/d	Treatment of inflammation and pain from osteoarthritis, rheumatoid arthritis, ankylosing spondylitis, gout, and dysmenorrhea. *Pregnancy category:* B; PB: UK; $t^1/_2$: 12-15 h
Ketorolac (Toradol, Acular)	A: PO: 10 mg q6h PRN; *max:* 40 mg/d IM: Initially 30-60 mg, then 15-30 mg q6h; *max:* 150 mg first d, 120 mg thereafter; IV: Initially 30 mg Elderly: PO: 5-10 mg q6h PRN; max 40 mg/d IM: Initially 30 mg, then 15 mg q6h IV: Initially 15 mg	Short-term treatment of pain *Pregnancy category:* B; PB: UK; $t^1/_2$: 4-6 h
Miscellaneous		
methotrimeprazine HCl (Levoprome)	*Sedative-analgesic:* A & C: >12 y: PO: 6-25 mg/d in divided doses with meals IM: 10-12 mg q4-6h PRN (deep IM) Elderly: IM: 5-10 mg q4-6h	Treatment of moderate to severe pain. May be used before and after surgery for pain and sedation. Has properties of phenothiazines, analgesia, and sedative-hypnotics. *Pregnancy category:* C; PB: UK; $t^1/_2$: 20 hr
tramadol (Ultram)	*Postanalgesia:* A & C: >12 y: IM: 2.5-7.5 mg q4-6h PRN A: PO: 50-100 mg q4-6 h, PRN; *max:* 400 mg/d Elderly: >75 y: *max:* 300 mg/d *Hepatic dysfunction:* 50 mg q12h *Renal disorder:* CL$_{cr}$ (CrCl) <30 ml/min: 50-100 mg q12h	Used for moderate to severe pain. Contraindicated in severe alcoholism or with use of narcotics. Nausea, vomiting, dizziness, constipation, headache, and anxiety may occur. *Pregnancy category:* C; PB: UK; $t^1/_2$: UK

the sap of seed pods of the opium poppy plant. Codeine is another drug obtained from opium. In the past 40 years, many synthetic and semisynthetic narcotics have been developed, with approximately 20 narcotics marketed for clinical use.

Narcotic analgesics (narcotics) act mostly on the central nervous system (CNS), whereas nonnarcotic analgesics (analgesics) act on the peripheral nervous system at the pain receptor sites. Narcotics not only suppress pain impulses but also suppress respiration and coughing by acting on the respiratory and cough centers in the medulla of the brainstem. One example of such a narcotic is morphine, a potent analgesic that can readily depress respirations. Codeine is not as potent as morphine ($\frac{1}{15}$ to $\frac{1}{20}$ as potent), but it also relieves mild to moderate pain and suppresses cough, which allows it also to be classified as an antitussive. Most opioids, with the exception of meperidine (Demerol), have an antitussive (cough suppression) effect. The opioids have two isomers (levo and dextro). The levo-isomers of opioids produce an analgesic effect only; however, both levo- and dextro-isomers possess an antitussive response. The dextro-isomers do not cause physical dependence, whereas the levo-isomers of opioids do. Synthetic cough suppressants are discussed in Chapter 38, Drugs for Common Upper Respiratory Disorders.

In addition to pain relief and antitussive effects, many narcotics possess antidiarrheal effects. Common side effects of most opioids include nausea and vomiting (particularly in ambulatory clients), constipation, a moderate decrease of blood pressure, and orthostatic hypotension with high doses. Opioids may also cause respiratory depression with high doses, urinary retention (usually in older adults), and antitussive effects (with the exception of meperidine).

Opioid Use in Children and Older Adults

Children

Pain management in children is complex because it is more difficult to determine their pain. Some children will not verbalize their discomfort when they are in severe pain and are fearful of treatments that relieve pain. Nurses should use their communication skills to determine the child's need for pain relief. The "ouch scale" illustrated in Figure 21-3 can be used to determine the pain level in many children. Also, the parent may help identify the presence and degree of the child's pain. Crying and whining may be indicators of the child's need for pain relief, or it may indicate other needs.

A child, like an adult, should be given medication before the pain becomes severe. The use of oral liquid medication for pain relief, if appropriate, is generally more acceptable to the child. The nurse, using drawings and pictures related to areas of pain in the body and pain relief with smiling faces, may alleviate the child's fear and help with drug compliance.

Older Adults

Usually, older adults who are 65 years of age or older require adjustment to drug doses to avoid severe side effects. Merely decreasing the doses of narcotic analgesic is not always the answer for older adults. Many older adults take many medications for health problems, thus increasing the possibility of drug interactions and drug side effects. In older adults, side effects from the use of narcotics become more pronounced. The nurse needs to closely monitor adverse reactions in older adults who take narcotic analgesics. As a person ages, the liver and renal functions decrease, causing the metabolism and excretion of the drug to decrease. As a result, drug accumulation can occur.

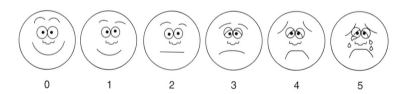

| 0 | 1 | 2 | 3 | 4 | 5 |

1. Explain to the child that each face is for a person who feels happy because he has no pain (hurt, or whatever word the child uses) or feels sad because he has some or a lot of pain.

2. Point to the appropriate face and state, "This face is . . ."
   0-"very happy because he doesn't hurt at all."
   1-"hurts just a little bit."
   2-"hurts a little more."
   3-"hurts even more."
   4-"hurts a whole lot."
   5-"hurts as much as you can imagine, although you don't have to be crying to feel this bad."

3. Ask the child to choose the face that best describes how he feels. Be specific about which pain (e.g., "shot" or incision) and what time (e.g., now? earlier? before lunch?).

FIGURE 21–3   A scale used to rate the intensity of pain in children. (From Hockenberry M: *Wong's essentials of pediatric nursing*, ed 7, St Louis, 2005, Mosby.)

Drugs that tend to be more toxic in older adults include meperidine (Demerol), pentazocine (Talwin), and propoxyphene (Darvon). Chronological age is one of several factors that influence medication use and dosage. Comorbidity must also be considered.

Morphine

Morphine, an extraction from opium, is a potent narcotic analgesic (Prototype Drug Chart 21–2). Morphine is effective against acute pain resulting from acute myocardial infarction (AMI), cancer, and dyspnea resulting from pulmonary edema. It may be used as a preoperative medication. Although it is effective in relieving severe pain,

it can cause respiratory depression, orthostatic hypotension, miosis, urinary retention, constipation resulting from reduced bowel motility, and cough suppression. An antidote for morphine excess or overdose is the narcotic antagonist naxolone (Narcan).

Pharmacokinetics

Morphine may be taken orally, although GI absorption can be somewhat erratic. For severe pain, such as with AMI, it is given intravenously (IV). Morphine is 30% protein bound. Oral morphine undergoes first hepatic pass; thus the liver metabolizes the oral drug before use. Only a small amount of morphine crosses the blood-brain barrier to produce an analgesic effect. It has a short half-life, and 90% is excreted in the urine. Morphine crosses the placenta and is present in a mother's breast milk.

PROTOTYPE DRUG CHART 21–2

MORPHINE SULFATE

Drug Class

Narcotic
Trade Names: Duramorph, MS Contin, Roxanol SR, Epimorph, Statex
CSS II
Pregnancy Category: B

Dosage

A: PO: 10-30 mg q4h PRN
SR: 15-30 mg, q8-12h PRN
IM/subQ: 5-15 mg PRN
IV: 4-10 mg q4h PRN: diluted; inject over 5 min
Epidural: 2-10 mg over 24h
C: IM/subQ: 0.1-0.2 mg/kg PRN; *max:* <15 mg/dose
Neonate: subQ/IM/IV: 0.05 mg/kg q4-8h; *max:* 0.1 mg/kg

Contraindications

Asthma with respiratory depression, increased intracranial pressure, shock
Caution: Respiratory, renal, or hepatic diseases; myocardial infarction; older adults; very young

Drug-Lab-Food Interactions

Drug: Increase effects of alcohol, sedatives-hypnotics, antipsychotic drugs, muscle relaxants
Lab: Increase AST, ALT

Pharmacokinetics

Absorption: PO: varies; IV: rapid
Distribution: PB: UK; crosses placenta, in breast milk
Metabolism: t½: 2.5-3 h
Excretion: 90% in urine

Pharmacodynamics

PO: Onset: variable
  Peak: 1-2 h
  Duration: 4-5 h; SR: 8-12 h
subQ/IM: Onset: 15-30 min
  Peak: SC: 50-90 min
  IM: 0.5-1 h
  Duration: 3-5 h
IV: Onset: rapid
  Peak: 20 min
  Duration: 3-5 h

Therapeutic Effects/Uses

To relieve severe pain
Mode of Action: Depression of the CNS; depression of pain impulses by binding with the opiate receptor in the CNS

Side Effects

Anorexia, nausea, vomiting, constipation, drowsiness, dizziness, sedation, confusion, urinary retention, rash, blurred vision, bradycardia, flushing, euphoria, pruritus

Adverse Reactions

Hypotension, urticaria, seizures
Life-threatening: Respiratory depression, increased intracranial pressure

---

A, Adult; *ALT,* alanine aminotransferase; *AST,* aspartate aminotransferase; *C,* child; *CNS,* central nervous system; *CSS,* Controlled Substances Schedule; *h,* hour; *IM,* intramuscular; *IV,* intravenous; *min,* minute; *PB,* protein binding; *PO,* by mouth; *PRN,* as necessary; *subQ,* subcutaneous; *SR,* sustained-release; *t½,* half-life; *UK,* unknown; <, less than; , Canadian drug names.

Pharmacodynamics

Morphine binds with the opiate receptor in the CNS. Parenterally, the onset of action is rapid, especially IV. Onset of action is slower for subcutaneous (subQ) and intramuscular (IM) injections. Duration of action with all types of drug administration is 3 to 5 hours except with sustained-release products such as MS Contin, which has a duration of action of 8 to 12 hours.

Patient-controlled analgesia (PCA) is an alternative route for morphine administration for pain relief. Within predetermined limits, the client controls the release of narcotic analgesic, depending on the amount of pain. To receive the narcotic, the client pushes a button on the PCA device, which releases a specific dose of analgesic into the IV line. The health care provider titrates the narcotic analgesic dose by regulating the time intervals (every several minutes) at which the drug can be received. A lockout mechanism on the PCA machine prevents the client from constantly pushing the button and causing a drug overdose. Meperidine (Demerol) and hydromorphone (Dilaudid) may also be given via PCA.

Nursing Process

Narcotic Analgesic I: Morphine Sulfate

ASSESSMENT

■ Obtain a medical history. Contraindications for morphine include severe respiratory disorders, increased intracranial pressure, and severe renal disease. Morphine may cause seizures.

■ Determine a drug history. Report if a drug-drug interaction is probable. Morphine increases the effects of alcohol, sedatives or hypnotics, antipsychotic drugs, and muscle relaxants and might cause respiratory depression.

■ Assess vital signs and urinary output. Note the depth and rate of respirations. Morphine can cause urinary retention.

NURSING DIAGNOSES

■ Pain related to surgery, tissue injury
■ Ineffective breathing patterns related to excess morphine dosage

PLANNING

■ Client will be free of pain, or the intensity of pain will be lessened.

NURSING INTERVENTIONS

■ Administer the narcotic before pain reaches its peak to maximize the effectiveness of the drug.

■ Monitor vital signs at frequent intervals to detect respiratory changes. Respirations of <10/min can indicate respiratory distress.

■ Record client's urine output; urine output should be at least 600 ml/day.

■ Check bowel sounds for decreased peristalsis, a cause of constipation caused by morphine. Dietary change or mild laxative might be needed.

■ Check for pupil changes and reaction. Pinpoint pupils can indicate morphine overdose.

■ Have naloxone (Narcan) available as an antidote if morphine overdose occurs.

■ Validate child's dose of morphine before its administration. The recommended dose is 0.1 to 0.2 mg/kg/q4h, intramuscularly or subcutaneously; maximum dose is 15 mg/dose.

Client Teaching

General

• Encourage client not to use alcohol or CNS depressants with any narcotic analgesics such as morphine. Respiratory depression can result.

• Suggest nonpharmacologic measures to relieve pain as client recuperates from surgery. If necessary, a non-narcotic analgesic may be prescribed.

Side Effects

• Alert client that with continuous use, narcotics such as morphine can become addicting. If addiction occurs, inform client about methadone treatment programs and other resources in the area.

• Instruct client to report dizziness or difficulty in breathing while taking morphine. Dizziness could be because of orthostatic hypotension. Advise the client to ambulate with caution or only with assistance.

Cultural Considerations ⊕

• When offering a prescription, instructions, or pamphlets to Asian and Pacific Islanders, use both hands, which shows respect.

EVALUATION

■ Evaluate the effectiveness of morphine in lessening or alleviating the pain.

■ Determine the stability of vital signs. Report any decrease in blood pressure and respiration.

HERBAL ALERT 21–1

Morphine and Herbs

🍃 Morphine taken with kava kava, valerian, and St. John's wort may increase sedation.

Meperidine

One of the first synthetic narcotics, meperidine (Demerol), became available in the mid-1950s. It is classified as a schedule II drug according to the Controlled Substances Act. Meperidine has a shorter duration of action than morphine, and its potency varies according to the dosage. Meperidine, which can be given orally, IM, and IV, is primarily effective in GI procedures. It does not have the antitussive property of opium preparations.

During pregnancy, meperidine is preferred to morphine because it does not diminish uterine contractions and causes less neonatal respiratory depression. Meperidine causes less constipation and urinary retention than morphine. Meperidine is not indicated for clients with chronic pain, severe liver dysfunction, sickle cell disease, a history of seizures, severe coronary artery disease (CAD), and cardiac dysrhythmias. When older adults and clients with advanced cancer receive large doses of meperidine, neurotoxicity (e.g., nervousness, tremors, agitation, irritability, seizures) have been reported. Meperidine should not be prescribed for long-term use; the dose is frequently limited to 600 mg in a 24-hour period for no longer than 48 to 72 hours.

Meperidine is metabolized in the liver to an active metabolite; therefore the dose should be decreased for clients with hepatic or renal insufficiency. It is excreted in the urine in a metabolite form called *normeperidine*. Meperidine should not be taken with alcohol or sedative-hypnotics because the combination of these drugs causes an additive CNS depression. A major side effect of meperidine is a decrease in blood pressure, which should be monitored, especially if the client is an older adult.

Table 21–3 lists narcotics and their dosages, uses, and considerations.

Hydromorphone

Hydromorphone (Dilaudid) is a semisynthetic narcotic similar to morphine. The analgesic effect is approximately six times more potent than morphine with fewer hypnotic effects and less GI distress. This narcotic has a faster onset and shorter duration of action than morphine. Hydromorphone is classified as a schedule II drug according to the Controlled Substances Act. Tolerance to hydromorphone increases gradually.

This drug is given orally, rectally, subQ, IM, and IV, and it may be administered by PCA for the relief of moderate to severe pain. When given IV, dilution of each dose with 5 ml of sterile water or normal saline is preferred. Direct IV administration of 2 mg or less should be given over 2 to 5 minutes. Hydromorphone is readily absorbed in the body and excreted in the urine. Respirations should be monitored closely and adequate hydration should be provided.

Drug data related to hydromorphone are covered in Prototype Drug Chart 21–3.

PREVENTING MEDICATION ERRORS

Do not confuse...

- **meperidine** with **morphine, meprobamate,** or **hydromorphone.**

- **Demerol** with **Desyrel, Dilaudid,** or **Temaril.** These drug names look alike, but the drugs are different.

Side Effects and Adverse Reactions

Many side effects are known to accompany the use of narcotics. Of particular importance are signs of respiratory depression (respiration <10/min). Other side effects include **orthostatic hypotension** (decrease in blood pressure when rising from sitting or lying position), tachycardia, drowsiness and mental clouding, constipation, and urinary retention. In addition, pupillary constriction (a sign of toxicity), tolerance, and psychological and physical dependence may occur with prolonged use.

Increased metabolism of narcotics contributes to tolerance, which causes an increased need for higher doses of the narcotic. If chronic use of the narcotic is discontinued, withdrawal symptoms (called **abstinence syndrome**) usually occur within 24 to 48 hours after the last narcotic dose. Abstinence syndrome is caused by physical dependence. Irritability, diaphoresis (sweating), restlessness, muscle twitching, and an increase in pulse rate and blood pressure are examples of withdrawal symptoms. Withdrawal symptoms from narcotics are unpleasant but are not so severe or life-threatening as those that accompany withdrawal from sedative-hypnotics—a process that may lead to convulsions.

Contraindications

Use of narcotic analgesics is contraindicated for clients with head injuries. Narcotics decrease respiration, thus causing an accumulation of carbon dioxide (CO_2). With an increase in carbon dioxide retention, blood vessels dilate (vasodilation), especially cerebral vessels, which causes increased intracranial pressure.

Narcotic analgesics given to a client with a respiratory disorder only intensify the respiratory distress. In the client with asthma, opiates decrease respiratory drive while simultaneously increasing airway resistance.

Narcotics may cause hypotension and are not indicated for clients in shock or for those who have very low blood pressure. If a narcotic is necessary, the dosage needs to be adjusted accordingly; otherwise, the hypotensive state may worsen. For an older adult or a person who is debilitated, the narcotic dose usually needs to be decreased.

Table 21–3

Narcotics: Opium and Synthetics

Generic (Brand)	Route and Dosage	Uses and Considerations
codeine (sulfate, phosphate) CSS II	A: PO/subQ/IM: 15-60 mg q4-6h PRN C: PO/subQ/IM: 0.5-1 mg/kg q4-6h	Effective for mild to moderate pain. Can be used with a nonnarcotic (acetaminophen) for pain relief. Has antitussive properties. Can decrease respiration and cause physical dependence and constipation. *Pregnancy category:* C; PB: 70%, $t^1/_2$: 2.5 h
hydrocodone bitartrate (Hycodan, Vicodin with acetaminophen) CSS II	*Analgesic:* A: C > 12 y: PO: 5-10 mg q4-6h C: 2-12 y: PO: 1.25-5 mg q4-6h Elderly: PO: 2.5-5 mg q4-6h *Extended-release:* A: PO: 10 mg q12h C: 6-12 y: PO: 5 mg q12h	Treatment of moderate to moderately-severe pain. Combination with acetaminophen (Lortab, Vicodin), aspirin (Lortab ASA), ibuprofen (Vicoprofin), and chlorpheniramine (Tussionex). Can be prescribed for analgesic and antitussive purposes. *Pregnancy category:* C; PB: UK; t: 4 h (longer $t^1/_2$: in older adults)
hydromorphone HCl (Dilaudid) CSS II	See Prototype Drug Chart 21–3.	
levorphanol tartrate (Levo-Dromoran) CSS II	A: PO/subQ: Initially: 2 mg PO/subQ: 2-3 mg q6-8h PRN	For moderate to severe pain. Has side effects similar to morphine. *Pregnancy category:* B; PB: 50%-60%; $^1/_2$: 1.2 h
meperidine (Demerol) CSS II	A: PO/subQ/IM/IV: 50-150 mg q3-4h PRN C: PO/subQ/IM/IV: 1-1.5 mg/kg q3-4h PRN; *max:* <100 mg q4h for children	For relief of moderate to severe pain, GI procedures, and preoperative sedation. *Pregnancy category:* B; PB: 60%-80%; $t^1/_2$: 3-8 h
morphine sulfate CSS II	See Prototype Drug Chart 21-2.	
oxycodone HCl (OxyContin) CSS II	A: PO: 5-10 mg q6h PRN C: >12 y: PO: 2.5 mg q6h PRN C: 6-12 y: PO: 1.25 mg q6h PRN	For relief of moderate to moderately severe pain including postoperative and postpartum pain. Avoid taking drug over an extended period of time. As potent as morphine. Take with food to avoid GI distress. *Pregnancy category:* B to D; PB: UK; $t^1/_2$: 2-3 h
oxycodone HCl with acetaminophen (Percocet) and oxycodone terephthalate with aspirin (Percodan) CSS II	A: PO: 5 mg q4-6h PRN or 5-10 mg q6h PRN C: 6-12 y: 1.25 mg q6h PRN C: 12-17 y: 2.5 mg q6h PRN	For moderate to severe pain. Percocet contains acetaminophen. Percodan contains aspirin and can cause gastric irritation, so it should be taken with food or plenty of liquids. *Pregnancy category:* B; PB: UK; $t^1/_2$: 2-3 h
propoxyphene HCl (Darvon) CSS IV propoxyphene napsylate (Darvon-N) CSS IV	A: PO: HCl: 65 mg q4h PRN; *max:* 390 mg/d A: PO: napsylate: 100 mg q4h PRN; *max:* 600 mg/d	For mild pain. Weak analgesic. Darvon-compound contains aspirin, and Darvocet-N contains acetaminophen. Is not a constipating drug; has little effect on physical dependence. *Pregnancy category:* C; PB: >90%; $t^1/_2$: 12 h
alfentanil (Alfenta) CSS II	A: IV: 8-40 mcg/kg for surgery Continuous infusion: 0.5-1 mcg/kg/min Total dose: 8-40 mcg/kg	An opioid analgesic with a rapid onset of action. It may be given to induce anesthesia or administered by continuous infusion with nitrous oxide and oxygen. *Pregnancy category:* C; PB: UK; $t^1/_2$: UK
fentanyl (Duragesic, Sublimaze) CSS II	A: IM: 50-100 mcg q1-2h PRN C: 2-12 y: IM: 1.7-3.3 mcg q1-2h PRN *Lozenge:* A: Suck on 400-mcg lozenge until sedated C: 35-40 kg: Suck on 400-mcg lozenge until sedated C: 25-35 kg: Suck on 400-mcg lozenge until sedated *Transdermal patch:* A: Initially 25 mcg/h patch q3d	Short-acting potent narcotic analgesic. It may be used with short-term surgery. Dose varies according to age. Also, drug is available as a transdermal patch for controlling chronic pain. *Pregnancy category:* C; PB: 80%-89%; $t^1/_2$: 3.6 h
sufentanil citrate (Sufenta) CSS II	*Primary anesthetic:* A: IV: 8-30 mcg/kg with 100% oxygen and muscle relaxant C: IV: 10-25 mcg/kg with 100% oxygen and muscle relaxant *Adjunct to anesthesia:* IV: 1-8 mcg/kg	It is a potent synthetic narcotic and is used as part of the balanced anesthesia group. Also may be used as a primary anesthetic. *Pregnancy category:* C; PB: 93%; $t^1/_2$: 1-3 h

A, Adult; *C,* child; *CSS,* Controlled Substances Schedule; *GI,* gastrointestinal; *h,* hour; *IM,* intramuscular; *IV,* intravenous; *max,* maximum; *min,* minute; *PB,* protein-binding; *PO,* by mouth; *PRN,* as necessary; *subQ,* subcutaneous; $t^1/_2$, half-life; *UK,* unknown; *y,* year.

Table 21-3

Narcotics: Opium and Synthetics—cont'd

Generic (Brand)	Route and Dosage	Uses and Considerations
remifentanil (Ultiva) CSS II	A: IV: Infusion rate: 0.05-2 mcg/min IV: Postop: 0.025-0.2 mcg/min	The newest opioid analgesic. Rapid onset of action; short-acting duration (5-10 min). Can cause respiratory depression, hypotension, and bradycardia. *Pregnancy category:* UK; PB: UK; $t^1/_2$: UK
methadone (Dolophine) CSS II	*Moderate to severe acute pain:* A: PO/subQ/IM: 2.5-10 mg q3-4h PRN C: PO/IV: 0.1 mg/kg q4h for 2-3 doses, then q6-12h PRN; *max:* 10 mg/dose *Detoxification:* A: PO/subQ/IM:15-40 mg/d; *max:* 120 mg/d Neonate: PO/IV: 0.05-0.2 mg/dk q12-24h; taper dose by 10%-20%/wk over 1-1$1/_2$ mo	Similar to morphine but has a longer duration of action. Used in drug abuse programs. Helps to alleviate craving for opioids. Peak action occurs in 30-60 min. *Pregnancy category:* C; PB: UK; $t^1/_2$: 15-25 h
For Narcotic Addiction levomethadyl acetate HCl (ORLAMM)	A: IM: Initially: 10-40 mg 3/wk: maint: 60-90 mg 3/wk; *max:* 140 mg (Mon, Wed, Fri regimen)	To manage narcotic addiction. *Pregnancy category:* UK; PB: UK; $t^1/_2$: UK

PROTOTYPE DRUG CHART 21-3

HYDROMORPHONE

Drug Class

Hydromorphone: Narcotic
Trade Name: Dilaudid
CSS II
Pregnancy Category: C

Dosage

A: PO/subQ/IM/IV: 1-4 mg q4-6h PRN
A: Rectal: 3 mg, q4-6h
C: PO: 0.03-0.08 mg/kg q4-6h; *max:* 5 mg/dose
C: IV: 0.015 mg/kg q4-6h

Contraindications

Opiate agonist intolerance
Caution: Pregnancy, children

Drug-Lab-Food Interactions

Drug: CNS depression is potentiated with alcohol or other CNS depressants
Lab: None known
Food: None known

Pharmacokinetics

Absorption: Readily absorbed
Distribution: PB: UK
Metabolism: $t^1/_2$: UK
Excretion: In urine

Pharmacodynamics

PO: Onset: 15-30 min
Peak: 30-90 min
Duration: 4-5 h

Therapeutic Effects/Uses

To relieve moderate to severe pain
Mode of Action: Semisynthetic derivative similar to morphine, depression of pain impulses by binding to the opiate receptor in the CNS

Side Effects

Drowsiness, dizziness, euphoria, sedation, blurred vision, nausea, vomiting, constipation, hypotension

Adverse Reactions

Bradycardia, tachycardia
Life-threatening: Respiratory depression

CNS, Central nervous system; *CSS,* Controlled Substances Schedule; *IM,* intramuscular; *IV,* intravenous; *max,* maximum; *min,* mininum; *PB,* protein-binding; *PO,* by mouth; *PRN,* as necessary; *subQ,* subcutaneous; *t¹/₂,* half-life; *UK,* unknown.

Nursing Process

Narcotic Analgesic II: Hydromorphone (Dilaudid)

ASSESSMENT

■ Obtain drug history from client of drugs he or she currently takes. Report if a drug-drug interaction is probable. CNS depressants enhance the action of hydromorphone; thus respiratory depression can occur.

■ Record baseline vital signs for future comparisons. Hydromorphone tends to decrease systolic blood pressure.

■ Assess type of pain, location, and duration before giving meperidine.

NURSING DIAGNOSIS

■ Pain related to surgery or injury

PLANNING

■ Client's pain will be decreased or alleviated. Drug dosing may need repeating.

NURSING INTERVENTIONS

■ Administer hydromorphone before the pain reaches its peak to maximize the effectiveness of the drug. The dose should be closely monitored to avoid neurotoxicity.

■ Monitor vital signs to compare blood pressure with baseline pressure. Hypotension is a side effect of hydromorphone. Note whether the client has any breathing dysfunction.

■ Have naloxone (Narcan) available, which can reverse respiratory depression resulting from narcotic overdose.

■ Determine urine output and bowel sounds. Urinary retention and constipation are side effects of hydromorphone.

■ Check older adults for side effects of hydromorphone. Confusion may occur, so use of side rails and other precautions should be taken. Dosage may need to be decreased.

Client Teaching

General

• Instruct client not to use alcohol or CNS depressants with hydromorphone because of increased depression of the CNS and of respirations.

• Inform client that drug dependence could occur with continual use of hydromorphone. If severe pain is still present, another narcotic analgesic or analgesic may be prescribed.

Side Effects

• Teach client to report side effects such as headaches, dizziness resulting from orthostatic hypotension, constipation, blurred vision, or decreased urine output. Report findings to the health care provider.

Cultural Considerations ⊕

• Respect cultural and religious beliefs concerning refusal of narcotic analgesics.

• Accept Asian and other cultural groups' use of alternative measures to relieve pain.

EVALUATION

■ Evaluate the effectiveness of the narcotic analgesic to lessen or alleviate the pain. If pain persists after several days, the cause should be determined or the narcotic should be changed.

■ Determine the stability of vital signs. Abnormal signs, such as decreased blood pressure, should be reported.

Combination Drugs

To treat moderate to severe pain, combination drugs of an analgesic and a narcotic analgesic may be used. Examples are hydrocodone and ibuprofen (Vicoprofin), which is a combination of an NSAID and an opioid. Another combination for the treatment of mild to moderate pain is acetaminophen and codeine. Using a combination of drugs for pain helps to decrease drug dependency that may result from possible long-time use of a narcotic agent.

Transdermal Opioid Analgesics

Transdermal opioid analgesics provide a continuous "around the clock" pain control that is helpful to clients who suffer from chronic pain. The transdermal method is not useful for acute or postoperative pain. An example of a transdermal opioid analgesic is fentanyl (Duragesic), which is administered via a transdermal patch. This patch comes in various strengths—25, 50, 75, and 100 mcg/hour. Maximum serum fentanyl levels occur within 24 hours when the patch is first applied. Fentanyl is also available for IM and IV use. Fentanyl is more potent than morphine. For older adults, the use of a lower fentanyl transdermal dose is usually suggested. Exercise caution when prescribing fentanyl for clients who weigh less than 110 pounds.

Narcotic Agonist-Antagonists

In the past 20 years, **mixed narcotic agonist-antagonists,** medications in which a narcotic antagonist (e.g., naloxone [Narcan]) is added to a narcotic agonist, were developed in hopes of decreasing narcotic abuse. Pentazocine (Talwin), the first mixed narcotic analgesic, can be given orally (tablet) and by injection (subQ, IM, and IV). Pentazocine

PROTOTYPE DRUG CHART 21–4

NALBUPHINE

Drug Class	Dosage
Nalbuphine HCl: Narcotic (agonist-antagonist) Trade Name: Nubain *Pregnancy Category:* B	A: IV/IM/subQ: 10-20 mg q3-6h; *max:* 160 mg/d C: IV/IM/subQ: 0.1-0.15 mg/kg q3-6h
Contraindications	**Drug-Lab-Food Interactions**
Hypersensitivity *Caution:* History of drug abuse or emotional instability, impaired respirations, head injury, increased intracranial pressure, MI, biliary tract surgery, renal or hepatic dysfunction	*Drug:* CNS depression is potentiated with alcohol or other CNS depressants
Pharmacokinetics	**Pharmacodynamics**
Absorption: Distribution: PB Metabolism: $t\frac{1}{2}$: 5 h Excretion: In urine	PO: Onset: 2-3 min IV; 15 minutes IM Peak: 30 min IV Duration: 3-6 h

Therapeutic Effects/Uses

To relieve moderate to severe pain
Mode of Action: Inhibition of pain impulses transmitted in the CNS by binding with the opiate receptor and increasing the pain threshold

Side Effects	Adverse Effects
Dizziness, confusion, hallucinations, blurred vision, headache, flushing, sedation, nervousness, restlessness, euphoria, depression, crying, dysphoria, unusual dreams, dry mouth, bitter taste, nausea, vomiting, abdominal cramps, clammy skin, urinary urgency	Bradycardia, tachycardia, hypotension, hypertension, dyspnea **Life-threatening:** Respiratory depression

CNS, Central nervous system; *d*, day; *h*, hour; *IM*, intramuscular; *IV*, intravenous; *max*, maximum; *MI*, myocardial infarction; *min*, minute; *PB*, protein-binding; *subQ*, subcutaneous; *t½*, half-life.

is classified as a schedule IV drug. Butorphanol tartrate (Stadol), buprenorphine (Buprenex), and nalbuphine hydrochloride (Nubain) are examples of other mixed narcotic agonist-antagonist analgesics. Reports are that pentazocine and butorphanol can cause dependence. These drug agents are considered safe for use during labor; however their safety when taken during early pregnancy has not been established.

Prototype Drug Chart 21–4 details the pharmacologic behavior of nalbuphine, and Table 21–4 lists the various narcotic agonist-antagonists.

PREVENTING MEDICATION ERRORS

Do not confuse...

• Do not confuse **Nubain** with **Nebcin** or **Nuprin**. These two drug names look alike, but the drugs are different.

Pharmacokinetics

Nalbuphine can be administered orally, IM, subQ, or IV. It is rapidly absorbed parenterally. Nalbuphine has a short half-life. It is metabolized in the liver and excreted in the urine.

Pharmacodynamics

Nalbuphine is effective in alleviating moderate to severe pain. Onset of action is rapid, and peak time occurs within 30 minutes with IV administration. Duration of action is the same for all routes of administration: approximately 5 hours.

Nursing Process

Mixed Narcotic Analgesic: Nalbuphine (Nubain)

ASSESSMENT

■ Obtain a drug history from client. Report if a drug-drug interaction is probable. When taken with nalbuphine, CNS depressants can cause respiratory depression.

■ Note baseline vital signs for future comparison.

■ Assess the type of pain, duration, and location before giving the drug.

NURSING DIAGNOSIS

■ Pain related to surgery or trauma

PLANNING

■ Client will be free of pain, or the intensity of pain will be lessened.

NURSING INTERVENTIONS

■ Monitor vital signs. Note any changes in respirations.

■ Check bowel sounds and date of last bowel movement to identify constipation. Decreased peristalsis may result in constipation. A mild laxative may be necessary.

■ Determine urine output. Report if urine output is <30 ml/hour or <600 ml/day.

■ Administer IV nalbuphine undiluted. Do not mix with barbiturates.

Client Teaching

General

• Instruct client not to use alcohol or CNS depressants while taking nalbuphine. Respiratory depression can occur.

• Suggest nonpharmacologic methods for lessening pain, such as changing position or ambulation.

Side Effects

• Direct client to report side effects to nalbuphine, such as dizziness, headaches, constipation, dysuria, rash, or blurred vision. Hallucinations, tachycardia, and respiratory depression are adverse reactions that might occur.

Cultural Considerations ⊕

• Accept various cultural groups' use of alternative methods in relief of pain.

EVALUATION

■ Evaluate the effectiveness of nalbuphine in relieving pain. If ineffective, another narcotic analgesic may be ordered.

■ Determine the stability of the vital signs. Note whether there is a change in respirations, pulse rate, or blood pressure. Report abnormal findings.

Narcotic Antagonists

Narcotic antagonists are antidotes for overdoses of narcotic analgesics. The narcotic antagonists have a higher affinity to the opiate receptor site than the narcotic being taken. The narcotic antagonist blocks the receptor and

---

Table 21–4

Narcotics: Agonist-Antagonists		
Generic (Brand)	**Route and Dosage**	**Uses and Considerations**
buprenorphine HCl (Buprenex) CSS V	A: IM/IV: Initially: 0.3 mg q6h; may increase to 0.6 mg q6h PRN; IV infusion: 25-50 mcg/h	For moderate to severe pain associated with surgery, cancer, ureteral calculi, myocardial infarction, and trauma. Avoid alcohol and CNS depressants. *Pregnancy category:* C; PB: 96%; $t^1/_2$: 2-3 h
butorphanol tartrate (Stadol) CSS IV	A: IM: 1-4 mg q3-4h PRN IV: 0.5-2 mg q3-4h PRN Nasal spray: 1 mg (1 spray) q3-4h	Management of moderate to severe pain for cancer, renal calculi, labor, musculoskeletal, and burns. *Pregnancy category:* C; PB: >90%; $t^1/_2$: 2.5-4 h
dezocine (Dalgan) CSS IV	A: IM: 5-20 mg q3-6h PRN; *max:* 120 mg/d IV: 2.5-10 mg q3-6h PRN	To control moderate to severe pain. *Pregnancy category:* C; PB: UK; $t^1/_2$: 2.2-2.6 h
nalbuphine HCl (Nubain) CSS IV	See Prototype Drug Chart 21-4.	
pentazocine lactate (Talwin) CSS IV	A: PO: 50-100 mg q3-4h PRN; *max:* 360 mg/d A: subQ/IM/IV: 30 mg q3-4 h PRN; *max:* 360 mg/d Elderly: PO: 50 mg q4h Elderly: IM: 30 mg q4h	To control moderate to severe pain. *Pregnancy category:* C; PB: 60%; $t^1/_2$: 2-3 h

A, Adult; *CNS,* central nervous system; *CSS,* Controlled Substances Schedule; *d,* day; *h,* hour; *IM,* intramuscular; *IV,* intravenous; *max,* maximum; *PB,* protein-binding; *PO,* by mouth; *PRN,* as needed; *subQ,* subcutaneous; $t^1/_2$, half-life; *UK,* unknown.

Table 21–5

Narcotic Antagonists

Generic (Brand)	Route and Dosage	Uses and Considerations
nalmefene (Revex)	A: IM/IV: 0.25 mcg/kg initially; repeat 0.25 mcg/kg at 2- to 5-min intervals PRN	Reverses opioid overdose and respiratory depression. Long half-life. Naloxone has a shorter half-life with shorter withdrawal effects. *Pregnancy category:* UK; PB: UK; $t^{1}/_{2}$: UK
naloxone HCl (Narcan)	Opiate overdose; *Narcotic-induced respiratory distress:* A: IV: 0.4-2 mg; may repeat q2-3min; *max:* 10 mg C: IV: 0.01-0.1 mg/kg; may repeat q2-3min; *max:* 10 mg *Postoperative respiratory depression:* A: IV: 0.1-0.2 mg; may repeat q2-3min PRN C: IV/IM: 0.005-0.01 mg/kg; may repeat q2-3min PRN	To treat narcotic overdose. May be given rapidly IV in small amounts with repeats at 2- to 3-min intervals PRN. Approved for use in neonates to reverse respiratory depression induced by maternal opioid use. *Pregnancy category:* B; PB: UK; $t^{1}/_{2}$: 1-1.5 h
naltrexone HCl (Trexan, ReVia)	A: PO: 25 mg/d; repeat 25 mg in 1 h if no withdrawal response	Treatment of opioid abuse and alcohol abuse. Three to five times more potent than naloxone. Long duration of action. Decreases but does not prevent the craving for opioids. Use after the client is off opioids for 7 or more days. Do not give if client is in opiate withdrawal; it can precipitate a withdrawal reaction. High doses can cause hepatotoxicity. *Pregnancy category:* C; PB: UK; $t^{1}/_{2}$: 4-13 h

A, Adult; *C*, child; *h*, hour; *IM*, intramuscular; *IV*, intravenous; *max*, maximum; *min*, minute; *PB*, protein-binding; *PO*, by mouth; *PRN*, as needed; $t^{1}/_{2}$, half-life; *UK*, unknown.

displaces any narcotic that would normally be at the receptor, thus inhibiting the narcotic action. Naloxone (Narcan), administered IM or IV; naltrexone hydrochloride (ReVia), administered orally by tablet or liquid; and nalmefene (Revex) are pure narcotic antagonists. These drugs reverse the respiratory and CNS depression caused by the narcotics and are perfect examples of pharmacologic antagonists. Table 21–5 lists the narcotic antagonists.

Treatment for Narcotic-Addicted Persons

Throughout the country there are many treatment programs that help the narcotic-addicted person withdraw from heroin or similar narcotics without causing withdrawal symptoms. One type of program is the **methadone treatment program.** This program works by replacing the narcotics with methadone, also a narcotic but one that causes less dependency than the narcotics it replaces. The half-life of methadone is longer than most narcotics, so it needs to be given only once a day. The dosage is from 15 to 40 mg daily; the maximum dosage is 120 mg daily.

The two types of methadone treatment programs are weaning programs and maintenance programs. In a

weaning program, the person receives a dose of methadone for the first 2 days that is approximately the same as the dose of the "street" drug to which she or he is addicted. After 2 days, the methadone dose may be decreased by 5 to 10 mg daily or as indicated until the person is completely weaned from methadone. In a maintenance program, the person is given the same methadone dose every day. The dose may be less than that of the street drug, but it remains consistent throughout the course of treatment.

WEBSITES

For further information on *Drugs for Pain Management,* visit these Internet resources:

Information on fentanyl:
www.rxlist.com/cgi/generic2/fentanyl.htm

Information about vicodin:
www.drugs.com/vicodin.html

Information about Toradol:
www.rxlist.com/cgi/generic/ketor.htm

Critical Thinking Case Study

R.J., 79 years old, had abdominal surgery for colon resection. The narcotic analgesic meperidine (Demerol), 75 mg, every 3 to 4 hours, was prescribed after the surgery. R.J. did not ask for "pain medication" because he thought he might become addicted to the narcotic. The nurse noted that he was restless and grimacing when he moved in bed. He refused to breathe deeply or cough when instructed to do so. The nurse compared his vital signs to his baseline findings. His pulse rate had increased and his systolic blood pressure had decreased by 6 mm Hg.

1. Should the nurse give meperidine? Explain.

2. What would your reaction be to R.J. in regard to his restlessness, grimacing, and refusal to deep breathe and cough?

3. What is the significance of the changes in the vital signs?

4. What classic side effects of narcotic analgesics should the nurse assess?

5. What are some possible nonpharmacologic measures that might be helpful to R.J. for decreasing his pain?

After the first day postoperatively, R.J. asked for meperidine every 3 hours. On the fifth day after surgery, the health care provider discontinued the meperidine and prescribed acetaminophen with codeine.

6. Why was the narcotic analgesic order changed?

7. R.J. does not want to ambulate. What is an appropriate nursing response?

Study Questions

1. A client has had major surgery. What type of analgesic best meets the client's needs? Explain.

2. A client complains of flu symptoms and takes aspirin to reduce fever and relieve the achiness associated with the flu. What is an appropriate intervention? Why?

3. Aspirin is a mild nonnarcotic analgesic. In what drug categories is aspirin used? Explain.

4. What is the most common side effect of nonnarcotics? What nursing measures decrease or alleviate this side effect?

5. What are the advantages and disadvantages of acetaminophen?

6. A client is physically dependent on a "street" narcotic. What type of program could be helpful to decrease or eliminate the drug addiction? How would you explain the program to the client?

7. A child took approximately 20 acetaminophen tablets. What should the parent do? What is the serious toxic effect of acetaminophen?

8. What are the serious side effects of narcotic analgesics?

9. When do withdrawal symptoms occur? Describe the symptoms.

22 Anticonvulsants

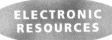

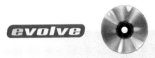

ELECTRONIC RESOURCES

Additional information can be found on the companion website at *http://evolve.elsevier.com/KeeHayes/pharmacology/* or on the companion CD-ROM, which includes:

- *NCLEX-style examination review questions*
- *Pharmacology animations*
- *Medication error and IV therapy checklists*
- *Medication calculation problems*
- *Electronic calculators*

OBJECTIVES

- Describe the two international classifications of seizures and give examples of types of seizures.
- Differentiate between the types of seizures.
- Give the pharmacokinetics, side effects and adverse reactions, therapeutic plasma phenytoin level, contraindications for use, and drug interactions of the hydantoin, phenytoin (Dilantin).
- Describe the uses for hydantoins, long-acting barbiturates, succinimides, oxazolidones, benzodiazepines, carbamazepine, and valproate.
- Explain the nursing interventions, including client teaching, related to the use of hydantoins and other anticonvulsants.

TERMS

anoxia
anticonvulsants
atonic seizure
clonic seizure
electroencephalogram (EEG)

gingival hyperplasia
grand mal
hydantoin
idiopathic
petit mal

psychomotor
status epilepticus
teratogenic
tonic seizure

Introduction

Epilepsy, a seizure disorder, occurs in approximately 1% of the population. The seizure associated with epilepsy results from abnormal electric discharges from the cerebral neurons and is characterized by a loss or disturbance of consciousness and usually by a convulsion (abnormal motor reaction). The **electroencephalogram (EEG)**, computerized tomography (CT), and magnetic resonance imaging (MRI) are useful in diagnosing epilepsy. The EEG records abnormal electric discharges of the cerebral cortex. Of all epilepsy cases, 50% are considered to be primary, or **idiopathic** (of unknown cause), and 50% are considered to be secondary to trauma, brain **anoxia**, infection, or cerebrovascular disorders (e.g., cerebrovascular accidents or stroke).

Epilepsy is a chronic, usually lifelong, disorder. Approximately 75% of persons with seizures had their first seizure before 18 years of age. Isolated seizures could result from fever, hypoglycemic reaction, electrolyte imbalance (hyponatremia), acid-base imbalance (acidosis or alkalosis), and alcohol or drug withdrawal. When these conditions are corrected, the seizures cease. Recurrent seizures may result from birth and perinatal injuries, head trauma, congenital malformations, neoplasms (tumors), and idiopathic or unknown causes.

International Classification of Seizures

There are various types and names of seizures, such as **grand mal** (tonic-clonic), **petit mal** (absence), and **psychomotor**. The international classification of seizures (Table 22–1) describes two categories of seizure: generalized and partial. A person may have more than one type of seizure.

Anticonvulsants

Drugs used for epileptic seizures are called **anticonvulsants**, or antiepileptics. Anticonvulsant drugs suppress the abnormal electric impulses from the seizure focus to other cortical areas, thus preventing the seizure but *not* eliminating the cause of the seizure. Anticonvulsants are classified as central nervous system (CNS) depressants.

With the use of anticonvulsants, 75% of persons with epilepsy are free of seizures. Anticonvulsants are usually taken throughout the person's lifetime. In some cases, the health care provider might discontinue the anticonvulsant if there has not been a seizure in the past 3 to 5 years.

Before 1850 there were various remedies for control of seizures. In 1857 potassium bromide was the first treat-

Table 22–1

International Classification of Seizures

Category	Characteristics
Generalized Seizures	Convulsive and nonconvulsive; involve both cerebral hemispheres of the brain
Tonic-clonic seizure	Also called *grand mal seizure;* most common form of seizures. In the tonic phase, the skeletal muscles contract or tighten in a spasm, lasting 3 to 5 seconds. In the clonic phase, there is a dysrhythmic muscular contraction, or jerkiness, of the legs and arms, lasting 2 to 4 minutes
Tonic seizure	Sustained muscle contraction
Clonic seizure	Dysrhythmic muscle contraction
Absence seizure	Also called *petit mal seizure;* brief loss of consciousness, lasting less than 10 seconds; fewer than three spike waves on the electroencephalogram (EEG) printout; usually occurs in children
Myoclonic seizure	Isolated clonic contraction or jerks lasting 3 to 10 seconds; may be limited to one limb (focal myoclonic) or involve the entire body (massive myoclonic); may be secondary to a neurologic disorder, such as encephalitis or Tay-Sachs disease
Atonic seizure	Head drop; loss of posture; sudden loss of muscle tone. If the lower limbs are involved, this could cause the client to collapse
Infantile spasms	Muscle spasm
Partial Seizures	Involve one hemisphere of the brain. There is no loss of consciousness in simple partial seizures, but there is a loss of consciousness in complex partial seizures
Simple seizure	Occurs in motor, sensory, autonomic, and psychic forms; no loss of consciousness
Motor	Formerly called the *jacksonian seizure;* involves spontaneous movement that spreads; can develop into a generalized seizure
Sensory	Visual, auditory, or taste hallucinations
Autonomic response	Paleness, flushing, sweating, or vomiting
Psychologic	Personality changes
Complex seizure	There is a loss of consciousness. Client does not recall behavior immediately before, during, and immediately after the seizure
Psychomotor	Complex symptoms: automatisms (repetitive behavior such as chewing or swallowing motions), behavioral changes, and motor seizures
Cognitive	Confusion or memory impairment
Affective	Bizarre behavior
Compound	May lead to generalized seizures such as tonic-clonic, tonic

ment to successfully control seizures. Bromide was the primary anticonvulsant used for years, although the drug was habit forming and caused side effects. Phenobarbital was introduced in 1918 and phenytoin (Dilantin) in 1938. Both are still used for seizure disorders.

There are many types of anticonvulsants used to treat epilepsy, including the hydantoins (phenytoin, mephenytoin, ethotoin), long-acting barbiturates (phenobarbital, mephobarbital, primidone), succinimides (ethosuximide), oxazolidones (trimethadione), benzodiazepines (diazepam, clonazepam), carbamazepine, and valproate (valproic acid). Anticonvulsants are not used for all types of seizures. For example, the hydantoin *phenytoin* is effective in treating grand mal (tonic-clonic) seizures and psychomotor seizures but is not effective in treating petit mal (absence) seizures.

Pharmacophysiology: Action of Anticonvulsants

The anticonvulsant drugs work in one of three ways: (1) by suppressing sodium influx through the drug binding to the sodium channel when it is inactivated, thus prolonging the channel inactivation and thereby preventing neuron firing; (2) by suppressing the calcium influx, thus preventing the electric current generated by the calcium ions to the T calcium channel; and (3) by increasing the action of gamma-aminobutyric acid (GABA), which inhibits neurotransmitter throughout the brain. The drugs that suppress sodium influx are phenytoin, fosphenytoin, carbamazepine, oxcarbazepine, valproic acid, topiramate, zonisamide, and lamotrigine. Valproic acid and ethosuximide are examples of drugs that suppress calcium influx. Examples of drug groups that enhance the action of GABA are barbiturates, benzodiazepines, and tiagabine. Gabapentin promotes GABA release. A new anticonvulsant, vigabatrin, inhibits the degradation of GABA from enzyme action.

Hydantoins

The first anticonvulsant used to treat seizures was phenytoin, a **hydantoin** discovered in 1938 that is still the most commonly used drug for controlling seizures. It has the least toxic effects, has a small effect on general sedation, and is nonaddicting. However, this drug should not be used during pregnancy because it can have a **teratogenic** effect on the fetus.

Drug dosage for phenytoin as well as for other anticonvulsants varies according to the age of the client. Newborns, persons with liver disease, and older adults require a lower dosage because of a decrease in metabolism resulting in more available drug. Children and young and middle-aged adults have an increased metabolism rate. The drug dosage is adjusted according to the therapeutic plasma or serum level. Phenytoin has a narrow therapeutic range of 10 to 20 mcg/ml. The benefits of an anticonvulsant become apparent when the serum drug level is within the therapeutic range; if, however, the drug level is below the desired range, the client is not receiving the required drug dosage to pre-

PREVENTING MEDICATION ERRORS

Do not confuse...

- **Cerebyx** (hydantoin anticonvulsant) with **celebrex** (nonsteroid antiinflammatory drug). These drugs look and sound alike but are different in their pharmacology.

vent seizures. In addition, if the drug level is above the desired range, drug toxicity may result. Monitoring the therapeutic serum drug range is of utmost importance to ensure drug effectiveness. Prototype Drug Chart 22–1 lists the pharmacologic data associated with phenytoin.

Pharmacokinetics

Phenytoin is slowly absorbed from the small intestine. It is a highly protein-bound (85% to 95%) drug; a decrease in serum protein or albumin can increase the free phenytoin serum level. With a small to average drug dose, the half-life of phenytoin is approximately 22 hours; however, the range can be from 6 to 45 hours. Phenytoin is metabolized to inactive metabolites, and that portion is excreted in the urine.

Pharmacodynamics

The pharmacodynamics of orally administered phenytoin include onset of action within 30 minutes to 2 hours, peak serum concentration in 1.5 to 3 hours, steady state of serum concentration in 7 to 10 days, and a duration of action dependent on the half-life. Oral phenytoin is most commonly ordered as a sustained-release capsule. The peak concentration time is 4 to 12 hours (sustained-release).

Intravenous (IV) infusion of phenytoin should be administered by direct injection into a large vein. The drug may be diluted in saline solution; however, dextrose solution should be avoided because of drug precipitation. Continuous IV infusion of phenytoin should not be used. IV phenytoin, 50 mg or fraction thereof, should be administered over a period of 1 minute for adults and, when the client is elderly, at a rate of 25 mg per minute. Infusion rates of more than 50 mg per minute may cause hypotension or cardiac dysrhythmias, especially with older and debilitated clients. Local irritation at the injection site may be noted, and sloughing may occur. Intramuscular (IM) injection of phenytoin irritates tissues and may cause damage. For this reason and because of its erratic absorption rate, IM administration of phenytoin is discouraged.

Mephenytoin is a potent hydantoin and much more toxic than phenytoin. It is used for severe grand mal or psychomotor seizures that do not respond to phenytoin or other anticonvulsant therapy. The newest hydantoin, ethotoin, produces similar responses as phenytoin and has a shorter half-life of 3 to 6 hours; therefore the chance of cumulative drug effects decreases.

Side Effects and Adverse Reactions

The severe side effects of hydantoins include **gingival hyperplasia**, or overgrowth of the gum tissues (reddened gums that bleed easily); neurologic and psychiatric effects, such as slurred speech, confusion, depression, and thrombocytopenia (low platelet count); and leukopenia (low white blood cell count). Clients on hydantoins for long periods might have an elevated blood sugar (hyperglycemia), which results from the drug inhibiting the release of insulin. Less severe side effects include nausea, vomiting, con-

PROTOTYPE DRUG CHART 22–1

PHENYTOIN

Drug Class

Anticonvulsant, hydantoin
Trade Name: Dilantin
Pregnancy Category: D

Dosage

A: PO: 100 mg, t.i.d., q.i.d.
IV: LD: 10-15 mg/kg/d; infusion <50 mg/min; *max:* 300 mg/d in divided doses
C: Initially 5 mg/kg/d in 2-3 divided doses; 4-8 mg/kg/d in divided doses
Therapeutic serum range: 10-20 mcg/ml
Toxic level: 30-50 mcg/ml

Contraindications

Hypersensitivity, heart block, psychiatric disorders, pregnancy

Drug-Lab-Food Interactions

Drug: Increase effects with cimetidine, isoniazid, chloramphenicol; *decrease* effects with cisplatin, folic acid, and vinblastine
Decrease effects of anticoagulants, oral contraceptives, antihistamines, corticosteroids, theophylline, cyclosporin, quinidine, dopamine, rifampin
Food: Decreased effects of folic acid, calcium, and vitamin D absorption by phenytoin

Pharmacokinetics

Absorption: PO: Slowly absorbed; IM: Erratic rate of absorption
Distribution: PB: 85%-95%
Metabolism: t½: 6-45 h; average: 22 h
Excretion: In urine, small amount; in bile and feces, moderate amount

Pharmacodynamics

PO: Onset: 0.5-2 h
Peak: 1.5-3 h
Duration: 6-12 h
IV: Onset: within min-1 h
Peak: 2 h
Duration: >12 h

Therapeutic Effects/Uses

To prevent grand mal and complex partial seizures
Mode of Action: Reduces motor cortex activity by altering transport of ions

Side Effects

Headache, diplopia, confusion, dizziness, sluggishness, decreased coordination, ataxia, slurred speech, rash, anorexia, nausea, vomiting, hypotension (IV), pink-red/brown discoloration of urine

Adverse Reactions

Leukopenia, hepatitis, depression, gingival hyperplasia, gingivitis, nystagmus, hirsutism
Life-threatening: Aplastic anemia, thrombocytopenia, agranulocytosis, Stevens-Johnson syndrome, hypotension, ventricular fibrillation

A, Adult; *C,* child; *d,* day; *h,* hour; *IM,* intramuscular; *IV,* intravenous; *LD,* loading dose; *max,* maximum; *min,* minute; *PB,* protein-binding; *PO,* by mouth; *q.i.d.,* four times a day; *t½,* half-life; *t.i.d.,* three times a day; >, greater than; <, less than.

stipation, drowsiness, headaches, alopecia, hirsutism, and nystagmus.

Drug-Drug Interactions

Drug-drug interaction is common with hydantoins because they are highly protein bound. Hydantoins compete with other drugs, such as anticoagulants and aspirin, for plasma protein-binding sites. The hydantoins displace the anticoagulants and aspirin, causing more free drug and increasing their activity. Barbiturates, rifampin, and a chronic ingestion of ethanol increase hydantoin metabolism. Drugs such as sulfonamides and cimetidine (Tagamet) can increase the action of hydantoins by inhibiting liver metabolism, which is necessary for drug excretion. Absorption of hydantoins

can be decreased by antacids, calcium preparations, sucralfate (Carafate) and antineoplastic drugs. Antipsychotics and certain herbs can lower the seizure threshold and can increase seizure activity. (See Herbal Alert 22–1.) The client should be closely monitored for seizure occurrence.

HERBAL ALERT 22-1

Anticonvulsants

❧ Evening primrose and borage may lower seizure threshold when these herbs are taken with anticonvulsants. The anticonvulsant dose may need modification.
❧ Ginkgo may decrease phenytoin effectiveness.

Barbiturates

Phenobarbital, a long-acting barbiturate, is still prescribed to treat grand mal seizures and acute episodes of **status epilepticus** seizures (rapid succession of epileptic seizures), meningitis, toxic reactions, and eclampsia. Possible teratogenic effects and other side effects related to phenytoin are less pronounced with phenobarbital. Problems associated with phenobarbital include its cause of general sedation and client tolerance to the drug. Discontinuance of phenobarbital should be gradual to avoid recurrence of seizures.

Succinimides

The succinimide drug group is used to treat absence or petit mal seizures, and it may be used in combination with other anticonvulsants to treat such seizures. Ethosuximide (Zarontin) is the succinimide of choice; the other formulations, methsuximide (Celontin) and phensuximide (Milontin), are used mainly for petit mal refractory seizures.

Oxazolidones/Oxazolidinedione

The oxazolidones, trimethadione and paramethadione, are also prescribed to treat petit mal seizures. Trimethadione was the first drug developed for petit mal; therefore it is prescribed more frequently than paramethadione. There are many severe side effects associated with this group of anticonvulsants. Trimethadione may be used in combination with other drugs or singly to treat refractory petit mal seizures.

Benzodiazepines

The three benzodiazepines that have anticonvulsant effects are clonazepam, clorazepate dipotassium, and diazepam. Clonazepam is effective in controlling petit mal (absence) seizures; however, tolerance may occur 6 months after drug therapy starts, and consequently clonazepam dosage has to be adjusted. Clorazepate dipotassium is frequently administered in adjunctive therapy for treating partial seizures.

Diazepam is primarily prescribed for treating acute status epilepticus and must be administered IV to achieve the desired response. The drug has a short-term effect; thus other anticonvulsants, such as phenytoin or phenobarbital, need to be given during or immediately after administration of diazepam.

Iminostilbenes

Carbamazepine, an iminostilbene, is effective in treating refractory seizure disorders that have not responded to other anticonvulsant therapies. It is used to control grand mal and partial seizures and a combination of these seizures.

Carbamazepine is also used for psychiatric disorders (e.g., bipolar disease), trigeminal neuralgia (as an analgesic), and alcohol withdrawal. However, the drug has not been approved by the Food and Drug Administration (FDA) for treatment of the aforementioned disorders.

An interaction may occur when grapefruit juice is taken with carbamazepine (Tegretol), causing possible toxicity. Therefore drug concentrations must be monitored carefully.

Valproate

Valproic acid has been prescribed for petit mal, grand mal, and mixed types of seizures. Care should be taken when giving this drug to very young children and clients with liver disorders because hepatotoxicity is one of the possible adverse reactions. Liver enzymes should be monitored. The FDA has approved divalproex sodium (Depakote) for treatment of manic episodes associated with bipolar disorder.

Table 22-2 lists the various anticonvulsants and their dosages, uses, and considerations. Table 22-3 lists selected anticonvulsants that are frequently prescribed to treat seizure disorders.

Anticonvulsant dosages usually start low and gradually increase over a period of weeks until the serum drug level is within therapeutic range or the seizures stop. Serum anticonvulsant drug levels should be closely monitored to prevent toxicity.

Anticonvulsants and Pregnancy

During pregnancy, seizure episodes increase 25% in women with epilepsy. Hypoxia that may occur during seizures places a pregnant woman with epilepsy and her fetus at risk.

Many anticonvulsant drugs have teratogenic properties that increase the risk for fetal malformations; however, many women with epilepsy give birth to normal infants. Phenytoin and carbamazepine have been linked to fetal anomalies such as cardiac defects and cleft lip and palate. Trimethadione should not be given to women of childbearing age because of its strong teratogenic effect. It has been reported that valproic acid is known to cause neural tubal defects (spina bifida) in 2% to 3% of pregnant women who take the drug. As expected, the highest incidence of birth defects occurs when the woman takes combinations of anticonvulsant drugs.

Anticonvulsant drugs increase the loss of folate (folic acid) in pregnant women; thus daily folate supplements should be taken. Anticonvulsants tend to act as inhibitors of vitamin K, which contributes to hemorrhaging in infants shortly after birth. Frequently, pregnant women taking anticonvulsants are given an oral vitamin K supplement during the last week or 10 days of the pregnancy, or vitamin K is administered to the infant soon after birth.

Anticonvulsants and Febrile Seizures

Seizures associated with fever usually occur in children between the ages of 3 months and 5 years. Epilepsy develops in approximately 2.5% of children who have had one or more febrile seizures. Prophylactic anticonvulsant treatment such as phenobarbital or diazepam may be indicated for high-risk clients. Valproic acid should not be given to children because of its possible hepatotoxic effect.

Table 22–2

Anticonvulsants

Generic (Brand)	Route and Dosage	Uses and Considerations
Barbiturates		
amobarbital (Amytal) CSS II	*Status epilepticus:* A: IM/IV: 75-500 mg; *max:* IM: 500 mg; IV: 1000 mg Therapeutic serum range: 1-5 mcg/ml	For acute convulsive episode and to control status epilepticus. Infusion rate should not exceed 100 mg/min for adult and 60 mg/m^2/min for children. *Pregnancy category:* D; PB: 50%-60%; t$^1/_2$: 20-25 h
mephobarbital (Mebaral) CSS II	A: PO: 400-600 mg/d in divided doses C: PO: 6-12 mg/kg/d in divided doses or C: ≥ 5 y: 32-64 mg t.i.d./q.i.d. C: <5 y: 16-32 mg t.i.d./q.i.d. Therapeutic serum range: 15-40 mcg/ml	For grand mal and petit mal (absence) seizures. May be used in combination with other anticonvulsants. Also used to manage delirium tremens. May cause drowsiness and dizziness. *Pregnancy category:* D; PB: UK; t$^1/_2$: 34 h
phenobarbital (Luminal) CSS IV	*Status epilepticus:* Neonate: IV: LD: 15-20 mg/kg single or divided dose A & C: IV: 15-18 mg/kg; *max:* 30 mg/kg *Maintenance:* Neonate: PO/IV: 3-4 mg/kg/d in 1-2 divided doses Infant: 5-6 mg/kg/d in 1-2 divided doses C: 1-5 y: PO: 6-8 mg/kg/d in 1-2 divided doses C: 6-12 y: PO: 4-6 mg/kg/d in 1-2 divided doses A: PO: 1-3 mg/kg/d; 100-300 mg/d in divided doses Therapeutic serum range: 15-40 mcg/ml	Long-acting barbiturate. Used for grand mal (tonic-clonic), partial seizures, and to control status epilepticus. May be used in combination with phenytoin. High doses given to older adults or children may cause confusion, depression, irritability. Long-term use with high doses could cause physical dependence. *Pregnancy category:* D; PB: 20%-40%; t$^1/_2$: A: 50-140 h; C: 35-75 h
primidone (Mysoline)	A: PO: 125-250 mg b.i.d./q.i.d.; max: 2 g/d C: <8 y: PO: $^1/_2$ of adult dose Therapeutic serum range: 5-10 mcg/ml	Barbiturate-like drug. Used to manage grand mal and psychomotor seizures. Take with food if the drug causes GI distress. *Pregnancy category:* D; PB: 99%; t$^1/_2$: 10-24 h
Benzodiazepines (Anxiolytics)		
clonazepam (Klonopin) CSS IV	A: PO: 0.5-1 mg t.i.d.; gradually increase dose q3d until seizures are controlled C: PO: 0.01-0.03 mg/kg/d; gradually increase Therapeutic serum range: 20-80 ng/ml	For petit mal, myoclonus, and status epilepticus. May be used when petit mal (absence) seizures are refractory to succinimides or valproic acid. *Pregnancy category:* C; PB: 85%; t$^1/_2$: A: 20-50 h; C: 24-36 h
clorazepate (Tranxene) CSS IV	A: PO: 7.5 mg t.i.d. C: >9 y: PO: 7.5 mg b.i.d.	May be used for partial seizures and as adjunctive therapy for seizures. *Pregnancy category:* D; PB: 97%; t$^1/_2$: 48 h
diazepam (Valium) CSS IV	*Status epilepticus:* A: IV: 5-10 mg; repeat if needed at 10- to 15-min intervals; *max:* 30 mg C <5 y: IV: 0.2-0.5 mg over 2-5 min; *max:* 5 mg C >5 y: IV 1 mg slowly; repeat if needed	For status epilepticus (drug of choice). Administer IV and repeat q10-15 min up to 30 mg PRN; then q2-4h PRN. *Pregnancy category:* D; PB: 98%; t$^1/_2$: 20-50 h
lorazepam (Ativan) CSS IV	*Status epilepticus:* Neonate: IV: 0.05 mg/kg over 2-5 min; may repeat in 10-15 min Infants & C: 0.1 mg/kg over 2-5 min; *max:* 4 mg/single dose A: IV: 4 mg over 2-5 min; *max:* 8 mg; may repeat in 10-15 min for all ages Therapeutic serum range: 50-240 ng/ml	To control status epilepticus. Infusion rate should not exceed 2 mg/min. *Pregnancy category:* D; PB: 85%; t$^1/_2$: 10-16 h

A, Adult; *b.i.d.,* twice a day; *C,* child; *CNS,* central nervous system; *CSS,* Controlled Substances Schedule; *d,* day; *h,* hour; *IM,* intramuscular; *inf,* infusion; *IV,* intravenous; *LD,* loading dose; *max,* maximum; *min,* minute; *PB,* protein-binding; *PE,* phenytoin equivalents; *PO,* by mouth; *PRN,* as needed; *q.i.d.,* four times a day; *t$^1/_2$,* half-life; *UK,* unknown; *y,* year; *>,* greater than; *<,* less than.

Table 22–2

Anticonvulsants—cont'd

Generic (Brand)	Route and Dosage	Uses and Considerations
Hydantoins		
fosphenytoin (Cerebyx)	A: IV: LD: 10-20 mg PE/kg *Maintenance:* 4-6 mg PE/kg/d *Status epilepticus:* IV: LD: 15-20 mg PE/kg infused at 100-150 mg PE/min	To treat grand mal seizures, complex partial seizures, and status epilepticus. Decreases sodium and calcium ion influx in the neurons. Converts to phenytoin. Dilute in D_5W or 0.9% NaCl. *Pregnancy category:* D; PB: UK; t½: 8-15 min
mephenytoin (Mesantoin)	A: PO: Initially: 50-100 mg; 100-200 mg t.i.d. C: PO: Initially: 50-100 mg; 100-400 mg/d in 3 divided doses or 3-15 mg/kg/d in 3 divided doses Therapeutic serum range: 25-40 mcg/ml	For grand mal, psychomotor, focal (simple) seizures. Severe adverse reaction may include blood dyscrasias. *Pregnancy category:* C; PB: UK; t½: 7 h; metabolite: 100-144 h
phenytoin (Dilantin)	See Prototype Drug Chart 22-1.	
Iminostilbene		
carbamazepine (Tegretol)	A: PO: 200 mg b.i.d.; increasing doses as needed C: PO: 10-20 mg/kg/d in divided doses or 100 mg b.i.d. Therapeutic serum range: 5-12 mcg/ml	For grand mal, psychomotor, mixed seizures. Used in treating seizures that do not respond to other anticonvulsants. *Pregnancy category:* C; PB: 75%-90%; t½: 15-30 h
oxcarbazepine (Trileptal)	A: PO: 300 mg b.i.d.; increase to 1200-2400 mg/d C: PO: 8-10 mg/kg; *max:* 600 mg/d	To control refractory partial seizures as monotherapy. Can be used for generalized tonic-clonic seizures. It blocks the sodium channel. Less severe side effects as carbamazepine. *Pregnancy category:* D; PB: UK; t½: 8-10 h.
Oxazolidones		
paramethadione (Paradione)	A: PO: 300-600 mg t.i.d./q.i.d. C: PO: 13 mg/kg t.i.d. or 335 mg/m² t.i.d. or 300-900 mg/d in divided doses	For petit mal (absence) seizures. May be used when refractory to other anticonvulsants. *Pregnancy category:* D; PB: UK; t½: 1-4 h
trimethadione (Tridione)	Same as paramethadione	For petit mal seizures. May be used when refractory to other anticonvulsants. It has many side effects. After prolonged use, drug should be withdrawn gradually. *Pregnancy category:* D; PB: <10%; t½: 6-12 d
Succinimides		
ethosuximide (Zarontin)	A: PO: 250 mg b.i.d.; increase dose gradually C: 3-6 y: PO: 250 mg/d Therapeutic serum range: 40-100 mcg/ml	For petit mal and myoclonic seizures. Gastric irritation is common; may take with food. *Pregnancy category:* C; PB: UK; t½: A: 50-60 h, C: 25-30 h
methsuximide (Celontin)	A & C: PO: Initially: 300 mg/d for 1 wk; may increase at intervals	For petit mal (absence) seizures when refractory to other drugs. High occurrence of toxicity; more so than ethosuximide. *Pregnancy category:* C; PB: UK; t½: 2-4 h
phensuximide (Milontin)	A & C: PO: 0.5-1 g, b.i.d., t.i.d.	Similar to methsuximide. *Pregnancy category:* C; PB: UK; t½: 5-12 h
Valproate		
valproic acid (Depakene) Divalproex Na (Depakote)	A & C: PO: 15 mg/kg; *max:* 60 mg/kg/d in divided doses Therapeutic serum range: 40-100 mcg/ml	For grand mal, petit mal, psychomotor, and myoclonic seizures. Doses may be increased weekly by 5-10 mg/kg/d until seizures are controlled. Avoid during pregnancy. *Pregnancy category:* D; PB: 90%; t½: 6-16 h
Miscellaneous		
acetazolamide (Diamox)	Commonly used with other anticonvulsants: A: PO/IM/IV: 375 mg/d; *max:* 250 mg q.i.d. or PO SR: 250-500 mg daily or b.i.d. C: PO: 8-30 mg/kg in divided doses; *max:* 1.5 g/d	For grand mal, petit mal (absence), and focal seizures. Adequate fluid intake should be maintained to prevent kidney stones. *Pregnancy category:* D; PB: 90%; t½: 2.5-6 h

Continued

Table 22–2

Anticonvulsants—cont'd

Generic (Brand)	Route and Dosage	Uses and Considerations
Miscellaneous—cont'd		
gabapentin (Neurontin)	*Adjunctive therapy for partial seizures:* A: PO: 900-1800 mg/d in 3 divided doses; max time between doses: 12 h; *max:* 2400 mg/d in divided doses	Used as adjunctive therapy for partial seizures. It promotes GABA release. To avoid GI upset, give drug with food. If drug is discontinued, dose should be gradually reduced to avoid occurrence of seizures. *Pregnancy category:* C; PB: <3%; t½: 5-7 h
felbamate (Felbatol)	A: PO: 1200 mg/d in divided doses C: >2 y: PO: 45 mg/kg/d in divided doses	To treat partial and secondary generalized seizures. Also used in adjunctive therapy for the treatment of Lennox-Gastaut syndrome in children. Weak inhibitory effect on GABA-receptor binding. CONTRAINDICATIONS: Client with a blood disorder (reported incidences of aplastic anemia from use of the drug). *Pregnancy category:* C; PB: UK; t½: UK
lamotrigine (Lamictal)	A: PO: Initially: 25-50 mg/d for 2 wk; then 50 mg b.i.d. for 2 wk *Maintenance:* 300-500 mg/d in 2 divided doses; if used with valproic acid, daily doses need to be reduced	Used for partial seizures and in adjunctive anticonvulsant therapy. Also to treat tonic-clonic, absence, atypical absence, myoclonic seizures, and for the treatment of Lennox-Gastaut syndrome in infants and children. It blocks the sodium influx. May be given with other anticonvulsants. *Pregnancy category:* C; PB: UK; t½: 12.5-25 h (half-life is increased when given with other anticonvulsants)
levetiracetam (Keppra)	A: PO: 500 mg b.i.d.; may increase dose by 1000 mg/d; *max:* 3000 mg/d	To treat complex partial seizures. For adjunctive and monotherapy. Unlikely to cause drug interactions. *Pregnancy category:* UK; PB: 0%; t½: 6-8 h
tiagabine (Gabitril)	A: PO: 4 mg/d; may increase by 4-8 mg/d; *max:* 56 mg/d C: 12-18 y: PO: 4 m/g/d; may increase by 4-8 mg; *max:* 32 mg/d	For partial seizures as adjunctive therapy. Increases GABA levels. *Pregnancy category:* UK; PB: UK; t½: UK
topiramate (Topamax)	A: PO: 25-50 mg/d; *max:* 400 mg/d; may be increased by weekly increment C: 2-16 y: PO: Initially 25 mg/d; increase 1-3 mg/kg/d to 5-9 mg/kg/d in divided doses	For partial seizures and generalized tonic-clonic seizures. Inhibits sodium or calcium channels and increases action of GABA. Older adults can take adult dose. *Pregnancy category:* UK; PB: UK; t½: UK.
vigabatrin (Sabril)	A: PO: 1-4 g/d in divided doses C: PO: 50-150 mg/d in divided doses	To treat complex partial seizures and used in adjunctive anticonvulsant therapy. It permits more GABA in the brain. Inhibits the enzyme that destroys GABA. New anticonvulsant drug. *Pregnancy category:* UK; PB: UK; t½: UK
zonisamide (Zonegran)	A & C >16 y: PO: 100 mg/d for 2 wk; may increase 100 mg/d at intervals of 2 wk; *max:* 400 mg/d	For adjunctive treatment of partial seizures. It blocks sodium and calcium channels. Does not affect the serum levels of phenytoin or valproic acid. Contraindicated if sensitive to sulfonamides. *Pregnancy category:* X; PB: UK; t½: 60 h
magnesium sulfate	*Preeclampsia or eclampsia:* A: IV: Initially: 4 g in 250 ml D_5W; then 4 g IM: follow with 4 g IM q4h PRN or Inf: 1-4 g/h *Hypomagnesemic seizures:* A: IV: 1-2 g (19% sol) over 20 min; follow with 1 g IM q4-6h based on blood levels	To control seizures in toxemia of pregnancy caused by eclampsia or preeclampsia. *Pregnancy category:* B; PB: UK; t½: UK

GABA, Gamma aminobutyric acid; *GI,* gastrointestinal; *inf,* infusion; *sol,* solution; *SR,* sustained release.

Table 22-3

Selected Anticonvulsants for Seizure Disorders

Seizure Disorder	Drug Therapy
Tonic-Clonic (Grand Mal)	phenytoin
	carbamazepine
	fosphenytoin
	valproic acid
	lamotrigine
	primidone
	phenobarbital
Partial (Complex-Secondarily Generalized)	phenytoin
	carbamazepine
	oxcarbazepine
	levetiracetam
	primidone
	phenobarbital
	tiagabine
	topiramate
	zonisamide
Absence (Petit Mal)	ethosuximide
	valproic acid
	lamotrigine
	clonazepam
Myoclonic, Atonic, Atypical Absence	valproic acid
	lamotrigine
	clonazepam
Status Epilepticus	diazepam
	fosphenytoin
	lorazepam
	phenytoin

Nursing Process

Anticonvulsants: Phenytoin

ASSESSMENT

■ Obtain a drug history of the current drugs and herbs client is taking. Report if a drug-drug or herb-drug interaction is probable.

■ Check urinary output to determine if adequate (>600 ml/d).

■ Determine laboratory values related to renal and liver function. If both BUN and creatinine levels are elevated, a renal disorder should be suspected. Elevated serum liver enzymes, such as alkaline phosphatase, alanine aminotransferase, gamma-glutamyl transferase, and/or 5'-nucleotidase, indicate a hepatic disorder.

NURSING DIAGNOSES

■ Risk for injury
■ Impaired oral mucous membranes

PLANNING

■ Client will be free of seizures and will adhere to anticonvulsant therapy.
■ Client's side effects from phenytoin will be minimal.

NURSING INTERVENTIONS

■ Monitor serum drug levels of anticonvulsant to determine overdosing or underdosing of drug; promote compliance to regimen.

■ Protect client from hazards in the environment, such as sharp objects and table corners, during a seizure.

■ Determine whether client is receiving adequate nutrients. Phenytoin may cause anorexia, nausea, and vomiting.

■ Women taking oral contraceptives and anticonvulsants may need to use an additional contraceptive method.

Client Teaching

General

• Instruct client to shake the suspension form well before pouring.

• Advise client not to drive or perform other hazardous activities when beginning anticonvulsant therapy. Until client adapts to drug dosage, drowsiness is likely to occur.

• Alert female clients contemplating pregnancy to consult with the health care provider because phenytoin and valproic acid may have a teratogenic effect.

• During pregnancy, seizures frequently increase because of increased metabolism rates, and serum phenytoin levels should be closely monitored. Most anticonvulsants are classified pregnancy category D.

• Inform client that alcohol and other CNS depressants can cause an added depressive effect on the body and should be avoided.

• Explain to client that certain herbs can interact with an anticonvulsant drug (see Herbal Alert 22-1). The anticonvulsant dose may need to be adjusted.

• Encourage client to obtain a medical alert identification card, medic alert bracelet, or tag that indicates the health problem and the drug taken.

• Teach client not to abruptly stop the drug therapy but rather to withdraw the prescribed drug gradually under medical supervision to prevent seizure rebound (recurrence of seizures).

• Counsel client of the need for preventive dental check-ups.

• Warn client to take the prescribed anticonvulsant, get laboratory tests as ordered, and to keep follow-up visits with the health care provider.

• Teach client not to self-medicate with OTC drugs without first consulting the health care provider.

• Instruct client with diabetes to monitor serum glucose levels more closely than usual because phenytoin may inhibit insulin release, thus causing an increase in glucose level.

• Inform client of the existence of national, state, and local associations that provide resources, current information, and support for persons with epilepsy.

Diet

- Educate client to take the anticonvulsant at the same time every day with food or milk. If liquid form is used, shake well before ingesting the drug.

Side Effects

- Tell client that urine may be a harmless pinkish red or reddish brown.
- Instruct the client to maintain good oral hygiene and to use a soft toothbrush to prevent gum irritation and bleeding.
- Teach client to report symptoms of sore throat, bruising, and nosebleeds, which may indicate a blood dyscrasia.
- Encourage client to inform the health care provider of adverse reactions such as gingivitis, nystagmus (involuntary movement of the eyeball), slurred speech, rash, and dizziness.

Cultural Considerations ⊕

- There may be a lack of understanding among certain cultural groups, such as Hispanics, Asians, and first-generation Europeans, related to the importance of taking anticonvulsants on a daily basis for life.
- A written drug schedule may be needed for members of cultural groups who do not understand the importance of the prescribed drug regimen.
- Follow-up by a community nurse may be needed to determine client's compliance to the drug regimen.
- When language barriers exist, use videos and literature in the client's preferred language and pictures of that group may help compliance with health interventions.

EVALUATION

- Evaluate the effectiveness of the drug in controlling seizures.
- Continue to monitor phenytoin serum levels to determine whether they are within the desired range. High serum levels of phenytoin are frequently indicators of phenytoin toxicity.
- Monitor client for hydantoin overdose, such as nystagmus and ataxia (impaired coordination) initially, later hypotension, unresponsive pupils, and coma. Respiratory and circulatory support, as well as hemodialysis are usually used in the treatment of phenytoin overdose.

Anticonvulsants and Status Epilepticus

Status epilepticus, a continuous seizure state, is considered a medical emergency. If treatment is not begun immediately, death could result. The choices of pharmacologic agents are diazepam (Valium) administered IV or lorazepam (Ativan) followed by IV administration of phenytoin (Dilantin). For continued seizures, midazolam (Versed) or propofol (Diprivan), then high-dose barbiturates are used. These drugs should be administered slowly to avoid respiratory depression.

Summary

The pharmacologic behavior of specified anticonvulsants is summarized in Table 22–4.

Table 22–4

Selected Anticonvulsants: Pharmacokinetics, Pharmacodynamics, and Therapeutic Ranges

| Drug | Pharmacokinetics | | | Pharmacodynamics | | | | |
	Protein-Binding (%)	t½	Excretion	PO Onset	Peak Time (h)	Duration of Action (h)	Therapeutic Serum Range
phenytoin (Dilantin)	85-95	6-45 h (average: 22 h)	Kidneys, bile, and GI	30 min-2 h	1.5-3	6-12	10-20 mcg/ml
phenobarbital	20-45	2-6 d	50%-75% in urine	30-60 min	8-12	6-24	15-40 mcg/ml
ethosuximide (Zarontin)	UK	60 h (adult) 30 h (child)	25% in urine unchanged	UK	>4	12-60	40-100 mcg/ml
clonazepam (Klonopin)	UK	20-50 h	Kidneys and feces	20-60 min	1-2	6-12	20-80 ng/ml
carbamazepine (Tegretol)	75	25-65 h	75% in urine, 25% in feces	Varies	4-7	6-12	5-12 mcg/ml
valproic acid (Depakene)	90	6-16 h	Kidneys	20-30 min	1-4	24	40-100 mcg/ml

d, Day; *GI*, gastrointestinal; *h*, hour; *min*, minute; *PO*, by mouth; *t½*, half-life; *UK*, unknown; >, greater than.

WEBSITES

For further information on *Anticonvulsants,* visit these Internet resources:

Information on phenytoin:
http://www.mentalhealth.com/drug/p30-d05.html

Information on carbamazepine:
http://www.personalhealthzone.com/drug_interactions/carbamazepine.html

Information on anticonvulsants:
http://www.giantegle.com/healthnotes/Drug/Anticonvulsants.htm

Critical Thinking Case Study

S.S., 26 years old, takes phenytoin (Dilantin) 100 mg, t.i.d., to control grand mal seizures. S.S. and her husband are contemplating starting a family.

1. What action should the nurse take in regard to client family planning?

S.S. complains of frequent "upset stomach" and "bleeding gums" when brushing her teeth.

2. To decrease GI distress, what can be suggested?
3. To alleviate bleeding gums, what client teaching for S.S. may be included?
4. The nurse checks S.S.'s serum phenytoin level. What are the indications of an abnormal serum level? What appropriate actions should be taken?

Study Questions

1. What are the differences between generalized and partial seizures according to the International Classification of Epileptic Seizures?
2. What are the implications of liver disease or kidney disease for a person taking anticonvulsants? Explain.
3. What is the therapeutic serum range of phenytoin? Is it considered to have a narrow or a wide range? Why should it be closely monitored?
4. What is gingival hyperplasia? Name the drug that might cause this. Give the nursing interventions that decrease this problem.

5. What are the drug-drug interactions between hydantoins and other drugs? Give examples.
6. What drugs are used to treat status epilepticus? By what route should these drugs be given?
7. What type of seizures are benzodiazepines effective in treating? What is another classification for benzodiazepines?

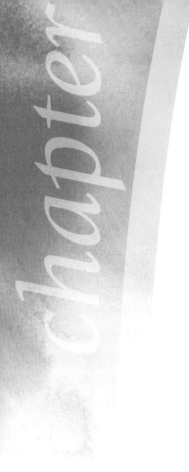

23 Drugs for Neurologic Disorders: Parkinsonism and Alzheimer's Disease

ELECTRONIC RESOURCES

evolve

Additional information can be found on the companion website at *http://evolve.elsevier.com/KeeHayes/pharmacology/* or on the companion CD-ROM, which includes:
- *NCLEX-style examination review questions*
- *Pharmacology animations*
- *Medication error and IV therapy checklists*
- *Medication calculation problems*
- *Electronic calculators*

OUTLINE

OBJECTIVES

- Define parkinsonism and Alzheimer's disease.
- Describe the actions of anticholinergics, dopaminergics, dopamine receptors, MAO-B inhibitor, and COMT inhibitors in the treatment of parkinsonism.
- Describe the side effects of antiparkinson drugs.
- Identify the drug group used to treat Alzheimer's disease.
- Describe the nursing interventions, including client teaching, for drugs used in the treatment of parkinsonism, and Alzheimer's disease.

TERMS

acetylcholinesterase (AChE) inhibitor

bradykinesia
dopamine agonists
dyskinesia

dystonic movement
parkinsonism

pseudoparkinsonism

Introduction

Parkinsonism (Parkinson's disease), a chronic neurologic disorder that affects the extrapyramidal motor tract (which controls posture, balance, and locomotion), is considered a syndrome (combination of symptoms) because of its three major features: rigidity, **bradykinesia** (slow movement), and tremors. Rigidity (abnormally increased muscle tone) increases with movement. Postural changes caused by rigidity and bradykinesia include the chest and head thrust forward with the knees and hips flexed, a shuffling gait, and the absence of arm swing. Other characteristic symptoms are masked facies (no facial expression), involuntary tremors of the head and neck, and pill-rolling motions of the hands. The tremors may be more prevalent at rest.

Alzheimer's disease is a chronic, progressive, neurodegenerative condition with marked cognitive dysfunction. Various theories exist as to the cause of Alzheimer's disease, such as neuritic plaques, degeneration of the cholinergic neurons, and deficiency in acetylcholine.

Parkinsonism

In 1817 Dr. James Parkinson described six clients as having "shaking palsy." Three symptoms were described by Parkinson: (1) involuntary tremors of the limbs, (2) rigidity of muscles, and (3) slowness of movement. In the United States there are approximately one million persons with parkinsonism, and 50,000 new cases are diagnosed each year. Because parkinsonism generally affects clients between the ages of 50 and 70 years and older, many consider the health problem to be part of the aging process caused by the loss of neurons. The three cardinal symptoms are rigidity, tremors, and bradykinesia. Normally the symptoms have a gradual onset and are usually mild and unilateral in the beginning.

There are different types of parkinsonism. **Pseudoparkinsonism** frequently occurs as an adverse reaction to many antipsychotic drugs, especially the phenothiazines. In addition, parkinsonism symptoms could result from poisons (e.g., carbon monoxide, manganese), arteriosclerosis, and Wilson's disease (hepatolenticular degeneration).

Nonpharmacologic Measures

Symptoms of parkinsonism can be lessened through the use of nonpharmacologic measures such as client teaching, exercise, nutrition, and group support. Exercise can improve mobility and flexibility; the client with Parkinson's disease should enroll in a therapeutic exercise program tailored to this disorder. A balanced diet with fiber and fluids helps prevent constipation and weight loss. Clients with Parkinson's disease and their family members should be encouraged to attend a support group; this helps all persons to cope with and understand parkinsonism.

Pathophysiology

Parkinsonism is caused by an imbalance of the neurotransmitters dopamine (DA) and acetylcholine (ACh). It is marked by degeneration of neurons that originate in the substantia nigra of the midbrain and terminate at the basal ganglia of the extrapyramidal motor tract. The reason for the degeneration of neurons is unknown.

There are two neurotransmitters within neurons of the striatum of the brain: dopamine, an inhibitory neurotransmitter, and acetylcholine, an excitatory neurotransmitter. Dopamine is released from the dopaminergic neurons; acetylcholine is released from the cholinergic neurons. Dopamine normally maintains control of acetylcholine and inhibits its excitatory response. In Parkinson's disease there is an unexplained degeneration of the dopaminergic neurons; thus an imbalance between dopamine and acetylcholine occurs. With less dopamine production, acetylcholine is unopposed, thereby causing the excitation and stimulation of the neurons that release gamma-aminobutyric acid (GABA). With the increased stimulation of GABA, the symptomatic movement disorders of parkinsonism occur.

By the time early symptoms of Parkinson's disease appear, 80% of the striatal dopamine has already been depleted. The remaining striatal neurons synthesize the dopamine from levodopa and release dopamine as needed. Before the next dose of levodopa, symptoms (e.g., slow walking, loss of dexterity) return or worsen; within 30 to 60 minutes of receiving a dose, the client's functioning is much improved.

Drugs used to treat parkinsonism reduce the symptoms or replace the dopamine deficit. These drugs fall into five categories: (1) *anticholinergics*, which block the cholinergic receptors; (2) *dopaminergics*, which convert to dopamine; (3) *dopamine agonists*, which stimulate the dopamine receptors; (4) *MAO-B inhibitor*, which inhibits the monoamine oxidase-B (MAO-B) enzyme that interferes with dopamine; and (5) *COMT inhibitors*, which inhibit the catechol-O-methyltransferase enzyme that inactivates dopamine. Table 23–1 compares the various parkinsonism drugs.

Anticholinergics

Anticholinergic drugs reduce the rigidity and some of the tremors characteristic of parkinsonism but have minimal effect on bradykinesia. The anticholinergics are parasym-

Table 23-1

Comparison of Drugs Used to Treat Parkinson's Disease

Drug	Purpose
Dopaminergics	
levodopa carbidopa-levodopa	Decrease symptoms of parkinsonism. Carbidopa, a decarboxylase inhibitor, permits more levodopa to reach the striatum nerve terminals (where levodopa is converted to dopamine). With the use of carbidopa, less levodopa is needed.
Dopamine Agonists	
amantadine	Amantadine was first used as an antiviral drug for influenza A. It decreases symptoms of parkinsonism. It can be given as an early treatment for Parkinson's disease, which could delay the necessity of levodopa. Amantadine is effective in treating drug-induced parkinsonism and has fewer side effects than anticholinergics.
bromocriptine	A D_2-dopamine receptor agonist. Bromocriptine may be used for early treatment of Parkinson's disease. With increasing motor symptoms, bromocriptine can be given with levodopa therapy.
pergolide	A D_1- and D_2-dopamine receptor agonist. It is more potent than bromocriptine and may be used for early treatment of Parkinson's disease. Pergolide can be used with levodopa.
pramipexole (Mirapex), ropinirole HCl (Requip)	D_2- and D_3-dopamine receptor agonists. These drugs can be used in combination with levodopa. They have fewer side effects than older dopamine agonists.
MAO-B Inhibitor	
selegiline	Inhibits the catabolic enzymes of dopamine. MAO-B inhibitor extends the action of dopamine. It can be given in the early phase of Parkinson's disease. If the drug is given with levodopa, the dosage of levodopa is usually decreased.
COMT Inhibitors	
entacapone (Comtan), tolcapone (Tasmar)	Inhibits the COMT enzyme; thus the concentration of levodopa is increased. These drugs are used in combination with levodopa-carbidopa (Sinemet). With COMT inhibitors, a smaller dose of levodopa is needed.
Anticholinergics; Antiparkinson	
	Anticholinergics were the first group of drugs used to treat Parkinson's disease before levodopa and dopamine agonists were introduced. Anticholinergics are useful in decreasing tremors related to Parkinson's disease. The major use of these agents currently is to treat drug-induced parkinsonism. Treatment should start with low dosages and then the dose should gradually be increased. Older adults are more susceptible to the many side effects of anticholinergics. Clients with memory loss or dementia should *not* be on anticholinergic therapy.

COMT, Catechol-O-methyltransferase; *MAO-B*, monoamine oxidase-B.

---

patholytics that inhibit the release of acetylcholine. Anticholinergics are still used to treat drug-induced parkinsonism, or pseudoparkinsonism, a side effect of the antipsychotic drug group phenothiazines. Examples of anticholinergics used for parkinsonism include trihexyphenidyl (Artane), benztropine (Cogentin), biperiden (Akineton), procyclidine (Kemadrin), ethopropazine (Parsidol), and orphenadrine (Norflex). The latter two drugs are the newest anticholinergics. Do not confuse Artane with Altace.

Diphenhydramine (Benadryl), an antihistamine, has similar anticholinergic properties. It is sometimes used to treat mild parkinsonism and for older adults who may not be able to tolerate levodopa or the dopamine agonist group of drugs.

Table 23-2 lists the anticholinergics and their dosages, uses, and considerations. Anticholinergics used to treat parkinsonism are also discussed in Chapter 18, Cholinergics and Anticholinergics.

Nursing Process

Antiparkinson: Anticholinergic Agent

ASSESSMENT

■ Obtain client's health history. Report if the client has a history of glaucoma, GI dysfunction, urinary retention, angina pectoris, or myasthenia gravis. All anticholinergics are contraindicated if the client has glaucoma.

■ Obtain a drug history. Report if a drug-drug interaction is probable. Phenothiazines, tricyclic antidepressants, and antihistamines increase the effect of trihexyphenidyl.

HERBAL ALERT 23-1

Orphenadrine Citrate

🌿 Valerian and kava kava potentiate sedation.

■ Assess baseline vital signs for future comparison. Pulse rate may increase.

■ Determine usual urinary output as a baseline for comparison. Urinary retention may occur with continuous use of anticholinergics.

NURSING DIAGNOSES

■ Impaired physical mobility
■ Risk for activity intolerance

PLANNING

■ Client will have decreased involuntary symptoms caused by parkinsonism or drug-induced parkinsonism.

NURSING INTERVENTIONS

■ Monitor vital signs, urine output, and bowel sounds. Increased pulse rate, urinary retention, and constipation are side effects of anticholinergics.
■ Observe for involuntary movements.

Client Teaching

General

• Advise client to avoid alcohol, cigarettes, caffeine, and aspirin to decrease gastric acidity.

Side Effects

• Suggest that client relieve dry mouth with hard candy, ice chips, or sugarless chewing gum. Anticholinergics decrease salivation.
• Suggest that client use sunglasses in direct sun because of possible photophobia.
• Advise client to void before taking the drug to minimize urinary retention. This is especially important if urine retention is present.
• Advise client who takes an anticholinergic to control symptoms of parkinsonism to have routine eye examinations to determine the presence of increased intraocular pressure, which indicates glaucoma. Clients who have glaucoma should *not* take anticholinergics.

Table 23–2

Antiparkinson Drugs: Anticholinergics

Generic (Brand)	Route and Dosage	Uses and Considerations
benztropine mesylate (Cogentin)	*Parkinsonism:* A: PO: Initially 0.5-1.0 mg/d in 1-2 divided doses (larger dose at bedtime); *maint:* 0.5-6 mg/d in 1-2 divided doses *Extrapyramidal syndrome:* A: PO: 1-4 mg/d in 1-2 divided doses IM/IV: 1-2 mg/d	For parkinsonism and drug-induced parkinsonism to reduce dystonia. May be taken with other antiparkinson drugs. Contraindicated in glaucoma, GI obstruction, severe ulcerative colitis, prostatic hypertrophy, myasthenia gravis. *Pregnancy category:* C; PB: UK; t½: UK
biperiden HCl (Akineton)	*Parkinsonism:* A: PO: 2 mg in 1-4 divided doses IM/IV: 2 mg every 30 min to 4 doses; *max:* 8 mg/d C: IM/IV: 0.04 mg/kg or 1.2 mg/m², repeat PRN	For parkinsonism and drug-induced parkinsonism (EPS). With prolonged use, drug tolerance may occur. Similar contraindications as benztropine. Avoid taking drug with alcohol or CNS depressants. Dry mouth, blurred vision, drowsiness, muscle weakness, and constipation may occur. *Pregnancy category:* C; PB: UK; t½: UK
ethopropazine HCl (Parsidol)	*Parkinsonism:* A: PO: Initially 50 mg daily/b.i.d.; *maint:* 100-400 mg/d in divided doses; *max:* 600 mg/d in divided doses	For all types of parkinsonism. A phenothiazine derivative with anticholinergic and antihistamine effects. Common side effects include dry mouth, drowsiness, dizziness, confusion, urinary retention, constipation. Contraindications: glaucoma, GU obstruction, prostatic hypertrophy. *Pregnancy category:* C; PB: UK; t½: UK
orphenadrine HCl or citrate (Disipal, Norflex, Banflex)	A: PO: 50 mg t.i.d. or 100 mg b.i.d.	For parkinsonism. It is an antihistamine with some anticholinergic effects. Has slight CNS stimulation and can cause euphoria. *Pregnancy category:* C; PB: UK; t½: 14 h
procyclidine HCl (Kemadrin)	*Parkinsonism:* A: PO: 2.5 mg pc t.i.d. *Extrapyramidal syndrome:* A: PO: Initially 2.5 mg p.c. t.i.d.; *maint:* 2.5-5 mg p.c. t.i.d.	For parkinsonism and drug-induced parkinsonism. Relieves rigidity more than tremors. May be taken with other antiparkinson drugs. Contraindicated in glaucoma. *Pregnancy category:* C; PB: UK; t½: UK
trihexyphenidyl HCl (Artane)	See Prototype Drug Chart 18–4.	

A, Adult; *b.i.d.,* two times a day; *C,* child; *CNS,* central nervous system; *d,* day; *EPS,* extrapyramidal symptoms; *GI,* gastrointestinal; *GU,* genitourinary; *h,* hour; *IM,* intramuscular; *IV,* intravenous; *min,* minute; *PB,* protein-binding; *p.c.,* after meals; *PO,* by mouth: *PRN,* as needed; *t½,* half-life; *t.i.d.,* three times a day; *UK,* unknown.

Diet
- Encourage client to ingest foods that are high in fiber and to increase fluid intake to prevent constipation.

Cultural Considerations
- Obtain an interpreter when necessary; do not rely on family members who may not fully disclose because of honor and shame.

EVALUATION

■ Evaluate client's response to trihexyphenidyl or benztropine mesylate to determine whether parkinsonism symptoms are controlled.

Dopaminergics

Levodopa

The first dopaminergic drug was levodopa (L-dopa), introduced in 1961. Levodopa is the most effective drug for diminishing the symptoms of Parkinson's disease. Its major benefit is increased mobility. Because dopamine cannot cross the blood-brain barrier, levodopa, a precursor of dopamine that *can* cross the blood-brain barrier, was developed. The enzyme dopa decarboxylase converts levodopa to dopamine in the brain. However, this enzyme is also found in the peripheral nervous system, thereby allowing 99% of levodopa to be converted to dopamine *before* it reaches the brain. Therefore about 1% of levodopa is converted to dopamine once it reaches the brain, large doses are needed to achieve a pharmacologic response. Because of these high doses, many side effects occur, including nausea, vomiting, dyskinesia, orthostatic hypotension, cardiac dysrhythmias, and psychosis. Levodopa has a short half-life (1 to 2 hours); therefore the drug is taken three to four times a day. The drug is initially administered in low doses for a week and then gradually increased over a period of weeks. It usually takes 2 to 4 months to achieve the drug's maximum effect.

Clients who have taken levodopa for 5 years or more may experience "on-off" fluctuations in its effectiveness. During the "on" time, the symptoms of parkinsonism are diminished or absent; however, symptoms return during the "off" time. As a result, the levodopa dose may need to be increased or a dopamine agonist or COMT inhibitor may be added to the levodopa regimen.

Carbidopa and Levodopa

Because of the side effects of levodopa and the fact that so much of the levodopa is metabolized before reaching the brain, an alternative drug, *carbidopa*, was developed to inhibit the enzyme dopa decarboxylase. By inhibiting the enzyme in the peripheral nervous system, more levodopa reaches the brain. The carbidopa is combined with levodopa in a ratio of 1 part carbidopa to 10 parts levodopa. Figure 23-1 illustrates the comparative action of levodopa and carbidopa-levodopa.

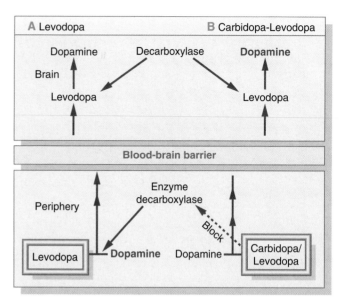

FIGURE 23–1 A, When levodopa is used alone, only 1% reaches the brain because 99% converts to dopamine while in the peripheral nervous system. **B,** By combining carbidopa with levodopa, carbidopa can inhibit the enzyme decarboxylase in the periphery, thereby allowing more levodopa to reach the brain.

The advantages of combining levodopa with carbidopa are the following:
- More dopamine reaches the basal ganglia.
- A single dose per day is administered instead of multiple doses.
- Smaller doses of levodopa are required to achieve the desired effect.

The disadvantage of the carbidopa-levodopa combination is that with more available levodopa, more side effects may be noted, including nausea, vomiting, **dystonic movement** (involuntary abnormal movement), and psychotic behavior. The peripheral side effects of levodopa are not as prevalent; however, cardiac dysrhythmia, palpitations, and orthostatic hypotension may occur. The carbidopa-levodopa combination is usually not used to treat drug-related parkinsonism. Prototype Drug Chart 23–1 lists the pharmacologic behavior of carbidopa-levodopa.

Nursing Process

Antiparkinson: Dopaminergic Agent: Carbidopa-Levodopa

ASSESSMENT

■ Obtain client's vital signs to use for future comparison.
■ Assess client for signs and symptoms of parkinsonism, including stooped forward posture, shuffling gait, masked facies, and resting tremors.
■ Obtain a history from client of glaucoma, heart disease, peptic ulcers, kidney or liver disease, and psychosis.

■ Report if drug-drug interaction is probable. Drugs that should be avoided or closely monitored are levodopa, bromocriptine, and anticholinergics.
■ Obtain a drug history.

NURSING DIAGNOSES

■ Impaired physical mobility
■ Risk for activity intolerance

PLANNING

■ Symptoms of parkinsonism will be decreased or absent after 1 to 4 weeks of drug therapy.

NURSING INTERVENTIONS

■ Monitor client's vital signs and electrocardiogram. Orthostatic hypotension may occur during early use of levodopa and bromocriptine. Instruct the client to rise slowly to avoid faintness.

■ Check for weakness, dizziness, or syncope, which are symptoms of orthostatic hypotension.
■ Administer carbidopa-levodopa (Sinemet) with low-protein foods. High-protein diets interfere with drug transport to the CNS.
■ Observe for symptoms of parkinsonism.

Client Teaching

General

● Advise client not to abruptly discontinue the medication. Rebound parkinsonism (increased symptoms of parkinsonism) can occur.
● Inform client that urine may be discolored and will darken with exposure to air. Perspiration also may be dark. Explain that both are harmless but that clothes may be stained.
● Advise client with diabetes that the blood sugar level should be checked with an OTC reagent strip (Hemastix or Chemstrip bG) and not done through

---

PROTOTYPE DRUG CHART 23–1

CARBIDOPA-LEVODOPA

Drug Class

Antiparkinson: dopaminergic
Trade Name: Sinemet
Pregnancy Category: C

Dosage

A: PO: 1:10 ratio; initially 10 carbidopa/100 levodopa
t.i.d.; *maint:* 25/250 mg t.i.d.

Contraindications

Narrow-angle glaucoma; severe cardiac, renal, or hepatic
  disease
Caution: Peptic ulcer, psychiatric disorders

Drug-Lab-Food Interactions

Drug: *Increase* hypertensive crisis with MAOIs
Decrease levodopa effect with anticholinergics, pheny-
  toin, tricyclic antidepressants, pyridoxine
Lab: May *increase* BUN, AST, ALT, ALP, LDH
Food: Avoid foods containing vitamin B_6 (pyridoxine)

Pharmacokinetics

Absorption: PO: Well absorbed
Distribution: PB: Carbidopa: 36%; levodopa: UK
Metabolism: $t\frac{1}{2}$: 1-2 h
Excretion: In urine as metabolites

Pharmacodynamics

PO: Onset: 15 min
  Peak: 1-3 h
  Duration: 5-12 h

Therapeutic Effects/Uses

To treat parkinsonism; to relieve tremors and rigidity
Mode of Action: Transmission of levodopa to brain cells for conversion to dopamine; carbidopa blocks the conversion
  of levodopa to dopamine in the peripheral nervous system

Side Effects

Anorexia, nausea, vomiting, dysphagia, fatigue, dizziness,
  headache, dry mouth, bitter taste, twitching, blurred
  vision, insomnia

Adverse Reactions

Involuntary choreiform movements, palpitations,
  orthostatic hypotension, urinary retention, psychosis,
  severe depression, hallucinations
Life-threatening: Agranulocytosis, hemolytic anemia,
  cardiac dysrhythmias, leukopenia

A, Adult; *ALP,* alkaline phosphatase; *ALT,* alanine aminotransferase; *AST,* aspartate aminotransferase; *BUN,* blood urea nitrogen;
h, hour; *LDH,* lactic dehydrogenase; *maint,* maintenance; *MAOIs,* monoamine oxidase inhibitors; *min,* minute; *PB,* protein-binding;
PO, by mouth; *t¹/₂,* half-life; *t.i.d.,* three times a day; *UK,* unknown.

urine testing. With Clinitest, a false-positive test result can occur; with Tes-Tape or Clinistix, a false-negative test result can occur.

Side Effects

- Instruct client to report side effects and symptoms of dyskinesia. Explain to client that it may take weeks or months before the symptoms are controlled.

Diet

- Suggest to client that taking levodopa with food may decrease GI upset; however, food will slow the drug absorption rate.
- Advise client to avoid vitamins that contain vitamin B_6 (pyridoxine) and foods rich in vitamin B_6, such as beans (lima, navy, kidney) and cereals.
- Advise client who takes high doses of selegiline to avoid foods high in tyramine, such as aged cheese, red wine, cream, yogurt, chocolate, bananas, and raisins. Encourage client to check with a dietitian regarding these foods.

Amantadine and Bromocriptine

- Suggest that client taking amantadine report any signs of skin lesions, seizures, or depression. A history of these health problems should have been previously reported to the health care provider.
- Advise client taking bromocriptine to report symptoms of lightheadedness when changing positions (a symptom of orthostatic hypotension).
- Advise client to avoid alcohol when taking bromocriptine.
- Teach client to check heart rate and to report changes in rate or irregularity. Client should know his or her baseline heart rate.
- Instruct client not to abruptly stop the drug without first notifying the health care provider. Any adverse reactions should be reported immediately.

Cultural Considerations 🕂

- Recognize that various cultural groups will need guidance in understanding the disease process of parkinsonism. Support client and family member who may be dismayed about the symptoms of parkinsonism and lack knowledge of the disease process.
- An interpreter may be needed for clients who speak little or no English to understand drug doses and schedules and to recognize severe side effects that need to be reported to the health care provider.

EVALUATION

- Evaluate the effectiveness of the drug therapy in controlling the symptoms of parkinsonism.
- Determine that there is an absence of side effects.

PREVENTING MEDICATION ERRORS

Do not confuse...

- **Symmetral** with **synthroid**.

- **Parlodel** with **pindolol**. These drug names look alike, but the pharmacology is different.

Dopamine Agonists

Other dopaminergics called **dopamine agonists** stimulate the dopamine receptors. For example, amantadine hydrochloride (Symmetrel) is an antiviral drug that acts on the dopamine receptors. It may be taken alone or in combination with levodopa or an anticholinergic drug. Initially, amantadine produces improvement in symptoms of parkinsonism in approximately two thirds of the clients; however, this improvement is usually not sustained because drug tolerance develops. Amantadine can also be used to treat drug-induced parkinsonism.

Bromocriptine mesylate (Parlodel) acts directly on the dopamine receptors in the central nervous system (CNS), cardiovascular system, and gastrointestinal (GI) tract. Bromocriptine is more effective than amantadine and the anticholinergics; however, it is not as effective as levodopa in alleviating parkinsonian symptoms. Clients who do not tolerate levodopa are frequently given bromocriptine. Bromocriptine may be given with levodopa or carbidopa-levodopa.

MAO-B Inhibitor

The enzyme monoamine oxidase-B (MAO-B) causes catabolism (breakdown) of dopamine. Selegiline inhibits MAO-B, thus prolonging the action of levodopa. It may be ordered for newly diagnosed clients with Parkinson's disease. The use of selegiline could delay levodopa therapy by a year. It decreases "on-off" fluctuations.

Large doses of selegiline may inhibit MAO-A, an enzyme that promotes the metabolism of tyramine in the GI tract. Ingestion of foods high in tyramine, such as aged cheese, red wine, and bananas, if they are not metabolized by MAO-A, can cause a hypertensive crisis. Severe adverse drug interactions can occur between selegiline and various tricyclic antidepressants (TCA) or selective serotonin reuptake inhibitors (SSRIs).

COMT Inhibitors

The enzyme catechol-O-methyltransferase (COMT) inactivates dopamine. When taken with a levodopa preparation, COMT inhibitors increase the amount of levodopa concentration in the brain. Tolcapone (Tasmar) was the first COMT inhibitor taken with levodopa for advanced Parkinson's disease. This drug can affect liver cell function; therefore serum liver enzymes should be closely moni-

Table 23-3

Antiparkinson: Dopaminergics

Generic (Brand)	Route and Dosage	Uses and Considerations
Dopaminergics		
carbidopa-levodopa (Sinemet) levodopa (or L-dopa) (Dopar, Larodopa)	See Prototype Drug Chart 23–1. A: PO: 0.5-1.0 g/d in 2-4 divided doses; increase dose gradually; average *maint*: 3-6 g/d with food, in divided doses; *max*: 8 mg/d	For parkinsonism. *Not* for drug-induced parkinsonism. Can cause GI upset; drug should be taken with food. Has many side effects, such as nausea, vomiting, orthostatic hypotension, cardiac dysrhythmias, and psychosis. *Pregnancy category*: C; PB: UK; t½: 1-3 h
Dopamine Agonists		
amantadine HCl; (Symmetrel)	*Parkinsonism:* A: PO: 100 mg b.i.d.; may increase dose; *max*: 400 mg/d	For early onset parkinsonism, drug-induced parkinsonism, and influenza A respiratory virus. Effective for rigidity and bradykinesia; less effective for decreasing tremors. May be used alone or in combination. Has fewer side effects than anticholinergic drugs. *Pregnancy category*: C; PB: 60%-70%; t½: 12-24 h
bromocriptine mesylate (Parlodel)	A: PO: Initially 1.25-2.5 mg/d; may gradually increase dose; *maint*: 30-60 mg/d in 3 divided doses; *max*: 100 mg/d	For parkinsonism. Response is better than amantadine. Can be taken in adjunct with levodopa or carbidopa-levodopa. Hypotension, lightheadedness, and syncope are major side effects. Initially, small doses are given and then gradually increased over several weeks. *Pregnancy category*: C; PB: 90%-96%; t½: 6-8 h; terminal phase: 50 h
pergolide mesylate (Permax)	A: PO: Initially 0.05 mg/d × 2 d; increase by 0.1-0.15 mg q3d × 12 d; *max*: 5 mg/d	For parkinsonism. Usually used as adjunct with levodopa or carbidopa-levodopa. It is more potent than bromocriptine. Same side effects as bromocriptine. *Pregnancy category*: B; PB: 90%; t½: UK
pramipexole dihydrochloride (Mirapex)	A: PO: Initially: 0.375 mg/d in 3 divided doses; *maint*: 1.5-4.5 mg/d in 3 divided doses	Stimulates dopamine receptors in striatum. *Pregnancy category*: C; PB: 15%; t½: 8-12 h
ropinirole HCl (Requip)	A: PO: Initially: 0.25 mg t.i.d.; *max*: 24 mg/d	Stimulates dopamine receptors in striatum. *Pregnancy category*: C; PB: 30%-40%; t½: 6 h
MAO-B Inhibitor		
selegiline HCl (Eldepryl)	A: PO: 10 mg/d in 2 divided doses	For early onset parkinsonism. May delay the use of levodopa therapy by 1 y. It can be given with levodopa preparations; dose of levodopa would need to be decreased. *Pregnancy category*: C; PB: >90%; t½: 2-20 h
COMT Inhibitors		
tolcapone (Tasmar)	A: PO: 50-200 mg t.i.d. Elderly: 50-100 mg t.i.d.	To potentiate dopamine activity by inhibiting the enzyme COMT. It is used in conjunction with levodopa-carbidopa (Sinemet) and prolongs the action of levodopa. *Pregnancy category*: UK; PB: 99%; t½: 2-3 h
entacapone (Comtan)	A: PO: 200 mg with each dose of levodopa-carbidopa; *max*: 2 g/d Elderly: same as adult	It is used in combination with levodopa-carbidopa. It prevents peripheral COMT; thus more levodopa reaches the brain. It prolongs the half-life of levodopa and decreases the "on-off" fluctuations. The levodopa dose should be decreased when it is taken with a COMT inhibitor. *Pregnancy category*: UK; PB: UK; t½: 1.5-3 h

A, Adult; *COMT*, catechol-O-methyltransferase; *d*, day; *GI*, gastrointestinal; *h*, hour; *max*, maximum; *PB*, protein-binding; *PO*, by mouth; *t½*, half-life; *t.i.d.*, three times a day; *UK*, unknown; >, greater than.

tored. Entacapone (Comtan), the newest COMT inhibitor approved by the Food and Drug Administration (FDA), does not affect liver function.

Table 23–3 lists dopaminergics, dopamine agonists, MAO-B inhibitor, and COMT inhibitors with their dosages, uses, and considerations.

Precautions for Drugs Used to Treat Parkinson's Disease

Side Effects and Adverse Reactions

The common side effects of anticholinergics include dry mouth and dry secretions, urinary retention, constipation, blurred vision, and an increase in pulse rate. Mental effects, such as restlessness and confusion, may occur in the older adult.

The side effects of levodopa are numerous. GI disturbances are common because dopamine stimulates the chemoreceptor trigger zone (CTZ) in the medulla, which stimulates the vomiting center. Taking the drug with food can decrease nausea and vomiting; however, food slows the absorption rate. **Dyskinesia** (impaired voluntary movement) may occur with high levodopa dosages. Cardiovascular side effects include orthostatic hypotension and increased heart rate during early use of levodopa. Cardiac dysrhythmias may occur as the levodopa dosages are increased. Psychosis (paranoia) and increased libido are additional side effects of increased levodopa dosages.

Amantadine has few side effects, but they can intensify when the drug is combined with other antiparkinson drugs. Orthostatic hypotension, confusion, urinary retention, and constipation are common side effects of amantadine.

Side effects from bromocriptine are more common than from amantadine. These include GI disturbances (nausea), orthostatic hypotension, palpitations, chest pain, edema in the lower extremities, nightmares, delusions, and confusion. If bromocriptine is taken with levodopa, usually the drug dosages are reduced and side effects and drug intolerance decrease.

Pramipexole (Mirapex) and ropinirole (Requip) can cause nausea, dizziness, somnolence, weakness, and constipation. These drugs intensify the dyskinesia and hallucination caused by levodopa. Do not confuse Mirapex with miraLax.

Large doses of selegiline (Eldepryl, Carbex) may inhibit MAO-A; thus hypertensive crisis might occur if foods high in tyramine, such as aged cheese, red wine, and bananas, are ingested.

Tolcapone (Tasmar) may cause severe liver damage. Clients with liver dysfunction should not take this drug. Entacapone (Comtan) is not known to affect liver function. With entacapone, the urine can be dark yellow to orange; with tolcapone, the urine can be bright yellow. Both tolcapone and entacapone can intensify the adverse reactions of levodopa (e.g., hallucinations, orthostatic hypotension, constipation, dizziness) because these drugs prolong the effect of levodopa.

Contraindications

Anticholinergics or any drugs that have anticholinergic effects are contraindicated for persons with glaucoma. Persons with severe cardiac, renal, or psychiatric health problems should avoid levodopa drugs because of adverse reactions. Clients with chronic obstructive lung diseases, such as emphysema, can have dry, thick mucous secretions caused by large doses of anticholinergic drugs.

Drug-Drug Interactions

Pyridoxine (vitamin B_6) increases dopa decarboxylase action, which metabolizes levodopa in the peripheral nervous system to dopamine. Foods rich in pyridoxine such as beans (lima, navy, kidney) and certain cereals therefore

Table 23–4

Prevalence of Alzheimer's Disease in the United States

Age (Years)	Percentage
45-65	2
65-74	3-5
75-84	19
>85	47

should be avoided. Antipsychotic drugs block the receptors for dopamine. Levodopa taken with a monoamine oxidase (MAO) inhibitor antidepressant can cause a hypertensive crisis.

Alzheimer's Disease

Alzheimer's disease is an incurable dementia illness characterized by chronic, progressive neurodegenerative conditions with marked cognitive dysfunction. The onset occurs between ages 45 and 65 (Table 23–4). It affects about four million Americans, and about 250,000 new cases are diagnosed annually. Approximately 50% of clients in nursing homes are admitted with Alzheimer's disease. This health problem is the fourth leading cause of death in adults. The annual cost for caring for clients with Alzheimer's disease is approximately $85 billion dollars.

Pathophysiology

Many physiologic changes contribute to Alzheimer's disease. Currently, the theories related to the changes that cause Alzheimer's disease include the following:

* Degeneration of the cholinergic neuron and deficiency in acetylcholine
* Neuritic plaques that form mainly outside the neurons and in the cerebral cortex
* Apolipoprotein E_4 (apo E_4) that promotes formation of neuritic plaques, which binds beta-amyloid in the plaques
* Beta-amyloid protein accumulation in high levels that may contribute to neuronal injury
* Presence of neurofibrillary tangles with twists inside the neurons

Figure 23–2 illustrates the normal neuron and the neuron affected by Alzheimer's disease. Other factors thought to influence the occurrence of Alzheimer's are genetic predisposition and a slow virus or infection that attacks brain cells.

Symptoms of Alzheimer's disease progress from confusion to memory loss to dementia (Table 23–5). With loss of memory, loss of logical thinking and judgment and time disorientation occur. As the disease progresses, memory loss becomes more severe; personality changes occur; and hyperactivity, hostility, paranoia, tendency to wander, and the inability to speak or express oneself result. Custodial care becomes necessary.

A Normal

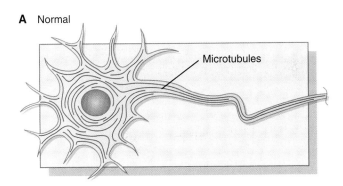

B Alzheimer's Disease

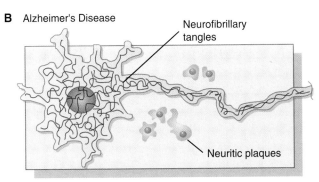

FIGURE 23-2 Histologic changes in Alzheimer's disease. **A,** Healthy neuron. **B,** Neuron affected by Alzheimer's disease showing characteristic neuritic plaques and cellular neurofibrillary tangles. (Modified from Lehne RA: *Pharmacology for nursing care,* ed 5, Philadelphia, 2004, Saunders.)

Acetylcholinesterase Inhibitors/ Cholinesterase Inhibitors

There are no known medications to cure Alzheimer's disease. The FDA has approved four medications to treat Alzheimer's disease: ergoloid mesylate (Hydergine), which has not been very successful for treating memory loss, and three AChE inhibitors. The AChE inhibitors are (1) tacrine (Cognex); (2) donepezil (Aricept); and (3) rivastigmine (Exelon), a new drug that permits more acetylcholine in the neuron receptors. Rivastigmine has effective penetration into the CNS; thus cholinergic transmission is increased. These AChE inhibitors increase cognitive function for clients with mild to moderate Alzheimer's disease.

Several drugs for treating Alzheimer's disease are under investigation. Some of these are certain nonsteroidal anti-inflammatory drugs (piroxicam, indomethacin), calcium channel blockers, MAO-B inhibitor (selegiline), serotonin antagonists, CNS stimulants (methylphenidate [Ritalin]), angiotensin-converting enzyme (ACE) inhibitors, and Vitamin E.

Tacrine

Tacrine (Cognex), an AChE inhibitor, is prescribed to improve cognitive function for clients with mild to moderate Alzheimer's disease (Prototype Drug Chart 23-2). This drug increases the amount of ACh at the cholinergic synapses. Tacrine tends to slow the disease process. Only 30% of clients have an effective response to tacrine, and even for those it has a short-lasting effect. Table 23-6 lists the drugs used to treat Alzheimer's disease. Do not confuse Cognex with Corgard.

Pharmacokinetics

Tacrine is absorbed faster through the GI tract without food. Because it has a relatively short half-life, tacrine is given four times a day, and the dose is gradually increased. The protein-binding power is average.

Pharmacodynamics

Tacrine has been somewhat successful in improving memory in the early phase of Alzheimer's disease. The onset of action is 0.5 to 1.5 hours; peak action is 2 hours. However, the duration of action is prolonged to 24 to 36 hours; thus side effects should be closely monitored. This drug is contraindicated for clients with liver disease because hepatotoxicity may occur. Cumulative drug effect is likely to occur in older adults and in clients with liver and renal dysfunction.

Table 23-5

Stages and Phases of Alzheimer's Disease

Stage	Clinical Phase	Symptoms
1	Mild (early confusion)	Early cognitive decline in one or more areas, memory loss, decreased ability to function in work situation, name-finding deficit, some decrease in social functioning, recall difficulties, anxiety
2	Moderate	Unable to perform complex tasks such as managing personal finances or planning a dinner party; unable to concentrate; no knowledge of current events
3	Moderately severe (early dementia)	Usually needs assistance for survival; need reminders to bathe, help in selecting clothes, and other daily functions; may be disoriented as to time and recent events although this can fluctuate; may become tearful
4	Severe (dementia)	Needs assistance with dressing, bathing, and toilet functions (e.g., flushing); may forget spouse, family, and caregivers' names, details of their personal life; generally unaware of their surroundings; incontinence of urine and feces may occur in this stage; increase in central nervous system disturbances such as agitation, delusions, paranoia, obsessive anxiety, and increased potential for violent behavior
5	Very severe (late dementia)	Unable to speak (speech limited to five words or less), person may scream or make other sounds; unable to ambulate, sit up, smile, or feed self; unable to hold head erect, will ultimately slip into stupor or coma

Data from McKenry LM, Salerno E: *Pharmacology in nursing,* ed 20, St Louis, 1998, Mosby, p. 469.

PROTOTYPE DRUG CHART 23–2

TACRINE

Drug Class	**Dosage**
Acetylcholinesterase inhibitor Trade Name: Cognex *Pregnancy Category:* C	**A: PO:** Initially: 10 mg q.i.d.; after 6 wk: 20 mg q.i.d.; after 12 wk: 30 mg q.i.d.; after 16 wk: 40 mg q.i.d.; *max:* 160 mg/d
Contraindications	**Drug-Lab-Food Interactions**
Liver and renal diseases	*Drug:* *Increase* effect of theophylline *Increase* effect with cimetidine *Lab:* *Increase* ALT, AST
Pharmacokinetics	**Pharmacodynamics**
Absorption: PO: Food decreases absorption rate **Distribution:** PB: 50% **Metabolism:** t½: 3 h **Excretion:** In urine	**PO:** Onset: 0.5 h Peak: 2 h Duration: 24-36 h
Therapeutic Effects/Uses	
Improves memory loss **Mode of Action:** Elevates acetylcholine concentration	
Side Effects	**Adverse Reactions**
Anorexia, nausea, vomiting, diarrhea, dizziness, headache, constipation, rhinitis, depression	**Life threatening:** Hepatotoxicity

A, Adult; *ALT,* alanine aminotransferase; *AST,* aspartate aminotransferase; *d,* day; *h,* hour; *max,* maximum; *PB,* protein-binding; *PO,*
by mouth; *q.i.d.,* four times a day; *t½,* half-life.

Table 23–6

Acetylcholinesterase (AChE) Inhibitors for Alzheimer's Disease

Generic (Brand)	Route and Dosage	Uses and Considerations
donepezil (Aricept)	A: PO: 5-10 mg/d	AChE inhibitor. To treat mild to moderate phase of Alzheimer's disease. *Pregnancy category:* C; PB: 90%; t½: 70 h
ergoloid mesylates (Hydergine)	A: PO: Initially, 1 mg	To increase cognitive function. The actual improvement is uncertain. *Pregnancy category:* C; PB: UK; t½: 3.5 h
rivastigmine (Exelon)	A: PO: Initial dose: 1.5 mg, b.i.d.; increase every 2 wk PRN; *max:* 6 mg b.i.d.	AChE inhibitor, To treat mild to moderate Alzheimer's disease. GI upset is common adverse effect. Weight loss may be a problem. This drug is not considered to cause hepatotoxicity. *Pregnancy category:* B; PB: UK; t½: 1.5 h
tacrine HCl (Cognex)	See Prototype Drug Chart 23–3.	
memantine (Namenda)	A: PO: 5 mg/d, may increase dose in 5 mg increments every week to 20 mg/d	Neurotransmitter inhibitor. To treat mild to severe Alzheimer's disease. *Pregnancy category:* B; PB: 45%; t½: 60-80 h
galantamine (Razadyne)	A: PO: 4 mg/twice daily, may increase 4 mg every 4 wk if well tolerated to 12 mg twice daily	Cholinesterase inhibitor. To treat mild to moderate dementia of Alzheimer's disease. *Pregnancy category:* B; PB: 18%; t½: 7 h

A, Adult; *b.i.d.,* twice a day; *d,* day; *GI,* gastrointestinal; *h,* hour; *max,* maximum; *PB,* protein-binding; *PO,* by mouth; *t½,* half-life; *UK,* unknown, *wk,* week.

Nursing Process

Drug Treatment for Alzheimer's Disease: Tacrine

ASSESSMENT

■ Record client's mental and physical abilities. Note limitation of cognitive function and self-care.
■ Obtain a history of liver or renal disease or dysfunction.
■ Assess for memory and judgment losses. Elicit from family members a history of behavioral changes, such as memory loss, declining interest in people or home, difficulty in following through with simple activities, and tendency to wander from home.
■ Observe for signs of behavioral disturbances such as hyperactivity, hostility, and wandering.
■ Check for signs of aphasia or difficulty in speech.
■ Note client's motor function.
■ Determine family members' ability to cope with client's mental and physical changes.

NURSING DIAGNOSES

■ Disturbed thought processes
■ Impaired physical mobility
■ Self-care deficit: dressing, feeding, toileting
■ Chronic confusion
■ Compromised family processes
■ Compromised family coping
■ Risk for injury
■ Imbalanced nutrition: less than body requirement

PLANNING

■ Client's loss of memory will proceed slower with the medication AChE inhibitor than without medication.
■ Client can maintain self-care of body functions with assistance.

NURSING INTERVENTIONS

■ Maintain consistency in care.
■ Assist client in ambulation and activity.
■ Check for side effects related to the continuous use of AChE inhibitors.
■ Record vital signs periodically. Note signs of bradycardia and hypotension.
■ Monitor client's behavioral changes and record improvement or decline.

Client Teaching

General

• Explain to client and family members the purpose for the prescribed drug therapy.
• Teach the time for drug dosing and the schedule for increasing drug dosing to the family member responsible for client's medications.
• Instruct the family member in techniques, such as placing obstacles away from client's foot path, so that client can avoid injury from wandering.
• Inform the family member of support groups that are available, such as Alzheimer's Disease and Related Disorders Association.

Side Effects

• Inform client and family member that client should rise slowly to avoid dizziness and loss of balance.

Diet

• Instruct family member about foods that may be prepared for client's consumption and tolerance.

Cultural Considerations

• Recognize that various cultural groups may need guidance in understanding the disease process of Alzheimer's disease.
• Explain to family members from various cultural backgrounds that their family member is not "crazy" but has a neurologic problem that may be part of the aging process. Explain how the symptoms may become more progressive.

EVALUATION

■ Evaluate the effectiveness of drug regimen by determining whether client's mental and physical status shows improvement from drug therapy.

WEBSITES

For further information on *Drugs for Neurologic Disorders*, visit these Internet resources:

Information on tacrine: *http://www.nlm.nih.gov/ medlineplus/druginfo/medmaster/a693039.html*

Critical Thinking Case Study

T.R., age 79, was diagnosed with Parkinson's disease 10 years ago. During his early treatment, he took levodopa. The drug dosage was increased to alleviate symptoms.

1. How does levodopa alleviate symptoms of parkinsonism?

2. What assessments should be made before and during the time T.R. takes levodopa?

Because T.R. developed numerous side effects and adverse reactions to levodopa, the health care provider changed the drug to carbidopa-levodopa (Sinemet). T.R. asks the nurse why the drug was changed.

3. What are the similarities and differences between levodopa and Sinemet? What would be an appropriate response to T.R.'s question about changing the drug for parkinsonism?

4. How does the dose for carbidopa-levodopa differ from that for levodopa? What are the advantages of carbidopa-levodopa?

T.R.'s family says they know a person with Parkinson's disease who takes the antiviral drug amantadine (Symmetrel). The family asks whether Symmetrel is the same as Sinemet and, if so, should T.R. take that drug instead of a drug containing levodopa.

5. What is the effect of amantadine on symptoms of parkinsonism?

6. What would be an appropriate response to the family's question concerning the use of Symmetrel for T.R.?

7. What are the uses for dopamine agonists and COMT inhibitors?

8. Certain anticholinergic drugs may be used to control parkinsonism symptoms. What is the action of these drugs and what are their side effects? These anticholinergic drugs are usually prescribed for parkinsonism symptoms resulting from what?

Study Questions

1. A 66-year-old man was recently diagnosed with Parkinson's disease. What are four physical characteristics associated with parkinsonism?

2. This same client was instructed to take 250 mg of levodopa three times a day. At what time of the day should the drug be taken? What are three side effects of the drug? Why should vitamin B_6 (pyridoxine) be avoided in foods and vitamin supplements?

3. Because of this client's side effects, the drug therapy was changed to bromocriptine. How do these two drugs differ? Explain.

4. Selected anticholinergics are prescribed to treat Parkinson's disease. What are the side effects of anticholinergics? What are their effects on symptoms of parkinsonism?

5. What is the action of COMT inhibitors? Give an example of a COMT inhibitor.

6. Why would levodopa and/or carbidopa be combined with an MAO-B inhibitor or COMT inhibitor for the treatment of parkinsonism?

7. AChE inhibitors are currently used to treat Alzheimer's disease. For what purpose are these agents used in the treatment of Alzheimer's disease, and how effective are they? What other drugs are being considered for treating Alzheimer's disease?

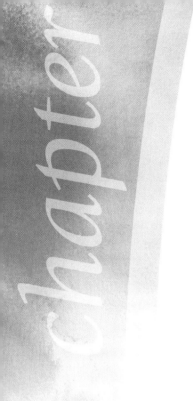

24 Drugs for Neuromuscular Disorders: Myasthenia Gravis, Multiple Sclerosis, and Muscle Spasms

ELECTRONIC RESOURCES

Additional information can be found on the companion website at *http://evolve.elsevier.com/KeeHayes/pharmacology/* or on the companion CD-ROM, which includes:

- *NCLEX-style examination review questions*
- *Pharmacology animations*
- *Medication error and IV therapy checklists*
- *Medication calculation problems*
- *Electronic calculators*

OBJECTIVES

- Define myasthenia gravis, multiple sclerosis, and muscle spasm.
- Identify the drug group used to treat myasthenia gravis.
- Explain the treatment strategies for multiple sclerosis.
- Differentiate between the muscle relaxants used for spasticity and those used for muscle spasms. Give an example of one drug used to treat spasticity and one drug used to treat general muscle spasms.
- Describe the nursing interventions, including client teaching, for drugs used in the treatment of myasthenia gravis and muscle spasms.

TERMS

acetylcholinesterase (AChE) inhibitor	cholinergic crisis	muscle relaxants	myasthenia crisis
	multiple sclerosis (MS)	muscle spasms	myasthenia gravis (MG)

Introduction

Myasthenia gravis (MG), a lack of nerve impulses and muscle responses at the myoneural (nerves in muscle endings) junction, causes fatigue and muscular weakness of the respiratory system, facial muscles, and extremities. Because of cranial nerve involvement, ptosis (drooping eyelid) and difficulty in chewing and swallowing occur. Respiratory arrest may result from respiratory muscle paralysis. MG is caused by an inadequate secretion of acetylcholine (ACh) or a loss of ACh because of an increase in the enzyme acetylcholinesterase, which destroys ACh at the myoneural junction.

The neuromuscular disorder **multiple sclerosis (MS)** attacks the myelin sheath of nerve fibers, causing lesions known as *plaques*. MS is difficult to diagnose; therefore pharmacologic treatment is necessary to control the symptoms of this disorder.

Muscle spasms have various causes, including injury or motor neuron disorders, resulting in conditions such as cerebral palsy, MS, spinal cord injuries (paraplegia [paralysis of the legs]), cerebral vascular accident (stroke), or hemiplegia (paralysis of one side of the body). Spasticity of muscles can be reduced with the use of skeletal **muscle relaxants.**

Myasthenia Gravis

Myasthenia gravis (MG) is mainly caused by an autoimmune disease that affects approximately 1 in 10,000 persons. MG can occur at any age; however, it occurs more commonly in women younger than 30 years and men older than 50. It is not a genetic disorder, but there can be a familial tendency.

Pathophysiology

MG results from a lack of acetylcholine (ACh) reaching the cholinergic receptors. This disorder involves an antibody response against an alpha subunit of the acetylcholine receptor (AChR) site in the skeletal muscle. Antibodies attack AChR sites, thus inhibiting normal neuromuscular transmission. The response leads to a degradation of the AChRs. Anti-acetylcholine antibodies accumulate at the neuromuscular synapse. About 90% of clients with MG have anti-acetylcholine antibodies that can be detected through serum testing. It has also been determined that clients with MG have about one third as many AChRs as normal, causing fewer binding sites for acetylcholine. The result is ineffective muscle contraction.

The thymus gland is involved in systemic immunity that is active during infancy and early childhood, but the gland shrinks during adulthood. Approximately 60% of MG clients have thymic hyperplasia. It has been suggested in some cases that if the thymus gland is removed during the early onset of MG, clinical symptoms are greatly decreased. Thymectomy has been an option for clients younger than 50 years of age.

Another theory for the cause of MG is that the decrease in acetylcholine is caused by the enzyme acetylcholinesterase (AChE) destroying the acetylcholine.

MG is characterized by weakness and fatigue of the skeletal muscles. Other characteristics of MG include muscle weakness, dysphagia, dysarthria, and respiratory muscle weakness. Early symptoms of MG are ptosis and diplopia.

The group of drugs used to control MG is the AChE inhibitors, also called *cholinesterase inhibitors* and *anticholinesterase*, which inhibit the action of the enzyme. As a result of this action, more acetylcholine activates the cholinergic receptors and promotes muscle contraction. The AChE inhibitors are classified as parasympathomimetics.

If muscle weakness persists after taking AChE inhibitors, the reason may be inadequate drug dosing. The client may be experiencing **myasthenia crisis.** If the muscle weakness remains untreated, death could result from paralysis of the respiratory muscle. Neostigmine, a fast-acting AChE inhibitor, can relieve myasthenia crisis. Overdosing with AChE inhibitors may cause **cholinergic crisis,** which is an acute exacerbation of symptoms. Cholinergic crisis results in severe muscle weakness, which can lead to respiratory paralysis and arrest.

Acetylcholinesterase Inhibitors/ Cholinesterase Inhibitors

The first drug used to manage MG was neostigmine (Prostigmin). It is a short-acting **acetylcholinesterase (AChE) inhibitor** with a half-life of 0.5 to 1 hour. The drug is given every 2 to 4 hours and must be given on time to prevent muscle weakness. The AChE inhibitor pyridostigmine bromide (Mestinon) has an intermediate action and is given every 3 to 6 hours. Ambenonium chloride (Mytelase) is a long-acting AChE inhibitor and is usually prescribed when the client does not respond to neostigmine or pyridostigmine. Prototype Drug Chart 24–1 presents drug data related to pyridostigmine. Table 24–1 lists the AChE inhibitors. The cholinesterase (AChE) inhibitors are discussed in Chapter 23, Drugs for Neurologic Disorders: Parkinsonism and Alzheimer's Disease.

Pharmacokinetics

Pyridostigmine is poorly absorbed from the GI tract. Half of the sustained-release capsule is absorbed readily, but the balance is poorly absorbed. The half-life of oral pyridostigmine is 3.5 to 4 hours; when given intravenously (IV), it is 2 hours. Because of its short half-life, pyridostigmine must be administered several times a day. The drug is metabolized by the liver and excreted in the urine.

Pharmacodynamics

Pyridostigmine increases muscle strength of clients with muscular weakness resulting from MG. The onset of action of oral preparations is 0.5 to 1 hour. The duration of action is longer with the sustained-release drug capsule. One thirtieth of the oral dose of pyridostigmine can be administered IV. Over-

PROTOTYPE DRUG CHART 24–1

PYRIDOSTIGMINE BROMIDE

Drug Class	**Dosage**
Cholinesterase inhibitor	A: PO: 60-120 mg t.i.d./q.i.d.; *max:* 1.5 g/d
Trade Name: Mestinon	SR: 180-540 mg q.d. or b.i.d.
Pregnancy Category: C	IM/IV: 2 mg q2-3h
	C: PO: 7 mg/kg/d in 5-6 divided doses
Contraindications	**Drug-Lab-Food Interactions**
GI and GU obstruction, severe renal disease	*Drug: Decrease* pyridostigmine effect with atropine,
Caution: Asthma, bradycardia, peptic ulcer, cardiac	muscle relaxants, antidysrhythmics, magnesium
dysrhythmias, pregnancy	
Pharmacokinetics	**Pharmacodynamics**
Absorption: PO: Poorly absorbed; SR: 50% absorbed	**PO:** Onset: 30-45 min
Distribution: PB: UK	Peak: UK
Metabolism: $t^{1}/_{2}$: PO: 3.5-4 h; IV: 2 h	Duration: 3-6 h
Excretion: In urine and by liver	**PO SR:** Onset: 0.5-1 h
	Peak: UK
	Duration: 6-12 h
	IM: Onset: 15 min
	Peak: UK
	Duration: 2-4 h
	IV: Onset: 2-5 min
	Peak: UK
	Duration: 2-3 h

Therapeutic Effects/Uses

To control and treat myasthenia gravis
Mode of Action: Transmission of neuromuscular impulses by preventing the destruction of acetylcholine

Side Effects	**Adverse Reactions**
Nausea, vomiting, diarrhea, headache, dizziness,	Hypotension, urticaria
abdominal cramps, sweating, rash, miosis	**Life-threatening:** Respiratory depression, bronchospasm,
	cardiac dysrhythmias, seizures

A, Adult; *ALP*, alkaline phosphatase; *ALT*, alanine aminotransferase; *AST*, aspartate aminotransferase; *b.i.d.*, twice a day; *BUN*, blood urea nitrogen; *C*, child; *d*, day; *GI*, gastrointestinal; *GU*, genitourinary; *h*, hour; *IM*, intramuscular; *IV*, intravenous; *LDH*, lactic dehydrogenase; *MAOIs*, monoamine oxidase inhibitors; *max*, maximum; *min*, minute; *PB*, protein-binding; *PO*, by mouth; *q.i.d.*, four times a day; *SR*, sustained-release; $t^{1}/_{2}$, half-life; *t.i.d.*, three times a day; *UK*, unknown.

dosing of pyridostigmine can result in signs and symptoms of **cholinergic crisis** (extreme muscle weakness; increased salivation, tears, sweating; miosis); thus the antidote, atropine sulfate, should be available. This crisis requires emergency medical intervention due to respiratory muscle weakness.

Clients who do not respond to AChE inhibitors may require prednisone or immunosuppressive drugs. Prednisone decreases MG symptoms and promotes remission; however, long-term use can cause adverse effects (see Chapter 48, Drugs for Dermatologic Disorders).

The immunosuppressive agent azathioprine (Imuran) can be used in conjunction with a lower dose of prednisone. With azathioprine, the white blood count (WBC) and liver enzymes should be closely monitored to avoid leukopenia and hepatotoxicity.

Overdosing and underdosing of AChE inhibitors have similar symptoms, such as muscle weakness, dyspnea (difficulty breathing), and dysphagia (difficulty swallowing). Ad-

ditional symptoms that may be present with overdosing are increased salivation (drooling), bradycardia, abdominal cramping, and increased tearing and sweating. All doses of AChE inhibitors should be administered *on time* because late administration of the drug could result in muscle weakness.

Underdosing can result in myasthenia crisis, and overdosing can result in cholinergic crisis. Edrophonium chloride (Tensilon) is a very short-acting AChE inhibitor that may be used to distinguish between myasthenia crisis and cholinergic crisis. These two different crises have a similar major symptom: severe muscle weakness. After edrophonium is administered, if the symptoms are alleviated because of an increase in ACh, the cause is myasthenia crisis. However, if the muscle weakness becomes more severe, the cause is cholinergic crisis caused by drug overdosing.

Edrophonium may also be used to diagnose MG. Its ultra-short duration of 5 to 20 minutes increases muscle

Table 24–1

Acetylcholinesterase (AChE) Inhibitors: Myasthenia Gravis

Generic (Brand)	Route and Dosage	Uses and Considerations
ambenonium (Mytelase)	A: PO: 2.5-5.0 mg t.i.d./q.i.d.; dose may be increased; *maint:* 5-40 mg t.i.d./q.i.d.	For myasthenia gravis. A long-acting AChE inhibitor. It is 6 times more potent than neostigmine. Frequently used when client cannot take neostigmine or pyridostigmine because of the bromide component. It can be taken in adjunct with glucocorticoid drug. *Pregnancy category:* C; PB: UK; t½: UK
edrophonium Cl (Tensilon)	A: IV 2 mg; then 8 mg if no response IM: 10 mg; may repeat with 2 mg in 30 min C: <34 kg: IV: 1 mg, repeat in 30-45 sec if no response; *max:* 5 mg C: >34 kg: IV: 2 mg, repeat with 1 mg if no response; *max:* 10 mg	For diagnosing myasthenia gravis. Ptosis should be absent in 1-5 min. Very short-acting drug. *Pregnancy category:* C; PB: UK; t½: 1.2-2 h
neostigmine bromide (Prostigmin) neostigmine methylsulfate (injectable form)	A: PO: 15-30 mg in 3-4 divided doses; *maint:* 150 mg/d in divided doses; *range:* 15-375 mg/d IM/IV: 0.5-2.5 mg PRN C: PO: 2 mg/kg/d in divided doses or 10 mg/m² q4h	For controlling myasthenia gravis. Must be given on time to prevent myasthenia crisis. Parenteral route is used if chewing, swallowing, and breathing are affected. Because of its short half-life, dose is usually given in 3 to 6 divided doses. Overdose can cause cholinergic reaction; nausea, abdominal cramps, excessive salivation, sweating. *Pregnancy category:* C; PB: 15%-25%; t½: 1-1.5 h
pyridostigmine bromide (Mestinon)	See Prototype Drug Chart 24–2.	

A, Adult; *C,* child; *d,* day; *h,* hour; *IM,* intramuscular; *IV,* intravenous; *PB,* protein-binding; *PO,* by mouth; *PRN,* as needed; *q.i.d.,* four times a day; *t½,* half-life; *t.i.d.,* three times a day; *UK,* unknown; <, less than; >, greater than.

strength immediately. If ptosis (droopy eyelids) is immediately corrected after administration of this drug, the diagnosis is most likely MG. Table 24–4 lists the AChE inhibitors.

Side Effects and Adverse Reactions

Side effects and adverse reactions of AChE inhibitors include GI disturbances (nausea, vomiting, diarrhea, abdominal cramps), increased salivation and tearing, miosis (constricted pupil of the eye), and possible hypertension.

Nursing Process

Drug Treatment for Myasthenia Gravis: Pyridostigmine (Mestinon)

ASSESSMENT

■ Obtain a drug history of drugs that the client currently takes. Report if a drug-drug interaction is likely. The client should avoid atropine, atropine-like drugs, and muscle relaxants.
■ Record baseline vital signs for future comparison.
■ Assess client for signs and symptoms of myasthenia crisis, such as muscle weakness with difficulty breathing and swallowing.

NURSING DIAGNOSES

■ Ineffective breathing pattern
■ Risk for activity intolerance
■ Anxiety related to possible recurrence of myasthenia crisis

PLANNING

■ Client's symptoms of muscle weakness and difficulty breathing and swallowing caused by myasthenia gravis will be eliminated or reduced in 2 to 3 days.

NURSING INTERVENTIONS

■ Monitor the effectiveness of drug therapy (acetylcholinesterase [AChE] inhibitors). Muscle strength should be increased. Both depth and rate of respirations should be assessed and maintained within normal range.
■ Administer pyridostigmine IV undiluted at rate of 0.5 mg/min. Do *not* add the drug to IV fluids.
■ Observe client for signs and symptoms of cholinergic crisis caused by overdosing, including muscle weakness; increased salivation, sweating, tearing; and miosis.
■ Have readily available an antidote for cholinergic crisis (atropine sulfate).

Client Teaching

General
- Instruct client to take the drugs as prescribed to avoid recurrence of symptoms.
- Encourage the client to wear a medical identification bracelet or necklace (e.g., MedicAlert) that indicates the health problem and the drugs taken.

Side Effects
- Advise client to report to the health care provider recurrence of symptoms of myasthenia gravis. Drug therapy may need to be modified.

Diet
- Inform client to take the drug before meals for best drug absorption. If gastric irritation occurs, take the drug with food.

Cultural Considerations ⊕
- Use simple and clear instructions. Ask family members to assist with translation only if an interpreter is not available. Do not use compound sentences.
- Many ethnocultural groups from countries outside the United States, and some people from within the United States as well, may be accustomed to not taking all of their medications as ordered, or they may use medicines prescribed for other people. Stress that medications need to be taken as prescribed; medications are ordered specifically for each ailment; unused drugs should be discarded; and the use of medications by individuals other than the intended may have serious consequences.

EVALUATION

- Evaluate the effectiveness of the drug therapy. Muscle strength should be maintained.
- Determine the absence of respiratory distress.

Multiple Sclerosis

Multiple sclerosis (MS) is an autoimmune disorder that attacks the myelin sheath of nerve fibers in the brain and spinal cord, causing lesions that are called *plaques*. In the United States MS affects approximately 300,000 persons (ages 20 to 40), mostly white women. It is uncommon in African and Asian populations. Onset of MS is usually slow. It is a condition in which there are remissions and exacerbations of multiple symptoms (sensory and cerebellar), such as diplopia, weakness in the extremities, or spasticity. MS is difficult to diagnose because there is no specific diagnostic test. Available laboratory tests that may suggest MS include elevated immunoglobulin G (IgG) in the cerebrospinal fluid, increased IgG/albumin ratio, and multiple lesions observable through magnetic resonance imaging (MRI). A study cited by Noronha and Arnason states that monthly MRI scans of clients with MS can readily identify new lesions before clients have clinical symptoms; however, this can be costly. Scheduling regular treatment protocols to avoid clinical MS attacks is not recommended because of the side effects of the drugs used, such as glucocorticoids.

There are treatment strategies for three types or phases of MS: the acute attack, remission-exacerbation, and chronic progressive MS. Table 24–2 describes these three

Table 24–2

Treatment Strategies for the Three Phases of Multiple Sclerosis

Phases of Multiple Sclerosis	Characteristics	Treatment Strategies

Acute attack	Fatigue; motor weakness; optic neuritis	• Tapering course of glucocorticoids (prednisone)
		• Adrenocorticotropic hormone (ACTH) stimulates the adrenal cortex to secrete cortisol
		• ACTH can be given IM or IV:
		  (1) Aqueous ACTH, 80 units in 500 ml of D_5W for 1-5 d
		  (2) Tapering doses of ACTH gel, IM for 25-30 d, starting with 40 units, b.i.d.
		• 6-alpha methylprednisolone sodium succinate (MP):
		  (1) MP 1 g/d, IV, for 5-7 d
		  (2) Tapering doses of oral glucocorticoid

Remission-exacerbation	Recurrence of clinical MS symptoms; spasticity	• Biologic (immune) response modifiers (BRM); see Chapter 37. Betaseron, an interferon-β (IFN-β), 0.25 mg (8 mIU) every other day. It reduces spasticity and improves muscle movement. Also, interferon β-1a includes Rebif (given subQ in doses of 44 mcg 3 times per week) and Avonex (given IM in doses of 30 mcg every week), used in relapsing forms of MS. • Immunosuppressant drug azathioprine (Imuran). Reduces exacerbation (relapses). Used for MS to decrease steroid use.

Chronic progressive	Progressive MS symptoms (wheelchair bound)	• Immunosuppressant cyclophosphamide (Cytoxan)
		Possible treatment protocol:
		  (1) Cytoxan 600 mg/m² in 250 ml of D_5W, every other day × 5 doses. Monitor WBC values.
		  (2) ACTH, tapering doses for 14 d. Starting with 40 units, IM, b.i.d.

b.i.d., Twice a day; *d,* day; *IM,* intramuscular; *IV,* intravenous; *WBC,* white blood count.

phases. Goals for treatment strategies are to decrease the inflammatory process of nerve fibers and to improve conduction of demyelinating axons.

Various drug regimens for treating MS are currently in research and development. It is known, however, that clients with MS avoid the following drugs: (1) histamine (H_2) blockers, such as cimetidine and ranitidine; (2) indomethacin (a nonsteroidal antiinflammatory drug [NSAID]); and (3) beta-blockers, such as propranolol.

Skeletal Muscle Relaxants

Muscle relaxants relieve muscular spasms and pain associated with traumatic injuries and spasticity from chronic debilitating disorders (e.g., MS, strokes [cerebrovascular accident], cerebral palsy, head and spinal cord injuries). Spasticity results from increased muscle tone from hyperexcitable neurons caused by increased stimulation from the cerebral neurons or lack of inhibition in the spinal cord or at the skeletal muscles. The centrally acting muscle relaxants depress neuron activity in the spinal cord or brain and act directly on the skeletal muscles.

Centrally Acting Muscle Relaxants

The mechanism of action of centrally acting muscle relaxants is not fully known. Centrally acting muscle relaxants are used for spasticity to suppress hyperactive reflex and for muscle spasms that do not respond to antiinflammatory agents, physical therapy, or other forms of therapy. The centrally acting muscle relaxants are described in Table 24–3. Prototype Drug Chart 24–2 gives the drug data for the centrally acting muscle relaxant carisoprodol (Soma).

Spasticity

Skeletal muscle spasticity is muscular hyperactivity that causes contraction of the muscles, resulting in pain and limited mobility. Centrally acting muscle relaxants act on the spinal cord. Examples of centrally acting muscle relaxants used to treat spasticity are baclofen (Lioresal), dantrolene (Dantrium), and tizanidine (Zanaflex). Diazepam (Valium), a benzodiazepine, has also been effective for treating spasticity.

Muscle Spasms

Various centrally acting muscle relaxants are used for muscle spasm to decrease pain and increase range of motion. They have a sedative effect and should not be taken concurrently with CNS depressants such as barbiturates, nar-

PREVENTING MEDICATION ERRORS

Do not confuse...

• **baclofen** (skeletal muscle relaxant) with **Bactroban** (topical antibacterial) or **Beclovent** (corticosteroid inhalant). These drug names look alike, but the actions and pharmacology are very different.

---

cotics, and alcohol. These agents, with the exception of cyclobenzaprine, can cause drug dependence. In addition, dizziness and drowsiness are common side effects. Examples of this group of centrally acting muscle relaxants are carisoprodol (Soma), chlorphenesin carbamate (Maolate), chlorzoxazone (Paraflex), cyclobenzaprine (Flexeril), metaxalone (Skelaxin), methocarbamol (Robaxin), and orphenadrine citrate (Norflex).

Pharmacokinetics

Carisoprodol is well absorbed from the GI tract, and its half-life is moderate. The protein-binding percentage for carisoprodol is unknown. Carisoprodol is metabolized in the liver and excreted in the urine.

Pharmacodynamics

Carisoprodol alleviates muscle spasm associated with acute painful musculoskeletal conditions. When carisoprodol is taken with alcohol, sedative-hypnotics, barbiturates, or tricyclic antidepressants (TCAs), increased central nervous system (CNS) depression occurs. The onset of action, peak concentration time, and duration of action for carisoprodol is short.

Side Effects and Adverse Reactions

The side effects from centrally acting muscle relaxants include drowsiness; dizziness; lightheadedness; headaches; and occasional nausea, vomiting, diarrhea, and abdominal distress. Cyclobenzaprine and orphenadrine have anticholinergic effects.

Nursing Process

Muscle Relaxant: Carisoprodol

ASSESSMENT

■ Collect medical history. Carisoprodol is contraindicated if client has severe renal or liver disease.
■ Obtain baseline vital signs for future comparison.
■ Secure client's health history to identify the cause of muscle spasm and to determine whether it is acute or chronic.
■ Gather a drug history. Report if a drug-drug interaction is probable.
■ Note if there is a history of narrow-angle glaucoma or myasthenia gravis. Cyclobenzaprine and orphenadrine are contraindicated with these health problems.

NURSING DIAGNOSES

■ Impaired physical mobility
■ Activity intolerance

Table 24–3

Muscle Relaxants (Skeletal)

Generic (Brand)	Route and Dosage	Uses and Considerations
Anxiolytics		
diazepam (Valium) CSS IV	A: PO: 2-10 mg b.i.d./q.i.d. IM/IV: 5-10 mg; may repeat	Diazepam has many uses, one of which is to relieve muscle spasms associated with paraplegia and cerebral palsy. Contraindicated in narrow-angle glaucoma. *Pregnancy category:* D; PB: 98%; t½: 20-50 h
meprobamate (Equanil, Miltown) CSS IV	A: PO: 400 mg-1.2 g/d in divided doses	This anxiolytic has a muscle relaxant effect. *Pregnancy category:* D; PB: UK; t½: 10-12 h
Muscle Relaxants		
Spasticity (Centrally Acting)		
baclofen (Lioresal)	A: PO: Initially 5 mg t.i.d.; may increase dose; *maint:* 10-20 mg t.i.d./q.i.d.; *max:* 80 mg/d	For muscle spasms caused by MS and spinal cord injury. Overdose may cause CNS depression. Drowsiness, dizziness, nausea, hypotension may occur. *Pregnancy category:* C; PB: 30%; t½: 3-4 h
tizanidine (Zanaflex)	A: PO: 4 mg q6-8h; adjust dose by 2 mg PRN; *max:* single dose of 12 mg	To manage spasticity especially for spinal cord injury and multiple sclerosis. *Pregnancy category:* C; PB: UK; t½: 2.5 h (half-life is longer for metabolites)
Spasticity (Direct Acting)		
dantrolene sodium (Dantrium)	A: PO: Initially 25 mg/d; increase gradually; *maint:* 100 mg b.i.d.-q.i.d. C: PO: Initially 0.5 mg/kg b.i.d.; increase dose gradually by 0.5 mg/kg t.i.d./q.i.d.; *max:* 100 mg q.i.d.	For chronic neurologic disorders causing spasms such as spinal cord injuries, stroke, MS. Start with low doses and increase every 4 to 7 d. Avoid taking with alcohol and CNS depressants. *Pregnancy category:* C; PB: 95%; t½: 8 h
Centrally Acting Muscle Relaxants		
carisoprodol (Soma)	See Prototype Drug Chart 24–4.	
chlorzoxazone (Paraflex, Parafon forte)	A: PO: 250-500 mg t.i.d./q.i.d.; *max:* 3 g/d C: PO: 20 mg/kg/d or 600 mg m²/d in 3-4 divided doses	For acute or severe muscle spasms. Not effective for cerebral palsy. Take with food to decrease GI upset. *Pregnancy category:* C; PB: UK; t½: 1 h
cyclobenzaprine HCl (Flexeril, Cycoflex)	A: PO: 10 mg t.i.d.; may increase dose; *maint:* 20-40 mg/d in 2-4 divided doses; *max:* 60 mg/d	For short-term treatment of muscle spasms. Not effective for relieving cerebral or spinal cord disease. Take with food or milk to decrease GI upset. *Pregnancy category:* B; PB: 93%; t½: 1-3 d
methocarbamol (Robaxin, Marbaxin)	A: PO: Initially 1.5 g q.i.d.; *maint:* 1 g q.i.d. IM/IV: 0.5-1 g q8h; *max:* 3 g/d	For acute muscle spasms; drug used for treatment of tetanus. Has CNS depressant effects (sedation). Avoid taking alcohol or CNS depressants. Urine may be green, brown, or black. Drowsiness that may occur usually decreases with continued drug use. *Pregnancy category:* C; PB: UK; t½: 1-2 h
orphenadrine citrate (Norflex, Flexon)	A: PO: 100 mg b.i.d. IM/IV: 60 mg; may repeat in 12 h	For acute muscle spasm. It can be toxic with a mild overdose. Used in combination with aspirin and caffeine (Norgesic). *Pregnancy category:* C; PB: <20%; t½: 14 h
Depolarizing Muscle Relaxants (Adjunct to Anesthesia)		
pancuronium bromide (Pavulon)	A: IV: 0.04-0.1 mg/kg; then 0.01 mg/kg every 30-60 min PRN C: >10 y: same as for adult	Used in surgery for relaxation of skeletal muscle (e.g., abdominal wall). It is considered to be five times as potent as tubocurarine chloride. It does not cause hypotension or bronchospasm. *Pregnancy category:* C; PB: <10%; t½: 2 h
succinylcholine Cl (Anectine Cl, Quelicin, Sucostrin)	A: IM: 2.5-4 mg/kg; *max:* 150 mg; IV: 0.3-1.1 mg/kg; *max:* 150 mg C: IM/IV: 1-2 mg/kg; *max:* IM: 150 mg	Used in surgery with anesthesia for skeletal muscle relaxation. Also used in endoscopy and intubation. *Pregnancy category:* C; PB: UK; t½: UK
vecuronium bromide (Norcuron)	A & C > 9 y: IV: Initially 0.04-0.1 mg/kg/dose, then 0.05-0.1 mg/kg/h PRN	Use is similar as succinylcholine chloride. It can be used for clients with asthma, renal disease, or limited cardiac reserve. Given after general anesthesia has been started. *Pregnancy category:* C; PB: 60%-80%; t½: 0.5-1.5 h
tubocurarine Cl	*Anesthesia intubation:* A: IV: Initially: 6-9 mg, followed by 3-4.5 mg in 3-5 min if needed C: IV: 0.2-0.5 mg/kg	Adjunct to general anesthesia. To induce skeletal muscle relaxation. *Pregnancy category:* C; PB: UK; t½: 1-3 h

A, adult; *b.i.d.,* twice a day; *C,* child; *CNS,* central nervous system; *CSS,* Controlled Substances Schedule; *d,* day; *GI,* gastrointestinal; *h,* hour; *IM,* intramuscular; *IV,* intravenous; *MS,* multiple sclerosis; *PB,* protein-binding; *PO,* by mouth; *PRN,* as needed; *q.i.d.,* four times a day; *t½,* half-life; *t.i.d.,* three times a day; *UK,* unknown; *y,* year; >, greater than; <, less than.

PLANNING

■ Client will be free of muscular pain within 1 week.

NURSING INTERVENTIONS

■ Monitor serum liver enzyme levels of clients taking dantrolene and carisoprodol. Report elevated levels of liver enzymes, such as alkaline phosphatase (ALP), alanine aminotransferase (ALT), and gamma-glutamyl transferase (GGT).
■ Record vital signs. Report abnormal results.
■ Observe for CNS side effects (e.g., dizziness).

Client Teaching

General
* Instruct client that the muscle relaxant should not be abruptly stopped. Drug should be tapered over 1 week to avoid rebound spasms.
* Advise the client not to drive or operate dangerous machinery when taking muscle relaxants. These drugs have a sedative effect and can cause drowsiness.
* Inform client that most of the centrally acting muscle relaxants for acute spasms are usually taken for no longer than 3 weeks.

* Teach client to avoid alcohol and CNS depressants. If muscle relaxants are taken with these drugs, CNS depression may be intensified.
* Warn client that these drugs are contraindicated for pregnant women or nursing mothers. Check with the health care provider.

Side Effects
* Tell client to report side effects of the muscle relaxant, such as nausea, vomiting, dizziness, faintness, headache, and diplopia. Dizziness and faintness are most likely caused by orthostatic (postural) hypotension.

Diet
* Educate the client to take muscle relaxants with food to decrease gastrointestinal upset.

Cultural Considerations ⊕
* When offering a prescription, instructions, or pamphlets to Asian and Pacific Islanders, use both hands, which shows respect.

EVALUATION

■ Evaluate the effectiveness of the muscle relaxant to determine whether the client's muscular pain has decreased or disappeared.

PROTOTYPE DRUG CHART 24–2

CARISOPRODOL

Drug Class

Centrally acting muscle relaxants
Trade Name: Soma, Soprodol
Pregnancy Category: C

Dosage

A: PO: 350 mg t.i.d. at bedtime
C: >5y: PO 25 mg/kg/d in 4 divided doses

Contraindications

Severe liver or renal disease

Drug-Lab-Food Interactions

Drug: Increase CNS depression with alcohol, narcotics, sedative-hypnotics, antihistamines, tricyclic antidepressants
May *increase* risk of ventricular fibrillation with calcium channel blockers

Pharmacokinetics

Absorption: PO: Well absorbed
Distribution: PB: UK
Metabolism: $t_{1/2}$: 8 h
Excretion: In urine

Pharmacodynamics

PO: Onset: 30 min
   Peak: 3-4 h
   Duration: 4-6 h

Therapeutic Effects/Uses

To relax skeletal muscles. Baclofen, dantrolene, and tizanidine are used to treat spasticity associated with stroke, spinal cord injury, multiple sclerosis, cerebral palsy
Mode of Action: Blocks interneuronal activity.

Side Effects

Nausea, vomiting, dizziness, weakness, insomnia

Adverse Reactions

Asthmatic attack, tachycardia, hypotension, diplopia

A, Adult; *C,* child; *CNS,* central nervous system; *d,* day; *h,* hour; *min,* minute; *PB,* protein-binding; *PO,* by mouth; $t_{1/2}$, half-life; *t.i.d.,* three times a day; *UK,* unknown; >, greater than.

WEBSITES

For further information on *Drugs for Neuromuscular Disorders,* visit these Internet resources:

Information on pyridostigmine:
*http://www.nlm.nih.gov/medlineplus/druginfo/
medmaster/a682229.html*

Critical Thinking Case Study

F.R., age 29, was diagnosed with myasthenia gravis 2 years ago. She is managed with pyridostigmine 120 m t.i.d. Last evening an automobile accident prevented F.R. from getting home from work. She was taken to the emergency room unconscious and missed two evening does of pyridostigmine.

1. How does pyridostigmine alleviate the symptoms of myasthenia gravis?

2. What are the potential side effects and adverse effects of pyridostigmine?

3. What problems are likely to develop following delayed pyridostigmine dosing?

F.R. is scheduled for surgery to repair a fractured femur, which was acquired in the accident. During surgery F.R. develops bradycardia.

4. What medications may lead to drug interactions with pyridostigmine?

5. What problems may develop from pyridostigmine overdosing?

6. What are the similarities between myasthenia crisis and cholinergic crisis?

Study Questions

1. A 56 year-old male was recently diagnosed with myasthenia gravis. What medications are used in the treatment of myasthenia gravis? What is the action of these medications?

2. What client teaching should be included concerning drug compliance and drug-dose intervals?

3. The client with multiple sclerosis has muscle spasms. What are two muscle relaxants used to reduce spasticity?

4. Which medications should be avoided for the client with multiple sclerosis?

5. Identify the different types of muscle relaxants with examples of each.

6. Centrally acting muscle relaxants are used for the treatment of what conditions? What is the major side effect of this group of drugs?

7. What client teaching should be included for the client taking carisoprodol?

8. What side effects and adverse effects should the client report when taking carisoprodol?

Seven

Psychiatric Agents

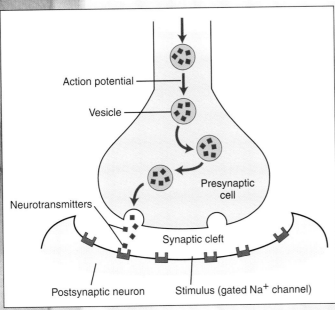

Action potential

Vesicle

Neurotransmitters

Presynaptic cell

Synaptic cleft

Postsynaptic neuron

Stimulus (gated Na$^+$ channel)

People normally experience moods and emotions such as excitement, anxiety, and depression. However, *pathology* may develop when moods and emotions become extreme. This imbalance may affect the performance of daily activities, perception of reality, ability to carry out responsibilities, fulfillment of work requirements, and establishment of interpersonal relationships.

From moods and emotions flow the various thoughts, feelings, and actions of individuals, which are communicated throughout the central nervous system (CNS) by chemical neurotransmitters. An impulse is communicated by traveling through the presynaptic neuron across the synaptic cleft and binding to a receptor on the postsynaptic neuron, as illustrated in the figure.

Neurotransmitters (chemicals in the body) are synthesized in the cytoplasm in the presynaptic neuron and stored in vesicles. The vesicle safeguards neurotransmitters from being destroyed by enzymes. When an impulse arrives by way of an action potential at a presynaptic neuron, vesicles are triggered to move to the cell membrane wall and release the transmitter into the synaptic cleft.

Neurotransmitters function with the help of receptors, which are embedded in the membrane of the postsynaptic neuron. Receptors are configured in size and shape to interlock with specific transmitters. Immediately upon connection of neurotransmitters to receptors, an action is exerted and the transmitter is removed. Once released, transmitters can be broken down into inactive substances by enzymes, diffused away from the synapse into intracellular fluid, or returned to the presynaptic neuron in a process called *reuptake*.

The major neurotransmitters affecting psychopathology include gamma-aminobutyric acid (GABA), serotonin, dopamine, norepinephrine, and acetylcholine. The GABA neurotransmitter is associated with the regulation of anxiety. When the level of GABA neurotransmitters is reduced, anxiety disorders may result. Benzodiazepines (antianxiety drugs) act by binding to a GABA receptor site making the postsynaptic receptor more sensitive to GABA and its neurotransmission. This connection decreases signs and symptoms of anxiety.

Serotonin neurotransmission is associated with arousal and general activity levels of the CNS. Serotonin functions to regulate sleep, wakefulness, and mood, as well as the delusions, hallucinations, and withdrawal of schizophrenia. Antidepressants block the reuptake of serotonin into the presynaptic neuron. A structurally specific drug is more likely to affect only the specific receptors for which it is intended and not the receptors specific for other neurochemicals, which would produce unintended effects or side effects. Selective serotonin reuptake inhibitor (SSRI) drugs are specific and generally produce fewer side effects in the treatment of depression than older antidepressants such as monamine oxidase inhibitors (MAOIs).

Dopamine-containing neurons are thought to be involved in regulation of cognition, emotional responses, and motivation, and dopamine neurotransmitters are associated with schizophrenia and other psychoses. Antipsychotic drugs block dopamine receptors in the postsynaptic neuron.

Norepinephrine is associated with control of arousal, attention, vigilance, mood, affect, and anxiety. This transmitter is involved with thinking, planning, and interpreting. Tricyclic antidepressants block the reuptake of norepinephrine into the presynaptic neuron and effectively treat depressive disorders. MAOIs inactivate norepinephrine, dopamine, and serotonin by inhibiting the monoamine oxidase enzyme to relieve signs and symptoms of depression.

Acetylcholine plays a role in sleep and wakefulness. Alzheimer's disease is associated with a reduction of acetylcholine.

A faulty release, reuptake, or elimination of neurotransmitters may lead to an imbalance of neurotransmission and pathology. Mental disorders can then develop, which affect an individual's thoughts, feelings, and behaviors.

Knowledge of psychopharmacology is essential to psychiatric mental health nursing. A basic understanding of the actions of psychotropic drugs will help nurses rapidly comprehend and apply information and enhance the effectiveness of pharmacologic treatment. Essential responsibilities of the psychiatric mental health nurse in administering psychotropic medications are to assess behavior, monitor for side effects, and educate the client and family. These actions are crucial to successful psychopharmacologic therapy.

This unit discusses drugs used to treat psychoses and anxiety in Chapter 25, Antipsychotics and Anxiolytics. Antidepressants and mood stabilizers are discussed in Chapter 26, Antidepressants and Mood Stabilizers.

25 Antipsychotics and Anxiolytics

ELECTRONIC RESOURCES

Additional information can be found on the companion website at *http://evolve.elsevier.com/KeeHayes/pharmacology/* or on the companion CD-ROM, which includes:

- *NCLEX-style examination review questions*
- *Pharmacology animations*
- *Medication error and IV therapy checklists*
- *Medication calculation problems*
- *Electronic calculators*

OBJECTIVES

- Differentiate between the two groups of drugs: antipsychotics and anxiolytics.
- Differentiate between the traditional/typical and the atypical antipsychotics.
- Name the general side effects associated with antipsychotics (typical and atypical) and anxiolytics.
- Give the nursing interventions, including client teaching, for antipsychotics and anxiolytics.

TERMS

acute dystonia
akathisia
antiemetic
antipsychotics
anxiolytics
atypical antipsychotics
blood dyscrasias
dopamine

dystonia
extrapyramidal symptoms (EPS)/extrapyramidal reactions
neuroleptic
neuroleptic malignant syndrome
orthostatic hypotension

parkinsonism
phenothiazines
psychosis
schizophrenia
tardive dyskinesia
typical antipsychotics

Introduction

This chapter discusses the CNS depressants antipsychotics and anxiolytics, which are used to manage symptoms of psychosis and anxiety disorders. Antipsychotics are also known as *neuroleptics* or *psychotropics*. The preferred name for this group is either antipsychotics or neuroleptics. **Neuroleptic** refers to any drug that modifies psychotic behavior thus exerting an antipsychotic effect. Anxiolytics are also called *antianxiety drugs* or *sedative-hypnotics*. Certain anxiolytics are used to treat sleep disorders, seizures, and withdrawal symptoms from alcohol intoxication. Some of these drugs are also used for conscious sedation and anesthesia supplement. However, the anxiolytics described in this chapter are used specifically to treat anxiety.

Psychosis

Psychosis is symptomatic in a variety of mental or psychiatric disorders. Psychosis is usually characterized by more than one symptom, such as difficulty in processing information and coming to a conclusion, delusions, hallucinations, incoherence, catatonia, and aggressive or violent behavior. **Schizophrenia,** a chronic psychotic disorder, is the major category of psychosis in which many of these symptoms are manifested.

Schizophrenia usually occurs in adolescence or early adulthood. The symptoms of this psychotic disorder are divided into two groups: those with positive symptoms and those with negative symptoms. The positive symptoms may be characterized by exaggeration of normal function (e.g., agitation), incoherent speech, hallucination, delusion, and paranoia. The negative symptoms are characterized by a decrease or loss in function and motivation. There is a poverty of speech content, poor self-care, and social withdrawal. The negative symptoms tend to be more chronic and persistent. The typical or traditional group of antipsychotics is more helpful for managing positive symptoms than the negative symptoms. Since 1984 a new group of antipsychotics, called *atypical,* have been found to be more useful in treating both the positive and negative symptoms of schizophrenia.

Antipsychotics comprise the largest group of drugs used to treat mental illness. Specifically, these drugs improve the thought processes and behavior of clients with psychotic symptoms, especially those with schizophrenia and other psychotic disorders. They are not used to treat anxiety or depression. The theory is that psychotic symptoms result from an imbalance in the neurotransmitter **dopamine** in the brain. Sometimes these antipsychotics are called *dopamine antagonists.* Antipsychotics block D_2 dopamine receptors in the brain, thereby reducing the psychotic symptoms. Many of the antipsychotics block the chemoreceptor trigger zone and vomiting (emetic) center in the brain, producing an **antiemetic** effect. By blocking dopamine, **extrapyramidal symptoms (EPS)/extrapyramidal reactions** of **parkinsonism,** such as tremors, masklike facies, rigidity, and shuffling gait, may occur. Many clients who take high-potency antipsychotic drugs may require long-term medication for parkinsonian symptoms.

Antipsychotic Agents

Antipsychotics are divided into two major categories: *typical* (or *traditional*) and *atypical.* The **typical antipsychotics,** introduced in 1952, are subdivided into phenothiazines and nonphenothiazines, which include butyrophenones, dibenzoxazepines, dihydroindolones, and thioxanthenes. The phenothiazines and thioxanthenes block norepinephrine, causing sedative and hypotensive effects early in treatment. The butyrophenones block only the neurotransmitter dopamine.

The second category of antipsychotics is the atypical agents. Clozapine, discovered in the 1960s and made available in Europe in 1971, was the first atypical antipsychotic agent. It was not marketed in the United States until 1990 because of adverse hematologic reactions. Atypical antipsychotics are effective for treating schizophrenia and other psychotic disorders for clients who do not respond to or are intolerant of typical antipsychotics. Because of the decreased side effects, atypical antipsychotics may be used as first-line therapy instead of traditional typical antipsychotics.

Pharmacophysiologic Mechanisms of Action

Antipsychotics block the actions of dopamine and thus may be classified as dopaminergic antagonists. There are five subtypes of dopamine receptors: D_1 through D_5. All antipsychotics block the D_2 (dopaminergic) receptor, which in turn promotes the presence of EPS, resulting in pseudoparkinsonism. The atypical antipsychotics have a weak affinity for D_2 receptors and a stronger affinity to D_4 receptors, and they block the serotonin receptor. These agents cause fewer EPS than the typical (phenothiazines) antipsychotic agents, which have a strong affinity to the D_2 receptors.

Adverse Reactions

Extrapyramidal Syndrome

Pseudoparkinsonism, which resembles symptoms of Parkinson's disease, is a major side effect of typical antipsychotic drugs. Symptoms of pseudoparkinsonism or EPS include stooped posture, masklike facies, rigidity, tremors at rest, shuffling gait, pill-rolling motion of the hand, and bradykinesia. When clients take high-potency typical antipsychotic drugs, these symptoms are more pronounced. Clients who take low-strength antipsychotics, such as chlorpromazine (Thorazine), are not as likely to have symptoms of pseudoparkinsonism as those who take fluphenazine (Prolixin).

During early treatment with typical antipsychotic agents for schizophrenia and other psychotic disorders, two adverse extrapyramidal reactions that may occur are **acute dystonia** and **akathisia. Tardive dyskinesia** is a later phase of extrapyramidal reaction to antipsychotics. Use of anticholinergic drugs helps to decrease pseudoparkinsonism symptoms and the symptoms of acute dystonia and akathisia. They have little effect for alleviating tardive dyskinesia.

The symptoms of *acute dystonia* usually occur in 5% of clients within days of taking typical antipsychotics. Characteristics of the reaction include muscle spasms of face, tongue, neck, and back; facial grimacing; abnormal or involuntary upward eye movement; and laryngeal spasms that can impair respiration. This condition is treated with anticholinergic/antiparkinsonism drugs, such as benztropine (Cogentin). The benzodiazepine lorazepam (Ativan) may also be prescribed.

Incidence of *akathisia* occurs in approximately 20% of clients who take a typical antipsychotic drug. With this reaction, the client has trouble standing still. The client is restless, paces the floor, and is in constant motion (e.g., rocks back and forth). This condition is best treated with a benzodiazepine (e.g., lorazepam) or a beta-blocker (e.g., propranolol).

Tardive dyskinesia is a serious adverse reaction occurring in clients who have taken a typical antipsychotic drug for more than a year. The prevalence for developing tardive dyskinesia depends on the dose and duration of the antipsychotic factor. Characteristics of tardive dyskinesia include protrusion and rolling of the tongue, sucking and smacking movements of the lips, chewing motion, and involuntary movement of the body and extremities. In older adults, these reactions are more frequent and severe. The antipsychotic drug should be stopped in all who experience tardive dyskinesia. Other benzodiazepines, calcium channel blockers, or beta-blockers are helpful in some cases in decreasing tardive dyskinesia. No one agent is effective for all clients. High doses of vitamin E may be helpful, and its use to treat tardive dyskinesia is currently under investigation. Clozapine has also been effective for treating tardive dyskinesia. Figure 25–1 shows the characteristics of pseudoparkinsonism, acute dystonia, akathisia, and tardive dyskinesia.

Neuroleptic Malignant Syndrome

Neuroleptic malignant syndrome (NMS) is a rare but potentially fatal condition that is associated with antipsychotic drugs. NMS symptoms involve muscle rigidity, sudden high fever, altered mental status, blood pressure fluctuations, tachycardia, dysrhythmias, seizures, rhabdomyolysis, acute renal failure, respiratory failure, and coma. Treatment of NMS involves immediate withdrawal of antipsychotics, adequate hydration, hypothermic blankets, and administration of antipyretics, benzodiazepines, and muscle relaxants, such as dantrolene (Dantrium).

Phenothiazines

In 1952 chlorpromazine hydrochloride (Thorazine) was the first phenothiazine introduced for treating psychotic behavior in clients in psychiatric hospitals. The **phenothiazines** are subdivided into three groups: aliphatic, piperazine, and piperidine, which differ mostly in their side effects.

The *aliphatic phenothiazines* produce a strong sedative effect, decreased blood pressure, and may cause moderate EPS (pseudoparkinsonism). Chlorpromazine (Thorazine) is in the aliphatic group and may produce pronounced **orthostatic hypotension**.

The *piperazine phenothiazines* produce a low sedative and a strong antiemetic effect, and they have little effect on blood pressure. They also cause more EPS than the other phenothiazines. Examples of piperazine phenothiazines include fluphenazine (Prolixin) and perphenazine (Trilafon).

The *piperidine phenothiazines* have a strong sedative effect, cause few EPS, have a low to moderate effect on blood pressure, and have no antiemetic effect. Thioridazine (Mellaril)

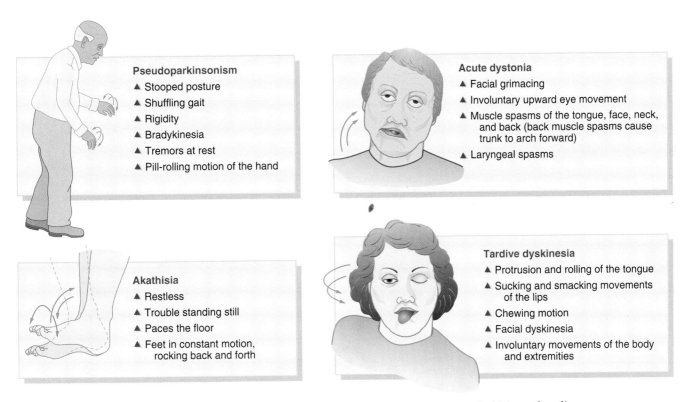

FIGURE 25–1 Characteristics of pseudoparkinsonism, acute dystonia, akathisia, and tardive dyskinesia.

and mesoridazine (Serentil) are examples of piperidine phenothiazines. Mesoridazine is a metabolite of thioridazine. Table 25–1 summarizes the effects of the phenothiazines.

Most antipsychotics can be given orally (tablet or liquid), intramuscularly (IM), or intravenously (IV). For oral use, the liquid form might be preferred because some clients hide tablets to avoid taking them. In addition, the absorption rate is faster with the liquid form. The peak serum drug level occurs in 2 to 3 hours. The antipsychotics are highly protein bound (>90%), and the excretion of the drug and its metabolites is slow. The drug is metabolized by the liver enzymes to phenothiazine metabolites. The metabolites can be detected in the urine several months after the medication has been discontinued. Phenothiazine metabolites may cause a harmless pinkish to red-brown urine color. The *full* therapeutic effects of antipsychotics may not be evident for 3 to 6 weeks following initiation of therapy; however, an observable therapeutic response may be apparent after 7 to 10 days.

Noncompliance with antipsychotics is common. Many ethnocultural groups from countries outside the United States, and some people from within the United States as well, may be accustomed to not taking all of their medications as ordered or use medicines prescribed for other people. Encourage the client to take the medication as prescribed. Also, explain and reexplain essential information to compensate for client's knowledge deficit or language limitations.

Prototype Drug Chart 25–1 illustrates the drug characteristics of fluphenazine (Prolixin), a phenothiazine antipsychotic used to manage psychosis.

Pharmacokinetics

The oral absorption of fluphenazine is rapid and is not affected by food. This drug is strongly protein bound and has a long half-life; therefore, the drug may accumulate. Fluphenazine is metabolized by the liver, crosses the blood-brain barrier and placenta, and is excreted as metabolites primarily in the urine. With hepatic dysfunction, the phenothiazine dose may need to be decreased because of lack of drug metabolism in the liver thus causing an elevation in drug level.

Pharmacodynamics

Fluphenazine is prescribed primarily for psychotic disorders. This drug has anticholinergic properties and should be cautiously administered to clients with glaucoma, especially narrow-angle glaucoma. Because hypotension is a side effect of these phenothiazines, any antihypertensives that are simultaneously administered can cause an additive hypotensive effect. Narcotics and sedative-hypnotics administered simultaneously with these phenothiazines can cause an additive CNS depression. Antacids decrease the absorption rate of both drugs and all phenothiazines; therefore they should be given 1 hour before or 2 hours after administering a phenothiazine.

The onset of action for fluphenazine hydrochloride is 1 hour, with a duration rate of 6 to 8 hours. Fluphenazine decanoate has delayed absorption with the onset of action 24 to 72 hours and duration of 1 to 6 weeks.

Nonphenothiazines

The many groups of nonphenothiazine antipsychotics include butyrophenone, dibenzoxazepines, dihydroindolone, and thioxanthene.

In the *butyrophenone* group, a frequently prescribed nonphenothiazine is haloperidol (Haldol), whose pharmacologic behavior is similar to that of the phenothiazines. Haloperidol is a potent antipsychotic drug in which the equivalent prescribed dose is smaller than drugs of lower potency (e.g., chlorpromazine). The drug dose for haloperidol is 0.5 to 5 mg, whereas the drug dose for chlorpromazine is 10 to 25 mg. Long-acting preparations, such as haloperidol decanoate (Haldol) and fluphenazine decanoate (Prolixin), are given for slow release via injection every 2 to 4 weeks. Administration precautions should be taken to prevent soreness and inflam-

---

HERBAL ALERT 25-1

Antipsychotic Agents

🍃 Kava kava may increase the risk and severity of dystonic reactions when taken with phenothiazines.
🍃 Kava kava may increase the risk and severity of dystonia when taken concurrently with fluphenazine.

Table 25–1

Effects of Phenothiazines (Varies Within Class)

Group	Sedation	Hypotension	EPS	Antiemetic
Aliphatic chlorpromazine and triflupromazine	+++	+++	++	++ / +++
Piperazine	++	+	+++	+++
Piperidine	+++	+++	+	—
Nonphenothiazines haloperidol	+	+	+++	++
loxapine	++	++	+++	—
molindone	+/++	+	+++	—
thiothixene	+	+	+++	—
Atypical antipsychotics risperidone	+	+	+/0	—

—, No effect; +, mild effect; ++, moderate effect; +++, severe effect; *EPS*, extrapyramidal symptoms.

PROTOTYPE DRUG CHART 25–1

FLUPHENAZINE

Drug Class	**Dosage**
Antipsychotic (neuroleptic)	*Psychoses*
Fluphenazine: piperazine phenothiazine	**A: PO:** 0.5-10 mg/d
Trade names:	*Max:* 20 mg/d
Prolixin, Permitil, 🍁 Moditen HCl	**IM/subQ:** HCl 2.5-10 mg/d q6-8h
Pregnancy Category: C	*Max:* 10 mg/d
	Elderly: 1-2.5 mg/d
	Decanoate 12.5-25 mg q1-4wk
Contraindications	**Drug-Lab-Food Interactions**
Hypersensitivity, subcortical brain damage, blood dyscrasias, renal or liver damage, coma	***Drug:*** Increase depressive effects when taken with alcohol or other CNS depressants
	Food: Kava kava may increase dystonia
Pharmacokinetics	**Pharmacodynamics**
Absorption: Rapidly absorbed	**PO: HCl:** Onset: 1 h
Distribution: PB 90%	Peak: 0.5 h
Metabolism: t½ 5-15 h	Duration: 6-8 h
Excretion: In urine	**IM:** Peak: 1.5-2 h
	IM: Decanoate: Onset: 24-72 h
	Duration: 1-6 wk

Therapeutic Effects/Uses

To manage symptoms of psychosis including schizophrenia
Mode of Action: Blocks dopamine receptors in the brain and controls psychotic symptoms.

Side Effects	**Adverse Reactions**
Sedation, dizziness, headache, dry mouth, nasal congestion, blurred vision, photosensitivity, nausea, constipation, urinary retention, polyuria, peripheral edema	Hypertension, hypotension, tachycardia, tardive dyskinesia, impaired thermoregulation, extrapyramidal symptoms, convulsions
	Life-threatening: Agranulocytosis

A, Adult; *CNS,* central nervous system; *d,* day; *h,* hour; *IM,* intramuscular; *max,* maximum; *PB,* protein-binding; *PO,* by mouth; *t½,* half-life; *wk,* week; 🍁, Canadian drug names.

Symptoms and Suggested Treatment for Overdose of Phenothiazines

Symptoms

- Unable to arouse, blood pressure fluctuations, tachycardia, agitation, delirium, convulsions, dysrhythmias, neuroleptic malignant syndrome, extrapyramidal symptoms, and renal, cardiac, and respiratory failure.

Treatment

- Maintain airway, gastric lavage, activated charcoal administration, adequate hydration, anticholinergics, and norepinephrine.

mation at the injection site. Because of the viscous, liquid medication, a dry, large-gauge needle (e.g., 21-gauge) should be used for administration in a deep muscle with the Z-track method. See Chapter 3 (Principles of Drug Administration, Figure 3–25) for further explanation of Z-track method of injection. The injection site should not be massaged and sites should be rotated. These medications should not remain in a plastic syringe longer than 15 minutes. Prototype Drug Chart 25–2 provides the drug data related to haloperidol.

Pharmacokinetics

Haloperidol is absorbed well through the gastrointestinal (GI) mucosa. It has a long half-life and is highly protein bound, so the drug may accumulate. Haloperidol is metabolized in the liver and is excreted in the urine and feces.

Pharmacodynamics

Haloperidol alters the effects of dopamine by blocking the dopamine receptors; thus sedation and EPS may occur. The drug is used to control psychoses and decrease signs of agitation in adults and children. Dosages need to be decreased in older adults because of decreased liver function and potential side effects. It may be prescribed for children with hyperactive behavior. Haloperidol has anticholinergic activity; thus care should be taken when administering it to clients with a history of glaucoma.

PROTOTYPE DRUG CHART 25–2

HALOPERIDOL AND HALOPERIDOL DECANOATE

Drug Class

Antipsychotic, neuroleptic (nonphenothiazine)
Trade Name: Haldol, ♣ Peridol
Pregnancy Category: C

Dosage

A: PO: 0.5-5 mg b.i.d.-t.i.d.
IM: 2-5 mg q4h PRN
IM: Decanoate: 50-100 mg q4wk
C: PO: 0.05-0.15 mg/kg/d in divided doses; 0.5 mg/d in 2-3 divided doses (not for child <3 y)
Elderly: Decreased doses PO: 0.5-2 mg b.i.d.-t.i.d.

Contraindications

Narrow-angle glaucoma; severe hepatic, renal, and cardiovascular diseases; bone marrow depression; Parkinson's disease; blood dyscrasias; CNS depression; subcortical brain damage

Drug-Lab-Food Interactions

Drug: Increase sedation with alcohol, CNS depressants; *increase* toxicity with anticholinergics, CNS depressants, lithium; *decrease* effects with phenobarbital, carbamazepine; *decrease* effects with caffeine

Pharmacokinetics

Absorption: PO: 60% absorbed
Distribution: PB: 80%-90%
Metabolism: t½: 15-35 h
Excretion: In urine and feces

Pharmacodynamics

PO: Onset: erratic
  Peak: 2-6 h
  Duration: 24-72 h
IM: Onset: 15-30 min
  Peak: 30-45 min
  Duration: 4-8 h
IM: Decanoate: Onset: UK
  Peak: 6-7 d
  Duration: 3-4 wk

Therapeutic Effects/Uses

To treat acute and chronic psychoses, to treat children with severe behavior problems who are combative, to suppress narcotic withdrawal symptoms, to treat schizophrenia resistant to other drugs, to treat Tourette's syndrome, to treat symptoms of dementia in older adults
Mode of Action: Alteration of the effect of dopamine on CNS; mechanism for antipsychotic effects are unknown

Side Effects

Sedation, extrapyramidal symptoms, orthostatic hypotension, headache, photosensitivity, dry mouth and eyes, blurred vision

Adverse Reactions

Tachycardia, seizures, urinary retention, tardive dyskinesia
Life-threatening: Laryngospasm, respiratory depression, cardiac dysrhythmias, neuromalignant syndrome

A, Adult; *b.i.d.,* twice a day; *C,* child; *CNS,* central nervous system; *d,* day; *h,* hour; *IM,* intramuscular; *min,* minute; *PB,* protein-binding; *PO,* by mouth; *PRN,* as needed; *t¹/₂,* half-life; *t.i.d.,* three times a day; *UK,* unknown; *wk,* week; *y,* year; <, less than; ♣, Canadian drug name.

Haloperidol has a similar onset of action, peak time of concentration, and duration of action as phenothiazines. It has strong EPS effects. Skin protection is necessary for prolonged use because of the possible side effect of photosensitivity.

From the *dibenzoxazepine* group, loxapine (Loxitane) is a moderate potent agent. It has moderate sedative and orthostatic hypotensive effects and a strong EPS effect.

The typical antipsychotic molindone hydrochloric acid (Moban) from the *dihydroindolone* group is a moderately potent agent. It has low sedative and orthostatic hypotensive effects and a strong EPS effect.

In the nonphenothiazine group, known as *thioxanthenes,* is thiothixene (Navane), a highly potent typical antipsychotic drug. It has side effects similar to those of molindone with low sedative and orthostatic hypotensive effects and a strong EPS effect.

Side Effects and Adverse Reactions

There are several common side effects associated with antipsychotics. The most common side effect for all antipsychotics is drowsiness. Many of the antipsychotics have some anticholinergic effects, such as dry mouth, increased heart rate, urinary retention, and constipation. Blood pressure decreases with the use of antipsychotics; aliphatics and piperidines cause a greater decrease in blood pressure than the others.

EPS are most prevalent with the phenothiazines, butyrophenones, and thioxanthenes and include pseudoparkinsonism, akathisia, **dystonia,** and tardive dyskinesia. Tardive dyskinesia may develop in 20% of clients taking antipsychotics for long-term therapy. Most antiparkinsonian anticholinergics are not always effective for treating tardive dyskinesia. EPS can begin 5 to 30 days after initiation of antipsychotic therapy. Anticholinergic drugs may be given to control EPS.

High dosing or long-term use of some antipsychotics can cause **blood dyscrasias** (blood cell disorders), such as agranulocytosis. White blood cell (WBC) count should be closely monitored and reported if there is an extreme decrease in the WBCs.

Dermatologic side effects seen early in drug therapy are pruritus and marked photosensitivity. Clients are urged to use sunscreen, hats, and protective clothing and to stay out of the sun.

Drug Interactions

Because phenothiazine lowers the seizure threshold, dosage adjustment of an anticonvulsant may be necessary. If either aliphatic phenothiazine or the thioxanthene group is administered, a higher dose of anticonvulsant might be necessary to prevent seizures.

Antipsychotics interact with alcohol, hypnotics, sedatives, narcotics, and benzodiazepines to potentiate the sedative effects of antipsychotics. Atropine counteracts the EPS and potentiates antipsychotic effects. Use of antihypertensives can cause an additive hypotensive effect.

Antipsychotics should *not* be given with other antipsychotic or antidepressant drugs except to control psychotic behavior for selected individuals who are refractory to drug therapy. Usually if one antipsychotic drug is ineffective, then another one is prescribed. Individuals should *not* take alcohol or other CNS depressants (e.g., narcotic analgesics, barbiturates) with antipsychotics because additive depression is likely to occur.

When discontinuing antipsychotics, the drug dosage should be reduced gradually to avoid sudden recurrence of psychotic symptoms. Table 25–2 lists common antipsychotic drugs (phenothiazines and nonphenothiazines) and their dosages, uses, and considerations.

Antipsychotic Dosage for Older Adults

Usually older adults require smaller doses of antipsychotics, from 25% to 50% less than young and middle-aged adults. Regular to high doses of antipsychotics increase the risk of severe side effects. Dosage amounts need to be individualized according to the client's age and physical status. In addition, dosage changes may be necessary during antipsychotic therapy.

Atypical (Serotonin/Dopamine Antagonists) Antipsychotics

A new category for antipsychotics was marketed in the United States in the early 1990s. This group, **atypical antipsychotics,** differs from the typical/traditional antipsychotics because the atypical agents are effective in treating both positive and negative symptoms of schizophrenia. The typical antipsychotics have not been effective in the treatment of negative symptoms. Two advantages of the atypical agents are that (1) they are effective in treating negative symptoms, and (2) they are not likely to cause EPS or tardive dyskinesia. The four atypical drugs available include clozapine (Clozaril), risperidone (Risperdal), olanzapine (Zyprexa), and quetiapine (Seroquel). These agents have a greater affinity for blocking serotonin and dopaminergic D_4 receptors than primarily blocking the dopaminergic D_2 receptor that is responsible for mild and severe EPS. Weight gain is a common side effect of atypical antipsychotics.

Clozapine (Clozaril) was the first atypical antipsychotic agent used to treat schizophrenia and other psychoses. It does not cause acute EPS, although tremors and occasional rigidity have been reported. The serious adverse reaction of clozapine is agranulocytosis, a decrease in the production of granulocytes, which results in a decrease in the body's defense mechanism and seizures. Currently it is only indicated for the treatment of severely ill schizophrenic clients who have not responded to traditional antipsychotic drugs. The WBC count needs to be closely monitored; if the WBC (leukocytes) level falls below 3000 mm^3, clozapine should be discontinued. Seizures have been reported in 3% of clients taking the drug. Dizziness, sedation, tachycardia, orthostatic hypotension, and constipation are common side effects.

Another atypical agent used to treat positive and negative symptoms of schizophrenia is risperidone (Risperdal). Its action is similar to that of clozapine, and the occurrence of EPS and tardive dyskinesia is low. It does not cause agranulocytosis.

The atypical antipsychotic olanzapine (Zyprexa), like clozapine and risperidone, is effective for treating positive and negative symptoms of schizophrenia. It does not cause agranulocytosis.

Quetiapine (Seroquel), like all the other atypical antipsychotics, is less likely to cause EPS. Tardive dyskinesia for long-term use has not been determined.

Ziprasidone (Geodon) was approved by the Food and Drug Administration (FDA) in 2001, and aripiprazole (Abilify) was FDA approved in 2002. Ziprasidone may lead to prolonged QT interval; therefore this drug may be contraindicated in clients with a history of prolonged QT interval or with other concurrent drugs known to prolong QT interval. Clients taking quetiapine, clozapine, risperidone, olanzapine, ziprasidone, and aripiprazole should be monitored for hyperglycemia and other symptoms of diabetes mellitus. Prototype Drug Chart 25–3 illustrates drug characteristics of risperidone (Ativan), an atypical antipsychotic.

When anxiety, hallucination, agitation, mania, confusion, or depression and other symptoms are noted, the health care provider should check the medications that the client is taking.

PREVENTING MEDICATION ERRORS

Do not confuse...

- **Seroquel** with **Serzone** (an antidepressant). Seroquel may also be confused with **sertindole (Serlect)** or mesoridazine besylate **(Serentil)** because the words look alike.

Nursing Process

Phenothiazine and Nonphenothiazine

ASSESSMENT

■ Record baseline vital signs for use in future comparison.

■ Obtain a health history from client of present drug therapy. If client is taking an anticonvulsant, the drug dose might need to be increased because antipsychotics tend to lower seizure threshold.

■ Assess mental status and cardiac, eye, and respiratory disorders before start of drug therapy and continue daily assessment.

NURSING DIAGNOSES

■ Disturbed thought processes

Table 25–2

Phenothiazines and Nonphenothiazines

Generic (Brand)	Drug Potency	Route and Dosage	Uses and Considerations
Phenothiazines			
Aliphatics			
chlorpromazine HCl (Thorazine)	Low	A: PO: 25-100 mg t.i.d. or q.i.d. A: IM/IV: 25-50 mg q4-6h A: PR: 50-100 mg q6-8h C: PO: >6 mo: 0.55 mg/kg q4-6h C: IM/IV: >6 mo: 0.55 mg/kg q6-8h C: PR: >6 mo: 1 mg/kg q6-8h	For psychosis, schizophrenia, intractable hiccups, preoperative sedation, behavioral problems in children, nausea, and vomiting. *Pregnancy category:* C; PB: 95%; t½: 8-30 h
Piperazines			
fluphenazine HCl (Prolixin)	High	See Prototype Drug Chart 25–1.	
perphenazine (Trilafon)	Moderate	A: PO: 4-16 mg b.i.d., t.i.d., or q.i.d.	For psychotic disorders; control severe nausea and vomiting; and treat intractable hiccups. Used also before chemotherapy to prevent nausea. *Pregnancy category:* C; PB: ≥90%; t½: 9.5 h
Piperidines			
mesoridazine besylate (Serentil)	Low-Moderate	A: PO: 10-50 mg b.i.d.-t.i.d.; gradually increase Optimal response: 100-400 mg/d A: IM: 25 mg; may repeat Elderly: ⅓-½ adult dose	For psychosis and schizophrenia, severe anxiety, chronic brain syndrome (smaller doses). Few EPS. Can cause hypotensive effects. *Pregnancy category:* C; PB: 92%-99%; t½: 24-48 h
thioridazine HCl (Mellaril)*	Low	A: PO: 50-100 mg t.i.d.; *max:* 800 mg/d Elderly: ⅓-½ adult dose	For psychosis. Higher doses for severe psychosis. Lower doses (10-50 mg t.i.d.) for marked depression, alcohol withdrawal, intractable pain. Few EPS. Little antiemetic effect. Can cause orthostatic hypotension. *Pregnancy category:* C; PB: ≥90%; t½: 24-34 h
Nonphenothiazines			
Butyrophenone			
haloperidol (Haldol)	High	See Prototype Drug Chart 25–2.	
Dibenzoxazepine			
loxapine (Loxitane)	Moderate	A: PO: Initially: 10 mg b.i.d.; then may increase to 50-100 mg/d in 2-4 divided doses Elderly: ⅓-½ regular adult dose A: IM: 12.5-50 mg q4-6h	For acute psychosis and schizophrenia. Likely to cause EPS. Overdose can cause cardiac toxicity or neurotoxicity. *Pregnancy category:* C; PB: 95%; t½: 5 h
Dihydroindolone			
molindone HCl (Moban)	Moderate	A: PO: Initial: 50-75 mg in 3-4 divided doses A: PO: 5-50 mg t.i.d.-q.i.d.; *max:* 225 mg/d Elderly: ⅓-½ adult dose	Management of schizophrenia. Can cause EPS. Has less sedative effect. *Pregnancy category:* C; PB: UK; t½: 1.5 h

A, Adult; *b.i.d.*, twice a day; *C*, child; *d*, day; *EPS*, extrapyramidal symptoms; *h*, hour; *IM*, intramuscular; *IV*, intravenous; *max*, maximum; *mo*, month; *PB*, protein-binding; *PO*, by mouth; *PR*, rectally; *q.i.d.*, four times a day; *t½*, half-life; *t.i.d.*, three times a day; *UK*, unknown; >, greater than; ≥, greater than or equal to.

*Avoid spilling liquid on skin. Contact dermatitis could result.

- Activity intolerance
- Disturbed sensory-perceptual
- Self-care deficit
- Noncompliance

PLANNING

- Client's psychotic behavior will improve with drug(s) and psychotherapy.

NURSING INTERVENTIONS

- Monitor vital signs. Orthostatic hypotension is likely to occur.
- Remain with client while he or she takes the medication to ensure compliance because some clients hide drugs.
- Avoid skin contact with liquid concentrates to prevent contact dermatitis. Liquid must be protected from light and should be diluted with fruit juice.
- Administer oral doses with food or milk to decrease gastric irritation.

- Administer by IM route deep into the muscle because the drug irritates fatty tissue. Do *not* inject into subQ tissue. Check blood pressure for marked decrease 30 minutes after drug is injected.
- Do *not* mix in same syringe with heparin, pentobarbital, cimetidine, or dimenhydrinate.
- Chill suppository in the refrigerator for 30 minutes before removing foil wrapper.
- Observe for extrapyramidal syndrome (EPS): *acute dystonia* (spasms of the tongue, face, neck, and back), *akathisia* (restlessness, inability to sit still, foot-tapping), *pseudoparkinsonism* (muscle tremors, rigidity, shuffling gait), and *tardive dyskinesia* (lip smacking, protruding and darting tongue, and constant chewing movement). Report these promptly to the health care provider.
- Assess for symptoms of neuroleptic malignant syndrome (NMS): increased fever, pulse, and blood pressure; muscle rigidity; increased creatine phosphokinase and WBC count; altered mental status; acute renal failure; varying levels of consciousness; pallor; diaphoresis; tachycardia; and dysrhythmias.

Table 25-2

Phenothiazines and Nonphenothiazines—cont'd

Generic (Brand)	Drug Potency	Route and Dosage	Uses and Considerations
Thioxanthenes			
thiothixene HCl (Navane)	High	A: PO: 2 mg t.i.d.; *max:* 60 mg/d; IM: 4 mg b.i.d.-q.i.d.; *max:* 30 mg/d	Management of psychotic disorders, especially acute and chronic schizophrenia. Can cause EPS. *Pregnancy category:* C; PB: ≥90%; $t^1/_2$: 24-34 h
Atypical Antipsychotics			
clozapine (Clozaril)	Low	A: PO: Initially: 25-50 mg/d; if tolerated, gradually increase to 300-450 mg/d in divided doses; *max:* 900 mg/d	For severely ill schizophrenic clients, especially those who do not respond to other antipsychotics. With long-term use, monitor white blood cell count. *Pregnancy category:* B; PB: 95%; $t^1/_2$: 8-12 h
olanzapine (Zyprexa)	UK	A: PO: 5 mg/d initially, 5-10 mg/d thereafter	Effective in treating positive and negative symptoms of schizophrenia. Does not cause EPS symptoms. May cause headaches, dizziness, agitation, insomnia, and somnolence. *Pregnancy category:* C; PB: UK; $t^1/_2$: 27-30 h
quetiapine (Seroquel)	UK	A: PO: 25 mg/d initially, 25-50 mg b.i.d. first week; *max:* 400 mg/d	Effective in treating positive and negative symptoms of schizophrenia. Is not likely to cause EPS. May cause dizziness, headache, insomnia. *Pregnancy category:* UK; PB: UK; $t^1/_2$: UK
risperidone (Risperdal)	Low	See Prototype Drug Chart 25-3.	
sertindole (Serlect)	UK	A: PO: 4 mg/d initially, then 20 mg/d	Improves positive and negative symptoms of schizophrenia. May cause little EPS. May cause dizziness, headache, constipation, ejaculatory disturbances. *Pregnancy category:* UK; PB: UK; $t^1/_2$: UK
ziprasidone (Geodon)	UK	A: PO: 20 mg b.i.d. may increase q 2 d; *max:* 80 mg b.i.d. A: IM: 10 mg q 2 h or 20 mg q 4 h; *max:* 40 mg/day	For management of schizophrenia. *Pregnancy category:* C; PB: 99%; $t^1/_2$: 7 h
aripiprazole (Abilify)	UK	A: PO: 10-15 mg/day may increase q 2 wk; *max:* 30 mg q day	For management of schizophrenia. *Pregnancy category:* C; PB: 99%; $t^1/_2$: 75 h

- Record urine output. Urinary retention may result.
- Monitor serum glucose level.

Client Teaching

General

- Instruct client to take the drug exactly as ordered. In schizophrenia and other psychotic disorders, antipsychotics do not cure the mental illness but do prevent symptoms. Many clients on medication can function outside the institution setting. Compliance with drug regimen is extremely important.
- Inform client that medication may take 6 weeks or longer to achieve full clinical effect.
- Caution client not to consume alcohol or other CNS depressants such as narcotics; these drugs intensify the depressant effect on the body.
- Recommend client not to abruptly discontinue the drug. Seek advice from the health care provider before making any changes in dosage.

- Encourage client to read labels on OTC preparations. Some are contraindicated when taking antipsychotics.
- Teach smoking cessation because smoking increases the metabolism of some antipsychotics.
- Guide client to maintain good oral hygiene by frequently brushing and flossing teeth.
- Encourage client to talk with the health care provider regarding family planning. The effect of antipsychotics on the fetus is not fully known; however, there may be teratogenic effects on the fetus.
- Explain to client that phenothiazine passes into breast milk. This could cause drowsiness and unusual muscle movement in the baby.
- Instruct client on the importance of routine follow-up examinations.
- Encourage client to obtain laboratory tests on schedule. WBCs are monitored for 3 months, especially during the start of drug therapy. Leukopenia, or decreased WBCs, may occur. Be alert to symptoms of

---

PROTOTYPE DRUG CHART 25–3

RISPERIDONE

Drug Class

Nonphenothiazine
Risperidone: Atypical Antipsychotic
Trade name: Risperdol
Pregnancy Category: C

Dosage

Psychosis
A: PO: 1 mg b.i.d.; increase by 1 mg b.i.d. daily to initial target of 3 mg b.i.d.; *max:* 8 mg/d
Elderly: PO: 0.5 mg b.i.d.; increase by 0.5 mg b.i.d. daily to initial target of 1.5 mg/d; *max:* 4 mg/d

Contraindications

Hypersensitivity, lactation, dysrhythmias, blood dyscrasias, liver damage

Drug-Lab-Food Interactions

Drug: Increased effects of antihypertensives; decreased risperidone levels with concurrent use of carbamazepine; concurrent use of cisapride may cause dysrhythmias
Lab: Increased AST, ALT, and ALP

Pharmacokinetics

Absorption: Rapidly absorbed
Distribution: PB: 90%
Metabolism: $t\frac{1}{2}$: 24 h
Excretion: In urine 70% and feces 14%

Pharmacodynamics

PO: Onset: UK
Peak: 1-2 h
Duration: UK

Therapeutic Effects/Uses

To manage symptoms of psychosis including schizophrenia
Mode of Action: Interferes with the binding of dopamine to dopamine (D_2) and serotonin 5-hydroxytryptamine (5-HT_2) receptors

Side Effects

Sedation, weight gain, headaches, dry mouth, photosensitivity, urinary retention, sexual dysfunction

Adverse Reactions

Orthostatic hypotension, tachycardia, EPS, ECG changes, convulsions
Life-threatening: Neuroleptic malignant syndrome

A, Adult; *ALP,* alkaline phosphatase; *ALT,* alanine aminotransferase; *AST,* aspartate aminotransferase; *b.i.d.,* twice a day; *d,* day; *ECG,* electrocardiogram; *EPS,* extrapyramidal symptom; *h,* hour; *max,* maximum; *PB,* protein-binding; *PO,* by mouth; $t^1/_2$, half-life; *UK,* unknown.

malaise, fever, and sore throat, which may be an indication of agranulocytosis, a serious blood dyscrasia. Report this promptly to the health care provider, especially when client is taking clozapine.

- Advise client to wear an identification bracelet indicating the medication taken.
- Inform client that tolerance to sedative effect develops over a period of days or weeks.

Side Effects

- Direct client to avoid potentially dangerous situations, such as driving, until drug dosing has been stabilized.
- Inform client about EPS; instruct the client to promptly report symptoms to the health care provider.
- Instruct client to avoid direct sunlight to prevent photosensitivity and to use sunscreen and protective clothing to prevent a skin rash.
- Advise client of orthostatic hypotension and possible dizziness.
- Teach client who is taking aliphatic phenothiazines, such as chlorpromazine, that the urine might be pink or red-brown; this discoloration is harmless.
- Inform client that changes may occur related to sexual functioning and menstruating. Women could have irregular menstrual periods or amenorrhea, and men might experience impotence and gynecomastia (enlargement of breast tissue).
- Suggest lozenges or hard candy if mouth dryness occurs. Advise client to consult the health care provider if dry mouth persists for more than 2 weeks.
- Encourage client to avoid extremes in temperatures and increased exercise.
- Advise client to rise slowly from sitting or lying to standing to prevent a sudden decrease in blood pressure.

Cultural Considerations

- Recognize that various cultural groups may have difficulty in accepting the client's mental disorder.

EVALUATION

- Evaluate the effectiveness of the drug and whether the client has acceptably reduced psychotic symptoms at the *lowest* dose possible.
- Ascertain whether client can cope with everyday living situations and attend to activities of daily living.
- Determine if any side effects of or adverse reactions to the drug have occurred.

Anxiolytics

Anxiolytics, or *antianxiety drugs,* are primarily used to treat anxiety and insomnia. The major group of anxiolytics are the benzodiazepines (a minor tranquilizer group). Long before benzodiazepines were prescribed for anxiety and insomnia, barbiturates were used. Benzodiazepines are considered more effective than barbiturates because they enhance the action of gamma-aminobutyric acid (GABA), an inhibitory

neurotransmitter within the CNS. Benzodiazepines have fewer side effects and may be less dangerous in overdosing. Long-term use of barbiturates causes drug tolerance and dependence and may cause respiratory distress. Currently, barbiturates are not the drug of choice to treat anxiety.

Table 25–3 lists the approved uses for benzodiazepines. Drugs used to treat insomnia, which include the benzodiazepines, are discussed in Chapter 20, Central Nervous System Depressants.

A certain amount of anxiety may make one more alert and energetic; however, when the anxiety is excessive, it could be disabling, and anxiolytics may be prescribed. The action of anxiolytics resembles that of the sedative-hypnotics but *not* that of the antipsychotics.

There are two types of anxiety—primary and secondary. *Primary anxiety* is not caused by a medical condition or by drug use; *secondary anxiety* is related to selected drug use or medical or psychiatric disorders. The anxiolytics are not usually given for secondary anxiety unless the medical problem is untreatable, severe, and causes disability. In this case, an anxiolytic could be given for a short period to alleviate any acute anxiety attacks. These agents treat the symptoms but do not cure them. Long-term use of anxiolytics is discouraged because tolerance develops within weeks or months, depending on

Table 25–3

Approved Uses for Benzodiazepines

Prescribed Uses	Drugs
Anxiety	alprazolam (Xanax) chlordiazepoxide (Librium) chlorazepate (Tranxene) diazepam (Valium) halazepam (Paxipam) ketazolam (Loftan) lorazepam (Ativan) prazepam (Centrax)
Anxiety Associated with Depression	alprazolam (Xanax) clonazepam (Klonopin) lorazepam (Ativan)
Insomnia: Short-Term Use	estazolam (Prosom) flurazepam (Dalmane) quazepam (Doral) temazepam (Restoril) triazolam (Halcion)
Seizures and Status Epilepticus	clonazepam (Klonopin) clorazepate (Tranxene) diazepam (Valium)—status epilepticus lorazepam (Ativan)—status epilepticus
Alcohol Withdrawal	clorazepate (Tranxene) chlordiazepoxide (Librium) diazepam (Valium)
Skeletal Muscle Spasms Preoperative Medications	diazepam (Valium) chlordiazepoxide (Librium) diazepam (Valium) lorazepam (Ativan) midazolam (Versed)

the agent. Drug tolerance can occur in less than 2 to 3 months in clients who take meprobamate or phenobarbital.

Nonpharmacologic Measures

Some of the symptoms of a severe or panic attack of anxiety include dyspnea (difficulty in breathing), choking sensation, chest pain, heart palpitations, dizziness, faintness, sweating, trembling and shaking, and fear of losing control. *Nonpharmacologic measures should be used for decreasing anxiety before giving anxiolytics.* These measures might include using a relaxation technique, psychotherapy, or support groups.

Benzodiazepines

Benzodiazepines have multiple uses, such as anticonvulsants, sedative-hypnotics, preoperative drugs, and anxiolytics. Most of the benzodiazepines are used mainly for severe or prolonged anxiety; examples include chlordiazepoxide (Librium), diazepam (Valium), clorazepate dipotassium (Tranxene), lorazepam (Ativan), alprazolam (Xanax), prazepam (Centrax), and halazepam (Paxipam). The most frequently prescribed benzodiazepine is lorazepam (Ativan). Table 25–4 describes the various uses for benzodiazepines. Many of the benzodiazepines are used for more than one purpose.

Benzodiazepines are lipid soluble and are absorbed readily from the GI tract. They are highly protein bound (80% to 98%). Benzodiazepines are primarily metabolized by the liver and excreted in urine, so the drug dosage for clients with liver or renal disease should be lowered accordingly to avoid possible cumulative effects. Traces of benzodiazepine metabolites could be present in the urine for weeks or months after the person has stopped taking the drug. These are controlled substance schedule IV (CSS IV) drugs.

In 1962 the first benzodiazepine, chlordiazepoxide (Librium), became widely used for its sedative effect. Diazepam (Valium) was the most frequently prescribed drug in the early 1970s and was called a miracle drug by many. Lorazepam (Ativan) is the prototype drug of benzodiazepine and is described in Prototype Drug Chart 25–4.

Pharmacokinetics

Lorazepam is highly lipid-soluble, and the drug is rapidly absorbed from the GI tract. The drug is highly protein-bound, and the half-life is 10 to 20 hours. The drug is excreted primarily in the urine.

Pharmacodynamics

Lorazepam acts on the limbic, thalamic, and hypothalamic levels of the CNS. The onset of action is 15 to 30 minutes by mouth and 1 to 5 minutes by IV. The serum levels of most oral doses of benzodiazepines peak in 2 hours. Oxazezpam levels peak in 3 hours, and prazepam levels peak in 6 hours. Duration of action varies. The average is 2 to 3 hours when given orally; when given IV, the longest duration of action is 1 hour.

It is recommended that benzodiazepines be prescribed for no longer than 3 to 4 months. Beyond 4 months, the effectiveness of the drug lessens. Table 25–4 lists the anxiolytics and their dosages, uses, and considerations.

HERBAL ALERT 25-2

Benzodiazepines

🍂 Kava kava should not be combined with benzodiazepines because it increases the sedative effect.

Miscellaneous Anxiolytics

The anxiolytic buspirone hydrochloride (BuSpar) might not become effective until 1 to 2 weeks after continuous use. It does not have many of the side effects associated with benzodiazepines, such as sedation and physical and psychologic dependency. Buspirone has an interaction with grapefruit juice that leads to possible toxicity. To avoid this interaction, it is recommended to limit daily intake of grapefruit juice to 8 oz daily or half of a fresh grapefruit.

Side Effects and Adverse Reactions

The side effects associated with benzodiazepines are sedation, dizziness, headaches, dry mouth, blurred vision, rare urinary incontinence, and constipation. Adverse reactions include leukopenia (decreased WBC count) with symptoms of fever, malaise, and sore throat; tolerance to the drug dosage with continuous use; and physical dependency. Box 25–1 lists guidelines for treating benzodiazepine overdose.

Benzodiazepines should not be abruptly discontinued because withdrawal symptoms are likely to occur. Withdrawal symptoms caused by short-term benzodiazepine use are similar to those from the sedative-hypnotics (agitation, nervousness, insomnia, tremor, anorexia, muscular cramps, sweating); however, they are slow to develop, taking 2 to 10 days and perhaps lasting several weeks, depending on the benzodiazepine's half-life. When discontinuing a benzodiazepine, the drug dosage should be gradually decreased over a period of days, depending on dose or length of time on the drug. Withdrawal symptoms from long-term, high-dose benzodiazepine therapy include paranoia, delirium, panic, hypertension, and status

---

BOX 25–1

Suggested Treatment for Overdose of Benzodiazepines

1. Administer an emetic and follow with activated charcoal if the client is conscious; use gastric lavage if the client is unconscious.
2. Administer the benzodiazepine antagonist flumazenil (Romazicon) IV if required.
3. Maintain an airway, give oxygen as needed for decreased respirations, and monitor vital signs.
4. Give IV vasopressors for severe hypotension.
5. Request a mental health consultation for the client.

NOTE: Dialysis has little value in removing benzodiazepine from the bloodstream.

Table 25–4

Anxiolytics

Generic (Brand)	Route and Dosage	Uses and Considerations
Benzodiazepines		
alprazolam (Xanax) CSS IV	A: PO: 0.25-0.5 mg t.i.d. Elderly: 0.125-0.25 mg b.i.d.; *max*: 4 mg/d	Management of anxiety and panic disorders and anxiety associated with depression. Side effects include drowsiness, dry mouth, and light-headedness. *Pregnancy category*: D; PB: 80%; $t^1/_2$: 12-15 h
chlordiazepoxide HCl (Librium) CSS IV	*Anxiety disorders:* A: PO: 5-25 mg t.i.d.-q.i.d. C: PO: 5 mg b.i.d.-q.i.d. *Acute alcohol withdrawal:* A: PO/IM/IV: 50-100 mg; *max*: 300 mg/d Elderly: $^1/_2$ adult dose	Effective for alcohol withdrawal syndrome (DTs), anxiety, and tension. Dose should be less for the older adult. *Pregnancy category*: D; PB: 90%-98%; $t^1/_2$: 6-30 h
clorazepate dipotassium (Tranxene) CSS IV	A: PO: 15-60 mg/d in divided doses (daily dose range) Elderly: 7.5 mg b.i.d. or at bedtime	For anxiety, alcohol withdrawal syndrome, and partial seizures. Avoid taking alcohol or CNS depressants with clorazepate. Drowsiness and dizziness may occur. *Pregnancy category*: C; PB: 80%-90%; $t^1/_2$: 0.5-1 h
diazepam (Valium) CSS IV	*Anxiety, muscle spasm, and alcohol withdrawal:* A: PO/IM/IV: 2-10 mg b.i.d.-q.i.d. Elderly: PO: 1-2 mg qd-b.i.d.; *max*: 10 mg/d C: >6 mo: PO: 1-2.5 mg b.i.d-t.i.d. *Preoperative sedation:* A: IV: 5-15 mg 15 min prior to surgery/procedure *Status epilepticus:* A: IV: 5-10 mg q10-20 min, *max*: 30 mg C: <6 yr: IV: 0.2-0.5 mg/kg q15-30min; *max*: 5 mg C: >6 yr: IV: 0.2-0.5 mg/kg q15-30min; *max*: 10 mg	Management of anxiety, muscle spasms, alcohol withdrawal, status epilepticus, and preoperative sedation. *Pregnancy category*: D; PB: 98%; $t^1/_2$: 25-50 h
halazepam (Paxipam) CSS IV	A: PO: 20-40 mg t.i.d.-q.i.d. Elderly: 20 mg daily/b.i.d.	Management of anxiety disorders. Drowsiness, sedation, confusion, headaches, and hypotension may occur. *Pregnancy category*: D; PB: 97%; $t^1/_2$: 14 h
lorazepam (Ativan) CSS IV	See Prototype Drug Chart 25-4.	For mild to moderate anxiety. To control alcohol syndrome. Drowsiness, dizziness may occur. *Pregnancy category*: C; PB: 85%-95%; $t^1/_2$: 3.5-21 h
Azapirones		
buspirone HCl (BuSpar)	A: PO: Initial: 5 mg b.i.d.-t.i.d. A: PO: 15-30 mg/d in divided doses; *max*: 60 mg/d Elderly: *max*: 30 mg/d	For anxiety and anxiety-related depression. Takes several weeks before anxiolytic effects occur. Common side effects include drowsiness, dizziness, headache, nausea. *Pregnancy category*: B; PB: 95%; $t^1/_2$: 2-3 h
Benzodiazepine Antagonist		
flumazenil (Romazicon)	A: IV: 0.2 mg over 15-30 sec; repeat 0.2 mg at 1-min intervals; *max*: 1 mg	Used to partially or completely reverse benzodiazepine dose from sedation, anesthesia, and overdose. It should not be used with antipsychotics or antidepressants. *Pregnancy category*: C; PB: UK; $t^1/_2$: UK

A, Adult; *b.i.d.*, twice a day; *C*, child; *CNS*, central nervous system; *CSS*, Controlled Substances Schedule; *d*, day; *h*, hour; *IM*, intramuscular; *IV*, intravenous; *max*, maximum; *min*, minute; *PB*, protein-binding; *PO*, by mouth; *q.i.d.*, four times a day; $t^1/_2$, half-life; *t.i.d.*, three times a day; *UK*, unknown.

epilepticus. Convulsions during withdrawal may be prevented with simultaneous substitution of an anticonvulsant. Alcohol and other CNS depressants should *not* be taken with benzodiazepines because respiratory depression could result. Tobacco, caffeine, and sympathomimetics decrease the effectiveness of benzodiazepines. Benzodiazepines are contraindicated during pregnancy because of the possible teratogenic effects on the fetus.

Nursing Process

Benzodiazepines

ASSESSMENT

- Assess for suicidal ideation.
- Obtain a history of client's anxiety reaction.

■ Determine client's support system (family, friends, groups), if any.
■ Obtain client's drug history. Report possible drug-drug interaction.

NURSING DIAGNOSES

■ Anxiety
■ Impaired physical mobility

PLANNING

■ Client's anxiety and stress will be reduced through nonpharmacologic methods, anxiolytic drugs, or support/group therapy.

NURSING INTERVENTIONS

■ Observe client for side effects of anxiolytics. Recognize that drug tolerance and physical and psychologic dependency can result with most anxiolytics.
■ Recognize that anxiolytic dosages should be less for older adults, children, and debilitated persons than for middle-age adults.
■ Monitor vital signs, especially blood pressure and pulse; orthostatic hypotension may occur.
■ Encourage the family to be supportive of client.

PROTOTYPE DRUG CHART 25–4

LORAZEPAM

Drug Class	**Dosage**
Anxiolytic	*Anxiety:*
Lorazepam (benzodiazepine)	**A: PO:** 2-6 mg/d
Trade name: Ativan	*Max:* 10 mg/d
Pregnancy Category: D	**C: PO/IV:** 0.05 mg/kg q4-8 h
	Max: 2 mg per dose
	Elderly: PO: 0.5-1 mg/d
	Max: 2 mg/d

Contraindications	**Drug-Lab-Food Interactions**
Hypersensitivity, CNS depression, shock, coma, narrow-angle glaucoma, pregnancy, lactation	*Drug:* Increases CNS depression when taken with alcohol, CNS depressants, and anticonvulsants, cimetidine increases lorazepam plasma levels, increases phenytoin levels, decreases levodopa effects, smoking decreases antianxiety effects
Caution: Hepatic or renal dysfunction, suicidal	*Food:* Kava kava may potentiate sedation

Pharmacokinetics	**Pharmacodynamics**
Absorption: Rapid from GI tract	**PO:** Onset: UK
Distribution: PB: 90%	Peak: 2 h
Metabolism: t½: 10-20 h	Duration: 12-24 h
Excretion: In urine	**IM:** Onset: 15-30 min
	Peak: 60-90 min
	Duration: UK
	IV: Onset: 1-5 min
	Peak: UK
	Duration: UK

Therapeutic Effects/Uses

To control anxiety, preoperative sedation, and to treat status epilepticus
Mode of Action: Potentiate gamma-aminobutyrate (GABA) effects by binding to specific benzodiazepine receptors and inhibiting GABA neurotransmission

Side Effects	**Adverse Reactions**
Drowsiness, dizziness, weakness, confusion, blurred vision, nausea, vomiting, anorexia, sleep disturbance, restlessness, hallucinations	Hypertension, hypotension

A, Adult; *C,* child; *CNS,* central nervous system; *d,* day; *GI,* gastrointestinal; *h,* hour; *IM,* intramuscular; *IV,* intravenous; *max,* maximum; *min,* minute; *PO,* by mouth; *PB,* protein-binding; *t½,* half-life; *UK,* unknown.

Client Teaching

General

- Advise client not to drive a motor vehicle or operate dangerous equipment when taking anxiolytics because sedation is a common side effect.
- Instruct client not to consume alcohol or CNS depressants such as narcotics while taking an anxiolytic.
- Teach client ways to control excess stress and anxiety, such as relaxation techniques.
- Inform client that effective response may take 1 to 2 weeks.
- Encourage client to follow drug regimen and not to abruptly stop taking the drug after prolonged use because withdrawal symptoms can occur. Drug dose is usually tapered when the drug is discontinued.

Side Effects

- Instruct client to arise slowly from the sitting to standing position to avoid dizziness from orthostatic hypotension.

Cultural Considerations

- Use simple and clear instructions. Ask family members to assist with translation only if an interpreter is not available. Do not use compound sentences.

EVALUATION

- Evaluate the effectiveness of drug therapy by determining if client is less anxious and more able to cope with stresses and anxieties.
- Determine if client is taking the anxiolytic drug as prescribed and is adhering to client teaching instructions.

WEBSITES

For further information on *Antipsychotics and Anxiolytics,* visit these Internet resources:

Information on risperidone: *http://www.risperdal.com*

More information on risperidone: *http://www.psyweb.com/Drughtm/risper.html*

Information on antipsychotics, antidepressants, mood stabilizers, and anxiolytics: *http://www.psych.uic.edu/education/courses/brain/Janicak*

 ## Critical Thinking Case Study

F.S., 75 years old, is receiving risperidone, 3 mg b.i.d., to control a psychotic disorder. She has taken the drug for 6 months. She has become agitated and is complaining of insomnia.

1. What is the relation between F.S.'s drug dose and her complaints? Explain.

2. What further assessment should be made concerning F.S. and the drug regimen?

3. How does the risperidone compare with other antipsychotics such as chlorpromazine and haloperidol regarding actions and adverse effects?

 ## Study Questions

1. Your client is taking the phenothiazine promazine (Sparine). What side effects associated with phenothiazines are similar to the side effects from anticholinergics and pseudoparkinsonism? Why should the blood pressure be closely monitored? What do you tell the client about the color of the urine?

2. What group of drugs has antiemetic properties? What is the route of administration for a client who is vomiting?

3. Haloperidol (Haldol) is a drug frequently used in psychiatry. How is it different from other antipsychotics?

4. How do the typical/traditional and atypical antipsychotics differ? Explain their therapeutic effects.

5. What is the major group of anxiolytics called? A client receiving a drug from this category should be observed for what side effects? Client teaching is important regarding the use of alcohol or over-the-counter drugs and discontinuing the anxiolytic. Why?

26 Antidepressants and Mood Stabilizer

ELECTRONIC RESOURCES

Additional information can be found on the companion website at *http://evolve.elsevier.com/KeeHayes/pharmacology/* or on the companion CD-ROM, which includes:

- *NCLEX-style examination review questions*
- *Pharmacology animations*
- *Medication error and IV therapy checklists*
- *Medication calculation problems*
- *Electronic calculators*

OUTLINE

OBJECTIVES

- Define the various categories of antidepressants. Give examples of their prototype drugs.
- Name the side effects and adverse reactions of antidepressants.
- Give the nursing interventions, including client teaching, for antidepressants (tricyclics, monoamine oxidase inhibitors [MAOIs], and selective serotonin reuptake inhibitors [SSRIs]).
- Explain the uses of lithium and its serum/plasma therapeutic ranges, side effects and adverse reactions, and nursing interventions.

TERMS

antidepressants
atypical (heterocyclic) antidepressants
bipolar affective disorder
depression
dysphoria

electroconvulsive therapy (ECT)
manic-depressive illness
monoamine oxidase inhibitors (MAOIs)
reactive depression

selective serotonin reuptake inhibitors (SSRIs)
tricyclic antidepressants (TCAs)

Introduction

Antidepressants have been called *mood elevators*. They are used for depressive episodes that are accompanied by feelings of hopelessness and helplessness. There are various drug categories of antidepressants that can be prescribed for more than 1 month to 12 months and perhaps longer.

The mood-stabilizer agents, such as lithium, are effective for **bipolar affective disorder (manic-depressive illness)**. Drug therapy for treating reactive, unipolar, and bipolar disorders is discussed in this chapter.

Depression

Depression is the most common psychiatric problem, affecting approximately 10% to 20% of the population. Only one third of depressed persons receive medical or psychiatric help. Women between the ages of 25 and 45 are two to three times more likely to experience major depression than men are. Depression is characterized primarily by mood changes and loss of interest in normal activities. It is second to hypertension as the most common chronic clinical condition.

Contributing causes of depression include genetic predisposition, social and environmental factors, and biologic conditions. Some signs of major depression include loss of interest in most activities, depressed mood, weight loss or gain, insomnia or hypersomnia, loss of energy, fatigue, feelings of despair, decreased ability to think or concentrate, and suicidal thoughts. Approximately two thirds of all suicides are related to depression. Depressed men, especially older white men, are more likely to commit suicide than depressed women. Antidepressants can mask suicidal tendencies.

The three types of depression are (1) *reactive*, (2) *major*, and (3) *bipolar affective disorder* (previously referred to as *manic-depressive*). **Reactive depression** usually has a sudden onset resulting from a precipitating event (e.g., depression resulting from a loss, such as death of a loved one). The client *knows* why he or she is depressed. The person may call this the "blues." Usually this type of depression lasts for months. A benzodiazepine agent may be prescribed. *Major depression* is characterized by loss of interest in work and home, inability to complete tasks, and deep depression **(dysphoria)**. Major depression can be either primary (i.e., not related to other health problems) or secondary to a health problem (e.g., physical or psychiatric disorder or drug use). Antidepressants have been effective in treating major depression. *Bipolar affective disorder* involves swings between two moods, the manic (euphoric) and the depressive (dysphoria). Lithium is the drug of choice for treating this type of disorder. Also, divalproex sodium (Depakote) is used for bipolar disorder by some health care providers.

Electroconvulsive therapy (ECT) was used to treat psychosis and depression before the introduction of antipsychotics and antidepressants. ECT is still used, although not as frequently as in the past, for clients who are extremely depressed, suicidal, or do not respond to antidepressant ther-apy. ECT is not as traumatic as it once was. The use of thiopental (short-acting anesthetic) and succinylcholine (short-acting neuromuscular blocking agent), which reduces the severe convulsive movements, has made ECT a more safe and desirable method for treating depression. The use of ECT does not affect the person's intellectual function and may affect short-term memory only temporarily.

Pathophysiology

There are many theories as to the cause of major depression. A common one suggests an insufficient amount of brain monoamine neurotransmitters (i.e., norepinephrine, serotonin, perhaps dopamine). It is thought that decreased levels of serotonin permit depression to occur and decreased levels of norepinephrine cause depression. However, there can be other physiologic causes of depression as well as social and environmental factors.

Herbal Supplements for Depression

St. John's wort and gingko biloba have been suggested for the management of mild depression. St. John's wort can decrease reuptake of the neurotransmitters: serotonin, norepinephrine, and dopamine. The use of these and many herbal products should be discontinued 1 to 2 weeks before surgery. The client should check with the health care provider regarding herbal treatments (Herbal Alert 26–1).

Antidepressant Agents

The antidepressants are divided into four groups: (1) tricyclic antidepressants (TCAs), or tricyclics; (2) selective serotonin reuptake inhibitors (SSRIs); (3) atypical antidepressants that affect various neurotransmitters; and (4) monoamine oxidase inhibitors (MAOIs). The tricyclics and MAOIs were marketed in the late 1950s, and many of the SSRIs and atypical antidepressants were available in the 1980s. The SSRI agents are popular antidepressants because they do not cause sedation, hypotension, anticholinergic effects, or cardiotoxicity as do many of the TCAs. Many of the SSRIs can cause sexual dysfunction, which can be managed.

Tricyclic Antidepressants

The **tricyclic antidepressants (TCAs)** are used to treat major depression because they are effective and less expensive than the SSRIs and other drugs. Imipramine was the first TCA marketed in the 1950s.

HERBAL ALERT 26–1

Selective Serotonin Reuptake Inhibitors (SSRIs)

🍃 Feverfew may interfere with SSRI antidepressants, such as fluoxetine (Prozac).

🍃 St. John's wort interacts with SSRIs, which may cause serotonin syndrome (dizziness, headache, sweating, and agitation).

PROTOTYPE DRUG CHART 26–1

AMITRIPTYLINE HCl

Drug Class

Antidepressant
amitriptyline HCl: Tricyclic antidepressant
Trade Name: Elavil, ✤ Apo-Amitriptyline, Novotriptyn
Pregnancy Category: D

Dosage

A: PO: 25 mg b.i.d.-q.i.d.; increase to 150-200 mg/d; dose may be given as a single at bedtime dose
IM: 20-30 mg q.i.d.
C: >13 y: PO: 10 mg t.i.d. and 20 mg at bedtime
Elderly: PO: 10 mg t.i.d., 10-25 mg at bedtime
Therapeutic serum range: 100-200 ng/ml

Contraindications

Acute myocardial infarction (AMI), taking MAOIs
Caution: Severe depression with suicidal tendency, severe liver or kidney disease
Narrow-angle glaucoma, seizures, prostatic disease

Drug-Lab-Food Interactions

Drug: Increase effects of CNS, respiratory depression, and hypotensive effect with alcohol and CNS depressants
Increase sedation, anticholinergic effects with phenothiazines, and haloperidol; *increase* toxicity with cimetidine; *decrease* effect of clonidine, guanethidine
Hypertensive crisis and death may occur with MAOIs.
Lab: Altered ECG readings

Pharmacokinetics

Absorption: PO: well absorbed
Distribution: PB: 95%
Metabolism: t½: 10-50 h
Excretion: Excreted primarily in urine

Pharmacodynamics

PO: Onset: 1-3 wk
Peak: 2-6 wk
Duration: UK

Therapeutic Effects/Uses

To treat depression with or without melancholia, manic and depressive phases of bipolar disorder, depression associated with organic disease, alcoholism, migraine headaches, mixed symptoms of anxiety and depression, or urinary incontinence
Mode of Action: Serotonin and norepinephrine are increased in nerve cells because of blockage from nerve fibers.

Side Effects

Sedation, drowsiness, blurred vision, dry mouth and eyes, urinary retention, constipation, weight gain, dizziness, nervousness nausea, anorexia, sexual dysfunction

Adverse Reactions

Orthostatic hypotension, cardiac dysrhythmias, extrapyramidal syndrome (EPS)
Life threatening: Agranulocytosis, thrombocytopenia, leukopenia, seizures

A, Adult; *b.i.d.,* twice a day; *C,* child; *CNS,* central nervous system; *d,* day; *ECG,* electrocardiogram; *h,* hour; *IM,* intramuscular; *MAOI,* monoamine oxidase inhibitor; *PB,* protein-binding; *PO,* by mouth; *q.i.d.,* four times a day; *t½,* half-life; *t.i.d.,* three times a day; *UK,* unknown; *wk,* week; *>,* greater than; ✤, Canadian drug names.

TCAs block the uptake of the neurotransmitters norepinephrine and serotonin in the brain. The clinical response of TCAs occurs after 2 to 4 weeks of drug therapy. If there is no improvement after 2 to 4 weeks, the antidepressant is slowly withdrawn and another antidepressant is prescribed. *Polydrug therapy,* the practice of giving several antidepressants or antipsychotics together, should be avoided because of possible serious side effects.

TCAs have been effective for treating *major depression.* This group of drugs elevates mood, increases interest in daily living and activity, and decreases insomnia. For agitated depressed persons, amitriptyline (Elavil), doxepin (Sinequan), or trimipramine (Surmontil) may be pre-scribed because of their highly sedative effect. Frequently, TCAs are given at night to minimize the problems caused by their sedative action. When discontinuing TCAs, the drugs should gradually be decreased to avoid withdrawal symptoms, such as nausea, vomiting, anxiety, and akathisia. Imipramine hydrochloride (Tofranil) is used for the treatment of enuresis (involuntary discharge of urine during sleep in children).

The TCA drugs include amitriptyline, imipramine, trimipramine, doxepin, desipramine, nortriptyline, and protriptyline. The TCA drugs desipramine and nortriptyline are major metabolites of imipramine and amitriptyline. Prototype Drug Chart 26–1 describes the drug characteristics of amitriptyline.

Pharmacokinetics

Amitriptyline is strongly protein-bound. The half-life is 10 to 50 hours, and a cumulative drug effect may result. Amitriptyline is primarily excreted in urine.

Pharmacodynamics

Amitriptyline is well absorbed, but antidepressant effects develop slowly over several weeks. The onset of the antidepressant effect of amitriptyline is 1 to 4 weeks, and the peak concentration is 2 to 12 hours. Drug doses are decreased for elderly clients to reduce side effects.

Side Effects and Adverse Reactions

The TCAs have many side effects, such as orthostatic hypotension, sedation, anticholinergic effects, cardiac toxicity, and seizures. Rising from a sitting position too rapidly can cause dizziness and light-headedness; thus the client should be instructed to rise to an upright position slowly to avoid *orthostatic hypotension*. This group of antidepressants blocks the histamine receptors; thus sedation is likely to occur initially but decreases with continuous use of the drug. TCAs block the cholinergic receptors that can cause anticholinergic effects, such as tachycardia, urinary retention, constipation, dry mouth, and blurred vision. Other side effects of TCAs include allergic reactions (skin rash, pruritus, and petechiae) and sexual dysfunction (impotence and amenorrhea). Most TCAs can cause blood dyscrasias (leucopenia, thrombocytopenia, and agranulocytosis) requiring close monitoring of blood cell counts. Amitriptyline may lead to extrapyramidal symptoms (EPS). Clomipramine may cause neuroleptic malignant syndrome (NMS). TCAs decrease seizure threshold; therefore clients with seizure disorders may need to have the TCA dose adjusted. The most serious adverse reaction to TCAs is cardiac toxicity, such as dysrhythmias that may result from high doses of the drug.

Drug Interactions

Alcohol, hypnotics, sedatives, and barbiturates potentiate central nervous system (CNS) depression when taken with TCAs. Concurrent use of MAOIs with amitriptyline may lead to cardiovascular instability and toxic psychosis. Antithyroid medications taken with amitriptyline may increase the risk of dysrhythmias.

Selective Serotonin Reuptake Inhibitors

In the late 1980s a group of antidepressants that did not have TCA chemical structure were identified. This group was first classified as second-generation antidepressants. Today they have been reclassified as **selective serotonin reuptake inhibitors (SSRIs).** The SSRIs block the reuptake of serotonin into the nerve terminal of the CNS, thereby enhancing its transmission at the serotonergic synapse. SSRIs do not block the uptake of dopamine or norepinephrine, and they do not block cholinergic and alpha$_1$-adrenergic receptors. SSRIs are more commonly used to treat depression than are the TCAs, although they are more costly. SSRIs have fewer side effects than TCAs.

The primary use of SSRIs is for major depressive disorders. They are also effective for treating anxiety disorders such as obsessive-compulsiveness, panic, phobias, post-traumatic stress disorders, and other forms of anxiety. Fluvoxamine (Luvox) is useful for treating obsessive-compulsive disorders in children and adults. SSRIs have also been used to treat eating disorders and selected drug abuses. Miscellaneous uses for SSRIs include decreasing premenstrual tension syndrome, preventing migraine headaches, and preventing or minimizing aggressive behavior in clients with borderline personality disorder.

The SSRIs include fluoxetine (Prozac), fluvoxamine (Luvox), sertraline (Zoloft), paroxetine (Paxil), citalopram (Celexa), and escitalopram (Lexapro). Fluoxetine (Prozac) has been effective in 50% to 60% of clients who fail to respond to TCA therapy (TCA-refractory depression). Of all the SSRIs, sertraline (Zoloft) is the most commonly prescribed antidepressant. The Food and Drug Administration (FDA) approved of a weekly fluoxetine dose of 90 mg. However before taking the weekly dose, the client should respond to a daily maintenance dose of 20 mg per day without serious effects. It has been reported that there are some side effects to the weekly 90 mg fluoxetine dose. Many SSRIs have an interaction with grapefruit juice that can lead to possible toxicity. It is recommended that daily intake be limited to 8 oz of grapefruit juice or one half a grapefruit. Do not confuse Celexa with Celebrex (anti-inflammatory) because the names look similar. Prototype Drug Chart 26–2 describes drug characteristics of the SSRI fluoxetine (Prozac). Table 26–1 lists the side effects of the various antidepressants.

Pharmacokinetics

Fluoxetine is strongly protein bound. The half-life is 2 to 3 days; therefore a cumulative drug effect may result from long-term use. Fluoxetine is metabolized and excreted by the kidneys.

Pharmacodynamics

Fluoxetine is well absorbed; however, its antidepressant effect develops slowly over several weeks. The onset of antidepressant effect of fluoxetine is between 1 and 4 weeks; however, the peak concentration times of fluoxetine is 4 to 8 hours. The drug dose for older adults should be decreased to reduce side effects.

Side Effects and Adverse Reactions

Fluoxetine produces common side effects, such as dry mouth, blurred vision, insomnia, headache, nervousness, anorexia, nausea, diarrhea, and suicidal ideation. Fluoxetine has fewer side effects than amitriptyline. See Table 26–1 for side effects of antidepressants.

Some clients may experience sexual dysfunction when taking SSRIs. Men have discontinued taking fluoxetine (Prozac) after experiencing a decrease in sexual arousal. Some women have become anorgasmic when taking paroxetine HCl (Paxil). The side effects often decrease or cease over the 2- to 4-week period of waiting for the therapeutic effect to emerge.

Atypical Antidepressants

Atypical (heterocyclic) antidepressants, or *second-generation antidepressants,* became available in the 1980s and have been used for major depression, reactive de-

PROTOTYPE DRUG CHART 26–2

FLUOXETINE

Drug Class	**Dosage**
Antidepressant Selective serotonin reuptake inhibitor Trade Name: Prozac *Pregnancy Category:* B	**A: PO:** 20 mg in AM *max:* 80 mg/d in divided doses **Elderly:** 10 mg/d initially; may increase by 10-20 mg q2wk **Therapeutic range:** 90-300 ng/ml
Contraindications	**Drug-Lab-Food Interactions**
Acute myocardial infarction (AMI), taking MAOIs *Caution:* Severe depression with suicidal tendency, severe liver or kidney disease	*Drug: Increase* effects of CNS, respiratory depression, and hypotensive effect with alcohol and CNS depressants *Lab:* Altered ECG readings
Pharmacokinetics	**Pharmacodynamics**
Absorption: PO: well absorbed **Distribution:** PB: 95% **Metabolism:** *fluoxetine:* t½: 2-3 d **Excretion:** Excreted primarily in urine	**PO:** Onset: 2-4 wk Peak: 2-4 wk Duration: weeks

Therapeutic Effects/Uses

To treat depression with or without melancholia, manic and depressive phases of bipolar disorder, depression associated with organic disease, alcoholism, migraine headaches, mixed symptoms of anxiety and depression, or urinary incontinence
Mode of Action: Serotonin is increased in nerve cells because of blockage from nerve fibers.

Side Effects	**Adverse Reactions**
Headache, nervousness, restlessness, insomnia, tremors, GI distress, sexual dysfunction	Seizures

A, Adult; *CNS,* central nervous system; *d,* day; *ECG,* electrocardiogram; *GI,* gastrointestinal; *MAOI,* monoamine oxidase inhibitor; *max,* maximum; *PB,* protein-binding; *PO,* by mouth; *t½,* half-life; *wk,* week.

---

pression, and anxiety. They affect one or two of the three neurotransmitters: serotonin, norepinephrine, and dopamine. One of the first atypical antidepressants marketed was amoxapine (Asendin), and others include bupropion (Wellbutrin), maprotiline (Ludiomil), nefazodone (Serzone), trazodone (Desyrel), mirtazapine (Remeron), venlafaxine (Effexor), and reboxetine (Vestra). Amoxapine and maprotiline are sometimes considered to be TCAs because of their pharmacologic similarities. Atypical antidepressant agents should not be taken with MAOIs and should not be used within 14 days after discontinuing MAOIs. Trazodone may have a potential drug interaction with ketoconazole, ritonavir, and indinavir that may lead to increased trazodone levels and adverse effects. Table 26–2 lists the drugs and how each affects the various neurotransmitters.

Monoamine Oxidase Inhibitors

The fourth group of antidepressants is the **monoamine oxidase inhibitors (MAOIs).** The enzyme monoamine oxidase inactivates norepinephrine, dopamine, epineph-

rine, and serotonin. By inhibiting monoamine oxidase, the levels of these neurotransmitters rise. In the body there are two forms of monoamine oxidase (MAO) enzyme: MAO-A and MAO-B. These enzymes are found primarily in the liver and brain. MAO-A inactivates dopamine in the brain, whereas MAO-B inactivates norepinephrine and serotonin. The MAOIs are nonselective; thus they inhibit both MAO-A and MAO-B. Inhibition of MAO by MAOIs is thought to relieve the symptoms of depression. Three MAOIs are currently prescribed: tranylcypromine sulfate (Parnate), isocarboxazid (Marplan), and phenelzine sulfate (Nardil). These MAOIs are discussed in Table 26–2.

MAOIs are as effective as TCAs for treating depression, but because of adverse reactions, such as the risk of hypertensive crisis resulting from food and drug interactions, only 1% of clients taking antidepressants take an MAOI. Currently, MAOIs are usually prescribed when the client does not respond to TCAs or second-generation antidepressants. MAOIs are not the antidepressants of choice. However, MAOIs are used for mild, reactive, and atypical depression (chronic anx-

Table 26–1

Side Effects of Antidepressants

Antidepressant Category	Anticholinergic Effect	Sedation	Hypotension	GI Distress	Cardiotoxicity	Seizures	Insomnia/ Agitation
Tricyclic Antidepressants							
amitriptyline (Elavil)	++++	++++	+++	—	++++	+++	—
clomipramine (Anafranil)	++++	++++	++	—	++++	++	—
desipramine (Norpramin)	+	++	++	—	++	++	+
doxepin (Sinequan)	+++	++++	++	—	++	++	—
imipramine (Tofranil)	+++	+++	+++	+	++++	++	+
nortriptyline (Aventyl)	+	+++	+	—	+++	++	—
protriptyline (Vivactil)	+++	+	++	—	+++	++	+
trimipramine (Surmontil)	+++	++++	+++	—	++++	++	—
Selective Serotonin Reuptake Inhibitors							
citalopram (Celexa)	+	0	0	++	—	—	+
fluoxetine (Prozac)	—	+	—	+++	—	0/+	++
fluvoxamine (Luvox)	—	++	—	+++	—	—	++
paroxetine (Paxil)	—	+	—	+++	—	—	++
sertraline (Zoloft)	—	+	—	+++	—	—	++
Atypical (Heterocyclic) Antidepressants							
amoxapine (Asendin)	+++	++	+	—	+	+++	++
bupropion (Wellbutrin)	++	—	0/+	+	+	++++	++
trazodone (Desyrel)	—	+++	++	+	+	+	—
maprotiline (Ludiomil)	+++	+++	+	—	++	+++	—
venlafaxine (Effexor)	0	0	0	0	0/+	+	—
Monoamine Oxidase Inhibitors (MAOIs)	—	+	++	+	—	—	++

—, No effect; +, mild effect; ++, moderate effect; +++, strong effect; ++++, severe effect.

iety, hypersomnia, fear). MAOIs and TCAs should *not* be taken together when treating depression.

Drug and Food Interactions

Certain drug and food interactions with MAOIs can be fatal. Any drugs that are CNS stimulants or sympathomimetics, such as vasoconstrictors and cold medications containing phenylephrine and pseudoephedrine, can cause a hypertensive crisis when taken with an MAOI. In addition, foods that contain tyramine, such as cheese (cheddar, Swiss, bleu), cream, yogurt, coffee, chocolate, bananas, raisins, Italian green beans, liver, pickled herring, sausage, soy sauce, yeast, beer, and red wines, have sympathomimetic-like effects and can cause a hypertensive crisis (Table 26–3). These types of food and drugs *must be avoided*. Frequent blood pressure monitoring is essential when a client takes MAOIs. Client teaching regarding foods and over-the-counter (OTC) drugs to avoid is an important nursing responsibility. Because of the danger associated with a hypertensive crisis, many psychiatrists will not prescribe MAOIs for depression unless they sense the client's ability to comply with the drug and food regimen. However, if properly taken, this group of drugs is effective for treating depression.

In teaching clients about the foods and drugs to avoid when taking MAOIs, some individuals respond better to verbal instructions and education with reinforcement from videos than to printed communications. See Herbal Alert 26–2 for herb interactions with MAOIs.

Side Effects and Adverse Reactions

Side effects of MAOIs include CNS stimulation (agitation, restlessness, insomnia), orthostatic hypotension, and anticholinergic effects.

HERBAL ALERT 26–2

Monoamine Oxidase Inhibitors (MAOIs)

🌸 Ginseng, ephedra, ma-huang, and St. John's wort may lead to palpitations, heart attack, and hypertensive crisis when taken with antidepressant MAOIs.

🌸 Ginseng may lead to manic episodes when given in combination with MAOIs, such as tranylcypromine sulfate.

🌸 Excessive dose of anise may interfere with MAOIs.

🌸 An increase use of brewer's yeast with MAOIs can increase the blood pressure.

Table 26-2

Antidepressants

Generic (Brand)	Route and Dosage	Uses and Considerations
Tricyclic Antidepressants		
amitriptyline HCl (Elavil, Endep, Enovil)	See Prototype Drug Chart 26–1. *Therapeutic serum range:* 100-200 ng/ml	
clomipramine HCl (Anafranil)	A: PO: 25-100 mg/d in divided doses; *max:* 250 mg/d; after titration, entire dose may be given at bedtime Elderly: 20-30 mg/d C: >10 y: PO: 25-100 mg/d in divided doses or 3 mg/kg/d	To treat obsessive-compulsive disorder. May be used to alleviate anxiety or panic disorder. Tremor, dizziness, weight gain, and dry mouth are common side effects. *Pregnancy category:* C; PB: 97%; t½: 20-30 h
desipramine HCl (Norpramin, Pertofrane)	A: PO: 25 mg t.i.d. or 75 mg at bedtime; increase to 200 mg/d; *max:* 300 mg/d Elderly: 25-50 mg/d in divided doses; *max:* 150 mg/d *Therapeutic serum range:* 150-250 ng/ml	For depression. Has been used for attention deficit/hyperactivity disorder (ADHD). Take with food if GI distress occurs. Common side effects include drowsiness, dry mouth, increased appetite, urinary retention, and postural hypotension. *Pregnancy category:* D; PB: 90%-95%; t½: 12-60 h
doxepin HCl (Sinequan, Zonalcon)	A: PO: 75-100 mg/d at bedtime or in divided doses; *max:* 300 mg/d Elderly: 25-50 mg/d *Therapeutic serum range:* 30-50 ng/ml	For depression and anxiety related to involutional depression or manic-depressive disorder. Has less effect on cardiac status than other drugs in this group. *Pregnancy category:* C; PB: 80%-85%; t½: 6-8 h
imipramine HCl (Tofranil)	A: PO: 75 mg/d (at bedtime or 25 mg t.i.d.); *max:* 300 mg/d IM: Initially: *max:* 100 mg/d in divided doses Elderly: 25-100 mg in divided doses C: <12 y: PO: 25-50 mg at bedtime C: >12 y: PO: 75 mg at bedtime *Therapeutic serum range:* 150-250 ng/ml	For depression. Can be taken at bedtime to lessen dangers from sedative effect. Take with food if GI distress occurs. Avoid taking with alcohol or CNS depressants. Common side effects include drowsiness, dry mouth, hypotension, delayed micturition. *Pregnancy category:* D; PB: 90%-95%; t½: 8-15 h
nortriptyline HCl (Aventyl)	A: PO: 25 mg t.i.d.-q.i.d.; *max:* 150 mg/d Elderly: 30-50 mg/d in divided doses or 10-25 mg at bedtime *Therapeutic serum range:* 50-150 ng/ml	For depression. Similar to imipramine HCl. *Pregnancy category:* D; PB: 90%-95%; t½: 18-28 h
protriptyline HCl (Vivactil)	A: PO: 15-40 mg/d in divided doses; increase gradually; *max:* 60 mg/d Elderly: 5 mg t.i.d.; *max:* 20 mg/d *Therapeutic serum range:* 70-250 ng/ml	For depression. Has little sedative effect. Effects are similar to imipramine HCl. *Pregnancy category:* C; PB: 92%; t½: 60-98 h
trimipramine maleate (Surmontil)	A: 75-150 mg/d in divided doses or at bedtime; *max:* 200 mg/d Elderly: *max:* 100 mg/d	For depression. Similar to imipramine HCl. *Pregnancy category:* C; PB: 95%; t½: 20-26 h
Selective Serotonin Reuptake Inhibitors (SSRIs)		
citalopram (Celexa)	A: PO: 20-40 mg/d; *max:* 80 mg/d Elderly: 10-20 mg/d	For depression, panic disorder, obsessive-compulsive disorder. Wait 14 days after stopping MAOIs. May cause sexual dysfunction, insomnia, nausea, and dry mouth. *Pregnancy category:* C; PB: UK; t½: 35 h
fluoxetine HCl (Prozac)	See Prototype Drug Chart 26–2.	
paroxetine HCl (Paxil)	*Depression:* A: PO: 10-50 mg/d; *max:* 80 mg/d Elderly: PO: Initially: 10 mg/d; *max:* 40 mg/d *Obsessive-compulsive disorder:* A: PO: 20-60 mg/d *Panic attack:* A: PO: 40 mg/d	For depression and obsessive-compulsive disorders. Lower dose for older adults and those with renal and hepatic disorders. Side effects include dizziness, insomnia, headache, nausea, dry mouth, tremors, postural hypotension. *Pregnancy category:* B; PB: 90%-95%; t½: 21 h, elderly: 68 h
sertraline HCl (Zoloft)	A: PO: 50 mg/d; *max:* 200 mg/d Elderly: 25 mg/d; dose may be increased	Management of major depression disorders. Do *not* take with MAOIs or TCAs. Take with food if GI distress occurs. Urine may be pink-red-brown color. *Pregnancy category:* B; PB: 98%; t½: 26 h

A, Adult; *b.i.d.,* twice a day; *C,* child; *CNS,* central nervous system; *d,* day; *EPS,* extrapyramidal symptoms; *GI,* gastrointestinal; *h,* hour; *IM,* intramuscular; *maint,* maintenance; *MAOIs,* monoamine oxidase inhibitors; *max,* maximum; *PB,* protein-binding; *PO,* by mouth; *q.i.d.,* four times a day; *t½,* half-life; *t.i.d.,* three times a day; *TCAs,* tricyclic antidepressants; *UK,* unknown; *y,* year; <, less than; >, greater than.

Table 26–2

Antidepressants—cont'd

Generic (Brand)	Route and Dosage	Uses and Considerations
Selective Serotonin Reuptake Inhibitors (SSRIs)—cont'd		
fluvoxamine (Luvox)	A: PO: 50 mg at bedtime, increase by 50 mg in 5 to 7 d; *max:* 300 mg/d C: 8-18 y: PO: 25 mg at bedtime, increase by 25 mg; *max:* 200 mg/d Elderly: decrease dose	To treat obsessive-compulsive disorder and depression. Caution: Do not use in renal or hepatic disorder. *Pregnancy category:* C; PB: UK; t$^1/_2$: 13-15 h
escitalopram (Lexapro)	A: PO: 10 mg/d, may increase to 20 mg/d after 1 wk Elderly: 10 mg/d	For management of depression. *Pregnancy category:* C; PB: 89%; t$^1/_2$: 25 h
Atypical (Heterocyclic or Second Generation) Antidepressants		
amoxapine (Asendin)	A: PO: 25 mg b.i.d.-q.i.d.; increase 150-200 mg/d; dose may be given as a single one	For depression with anxiety and reactive depression. Do not take with MAOIs. Side effects include drowsiness, dizziness, EPS, postural hypotension, increased appetite, urinary retention. *Pregnancy category:* C; PB: >90%; t$^1/_2$: 8 h
maprotiline HCl (Ludiomil)	A: PO: 75 mg at bedtime or in divided doses; *max:* 150 mg/d in single or divided doses Elderly: 25 mg at bedtime; *max:* 75 mg/d	Same as amoxapine. Can be taken at bedtime. *Pregnancy category:* B; PB: 88%; t$^1/_2$: 21-25 h
trazodone HCl (Desyrel)	A: PO: 75 mg at bedtime or 50 mg t.i.d.-q.i.d.; *max:* 600 mg/d	For depression. Can be taken at bedtime to lessen dangers from sedative effect. Drowsiness, light-headedness, orthostatic hypotension, and dry mouth might occur. Take with food to decrease GI distress. *Pregnancy category:* C; PB: 85%-95%; t$^1/_2$: 5-10 h
Norepinephrine and Dopamine Reuptake Inhibitors (NDRIs)		
bupropion HCl (Wellbutrin)	A: PO: Initially: 200 mg/d as b.i.d.; increase gradually to 300 mg/d in divided doses; *max:* 450 mg/d	For depression. May cause increased risk of seizures. Avoid with a history of seizures. Many side effects. *Pregnancy category:* B; PB: >80%; t$^1/_2$: 50 h
Serotonin Antagonists		
mirtazapine (Remeron)	A: PO: 15-30 mg at bedtime; *maint:* 15-45 mg at bedtime; *max:* 60 mg/d	For depression, anxiety, and insomnia. It increases both norepinephrine and serotonin neurotransmitters. It has low anticholinergic activity. *Pregnancy category:* C/D; PB: UK; t$^1/_2$: 20-40 h
Serotonin and Norepinephrine Reuptake Inhibitors		
venlafaxine (Effexor)	A: PO: 75-150 mg/d in 2-3 divided doses; *max:* 375 mg/d in 3 divided doses	For depression, feelings of guilt, worthlessness, and anxiety. Dose decreased with renal and hepatic disorders and for anxiety. Does not cause cardiovascular problems or sedation. *Pregnancy category:* C; PB: UK; t$^1/_2$: 3-7 h, metabolites 9-13 h.
Selective Norepinephrine Reuptake Inhibitors (SNRIs)		
reboxetine (Vestra)	A: PO: Initially: 4 mg/d; *maint:* 4-12 mg/d	For depression. New antidepressant agent. Blood pressure should be monitored. *Pregnancy category:* UK; PB: UK; t$^1/_2$: 12-16 h
Monoamine Oxidase Inhibitors (MAOIs)		
isocarboxazid (Marplan)	A: PO: 10-20 mg/d; *max:* 60 mg/d	For depression that is refractory to TCAs. Avoid certain foods such as cheese, beer, figs, shrimp, bananas, and chocolate and avoid drugs (e.g., TCAs). *Pregnancy category:* C; PB: UK; t$^1/_2$: UK
phenelzine sulfate (Nardil)	A: PO: 15 mg t.i.d.; 1 mg/kg in divided doses; *max:* 90 mg/d Elderly: *max:* 45-60 mg/d	For depression. Avoid certain foods and drugs (see isocarboxazid). *Pregnancy category:* C; PB: UK; t$^1/_2$: UK
tranylcypromine sulfate (Parnate)	A: PO: 30 mg/d in 2 divided doses (20 mg in AM and 10 mg in PM); *max:* 60 mg/d Elderly: *max:* 45 mg/d	Same as isocarboxazid and phenelzine sulfate.
Mood Stabilizer		
lithium carbonate: lithium citrate	See Prototype Drug Chart 21–3.	

Table 26–3

Foods that Can Cause a Hypertensive Crisis When Taken with Monoamine Oxidase Inhibitors

Foods	Effects
Cheese (cheddar, Swiss, bleu)	Sweating, tremors
Bananas, raisins	Bounding heart rate
Pickled foods	Increased blood pressure
Red wine, beer	Increased temperature
Cream, yogurt	
Chocolate, coffee	
Italian green beans	
Liver	
Yeast	
Soy sauce	

*Avoid taking barbiturates, tricyclic antidepressants, antihistamines, central nervous system depressants, and over-the-counter cold medications with monoamine oxidase inhibitors.

Nursing Process

Antidepressants

ASSESSMENT

■ Record client's baseline vital signs and weight for future comparison.

■ Check client's liver and renal function by assessing urine output (>600 ml/d), blood urea nitrogen (BUN), and serum creatinine and liver enzyme levels.

■ Obtain a health history of episodes of depression; assess mental status and assess for suicidal tendencies.

■ Secure a drug history of the current drugs and herbs client is taking. CNS depressants can cause an additive effect. Antidepressants that cause anticholinergic-like symptoms are contraindicated if client has glaucoma.

■ Assess for tardive dyskinesia and neuroleptic malignant syndrome (NMS), including hyperpyrexia, muscle rigidity, tachycardia, and cardiac dysrhythmias.

NURSING DIAGNOSES

■ Potential for violence and injury
■ Anxiety
■ Social isolation
■ Ineffective coping
■ Altered mood
■ Hopelessness
■ Knowledge deficit
■ Ineffective health maintenance

PLANNING

■ Client's depression or manic-depressive behavior will be decreased.

NURSING INTERVENTIONS

■ Observe client for signs and symptoms of depression: mood changes, insomnia, apathy, or lack of interest in activities.

■ Check client's vital signs. Orthostatic hypotension is common. Check for anticholinergic-like symptoms: dry mouth, increased heart rate, urinary retention, or constipation. Check weight two or three times per week.

■ Monitor client for suicidal tendencies when marked depression is present.

■ If client is taking an anticonvulsant, observe client for seizures; antidepressants lower the seizure threshold. The anticonvulsant dose might need to be increased.

■ Provide the client with a list of foods to avoid, especially when taking monoamine oxidase inhibitors (MAOIs). These include cheese, red wine, beer, liver, bananas, yogurt, sausage, and others.

■ Check client for extremely high blood pressure when taking MAOIs. Sympathomimetic-like drugs and foods containing tyramine may cause a hypertensive crisis if taken with MAOIs.

Client Teaching

General

• Teach client to take the medication as prescribed. Compliance is important.

• Inform client that the full effectiveness of the drug may not be evident until 1 to 2 weeks after the start of therapy.

• Encourage client to keep medical appointments.

• Instruct client not to consume alcohol or any CNS depressants because of their addictive effect.

• Inform client that many herbal products interact with antidepressants, especially MAOIs and selective serotonin reuptake inhibitors (SSRIs). Herbs may need to be discontinued or the antidepressant drug dosage may need modification. See Herbal Alert 26–1 and 26–2.

• Teach client not to drive or be involved in potentially dangerous mechanical activity until stabilization of drug dose has been established.

• Instruct client not to abruptly stop taking the drug. Drug dose should be gradually decreased.

• Encourage client who is planning pregnancy to consult with the health care provider about possible teratogenic effects of the drug on the fetus.

• Take with food if GI distress occurs.

Side Effects

• Advise client that antidepressants may be taken at bedtime to decrease the dangers from the sedative effect. Have client check with the health care provider. Transient side effects include nausea, drowsiness, headaches, and nervousness.

Cultural Considerations ⊡

• If Asian client is taking an antipsychotic, such as tricyclic antidepressant (TCA) or lithium, the drug dose may need to be decreased. Explain this to client.

- Explain to Hispanic client that the dose for the antidepressant drug may be lower than is required for other cultural groups.

EVALUATION

■ Evaluate the effectiveness of the drug therapy regarding whether client's depression is controlled or has ceased.

Mood Stabilizer: Lithium for Bipolar Disorder

The last antidepressant drug to be discussed in this chapter is lithium, which is used to treat bipolar affective disorder. Lithium was first used as a salt substitute in the 1940s, but because of lithium poisoning, it was banned from the market. Some refer to lithium as an antimania drug that is effective in controlling manic behavior that arises from underlying depression. It is most effective in controlling the manic phase. Lithium has a calming effect without impairing intellectual activity. It controls any evidence of flight of ideas and hyperactivity. If the person stops taking lithium, manic behavior may return.

Lithium is an inexpensive drug that must be closely monitored. Lithium has a narrow therapeutic serum range: 0.5 to 1.5 mEq/L. Serum lithium levels greater than 1.5 to 2 mEq/L are toxic. The serum lithium level should be monitored biweekly until the therapeutic level has been obtained and then monitored monthly on the maintenance dose. Serum sodium levels also need to be monitored because lithium tends to deplete sodium. Use lithium with caution, if at all, in clients taking diuretics. Prototype Drug Chart 26–3 lists the pharmacologic behavior of lithium.

Pharmacokinetics

More than 95% of lithium is absorbed through the gastrointestinal (GI) tract. The average half-life of lithium is 24 hours; however, in older adults the half-life can be up to 36 hours. Because of its long half-life, cumulative drug action may result. Lithium is metabolized by the liver, and most of the drug is excreted unchanged in the urine.

PROTOTYPE DRUG CHART 26–3

LITHIUM

Drug Class

Mood stabilizer
Trade Name: Eskalith, Lithane, Lithonate, Lithobid,
🍁 Carbolith, Lithizine
Pregnancy Category: D

Contraindications

Liver and renal disease, pregnancy, lactation, severe cardiovascular disease, severe dehydration, brain tumor or damage, sodium depletion, children <12 y of age
Caution: Thyroid disease

Dosage

A: PO: 300-600 mg t.i.d.; *maint:* 300 mg t.i.d.-q.i.d.; *max:* 2.4 g/d
Elderly: Lower dosage
Therapeutic drug range: 0.5-1.5 mEq/L

Drug-Lab-Food Interactions

Drug: May *increase* lithium level with thiazide diuretics, methyldopa, haloperidol, NSAIDs, antidepressants, carbamazepine, theophylline, aminophylline, sodium bicarbonate, phenothiazines
Lab: *Increase* urine and blood glucose, protein; decrease serum sodium level
Food: *Increase* sodium intake; lithium may cause sodium depletion

Pharmacokinetics

Absorption: PO: well absorbed
Distribution: PB: UK
Metabolism: t½: 21-30 h; >36 h with renal impairment or in elderly
Excretion: 98% in urine, mostly unchanged

Pharmacodynamics

PO: Onset: UK
Peak: 2-4 h
Duration: 24 h

Therapeutic Effects/Uses

To treat bipolar manic-depressive psychosis, manic episodes
Mode of Action: Alteration of ion transport in muscle and nerve cells; increased receptor sensitivity to serotonin

Side Effects

Headache, lethargy, drowsiness, dizziness, tremors, slurred speech, dry mouth, anorexia, vomiting, diarrhea, polyuria, hypotension, abdominal pain, muscle weakness, restlessness

Adverse Reactions

Urinary incontinence, clonic movements, stupor, azotemia, leukocytosis, nephrotoxicity
Life-threatening: Cardiac dysrhythmias, circulatory collapse

A, Adult; *C,* child; *d,* day; *h,* hour; *max,* maximum; *NSAIDs,* nonsteroidal antiinflammatory drugs; *PB,* protein-binding; *PO,* by mouth; *q.i.d.,* four times a day; *SR,* sustained release; *t.i.d.,* three times a day; *t½* half-life; *UK,* unknown; <, less than; 🍁, Canadian drug names.

Pharmacodynamics

Lithium is prescribed mostly for the stabilization of bipolar affective disorder. The onset of action is fast, but the client may not achieve the desired effect for 5 to 6 days. Increased sodium intake increases renal excretion, so the sodium intake needs to be closely monitored. Increased urine output can result in body fluid loss and dehydration. Adequate fluid intake of 1 to 2 L should be maintained daily.

Anticonvulsants such as carbamazepine (Tegretol) and valproic acid (Depakote) have been used in place of lithium for some clients. The drug olanzapine (Zyprexa) is used for treating acute mania and maintenance therapy; lamotrigine (Lamictal) is now used for maintenance therapy to treat bipolar disorder. Also, a combination of olanzapine and fluoxetine HCl (Symbyax) is now used for depressive episodes associated with bipolar disorder.

Side Effects and Adverse Reactions

Many side effects from taking lithium, such as dry mouth, thirst, increased urination (loss of water and sodium), weight gain, bloated feeling, metallic taste, and edema of the hands and ankles, can be annoying to the client. If taken during pregnancy, lithium may have teratogenic effects on the fetus.

Lithium and nonsteroidal antiinflammatory drugs (NSAIDs) should not be given together on a continuous basis and should not be prescribed for clients who have a cardiac sick sinus syndrome. If the client has taken lithium for a long period, laboratory tests to determine thyroid function should be closely monitored.

Nursing Process

Mood Stabilizer: Lithium

ASSESSMENT

■ Assess for suicidal ideation.
■ Record client's baseline vital signs for future comparison.
■ Evaluate client's neurologic status, including gait, level of consciousness, reflexes, and tremors.
■ Check client's hepatic and renal function by assessing urine output (>600 ml/d) and whether blood urea nitrogen (BUN) and serum creatinine and liver enzyme levels are within normal range. Assess for toxicity. Draw weekly blood levels initially and then every 1 to 2 months. Therapeutic serum levels for acute mania are 1 to 1.5 mEq/L; for maintenance, levels are 0.5 to 1.5 mEq/L. Signs and symptoms of toxicity at serum levels of 1.5 to 2 mEq/L are persistent nausea and vomiting, severe diarrhea, ataxia, blurred vision, and tinnitus. At 2 to 3.5 mEq/L, signs and symptoms of toxicity are excessive output of dilute urine, increasing tremors, muscular irritability, psychomotor retardation, mental confusion, and giddiness. At >3.5 mEq/L, levels are life

threatening and may result in impaired consciousness, nystagmus, seizures, coma, oliguria/anuria, cardiac dysrhythmias, myocardial infarction, and cardiovascular collapse. Withhold medications and notify health care provider immediately if any of these occur.
■ Obtain a health history of episodes of depression or manic-depressive behavior.
■ Obtain client's drug history. Diuretics, nonsteroidal antiinflammatory drugs (NSAIDs) (e.g., ibuprofen), tetracyclines, methyldopa, and probenecid decrease renal clearance of lithium thus causing lithium accumulation.

NURSING DIAGNOSES

■ Potential for injury or violence related to excessive hyperactivity
■ Ineffective individual coping
■ Noncompliance

PLANNING

■ Client's manic-depressive behavior will be decreased.

NURSING INTERVENTIONS

■ Observe client for signs and symptoms of depression: mood changes, insomnia, apathy, or lack of interest in activities.
■ Record client's vital signs. Orthostatic hypotension is common.
■ When drawing blood to check for lithium levels, draw samples immediately before the next dose (8 to 12 hours after the previous dose). Monitor for signs of lithium toxicity. Report high (>1.5 mEq/L) or toxic (>2 mEq/L) serum lithium levels immediately to the health care provider.
■ Monitor client for suicidal tendencies when marked depression is present.
■ Evaluate client's urine output and body weight. Fluid volume deficit may occur as a result of polyuria.
■ Observe client for fine and gross motor tremors and presence of slurred speech, which are signs of adverse reaction.
■ Check client's cardiac status. Loss of fluids and electrolytes may cause cardiac dysrhythmias.
■ Monitor client's serum electrolytes. Report abnormal findings.

Client Teaching
General
• Teach client to take lithium as prescribed. Emphasize the importance of adherence to the therapy, laboratory tests, and follow-up visits with the health care provider. If lithium is stopped, manic symptoms will reappear.
• Encourage client to keep medical appointments. Have client check with the health care provider before taking OTC preparations.

- Instruct client not to drive a motor vehicle or be involved in potentially dangerous mechanical activity until stable lithium level is established.
- Advise client to maintain adequate fluid intake: 2 to 3 L/d initially and 1 to 2 L/d maintenance. Fluid intake should increase in hot weather.
- Teach client to take the lithium with meals to decrease gastric irritation.
- Inform client that the effectiveness of the drug may not be evident until 1 to 2 weeks after the start of therapy. Compliance in taking the prescribed lithium doses on a daily basis is a major problem with bipolar clients. When client has a period of emotional stability, he or she does not believe that the drug is needed; thus, client stops taking the lithium.
- Advise client who is planning pregnancy to consult with the health care provider about possible teratogenic effects of the drug on the fetus, especially during the first 3 months.
- Encourage client to wear or carry an identification tag or bracelet indicating the drug taken.

Diet
- Inform client to avoid caffeine products (coffee, tea, cola) because they can aggravate the manic phase of the bipolar disorder.
- Instruct client to maintain adequate sodium intake and to avoid crash diets that affect physical and mental health.

Side Effects
- Advise client to contact the health care provider for early symptoms of toxicity: diarrhea, drowsiness, loss of appetite, muscle weakness, nausea, vomiting, slurred speech, trembling; for late symptoms of toxicity: blurred vision, confusion, increased urination, convulsions, severe trembling, and unsteadiness.

Cultural Considerations

- Obtain an interpreter when necessary; do not rely on family members, who may not fully disclose because of honor and shame.

EVALUATION

- Evaluate the effectiveness of the drug therapy. Client is free of bipolar behavior.
- Allow client to verbalize understanding of symptoms of toxicity.
- Determine whether client demonstrates a subsiding or resolution of the symptoms.

WEBSITES

For further information on *Antidepressants and Mood Stabilizer,* visit these Internet resources:

Antidepressants:
http://www.nimh.nih.gov/publicat/medicate.cfm

Information on sertraline:
http://www.zoloft.com

Critical Thinking Case Study

S.T., 37 years old, is receiving fluoxetine (Prozac) 20 mg in the evening for depression. S.T. complains of insomnia and GI upset.

1. To avoid insomnia, what could you suggest to S.T.? Explain.
2. How might S.T. avoid GI upset when taking fluoxetine?

S.T. states that she does not think the fluoxetine is helping. She has heard that there are herbal supplements that may be taken for depression. In addition, she heard that fluoxetine can be taken weekly.

3. Is S.T.'s fluoxetine dose within normal dosage range? Explain.
4. How would you respond to S.T. about the use of certain herbal supplements for depression?
5. What would your response be concerning the use of fluoxetine in a weekly dose?

Study Questions

1. The client is receiving imipramine hydrochloride (Tofranil). Imipramine is from what drug category? Why do some clients take the drug at bedtime?

2. The client is taking tranylcypromine sulfate (Parnate), a monoamine oxidase inhibitor. What should the nurse teach the client regarding food and drugs? Explain.

3. What are the similarities and differences between SSRIs and atypical antidepressants?

4. Lithium is effective for what type of psychiatric disorder? What is the therapeutic serum lithium level? Why should the urinary output and vital signs be closely monitored?

5. What anticonvulsant(s) may be used in place of lithium? Explain.

Eight

Antiinflammatory and Antiinfective Agents

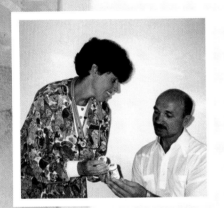

Introduction

Unit V discusses agents prescribed to alleviate an inflammatory process and combat disease-producing microorganisms (pathogens). Included in this unit are antiinflammatory drugs; antibacterials-antibiotics (penicillins, cephalosporins, macrolides, tetracyclines, aminoglycosides, and fluoroquinolones); sulfonamides; peptides; antitubercular, antifungal, antiviral, antimalarial and anthelmintic drugs; and urinary antiseptics.

Inflammation

Inflammation is a reaction to tissue injury caused by the release of chemical mediators that cause both a vascular response and the migration of fluid and cells (leukocytes, or white blood cells) to the injured site. The chemical mediators are (1) histamines, (2) kinins, and (3) prostaglandins. *Histamine,* the first mediator in the inflammatory process, causes dilation of the arterioles and increases capillary permeability, allowing fluid to leave the capillaries and flow into the injured area. *Kinins,* such as bradykinin, also increase capillary permeability and the sensation of pain. *Prostaglandins* are released, causing an increase in vasodilation, capillary permeability, pain, and fever. The antiinflammatory drugs, such as nonsteroidal antiinflammatory drugs (NSAIDs) and steroids (cortisone preparations), inhibit chemical mediators thus decreasing the inflammatory process. Figure VIII–1 illustrates the process of chemical mediators acting on the injured tissues. The five responses to tissue injury are called the *cardinal signs of inflammation:* redness, swelling, pain, heat, and loss of function.

Inflammation may or may not be the result of an infection. (Only a small percentage of inflammations are caused by infections.) Other causes of inflammation include trauma, surgical interventions, extreme heat or cold, and caustic chemical agents. Antiinflammatory drugs reduce fluid migration and pain thus lessening loss of function and increasing the client's mobility and comfort.

Infection

Disease-producing organisms may be gram-positive or gram-negative bacteria, viruses, or fungi. The degree to which they are pathogenic depends on the microorganism and its virulence.

The cell walls of bacteria differ in their structure: bacilli are elongated, cocci are spherical, and spirilla are helical.

Viruses are very small organisms that do not have an organized cellular structure. There are numerous families of virus, including herpesviruses, cytomegalovirus, adenovirus, papovavirus, and the human immunodeficiency virus (HIV). HIV agents are discussed in Chapter 34, HIV- and AIDS-Related Agents.

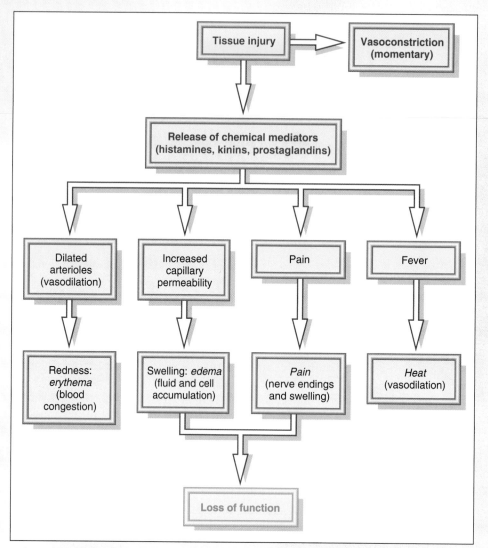

FIGURE VIII–1 Chemical mediator response to tissue injury.

The fungi are divided into yeasts and molds. The few fungi that produce disease usually affect the skin and subcutaneous tissues in conditions such as athlete's foot and ringworm. Serious fungal infections are systemic and usually need aggressive drug therapy. Opportunistic fungal infections commonly result from prolonged antibiotic and steroidal therapies and debilitating diseases, such as cancer. The yeast *Candida albicans* is a cause of common infections of the mucous membranes of the mouth, gastrointestinal tract, vagina, and skin. Candida, like most fungi, is resistant to penicillin-type antibiotics because of its rigid cell wall structure. Chapter 31, Antitubercular Drugs: Antifungal Drugs, Peptides, and Metronidazole, describes the variety of topical and systemic drugs used to treat yeast and mold infections.

Bioterrorism

Bioterroism is a current threat to humanity. In recent years, anthrax has been developed as a biological weapon, usually in a powder form for inhalation. While there are three types of anthrax affecting the skin, gastrointestinal systems, and lungs, inhalation is the most lethal form. An aerosol cloud of anthrax spores is colorless, odorless, and invisible, creating the same exposure for individuals indoors as those outside. The World Health Organization analyzed the release of aerosolized anthrax in 1970 and concluded that in appropriate weather and wind conditions, upwind, in a population of 5 million, approximately 250,000 individuals would be affected and with an expected mortality rate of 100,000.

Often the first sign of anthrax use as a biological weapon is the recognition of symptoms. Infectious symptoms of anthrax are fever, chills, headache, nausea, vomiting, nasal congestion, shortness of breath, cough, malaise, joint pain and stiffness, and chest pain. Onset of symptoms of anthrax may appear from 7 days to 8 weeks.

Anthrax may be prevented by a vaccination. The Centers for Disease Control and Prevention (CDC) is working with state and local officials to prepare for an anthrax attack. When appropriate antibiotics are not initiated before the development of symptoms, the mortality rate is approximately 90%. Anthrax is caused by the spore-forming *Bacillus anthracis*. This acute infectious disease can be treated with fluoroquinolones, such as ciprofloxacin (Cipro); tetracyclenes, such as doxycyclene (Vibramycin); or penicillins, such as Penicillin V.

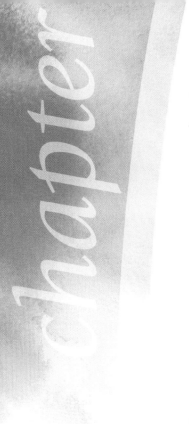

27 Antiinflammatory Drugs

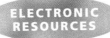
ELECTRONIC RESOURCES

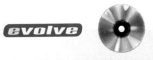

Additional information can be found on the companion website at *http://evolve.elsevier.com/KeeHayes/pharmacology/* or on the companion CD-ROM, which includes:

- *NCLEX-style examination review questions*
- *Pharmacology animations*
- *Medication error and IV therapy checklists*
- *Medication calculation problems*
- *Electronic calculators*

OUTLINE

OBJECTIVES

- Identify the five cardinal signs of inflammation.
- Describe the action of nonsteroidal antiinflammatory drugs (NSAIDs).
- List the major side effects of NSAIDs.
- Explain the use of disease-modifying antirheumatic drugs (DMARDs).
- Identify several side effects and adverse reactions of DMARDs.
- Differentiate between the nursing processes associated with NSAIDs and DMARDs, including client teaching.
- Compare the action of antigout medications.

TERMS

chrysotherapy
disease-modifying an-
 tirheumatic
 drugs (DMARDs)

gout
immunomodulators
immunosuppressives
infection

inflammation
nonsteroidal antiinflam-
 matory drugs (NSAIDs)

prostaglandins
uricosurics

Introduction

Inflammation is a response to tissue injury and infection. When the inflammatory process occurs, a vascular reaction takes place in which fluid, elements of blood, leukocytes (white blood cells [WBCs]), and chemical mediators accumulate at the injured tissue or infection site. The process of inflammation is a protective mechanism in which the body attempts to neutralize and destroy harmful agents at the site of injury and to establish conditions for tissue repair.

Although there is a relationship between inflammation and infection, these terms should *not* be used interchangeably. **Infection** is caused by microorganisms and results in inflammation, but *not* all inflammations are caused by infections.

Pathophysiology

The five characteristics of inflammation, called the *cardinal signs of inflammation*, are redness, swelling (edema), heat, pain, and loss of function. Table 27–1 gives the description and explanation of the cardinal signs of inflammation. The two phases of inflammation are the *vascular phase*, which occurs 10 to 15 minutes after an injury, and the *delayed phase*. The vascular phase is associated with vasodilation and increased capillary permeability, during which blood substances and fluid leave the plasma and go to the injured site. The delayed phase occurs when leukocytes infiltrate the inflamed tissue.

Various chemical mediators are released during the inflammation process. Prostaglandins that have been isolated from the exudate at inflammatory sites are among them. **Prostaglandins** (chemical mediators) have many effects, including vasodilation, relaxation of smooth muscle, increased capillary permeability, and sensitization of nerve cells to pain.

The cyclo-oxygenase (COX) is the enzyme responsible for converting arachidonic acid into prostaglandins and their products. COX promotes the synthesis of prostaglandins causing inflammation and pain at the tissue injury site. There are two enzyme forms of cyclo-oxygenase: COX-1 and COX-2. COX-1 protects the stomach lining and regulates blood platelets, and COX-2 triggers inflammation and pain. Chapter 21, Drugs for Pain Management: Nonnarcotic and Narcotic Analgesics, discusses COX-1 and COX-2 and their physiologic effects on the body, including pain and inflammation.

Antiinflammatory Agents

Drugs such as aspirin inhibit the biosynthesis of prostaglandin and therefore are called *prostaglandin inhibitors*. Because prostaglandin inhibitors affect the inflammatory process, they are also called *antiinflammatory agents*.

Antiinflammatory agents have additional properties, such as relief of pain (analgesic), reduction of an elevated body temperature (antipyretic), and inhibition of platelet

Table 27–1

Cardinal Signs of Inflammation

Signs	Description and Explanation
Erythema (redness)	Redness occurs in the first phase of inflammation. Blood accumulates in the area of tissue injury because of the release of the body's chemical mediators (kinins, prostaglandins, and histamine). Histamine dilates the arterioles.
Edema (swelling)	Swelling is the second phase of inflammation. Plasma leaks into the interstitial tissue at the injury site. Kinins dilate the arterioles, increasing capillary permeability.
Heat	Heat at the inflammatory site can be caused by increased blood accumulation and may result from pyrogens (substances that produce fever) that interfere with the temperature-regulating center in the hypothalamus.
Pain	Pain is caused by tissue swelling and the release of chemical mediators.
Loss of function	Function is lost because of the accumulation of fluid at the tissue injury site and because of pain, which decreases mobility at the affected area.

aggregation (anticoagulant). Aspirin is the oldest antiinflammatory drug, but it was first used for its analgesic and antipyretic properties. As a result of searching for a more effective drug with fewer side effects, many other antiinflammatory agents, or prostaglandin inhibitors, have been discovered. Although these drugs have potent antiinflammatory effects that mimic the effects of corticosteroids (cortisone), they are *not* chemically related and therefore are called **nonsteroidal antiinflammatory drugs (NSAIDs)**. Most NSAIDs are used to decrease the inflammation and pain for clients who have some type of arthritic condition.

Nonsteroidal Antiinflammatory Drugs

NSAIDs are aspirin and aspirin-like drugs that inhibit the enzyme COX, which is needed for the biosynthesis of prostaglandins (see Chapters 21, Drugs for Pain Management: Nonnarcotic Analgesics, and 43, Anticoagulants, Antiplatelets, and Thrombolytics and Figure 21–1). These drugs may be called prostaglandin inhibitors, with varying degrees of analgesic and antipyretic effects, but they are used primarily as antiinflammatory agents to relieve inflammation and pain. When administering NSAIDs for pain relief, the dosage is usually higher than for treatment of inflammation. Their antipyretic effect is less than their antiinflammatory effect. With the exceptions of aspirin and ibuprofen, NSAID preparations are not suggested for use in alleviating mild headaches and mild elevated temperature. The choice of drugs for headaches and fever are aspirin, acetaminophen, and ibuprofen (given to children and adults with high fever). NSAIDs are more appropriate for reducing swelling, pain, and stiffness in joints.

NSAIDs cost more than aspirin. Other than aspirin, the only NSAIDs that can be purchased over-the-counter (OTC) are ibuprofen (Motrin, Nuprin, Advil, Medipren) and naproxen (Aleve). Ibuprofen is also available in the generic form of 200 mg per tablet or capsule. All other NSAIDs must be ordered with a prescription. Examples of prescription products on the market that contain NSAIDs include Anaprox, Celebrex, Clinoril, Daypro, Equagesic, Naprosyn, Percodan, Relafen, Soma Compound, Talwin, and Toradol. If a client can take aspirin for the inflammatory process without gastrointestinal (GI) upset, salicylate products are usually recommended.

There are seven groups of NSAIDs:
1. Salicylates related to aspirin (see Chapter 21, Drugs for Pain Management: Nonnarcotic and Narcotic Analgesics)
2. *Para*-chlorobenzoic acid derivatives, or indoles
3. Phenylacetic acids
4. Propionic acid derivatives
5. Fenamates
6. Oxicams
7. Selective COX-2 inhibitors

The first seven NSAIDs are now known as *first-generation NSAIDs,* and the COX-2 inhibitors are called *second-generation NSAIDs.*

Table 27–2 provides dosage information and considerations for use for the most commonly used NSAIDs. The half-lives of NSAIDs differ greatly—some have a short half-life, yet others have a moderate to long half-life with a general range of 8 to 24 hours. Aspirin should *not* be taken with an NSAID because of the side effects. In addition, combined therapy does *not* increase effectiveness.

Salicylates

Aspirin comes from the family of salicylates derived from salicylic acid. Aspirin is also called acetylsalicylic acid (ASA) after the acetyl group used in the composition of aspirin. The abbreviation frequently used for aspirin is ASA.

Aspirin was developed in 1899 by Adolph Bayer, making it the oldest antiinflammatory agent. It was the most frequently used antiinflammatory agent before the introduction of ibuprofen. Aspirin is a prostaglandin inhibitor that decreases the inflammatory process. It is also considered an antiplatelet drug for clients with cardiac or cerebrovascular disorders; aspirin decreases platelet aggregation, and thus blood clotting is decreased. Because high doses of aspirin are usually needed to relieve inflammation, gastric distress is a common problem. In such cases, enteric-coated (EC) tablets may be used. Aspirin should *not* be taken with other NSAIDs because it decreases the blood level and the effectiveness of NSAIDs.

Aspirin and other NSAIDs inhibit COX-1, which decreases the protection of the stomach lining, and COX-2, which decreases inflammation and pain. As a result of the inhibition of COX-1, stomach ulcers and bleeding may occur. Aspirin is the drug of choice for alleviating inflammation and pain in arthritic conditions, but when given in high doses, severe GI problems develop in approximately 20% of clients. Some pharmaceutical companies have developed antiinflammatory and analgesic drugs that inhibit only COX-2. The COX-2 inhibitors were developed to eliminate the GI side effects associated with aspirin and other NSAIDs.

Pharmacokinetics

Aspirin is well absorbed from the GI tract (Prototype Drug Chart 27–1). It can cause GI upset; therefore it should be taken with water, milk, or food. The EC or buffered form can decrease gastric distress. EC tablets should not be crushed or broken.

Aspirin has a short half-life. It should not be taken during the last trimester of pregnancy because it could cause premature closure of ductus arteriosus in the fetus. Aspirin should not be taken by children with flu symptoms because it may cause the potentially fatal Reye syndrome.

Pharmacodynamics

Aspirin, like other NSAIDs, inhibits prostaglandin synthesis by inhibiting COX-1 and COX-2; thus it decreases inflammation and pain. The onset of action for aspirin is within 30 minutes. It peaks in 1 to 2 hours, and the duration of action is an average of 4 to 6 hours. The action for the rectal preparation of aspirin can be erratic because of blood supply and fecal material in the rectum; it may take a week or longer for a therapeutic antiinflammatory effect.

Table 27–2

Antiinflammatory: Nonsteroidal Antiinflammatory

Generic (Brand)	Route and Dosage	Uses and Considerations
First-Generation NSAIDs		
Salicylates		
aspirin (ASA, Bayer, Ecotrin)	See Prototype Drug Chart 27–1.	
diflunisal (Dolobid)	A: PO: Initially: 1 g (1000 mg); *maint:* 500 mg q8-12h	Relief of mild to moderate pain; used to treat osteoarthritis and rheumatoid arthritis. Acts by inhibiting prostaglandin synthesis. Avoid if hypersensitive to aspirin. Do not use during third trimester of pregnancy. *Pregnancy category:* C; PB: 99%; t$\frac{1}{2}$: 8-12 h
Salicylate Derivatives		
olsalazine sodium (Dipentum)	A: PO: 500 mg q12h; may increase dose every 2 to 4 wk; *max:* 3 g/d in divided doses	To treat inflammatory bowel disease especially ulcerative colitis. Excretion is mainly in feces as 5-ASA. *Pregnancy category:* C; PB: UK; t$\frac{1}{2}$: 6 h
sulfasalazine (Azulfidine)	A: PO: 0.5 g daily initially then 2 g daily in divided doses; *max:* 75 mg/kg/d C: PO: 40-50 mg/kg/d in 4 divided doses	For treatment of ulcerative colitis and rheumatoid arthritis. Avoid if allergic to sulfonamides or aspirin. *Pregnancy category:* B (D if near term); PB: UK; t$\frac{1}{2}$: 5-10 h
Acetic Acid Group Para-Chlorobenzoic Acid (Indoles)		
indomethacin (Indocin)	A: PO: 25-50 mg b.i.d./t.i.d. with food; SR: 75 mg daily/b.i.d.; *max:* 200 mg/d C: PO: 1-2 mg/kg/d in 2-4 divided doses; may increase to 4 mg/kg/d; *max:* 150-200 mg/d	For moderate to severe arthritic conditions. Potent drug. GI upset and ulceration are common. Take drug with food. Avoid indomethacin if allergic to aspirin. *Pregnancy category:* B (D near term); PB: 90%-99%; t$\frac{1}{2}$: 3-120 h
sulindac (Clinoril)	A: PO: 150-200 mg b.i.d.	For acute and chronic arthritis, bursitis, and tendinitis. Not as potent as indomethacin. Give with food. *Pregnancy category:* C; PB: 93%; t$\frac{1}{2}$: 7-18 h
tolmetin (Tolectin)	A: PO: Initially: 400 mg t.i.d.; *maint:* 600-1800 mg/d in divided doses; *max:* 2 g/d C: >2 y: PO: 20 mg/kg/d in divided doses; *max:* 30 mg/kg/d	For acute and chronic arthritis, including juvenile rheumatoid arthritis. Less potent than indomethacin; more effective than aspirin. Take drug with food. *Pregnancy category:* B (D near term); PB: 90%-99%; t$\frac{1}{2}$: 1-1.5 h
Phenylacetic Acid		
diclofenac sodium (Voltaren)	A: PO: 25-50 mg t.i.d./q.i.d. or 75 mg b.i.d.	For rheumatoid arthritis, osteoarthritis, and spondylitis. Also for acute gout, juvenile rheumatoid arthritis, bursitis, and tendinitis. If GI distress occurs, take with food. *Pregnancy category:* B; PB: 90%-99%; t$\frac{1}{2}$: 2 h
etodolac (Lodine)	A: PO: 600-1200 mg/d in 2-4 divided doses PRN; *max:* 1200 mg/d *Rheumatoid arthritis:* A: PO: 500 mg b.i.d.	Used for acute pain, rheumatoid arthritis, and osteoarthritis. Take with food or antacid to avoid GI distress. *Pregnancy category:* C; PR: 99%; t$\frac{1}{2}$: 6-7 h
ketorolac tromethamine (Toradol)	A: <50 kg: IM: LD: 30 mg; *maint:* 15 mg q6h A: >50 kg: IM: LD: 30-60 mg; *maint:* 15-30 mg PRN	First injectable NSAID. For short-term management of pain. Also available for ophthalmic use to relieve itching caused by allergic conjunctivitis. *Pregnancy category:* B; PB: 99%; t$\frac{1}{2}$: 3-8 h; increase in elderly
Propionic Acid		
fenoprofen calcium (Nalfon)	A: PO: 300-600 mg t.i.d./q.i.d.; *max:* 3.2 g/d C: PO: 900 mg/m² in divided doses	Treatment of mild to moderate pain. Also for arthritic conditions. Most effective after 2-3 wk of therapy. Take with food. *Pregnancy category:* B (D at term); PB: 90%-99%; t$\frac{1}{2}$: 3 h

A, Adult; *b.i.d.,* twice a day; *C,* child; *d,* day; *GI,* gastrointestinal; *h,* hour; *IM,* intramuscular; *LD,* loading dose; *maint,* maintenance; *max,* maximum; *NSAID,* nonsteroidal antiinflammatory drug; *OTC,* over the counter; *PB,* protein-binding; *PO,* by mouth; *PRN,* as needed; *q.i.d.,* four times a day; *sol,* solution; *SR,* sustained-release; *t$\frac{1}{2}$,* half-life; *t.i.d.,* three times a day; *UK,* unknown; *wk,* week; *y,* year; *>,* greater than; *<,* less than.

Table 27–2

Antiinflammatory: Nonsteroidal Antiinflammatory—cont'd

Generic (Brand)	Route and Dosage	Uses and Considerations
First-Generation NSAIDs—cont'd		
Propionic Acid—cont'd		
flurbiprofen sodium (Ansaid, Ocufen)	A: PO: 50-300 mg/d in 2-4 divided doses; *max:* 300 mg/d *Ophthalmic use:* 0.03% sol	Treatment of acute and chronic arthritis. Take drug with food. *Pregnancy category:* C; PB: UK; t: 5 h
ibuprofen (Motrin, Advil, Nuprin, Medipren)	See Prototype Drug Chart 27–2.	
ketoprofen (Orudis, Actron)	*Inflammatory:* A: PO: *maint:* 150-300 mg/d in 3-4 divided doses; *max:* 300 mg/d *Mild to moderate pain:* A: PO: 25-50 mg q6-8h PRN; *max:* 300 mg/d	Relief of mild to moderate pain and acute and chronic arthritis. Take with food or 8 ounces of water to avoid GI upset. *Pregnancy category:* B (D at term); PB: 99%; t½: 3-4 h
naproxen (Naprosyn)	A: PO: 250-500 mg b.i.d. C: PO: 5-10 mg/kg/d in 2 divided doses	Relief of mild to moderate pain. Also for arthritic, gout, bursitis conditions. Similar OTC drug: Aleve. Take with food or with a full glass of water. *Pregnancy category:* B; PB: 99%; t½: 10-15 h
oxaprozin (Daypro)	A: PO: Initially: 1200 mg/d; *maint:* 600 mg/d; *max:* 1800 mg/d in divided doses	Treatment of acute and chronic arthritis. Take with food for GI discomfort. *Pregnancy category:* C; PB: 99%; t½: 40 h
Anthranilic Acids (Fenamates)		
meclofenamate (Meclomen)	A: PO: 200-400 mg in 3-4 divided doses	For acute and chronic arthritis. GI symptoms can be severe. Used when other NSAIDs are not effective. Take with food to avoid GI upset. *Pregnancy category:* B (D at term); PB: 99%; t½: 3 h
mefenamic acid (Ponstel)	A: PO: Initially: 500 mg; then 250 mg q6h PRN; *max:* 1 g/d	For acute and chronic arthritis. Diarrhea is a common problem. Usually discontinued after 7 days. *Pregnancy category:* C; PB: 90%; t½: 2-4 h
Oxicams		
piroxicam (Feldene)	A: PO: 10 mg b.i.d. or 20 mg daily	For arthritic conditions. Long half-life; effective at 2 weeks. GI upset may occur. *Pregnancy category:* C; PB: 99%; t½: 30-86 h
COX-2 Inhibitors (Second-Generation NSAIDs)		
celecoxib (Celebrex)	A: PO: 100-200 mg/d Elderly: Same dose	To treat arthritic-type pain. Relieves inflammation and pain without causing GI distress. Should not be used like aspirin for cardiac precautions. Avoid at third trimester of pregnancy. *Pregnancy category:* C (D at late pregnancy); PB: 97%; t½: 11 h
meloxicam (Mobic)	A: PO: 7.5-15 mg daily	For treatment of osteoarthritis. Some COX-2 selectivity. *Pregnancy category:* C (first and second trimester), D (third trimester); PB: 99%; t½: 15-20 h
nabumetone (Relafen)	A: PO: 500-1000 mg/d or in 2 divided doses	To treat chronic inflammation and pain especially for arthritic conditions, such as rheumatoid arthritis. Inhibits cyclooxygenase, particularly COX-2 more than COX-1 therefore causing fewer GI problems. *Pregnancy category:* C; PB: 99%; t½: 22-30 h

Hypersensitivity to Salicylate Products

Clients may be hypersensitive to aspirin. Tinnitus (ringing in the ears), vertigo (dizziness), and bronchospasm—especially in asthmatic clients—are symptoms of aspirin overdose or hypersensitivity to aspirin. Clients should not take diflunisal if they are hypersensitive to aspirin. Diflunisal is a derivative of salicylic acid, although it is not converted to salicylic acid in the body.

Salicylates are present in numerous foods (e.g., prunes, raisins, licorice) and in spices (e.g., curry powder, paprika).

PROTOTYPE DRUG CHART 27–1

ASPIRIN

Drug Class

Analgesic and antiinflammatory drug
Trade Name: ASA, Bayer, Ecotrin, Alka Seltzer (in some),
    Empirin, ✿ Astrin, Entrophen, Novasen
Pregnancy Category: D

Dosage

Analgesic:
A: PO: 325-650 mg q4h PRN; *max:* 4 g/d
C: PO: 40-65 mg/d or 10-15 mg/kg in 4-6 divided doses;
    max: 3.5 g/d
TIA and thromboembolic condition:
A: PO: 325-650 mg/d or b.i.d.
Arthritis:
A: PO: 3.6-5.4 g/d in divided doses
Therapeutic drug monitoring: 15-30 mg/dl;
    150-300 mcg/ml

Contraindications

Hypersensitivity to salicylates or NSAIDs, flu or virus
    symptoms in children, third trimester of pregnancy
Caution: Renal or hepatic disorders

Drug-Lab-Food Interactions

Drug: Increase risk of bleeding with anticoagulants; *increase* risk of hypoglycemia with oral hypoglycemic
drugs; *increase* ulcerogenic effect with glucocorticoids
Lab: Decrease cholesterol and potassium, T_3, T_4 levels;
    increase PT, bleeding time, uric acid

Pharmacokinetics

Absorption: PO: 80%-100%
Distribution: PB: 59%-90%, crosses placenta
Metabolism: $t^{1/2}$: 2-3 h (low dose); 2-20 h (high dose)
Excretion: 50% in urine

Pharmacodynamics

PO: Onset: 15-30 min
    Peak: 1-2 h
    Duration: 4-6 h
PR: Onset: 1-2 h
    Peak: 3-5 h
    Duration: 4-7 h

Therapeutic Effects/Uses

To reduce pain and inflammatory symptoms; to decrease body temperature; to inhibit platelet aggregation
Mode of Action: Inhibition of prostaglandin synthesis, inhibition of hypothalamic heat-regulator center

Side Effects

Anorexia, nausea, vomiting, diarrhea, dizziness, confusion,
    hearing loss, heartburn, rash, stomach pains, drowsiness

Adverse Reactions

Tinnitus, urticaria, ulceration
Life-threatening: Agranulocytosis, hemolytic anemia,
    bronchospasm, anaphylaxis, thrombocytopenia,
    hepatotoxicity, leukopenia

A, Adult; *ASA,* acetylsalicylic acid; *b.i.d.,* two times a day; *C,* child; *d,* day; *h,* hour; *max,* maximum; *min,* minute; *NSAIDs,* nonsteroidal
antiinflammatory drugs; *PB,* protein-binding; *PO,* by mouth; *PR,* per rectum; *PRN,* as necessary; *PT,* prothrombin; *t¹/₂,* half-life; *TIA,* transient ischemic attack; ✿ , Canadian drug names.

Nursing Process

Analgesic and Antiinflammatory Drug: Aspirin

ASSESSMENT

■ Determine a medical history. Determine whether
there is any history of gastric upset, gastric bleeding, or
liver disease. Aspirin can cause gastric irritation. It prolongs bleeding time by inhibiting platelet aggregation.
■ Obtain a drug history. Report if a drug-drug interaction is probable.

NURSING DIAGNOSES

■ Risk for injury
■ Pain

PLANNING

■ Client will be free of mild pain in 12 to 24 hours and
mild inflammation within 1 week. Aspirin may be ordered for mild to severe arthritic condition, pain relief,
antiinflammatory effects, fever reduction, and inhibition of platelet aggregation.

NURSING INTERVENTIONS

■ Monitor serum salicylate (aspirin) level when client takes high doses of aspirin for chronic conditions such as arthritis. The normal therapeutic range is 15 to 30 mg/dl. Mild toxicity occurs at serum level of >30 mg/dl, and severe toxicity occurs at >50 mg/dl.

■ Observe client for signs of bleeding, such as dark (tarry) stools, bleeding gums, petechiae (round red spots), ecchymosis (excessive bruising), and purpura (large red spots) when client takes high doses of aspirin.

Client Teaching

General

- Advise client not to take aspirin with alcohol or drugs that are highly protein-bound, such as the anticoagulant warfarin (Coumadin). Aspirin displaces drugs such as warfarin from the protein-binding site, causing more free anticoagulant.
- Suggest that client inform the dentist before a dental visit if taking high doses of aspirin.
- With the health care provider's approval, instruct client to discontinue aspirin 3 to 7 days before surgery to reduce the risk of bleeding.
- Keep the aspirin bottle out of the reach of small children.
- Educate the parent to call the poison control center immediately if a child has taken a large or unknown amount of aspirin (also acetaminophen).
- Warn client *not* to administer aspirin for virus or flu symptoms in children. Reye syndrome (vomiting, lethargy, delirium, and coma) has been linked with aspirin and viral infections. Acetaminophen is usually prescribed for cold and flu symptoms.
- Inform client that aspirin tablets can cause GI distress.
- Inform client with dysmenorrhea to take acetaminophen instead of aspirin 2 days before and during the first 2 days of the menstrual period.

Side Effects

- Direct client to report side effects such as drowsiness, tinnitus (ringing in the ears), headaches, flushing, dizziness, GI symptoms (bleeding, heartburn), visual changes, and seizures.

Diet

- Instruct client to take aspirin (also ibuprofen) with food, at mealtime, or with plenty of fluids. Enteric-coated aspirin avoids GI disturbance.

Cultural Considerations ⊕

- Do not misunderstand loud voice volume as necessarily reflecting anger among some African Americans and Arabs, who may be merely expressing their thoughts in a dynamic manner.

EVALUATION

■ Evaluate the effectiveness of aspirin in relieving pain. If pain persists, another analgesic such as ibuprofen may be prescribed.

■ Determine whether client has any side effects to aspirin.

Para-Chlorobenzoic Acid

One of the first NSAIDs introduced was indomethacin (Indocin), a *para*-chlorobenzoic acid. It is used for rheumatoid arthritis, gouty arthritis, and osteoarthritis and is a potent prostaglandin inhibitor. It is highly protein bound (90%) and displaces other protein-bound drugs, resulting in potential toxicity. It has a moderate half-life (4 to 11 hours). Indomethacin is very irritating to the stomach and thus should be taken with food.

Two other *para*-chlorobenzoic acid derivatives—sulindac (Clinoril) and tolmetin (Tolectin)—produce less severe adverse reactions than indomethacin. Tolmetin is not as highly protein-bound as indomethacin, and sulindac and has a short half-life. This group of NSAIDs may cause sodium and water retention as well as increased blood pressure.

Phenylacetic Acid Derivatives

Diclofenac sodium (Voltaren), a phenylacetic acid derivative, has a plasma half-life of 8 to 12 hours. Its analgesic and antiinflammatory effects are similar to those of aspirin, but it has minimal to no antipyretic effects. It is indicated for rheumatoid arthritis, osteoarthritis, and ankylosing spondylitis. Adverse reactions are similar to those of other NSAIDs.

Ketorolac (Toradol), another phenylacetic acid derivative, is the first injectable NSAID. Like other NSAIDs, it inhibits prostaglandin synthesis, but it has greater analgesic properties than other antiinflammatory agents. Ketorolac is recommended for short-term management of pain. For postsurgical pain it has shown analgesic efficacy equal or superior to that of opioid analgesics. It is administered intramuscularly in doses of 30 to 60 mg every 6 hours for adults.

Propionic Acid Derivatives

The propionic acid group is a relatively new group of NSAIDs. These drugs are aspirin-like but have stronger effects and create less GI irritation. Drugs in this group are highly protein-bound so drug interactions might occur, especially when given with another highly protein-bound drug. Propionic acid derivatives are better tolerated than other NSAIDs. Gastric upset occurs, but it is not as severe as it is with aspirin and indomethacin. Severe adverse reactions, such as blood dyscrasias, are *not* frequently seen. Ibuprofen (Motrin) is the most widely used NSAID, and it may be purchased OTC in lower doses (200 mg). Prototype Drug Chart 27–2 details the phar-

PROTOTYPE DRUG CHART 27–2

IBUPROFEN

Drug Class

Nonsteroidal antiinflammatory drug, propionic acid
  derivative
Trade Name: Motrin, Advil, Nuprin, Medipren,
  Rufen, ♣ Amersol
Pregnancy Category: B

Dosage

A: PO: 200-800 mg t.i.d./q.i.d.; *max:* <3.2 g/d (<3200
  mg/d)
C: PO: Average: 5-10 mg/kg/d; *max:* 40 mg/kg/d
1-4 y or <20 kg: 400 mg/d in divided doses
5-7 y or 20-30 kg: 600 mg/d in divided doses
>8 y or 30-40 kg: 800 mg/d in divided doses

Contraindications

Severe renal or hepatic disease, asthma, peptic ulcer
Caution: Bleeding disorders, early pregnancy, lactation,
  systemic lupus erythematosus

Drug-Lab-Food Interactions

Drug: Increase bleeding time with oral anticoagulants;
  increase effects of phenytoin, sulfonamides, warfarin;
  decrease effect with aspirin; may *increase* severe side
  effects of lithium

Pharmacokinetics

Absorption: PO: Well absorbed
Distribution: PB: 98%
Metabolism: $t\frac{1}{2}$: 2-4 h
Excretion: In urine, mostly as inactive metabolites;
  some in bile

Pharmacodynamics

PO: Onset: 0.5 h
  Peak: 1-2 h
  Duration: 4-6 h

Therapeutic Effects/Uses

To reduce inflammatory process; to relieve pain; antiinflammatory effect for arthritic conditions; to reduce fever
Mode of Action: Inhibition of prostaglandin synthesis, thus relieving pain and inflammations

Side Effects

Anorexia, nausea, vomiting, diarrhea, edema, rash,
  purpura, tinnitus, fatigue, dizziness, lightheadedness,
  anxiety, confusion

Adverse Reactions

GI bleeding
Life-threatening: Blood dyscrasias, cardiac dysrhythmias,
  nephrotoxicity, anaphylaxis

A, Adult; *C*, child; *d*, day; *GI*, gastrointestinal; *h*, hour; *max*, maximum; *PB*, protein-binding; *PO*, by mouth; *q.i.d.*, four times a day;
t½, half-life; *t.i.d.*, three times a day; *y*, year; <, less than; >, greater than; ♣, Canadian drug name.

macologic behavior of ibuprofens. Six other propionic acid agents are fenoprofen calcium (Nalfon), naproxen (Naprosyn), suprofen (Profenal), ketoprofen (Orudis), flurbiprofen (Ansaid), and oxaprozin (Daypro).

Pharmacokinetics

Ibuprofens are well absorbed from the GI tract. These drugs have a short half-life but are highly protein bound. If ibuprofen is taken with another highly protein-bound drug, severe side effects may occur. The drug is metabolized in the liver to inactivate metabolites and is excreted as inactive metabolites in the urine.

Pharmacodynamics

Ibuprofens inhibit prostaglandin synthesis and are therefore effective in alleviating inflammation and pain. They have a short onset of action, peak concentration time, and duration of action. It may take several days for the antiinflammatory effect to be evident.

There are many drug interactions associated with ibuprofen. It can increase the effects of warfarin (Coumadin), sulfonamides, many of the cephalosporins, and phenytoin. When taken with aspirin, its effect can be decreased. Hypoglycemia may result when ibuprofen is taken with insulin or an oral hypoglycemic drug. There is a high risk of toxicity when ibuprofen is taken concurrently with calcium blockers.

Fenamates

The fenamate group includes potent NSAIDs used for acute and chronic arthritic conditions. Like most NSAIDs, gastric irritation is a common side effect of fenamates, and clients with a history of peptic ulcer should avoid taking this group of drugs. Other side effects include edema, dizziness, tinnitus, and pruritus. Two fenamates are meclofen-amate sodium monohydrate (Meclomen) and mefenamic acid (Ponstel).

Oxicams

Piroxicam (Feldene), an oxicam, is indicated for long-term arthritic conditions such as rheumatoid arthritis and osteoarthritis. It too can cause gastric problems, such as ulceration and epigastric distress, but the incidence is lower than for some other NSAIDs. It is well tolerated, and its major advantage over other NSAIDs is its long half-life, which allows it to be taken only once daily.

Full clinical response to piroxicam may take 1 to 2 weeks. This drug is also highly protein bound and may interact with another highly protein-bound drug if taken together. Piroxicam should not be taken with aspirin or other NSAIDs.

General Side Effects and Adverse Reactions for First-Generation NSAIDs

Most NSAIDs tend to have fewer side effects than aspirin when taken at antiinflammatory doses, but gastric irritation is still a common problem when NSAIDs are taken without food. In addition, sodium and water retention may occur. Alcoholic beverages consumed with NSAIDs may increase gastric irritation and should be avoided.

Nursing Process

Antiinflammatory: Nonsteroidal Antiinflammatory Drugs (NSAIDs)

ASSESSMENT

■ Check client's history of allergy to NSAIDs, including aspirin. If an allergy is present, notify the health care provider.
■ Obtain a drug and herbal history and report any possible drug-drug or herb-drug interactions. NSAIDs can increase the effects of phenytoin (Dilantin), sulfonamides, and warfarin. Most NSAIDs are highly protein-bound and can displace other highly protein-bound drugs, such as warfarin (Coumadin).
■ Determine a medical history. NSAIDs are contraindicated if client has a severe renal or liver disease, peptic ulcer, or bleeding disorder.
■ Assess client for GI upset and peripheral edema, which are common side effects of NSAIDs.

NURSING DIAGNOSES

■ Impaired tissue integrity
■ Risk for activity intolerance

PLANNING

■ The inflammatory process will subside in 1 to 3 weeks.

NURSING INTERVENTIONS

■ Observe client for bleeding gums, petechiae, ecchymoses, or black (tarry) stools. Bleeding time can be prolonged when NSAIDs are taken, especially with a highly protein-bound drug such as warfarin (anticoagulant).
■ Report if client has GI discomfort. Administer the NSAIDs at mealtime or with food to prevent GI upset.
■ Monitor vital signs and check for peripheral edema, especially in the morning.

■ Do not give directions such as take one "blue" pill at a specified time. Instead, provide the name and dosage of the medication.

Client Teaching

General
• Inform client not to take aspirin and acetaminophen with NSAIDs. Taking an NSAID with aspirin could cause GI upset and possible GI bleeding.
• Inform client to avoid alcohol when taking NSAIDs. GI upset or gastric ulcer may result.
• Alert client that many herbal products may interact with NSAIDs and could cause bleeding. Doses of NSAIDs and/or herbs may need to be modified to avoid possible bleeding occurrence. See Herbal Alert 27–1.
• Direct client to inform the dentist or surgeon before a procedure when taking ibuprofen or other NSAIDs for a continuous period.
• Warn women not to take NSAIDs 1 to 2 days before menstruation to avoid heavy menstrual flow. If discomfort occurs, acetaminophen is usually prescribed.
• Guide women in the third trimester of pregnancy to avoid NSAIDs. If delivery occurs, excess bleeding might result from use of NSAIDs.
• Tell client that it may take several weeks to experience the desired drug effect of some NSAIDs and disease-modifying antirheumatic drugs (DMARDs).

Side Effects
• Educate client of the common side effects of NSAIDs. Nausea, vomiting, peripheral edema, GI upset, purpura or petechiae, or dizziness might occur. Report occurrences of side effects.

Diet
• Advise client to take NSAIDs with meals or food to reduce GI upset.

Cultural Considerations
• Recognize that clients from various cultural backgrounds respond to pain and inflammation in various ways. In some cultures, the use of drugs to alleviate pain and inflammation is not acceptable. Herbal medicine and acupuncture may be used to alleviate pain.
• Be supportive of client's methods for pain control. Explain the purpose of medications and their action and side effects.

HERBAL ALERT 27–1

NSAIDs
Dong quai, feverfew, garlic, ginger, and ginkgo when taken with nonsteroidal antiinflammatory drugs (NSAIDs) may cause bleeding.

PROTOTYPE DRUG CHART 27–3

CELECOXIB

Drug Class

Nonsteroidal antiinflammatory: COX-2 inhibitor
Trade Name: Celebrex
Pregnancy Category: C (first and second trimester),
D (third trimester)

Dosage

Arthritis:
A: PO: 100-200 mg daily or b.i.d.
Dysmenorrhea:
A: PO: 400 mg first dose, follow with 200 mg same day
if needed, then 200 mg twice daily PRN

Contraindications

Hypersensitivity, advanced renal disease, severe hepatic
failure, anemia, concurrent use of diuretics and ACE
inhibitors
Caution: Renal or hepatic dysfunction, hypertension,
fluid retention, heart failure, infection, history of GI
bleeding or ulceration, concurrent anticoagulant therapy,
steroids, or alcohol use

Drug-Lab-Food Interactions

Drug: Decrease effect of ACE inhibitors, increased INR
and GI bleeding with warfarin, may increase toxicity
with lithium, fluconazole increases celecoxib levels

Pharmacokinetics

Absorption: Well absorbed in GI tract
Distribution: PB: 97%
Metabolism: $t\frac{1}{2}$: 11.2 h
Excretion: Primarily in feces

Pharmacodynamics

PO: Onset: UK
Peak: 3 h
Duration: UK

Therapeutic Effects/Uses

To treat osteoarthritis and rheumatoid arthritis, and relieve dysmenorrhea
Mode of Action: Inhibits COX-2, which normally promotes prostaglandin synthesis and inflammatory response,
but does not inhibit COX-1

Side Effects

Headache, dizziness, sinusitis, nausea, flatulence,
diarrhea, rash

Adverse Reactions

Peripheral edema

A, Adult; *ACE,* angiotensin-converting enzyme; *b.i.d.,* twice a day; *COX,* cyclooxygenase; *GI,* gastrointestinal; *h,* hour; *INR,* international
normalized ratio; *PB,* protein-binding; *PO,* by mouth; *PRN,* as needed; *t½,* half-life; *UK,* unkown.

EVALUATION

■ Evaluate the effectiveness of the drug therapy, such as
a decrease in pain and in swollen joints and an increase
in mobility.

Selective COX-2 Inhibitors (Second-Generation NSAIDs)

COX-2 inhibitors became available in the last several years to
decrease inflammation and pain. Most NSAIDs are nonselective inhibitors that inhibit COX-1 and COX-2. By inhibiting COX-1, protection of the stomach lining is decreased and the clotting time is also decreased, which may
benefit the client with cardiovascular or coronary artery disease (CAD). The selected COX-2 inhibitors are the drug of
choice for clients with severe arthritic conditions who need
high doses of an antiinflammatory drug. However, large
doses of NSAIDs may cause peptic ulcer and gastric bleeding.

In the next few years, more COX-2 inhibitors will become available. [Currently there is one drug, celecoxib
(Celebrex), that is classified as a COX-2 inhibitor. Nabume-

tone (Relafen) is another drug that can be used; however it
is not considered a "true" COX-2 inhibitor. Nabumetone
inhibits COX-2 more than COX-1.] See Prototype Drug
Chart 27–3 for more information on celecoxib.

Use of NSAIDs in Older Adults

Older adults use NSAIDs frequently to treat pain associated with inflammation caused by osteoarthritis, rheumatoid arthritis, and neuromuscular-skeletal disorders. As
older adults age, the number of drugs taken daily increases;
therefore drug interactions are more common, especially

PREVENTING MEDICATION ERRORS

Do not confuse...

• **Celebrex** (COX-2 inhibitor) with **Celexa** (selective
serotonin-reuptake inhibitor or antipsychotic).
These names look alike, but the drug class and action are very different.

when numerous drugs are taken with NSAIDs. With the use of NSAIDs, GI distress (including ulceration) is four times more common in older adults; hospitalization is often necessary.

The introduction of COX-2 inhibitors (second-generation NSAIDs) has decreased GI problems associated with their use; however, edema is likely to occur. Renal function should be evaluated, and older adults should increase their fluid intake for adequate hydration. To decrease possible complications, the NSAID dose should be lowered.

Corticosteroids

Corticosteroids, such as prednisone, prednisolone, and dexamethasone, are frequently used as antiinflammatory agents. This group of drugs controls inflammation by suppressing or preventing many of the components of the inflammatory process at the injured site. Corticosteroids have been widely prescribed for arthritic conditions, and, although they are not the drug of choice for arthritis because of their numerous side effects, they are frequently used to control arthritic flare-ups.

The half-life of corticosteroids is long (greater than 24 hours), and it is administered once a day in a large prescribed dose. When discontinuing steroid therapy, the dosage should be tapered over a period of 5 to 10 days. Steroids are discussed in more detail in Chapter 49, Endocrine Pharmacology: Pituitary, Thyroid, Parathyroids, and Adrenals.

Disease-Modifying Antirheumatic Drugs

When NSAIDs do not control immune-mediated arthritic disease sufficiently, other drugs, although more toxic, can be prescribed to alter the disease process. The **disease-modifying antirheumatic drugs (DMARDs)** include gold drug therapy, immunosuppressive agents, immunomodulators, and antimalarials. DMARDs help to alleviate the symptoms of rheumatoid arthritis for the 2 million persons in the United States affected by the disorder.

Gold

Gold drug therapy, called **chrysotherapy** or heavy metal therapy, is the most frequently used DMARD. It is used to arrest progression of rheumatoid arthritis and to prevent deformities caused by the disease. It depresses migration of leukocytes and suppresses prostaglandin activity. Gold preparations are thought to inhibit destructive lysosomal enzymes that are contained in leukocytes, which are released in the joints. The effect of gold on the immune mechanism is limited.

Gold is not used in the early stages of arthritis unless the illness is progressing rapidly and is unresponsive to other therapy, nor is it used in far-advanced arthritis. It is used for palliative (relief of symptoms), not curative, effects. Response in alleviating symptoms is slow. With injectable gold, results may take up to 2 months; oral dosages could take 3 to 6 months for clinical response. The half-life of gold is 7 to 25 days, and gold drugs are highly protein bound. Blood should be monitored for blood dyscrasia before and during parenteral or oral gold therapy.

The gold salt auranofin (Ridaura) is the only gold preparation that can be administered orally. The two parenteral gold salts are aurothioglucose (Solganal) and gold sodium thiomalate (Myochrysine). Oral gold may be absorbed erratically; thus parenteral gold may be advisable. Switching from parenteral to oral gold preparations may be necessary for long-term use. Prototype Drug Chart 27–4 presents drug data for the gold preparation auranofin (Ridaura).

Pharmacokinetics

The GI tract absorbs 25% of auranofin. It is moderately highly protein bound. Its half-life is long, both in the blood (26 days) and in the body tissues (40 to 120 days). Although 60% of auranofin is excreted in the urine, the drug may be present in the urine for up to 15 months after chrysotherapy has been discontinued.

Pharmacodynamics

Auranofin is prescribed to relieve inflammation and pain from rheumatoid arthritis when NSAIDs and other measures are ineffective. The therapeutic effect may take 3 to 6 months; steady state (the average therapeutic effect that is maintained) of the drug is achieved after 2 to 4 months. Side effects and adverse reactions need to be closely monitored.

Table 27–3 details the dosages and considerations for the three gold drugs used as antiinflammatory agents for rheumatoid arthritis.

Side Effects and Adverse Reactions

Approximately 25% to 45% of clients receiving gold therapy experience side effects. The side effects may occur anytime during or several months after therapy. The numerous possible side effects include dermatitis, urticaria (hives), erythema, alopecia (loss of hair), stomatitis (mouth ulcers), pharyngitis, gastritis, colitis, hepatitis, severe blood dyscrasias (agranulocytosis, aplastic anemia), and even anaphylactic shock.

Contraindications

Gold therapy is contraindicated for clients with eczema, urticaria, colitis, hemorrhagic conditions, and systemic lupus erythematosus.

Nursing Process

Antiinflammatory: Gold

ASSESSMENT

■ Determine client's health history. Usually, gold drugs such as auranofin are contraindicated if there is renal or hepatic dysfunction, marked hypertension, congestive heart failure, systemic lupus erythematosus, or uncontrolled diabetes mellitus.

■ Check for proteinuria and hematuria before giving initial gold dose and during gold therapy.

■ Observe client for 30 minutes after gold injection for possible allergic reaction after the first and second

injections. It takes approximately 10 to 15 minutes for a serious allergic reaction (anaphylaxis) to occur.
■ Obtain baseline vital signs and hematology laboratory findings for future comparison.

NURSING DIAGNOSES

■ Impaired physical mobility
■ Pain, chronic
■ Risk for impaired skin integrity

PLANNING

■ Client will have reduced inflammation and pain while taking the gold treatment without adverse drug reaction.

NURSING INTERVENTIONS

■ Record client's vital signs. Report abnormal findings.
■ Monitor laboratory tests (e.g., complete blood count). Report abnormal findings.
■ Check periodically for signs of side effects and adverse reactions to gold therapy. Side effects may include anorexia, nausea, vomiting, diarrhea, gingivitis, stomatitis,

rash, itching, and decreased urine output. Most gold drugs have a long half-life; thus a cumulative effect can result. Auranofin causes less severe adverse reactions than other gold preparations.

Client Teaching
General

● Instruct client to perform frequent dental hygiene, including brushing the teeth with a soft toothbrush and flossing to prevent or control gingivitis and stomatitis. Use of diluted hydrogen peroxide can be helpful in mild stomatitis.
● Advise client to adhere to scheduled laboratory blood tests and appointments with the health care provider so any adverse reactions can be monitored.
● Inform client that the desired therapeutic effect may take as long as 3 to 4 months to occur.

Side Effects

● Direct client to report early symptoms of possible gold toxicity such as a metallic taste or pruritus. A rash may occur. These symptoms should be reported to the health care provider.

PROTOTYPE DRUG CHART 27–4

GOLD

Drug Class	**Dosage**
Disease-modifying antirheumatic drug Trade Name: Ridaura *Pregnancy Category:* C	A: PO: 6 mg/d in single or divided doses; may increase dose to 9 mg/d C: Initial: 0.1 mg/kg/d in 1-2 divided doses; *maint:* 0.15 mg/kg/d in 1-2 divided doses; *max:* 0.2 mg/kg/d in 1-2 divided doses
Contraindications	**Drug-Lab-Food Interactions**
Severe renal or hepatic disease, colitis, systemic lupus erythematosus, pregnancy, blood dyscrasias *Caution:* Diabetes mellitus, congestive heart failure	*Drug:* With anticancer drugs, may cause bone marrow depression *Lab:* Slightly *increase* liver enzyme tests
Pharmacokinetics	**Pharmacodynamics**
Absorption: PO: 25% absorbed **Distribution:** PB: 60% **Metabolism:** t½: 26 d in blood; 40-120 d in tissue **Excretion:** >60% in urine (may appear for 15 mo); in feces	PO: Onset: UK Peak: 1-2 h Duration: Months

Therapeutic Effects/Uses

To alleviate inflammation and pain of rheumatoid arthritis
Mode of Action: Inhibition of prostaglandin synthesis and decreased phagocytosis

Side Effects	**Adverse Reactions**
Anorexia, nausea, vomiting, diarrhea, stomatitis, abdominal cramps, pruritus, dizziness, headache, metallic taste, rash, dermatitis, photosensitivity	Corneal gold deposits, urticaria, hematuria, proteinuria, bradycardia **Life-threatening:** Nephrotoxicity, agranulocytosis, thrombocytopenia, interstitial pneumonitis

A, Adult; *C,* child; *d,* day; *h,* hour; *maint,* maintenance; *max,* maximum; *mo,* month; *PB,* protein-binding; *PO,* by mouth; *t½,* half-life; *UK,* unknown; >, greater than.

- Teach client the side effects and to report them immediately. (See Prototype Drug Chart 27–4 for a list of side effects and adverse reactions.)
- Warn client to avoid direct sunlight because the gold drug may cause photosensitivity. Use of sun block is necessary.
- Alert client to report skin conditions such as dermatitis, bruising, and petechiae. Bleeding gums and blood in the stools should be reported to the health care provider.

Diet
- Suggest high-fiber diet or antidiarrheal drugs to control diarrhea. If diarrhea is continuous or severe for a prolonged time, the gold drug is usually discontinued.

Cultural Considerations

- Use simple, clear instructions. Ask family members to assist with translation only if an interpreter is not available. Do not use compound sentences.

EVALUATION

- Determine the effectiveness of the gold therapy by determining whether client has less pain and inflammation.

- Evaluate client for present or repeated side effects. The gold therapy regimen may need to be changed or discontinued.

Immunosuppressive Agents

Immunosuppressives are used to treat refractory rheumatoid arthritis (i.e., arthritis that does not respond to antiinflammatory drugs). In low doses, selected immunosuppressive agents have been effective in the treatment of rheumatoid arthritis. Drugs such as azathioprine (Imuran), cyclophosphamide (Cytoxan), and methotrexate (Mexate), primarily used to suppress cancer growth and proliferation, might be used to suppress the inflammatory process of rheumatoid arthritis when other treatments fail. In one study of clients receiving cyclophosphamide, few new erosions of joint cartilage were present, which suggests that the disease process is not active. These agents are not the first or second choice for treatment of rheumatoid arthritis.

Immunomodulators

Immunomodulators treat moderate to severe rheumatoid arthritis by disrupting the inflammatory process and delaying the disease progression. Interleukin (IL-1) receptor

Table 27–3

Antiinflammatory Drugs: DMARDs

Generic (Brand)	Route and Dosage	Uses and Considerations
auranofin (Ridaura) aurothioglucose (Solganal)	See Prototype Drug Chart 27–3. Increase dose weekly: A: IM: 10, 25, 50 mg (sol in oil) C: IM: 6-12 y: 0.25 mg-1 mg	For rheumatoid arthritis when unresponsive to NSAIDs. Start with low dose. Check laboratory values, especially white blood cell count, hemoglobin, and hematocrit. Check renal and liver function. *Pregnancy category:* C; PB: 95%; $t^{1}/_{2}$: 3-27 d
gold sodium thiomalate (Myochrysine)	Increase dose weekly: A: IM: 10, 25, 50 mg (aqueous sol) until 1 g cumulative dose; maint: 25-50 mg q2-3 wk; *max:* 1 g/wk C: TD: 10 mg, followed by 1 mg/kg/wk × 20 wk; *maint:* 1 mg/kg/dose every 2-4 wk; *max:* 50/kg/dose	Same considerations as aurothioglucose. Contains 50% gold. *Pregnancy category:* C; PB: 95%; $t^{1}/_{2}$: 3-27 d
anakinra (Kineret)	A: subQ: 100 mg daily	For treatment of rheumatoid arthritis unresponsive to other DMARDs. *Pregnancy category:* B; PB: UK; $t^{1}/_{2}$: 4-6 h
etanercept (Enbrel)	A: subQ: 25 mg 2 times/wk C: >4 y: subQ: 0.4 mg/kg 2 times/wk; *max:* 25 mg/dose	For treatment of rheumatoid arthritis unresponsive to other DMARDs. *Pregnancy category:* B; PB: UK; $t^{1}/_{2}$: 115 h
infliximab (Remicade)	*Rheumatoid arthritis* A: IV: 3 mg/kg over 2 h, then 2 mg/kg on wk 2 and 6 *Crohn's disease* A: IV: 5 mg/kg over 2 h, then 2 mg/kg on wk 2 and 6	For treatment of moderate to severe rheumatoid arthritis and Crohn's disease. *Pregnancy category:* C; PB: UK; $t^{1}/_{2}$: 9.5 d
adalimumab (Humira)	A: subQ: 40 mg every 2 wk	For treatment of rheumatoid arthritis unresponsive to other DMARDs. *Pregnancy category:* X; PB: UK; $t^{1}/_{2}$: 16.5 d
leflunomide (Arava)	A: PO: 100 mg/d for 3 d initially, then 20 mg daily	For treatment of rheumatoid arthritis unresponsive to other DMARDs. *Pregnancy category:* X; PB: 99%; $t^{1}/_{2}$: 19 d

A, Adult; *C,* child; *d,* day; *DMARDs,* disease-modifying antirheumatic drugs; *h,* hour; *IM,* intramuscular; *IV,* intravenous; *maint,* maintenance; *NSAIDs,* nonsteroidal antiinflammatory drugs; *PB,* protein-binding; *sol,* solution; *subQ,* subcutaneous; $t^{1}/_{2}$, half-life; *TD,* test dose; *UK,* unknown; *wk,* week; *y,* year; *>,* greater than.

PROTOTYPE DRUG CHART 27–5

INFLIXIMAB

Drug Class	**Dosage**
Immunomodulator: Tumor necrosis factor blocker	*Rheumatoid arthritis:*
Trade Name: Remicade	A: IV: 3 mg/kg wk 1 then 2 mg/kg wk 2 and 6 then
Pregnancy Category: C	2 mg/kg q8 wk
	Crohn's disease:
	A: IV: 5 mg/kg wk 1 may repeat wk 2 and 6
Contraindications	**Drug-Lab-Food Interactions**
Hypersensitivity, heart failure	*Drug:* May decrease effectiveness of vaccines
Caution: Renal or hepatic dysfunction, immuno-suppression, multiple sclerosis, elderly	
Pharmacokinetics	**Pharmacodynamics**
Absorption: UK	IV: Onset: UK
Distribution: UK	Peak: UK
Metabolism: t½: 9.5 d	Duration: UK
Excretion: UK	

Therapeutic Effects/Uses

To treat moderate to severe rheumatoid arthritis and Crohn's disease

Side Effects	**Adverse Reactions**
Headache, dizziness, coughing, fatigue, chills, hot flashes, anxiety, insomnia, depression, nausea, vomiting, diarrhea, constipation, flatulence, rash, alopecia, dry skin, urinary frequency	Severe infections, chest pain, hypotension, hypertension, increased hepatic enzymes

A, Adult; *d,* day; *IV,* intravenous; *t½,* half-life; *UK,* unknown; *wk,* week.

antagonists and tumor necrosis factor (TNF) blockers are two groups of drugs classified as immunomodulators.

Anakinra (Kineret), an IL-1 receptor antagonist, blocks activity of IL-1 by inhibiting IL-1 from binding to interleukin receptors located in cartilage and bone. IL-1 is a proinflammatory cytokine that contributes to synovial inflammation and joint destruction. Anakinra is administered subcutaneously. The peak is 3 to 7 hours, and the half-life is 6 hours.

The TNF blockers bind to the TNF and block it from attaching to TNF receptors on the synovial cell surfaces. By neutralizing TNF, a contributor to synovitis, inflammatory disease process is delayed. Etanercept (Enbrel) was the first TNF blocker developed and is administered subcutaneously. The peak half-life is 115 hours. Signs and symptoms of rheumatoid arthritis are suppressed rapidly with etanercept therapy but reappear if the drug is discontinued. Other TNF blockers include infliximab (Remicade), adalimumab (Humira), and leflunomide (Arava). Infliximab is administered intravenously (IV) over at least 2 hours, adalimumab is administered subcutaneously, and leflunomide is administered orally. (See Prototype Drug Chart 27–5 for information on Infliximab.)

Both IL-1 receptor antagonists and TNF blockers predispose the client to severe infections; therefore are contraindicated in active infection and should be discontinued when an infection occurs. Immunomodulators are usually very expensive: approximately $14,000 to $37,000 per year.

Antimalarials

Antimalarial drugs may be used to treat rheumatoid arthritis when other methods of treatment fail. The mechanism of action of antimalarials in suppression of rheumatoid arthritis is unclear. The effect may take 4 to 12 weeks to become apparent, and antimalarials are usually used in combination with NSAIDs in clients whose arthritis is not under control.

Antigout Drugs

Gout has been called the "disease of kings" because, in the past, royalty ate rich foods, drank wine and alcohol, and suffered from gout. It was also called the "unwalkable disease." Hippocrates (460–357 BC) referred to gout as *podagra* (foot seizure). He recognized gout as affecting other joints of the large toe, hand, elbow, knee, and shoulder. Hippocrates' recommendation of treatment included purgatives (strong laxatives). Galen (131–200 AD) attributed gout to "intemperance" and heredity.

Gout is an inflammatory condition that attacks joints, tendons, and other tissues. It may be called *gouty arthritis.* The most common site of acute gouty inflammation is at the joint of the big toe. Gout is characterized by a uric acid metabolism disorder and a defect in purine (products of certain proteins) metabolism, resulting in an increase in urates (uric acid salts) and an accumulation of uric acid (hyperuricemia) or an ineffective clearance of uric acid by the kidneys. Uric acid solubility is poor in acid urine and urate crystals may form, causing urate calculi. Gout may appear as bumps, or *tophi,* in the subcutaneous tissue of earlobes, elbows, hands, and the base of the large toe. In addition to tophi, the complications of untreated or prolonged periods of gout include gouty arthritis, urinary calculi, and gouty nephropathy.

Fluid intake should be increased while taking antigout drugs, and the urine should be alkaline. Foods rich in purine (e.g., wine, alcohol, organ meats, sardines, salmon, gravy) should be avoided. Acetaminophen should be taken for discomfort instead of aspirin (salicylic acid) to reduce acidity.

Antiinflammatory Gout Drug: Colchicine

The first drug used to treat gout was colchicine, introduced in 1936. The antiinflammatory drug colchicine inhibits the migration of leukocytes to the inflamed site. It is effective in alleviating acute symptoms of gout, but it is not effective in decreasing inflammation occurring in other inflammatory disorders. It does not inhibit uric acid synthesis and does not promote uric acid excretion. It should not be used if the client has a severe renal, cardiac, or GI problem. Gastric irritation is a common problem; therefore colchicine should be taken with food. With high doses of colchicine, nausea, vomiting, diarrhea, or abdominal pain occurs in approximately 75% of clients taking the drug.

Colchicine is well absorbed in the GI tract, and its peak concentration time is within 2 hours. Most of the drug is excreted in the feces, but 10% to 20% is excreted in the urine.

Uric Acid Inhibitor

Allopurinol (Zyloprim), marketed in 1963, is not an antiinflammatory drug; instead, it inhibits the final steps of uric acid biosynthesis and therefore lowers serum uric acid levels, preventing the precipitation of an attack. This drug is frequently used as a prophylactic to prevent gout. It is a choice drug for clients with chronic tophaceous gout. Allopurinol is also indicated for gout clients with renal impairment. It is useful for clients who have renal obstructions caused by uric acid stones and for clients with blood disorders such as leukemia and polycythemia vera. It is also given to clients who do not respond well to uricosuric drugs such as probenecid. Increased fluid intake is recommended to promote diuresis and prevent alkalinization of the urine. Prototype Drug Chart 27–6 presents the pharmacologic behavior of allopurinol.

Pharmacokinetics

Eighty percent of allopurinol is absorbed from the GI tract. Biosynthesis of uric acid occurs in the liver in pure form and active metabolites. The half-life of the drug itself is 2 to 3 hours and 20 to 24 hours for its active metabolites. The protein-binding percentage is unknown. Most of the drug and its metabolites are excreted in feces and some in urine.

Pharmacodynamics

Allopurinol inhibits the production of uric acid by inhibiting the enzyme xanthine oxidase, which is needed in the synthesis of uric acid. Allopurinol also improves the solubility of uric acid. Its onset of action occurs

within 30 to 60 minutes; its peak time averages 2 to 4 hours. Allopurinol has a long duration of action.

Alcohol, caffeine, and thiazide diuretics increase the uric acid level. Use of ampicillin or amoxicillin with allopurinol increases the risk of rash formation. Allopurinol can increase the effect of warfarin (Coumadin) and oral hypoglycemic drugs.

Uricosurics

Uricosurics increase the rate of uric acid excretion by inhibiting its reabsorption. These drugs are effective in alleviating chronic gout, but they should *not* be used during acute attacks. Probenecid (Benemid) is a uricosuric that has been available since 1945. It blocks the reabsorption of uric acid and promotes its excretion. Probenecid can be taken with colchicine. To begin initial therapy for relieving symptoms of gout and inhibiting uric acid reabsorption, small doses of colchicine should be given before adding probenecid. If gastric irritation occurs, probenecid should be taken with meals. It has an average half-life of 8 to 10 hours and is 85% to 95% protein bound. Use caution when administering this drug with other highly protein-bound drugs.

Another uricosuric is sulfinpyrazone (Anturane). This drug is a metabolite of phenylbutazone and is more potent than probenecid. Sulfinpyrazone should be taken with meals or with antacids to prevent gastric irritation. Severe blood dyscrasias might occur, especially in clients with a history of blood dyscrasia. Table 27–4 gives dosages and considerations for the commonly used antigout drugs.

Side Effects and Adverse Reactions

Side effects may include flushed skin, sore gums, and headache. Kidney stones, resulting from the uric acid, could be prevented by increasing water intake and maintaining a urine pH above 6. Blood dyscrasias occur rarely. Aspirin use should be avoided because it causes uric acid retention.

Nursing Process

Antigout

ASSESSMENT

■ Determine a medical history from client of any gastric, renal, cardiac, or liver disorders. Antigout drugs are excreted via kidneys, so sufficient renal function is needed. Drug dosage and drug selection might need to be changed.

■ Obtain a drug history. Report possible drug-drug interactions. (See Drug-Lab-Food Interactions in Prototype Drug Chart 27–2.)

■ Assess the serum uric acid value for future comparison.

■ Record the urine output. Use the initial urine output for future comparison.

■ Check laboratory tests (e.g., blood urea nitrogen [BUN], serum creatinine, alkaline phosphatase [ALP], aspartate aminotransferase [AST], alanine aminotransferase

[ALT], lactate dehydrogenase [LDH]) and compare with future laboratory test results.

NURSING DIAGNOSES

■ Impaired tissue integrity
■ Pain, acute

PLANNING

■ Client's "gouty pain" is absent or controlled without side effects.

NURSING INTERVENTIONS

■ Report GI symptoms, gastric pain, nausea, vomiting, or diarrhea when taking antigout drugs. Take these drugs with food to alleviate gastric distress.
■ Record client's urine output. Because the drugs and uric acid are excreted through the urine, kidney stones might occur, so both water intake and urine output should be increased.

■ Monitor laboratory tests for renal and liver function (BUN, serum creatinine, ALP, AST, ALT).

Client Teaching

General
• Encourage client to keep medical appointments and to have regular scheduled laboratory tests for renal, liver, and complete blood count functions. Some antigout drugs may cause blood dyscrasias; blood tests should be monitored.
• Instruct client to increase fluid intake; it will increase drug and uric acid excretion.

Side Effects
• Inform client to report side effects of antigout drugs, such as anorexia, nausea, vomiting, diarrhea, stomatitis, dizziness, rash, pruritus, and metallic taste, to the health care provider.
• Advise client to have a yearly eye examination because visual changes can result from prolonged use of allopurinol.

PROTOTYPE DRUG CHART 27–6

ALLOPURINOL

Drug Class

Antigout: Uric acid biosynthesis inhibitor
Trade Name: Zyloprim, ✤ Alloprin, Apo-Allopurinol, Novopurinol
Pregnancy Category: C

Dosage

A: PO: Initially: 100 mg/dl, may increase; 200-300 mg/d (for mild gout); 400-600 mg/d (for severe gout); *max:* 800 mg/d
C: ≤10 y: PO: 10 mg/kg/d in 2-3 divided doses

Contraindications

Hypersensitivity, severe renal disease
Caution: Hepatic disorder

Drug-Lab-Food Interactions

Drug: Increase effect of warfarin, phenytoin, theophylline, anticancer drugs, ACE inhibitors; *increase* rash with ampicillin, amoxicillin; *increase* toxicity with thiazide diuretics; *decrease* allopurinol effect with antacids
Lab: Increase AST, ALT, BUN

Pharmacokinetics

Absorption: PO: 80% absorbed
Distribution: PB: UK
Metabolism: $t^{1/2}$: 2-3 h
Metabolite: 20-24 h
Excretion: 10%-20% in urine; 80%-90% in feces

Pharmacodynamics

PO: Onset: 0.5-1 h
Peak: 2-4 h
Duration: 18-30 h

Therapeutic Effects/Uses

To treat gout and hyperuricemia; prevent urate calculi
Mode of Action: Reduction of uric acid synthesis

Side Effects

Anorexia, nausea, vomiting, diarrhea, stomatitis, dizziness, headache, rash, pruritus, malaise, metallic taste

Adverse Reactions

Cataracts, retinopathy
Life-threatening: Bone marrow depression, aplastic anemia, thrombocytopenia, agranulocytosis, leukopenia

---

A, Adult; *ACE,* angiotensin-converting enzyme; *ALT,* alanine aminotransferase; *AST,* aspartate aminotransferase; *BUN,* blood urea nitrogen; *C,* child; *d,* day; *h,* hour; *max,* maximum; *PB,* protein-binding; *PO,* by mouth; $t^{1/2}$, half-life; *UK,* unknown; *y,* year; ≤, equal to or less than; ✤, Canadian drug names.

Diet

- Warn client to avoid alcohol and caffeine because they can increase uric acid levels.
- Suggest to client not to take large doses of vitamin C while taking allopurinol; kidney stones may occur.
- Tell client not to ingest foods that are high in purine content (e.g., organ meats, salmon, sardines, gravy, legumes). Purine foods increase the uric acid levels.
- Direct client to report any gastric distress. Encourage client to take antigout drugs with food or at mealtime.

Cultural Considerations

- Provide additional explanation as needed to clients and their families from various cultural groups related to the disease process and the purpose of the drug and its side effects.
- Suggest follow-up by a community health nurse to determine client's compliance to the drug regimen and the effectiveness of the prescribed drug therapy.

EVALUATION

■ Evaluate client's response to the antigout drug. If pain persists, the drug regimen may need modification.
■ Determine the presence of adverse reactions. Drug therapy for gout pain may need to be changed.

WEBSITES

For further information on *Antiinflammatory Drugs,* visit these Internet resources:

Information on Naproxen:
www.nlm.nih.gov/medlineplus/druginfo/medmaster/a681029.html

Information on Colchicine:
www.focusonarthritis.com/script/main/art.asp?li=MNI&ArticleKey=724

Information on allopurinol:
www.medicinenet.com/allopurinol/article.htm

Table 27–4

Antigout Drugs

Generic (Brand)	Route and Dosage	Uses and Considerations
Antiinflammatory Gout Drug		
colchicine (🍁 Novocolchine)	A: PO: Initially: 0.5-1.2 mg; then 0.5-0.6 mg q1-2h for pain relief; *max:* 4 mg/d; IV: Initially: 2 mg, then 0.5 mg q6h PRN; *max:* 4 mg/d	Treatment of acute gout and prophylaxis of recurrent gouty arthritis. Not for clients with renal or gastric disorders. Take with food. *Pregnancy category:* C; PB: 10%-30%; t$^{1/2}$: 20-30 min
Uric Acid Biosynthesis Inhibitor		
allopurinol (Zyloprim)	See Prototype Drug Chart 27–4.	
Uricosurics		
probenecid (Benemid)	A: PO: First week: 250 mg b.i.d.; *maint:* 500 mg b.i.d.; *max:* 2 g/d C: <50 kg: PO: 25-40 mg/kg/d in 4 divided doses	Treatment for hyperuricemia; promotes urinary excretion of uric acid. For gout and gouty arthritis. Alkaline urine helps prevent renal stones. Increase fluid intake. *Pregnancy category:* B; PB: 90%; t$^{1/2}$: 4-10 h
sulfinpyrazone (Anturane)	A: PO: First week: 100-200 mg b.i.d.; *maint:* 200-400 mg b.i.d.; may reduce to 200 mg/d; *max:* 800 mg/d	Used in the management of hyperuricemia; decreases gouty attacks. Can cause GI distress. Take with food. *Pregnancy category:* C; PB: 90%; t$^{1/2}$: 3 h

A, Adult; *b.i.d.,* twice a day; *C,* child; *d,* day; *GI,* gastrointestinal; *h,* hour; *IV,* intravenous; *maint,* maintenance; *max,* maximum; *min,* minute; *PB,* protein-binding; *PO,* by mouth; *PRN,* as needed; *t$^{1/2}$,* half-life; <, less than; 🍁, Canadian drug.

Critical Thinking Case Study

P.Q., age 72, had taken 650 mg of aspirin four times a day for 8 months to alleviate her chronic symptoms of pain and inflammation associated with arthritis. Four weeks ago, a peptic ulcer developed.

1. Explain the process in which P.Q. could have a peptic ulcer. How could this have been prevented?

2. Compare the similarities and differences in the side effects of salicylates with those of acetic acid agents, propionic acid agents, COX-2 inhibitors, and phenylacetic acid.

3. What client teaching points should P.Q. receive before and during the time she takes aspirin?

4. How would COX-2 inhibitors prevent the development of a peptic ulcer?

5. Would the DMARD group be more helpful to alleviate P.Q.'s symptoms? Explain your rationale.

6. Compare the differences in the various types of DMARDs.

Study Questions

1. What is the action of nonsteroidal antiinflammatory drugs (NSAIDs)? Give examples of common NSAIDs.

2. What are the major side effects of NSAIDs?

3. What are the advantages for the use of second-generation NSAIDs (COX-2 inhibitors) over traditional NSAIDs? Explain.

4. What are the uses of disease-modifying antirheumatic drugs (DMARDs)?

5. What are the side effects and adverse reactions of DMARDs?

6. What are the nursing interventions associated with the use of NSAIDs and DMARDs?

7. What drugs are used to treat gout? What are the nursing considerations?

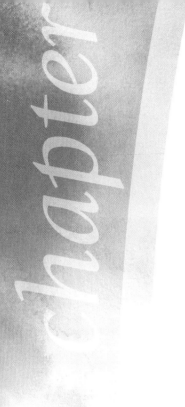

28 Antibacterials: Penicillins and Cephalosporins

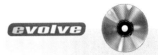

ELECTRONIC RESOURCES

Additional information can be found on the companion website at *http://evolve.elsevier.com/KeeHayes/pharmacology/* or on the companion CD-ROM, which includes:

- *NCLEX-style examination review questions*
- *Pharmacology animations*
- *Medication error and IV therapy checklists*
- *Medication calculation problems*
- *Electronic calculators*

OUTLINE

OBJECTIVES

- Explain the mechanisms of action of antibacterial drugs.
- Differentiate between bacteria that are naturally resistant and those that have acquired resistance to an antibiotic.
- Describe the three general adverse effects associated with antibacterial drugs.
- Differentiate between narrow-spectrum and broad-spectrum antibiotics.
- Give an example for each of the natural, broad-spectrum (extended), penicillinase-resistant, and antipseudomonal penicillins, and explain their effects.
- Explain the expected effects of first-, second-, third-, and fourth-generation cephalosporins.
- Explain the use of the nursing process in caring for clients receiving penicillins and cephalosporins.

TERMS

acquired resistance	bacteriostatic	inherent resistance	nephrotoxicity
antibacterials	broad-spectrum antibiotics	microorganisms	nosocomial infections
antimicrobials	cross-resistance	narrow-spectrum	superinfection
bactericidal	immunoglobulins	antibiotics	

Introduction

This chapter discusses the antibacterials and their effects, which include mechanisms of antibacterial action, body defenses, resistance to antibacterials, use of antibacterial combinations, general adverse reactions to antibacterials, and narrow- and broad-spectrum antibiotics. This chapter also covers two antibacterials: penicillin and cephalosporin.

Pathophysiology

Bacteria, known as *prokaryotes,* are single-cell organisms lacking a true nucleus and nucleus membrane. Most bacteria have a rigid cell wall. The structure of the cell wall determines the shape of the bacteria. A *bacillus* is a rod-shaped organism. Cocci are a spherical bacterium. When the cocci appear in clusters, it is called *staphylococci;* when the cocci divide into chains, it called *streptococci.* Bacteria reproduce by cell division about every 20 minutes.

Bacteria produce toxins that cause cell lysis (cell death). Many bacteria produce the enzyme beta-lactamase, which destroys the beta-lactam antibiotics such as penicillins and cephalosporins.

Antibacterial Drugs

Antibacterials/Antibiotics

Although the terms *antibacterial, antimicrobial,* and *antibiotic* are frequently used interchangeably, there are some subtle differences in meaning. **Antibacterials** and **antimicrobials** are substances that inhibit the growth of or kill bacteria and other **microorganisms** (microscopic organisms including viruses, fungi, protozoa, and rickettsiae). Technically, the term *antibiotic* refers to chemicals produced by one kind of microorganism that inhibits the growth of or kills another. For practical purposes, however, these terms may be used interchangeably. Several drugs, including anti-infective and chemotherapeutic agents, have actions similar to those of the antibacterial and antimicrobial agents. Antibacterial drugs do not act alone in destroying bacteria. Natural body defenses, surgical procedures to excise infected tissues, and dressing changes may be needed along with antibacterial drugs to eliminate the infecting bacteria.

Antibacterial drugs are either obtained from natural sources or manufactured. The use of moldy bread on wounds to fight infection dates back 3500 years. In 1928 Alexander Fleming, a British bacteriologist, noted that "mold" was contaminating the bacterial cultures and inhibiting the bacterial growth. The mold was called *Penicillium notatum;* thus Fleming called the substance *penicillin.*

In 1939 Howard Florey continued with Fleming's findings and purified the penicillin so it could be used commercially. Penicillin was used during World War II and was marketed in 1945. Sulfonamide, a synthetic antibacterial, was introduced in 1935. Sulfonamides are discussed in greater detail in Chapter 30, Antibacterials: Sulfonamides.

Bacteriostatic drugs inhibit the growth of bacteria, whereas **bactericidal** drugs kill bacteria. Some antibacterial drugs, such as tetracycline and sulfonamides, have a bacteriostatic effect, whereas other antibacterials, such as penicillins and cephalosporins, have a bactericidal effect. Depending on the drug dose and serum level, certain drugs can have both bacteriostatic and bactericidal effects.

Peaks and troughs of serum antibiotic levels are monitored for drugs with a narrow therapeutic index, such as aminoglycosides, to determine whether the drug is within the therapeutic range for its desired effect. If the serum peak level is too high, drug toxicity could occur. If the serum trough level, which is drawn minutes before administration of the next drug dose, is below the therapeutic range, the client is not receiving an adequate antibiotic dose to kill the microorganism.

Mechanisms of Antibacterial Action

Five mechanisms of antibacterial action are responsible for the inhibition of growth or destruction of microorganisms: (1) inhibition of bacterial cell-wall synthesis, (2) alteration of membrane permeability, (3) inhibition of protein synthesis, (4) inhibition of the synthesis of bacterial ribonucleic acid (RNA) and deoxyribonucleic acid (DNA), and (5) interference with metabolism within the cell (Table 28-1).

Pharmacokinetics

Antibacterial drugs must not only penetrate the bacterial cell wall in sufficient concentration but also must have an affinity to the binding sites on the bacterial cell. The time that the drug remains at the binding sites increases the effect of the antibacterial action. The time is controlled by the pharmacokinetics (distribution, half-life, and elimination) of the drug. Antibacterials that have a longer half-life usually maintain a greater concentration at the binding site; therefore frequent dosing is not required. Most antibacterials are not highly protein bound, with a few exceptions (e.g., oxacillin, ceftriaxone, cefoperazone, cefonicid, cefprozil, cloxacillin, nafcillin, clindamycin); thus protein binding does not have a major influence on the effectiveness of the drug dose. The steady state of the antibacterial drug occurs after the fourth to fifth half-lives, and the drug is eliminated from the body, mainly through urine, after the seventh half-life.

Pharmacodynamics

The drug concentration at the site or the exposure time for the drug plays an important role in bacteria eradication. Antibacterial drugs are used to achieve the minimum effective concentration (MEC) necessary to halt the growth of a microorganism. Many antibacterials have a bactericidal effect

Table 28-1

Mechanisms of Actions of Antibacterial Drugs

Action	Effect	Drugs
Inhibitions of cell wall synthesis	Bactericidal effect. Enzyme breakdown of the cell wall. Inhibition of the enzyme in the synthesis of the cell wall.	penicillin cephalosporins bacitracin vancomycin
Alteration in membrane permeability	Bacteriostatic or bactericidal effect. Membrane permeability is increased. The loss of cellular substances causes lysis of the cell.	amphotericin B nystatin polymyxin colistin
Inhibition of protein synthesis	Bacteriostatic or bactericidal effect. Interferes with protein synthesis without affecting normal cell. Inhibits the steps of protein synthesis.	aminoglycosides tetracyclines erythromycin lincomycins
Inhibition of synthesis of bacterial RNA and DNA	Inhibits synthesis of RNA and DNA in bacteria. It binds to the nucleic acid and to the enzymes, which are needed for nucleic acid synthesis.	fluoroquinolones
Interference with cellular metabolism	Bacteriostatic effect. Interferes with steps of metabolism within the cells.	sulfonamides trimethoprim isoniazid (INH) nalidixic acid rifampin

DNA, Deoxyribonucleic acid; *RNA,* ribonucleic acid.

against the pathogen when the drug concentration remains constantly above the MEC during the dosing interval. Duration of time for use of the antibacterial varies according to the type of pathogen, site of infection, and immunocompetence of the host. With some severe infections, a continuous infusion regimen is more effective than an intermittent dosing because of constant drug concentration and time exposure. Once-daily antibacterial dosing (e.g., aminoglycosides, macrolides, fluoroquinolones) has been effective in eradicating pathogens and, in most of those cases, has not caused severe adverse reactions (ototoxicity, nephrotoxicity). In addition, once- or twice-daily drug dosing increases the client's adherence to the drug regimen.

Figure 28–1 illustrates the effect of three methods of drug dosing. The drug dose is effective when it remains above the MEC.

Body Defenses

Body defenses and antibacterial drugs work together to stop the infectious process. The effect that antibacterial drugs have on an infection depends not only on the drug but also on the host's defense mechanisms. Factors such as age, nutrition, immunoglobulins, white blood cells (WBCs), organ function, and circulation influence the body's ability to fight infection. If the host's natural body defense mechanisms are inadequate, drug therapy might not be as effective. As a result, drug therapy may need to be closely monitored or revised. When circulation is impeded, an antibacterial drug may not be distributed properly to the infected area. In addition, **immunoglobulins,** such as IgG and IgM (a protein with antibody activity, part of the immune response system), and WBCs needed to combat infections may be depleted in individuals with poor nutritional status.

Resistance to Antibacterials

Bacteria may be sensitive or resistant to certain antibacterials. When bacteria are sensitive to the drug, the organism is inhibited or destroyed. If bacteria are resistant to an antibacterial, the organism continues to grow despite administration of that antibacterial drug.

Bacterial resistance may result naturally **(inherent resistance),** or it may be acquired. A natural, or inherent, resistance occurs without previous exposure to the antibacterial drug. For example, the gram-negative (non-gram-staining) bacterium *Pseudomonas aeruginosa* is resistant to penicillin G. An **acquired resistance** is caused by prior exposure to the antibacterial. For example, although *Staphylococcus aureus* was once sensitive to penicillin G, previous exposures have caused this organism to become resistant to it. Penicillinase, an enzyme produced by the microorganism, is responsible for causing penicillin resistance. This enzyme metabolizes penicillin G, causing the drug to be ineffective. Penicillinase-resistant penicillins that are effective against *S. aureus* are currently available.

Antibiotic resistance is a major problem. In the early 1980s pharmaceutical companies thought that enough an-

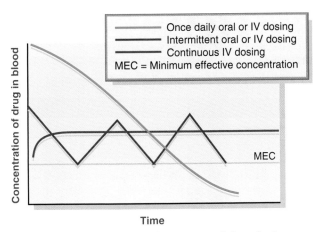

- Once daily oral or IV dosing
- Intermittent oral or IV dosing
- Continuous IV dosing
- MEC = Minimum effective concentration

Concentration of drug in blood

MEC

Time

FIGURE 28–1   Effects of concentrated drug dosing.

tibiotics were on the market, so these companies concentrated on developing antiviral and antifungal drugs. As a result, fewer new antibiotics were developed during the 1980s. Now pharmaceutical companies have developed many new antibiotics. Antibiotic resistance continues to occur, especially when antibiotics are used frequently. As the bacteria reproduce, some mutation occurs, and eventually the mutant bacteria survive the effects of the drug. One explanation is that the mutant bacteria strain may have grown a thicker cell wall.

In large health care institutions, there is a tendency toward drug resistance in bacteria. Mutant strains of organisms have developed, thus increasing the resistance to antibiotics that were once effective. Infections that are acquired while clients are hospitalized are called **nosocomial infections.** Many of these infections are caused by drug-resistant bacteria and can prolong hospitalization, which is costly to the client.

Another problem related to antibiotic resistance is that bacteria can transfer their genetic instruction to another bacterial species; thus the other bacterial species becomes resistant to that antibiotic as well. Bacteria can pass its high resistance to a more virulent and aggressive bacterium, such as *S. aureus* and enterococci. Many enterococcal strains are resistant to penicillin, ampicillin, gentamicin, streptomycin, and vancomycin. One of the biggest resistance problems is vancomycin-resistant enterococci (VRE), which can cause death in many persons with weakened immune systems. The incidence of VRE in hospitals increased from 0.3% in 1989 to 14.2% in 1996. Staphylococcal bacteria tend to be resistant to every drug except vancomycin. If VRE transfers to *Staphylococcus* its resistance to vancomycin, a major medical problem could result.

One antibiotic after another is ineffective against new resistant strains of bacteria. As new drugs are developed, drug resistance will probably develop as well. Pharmaceutical companies and biotechnical firms are working on new classes of drugs to "beat" the problem of bacterial resistance to antibiotics. Recently, the new everninomicin class antibiotic Ziracin has been approved. Another class of antibiotics, oxazolidinones, was discovered by a pharmaceutical company in 1988, but the company could not overcome toxicity problems in this class of drug. Another pharmaceutical company has taken the compound and made it less toxic. This new antibiotic, Linezolid, is effective against methicillin-resistant staphylococci, VRE, and penicillin-resistant streptococci. Quinupristin/dalfopristin (Synercid), two streptogramin antibacterials, is marketed in a combination of 30:70 for intravenous (IV) use against life-threatening infection caused by VRE and for treatment of bacteremia, *S. aureus*, and *Streptococcus pyogenes.*

Another way to attack antimicrobial resistance is to develop drugs that disable the antibiotic-resistant mechanism in the bacteria. Clients would take the antibiotic-resistance disabler along with the antibiotic already on the market, making it effective again. Developing bacterial vaccine is another way to combat bacteria and lessen the need for an-

tibiotics. The bacterial vaccine against pneumococcus has been effective in decreasing the occurrence of pneumonia and meningitis among various age groups. An important way to decrease antibiotic resistance is to prevent antibiotic abuse, a major problem. Consumer education is important because many clients "demand" antibiotics for viral conditions. Antibiotics are ineffective against viruses. However, viral infections that persist could decrease the body's immune system thus promoting a bacterial infection.

Cross-resistance can also occur between antibacterial drugs that have similar actions, such as the penicillins and cephalosporins. The organism causing the infection can be determined by culture, and the antibiotics sensitive to the organism are determined by culture and sensitivity (C & S). To determine the effect antibacterial drugs have on a specific microorganism, C & S or antibiotic susceptibility testing is performed. The susceptibility or resistance of one microorganism to several antibacterials can be determined by this method. Multiantibiotic therapy (daily use of several antibacterials) delays the development of microorganism resistance.

Use of Antibiotic Combinations

Combination antibiotics should not be routinely prescribed or administered except for specific uncontrollable infections. Usually a single antibiotic will successfully treat a bacterial infection. When there is a severe infection that persists and is of unknown origin or has been unsuccessfully treated with several single antibiotics, a combination of two or three antibiotics may be suggested. Before antibiotic therapy, a culture or cultures should be taken to identify the bacteria.

When two antibiotics are combined, the result is additive, potentiative, or antagonistic. The *additive* effect is equal to the sum of the effects of two antibiotics. The *potentiative* effect occurs when one antibiotic potentiates the effect of the second antibiotic, increasing their effectiveness. The *antagonistic* result is a combination of a drug that is bactericidal, such as penicillin, and a drug that is bacteriostatic, such as tetracycline. When these two drugs are used together, the desired effect may be greatly reduced.

General Adverse Reactions to Antibacterials

Three major adverse reactions associated with the administration of antibacterial drugs are allergic (hypersensitivity) reactions, superinfection, and organ toxicity. Table 28-2 describes these adverse reactions, all of which require close monitoring of the client.

Narrow-Spectrum and Broad-Spectrum Antibiotics

Antibacterial drugs are either narrow spectrum or broad spectrum. The **narrow-spectrum antibiotics** are primarily effective against one type of organism. For example, penicillin and erythromycin are used to treat infections caused by gram-positive bacteria. Certain **broad-spectrum antibiotics,** such as tetracycline and the cephalosporins, can be effective against both gram-positive and gram-negative or-

Table 28–2

General Adverse Reactions to Antibacterial Drugs

Type	Considerations
Allergy or hypersensitivity	Allergic reactions to drugs may be mild or severe. Examples of mild reactions are rash, pruritus, and hives. An example of a severe response is anaphylactic shock. Anaphylaxis results in vascular collapse, laryngeal edema, bronchospasm, and cardiac arrest. Shortness of breath is frequently the first symptom of anaphylaxis. Severe allergic reaction generally occurs within 20 minutes. Mild allergic reaction is treated with an antihistamine; anaphylaxis requires treatment with epinephrine, bronchodilators, and antihistamines.
Superinfection	Superinfection is a secondary infection that occurs when the normal microbial flora of the body are disturbed during antibiotic therapy. Superinfections can occur in the mouth, respiratory tract, intestine, genitourinary tract, or skin. Fungus infections frequently result in superinfections, although bacterial organisms, such as *Proteus, Pseudomonas,* and staphylococci may be the offending microorganisms. Superinfections rarely develop when the drug is administered for less than a week. They occur more commonly with the use of broad-spectrum antibiotics. For fungal infection of the mouth, nystatin is frequently used.
Organ toxicity	Organs, such as the liver and kidney, are involved in drug metabolism and excretion. Antibacterials may result in damage to these organs. For example, aminoglycosides can be ototoxic and nephrotoxic.

ganisms. Because narrow-spectrum antibiotics are selective, they are more active against those single organisms than the broad-spectrum antibiotics. Broad-spectrum antibiotics are frequently used to treat infections when the offending microorganism has not been identified by C & S.

Penicillins and Cephalosporins

Penicillins

Penicillin, a natural antibacterial agent obtained from the mold genus *Penicillium*, was introduced to the military during World War II and is considered to have saved many soldiers' lives. It became widely used in 1945 and was labeled a "miracle" drug. With the advent of penicillin, many clients survived who would have normally died from wound and severe respiratory infections.

Penicillin's beta-lactam structure (beta-lactam ring) interferes with bacterial cell-wall synthesis by inhibiting the bacterial enzyme that is necessary for cell division and cellular synthesis. The bacteria die of cell lysis (cell breakdown). The penicillins can be both bacteriostatic and bactericidal, depending on the drug and dosage. Penicillin G is primarily bactericidal.

Penicillins are mainly referred to as *beta-lactam antibiotics.* Bacteria can produce a variety of enzymes, beta-lactamases, that can inactivate penicillin and other beta-lactam antibiotics such as the cephalosporins. The beta-lactamases, which attack penicillins, are called *penicillinases.*

Penicillin G was the first penicillin administered orally and by injection. With oral administration, only about one third of the dose is absorbed. Because of its poor absorption, penicillin G given by injection (intramuscular [IM] and intravenous [IV]) is more effective in achieving a therapeutic serum penicillin level. Aqueous penicillin G has a short duration of action, and the IM injection is very

painful because it is an aqueous drug solution. As a result, a longer-acting form of penicillin, procaine penicillin (milky color), was produced to extend the activity of the drug. Procaine in the penicillin decreases the pain related to injection.

Penicillin V was the next type of penicillin produced. Although two thirds of the oral dose is absorbed by the gastrointestinal (GI) tract, it is a less potent antibacterial drug than penicillin G. Penicillin V is effective against mild to moderate infections, including anthrax as a biological weapon of bioterrorism.

Initially, penicillin was overused. It was first introduced for the treatment of staphylococcal infections, but after a few years, mutant strains of *Staphylococcus* developed that were resistant to penicillins G and V because of the bacterial enzyme penicillinase, which destroys penicillin. This led to the development of new broad-spectrum antibiotics with structures similar to penicillin to combat infections that are resistant to penicillins G and V.

Food may decrease the absorption of many penicillins that are taken orally; therefore those penicillins should be taken with a full glass of water 1 hour before food intake or 2 hours after mealtime. Amoxicillins and bacampicillin are penicillins that are unaffected by food.

Broad-Spectrum Penicillins (Aminopenicillins)

The broad-spectrum penicillins are used to treat both gram-positive and gram-negative bacteria. They are not, however, as "broadly" effective against all microorganisms as they were once considered to be. This group of drugs is costlier than penicillin and therefore should not be used when ordinary penicillins, such as penicillin G, are effective. The broad-spectrum penicillins are effective against some gram-negative organisms, such as *Escherichia coli, Haemophilus influenzae, Shigella dysenteriae, Proteus mirabilis,* and *Salmonella;* however, these drugs are not penicillinase resistant. They are readily

Table 28–3

Antibacterials: Penicillins

Generic (Brand)	Route and Dosage	Uses and Considerations
Basic Penicillins		
penicillin G procaine (Crysticillin, Wycillin)	A: IM: 600,000-1.2 million units/d in 1-2 divided doses C: IM: 300,000-600,000 units/d in 1-2 divided doses NB: IM: 50,000 units/kg/d	For moderately serious infections. Slow IM absorption with prolonged action. The solution is milky. *Pregnancy category:* B; PB: 65%; t^1/$_2$: 0.5 h
penicillin G benzathine (Bicillin)	A: IM: 1.2 million units as a single dose C: IM: >27 kg: 900,000 units/dose IM: <27 kg: 50,000 units/kg/dose or 300,000-600,000 units/dose	Long-acting penicillin when given by injection. Used as a prophylaxis for rheumatic fever. *Pregnancy category:* B; PB: 65%; t^1/$_2$: 1 h
penicillin G sodium/potassium (Pentids, Pfizerpen)	A: PO: 200,000-500,000 units q6h IM: 500,000-5 million units/d in divided doses IV: 4-20 million units/d in divided doses, diluted in IV fluids C: PO: 25,000-90,000 units/d in divided doses IV: 50,000-100,000 units/kg/d in divided doses	Poorly absorbed orally because of gastric acidity and food. Take before or after meals. Penicillin G is available in salts (potassium [K] and sodium [Na]). With high doses, electrolyte levels should be monitored. Injectable solution is clear. *Pregnancy category:* B; PB: 60%; t^1/$_2$: 0.5-1 h
penicillin V potassium (V-Cillin K, Veetids, Betapen VK)	A: PO: 125-500 mg q6h C: PO: 15-50 mg/kg/d in 3-4 divided doses	Acid-stable and less active than penicillin G against some bacteria. Not recommended in renal failure. Take drug after meals. *Pregnancy category:* B; PB: 80%; t^1/$_2$: 0.5 h
Broad-Spectrum Penicillins		
amoxicillin (Amoxil)	See Prototype Drug Chart 28–1.	
amoxicillin-clavulanate (Augmentin)	A: PO: 250-500 mg q8-12h C: PO: <40 kg: 20-40 mg/kg/d	Treatment of lower respiratory infections, otitis media, sinusitis, skin infections, and UTIs. *Pregnancy category:* B; PB: UK; t^1/$_2$: 1-3 h
ampicillin (Polycillin, Omnipen)	A: PO: 250-500 mg q6h IM/IV: 2-8 g/d in divided doses (250 mg-2 g q6h) C: PO: 25-50 mg/kg/d in 4 divided doses IM/IV: 25-100 mg/kg/d in 4 divided doses	First broad-spectrum penicillin. 50% of drug is absorbed by GI tract. Effective against gram-negative and gram-positive bacteria. Individuals with penicillin allergies may also be allergic to ampicillin. *Pregnancy category:* B; PB: 15%-28%; t^1/$_2$: 1-2 h
ampicillin-sulbactam (Unasyn)	A: IV: 1.5-3.0 g q6h C: IV: 100-300 mg/kg/d, divided q6h	Same as ampicillin. Sulbactam inhibits beta lactamase thus extending the spectrum. *Pregnancy category:* B; PB: 28%-38%; t^1/$_2$: 1-2 h
bacampicillin HCl (Spectrobid)	A: PO: 400-800 mg q12h C: PO: 12.5-25 mg/kg/d in 2 divided doses	Same as ampicillin. 90% is absorbed. It is hydrolyzed to ampicillin during absorption from the GI tract. *Pregnancy category:* B; PB: 17%-20%; t^1/$_2$: 1 h
Penicillinase-Resistant Penicillins		
cloxacillin (Tegopen)	A: PO: 250-500 mg q6h C: PO: <20 kg: 12.5-25 mg/kg q6h; *max:* 4 g/d	For most gram-positive bacterial infections. *Pregnancy category:* B; PB: 90-95%; t^1/$_2$: 30-60 min
dicloxacillin sodium (Dynapen)	See Prototype Drug Chart 28–1.	
methicillin (Staphcillin)	A: IM: 1 g q6h IV: 1-2 g q6h diluted in NSS C: IM/IV: 100-200 mg/kg/d in 4-6 divided doses	First penicillinase-resistant penicillin. Used to treat staphylococcal infection. *Pregnancy category:* B; PB: 25%-40%; t^1/$_2$: 0.5-1 h

A, Adult; *C,* child; *d,* day; *GI,* gastrointestinal; *h,* hour; *IM,* intramuscular; *IV,* intravenous; *max,* maximum; *NB,* newborn; *NSS,* normal saline solution; *PB,* protein-binding; *PO,* by mouth; *t^1/$_2$,* half-life; *UK,* unknown; *UTI,* urinary tract infection; *y,* year; *>,* greater than; *<,* less than.

inactivated by beta-lactamases, thus becoming ineffective against *S. aureus.* Examples of this group are ampicillin (Omnipen), amoxicillin (Amoxil), and bacampicillin (Spectrobid), bacampicillin (Table 28–3). Amoxicillin is the most prescribed penicillin derivative for adults and children.

Penicillinase-Resistant Penicillins (Antistaphylococcal Penicillins)

The penicillinase-resistant penicillins (antistaphylococcal penicillins) are used to treat penicillinase-producing *S. aureus.* Cloxacillin (Cloxapen) and dicloxacillin (Dy-

Table 28–3

Antibacterials: Penicillins—cont'd

Generic (Brand)	Route and Dosage	Uses and Considerations
Penicillinase-Resistant Penicillins—cont'd		
nafcillin (Nafcin, Unipen)	A: PO: 250 mg-1 g q4-6h IM: 250-500 mg q6h IV: 500 mg-2 g q4-6h C: PO: 25-100 mg/kg/d in 4 divided doses IM: 25 mg/kg b.i.d. IV: 50-300 mg/kg/d in 4-6 divided doses	Highly effective against penicillin G-resistant *Staphylococcus aureus*. Not recommended for oral use because of its instability in gastric juices. *Pregnancy category:* B; PB: 90%; $t^1/_2$: 0.5-1.5 h
oxacillin sodium (Prostaphlin, Bactocil)	A: PO: 250-1 g q4-6h IM/IV: 500 mg-2 g q4h; *max:* IM/IV: 12 g C: PO/IM/IV: 50-100 mg/kg/d in divided doses; IM/IV: 50-150 mg/kg/d in divided doses	For penicillin-resistant staphylococci. As effective as methicillin. *Pregnancy category:* B; PB: 95%; $t^1/_2$: 0.5-1 h
Extended-Spectrum Penicillins		
carbenicillin indanyl (Geocillin, Geopen)	A: PO: 382-764 mg q6h	The first penicillin-like drug developed to treat infections caused by *Pseudomonas aeruginosa* and *Proteus* spp. It contains large amounts of sodium. Use with caution when administering to clients with hypertension or congestive heart failure. *Pregnancy category:* B; PB: 50%; $t^1/_2$: 1-1.5 h
mezlocillin sodium (Mezlin)	A: IM/IV: 3-4 g q6h or 100-300 mg/kg/d in 4 divided doses; *max:* 24 g/d C: IM/IV: 50 mg/kg q4h	For serious infections, especially because of *Pseudomonas aeruginosa*. It can be given in combination with aminoglycosides and cephalosporins to obtain synergistic effect. *Pregnancy category:* B; PB: 30%-40%; $t^1/_2$: 1 h
piperacillin sodium (Pipracil)	A: IM/IV: 2-4 g q6h or 100-300 mg/kg/d in divided doses; *max:* 24 g/d C: <12 y: IM/IV: 100-300 mg/kg/d in 4-6 divided doses	For serious infections. Can be given before and after surgery. Primarily used for gram-negative organisms. Treatment for septicemia; bone, joint, respiratory, and urinary tract infections. *Pregnancy category:* B; PB: 16%-22%; $t^1/_2$: 0.6-1.5 h
piperacillin-tazobactam (Zosyn)	A: IV: 3.375 g, q6h over 30 min, 7-10 d Reduce for renal insufficiency	To treat severe appendicitis, skin infections, pneumonia, beta-lactamase-producing bacteria. Tazobactam is a beta-lactamase inhibitor. *Pregnancy category:* B; PB: UK; $t^1/_2$: 0.7-1.2 h
ticarcillin disodium (Ticar)	A: IM/IV: 1-2 g q6h C: IM/IV: 50-200 mg/kg/d in 4 divided doses *Systemic infections:* Dose is increased	Effective against gram-positive and gram-negative bacilli. Used to treat respiratory, urinary, reproductive, skin, and soft tissue infections. It can be given in combination with aminoglycosides for synergistic effect. *Pregnancy category:* C; PB: 45%-65%; $t^1/_2$: 1-1.5 h
ticarcillin-clavulanate (Timentin)	A: IV: 3.1 g q6h C: >12 y: IV: 200-300 mg/kg/d in 4-6 divided doses	Clavulanic acid protects ticarcillin from degradation by beta-lactamase enzymes. Effective for treating septicemia and lower respiratory tract, urinary tract, skin, bone, and joint infections. *Pregnancy category:* B; PB: 45%-65%; $t^1/_2$: 1.1-1.5 h

napen) are oral preparations of these antibiotics; nafcillin (Unipen) and oxacillin (Prostaphin) nafcillin and oxacillin are IM and IV preparations. This group of drugs is not effective against gram-negative organisms, and they are less effective than penicillin G against gram-positive organisms. Prototype Drug Chart 28–1 compares the similarities and differences of the broad-spectrum penicillin amoxicillin and the penicillinase-resistant penicillin dicloxacillin.

Extended-Spectrum Penicillins (Antipseudomonal Penicillins)

The antipseudomonal penicillins are a group of broad-spectrum penicillins. This group of drugs is effective against *Pseudomonas aeruginosa*, a gram-negative bacillus that is difficult to eradicate. These drugs are also useful against many gram-negative organisms such as *Proteus* spp., *Serratia* spp., *Klebsiella pneumoniae*, *Enterobacter* spp., and *Acinetobacter* spp. The antipseudomonal penicillins are

PROTOTYPE DRUG CHART 28–1

AMOXICILLIN AND DICLOXACILLIN

Drug Class

amoxicillin: broad-spectrum penicillin
dicloxacillin: penicillinase-resistant penicillin
Trade Name:
amoxicillin: Amoxil, ✚ Apo-Amoxi
Pregnancy Category: B
dicloxacillin: Dynapen, Dycill, Pathocil
Pregnancy Category: B

Dosage

amoxicillin:
A: PO: 250-500 mg q8h
C: PO: 20-40 mg/kg/d in 3 divided doses
dicloxacillin:
A: PO: 125-500 mg q6h
C: PO: 12.5-25 mg/kg/d q6h

Contraindications

amoxicillin/dicloxacillin: Allergic to penicillin
amoxicillin: Severe renal disorder
Caution: amoxicillin/dicloxacillin: Hypersensitivity to cephalosporins

Drug-Lab-Food Interactions

Drug: amoxicillin/dicloxacillin: Increase effect with aspirin, probenecid; *decrease* effect with tetracycline, erythromycin
Lab: *Increase* serum AST, ALT, BUN, and creatinine
Food: *Decrease* affect with acidic fruits or juices

Pharmacokinetics

Absorption: PO:
amoxicillin: >80% in intestine
dicloxacillin: 35%-76% in GI tract
Distribution: PB:
amoxicillin: 20%
dicloxacillin: 95%
Metabolism: t½:
amoxicillin: 1-1.5 h
dicloxacillin: 0.5-1 h
Excretion:
amoxicillin: 70% in urine; clavulanate: 30%-40% in urine
dicloxacillin: Excreted in bile and urine

Pharmacodynamics

amoxicillin:
PO: Onset: 0.5 h
  Peak: 1-2 h
  Duration: 6-8 h
dicloxacillin:
PO: Onset: 0.5 h
  Peak: 1 h
  Duration: 4-6 h

Therapeutic Effects/Uses

amoxicillin: To treat respiratory tract infection, urinary tract infection, otitis media, sinusitis
dicloxacillin: To treat *Staphylococcus aureus* infection
Mode of Action: *amoxicillin/dicloxacillin:* Inhibition of the enzyme in cell wall synthesis; bactericidal effect

Side Effects

amoxicillin/dicloxacillin: Nausea, vomiting, diarrhea, rash
amoxicillin: Edema, stomatitis
dicloxacillin: Abdominal pain, flatulence

Adverse Reactions

amoxicillin/dicloxacillin: Superinfections (vaginitis)
Life-threatening: *amoxicillin/dicloxacillin:* Blood dyscrasias, hemolytic anemia, bone marrow depression
amoxicillin: Respiratory distress
dicloxacillin: Eosinophilia, liver toxicity

A, Adult; *ALT,* alanine aminotransferase; *AST,* aspartate aminotransferase; *BUN,* blood urea nitrogen; *C,* child; *d,* day; *GI,* gastrointestinal; *h,* hour; *PB,* protein-binding; *PO,* by mouth; *t½,* half-life; >, greater than; ✚, Canadian drug name.

not penicillinase-resistant. Their pharmacologic action is similar to that of aminoglycosides, but they are less toxic than the aminoglycosides.

Table 28–3 lists the drugs in the four categories of penicillin-type drugs. The route of administration of various types of penicillins (oral, IM, IV) along with the cephalosporins are available on the Evolve website.

Beta-Lactamase Inhibitors

When a broad-spectrum antibiotic (e.g., amoxicillin) is combined with a beta-lactamase (enzyme) inhibitor (e.g., clavulanic acid), the resulting antibiotic (e.g., amoxicillin-clavulanic acid [Augmentin]) inhibits the bacterial beta-lactamases, thus making the antibiotic effective and extending its antimicrobial effect. There are three beta-lactamase inhibitors: clavulanic acid, sulbactam, and tazobactam. These inhibitors are not given alone but are combined with a penicillinase-sensitive penicillin such as amoxicillin, ampicillin, piperacillin, and ticarcillin. The combined drugs currently marketed include the following:

• *Oral use:* amoxicillin-clavulanic acid (Augmentin)
• *Parenteral use:* ampicillin-sulbactam (Unasyn), piperacillin-tazobactam (Zosyn), and ticarcillin-clavulanic acid (Timentin)

Pharmacokinetics

Amoxicillin is well absorbed from the GI tract, whereas cloxacillin is only partially absorbed. Protein-binding power differs between the two drugs—amoxicillin is 25% protein bound and cloxacillin is highly protein bound (>90%). Drug toxicity may result when other highly protein-bound drugs are used with cloxacillin. Both drugs have short half-lives. Seventy percent of amoxicillin is excreted in the urine; cloxacillin is excreted in the bile and urine.

Pharmacodynamics

Both amoxicillin and cloxacillin are penicillin derivatives and are bactericidal. These drugs interfere with bacterial cell-wall synthesis, causing cell lysis. Amoxicillin may be produced with or without clavulanic acid, an agent that prevents the breakdown of amoxicillin by decreasing resistance to the antibacterial drug. The addition of clavulanic acid intensifies the effect of amoxicillin. The amoxicillin-clavulanic acid preparation (Augmentin) and amoxicillin trihydrate (Amoxil) have similar pharmacokinetics and pharmacodynamics as well as similar side effects and adverse reactions. When aspirin and probenecid are taken with amoxicillin or cloxacillin, the serum antibacterial levels may be increased. The effects of amoxicillin and cloxacillin are decreased when taken with erythromycin and tetracycline. The onset of action, serum peak concentration time, and duration of action for amoxicillin and cloxacillin are very similar.

Geriatrics

Most beta-lactam antibiotics are excreted via the kidneys. With older adults, assessment of renal function is most important. Serum blood urea nitrogen (BUN) and serum creatinine should be monitored. With a decrease in renal function, the antibiotic dose is most likely decreased.

Side Effects and Adverse Reactions

Common adverse reactions to penicillin administration are hypersensitivity and **superinfection** (occurrence of a secondary infection when the flora of the body is disturbed) (see Table 28–2). Nausea, vomiting, and diarrhea are common GI disturbances. Rash is an indicator of a mild to moderate allergic reaction. Severe allergic reaction leads to anaphylactic shock. Allergic effects occur in 5% to 10% of persons receiving penicillin compounds; therefore close monitoring during the first dose and subsequent doses of penicillin is essential.

Drug Interactions

The broad-spectrum penicillins—amoxicillin and ampicillin—may decrease the effectiveness of oral contraceptives. Potassium supplements can increase the serum potassium levels when taking potassium penicillin G or V. When penicillin is mixed with an aminoglycoside in IV solution, the actions of both drugs are inactivated.

Nursing Process

Antibacterials: Penicillins

ASSESSMENT

■ Assess for allergy to penicillin or cephalosporins. Client who is hypersensitive to amoxicillin should not take any type of penicillin products. Severe allergic reaction could occur. A small percentage of clients who are allergic to penicillin could also be allergic to a cephalosporin product.

■ Check laboratory results, especially liver enzymes. Report elevated alkaline phosphatase, alanine aminotransferase, aspartate aminotransferase.

■ Record urine output. If the amount is inadequate (<30 ml/h or <600 ml/d), drug or drug dosage may need to be changed.

NURSING DIAGNOSES

■ Risk for infection
■ Risk for impaired tissue integrity
■ Noncompliance with drug regimen

PLANNING

■ Client's infection will be controlled and later eliminated.

NURSING INTERVENTIONS

■ Send a sample of material from the infected area to the laboratory for culture to determine antibiotic susceptibility (also known as *C & S*) before antibiotic therapy is started.

■ Check for signs and symptoms of superinfection, especially for clients taking high doses of the antibiotic for a prolonged time. Signs and symptoms include stomatitis (mouth ulcers), genital discharge (vaginitis), and anal or genital itching.

■ Examine client for allergic reaction to the penicillin product, especially after the first and second doses. This may be a mild reaction, such as a rash, or a severe reaction, such as respiratory distress or anaphylaxis.

■ Have epinephrine available to counteract a severe allergic reaction.

■ Do not mix aminoglycosides with a high-dose or extended-spectrum penicillin G because this combination may inactivate the aminoglycoside.

■ Check client for bleeding if high doses of penicillin are being given; a decrease in platelet aggregation (clotting) may result.

■ Monitor body temperature and infectious area.

■ Dilute the antibiotic for IV use in an appropriate amount of solution as indicated in the drug pamphlet.

Client Teaching

General

- Instruct client to take all of the prescribed penicillin product such as amoxicillin until the bottle is empty. If only a portion of the penicillin is taken, drug resistance to that antibacterial agent may develop in the future.
- Advise client who is allergic to penicillin to wear a medical alert (MedicAlert) bracelet or necklace and carry a card that indicates the allergy. Client should notify the health care provider of any allergy to penicillin when recording the health history.
- Keep drugs out of the reach of small children. Request childproof containers.
- Inform client to report any side effects or adverse reaction that may occur while taking the drug.
- Encourage client to increase fluid intake; fluids aid in decreasing the body temperature and in excreting the drug.
- Instruct client or child's parent that chewable tablets must be chewed or crushed before swallowing.

Diet

- Advise client to take medication with food if gastric irritation occurs and to take oral penicillin 1 hour before or 2 hours after meals to avoid delay in drug absorption.

Cultural Considerations

- Recognize that clients and family members from various cultural backgrounds have various alternatives for alleviating infections. Accept their alternative methods if they are not harmful to client. Explain the purpose of the antibiotic.
- If client does not speak English, request a translator to obtain a history of symptoms related to the infection and any allergies to antibiotics.

EVALUATION

- Evaluate the effectiveness of the antibacterial agent by determining whether the infection has ceased and whether any side effects, including superinfection, have occurred.

Cephalosporins

In 1948 a fungus called *Cephalosporium acremonium* was discovered in seawater at a sewer outlet off the coast of Sardinia. This fungus was found to be active against gram-positive and gram-negative bacteria and resistant to beta-lactamase (an enzyme that acts against beta-lactam structure of penicillin). In the early 1960s cephalosporins were used with clinical effectiveness. For the cephalosporins to be effective against numerous organisms, their molecules were chemically altered and semisynthetic cephalosporins were produced. Like penicillin,

Table 28–4

Activity of the Four Generations of Cephalosporins

Generation	Activity
First	Effective against gram-positive bacteria, such as streptococci and most staphylococci. Effective against most gram-negative bacteria, such as *Escherichia coli* and species of *Klebsiella, Proteus, Salmonella,* and *Shigella.*
Second	Same effectiveness as the first generation. These antibiotics possess a broader spectrum against other gram-negative bacteria, such as *Haemophilus influenzae, Neisseria gonorrhoeae, Neisseria meningitidis, Enterobacter* spp., and several anaerobic organisms.
Third	Same effectiveness as the first and second generations. Also effective against gram-negative bacteria, such as *Pseudomonas aeruginosa, Serratia* spp., and *Acinetobacter* spp. Less effective against gram-positive bacteria.
Fourth	Similar to the third generation. Resistant to most beta-lactamase bacteria. Has a broader gram-positive coverage than the third generations. Effective against *E. coli, Klebsiella, Proteus,* streptococci, certain staphylococci, and *P. aeruginosa.*

the cephalosporins have a beta-lactam structure and act by inhibiting the bacterial enzyme that is necessary for cell wall synthesis. Lysis to the cell occurs, and the bacterial cell dies.

First-, Second-, Third-, and Fourth-Generation Cephalosporins

Cephalosporins are a major antibiotic group used in hospitals and in health care offices. These drugs are bactericidal with action similar to penicillin. For antibacterial activity, the beta-lactam ring of cephalosporins is necessary.

Four groups of cephalosporins have been developed, identified as *generations*. Each generation is effective against a broader spectrum of bacteria (Table 28–4).

Not all cephalosporins are affected by the beta-lactamases. The first-generation cephalosporins are destroyed by beta-lactamases, but not all of the second generation is affected by beta-lactamases. Third-generation cephalosporins are resistant to beta-lactamases. Most of the third- and fourth-generation cephalosporins (e.g., aztreonam, imipenem-cilastatin) are effective in treating sepsis and many strains of gram-negative bacilli. The cephalosporins ceftazidime and cefepime, along with aztreonam and imipenem-cilastatin, are effective against most strains of *Pseudomonas aeruginosa.* Table 28–5 lists the other unclassified beta-lactam antibiotics.

Table 28–5

Other Beta-Lactam Antibiotics

Generic (Brand)	Route and Dosage	Uses and Considerations
aztreonam (Azactam)	*Severe infections:* A: IM/IV: 1.0-2.0 g q6-8 h; *max:* 8 g/d	For treatment of gram-negative infections of the lower respiratory tract, urinary tract, skin, and vagina. Not effective against gram-positive organisms. May be used in combination with other antibiotics. *Pregnancy category:* B; PB: 56%; $t^1/_2$: 1.7-2.1 h
imipenem-cilastatin (Primaxin)	A: IM: 500-750 mg q12h IV: 250 mg-1 g q6-8h C: IV: 15-25 mg/kg q6h	For treatment of septicemia and severe infections of the lower respiratory tract, urinary tract, skin, bones, and joints. Effective against most gram-negative organisms including *Pseudomonas aeruginosa*. *Pregnancy category:* C; PB: 20%; $t^1/_2$: 1 h
loracarbef (Lorabid)	A: PO: 200-400 mg q12h, × 7-10 d C: 6 mo-12 y: PO: 15 mg/kg q12h × 7 d C: >12 y: Same as adult Elderly: Same as adult	A synthetic beta-lactam antibiotic; a carbacephem class. For treatment of respiratory, urinary tract, and skin infections. Effective against gram-positive organisms (e.g., *Staphylococcus aureus, Streptococcus pneumoniae*) and gram-negative organisms (e.g., *E. coli, H. influenzae*). If creatinine clearance is <50 ml/min, drug dose is reduced by 50%. *Pregnancy category:* B; PB: UK; $t^1/_2$: 1.5 h
meropenem (Merrem)	A: IV: 1-2 g q8h C: >3 mo: 20-40 mg/kg q8h	A carbapenem antibiotic, similar to cephalosporins. Effective against most strains of gram-negative organisms, including *Pseudomonas aeruginosa*, and effective for complicated appendicitis, peritonitis, meningitis, and soft tissue infections. *Pregnancy category:* B; PB: UK; $t^1/_2$: 1 h

A, Adult; *C,* child; *d,* day; *h,* hour; *IM,* intramuscular; *IV,* intravenous; *max,* maximum; *min,* minute; *PB,* protein-binding; *PO,* by mouth; $t^1/_2$, half-life; *UK,* unknown; *y,* year; >, greater than; <, less than.

Approximately 10% of persons allergic to penicillin are also allergic to cephalosporins because both groups of antibacterials have similar molecular structures. If a client is allergic to penicillin and is taking a cephalosporin, the nurse should watch for a possible allergic reaction to the cephalosporin, although the likelihood of a reaction is small.

Only a few cephalosporins are administered orally. These include cephalexin (Keflex), cefadroxil (Duricef), cephradine (Velosef), cefaclor (Ceclor), cefuroxime axetil (Ceftin), cefuroxime sodium (Zinacef), cefdinir (Omnicef), ceftibuten (Cedax), and cefixime (Suprax). The rest of the cephalosporins are administered IM and IV. Prototype Drug Chart 28-2 compares the similarities of and differences between a first-generation cephalosporin, cefazolin sodium (Ancef, Kefzol), and a second-generation cephalosporin, cefaclor (Ceclor).

Pharmacokinetics
Cefazolin is administered IM and IV, and cefaclor is given orally. The protein-binding power of cefazolin is greater than that of cefaclor. The half-life of each drug is short, and the drugs are excreted 60% to 80% unchanged in the urine.

Pharmacodynamics
Cefazolin and cefaclor inhibit bacterial cell-wall synthesis and produce a bactericidal action. For IM and IV use of cefazolin, the onset of action is almost immediate; the peak concentration time is 5 to 15 minutes for IV

use. The peak concentration time for an oral dose of cefaclor is 30 to 60 minutes.

When probenecid is administered with either of these drugs, the urine excretion of cefazolin or cefaclor is decreased, which increases the action of the drug. The effects of cefazolin and cefaclor can be decreased if the drug is given with tetracyclines or erythromycin. These drugs can cause false-positive laboratory results for proteinuria and glucosuria, especially when they are taken in large doses.

Table 28-6 lists the cephalosporins in their designated generation, dosages, and considerations.

Side Effects and Adverse Reactions

The side effects and adverse reactions to cephalosporins include GI disturbances (nausea, vomiting, diarrhea), alteration in blood clotting time (increased bleeding) with administration of large doses, and **nephrotoxicity** (toxicity to the kidney) in individuals with a preexisting renal disorder.

Drug Interactions

Drug interactions can occur with certain cephalosporins and alcohol. For example, consuming alcohol while taking cefamandole, cefoperazone, or moxalactam may cause flushing, dizziness, headache, nausea and vomiting, and muscular cramps. Taking uricosuric drugs concurrently can decrease the excretion of cephalosporins, thereby greatly increasing serum levels.

PROTOTYPE DRUG CHART 28–2

CEFAZOLIN AND CEFACLOR

Drug Class

cefazolin: first-generation cephalosporin
cefaclor: second-generation cephalosporin
Trade Name:
cefazolin: Ancef, Kefzol
Pregnancy Category: B
cefaclor: Ceclor
Pregnancy Category: B

Dosage

cefazolin:
A: IM/IV: 250 mg-2 g q6-8h; *max:* 12 g/d
C: IM/IV: 25-100 mg/kg/d in 3 divided doses; *max:* 4 g/d
cefaclor:
A: PO: 250-500 mg q8h; *max:* 4 g/d
C: PO: 20-40 mg/kg/d in 3 divided doses; *max:* 1 g/d

Contraindications

cefazolin/cefaclor: Hypersensitivity to cephalosporins
Caution: cefazolin/cefaclor: Hypersensitivity to penicillins; renal disease, lactation

Drug-Lab-Food Interactions

Drug: *cefazolin/cefaclor: Increase* effect with probenecid; *increase* toxicity with loop diuretics, aminoglycosides, colistin, vancomycin; *decrease* effect with tetracyclines, erythromycin
Lab: May *increase* BUN, serum creatinine, AST, ALT, ALP, LDH, bilirubin

Pharmacokinetics

Absorption:
cefazolin: IM, IV
cefaclor: PO: Well absorbed
Distribution: PB:
cefazolin: 75%-85%
cefaclor: 25%
Metabolism: t½:
cefazolin: 1.5-2.5 h
cefaclor: 0.5-1 h
Excretion:
cefazolin: 70% excreted unchanged in urine
cefaclor: 60%-80% excreted unchanged in urine

Pharmacodynamics

cefazolin:
IM: Onset: rapid
 Peak: 0.5-2 h
 Duration: UK
IV: Onset: immediate
 Peak: 5-15 min
 Duration: UK
cefaclor:
PO: Onset: rapid
 Peak: 0.5-1 h
 Duration: UK

Therapeutic Effects/Uses

cefazolin/cefaclor: To treat respiratory, urinary, and skin infections
cefazolin: To treat bone and joint infection, genital infections, and endocarditis
cefaclor: To treat ear infection, ampicillin-resistant strains, and certain gram-negative organisms; *E. coli, Proteus, H. influenzae,* and gram-positive strains; *Streptococcus pneumoniae, S. pyogenes,* and *S. aureus*
Mode of Action: Inhibition of cell wall synthesis, causing cell death; bactericidal effect

Side Effects

cefazolin/cefaclor: Anorexia, nausea, vomiting, diarrhea, rash
cefazolin: Abdominal cramps, fever
cefaclor: Pruritus, headaches, vertigo, weakness

Adverse Reactions

cefazolin/cefaclor: Superinfections, urticaria
Life-threatening:
cefazolin: Seizures (high doses), anaphylaxis
cefaclor: Renal failure

A, Adult; *ALP,* alkaline phosphatase; *ALT,* alanine aminotransferase; *AST,* aspartate aminotransferase; *BUN,* blood urea nitrogen; *C,* child; *d,* day; *h,* hour; *IM,* intramuscular; *IV,* intravenous; *LDH,* lactic dehydrogenase; *max,* maximum; *min,* minute; *PB,* protein-binding; *PO,* by mouth; *t½,* half-life; *UK,* unknown.

Table 28-6

Antibacterials: Cephalosporins

Generic (Brand)	Route and Dosage	Uses and Considerations
First Generation		
cefadroxil (Duricef)	A: PO: 500 mg-2 g/d in 1-2 divided doses C: PO: 30 mg/kg/d in 2 divided doses	To treat urinary tract infections, beta-hemolytic streptococcal infections, and staphylococcal skin infection. It is well absorbed by the GI tract and is not affected by food. *Pregnancy category:* B; PB: 20%; $t^1/_2$: 1-2 h
cefazolin sodium (Ancef, Kefzol)	A: IM/IV: 250 mg-1 g q6-8h; *max:* 12 g/d C: IM/IV: 25-100 mg/kg/d in 3 divided doses; *max:* 6 g/d	Similar to cephalothin but more effective against *Escherichia coli* and *Klebsiella. Pregnancy category:* B; PB: 75%-85%; $t^1/_2$: 1.5-2.5 h
cephalexin (Keflex)	*Infection:* A: PO: 250-500 mg q6h C: PO: 25-50 mg/kg/d in 3-4 divided doses *Otitis media:* C: PO: 25-100 mg/kg/d in 4 divided doses	First acid-stable cephalosporin sufficiently absorbed from the GI tract. Useful for treating urinary tract infections. *Pregnancy category:* B; PB: 10%-15%; $t^1/_2$: 0.5-1.2 h
cephalothin (Keflin)	A: IM/IV: 500 mg-1 g q4-6h C: IM/IV: 20-40 mg/kg q6h	To treat respiratory, GI, genitourinary, bone, joint, skin, soft tissue infections; septicemia; endocarditis; meningitis. Cephalothin is the first cephalosporin used clinically. It is usually given IV. *Pregnancy category:* B; PB: 65%-80%; $t^1/_2$: 0.5-1 h
cephapirin sodium (Cefadyl)	A: IM/IV: 500 mg-1 g q4-6h; *max:* 12 g/d C: IM/IV: 40-80 mg/kg/d in 4 divided doses	Treatment is the same as for cephalothin. *Pregnancy category:* B; PB: 40%-50%; $t^1/_2$: 0.5-1 h
cephradine (Velosef)	A: PO: 250-500 mg q6h or 500 mg-1 g q12h IM/IV: 500 mg-1 g q6-12h C: PO: 25-50 mg/kg/d in 4 divided doses IM/IV: 50-100 mg/kg/d in 4 divided doses	Treatment is the same as for cephalothin. The oral drug is similar to cephalexin. Well absorbed from GI tract. *Pregnancy category:* B; PB: 20%; $t^1/_2$: 1-2 h
Second Generation		
cefaclor (Ceclor)	See Prototype Drug Chart 28-2.	
cefamandole (Mandol)	A: IM/IV: 500 mg-1 g q4-8h	Used to treat septicemia and infections of the bone, joint, and respiratory tract. *Pregnancy category:* B; PB: 60%-75%; $t^1/_2$: 1 h
cefmetazole sodium (Zefazone)	A: IV: 1-2 g q6-12h	For treatment of lower respiratory and urinary tract infections. Also used for preoperative prophylaxis for surgery. *Pregnancy category:* B; PB: 68%; $t^1/_2$: 1.5-3 h
cefonicid sodium (Monocid)	A: IM/IV: 500 mg-2 g/d single dose or b.i.d.	Similar to cefamandole. Also used for surgical prophylaxis. *Pregnancy category:* B; PB: 98%; $t^1/_2$: 4.5 h
ceforanide (Precef)	A: IM/IV: 500 mg-1 g q12h C: IM/IV: 20-40 mg/kg/d in 2 divided doses	For treatment of respiratory, urinary, skin, bone, and joint infections. Also used to treat septicemia, endocarditis, cardiovascular surgery, and prosthetic arthroplasty. *Pregnancy category:* B; PB: 80%; $t^1/_2$: 3 h
cefotetan (Cefotan)	A: IM/IV: 500 mg-2g q12h C: IM/IV: 40-80 mg/kg/d in 2 divided doses; *max:* 6 g/d	Effective against some gram-negative organisms, except *Pseudomonas aeruginosa. Pregnancy category:* B; PB: 85%; $t^1/_2$: 3-5 h
cefoxitin sodium (Mefoxin)	A: IM/IV: 1-2 g q6-8h; *max:* 12 g/d C: IM/IV: 80-160 mg/kg/d in divided doses	Used to treat severe infections and septicemia. *Pregnancy category:* B; PB: 70%; $t^1/_2$: 45 min-1 h
cefprozil monohydrate (Cefzil)	A: PO: 250-500 mg daily or q12h C: PO: 15 mg/kg q12h × 10 d	Effective against gram-positive bacilli including *Staphylococcus aureus.* With impaired renal function, dose is usually decreased by 50%. *Pregnancy category:* B; PB: 99%; $t^1/_2$: 1-2 h
cefuroxime (Ceftin, Zinacef)	A: PO: 250-500 mg q12h IM/IV: 750 mg-1.5 g q8h C: PO: 125-250 mg q12h IM/IV: 50-100 mg/kg/d in divided doses	Similar to cefamandole. Effective in treating meningitis and septicemia and for cardiothoracic procedures and surgical prophylaxis. *Pregnancy category:* B; PB: 50%; $t^1/_2$: 1.5-2 h

A, Adult; *b.i.d.,* two times a day; *C,* child; *d,* day; *GI,* gastrointestinal; *h,* hour; *IM,* intramuscularly; *IV,* intravenously; *PB,* protein-binding; *PO,* by mouth; $t^1/_2$, half-life; *UK,* unknown; <, less than.

Continued

Table 28–6

Antibacterials: Cephalosporins—cont'd

Generic (Brand)	Route and Dosage	Uses and Considerations
Third Generation		
cefdinir (Omnicef)	A: PO: 300 mg q12h or 600 mg/d C: PO: 7 mg/kg q12h or 14 mg/kg/d *Preferred:* q12h dosing because of short t¹/₂	New third-generation cephalosporin. To treat otitis media, acute sinusitis, chronic bronchitis, pharyngitis, pneumonia, and skin infections. Active for *Haemophilus influenzae, Neisseria gonorrhoeae,* and many strains of enteric gram-negative bacilli. Not active for *P. aeruginosa, Enterococcus, Legionella, Chlamydia. Pregnancy category:* B; PB: 60%-70%; t¹/₂: 1.7 h
cefixime (Suprax)	A: PO: 400 mg/d in 1-2 divided doses C: <12 y: PO: 8 mg/kg/d in 1-2 divided doses	Effective against most gram-positive and gram-negative bacilli: minimal effect against staphylococci and ineffective against *P. aeruginosa.* Food does not affect drug dose. *Pregnancy category:* B; PB: 65%; t¹/₂: 2.5-4 h
cefoperazone (Cefobid)	A: IM/IV: 2-4 g/d in 2 divided doses C: IV: 25-100 mg/kg q12h	To treat respiratory, urinary tract, and female genital tract infections. Most effective against pseudomonas. *Pregnancy category:* B; PB: 70%-80%; t¹/₂: 2.5 h
cefotaxime (Claforan)	A: IM/IV: 1-2 g q8-12h C: IM/IV: 50-200 mg/kg/d in 4-6 divided doses *Life-threatening infection:* 2 g q4	First of the third generation. Effective against *P. aeruginosa.* Also used in treating gram-negative meningitis. *Pregnancy category:* B; PB: 30%-40%; t¹/₂: 1-1.5 h
cefpodoxime (Vantin)	A: PO: 200 mg q12h × 1-2 wk C: 6 mo-12 y: PO: 10 mg/kg/d in 2 divided doses	To treat otitis media and respiratory and urinary tract infection. Food enhances drug absorption. *Pregnancy category:* B; PB: 20%-40%; t¹/₂: 2-3 h
ceftazidime (Fortaz, Tazicef)	A: IM/IV: 500 mg-2 g q8-12h C: IV: 30-50 mg/kg q8h; *max:* 6 g/d	Most effective against *Pseudomonas* spp. *Pregnancy category:* B; PB: 10%-17%; t¹/₂: 1-2 h
ceftriaxone (Rocephin)	A: IM/IV: 500 mg-2 g in single dose or q12h; *max:* 4 g/d C: IM/IV: 50-75 mg/kg/d in 2 divided doses	Similar to ceftizoxime and cefotaxime. It has a very long half-life so is given once or twice a day. It is used against neisseria and gonococcal infections and in the treatment of Lyme disease. *Pregnancy category:* B; PB: 85%-95%; t¹/₂: 8 h
ceftizoxime sodium (Cefizox)	A: IM/IV: 500 mg-2 g q8-12h C: IV: 50 mg/kg q6-8h; *max:* 200 mg/kg/d	For treatment of respiratory, urinary tract, skin, bone, and joint infections. For surgical prophylaxis. *Pregnancy category:* B; PB: 30%-60%; t¹/₂: 2 h
ceftibuten (Cedax)	A: PO: 400 mg/d × 10 d (for renal insufficiency, reduced dose) C: (6 mo-12 yr): PO: 9 mg/kg/d × 10 d; *max:* 400 mg/d	Treatment for chronic bronchitis, pharyngitis, and tonsillitis. Active against gram-positive and gram-negative bacteria, *H. influenzae, Streptococcus pneumoniae,* and *Streptococcus pyogenes.* Poor activity against staphylococci and pneumococci. *Pregnancy category:* B; PB: UK; t¹/₂: 1.5-3 h
moxalactam disodium (Moxam)	A: IM/IV: 2-6 g/d in 2-3 divided doses; *max:* 4 g q8h C: IM/IV: 50 mg/kg q6-8h	For lower respiratory, urinary tract, bone, and joint infection. Also for septicemia and meningitis. Less active against gram-positive cocci, *S. aureus,* and streptococci. Active against *E. coli, Klebsiella pneumoniae,* and *Serratia.* Variable activity for *P. aeruginosa.* Can be used with an aminoglycoside. *Pregnancy category:* C; PB: UK; t¹/₂: 2-3.5 h
cefditoren pivoxil (Spectracef)	A: PO: 200-400 mg b.i.d for 10 d	For chronic bronchitis, pharyngitis, tonsillitis, skin infections and other mild to moderate bacterial infections. *Pregnancy category:* B; PB: 88%; t¹/₂: 1.6 h
Fourth Generation		
cefepime (Maxipime)	A: IM/IV: 0.5-1g q12h *Severe infection:* A: IV: 2 g q12 h × 10 d	Similar to third-generation cephalosporins. Resistant to most beta-lactamase bacteria. Effective against pneumonia, *E. coli, Klebsiella, Proteus,* streptococci, certain staphylococci, and *P. aeruginosa.* It has a broader gram-positive coverage than the third-generation cephalosporins. *Pregnancy category:* B; PB: UK; t¹/₂: 2 h

Nursing Process

Antibacterials: Cephalosporins

ASSESSMENT

■ Assess for allergy to cephalosporins. If allergic to one type or class of cephalosporin, client should not receive any other type of cephalosporin.

■ Record vital signs and urine output. Report abnormal findings, which may include an elevated temperature or a decrease in urine output.

■ Check laboratory results, especially those that indicate renal and liver function, such as blood urea nitrogen, serum creatinine, aspartate aminotransferase, alanine aminotransferase, alkaline phosphatase, and bilirubin. Report abnormal findings. Use these laboratory results for baseline values.

NURSING DIAGNOSES

■ Risk for infection
■ Noncompliance with drug regimen

PLANNING

■ Client's infection will be controlled and later eliminated.

NURSING INTERVENTIONS

■ Culture the infected area before cephalosporin therapy is started. The organism causing the infection can be determined by culture, and the antibiotics sensitive to the organism are determined by culture and sensitivity (C & S). (Antibiotic therapy may be started before culture result is reported. The antibiotic may need to be changed after C & S test results are received.)

■ Check for signs and symptoms of a superinfection, especially if client takes high doses of a cephalosporin product for a prolonged period. Superinfection is usually caused by the fungal organism *Candida* in the mouth (mouth ulcers) or in the genital area, such as the vagina (vaginitis).

■ Refrigerate oral suspensions. For IV cephalosporins, dilute in an appropriate amount of IV fluids (50-100 ml) according to the drug pamphlet.

■ Administer IV cephalosporins over 30 to 45 minutes 2 to 4 times a day.

■ Monitor vital signs, urine output, and laboratory results. Report abnormal findings.

Client Teaching

General

• Keep drugs out of reach of small children. Request childproof containers.

• Instruct client to report signs of superinfection, such as mouth ulcers or discharge from the anal or genital area.

• Advise client to ingest buttermilk or yogurt to prevent superinfection of the intestinal flora with long-term use of a cephalosporin.

• Instruct client with diabetes to *not* use Clinitest tablets for urine glucose testing because false test results may occur. Tes-Tape or Clinistix may be used for urine testing, or Chemstrip bG may be used for blood glucose testing.

• Instruct client to take the complete course of medication even when symptoms of infection have ceased.

• Infuse all IV cephalosporins over 30 minutes or as ordered to prevent pain and irritation.

• Observe for hypersensitivity reactions.

Side Effects

• Instruct client to report any side effects from use of oral cephalosporin drugs; they may include anorexia, nausea, vomiting, headache, dizziness, itching, and rash.

Diet

• Advise client to take medication with food if gastric irritation occurs.

Cultural Considerations ⊕

• Failing to allow adequate time for information processing may result in an inaccurate response or no response. Allow time for people to respond to questions, especially for those who have language barriers. Speak clearly and slowly, giving time for translation. Obtain an interpreter if necessary.

EVALUATION

■ Evaluate the effectiveness of the cephalosporin by determining if the infection has ceased and no side effects, including superinfection, have occurred.

WEBSITES

For further information on *Antibacterials: Penicillins and Cephalosporins*, visit these Internet resources:

Information on ampicillin:
www.nlm.nih.gov/medlineplus/druginfo/medmaster/a685002.htm

Information on dicloxacillin:
www.mdadvice.com/library/drug/drug103.html

Critical Thinking Case Study

S.A., age 6, has otitis media. The health care provider ordered amoxicillin 250 mg every 8 hours. The nurse asks S.A.'s mother if S.A. is allergic to any drugs, and her mother says she is allergic to penicillin.

1. What are the similarities and differences of penicillin and amoxicillin? Explain.

2. What nursing action should the nurse take? Why? The health care provider changed the amoxicillin order to cefaclor (Ceclor) 250 mg every 8 hours. The therapeutic dosage for children is 20 to 40 mg/kg/d in three divided doses. S.A. weighs 40 pounds.

3. What are the similarities and differences of amoxicillin and cefaclor? Explain.

4. Is the prescribed cefaclor dosage for S.A. within safe parameters? Explain.

5. Explain the significance of the nurse asking about allergies to antibiotics such as penicillin. What is the relationship of penicillin and cefaclor in regard to allergies?

6. What should the nurse include in client teaching for S.A. and her mother?

Study Questions

1. What is the action of a bacteriostatic drug? What is the action of a bactericidal drug?

2. What is a nosocomial infection?

3. What is meant by cross-resistance? Give an example of how it can occur.

4. When do superinfections occur? What is the nurse's role?

5. Your client takes ampicillin. What drug category is ampicillin? Explain the drug effect against pathogens.

6. What is the severe adverse reaction associated with penicillin? What is an early symptom of such an adverse reaction? What emergency intervention is required?

7. Your client takes cephalexin (Keflex) for a urinary tract infection. What generation of cephalosporin is cephalexin? What is its route of administration?

8. What antibiotics are used as penicillin substitutes?

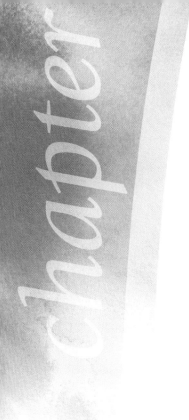

29 Antibacterials: Macrolides, Tetracyclines, Aminoglycosides, and Fluoroquinolones

ELECTRONIC RESOURCES

Additional information can be found on the companion website at *http://evolve.elsevier.com/KeeHayes/pharmacology/* or on the companion CD-ROM, which includes:

- *NCLEX-style examination review questions*
- *Pharmacology animations*
- *Medication error and IV therapy checklists*
- *Medication calculation problems*
- *Electronic calculators*

OBJECTIVES

- Describe the pharmacokinetics and pharmacodynamics of erythromycin.
- Explain the nursing process for tetracyclines, including the adverse reactions.
- Describe the nurse's role in detecting ototoxicity and nephrotoxicity associated with the administration of aminoglycosides.
- Discuss the reasons for ordering serum aminoglycosides for peak and trough concentration levels.
- Explain the mechanism of action of fluoroquinolones (quinolones).
- Describe the nursing interventions, including client teaching, for each of the drug categories: macrolides, tetracyclines, aminoglycosides, and fluoroquinolones.

Introduction

The groups of antibacterials discussed in this chapter include macrolides (erythromycin, clarithromycin, azithromycin, dirithromycin), lincosamides, vancomycin, ketolides, tetracyclines, aminoglycosides, and fluoroquinolones (quinolones). The macrolides, lincosamides, and tetracyclines are primarily **bacteriostatic** drugs and may be bactericidal, depending on the drug dose or **pathogen.** Vancomycin, aminoglycosides, and fluoroquinolones are **bactericidal** drugs.

Macrolides, Lincosamides, Vancomycin, and Ketolides

These four groups of drugs are discussed together because they have similar spectrums of antibiotic effectiveness to penicillin, although they differ in structure. Drugs from these groups are used as penicillin substitutes, especially in individuals who are allergic to penicillin. Erythromycin is the drug frequently prescribed if the client has a hypersensitivity to penicillin.

Macrolides

Macrolides, including azithromycin (Zithromax), clarithromycin (Biaxin), dirithromycin (Dynabac), and erythromycin (E-Mycin), are called *broad-spectrum antibiotics*, reflecting their large size. Erythromycin, the first macrolide, was derived from the funguslike bacteria *Streptomyces erythreus* and was first introduced in the early 1950s. Macrolides bind to the 50S ribosomal subunits and inhibit protein synthesis. At low to moderate drug doses, macrolides have a bacteriostatic effect, and with high drug doses, the effect is bactericidal. Macrolides can be administered orally or intravenously (IV) but not intramuscularly (IM) because it is too painful. Administration of IV macrolides should be infused slowly to avoid unnecessary pain (phlebitis).

Gastric acid destroys erythromycin in the stomach; therefore acid-resistant salts are added to erythromycin (e.g., ethylsuccinate, stearate, estolate) to decrease dissolution (breakdown in small particles) in the stomach. This allows the drug to be absorbed in the intestine. Normally food does not hamper the absorption of acid-resistant macrolides. Table 29-1 lists the dosages, uses, and considerations of macrolides.

Macrolides are active against most gram-positive bacteria and moderately active against some gram-negative bacteria. Resistant organisms may emerge during treatment. Macrolides are used to treat mild to moderate infections of

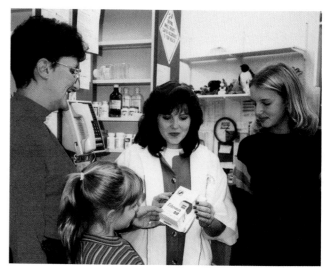

FIGURE 29-1 The pharmacist discusses the use of azithromycin with the family of an 8-year-old child for whom it was prescribed. What would be the recommended dosage for this child?

the respiratory tract, sinuses, gastrointestinal tract (GI), skin, and soft tissue, as well as diphtheria, impetigo contagiosa, and sexually transmitted diseases (STDs).

Erythromycin is the drug of choice for the treatment of mycoplasmal pneumonia and Legionnaire's disease. The first macrolide developed after the introduction of erythromycin was clarithromycin (Biaxin), which has been effective against many bacterial infections. Biaxin XL Pac is a new introduction of clarithromycin in a once-a-day extended-release tablet to be taken for 7 days. Azithromycin is frequently prescribed for upper and lower respiratory infections, STDs, and uncomplicated skin infections (Figure 29-1). Dirithromycin is usually prescribed to treat chronic bronchitis, community-acquired pneumonia, and uncomplicated skin infections. Table 29-1 lists the drugs developed from the derivatives of erythromycin. Prototype Drug Chart 29-1 details the pharmacologic behavior of azithromycin.

Pharmacokinetics

Clarithromycin, dirithromycin, and erythromycin are readily absorbed from the GI tract mainly by the duodenum. Azithromycin is incompletely absorbed from the GI tract, and only 37% reaches systemic circulation. Azithromycin and erythromycin are available IV, but intermittent infusions should be diluted in normal saline (NS) or in dextrose 5% in water (D_5W) to prevent phlebitis or burning sensations at the injection site. Azithromycin 500 mg should be diluted in 250 to 500 ml and erythromycin lactobionate 1 g should be diluted in 100 to 200 ml of fluid. Macrolides are excreted in bile, feces, and urine. Because only a small amount is excreted in the urine, renal insufficiency is not a contraindication for macrolide use.

Table 29-1

Antibacterials: Macrolides, Lincosamides, Vancomycin, and Ketolides

Generic (Brand)	Route and Dosage	Uses and Considerations
Macrolides		
azithromycin (Zithromax)	See Prototype Drug Chart 28–1.	
clarithromycin (Biaxin)	A: PO: 250-500 mg q12h × 7-14 d C: PO: 7.5 mg/kg/d in 2 divided doses	For treatment of upper and lower respiratory infections, skin and soft tissue infections, *Helicobacter pylori* and mycobacterial species, and gram-positive and negative organisms. Report persistent diarrhea. *Pregnancy category:* C; PB: 65%-75%; t$^1/_2$: 3-6 h
dirithromycin (Dynabac)	A: PO: 500 mg/d C: >12 y: PO: same as adult	To treat chronic bronchitis, pneumonia, pharyngitis, tonsillitis, and uncomplicated skin infections. Effective against *H. pylori, Legionella,* and *Chlamydia trachomatis.* Not effective against *Pseudomonas aeruginosa,* methicillin-resistant *S. aureus,* or *H. influenzae. Pregnancy category:* C; PB: UK; t$^1/_2$: 20-50 h
erythromycin base (E-Mycin, Ilotycin); erythromycin estolate (Ilosone); erythromycin ethylsuccinate (E.E.S., E-Mycin E, Pediamycin)	A: PO: 250-500 mg q6h C: PO: 30-100 mg/kg/d A, Elderly, & C: IV: 15-20 mg/kg/d; *max:* 4 g/d	For treatment of moderate to severe infections, such as pneumococcal pneumonia, acute pelvic inflammatory disease, intestinal amebiasis, Legionnaires' disease, and chlamydial infections. Report persistent diarrhea.
erythromycin lactobionate (Erythrocin Lactobionate IV) erythromycin stearate (Erythrocin)		For IV administration. Drug should not be dissolved in a solution that contains a preservative. *Pregnancy category:* B; PB: 65%; t$^1/_2$: PO: 1-2 h; IV: 3-5 h
Lincosamides		
clindamycin HCl (Cleocin)	A: PO: 150-450 mg q6-8h; *max:* 1800 mg/d	For serious infections. Available in capsule form. Taken with a full glass of water. Not affected by food. *Pregnancy category:* B; PB: 94%; t$^1/_2$: 2-3 h
clindamycin palmitate (Cleocin Pediatric)	C: PO: 25-40 mg/kg/d in 3-4 divided doses	Available in suspension for children and older adults. *Pregnancy category:* B; PB: 94%; t$^1/_2$: 2-3 h
clindamycin phosphate (Cleocin Phosphate)	A: IM/IV: 300-900 mg q6-8 h; *max:* 2700 mg/d C: IM/IV: 20-30 mg/kg/d in 3-4 divided doses	For treatment of serious infections, such as septicemia, caused by gram-negative organism. *Not to be given as a bolus. Pregnancy category:* B; PB: 94%; t$^1/_2$: 2-3 h
lincomycin (Lincocin)	A: PO: 500 mg q6-8h; *max:* 8 g/d IM: 600 mg daily-q12h IV: 600 mg-1 g q8-12h; dilute in 100 ml of IV fluids C: PO: 30-60 mg/kg/d in 3-4 divided doses IV: 10-20 mg/kg/d in 2-3 divided doses, dilute in IV fluids	In most situations, this drug has been replaced by clindamycin. *Pregnancy category:* B; PB: 70%-75%; t$^1/_2$: 4-6 h
Vancomycin		
vancomycin HCl (Vancocin)	A: IV: 500 mg q6 h or 1 g q12h C: IV: 40 mg/kg/d in 4 divided doses; dilute in IV fluids; run for 1-1.5 h	For *S. aureus*-resistant infections and cardiac surgical prophylaxis in clients with penicillin allergy. Adverse reactions include possible ototoxicity, nephrotoxicity, vascular collapse. *Pregnancy category:* C; PB: 10%; t$^1/_2$: 5-11 h
Ketolides		
telithromycin (Ketek)	A: PO: 400 mg twice daily	To treat acute chronic bronchitis, acute bacterial sinusitis, and community-acquired pneumonia. *Pregnancy category:* UK; PB: 60%-70%; t$^1/_2$: 10 h

A, Adult; *C,* child; *d,* day; *h,* hour; *IM,* intramuscular; *IV,* intravenous; *maint,* maintenance; *max,* maximum; *mo,* month; *PB,* protein-binding; *PO,* by mouth; *t$^1/_2$,* half-life; *UK,* unknown; *y,* year; >, greater than.

PROTOTYPE DRUG CHART 29–1

AZITHROMYCIN

Drug Class	**Dosage**
Antibacterial macrolide Trade Name: Zithromax *Pregnancy Category:* B	A: PO: 250-500 mg daily IV: 500 mg daily C: PO: 5-10 mg/kg/d
Contraindications	**Drug-Lab-Food Interactions**
Hypersensitivity *Caution:* Hepatic dysfunction, lactation, renal dysfunction	***Drug:*** *Increase* effect of digoxin, carbamazepine, theophylline, cyclosporine, warfarin, triazolam; *decrease* effect of penicillins, clindamycin
Pharmacokinetics	**Pharmacodynamics**
Absorption: PO: 37% absorbed **Distribution:** PB: 51% **Metabolism:** $t^1/_2$: 68 h **Excretion:** In bile and small amount in urine	**PO:** Onset: 1 h Peak: 2.5-5 h Duration: 24 h **IV:** Onset: UK Peak: UK Duration: UK

Therapeutic Effects/Uses

To treat gram-positive and some gram-negative organisms; for clients who are allergic to penicillin; to treat
respiratory infections, gonorrhea, skin infections
Mode of Action: Inhibition of the steps of protein synthesis; bacteriostatic or bactericidal effect

Side Effects	**Adverse Reactions**
Anorexia, nausea, vomiting, diarrhea, tinnitus, abdominal cramps, pruritus, rash	Superinfections, vaginitis, urticaria, stomatitis, hearing loss **Life-threatening:** Hepatotoxicity, anaphylaxis

A, Adult; *C,* child; *d,* day; *h,* hour; *IV,* intravenous; *PB,* protein-binding; *PO,* by mouth; *t¹/₂,* half-life; *UK,* unknown.

Pharmacodynamics

Macrolides suppress bacterial protein synthesis. The onset of action of oral preparations of erythromycin is 1 hour, peak concentration time is 4 hours, and the duration of action is 6 hours. New macrolides have a longer half-life and are administered less frequently. Clarithromycin is administered twice a day. Azithromycin (Zithromax) and dirithromycin (Dynabac) have up to 40- to 68-hour half-lives and are prescribed only once a day for 5 days.

Side Effects and Adverse Reactions

Side effects and adverse reactions to macrolides include GI disturbances such as nausea, vomiting, diarrhea, and abdominal cramping. Allergic reactions to erythromycin are rare. **Hepatotoxicity** (liver toxicity) can occur when erythromycin and azithromycin are taken in high doses with other hepatotoxic drugs, such as acetaminophen (high doses), phenothiazines, and sulfonamides. Erythromycin estolate (Ilosone) appears to have more toxic effects on the liver than the other erythromycins. Liver damage is usually reversible when the drug is discontinued. Erythromycin should not be taken with clindamycin or lincomycin because they compete for receptor sites.

Drug Interactions

Macrolides can increase the serum levels of theophylline (bronchodilator), carbamazepine (anticonvulsant), and warfarin (anticoagulant). If these drugs are given with

macrolides, their drug serum levels should be closely monitored. Erythromycin should not be used with other macrolides to avoid severe toxic effects. Azithromycin peak levels may be reduced by antacids when taken at the same time.

Extended Macrolide Group

New derivatives of erythromycin have been effective in the treatment of numerous organisms. Like erythromycin, they inhibit protein synthesis. Many of these macrolides have a longer half-life and are administered once a day. The first extended macrolide group developed after the introduction of erythromycin was clarithromycin (Biaxin), which has been effective against many bacterial infections. Clarithromycin is administered twice a day. Two other extended macrolides are azithromycin (Zithromax) and dirithromycin (Dynabac). These two drugs have long half-lives—up to 40 to 68 hours—therefore they are only prescribed once a day for 5 days. Elimination of these drugs is via bile and feces. Azithromycin is frequently prescribed for upper and lower respiratory infections, STDs, and uncomplicated skin infections.

When erythromycin is given concurrently with verapamil (Verelan, Isoptin), diltiazem (Cardizem), clarithromycin (Biaxin), fluconazole (Diflucan), ketoconazole (nizoral), and itraconazole (Sporanox), erythromycin blood concentration and the risk of sudden cardiac death increase (see Figure 29-1). Dirithromycin is usually prescribed to treat chronic bronchitis, community-acquired pneumonia, and uncomplicated skin infections. Table 29-1 lists the drugs developed from the derivatives of erythromycin.

Common side effects of clarithromycin and dirithromycin are nausea, diarrhea, and abdominal discomfort. With azithromycin, the side effects of nausea, diarrhea, and abdominal pain are uncommon.

Nursing Process

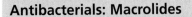

Antibacterials: Macrolides

ASSESSMENT

■ Assess vital signs and urine output. Report abnormal findings.
■ Check laboratory tests for liver enzyme values to determine liver function. Liver enzyme tests should be periodically ordered for clients taking large doses of azithromycin for a continuous period.
■ Obtain a history of drugs client currently takes. The peak level of azithromycin may be decreased by antacids.

NURSING DIAGNOSES

■ Risk for infection
■ Risk for impaired tissue integrity

PLANNING

■ Client's infection will be controlled and later eliminated.

NURSING INTERVENTIONS

■ Obtain a sample from the infected area and send to the laboratory for culture and sensitivity (C & S) test *before* starting azithromycin therapy. Antibiotic can be initiated after obtaining culture sample.
■ Monitor vital signs, urine output, and laboratory values, especially liver enzymes: alkaline phosphatase, alanine aminotransferase, aspartate aminotransferase, and bilirubin.
■ Monitor client for liver damage resulting from prolonged use and high dosage of macrolides, such as azithromycin. Signs of liver dysfunction include elevated liver enzyme levels and jaundice.
■ Administer oral azithromycin 1 hour before meals or 2 hours after meals. Give with a full glass of water and not fruit juice. Give the drug with food if GI upset occurs. Chewable tablets should be chewed and not swallowed whole.
■ For IV azithromycin, dilute in an appropriate amount of solution as indicated in the drug circular.
■ Administer antacids either 2 hours before or 2 hours after azithromycin.

Client Teaching

General
● Instruct client to take the full course of antibacterial agent as prescribed. Drug compliance is most important for all antibacterials (antibiotics).

Side Effects
● Instruct client to report side effects, including adverse reactions. Encourage client to report nausea, vomiting, diarrhea, abdominal cramps, and itching. Superinfection (a secondary infection resulting from drug therapy) such as stomatitis or vaginitis may occur.
● Instruct client to report onset of loose stools or diarrhea. Pseudomembranous colitis should be ruled out.

Cultural Considerations
● Recognize that client and family members from various cultural backgrounds may need a written drug schedule as to when the drug should be taken. The nurse should either give a detailed explanation or write out the possible side effects that should be reported to the health care provider.

EVALUATION

■ Evaluate the effectiveness of azithromycin by determining whether the infection has been controlled or has ceased and no side effects, including superinfection, have occurred.

Lincosamides

Like erythromycin, lincosamides inhibit bacterial protein synthesis and have both bacteriostatic and bactericidal actions, depending on drug dosage. Clindamycin (Cleocin) and lincomycin (Lincocin) are examples of lincosamides. Clindamycin is more widely prescribed than lincomycin because it is active against most gram-positive organisms, including *Staphylococcus aureus* and anaerobic organisms. It is not effective against the gram-negative bacteria, such as *Escherichia coli, Proteus,* and *Pseudomonas.* Clindamycin is absorbed better than lincomycin through the GI tract and maintains a higher serum drug concentration. Clindamycin is considered more effective than lincomycin and has fewer toxic effects. Table 29-1 lists the lincosamides.

Side Effects and Adverse Reactions
Side effects and adverse reactions to clindamycin and lincomycin include GI irritation, such as nausea, vomiting, and stomatitis. Rash may also occur. Severe adverse reactions include colitis and anaphylactic shock.

Drug Interactions
Clindamycin and lincomycin are incompatible with aminophylline, phenytoin (Dilantin), barbiturates, and ampicillin.

Vancomycin

Vancomycin (Vancocin), a glycopeptide bactericidal antibiotic, was widely used in the 1950s to treat staphylococcal infections. Its use was almost abandoned because of the many reports of nephrotoxicity and ototoxicity. **Ototoxicity** results in damage to the auditory or vestibular branch of cranial nerve VIII. Such damage can result in permanent hearing loss (auditory branch) or temporary or permanent loss of balance (vestibular branch). Vancomycin is still used against drug-resistant *S. aureus* and in cardiac surgical prophylaxis for individuals with penicillin allergies. Serum vancomycin levels should be monitored.

Vancomycin has become resistant for treating enterococci. Quinupristin/dalfopristin are two new combined antibacterials used to treat life-threatening vancomycin-resistant enterococci (VRE) infections. Antibiotic-resistant enterococci can cause endocarditis.

Ketolides

Ketolides are a new classification of antibiotics, which are structurally related to macrolides. The first drug in this class is telithromycin (Ketek) used for adults of 18 years and older to treat acute chronic bronchitis, acute bacterial sinusitis, and community-acquired pneumonia. These disorders are usually caused by *Streptococcus pneumoniae* and *Haemophilus influenza*.

Pharmacokinetics

Telithromycin is given orally and is well absorbed by the GI tract and not affected by food intake. Telithromycin is excreted in the feces and urine. It is 60% to 70% protein bound and the half-life is 10 hours.

Pharmacodynamics

Telithromycin blocks protein synthesis in microorganisms. The peak action is 1 hour.

Side Effects and Adverse Reactions

Side effects and adverse reactions to telithromycin include visual disturbances, stomatitis, glossitis, gastritis, nausea, vomiting, abdominal distention, flatulence, oral and vaginal candidiasis, constipation, and watery stools. Telithromycin may also lead to an exacerbation of myasthenia gravis.

Drug Interactions

When telithromycin is taken concurrently with antilipidemics (simvastatin, lovastatin, and atorvastatin), class 1A or class III antidysrhythmics, cisapride, or midazolam, the risk of adverse effects are increased. Blood levels of telithromycin are decreased when taken with rifampin, phenytoin, carbamazepine, or phenobarbital producing a subtherapeutic level. Concurrent use of ketolides (telithromycin) and macrolides may lead to acute ergot toxicity.

Tetracyclines

The tetracyclines, isolated from *Streptomyces aureofaciens* in 1948, were the first broad-spectrum antibiotics effective against gram-positive and gram-negative bacteria and many other organisms, such as mycobacteria, rickettsiae, spirochetes, and chlamydiae. Tetracyclines act by inhibiting bacterial protein synthesis and have a bacteriostatic effect.

Tetracyclines are not effective against *S. aureus* (except for the newer tetracyclines), *Pseudomonas*, or *Proteus*. They can be used against *Mycoplasma pneumoniae*. Tetracycline in combination with metronidazole and bismuth subsalicylate is useful in treating *Helicobacter pylori*, a bacterium in the stomach that can cause a peptic ulcer. For years, oral and topical tetracycline has been used to treat severe acne vulgaris. Low doses are usually prescribed to minimize the toxic effect of the drug.

Continuous use of tetracyclines has resulted in bacterial resistance to the drugs. Tetracycline resistance has increased in the treatment of pneumococci and gonococci infections; therefore tetracyclines are not as useful in treating these infections.

The tetracyclines are frequently prescribed for oral use, although they are also available for IM and IV use (Prototype Drug Chart 29–2). Because IM administration of tetracycline causes pain on injection and tissue irritation, this route of administration is seldom used. The IV route is used to treat severe infections. The newer oral preparations of tetracyclines, doxycycline, minocycline, and methacycline, are more rapidly and completely absorbed. Tetracyclines should not be taken with magnesium and aluminum preparations (antacids), milk products containing calcium, or iron-containing drugs because these substances bind with tetracycline and prevent absorption of the drug. It is suggested that tetracyclines, except for doxycycline and minocycline, be taken on an empty stomach 1 hour before or 2 hours after mealtime. The absorption of doxycycline and minocycline is improved with food ingestion. Table 29–2 describes the tetracycline preparations and their dosages, uses, and considerations. The tetracyclines are listed according to short-acting, intermediate-acting, and long-acting.

Although tetracyclines are widely used, they have numerous side effects, adverse reactions, toxicities, and drug interactions.

Side Effects and Adverse Reactions

GI disturbances such as nausea, vomiting, and diarrhea are side effects of tetracyclines. **Photosensitivity** (sunburn reaction) may occur in persons taking tetracyclines, especially demeclocycline (Declomycin). Pregnant women should not take tetracycline during the first trimester of pregnancy because of possible teratogenic effects. Women in the last trimester of pregnancy and children younger than 8 years should *not* take tetracycline because it irreversibly discolors the permanent teeth. Minocycline (Minocin) can cause damage to the vestibular part of the inner ear, which may result in difficulty maintaining balance. Outdated tetracyclines should always be discarded because the drug breaks down into a toxic by-product. **Nephrotoxicity** results when the tetracycline is given in high doses with other nephrotoxic drugs. **Superinfection**

PROTOTYPE DRUG CHART 29–2

DOXYCYCLINE

Drug Class

Antibacterial: tetracycline
Trade Name: Adoxa, Doryx, Doxy, Doxycin, Vibramycin,
   Vibea-Tabs
Pregnancy Category: D (includes child <8 y)

Dosage

Systemic infection:
A: PO: 100 mg q12h, IV: 100-200 mg q24h
C: >8 y: PO: 4.4 mg/kg/d in 1-2 divided doses
C: >8 y: IV: 4.4 mg/kg/d daily or b.i.d.

Contraindications

Hypersensitivity, pregnancy, severe hepatic or renal
   disease
Caution: History of allergies, renal and hepatic
   dysfunction, alcoholism, hypokalemia, antidysrhythmics,
   significant bradycardia

Drug-Lab-Food Interactions

Drug: May *increase* effects of digoxin; *decrease* doxycycline absorption with antacids, iron, and zinc; *decrease*
   effects of oral contraceptives; may alter lithium levels
Lab: *Decrease* serum potassium level
Food: Dairy products (milk, cheese) *decrease* effect

Pharmacokinetics

Absorption: PO: 100% absorbed
Distribution: PB: 25%-93%
Metabolism: $t\frac{1}{2}$: 14-24 h
Excretion: Unchanged in the urine

Pharmacodynamics

PO: Onset: 1-2 h
   Peak: 2-4 h
   Duration: 12 h
IV: Onset: Rapid
   Peak: 0.5-1 h
   Duration: 12 h

Therapeutic Effects/Uses

To treat infections caused by uncommon gram-positive and gram-negative organisms, respiratory and skin
   infections or disorders, chlamydial infection, gonorrhea, syphilis, rickettsial infection
Mode of Action: Inhibition of the steps of protein synthesis; bacteriostatic or bactericidal

Side Effects

Nausea, vomiting, diarrhea, rash, flatulence,
   abdominal discomfort, headache, photosensitivity,
   pruritus, epigastric distress, heartburn

Adverse Reactions

Superinfections (candidiasis)
Life-threatening: Blood dyscrasias, hepatotoxicity,
   nephrotoxicity, intracranial hypertension,
   pseudomembranous colitis, CNS toxicity

A, Adult; *b.i.d.*, twice a day; *C*, child; *CNS*, central nervous system; *d*, day; *h*, hour; *IV*, intravenous; *PB*, protein-binding; *PO*, by mouth;
t½, half-life; *y*, year; >, greater than; <, less than.

is another problem that might result because tetracycline
can disrupt the microbial flora of the body.

Drug Interactions

Antacids such as Maalox and iron-containing drugs can prevent the absorption of tetracycline from the GI tract. Milk
and drugs high in calcium can inhibit tetracycline absorption. To avoid drug interaction, these drugs should be taken
2 hours apart from tetracycline. The new lipid-soluble tetracyclines, doxycycline and minocycline, are absorbed from
the GI tract when taken with milk products and food.

   The desired action of oral contraceptives can be lessened when taken with tetracyclines. The activity of penicillins given with a tetracycline can be decreased. Tetracyclines could cause a bacterial resistance to the action of
penicillin. Administering tetracycline with an aminoglycoside may increase the risk of nephrotoxicity.

Nursing Process

Antibacterials: Tetracyclines

ASSESSMENT

■ Assess vital signs and urine output. Report abnormal
findings.

■ Check laboratory results, especially those that indicate renal and liver function, such as blood urea nitrogen, serum creatinine, aspartate aminotransferase, alanine aminotransferase, and bilirubin.

■ Obtain a history of dietary intake and drugs client currently takes. Dairy products, antacids, iron, calcium, and
magnesium decrease drug absorption. Digoxin absorption is increased, which may lead to digitalis toxicity.

NURSING DIAGNOSES

■ Risk for infection
■ Noncompliance with drug regimen
■ Risk for impaired skin integrity

PLANNING

■ Client's infection will be controlled and later eliminated.

NURSING INTERVENTIONS

■ Obtain a sample for culture from the infected area and send to the laboratory for a culture and sensitivity test. Antibiotic therapy can be started after the culture sample has been taken.
■ Administer tetracycline 1 hour before meals or 2 hours after meals for absorption.

■ Monitor laboratory values for liver and kidney functions; these include liver enzymes, blood urea nitrogen, and serum creatinine.
■ Record vital signs and urine output.

Client Teaching

General

• Instruct client to store tetracycline out of the light and extreme heat. Tetracycline decomposes in light and heat, causing the drug to become toxic.
• Advise client to check the expiration date on the bottle of tetracycline; out-of-date tetracycline can be toxic.
• Inform woman who is contemplating pregnancy who has an infection to tell her health care provider and to avoid taking tetracycline because of possible teratogenic effect.
• Warn parents that children less than 8 years old should not take tetracycline because it can cause discoloration of permanent teeth.

Table 29–2

Antibacterials: Tetracyclines

Generic (Brand)	Route and Dosage	Uses and Considerations
Short-Acting		
tetracycline (Achromycin, Tetracyn, Sumycin, Panmycin)	A: PO: 250-500 mg q6h IM: 250 mg daily C: >8y: PO: 25-50 mg/kg/d in 4 divided doses IM: 15-25 mg/kg/d in 2-3 divided doses; *max:* 250 mg/dose	Used for treatment of infections caused by gram-positive and gram-negative microorganisms, respiratory and skin disorders, chlamydial infection, gonorrhea, syphilis, and rickettsial infections. *Pregnancy category:* D; PB: 30%-60%; t$^1/_2$: 6-12 h
oxytetracycline HCl (Terramycin)	A: PO: 250-500 mg q6-12h IM: 200-300 mg/d in 2-3 divided doses IV: 250-500 mg in 2 divided doses C: >8 y: PO: 25-50 mg/kg/d in 4 divided doses IM: 15-25 mg/kg/d in 2-3 divided doses; *max:* 250 mg/dose IV: 10-20 mg/kg/d in 2 divided doses	Used for urinary tract infections. Administered primarily by the oral route. *Pregnancy category:* D; PB: 20%-40%; t$^1/_2$: 6-10 h
Intermediate-Acting		
demeclocycline HCl (Declomycin)	A: PO: 150 mg q6h or 300 mg q12h C: >8 y: PO: 8-12 mg/kg/d in 2-3 divided doses	Used for gram-positive and gram-negative bacteria. Photosensitivity may occur. *Pregnancy category:* D; PB: 35%-90%; t$^1/_2$: 10-17 h
methacycline HCl (Rondomycin)	A: PO: 600 mg q12h C: PO: 6-12 mg/kg	It is a costly tetracycline. It has similar actions as demeclocycline. The side effects are similar to other tetracyclines. *Pregnancy category:* UK; PB: UK; t$^1/_2$: UK
Long-Acting		
doxycycline hyclate (Vibramycin)	See Prototype Drug Chart 29–2.	
minocycline HCl (Minocin)	A: PO/IV: Initially: 200 mg; 100 mg q12h or 50 mg q6h C: >8 y: PO/IV: Initially: 4 mg/kg/d; 2 mg/kg q12h	Effective against bacterial infections and acne. Should not be administered to clients with renal insufficiency. Should take with food. *Pregnancy category:* D; PB: 55%-88%; t$^1/_2$: 11-20 h

A, Adult; *C,* child; *d,* day; *h,* hour; *IM,* intramuscular; *IV,* intravenous; *max,* maximum; *PB,* protein-binding; *PO,* by mouth; *t$^1/_2$,* half-life; *UK,* unknown; *y,* year; >, greater than.

- Direct client to take the complete course of tetracycline as prescribed.

Side Effects

- Encourage client to use sun block and protective clothing during sun exposure. Photosensitivity is associated with tetracycline.
- Instruct client to report signs of a superinfection (mouth ulcers, anal or genital discharge).
- Advise client to use additional contraceptive techniques and not to rely on oral contraceptives when taking drug because effectiveness may decrease.
- Teach client to use effective oral hygiene several times a day to prevent or alleviate mouth ulcers (stomatitis).

Diet

- Educate client to avoid milk products, iron, and antacids. Tetracycline should be taken 1 hour before meals or 2 hours after meals with a full glass of water. If gastrointestinal upset occurs, the drug can be taken with nondairy foods.

Cultural Considerations ⊕

- Recognize that client and family members from various cultural backgrounds may need a written drug schedule as to when the drug should be taken. Explain how dairy products should not be taken with specific tetracyclines but that food helps with the absorption of minocycline and doxycycline.
- Provide a detailed explanation orally or in written form of the possible side effects that should be reported to the health care provider.

EVALUATION

- Evaluate the effectiveness of tetracycline by determining whether the infection has been controlled or has ceased and that there are no side effects.

Aminoglycosides

Aminoglycosides act by inhibiting bacterial protein synthesis. The aminoglycoside antibiotics are used against gram-negative bacteria, such as *E. coli, Proteus* spp., and *Pseudomonas* spp. Some gram-positive cocci are resistant to aminoglycosides, so penicillins or cephalosporins may be used.

Streptomycin sulfate, derived from the bacterium *Streptomyces griseus* in 1944, was the first aminoglycoside available for clinical use and was used to treat tuberculosis. Because of its ototoxicity and the bacterial resistance that can develop, it is infrequently used today. Despite its toxicity, streptomycin is the drug of choice to treat tularemia and bubonic pneumonic forms of plague.

Aminoglycosides are for serious infections. Aminoglycosides cannot be absorbed from the GI tract and cannot cross into the cerebrospinal fluid. They cross the blood-brain barrier in children but not in adults. These agents are primarily administered IM and IV except for a few aminoglycosides (e.g., neomycin, paromomycin), which may be given orally to decrease bacteria and other organisms in the bowel. Neomycin is frequently used as a preoperative bowel antiseptic. Paromomycin is useful in treating intestinal amebiasis and tapeworm infestation.

The aminoglycosides currently used to treat *Pseudomonas aeruginosa* infection include gentamicin (1963), tobramycin (1970), amikacin (1970s), and netilmicin (1980s). Netilmicin is one of the latest aminoglycosides, and the occurrence of toxicities from this drug is not so frequent or intense as with other aminoglycosides. *P. aeruginosa* is sensitive to gentamicin. Amikacin (Amiken) may be used when there is bacterial resistance to gentamicin and tobramycin. Prototype Drug Chart 29–3 lists the drug data related to the aminoglycoside gentamicin (Garamycin).

Pharmacokinetics

Gentamicin and netilmicin are administered IM and IV. Both drugs have a short half-life, and the drug dose can be given three to four times a day. Netilmicin has a low protein-binding power. Excretion of these drugs is primarily unchanged in the urine.

Pharmacodynamics

Gentamicin and netilmicin inhibit bacterial protein synthesis and have a bactericidal effect. Although netilmicin is the newer aminoglycoside, its pregnancy category is D, whereas gentamicin has a pregnancy category of C. The onset of action for both drugs is similar (rapid or immediate). The peak action for netilmicin is 30 minutes faster than gentamicin.

To ensure a desired blood level, aminoglycosides are usually administered IV. They can be given with penicillins and cephalosporins but should not be mixed together in the same administered container. When combinations of antibiotics are given IV, the IV line is flushed after each antibiotic has been administered to ensure that the antibiotic was completely delivered.

Side Effects and Adverse Reactions

The serious adverse reactions to aminoglycosides include ototoxicity and nephrotoxicity. Nephrotoxicity might occur, depending on renal function, drug dose, and age. Careful drug dosing is especially important with younger and older clients. The nurse must assess changes in clients' hearing, balance, and urinary output. Prolonged use of aminoglycosides could result in a superinfection. Specific serum aminoglycoside levels should be closely monitored to avoid adverse reactions. Table 29–3 lists the aminoglycosides and their dosages, uses, and considerations.

Drug Interactions

When aminoglycosides are administered concurrently with penicillins, the desired effects of aminoglycosides are greatly decreased. Preferably, these drugs should be given several hours apart. The drug action of oral anticoagulants such as warfarin (Coumadin) can increase when taken simultaneously with aminoglycoside administration. The risk of ototoxicity increases when ethacrynic acid and aminoglycoside are given.

PROTOTYPE DRUG CHART 29–3

GENTAMICIN SULFATE

Drug Class

Antibacterial: aminoglycosides
Trade Name: Garamycin
Pregnancy Category: C

Dosage

A: IM: 3 mg/kg/d in 3-4 divided doses
IV: 3-5 mg/kg/d in 3 divided doses
C: IM/IV: 6-7.5 mg/kg q8h
TDM: 5-10 mcg/ml; peak: 10-12 mcg/ml; trough: 0.5-2 mcg/ml

Contraindications

Hypersensitivity, severe renal disease, pregnancy, and breastfeeding
Caution: Renal disease, neuromuscular disorders (myasthenia gravis, parkinsonism), heart failure, elderly, neonates

Drug-Lab-Food Interactions

Drug: Increase risk of ototoxicity with loop diuretics, methoxyflurane; *increase* risk of nephrotoxicity with amphotericin B, polymyxin, cisplatin, furosemide, vancomycin
Lab: Increase BUN, serum AST, ALT, LDH, bilirubin, creatinine; *decrease* serum potassium and magnesium

Pharmacokinetics

Absorption: IM, IV
Distribution: PB: UK
Metabolism: $t^{1}/_{2}$: 2 h
Excretion: Unchanged in urine

Pharmacodynamics

IM/IV: Onset: rapid
Peak: 1-2 h
Duration: 6-8 h

Therapeutic Effects/Uses

To treat serious infections caused by gram-negative organisms, such as *Pseudomonas aeruginosa, Proteus;* to treat pelvic inflammatory disease; effective against methicillin-resistant *Staphylococcus aureus* infections
Mode of Action: Inhibition of bacterial protein synthesis; bactericidal effect

Side Effects

Anorexia, nausea, vomiting, rash, numbness, visual disturbances, tremors, tinnitus, pruritus, muscle cramps or weakness, photosensitivity

Adverse Reactions

Oliguria, urticaria, palpitation, superinfection
Life-threatening: Ototoxicity, nephrotoxicity, thrombocytopenia, agranulocytosis, neuromuscular blockade, liver damage

A, Adult; *ALT,* alanine aminotransferase; *AST,* aspartate aminotransferase; *BUN,* blood urea nitrogen; *C,* child; *d,* day; *h,* hour; *IM,* intramuscular; *IV,* intravenous; *LDH,* lactic dehydrogenase; *PB,* protein-binding; *t¹/₂,* half-life; *TDM,* therapeutic drug monitoring; *UK,* unknown.

Nursing Process

Antibacterials: Aminoglycosides

ASSESSMENT

■ Record vital signs and urine output. Compare these results with future vital signs and urine output. An adverse reaction to most aminoglycosides is nephrotoxicity.

■ Assess laboratory results to determine renal and liver functions, including blood urea nitrogen, serum creatinine, alkaline phosphatase, alanine aminotransferase, aspartate aminotransferase, and bilirubin. Serum electrolytes should also be checked. Aminoglycosides may decrease the serum potassium and magnesium levels.

■ Obtain a medical history related to renal or hearing disorders. Large doses of aminoglycosides could cause nephrotoxicity or ototoxicity.

NURSING DIAGNOSES

■ Risk for infection
■ Risk for impaired tissue integrity
■ Risk for ineffective tissue perfusion: renal

PLANNING

■ Client's infection will be controlled and later eliminated.

NURSING INTERVENTIONS

■ Send a sample from the infected area to the laboratory for culture to determine organism and antibiotic sensitivity *before* aminoglycoside is started.

■ Monitor intake and output. Urine output should be at least 600 ml/d. Immediately report if urine output is decreased. Urinalysis may be ordered daily. Check results for proteinuria, casts, blood cells, or appearance.

■ Check for hearing loss. Aminoglycosides can cause ototoxicity.

■ Evaluate laboratory results and compare with baseline values. Report abnormal results.

■ Monitor vital signs. Note if body temperature has decreased.

■ For IV use, dilute the aminoglycoside in 50-200 ml of normal saline solution or dextrose 5% in water (D₅W) solution and administer in 30-60 minutes.

■ Check that therapeutic drug monitoring (TDM) has been ordered for peak and trough drug levels. The TDM for gentamicin is 5-10 mcg/ml. Blood should be drawn 45-60 minutes after drug has been administered for peak levels and minutes before the next drug dosing for trough levels. Drug peak values should be 10-12 mcg/ml, and trough values should be 0.5-2 mcg/ml.

■ Monitor for signs and symptoms of superinfection such as stomatitis (mouth ulcers), genital discharge (vaginitis), and anal or genital itching.

Client Teaching

General
• Unless fluids are restricted, encourage client to increase fluid intake.
• Instruct client never to take leftover antibiotics.

Side Effects
• Inform client to report side effects resulting from the aminoglycosides, including nausea, vomiting, tremors, tinnitus, pruritus, and muscle cramps.
• Direct client to use sun block and protective clothing during sun exposure. Photosensitivity can be caused by aminoglycosides.

Table 29–3

Antibacterials: Aminoglycosides

Generic (Brand)	Route and Dosage	Uses and Considerations
amikacin SO₄ (Amikin)	A & C: IM/IV: 15 mg/kg/d in 2 divided doses; *max:* 1.5 g/d C: IV: 5 mg/kg q8h or 7.5 mg/kg q12h TDM: Peak: 15-30 mg/ml; trough: 5-10 mg/ml	Synthetic derivative of kanamycin. Effective against *Pseudomonas* spp. Hearing changes should be monitored. *Pregnancy category:* C; PB: 4%-11%; t½: 2-3 h
gentamicin SO₄ (Garamycin)	See Prototype Drug Chart 29–3.	
kanamycin SO₄ (Kantrex)	A: PO: 1 g q6h *Hepatic coma:* 8-12 g/d in divided doses IM/IV: 15 mg/kg/d in 2 divided doses C: IV: Same as adult	Used orally for hepatic coma. Effective against gram-negative bacteria with the exception of *Pseudomonas aeruginosa.* Monitor for hearing loss and urinary output. *Pregnancy category:* D; PB: 10%; t½: 2-3 h
neomycin SO₄ (Mycifradin)	A: PO: GI surgery: 1 g qh for 4 doses; then 1 g q4h for 5 doses for 24 h or other regimens *Hepatic coma:* 4-12 g/d in divided doses for 5-6 d IM: 15 mg/kg/d in 4 divided doses; *max:* 1 g/d C: PO: 10 mg/kg q4-6h for 3 d	Decreases bacteria in the bowel and is used as a preoperative bowel antiseptic. It is also available as a topical antibiotic ointment. *Pregnancy category:* C; PB: 10%; t½: 2-3 h
netilmicin (Netromycin)	A: IM/IV: 3-6.5 mg/kg/d in 3 divided doses C: IM/IV: 2.5-4 mg/kg q12h TDM: Peak: 0.5-10 mcg/ml; trough: <4 mcg/ml	Used in treating moderate to severe gram-negative infections, such as those caused by *Enterobacter, Escherichia coli, Klebsiella, Proteus, Pseudomonas,* and *Serratia. Pregnancy category:* D; PB: 10%; t½: 2-2.5 h
paromomycin (Humatin)	*Intestinal amebiasis:* A & C: PO: 25-35 mg/kg/d in 3 divided doses for 5-10 d *Hepatic coma:* A: PO: 4 g/d in 2-4 divided doses for 5-6 d	Used in treating hepatic coma and parasitic infections. Hearing changes and urinary output should be monitored. Is not systemically absorbed. *Pregnancy category:* C; PB: UK; t½: UK
streptomycin SO₄	*Tuberculosis:* A: IM: 1 g daily for 2-3 mo; then 1 g × 3 wk *Endocarditis:* A: IM: 1 g q12h for 1 wk; dose may be decreased	First aminoglycoside. Used with antituberculosis drugs in treatment of tuberculosis. Ototoxicity is a major problem. *Pregnancy category:* C; PB: 30%; t½: 2-3 h
tobramycin SO₄ (Nebcin)	A: IM/IV: 3-5 mg/kg/d in 3 divided doses C: IM/IV: 3 mg/kg/d in 3 divided doses TDM: Peak: 10-12 mcg/ml; trough: 0.5-2 mcg/ml	Very effective against *Pseudomonas aeruginosa.* Hearing changes and urinary output should be monitored. Toxic effects are less than for other aminoglycosides. *Pregnancy category:* D; PB: 10%; t½: 2-3 h

A, Adult; *C,* child; *d,* day; *GI,* gastrointestinal; *h,* hour; *IM,* intramuscular; *IV,* intravenous; *max,* maximum; *PB,* protein-binding; *PO,* by mouth; *t½,* half-life; *TDM,* therapeutic drug monitoring; *UK,* unknown; *wk,* week.

- Do not give directions such as take one "blue" pill at a specified time. Instead, provide the name and dosage of the medication.

EVALUATION

■ Evaluate the effectiveness of the aminoglycoside by determining whether the infection has ceased and no side effects have occurred.

Fluoroquinolones (Quinolones)

The mechanism of action of fluoroquinolones is to interfere with the enzyme DNA gyrase, which is needed to synthesize bacterial deoxyribonucleic acid (DNA). Their antibacterial spectrum includes both gram-positive and gram-negative organisms. They are bactericidal. Nalidixic acid (NegGram) and cinoxacin (Cinobac) are the earliest derivatives of the fluoroquinolone group, which is prescribed primarily for urinary tract infection caused by common gram-negative organisms such as *E. coli*. The fluoroquinolones are effective against some gram-positive organisms, such as *Streptococcus pneumoniae*, and against *Haemophilus influenzae*, *P. aeruginosa*, *Salmonella*, and *Shigella*. This group of antibiotics is useful in the treatment of urinary tract, bone, and joint infections; bronchitis; pneumonia; gastroenteritis; and gonorrhea. Table 29–4 lists the various fluoroquinolones.

Ciprofloxacin (Cipro) and norfloxacin (Noroxin) are synthetic antibacterials related to nalidixic acid. These two fluoroquinolones have a broad spectrum of action on gram-positive and gram-negative organisms, including *P. aeruginosa*. Norfloxacin is indicated for urinary tract infections, and ciprofloxacin is approved for use for urinary tract infections; lower respiratory tract infections; and skin, soft tissue, bone, and joint infections.

The use of fluoroquinolones as urinary antibiotics is discussed in Chapter 32, Drugs for Urinary Tract Disorders. Prototype Drug Chart 29–4 lists the drug data related to levofloxacin. Levofloxacin's use is not limited to urinary tract infections.

The number of new fluoroquinolones has increased in the past few years. Levofloxacin (Levaquin), sparfloxacin (Zagam), and trovafloxacin (Trovan) are used primarily to treat respiratory problems, such as community-acquired

---

PROTOTYPE DRUG CHART 29–4

LEVOFLOXACIN

Drug Class

Antibacterials: quinolone, fluoroquinolone
Trade Name: Levaquin
Pregnancy Category: C (X at term), breastfeeding

Dosage

A: PO: 500 mg q24h
IV: 500 mg q24h, infused over 60 min
Moderate to severe infections

Contraindications

Severe renal disease, hypersensitivity to other quinolones, pregnancy and breastfeeding
Caution: Seizure disorders, renal disorders, children <14 y, elderly, clients receiving theophylline

Drug-Lab-Food Interactions

Drug: *Increase* effect of oral hypoglycemics and theophylline, caffeine; *decrease* drug absorption with antacids, iron
Lab: *Increase* AST, ALT

Pharmacokinetics

Absorption: PO: 95%-98% absorbed
Distribution: PB: 24%-30%
Metabolism: t½: 6.5-7.5 h
Excretion: 87% unchanged in urine

Pharmacodynamics

PO: Onset: 0.5-1 h
Peak: 1-2 h
Duration: UK

Therapeutic Effects/Uses

To treat lower respiratory tract, renal, bone, and joint infections
Mode of Action: Interference with the enzyme DNA gyrase, which is needed for bacterial DNA synthesis; bactercidal effect

Side Effects

Nausea, vomiting, diarrhea, abdominal cramps, flatulence, headache, dizziness, fatigue, restlessness, insomnia, rash, flushing, tinnitus, photosensitivity

Adverse Reactions

Stevens-Johnson syndrome, encephalopathy, seizures, pseudomembranous colitis, dysrhythmias

A, Adult; *ALT,* alanine aminotransferase; *AST,* aspartate aminotransferase; *DNA,* deoxyribonucleic acid; *h,* hour; *IV,* intravenous; *min,* minute; *PB,* protein-binding; *PO,* by mouth; *t½,* half-life; *UK,* unknown; *y,* year; <, less than.

Table 29–4

Antibacterials: Fluoroquinolones (Quinolones) and Unclassified Drugs

Generic (Brand)	Route and Dosage	Uses and Considerations
Fluoroquinolones		
cinoxacin (Cinobac)	A: PO: 1 g/d 2-4 divided doses for 1-2 wk C: >12 y: Same as adult	For acute and chronic UTIs. Effective against gram-negative organisms except for *Pseudomonas*. Absorbed in prostatic tissue. More effective than nalidixic acid. *Pregnancy category:* B; PB: 60%-80%; t^1/$_2$: 1.5 h
ciprofloxacin HCl (Cipro)	A: PO: 250-750 mg q12h IV: 200-400 mg q12h	To treat lower respiratory tract, renal, bone and joint, and skin infections. *Pregnancy category:* C; PB: 20%-40%; t^1/$_2$: 4-6 h
enoxacin (Penetrex)	A: PO: 200-400 mg b.i.d. 7-14 d	To treat UTI, including those caused by *Escherichia coli*, *Proteus*, *Pseudomonas*. *Pregnancy category:* C; PB: 40%; t^1/$_2$: 3-6 h
gatifloxacin (Tequin)	A: PO/IV: 400 mg/d for 7-10 days	To treat community-acquired pneumonia, acute sinusitis, UTIs. It is two to four times more active than levofloxacin against *Streptococcus pneumoniae* and is active against *Legionella pneumophila*, *Mycobacterium tuberculosis*, and *Haemophilus influenzae*. Has similar side effects as other fluoroquinolones. *Pregnancy category:* C; PB: UK; t^1/$_2$: 7-12 h
levofloxacin (Levaquin)	See Prototype Drug Chart 29–4.	
lomefloxacin HCl (Maxaquin)	A: PO: 200-400 mg/d 7-14 d	For complicated and uncomplicated UTIs, transurethral surgery, lower respiratory infections. Drug dose is reduced for clients with a low creatinine clearance. *Pregnancy category:* C; PB: UK; t^1/$_2$: 6-8 h
moxifloxacin (Avelox)	A: PO: 400 mg/d for 10 d	Treatment is similar to gatifloxacin. It is 4 to 8 times more active than levofloxacin against *S. pneumoniae*. Side effects are similar to other fluoroquinolones. *Pregnancy category:* PB: UK; t^1/$_2$: 7-12 h
nalidixic acid (NegGram)	A: PO: 1 g q.i.d. for 1-2 wk; 1 g b.i.d. for long-term use C: PO: 55 mg/kg/d in 4 divided doses for 1-2 wk; 33 mg/kg/d for long-term use	For acute and chronic UTIs. Drug resistance may occur. Is not distributed in prostatic fluid. *Pregnancy category:* B; PB: 95%; t^1/$_2$: 2-6 h
norfloxacin (Noroxin)	A: PO: 400 mg b.i.d., a.c. or p.c. for 1-3 wk	For acute and chronic UTIs. Most potent drug of the fluoroquinolone group. Food may inhibit drug absorption. *Pregnancy category:* C; PB: 10%-15%; t^1/$_2$: 3-4 h
ofloxacin (Floxin)	A: PO/IV: 200-400 mg q12h 7-10 d	For respiratory and UTIs, prostatitis, and skin infections. Not to be taken with meals. Superinfection may result. Avoid excessive sunlight. *Pregnancy category:* C; PB: 20%; t^1/$_2$: 5-8 h
sparfloxacin (Zagam)	A: PO: 400 mg for 1 d, 200 mg/d for day 2 to 10	To treat community-acquired pneumonia, chronic bronchitis, and skin disorders. Side effects include GI disturbances and photosensitivity. Clients should use sun block when in the sun. *Pregnancy category:* UK; PB: UK; t^1/$_2$: UK
trovafloxacin (Trovan)	A: PO: IV: 100-200 mg/d for 7-10 d	To treat acute sinusitis, chronic bronchitis, UTIs, and skin infections. *Pregnancy category:* UK; PB: UK; t^1/$_2$: UK
Unclassified Drugs		
chloramphenicol (Chloromycetin)	A & C: PO/IV: 50 mg/kg/d in 4 divided doses (q6h) NB: 25 mg/kg/d in 4 divided doses (q6h)	For treatment of severe infections. Drug can be toxic. *Pregnancy category:* C; PB: 50%-60%; t^1/$_2$: 1.5-4 h
quinupristin/dalfopristin (Synercid)	A: IV: 7.5 mg/kg given over 1 h, q8h × 10 days	For treatment of vancomycin-resistant *Enterococcus faecium*. Also effective against skin infected by *Staphylococcus aureus*. Adverse effects at infusion site; pain, inflammation, edema and thrombophlebitis. Central venous line is preferred. *Pregnancy category:* UK; PB: UK; t^1/$_2$: 1 h
spectinomycin HCl (Trobicin)	A: IM: 2 g as single dose or 2 g q12h for severe infection C: IM: 40 mg/kg as single dose	Has a bacteriostatic effect. Effective against *Neisseria gonorrhoeae*. Ineffective against syphilis. *Pregnancy category:* B; PB: 10%; t^1/$_2$: 1-3 h

A, Adult; *b.i.d.*, twice a day; *C*, child; *d*, day; *GI*, gastrointestinal; *h*, hour; *IM*, intramuscular; *IV*, intravenous; *max*, maximum; *NB*, newborn; *PB*, protein-binding; *PO*, by mouth; *q.i.d.*, four times a day; *t*^{1}/$_2$, half-life; *UK*, unknown; *UTI*, urinary tract infection; *wk*, week; *y*, year; *>*, greater than.

pneumonia, chronic bronchitis, acute sinusitis, urinary tract infections, and uncomplicated skin infections.

Gatifloxacin (Tequin) and moxifloxacin (Avelox) received Food & Drug Administration approval in 1999 and are available for once-a-day oral and parenteral dosing. These two drugs are prescribed to treat similar infections to other fluoroquinolones. Gatifloxacin and moxifloxacin are more active than levofloxacin against *S. pneumoniae*. They are also effective against some strains of *S. aureus* and enterococci but not VRE. The fluoroquinolones are included in Table 29–4.

Pharmacokinetics

Approximately 70% of levofloxacin (Levaquin) is absorbed from the GI tract. It has a low protein-binding effect and a moderately short half-life of 6.5 to 7.5 hours. More than 75% of the drug is excreted unchanged in the urine.

Pharmacodynamics

Levofloxacin inhibits bacterial DNA synthesis by inhibiting the enzyme DNA gyrase. The drug has a high tissue distribution. If possible, it should be taken before meals because food slows the absorption rate. Antacids also decrease absorption rate. Levofloxacin increases the effect of oral hypoglycemics, theophylline, and caffeine.

Levofloxacin has an average onset of action of 0.5 to 1 hour, and the peak concentration time is 1 to 2 hours. The duration of action is unknown.

Nursing Process

Antibacterials: Fluoroquinolones

ASSESSMENT

■ Record vital signs and intake and urine output. Compare these results with future vital signs and urine output. Fluid intake should be at least 2000 ml/d.

■ Assess laboratory results to determine renal function: blood urea nitrogen and serum creatinine.

■ Obtain a drug and diet history. Antacids and iron preparations decrease absorption of fluoroquinolones such as levofloxacin (Levoquin). Levofloxacin can increase the effects of theophylline and caffeine. Levofloxacin can increase the effects of oral hypoglycemics. When levofloxacin is taken with NSAIDs, CNS reactions including seizures may occur.

NURSING DIAGNOSES

■ Risk for infection
■ Risk for impaired tissue integrity
■ Noncompliance with drug regimen

PLANNING

■ Client's infection will be controlled and later eliminated.

NURSING INTERVENTIONS

■ Obtain specimen from the infected site and send to the laboratory for culture and sensitivity *before* initiating antibacterial drug therapy.

■ Monitor intake and output. Urine output should be at least 750 ml/d. Client should be well hydrated, and fluid intake should be >2000 ml/d to prevent crystalluria. Urine pH should be <6.7.

■ Record vital signs. Report abnormal findings.

■ Check laboratory results, especially blood urea nitrogen and serum creatinine. Elevated values may indicate renal dysfunction.

■ Administer levofloxacin 2 hours before or after antacids and iron products for absorption. Give with a full glass of water. If gastrointestinal distress occurs, the drug may be taken with food.

■ For IV levofloxacin, dilute the antibiotic in an appropriate amount of solution as indicated in the drug circular. Infuse over 60 minutes.

■ Check for signs and symptoms of superinfection such as stomatitis (mouth ulcers), furry black tongue, anal or genital discharge, and itching.

■ Monitor serum theophylline levels. Levofloxacin can increase theophylline levels. Check for symptoms of central nervous system stimulation: nervousness, insomnia, anxiety, and tachycardia.

■ Monitor blood sugar. Levofloxacin can increase the effects of oral hypoglycemics.

Client Teaching

General

• Teach client to drink at least 6 to 8 glasses (8 oz) of fluid daily.
• Encourage client to avoid caffeinated products.

Side Effects

• Direct client to avoid operating hazardous machinery or operating a motor vehicle while taking the drug or until drug stability has occurred because of possible drug-related dizziness.
• Inform client that photosensitivity is a side effect of most fluoroquinolones. Client should use sunglasses, sun block, and protective clothing when in the sun.
• Instruct client to report side effects, such as dizziness, nausea, vomiting, diarrhea, flatulence, abdominal cramps, tinnitus, and rash. Older adults are more likely to develop side effects.

Cultural Considerations ⊕

• To establish trust among Hispanics/Latinos and Appalachians, it is necessary to demonstrate an interest in client's family and other personal matters, drop hints instead of giving orders, and solicit client's opinions and advice.

EVALUATION

■ Evaluate the effectiveness of the fluoroquinolone by determining if the infection has ceased and the body temperature has returned within normal range.

Unclassified Antibacterial Drugs

Several antibacterials, such as chloramphenicol, spectinomycin, and quinupristin/dalfopristin, do not belong to any major drug group. Chloramphenicol (Chloromycetin) was discovered in 1947 and has a bacteriostatic action by inhibiting bacterial protein synthesis. Because of the toxic effects of chloramphenicol, including blood dyscrasias related to bone marrow suppression, it is used only to treat serious infections. It is effective against gram-negative and gram-positive bacteria and many other microorganisms, such as rickettsiae, *Mycoplasmas,* and *H. influenzae.*

Spectinomycin hydrochloride (Trobicin), introduced in 1971, is used against *Neisseria gonorrhoeae,* the microbe that causes gonorrhea. It is also prescribed for persons allergic to penicillins, cephalosporins, or tetracyclines. It is administered IM as a single dose.

Quinupristin/dalfopristin (Synercid) is effective for treating vancomycin-resistant *Enterococcus faecium* (VREF)

bacteremia and skin infected by *S. aureus* and *S. pyogenes.* It acts by disrupting the protein synthesis of the organism. When administering the drug through a peripheral IV line, pain, edema, and phlebitis may occur.

WEBSITES

For further information on *Antibacterials: Macrolides, Tetracyclines, Aminoglycosides, and Fluoroquinolones,* visit these Internet resources:

Information on levofloxacin:
www.nlm.nih.gov/medlineplus/druginfo/medmaster/a697040.html

Information on azithromycin:
www.drugs.com/zithromax.html

Critical Thinking Case Study

A.J.N., age 46, has a wound infection. The culture report stated that the infection was caused by *Pseudomonas aeruginosa.* A.J.N.'s temperature was 104° F (40° C). Amikacin sulfate (Amikin) is to be administered IV in 100 ml of D_5W over 45 minutes every 8 hours. Dosage is 15 mg/kg daily in three divided doses. A.J.N. weighs 165 pounds.

1. What is the drug classification of amikacin? How many milligrams of amikacin should A.J.N. receive every 8 hours?

2. What type of IV infusion should be used? What would be the IV flow rate?

3. When should a wound culture be obtained to determine the appropriate antibacterial agent? Give your rationale.

4. What are the similarities of amikacin to other aminoglycosides such as gentamicin? Would one aminoglycoside be preferred over another one? Explain.

The nurse assessed A.J.N. for hearing and urinary function before and during amikacin therapy.

5. What should a hearing assessment include?

6. A.J.N.'s urine output in the last 8 hours was 125 ml. Explain the possible cause for the amount of urine output. What nursing action should be taken?

7. What laboratory tests monitor renal function?

8. The health care provider requests peak and trough serum amikacin levels. When should the blood samples to determine peak serum level and trough serum level be drawn?

Study Questions

1. What two groups of drugs are classified as bacteriostatic drugs?

2. What antibacterial drugs are used as penicillin substitutes?

3. What is an example of a macrolide?

4. What is the nurse's role in client teaching about tetracycline?

5. What types of antibacterial drugs are aminoglycosides?

6. What two types of toxicities are related to aminoglycosides? What signs and symptoms should the nurse assess?

7. Fluoroquinolones are used to treat what health problems?

8. What are four GI problems associated with a fluoroquinolone such as levofloxacin?

30 Antibacterials: Sulfonamides

ELECTRONIC RESOURCES

Additional information can be found on the companion website at *http://evolve.elsevier.com/KeeHayes/pharmacology/* or on the companion CD-ROM, which includes:
* *NCLEX-style examination review questions*
* *Pharmacology animations*
* *Medication error and (IV) therapy checklists*
* *Medication calculation problems*
* *Electronic calculators*

OUTLINE

OBJECTIVES

- Differentiate between short-acting and intermediate-acting sulfonamides.
- Describe the uses, side effects, and adverse reactions to all the sulfonamides and co-trimoxazole.
- Explain the nursing interventions, including client teaching, related to sulfonamides.

TERMS

bacteriostatic
cross-sensitivity
crystalluria

erythema multiforme
exfoliative dermatitis

photosensitivity
synergistic effect

Introduction

Sulfonamides are one of the oldest antibacterial agents used to combat infection. When penicillin was initially marketed, the sulfonamide drugs were not widely prescribed because penicillin was considered the "miracle drug." However, use of sulfonamides has increased as a result of new sulfonamides and the combination drug of sulfonamide with an antibacterial agent in preparations such as trimethoprim-sulfamethoxazole (Bactrim, Septra).

Sulfonamides

Sulfonamides were first isolated from a coal tar derivative compound in the early 1900s and were produced for clinical use against coccal infections in 1935. It was the first group of drugs used against bacteria. Sulfonamides are not classified as an antibiotic because they were not obtained from biologic substances. The sulfonamides are **bacteriostatic** because they inhibit bacterial synthesis of folic acid, which is essential for bacterial growth. Humans do not synthesize folic acid but acquire it through the diet; therefore sulfonamides selectively inhibit bacterial growth without affecting normal cells. Folic acid (folate) is required by cells for biosynthesis of ribonucleic acid (RNA), deoxyribonucleic acid (DNA), and proteins.

The clinical usefulness of sulfonamides only, not in combination, has decreased because the availability and effectiveness of penicillin and other antibiotics has increased and bacterial resistance to some sulfonamides can develop. Sulfonamides may be used as an alternative drug for clients allergic to penicillin. They are still used to treat urinary tract and ear infections and may be used for newborn eye prophylaxis. Sulfonamides are approximately 90% effective against *Escherichia coli*; therefore they are frequently a preferred treatment for urinary tract infections, which are often caused by *E. coli*. They are also useful in the treatment of meningococcal meningitis and against the organisms *Chlamydia* and *Toxoplasma gondii*. Sulfonamides are not effective against viruses and fungi.

Pharmacokinetics

Sulfonamide drugs are well absorbed by the gastrointestinal (GI) tract and are well distributed to body tissues and the brain. The liver metabolizes the sulfonamide drug, and the kidneys excrete it.

Pharmacodynamics

Many sulfonamides are for oral administration because they are absorbed readily by the GI tract. They are also available in solution and ointment for ophthalmic use and in cream form, silver sulfadiazine (Silvadene) and mafenide acetate (Sulfamylon), for burns. Most of the early sulfonamides were highly protein bound and displaced other drugs by competing for protein sites. The following are two categories of sulfonamides, classified according to their duration of action:

- Short-acting sulfonamides (rapid absorption and excretion rate)
- Intermediate-acting sulfonamides (moderate to slow absorption and slow excretion rate)

Sulfisoxazole (Gantrisin) is a water-soluble sulfonamide that is effective in treating most uncomplicated urinary tract infections. It is also useful, along with sulfadiazine, in prophylactic treatment of streptococcal infections in clients with rheumatic fever who are hypersensitive to penicillin. Sulfadiazine is poorly soluble in urine and can cause crystallization, which could damage the kidneys if there is insufficient fluid and water intake. Sulfamethoxazole (Gantanol), an intermediate-acting sulfonamide, has a longer duration of action than other sulfonamides; however, it has poorer water solubility than sulfisoxazole. Table 30-1 lists the protein-binding, half-life, and solubility in urine of most drugs in the sulfonamide group.

The only combination of sulfonamides still marketed—but infrequently used—is trisulfapyrimidines. This triple sulfa drug is a combination of low doses of sulfadiazine, sulfamerazine, and sulfamethazine. The three drugs have an additive effect, which increases the potency of the drug. Trisulfapyrimidines have a longer duration of action than other sulfonamides and are considered to be poorly soluble in water. With the low doses of the three drugs, crystal formation in the urine is less likely to occur. Older sulfonamides (e.g., sulfadiazine) have low solubility and may cause crystallization in the urine. The current sulfonamides (e.g., sulfisoxazole) have greater water solubility; therefore crystal formations in the urine and renal damage are unlikely. Table 30-2 lists and describes the sulfonamides.

Table 30–1

Pharmacokinetics of Selected Sulfonamides

Drug	Protein-Binding (%)	Half-Life (Hour)	Solubility in Urine
Short-Acting			
sulfadiazine (Microsulfon)	20-60	17	+1
sulfamethizole (Thiosulfil)	90	2.5	+3
sulfisoxazole (Gantrisin)	90	5-7.5	+3
Intermediate-Acting			
sulfamethoxazole (Gantanol)	85-90	11	+1
sulfasalazine (Azulfidine)	99	5-10	+1
trimethoprim-sulfamethoxazole	50-65	8-12	+1-2

Table 30–2

Antibacterials: Sulfonamides

Generic (Brand)	Route and Dosage	Uses and Considerations
Short-Acting		
sulfadiazine (Microsulfon)	A: PO: LD: 2-4 g; then 2-4 g/d in 4-6 divided doses C: >2 mo: PO: LD: 75 mg/kg; then 150 mg/kg/d in 4-6 divided doses	For treatment of systemic infections. This drug could be classified as a short-immediate-acting sulfonamide. When taking this drug, increase the fluid intake to >2000 ml/d. *Pregnancy category:* C; PB: 20%-30%; t$^1/_2$: 8-12 h
sulfamethizole (Sulfasol, Thiosulfil Forte)	A: PO: 0.5-1 g in 3-4 divided doses C: PO: 30-45 mg/kg/d in 4 divided doses	For treatment of urinary tract infections. It is highly soluble. Fluid intake should be at least 2000 ml/d. *Pregnancy category:* C; PB: 90%; t$^1/_2$: 1.5 h
sulfisoxazole (Gantrisin)	A: PO: LD: 2-4 g; then 4-8 g/d in 4-6 divided doses C: >2 mo: PO: LD: 75 mg/kg; then 150 mg/kg/d in 4-6 divided doses; *max:* 6 g/d	Popular drug for treating urinary tract infections because it is more soluble in urine. Rapidly absorbed from GI tract. Used for treatment and prophylaxis of otitis media. Often ordered with a one-time initial loading dose. Fluid intake ≥2000 ml/d. *Pregnancy category:* C; PB: 85%-95%; t$^1/_2$: 4.5-7.5 h
Intermediate-Acting		
sulfamethoxazole (Gantanol)	A: PO: LD: 2 g; then 2-3 g/d in 2-3 divided doses for 7-10 d C: >2 mo: PO: LD: 50-60 mg/kg; then 25-30 mg/kg q12h; *max:* 75 mg/kg/d	For urinary tract infections, otitis media, and meningococcal A strain meningitis prophylaxis. Similar to Gantrisin, except it is absorbed and excreted slowly. Fluid intake should be at least 2000 ml/d. *Pregnancy category:* C; PB: 60%-70%; t$^1/_2$: 7-12 h
sulfasalazine (Azulfidine, Salazopyrin)	A: PO: Initially: 1 g q6-8h; maint: 2 g q6h C: >2 y: PO: Initially: 40-50 mg/kg/d in 4-6 divided doses; maint: 20-30 mg/kg/d in 4 divided doses; *max:* 2 g/d	For treatment of ulcerative colitis, Crohn's disease, rheumatoid arthritis (some cases). Take after eating. Side effects include nausea, vomiting, bloody diarrhea. *Pregnancy category:* C (near term: D); PB: 99%; t$^1/_2$: 5.5 h
trimethoprim-sulfamethoxazole: co-trimoxazole (Bactrim, Septra)	See Prototype Drug Chart 30–1.	

A, Adult; *C*, child; *d*, day; *h*, hour; *LD*, loading dose; *maint*, maintenance; *max*, maximum; *mo*, month; *PB*, protein-binding; *PO*, by mouth; *t$^1/_2$*, half-life; *y*, year; >, greater than; ≥, greater than or equal to.

Side Effects and Adverse Reactions

Side effects of sulfonamides may include an allergic response such as skin rash and itching. Anaphylaxis is not common. Blood disorders, such as hemolytic anemia, aplastic anemia, and low white blood cell and platelet counts, could result from prolonged use and high dosages. GI disturbances (anorexia, nausea, vomiting) may also occur. The early sulfonamides were insoluble in acid urine; thus **crystalluria** (crystals in urine) and hematuria were common problems. Crystalluria occurs less commonly with sulfisoxazole (Gantrisin) than it does with sulfadiazine and sulfamethoxazole. Increasing fluid intake dilutes the drug, which helps to prevent crystalluria from occurring. **Photosensitivity** can occur, so the client should avoid sunbathing and excess ultraviolet light. **Cross-sensitivity** might occur with the different sulfonamides but does not occur with other antibacterial drugs. Sulfonamides should be avoided during the third trimester of pregnancy.

Trimethoprim and Co-Trimoxazole

Trimethoprim (Proloprim, Trimpex) is an antibacterial agent that interferes with bacterial folic acid synthesis similarly to sulfonamides. Trimethoprim is classified as a urinary tract antiinfective that may be used alone for uncomplicated urinary tract infections. This drug is effective against the gram-negative bacteria *Proteus* spp., *Klebsiella* spp., and *E. coli*. In the 1970s it was combined with the sulfonamide sulfamethoxazole (an intermediate-acting sulfonamide) to prevent bacterial resistance to sulfonamide drugs and to obtain a better response against many organisms. Giving both drugs together in one compound form causes bacterial resistance to develop much more slowly than if only one of the drugs was used alone. This combination drug, trimethoprim-sulfamethoxazole (TMP-SMZ) (co-trimoxazole; Bactrim, Septra) is commonly used. The drug ratio is 1:5: one part trimethoprim and five parts sul-

PREVENTING MEDICATION ERRORS

Do not confuse...

• **Septra** (an antibacterial) with **Sectral** (a beta-adrenergic antagonist that is used to manage dysrhythmias). These two drugs look alike, but the actions and pharmacology are very different.

PROTOTYPE DRUG CHART 30–1

CO-TRIMOXAZOLE/TMP-SMZ

Drug Class

Antibacterials: sulfonamides
Trade Name: Bactrim, Septra
Pregnancy Category: C

Dosage

A: **PO:** 160/800 mg q12h (160 mg [TMP]/800 mg [SMZ])
IV: 8-10 mg/kg/d in 2-4 divided doses; infuse over 1 to 1.5 h
C: **PO:** <40 kg: 4 mg/kg/d in 2 divided doses
PO: >40 kg: same as adult
IV: >2 mo: same as adult
NOTE: Sulfa drugs should *not* be used in infants <2 months.
Dosage may vary according to the severity of the health problem.
Dosing is based on trimethoprim component.

Contraindications

Severe renal or hepatic disease, hypersensitivity to sulfonamides

Drug-Lab-Food Interactions

Drug: *Increase* anticoagulant effect with warfarin; *increase* hypoglycemic effect with an oral hypoglycemic drug
Lab: May *increase* BUN, serum creatinine, AST, ALT, ALP

Pharmacokinetics

Absorption: PO: Well absorbed
Distribution: PB: 50%-65%; crosses placenta
Metabolism: t½: 8-12 h
Excretion: In urine as metabolites

Pharmacodynamics

PO: Onset: 0.5-1 h
Peak: 2-4 h
Duration: UK
IV: Onset: Immediate
Peak: 0.5-1 h
Duration: UK

Therapeutic Effects/Uses

To treat urinary tract infection, otitis media, bronchitis, pneumonia, *Pneumocystis carinii* infection, rheumatic fever, burns
Mode of Action: Inhibition of protein synthesis of nucleic acids; bactericidal effect

Side Effects

Anorexia, nausea, vomiting, diarrhea, rash, stomatitis, fatigue, depression, headache, vertigo, photosensitivity

Adverse Reactions

Life-threatening: Leukopenia, thrombocytopenia, increased bone marrow depression, hemolytic anemia, aplastic anemia, agranulocytosis, Stevens-Johnson syndrome, renal failure

A, Adult; *ALP,* alkaline phosphatase; *ALT,* alanine aminotransferase; *AST,* aspartate aminotransferase; *BUN,* blood urea nitrogen; *C,* child; *d,* day; *h,* hour; *IV,* intravenous; *PB,* protein-binding; *PO,* by mouth; *SMZ,* sulfamethoxazole; *TMP,* trimethoprim; *t½,* half-life; *UK,* unknown; < greater than; > less than.

famethoxazole. The two drugs have a **synergistic effect**, increasing the desired drug response.

TMP-SMZ is effective in treating urinary, intestinal, and lower respiratory tract infections; otitis media; prostatitis; and gonorrhea; and in preventing *Pneumocystis carinii* in clients with acquired immunodeficiency syndrome (AIDS). Increased fluid intake is highly recommended to prevent any complications, such as crystallization in the urine. Prototype Drug Chart 30-1 describes the pharmacologic behavior of TMP-SMZ.

Pharmacokinetics

TMP-SMZ (Bactrim, Septra) is well absorbed from the GI tract and is moderately protein bound. Its half-life is 8 to 12 hours; thus it is administered twice a day. It is excreted as unchanged metabolites in the urine.

Pharmacodynamics

The combination of TMP-SMZ is generically called *co-trimoxazole* in many countries. Trimethoprim, a nonsulfonamide antibiotic, enhances the activity of the drug combination. Co-trimoxazole blocks steps in bacterial synthesis of protein and nucleic acid, producing a bactericidal effect.

Co-trimoxazole (TMP-SMZ) can be administered orally or intravenously (IV). Orally, the drug has a moderately rapid onset of action; the drug action is immediate via the IV route. Serum peak concentration time for oral use is 2 to 4 hours and 0.5 to 1 hour for IV use. Co-trimoxazole increases the hypoglycemic response when taken with an oral hypoglycemic agent sulfonylurea. It can also increase the activity of oral anticoagulants.

Side Effects and Adverse Reactions

Side effects of co-trimoxazole may include mild to moderate rashes, anorexia, nausea, vomiting and diarrhea, stomatitis, crystalluria, and photosensitivity. Serious adverse reactions are rare; however, agranulocytosis, aplastic anemia, and allergic myocarditis have been reported as possible life-threatening conditions. Clients with AIDS are more susceptible to TMP-SMZ toxicity.

Topical and Ophthalmic Sulfonamides

Sulfonamides can be administered for topical and ophthalmic uses. Topical use of sulfonamides can cause hypersensitivity reactions; therefore they are not frequently used. Mafenide acetate (Sulfamylon) is a sulfonamide derivative prescribed for second- and third-degree burns to prevent sepsis. Silver sulfadiazine (Silvadene) is another topical sulfonamide used to treat burns. Both of these drugs are discussed in more detail in Chapter 47, Drugs for Disorders of the Eye and Ear.

Sulfacetamide sodium (AK-Sulf, Cetamide, Isopto Cetamide, Sodium Sulamyd, Sulf-10) is a sulfonamide for ophthalmic and topical uses. For the ophthalmic preparations (liquid/drop and ointment), sulfacetamide sodium is used to treat conjunctivitis and corneal ulcers. It is used as prophylactic treatment after an eye injury or the removal of a foreign body. Do *not* use ointment for the eye unless it has "ophthalmic" printed on the drug label. Sulfacetamide sodium is discussed in more detail in Chapter 47, Drugs for Disorders of the Eye and the Ear.

Topical sulfacetamide sodium for the skin is an ointment and is used to treat seborrheic dermatitis and secondary bacterial skin infections. This form is *not* used for the eye.

Nursing Process

Antibacterials: Sulfonamides

ASSESSMENT

■ Assess client's renal function by checking urinary output (>600 ml/d), blood urea nitrogen (normal, 8 to 25 mg/dl), and serum creatinine (normal, 0.5 to 1.5 mg/dl).

■ Obtain a medical history from client. Sulfonamides such as co-trimoxazole (trimethoprim-sulfamethoxazole [Bactrim, Septra]) are contraindicated for clients with severe renal or liver disease.

■ Determine whether client is hypersensitive to sulfonamides. An allergic reaction can include rash, skin eruptions, and itching. A severe hypersensitivity reaction includes **erythema multiforme** (erythematous macular, papular, or vesicular eruption; if severe, can cover the entire body) or **exfoliative dermatitis** (desquamation, scaling, and itching of skin).

■ Obtain a drug history of drugs client currently takes. Oral antidiabetic drugs (sulfonylureas) with sulfonamides increase the hypoglycemic effect; the use of warfarin with sulfonamides increases the anticoagulant effect.

■ Assess baseline laboratory results, especially complete blood count (CBC). Blood dyscrasias may occur as a result of high doses of sulfonamides over a continuous period, causing life-threatening conditions.

NURSING DIAGNOSES

■ Risk for infection
■ Risk for impaired tissue integrity
■ Impaired urinary elimination

PLANNING

■ Client's infection will be controlled and later alleviated.

NURSING INTERVENTIONS

■ Administer sulfonamides with a full glass of water. Extra fluid intake can prevent crystalluria and kidney stone formation.

■ Record client's intake and output. Urine output should be at least 1200 ml/d to decrease the risk of crystalluria. The sulfonamides sulfadiazine and sulfamethoxazole are more likely to cause crystalluria than sulfisoxazole (Gantrisin) and combination drugs. Fluid intake should be at least 2000 ml/d.

■ Monitor vital signs. Note if client's temperature has decreased.

■ Observe client for hematologic reaction that may lead to life-threatening anemias. Early signs are sore throat, purpura, and decreasing white blood cell and platelet counts. Check client's CBC and compare with baseline findings.

■ Check for signs and symptoms of superinfection (secondary infection caused by a different organism than the primary infection). Symptoms include stomatitis (mouth ulcers), furry black tongue, anal or genital discharge, and itching.

Client Teaching

General

• Instruct client to drink several quarts of fluid daily while taking sulfonamides to avoid the complication of crystalluria.

• Advise pregnant woman to avoid sulfonamides during the last 3 months of pregnancy.

• Inform client not to take antacids with sulfonamides because antacids decrease the absorption rate.

• Warn client who has an allergy to one sulfonamide that all sulfonamide preparations should be avoided, with the health care provider's approval, because of the possibility of cross-sensitivity. Observe the client for rash or any skin eruptions.

Self-Administration

• Teach client to take the sulfonamide 1 hour before or 2 hours after meals with a full glass of water.

Side Effects

• Direct client to report bruising or bleeding that could be a result of drug-induced blood disorder. Advise the client to have blood cell count monitored on a regular basis.

• Advise client to avoid direct sunlight and to use sun block and protective clothing to decrease the risk of photosensitive reactions.

Cultural Considerations ⊕

- Respect cultural beliefs and values regarding alternative methods for treating infections. Explain the purpose of the drug therapy and how often the drug should be taken.
- Communicate that client should increase fluid intake to 10 to 12 glasses per day. Written instructions may be necessary if the client's cultural background prevents understanding of the health problem and drug regimen.

EVALUATION

- ▪ Evaluate the effectiveness of the sulfonamide by determining whether the infection has been alleviated and the blood cell count is within normal range.

WEBSITES

For further information on *Antibacterials: Sulfonimides,* visit these Internet resources:

Information on Bactrim:
www.infagra.com/b/bactrim.html

More information on Bactrim:
www.nlm.nih.gov/medlineplus/druginfo/uspdi/202781.html

Critical Thinking Case Study

R.M., age 46, has a severe urinary tract infection (UTI). She takes TMP-SMZ (co-trimoxazole) 160 mg/800 mg every 6 hours.

1. Is the dose within the recommended drug dose and dosing interval? What is the nurse's responsibility?
2. What are the similarities and differences between trimethoprim-sulfamethoxazole (co-trimoxazole) and sulfisoxazole?
3. What are the signs of thrombocytopenia, hemolytic anemia, and agranulocytosis for clients who take high doses of sulfonamides? Explain the assessment and nursing interventions regarding these severe adverse reactions to sulfonamides.

Client teaching is an important part of nursing interventions. Explain the nurse's role regarding client teaching concerning the following:

4. What is the required amount of daily fluid intake?
5. What are the cross-sensitive effects if a client is allergic to other sulfonamide preparations? What allergic reactions may occur?
6. What time of day should sulfonamides be taken?
7. Why should bruising and bleeding be reported?
8. What protective measures should be taken to prevent possible photosensitive reaction?

R.M. takes the anticoagulant Coumadin 7.5 mg a day.

9. What effect does co-trimoxazole have on warfarin (Coumadin), and what is the nursing responsibility? Should R.M.'s Coumadin dosage be increased or decreased? Explain.

Study Questions

1. Why would a nurse instruct a client taking a sulfonamide to increase fluid intake? Why is the use of sun block indicated for sun exposure for a client taking a sulfonamide drug?
2. If your client is allergic to a sulfonamide drug, what should you advise the client about the use of other sulfonamides?
3. What is the generic name for Gantrisin? What is its main clinical use? Is it classified as a short-acting, intermediate-acting, or long-acting sulfonamide?
4. What is the purpose of the drug trimethoprim-sulfamethoxazole/co-trimoxazole (Bactrim, Septra)?
5. Your client takes a sulfonylurea (oral hypoglycemic to promote insulin production). What effect may co-trimoxazole (TMP-SMZ) have on the sulfonylurea? What is the nurse's responsibility if the client receives both drugs?
6. What effects can co-trimoxazole (TMP-SMZ) have on the following laboratory tests: aspartate aminotransferase, alanine aminotransferase, alkaline phosphatase, blood urea nitrogen, serum creatinine?
7. What hematologic conditions can occur because of excessive or long-term use of sulfonamides such as co-trimoxazole (TMP-SMZ)?

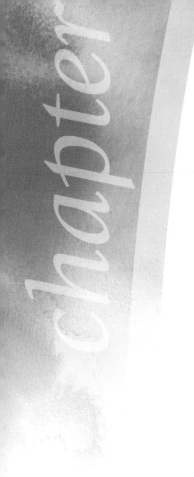

31 Antitubercular Drugs, Antifungal Drugs, Peptides, and Metronidazole

ELECTRONIC RESOURCES

Additional information can be found on the companion website at *http://evolve.elsevier.com/KeeHayes/pharmacology/* or on the companion CD-ROM, which includes:

- *NCLEX-style examination review questions*
- *Pharmacology animations*
- *Medication error and (IV) therapy checklists*
- *Medication calculation problems*
- *Electronic calculators*

OBJECTIVES

- Differentiate between first-line and second-line antitubercular drugs and give examples of each.
- Compare the five groups of antifungal drugs.
- Identify examples of polyenes and explain their uses.
- Differentiate between the adverse reactions of antitubercular, antifungal, and peptide drugs.
- Describe the nursing interventions, including client teaching, for clients taking antitubercular, antifungal, and peptide drugs.
- Give the uses for metronidazole.

TERMS

acquired immunodefi-
ciency syndrome (AIDS)
antifungal drugs
antimycotic drugs
antitubercular drugs

first-line drugs
hepatotoxicity
human immunodeficiency
virus (HIV)

neurotoxicity
opportunistic infection
paresthesias

peptides
prophylaxis
second-line drugs

Introduction

This chapter covers antitubercular, antifungal, and peptide drugs, as well as metronidazole. Although these drug categories differ from each other, they each contain drugs that inhibit or kill organisms that cause diseases.

Tuberculosis

Tuberculosis (TB) is caused by the acid-fast bacillus *Mycobacterium tuberculosis*. The pathogen is frequently called the *tubercle bacillus*. TB is one of the world's major health problems, and it kills more persons than any other infectious disease, including **acquired immunodeficiency syndrome (AIDS)**. More than 1.5 billion people in the world have TB, and many are unaware of their infection. Each year more than 8 million new cases of TB are diagnosed. Until the 1980s the occurrence of TB had decreased in the United States. This increase in TB can be attributed, in part, to the increase in persons with AIDS in whom active TB has developed because of their compromised immune systems. In addition, the increasing incidence is partly a result of increasingly crowded living conditions in urban areas. Clients susceptible to TB are those with alcohol addiction, AIDS, and debilitative conditions. Since 1993 the reported numbers of clients with active TB have declined slightly.

Pathophysiology

Tuberculosis is transmitted from one person to another by droplets dispersed in the air through coughing and sneezing. The organisms are inhaled into the alveoli (air sacs) of the lung. When the immune system is compromised, the tubercle bacilli can spread from the lungs to other organs of the body via the blood and lymphatic system. However, if the body's immune system is strong or intact, the phagocytes stop the multiplication of the tubercle bacilli. Dissemination of TB bacilli can be found in the liver, kidneys, spleen, and other organs. Symptoms of TB include anorexia, cough and sputum production, increased fever, night sweats, weight loss, and positive acid-fast bacilli in the sputum.

Antitubercular Drugs

Before 1944, many people died from TB because of the absence of drug therapy. Streptomycin, a parenteral antibiotic, was the first drug used to treat TB. Isoniazid (INH), discovered in 1952, was the first oral drug preparation effective against the tubercle bacillus. Isoniazid is a bactericidal drug that inhibits cell wall synthesis and blocks pyridoxine (vitamin B_6), which is used for intracellular enzyme production. When isoniazid is prescribed, usually pyridoxine is also prescribed to avoid possible occurrence of peripheral neuropathy. Group names for drugs used to treat TB include *antimycobacterial agents* and **antitubercular drugs.**

Prophylactic antitubercular therapy is suggested for persons who have been in close contact with persons with TB and for those who test positive for **human immunodeficiency virus (HIV)** who also have a positive TB skin test or are in close contact with someone who has TB. Clients who have converted from a negative to a positive TB skin test should be considered candidates for prophylactic isoniazid therapy. Young children who have been in contact with persons with active TB are at high risk and should receive prophylactic antitubercular therapy. When a person is diagnosed with TB, family members are usually given prophylactic doses of isoniazid for 6 months to 1 year. For HIV-positive clients with positive TB skin tests, a 2-month prophylactic treatment with rifampin and pyrazinamide may be recommended.

Prophylactic therapy is contraindicated for persons with liver disease. Isoniazid is the primary antitubercular drug used and may cause isoniazid-induced liver damage. Other antitubercular drugs may also cause liver damage if given in high doses over an extended period.

Single-drug therapy with isoniazid proved ineffective in treating TB because resistance to the drug developed in a short time. It was discovered that, when a combination of antitubercular drugs was used, bacterial resistance did not occur. In fact, the duration of treatment was reduced from 2 years to 6 to 9 months. Different combinations of drugs can be used, such as (1) isoniazid and rifampin; (2) isoniazid, rifampin, and ethambutol; or (3) isoniazid, rifampin, and pyrazinamide. Rifampin and ethambutol were discovered in the early 1960s, and neither drug is effective against the tubercle bacillus when given alone. In fact, if rifampin is taken alone, bacterial resistance occurs quickly. Prototype Drug Chart 31–1 lists the drug data for isoniazid. Figure 31–1 provides charts used to keep records of clients taking antitubercular drugs.

Multidrug therapy against TB is more effective. The treatment regimen is divided into two phases: the first or the initial phase is for 2 months, and the second phase is the next 4 to 7 months. The total treatment plan is for 6 to 9 months and depends on the response to the antituber-

PROTOTYPE DRUG CHART 31–1

ISONIAZID

Drug Class

Antitubercular drug
Trade Name: INH, Nydrazid, Laniazid, 🍁 Isotamine, PMS-Isoniazid
Pregnancy Category: C

Dosage

A: PO/IM: 5 mg/kg/d in single dose; *max:* 300 mg/d
Prophylaxis: 300 mg/d
C: PO/IM: 10-20 mg/kg/d in single dose; *max:* 300 mg/d
Prophylaxis: 10 mg/kg/d in a single dose or 15 mg/kg 3×/wk

Contraindications

Severe renal or hepatic disease, alcoholism, diabetic retinopathy

Drug-Lab-Food Interactions

Drug: Increase effect with alcohol, rifampin, cycloserine, and phenytoin; decreases GI absorption while taking aluminum antacids
Lab: Increase AST, ALT, bilirubin

Pharmacokinetics

Absorption: PO: Well absorbed
Distribution: PB: 10%
Metabolism: t½: 1-4 h
Excretion: 50% unchanged in urine

Pharmacodynamics

PO: Onset: 0.5 h
 Peak: 1-2 h
 Duration: 6-8 h
IM: Peak: 1-2 h
 Duration: 6 h

Therapeutic Effects/Uses

To treat tuberculosis; prophylactic measure against tuberculosis
Mode of Action: Inhibition of bacterial cell-wall synthesis

Side Effects

Drowsiness, tremors, rash, blurred vision, photosensitivity, tinnitus, dizziness, nausea, vomiting, dry mouth, constipation

Adverse Reactions

Psychotic behavior, peripheral neuropathy, vitamin B₆ deficiency
Life-threatening: Blood dyscrasias, thrombocytopenia, seizures, agranulocytosis, hepatotoxicity

A, Adult; *ALT,* alanine aminotransferase; *AST,* aspartate aminotransferase; *C,* child; *d,* day; *GI,* gastrointestinal; *h,* hour; *IM,* intramuscular; *max,* maximum; *PB,* protein-binding; *PO,* by mouth; *t½,* half-life; *wk,* week; 🍁, Canadian drug name.

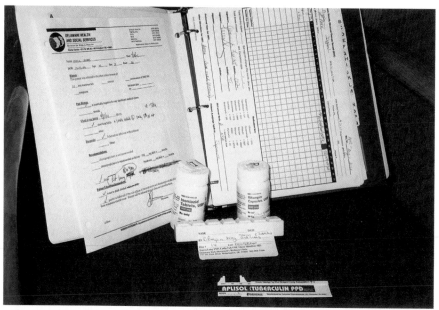

FIGURE 31–1 When giving multiple drugs for treatment of tuberculosis, such as isoniazid and rifampin, record keeping is essential to ensure that the client is taking the prescribed antituberculin drugs.

Table 31–1

Possible Drug Regimens for Tuberculosis

Phase	Example I	Example II	Example III	Example IV
First phase (2 mo)*	isoniazid, rifampin	isoniazid, rifampin, pyrazinamide	isoniazid, rifampin, streptomycin	isoniazid, rifampin, pyrazinamide, kanamycin or ciprofloxacin
Second phase (4-7 mo)	isoniazid, rifampin	isoniazid, rifampin, ethambutol	isoniazid, rifampin, capreomycin or cycloserine	isoniazid, rifampin, ethambutol, streptomycin or kanamycin or ciprofloxacin or clarithromycin or capreomycin

mo, Month.
*If there is bacterial resistance to isoniazid, the first phase of the drug regimen may be rifampin, ethambutol, and pyrazinamide. Adjust drug regimen according to drug susceptibility. The health care provider determines which antitubercular drug and how many combinations to use. Symptoms for drug toxicity should be closely monitored. Examples III and IV may be used in various combinations for multidrug resistance.

cular therapy. Table 31–1 gives examples of various drug regimens to treat TB.

If multidrug resistance to the tubercle bacilli persists, other antibacterial drugs such as the aminoglycosides (streptomycin, kanamycin, amikacin) or the fluoroquinolones (ciprofloxacin, ofloxacin) may be given as part of the multidrug therapy. Susceptibility testing to determine drug resistance should be performed before drug therapy. At times, susceptibility testing of the sputum and antitubercular drugs is performed only if the client has not responded to the drug therapy regimen.

Mycobacterium tuberculosis strains that are resistant to streptomycin can be sensitive to kanamycin. An aminoglycoside should not be taken if renal dysfunction is present. When antibacterial agents are used continuously or at high doses, the serum drug level should be closely monitored to avoid drug toxicity.

Pharmacokinetics

Isoniazid is well absorbed from the gastrointestinal (GI) tract. It can also be administered intramuscularly (IM). It has a very low protein-binding rate (10%), and its half-life is 1 to 4 hours. Isoniazid is metabolized by the liver, and 75% to 95% of the drug is excreted in the urine.

Pharmacodynamics

Isoniazid inhibits cell-wall synthesis of the tubercle bacillus. It is usually prescribed with other antitubercular agents. The onset of action and peak concentration time for oral and IM routes of isoniazid are the same. Peripheral neuropathy is an adverse reaction to isoniazid; thus pyridoxine (vitamin B6) is usually taken with isoniazid to decrease the probability of neuropathy. Alcohol ingestion with the drug can increase the incidence of peripheral neuropathy. If phenytoin is taken with isoniazid, the effect of phenytoin may be decreased. Antacids decrease isoniazid absorption.

Antitubercular drugs are divided into two categories: first-line and second-line drugs. **First-line drugs** (isoniazid, rifampin, rifabutin, rifapentine, pyrazinamide, ethambutol, and streptomycin) are considered more effective and less toxic than second-line drugs in treating TB. Rifapentine, analog of rifampin, is the newest first-line drug for treating TB. The client takes it only twice a week, unlike rifampin, which is given daily. To avoid resistance, rifapentine should be combined with another antitubercular drug. **Second-line drugs** (*para*-aminosalicylic acid, kanamycin, cycloserine, ethionamide, capreomycin, pyrazinamide, and others) are not as

effective as first-line drugs and some can be more toxic. Second-line drugs may be used in combination with first-line drugs, especially to treat disseminated TB. First-line drugs and some second-line drugs are described in Table 31–2.

Side Effects and Adverse Reactions

Side effects and adverse reactions differ according to the drug prescribed. For isoniazid, peripheral neuropathy can be a problem, especially for those who are malnourished, have diabetes mellitus, or are alcoholics. This condition can be prevented if pyridoxine (vitamin B6) is administered. **Hepatotoxicity** is an adverse reaction to isoniazid, from which hepatitis can result. Clients with liver disorders should not take isoniazid or isoniazid and rifampin unless liver enzymes are closely monitored. Rifampin can increase liver enzyme levels.

Nursing Process

Antitubercular Drugs

ASSESSMENT

■ Determine a history from client of any past instances of tuberculosis, last purified protein derivative (PPD) tuberculin test and reaction, last chest radiograph and result, and any allergies to the antitubercular drugs if taken previously.

■ Obtain a medical history from the client. Most antitubercular drugs are contraindicated if the client has a severe hepatic disease.

■ Check laboratory tests for liver enzyme values, bilirubin, blood urea nitrogen (BUN), and serum creatinine. These baseline values can be compared with future laboratory test results.

■ Evaluate client for signs and symptoms of peripheral neuropathy, such as numbness or tingling of the extremities.

■ Assess client for hearing changes if the antitubercular drug regimen includes streptomycin. Ototoxicity is an adverse reaction to streptomycin.

NURSING DIAGNOSES

■ Risk for infection
■ Risk for impaired tissue integrity

PLANNING

■ Client's sputum test for acid-fast bacilli will be negative 2 to 3 months after the prescribed antitubercular therapy.

NURSING INTERVENTIONS

■ Administer the commonly ordered antitubercular drug isoniazid (INH) 1 hour before or 2 hours after meals. Food decreases absorption rate.
■ Give pyridoxine (vitamin B₆) as prescribed with isoniazid to prevent peripheral neuropathy.
■ Monitor serum liver enzyme levels, especially if the client takes isoniazid or rifampin. Elevated levels may indicate liver toxicity.
■ Collect sputum specimens for acid-fast bacilli early in the morning. Usually three consecutive morning sputum specimens are sent to the laboratory, and the routine is repeated several weeks later.
■ Have eye examinations performed on clients taking isoniazid and ethambutol. Visual disturbances may result in clients taking these antitubercular drugs.
■ Emphasize the importance of complying with the drug regimen.

Client Teaching

General
- Instruct client to take the antitubercular drug such as isoniazid 1 hour before meals or 2 hours after meals for better absorption.
- Direct client to take the antitubercular drugs as prescribed. Ineffective treatment of tuberculosis might occur if the drugs are taken intermittently or discontinued when symptoms are decreased or when client is feeling better. Compliance with the drug regimen is a must.
- Teach client not to take antacids while taking antitubercular drugs because they decrease drug absorption. The client should also avoid alcohol because it may increase the risk of hepatotoxicity.
- Advise client to keep medical appointments and to participate in sputum testing. Sputum testing is important to determine the effectiveness of the drug regimen.
- Warn woman contemplating pregnancy to first check with her health care provider about taking the antitubercular drugs ethambutol and rifampin.

Side Effects
- Guide client to report any numbness, tingling, or burning of the hands and feet. Peripheral neuritis is a common side effect of isoniazid. Vitamin B₆ prevents peripheral neuropathy. Neuritis may not occur if client eats a balanced diet daily.

- Encourage client to avoid direct sunlight to decrease the risk of photosensitivity. Client should use sun block while in the sun.
- Inform client taking rifampin that urine, feces, saliva, sputum, sweat, and tears may be a harmless red-orange color. Soft contact lenses may be permanently stained.
- Alert client receiving ethambutol to take daily single doses to avoid visual problems. Divided doses of ethambutol may cause visual disturbances.

Cultural Considerations ⊕
- Explain to clients from various cultural backgrounds who have active tuberculosis that their family members should get a tubercular skin test and may receive a prophylactic drug for 6 months to 1 year. Emphasize the importance of their family members seeking medical care.
- Provide a written sheet for their drug and treatment regimens. Explain the importance of good hygiene, such as discarding tissues that contain sputum, separating dishes, and using a dishwasher to clean dishes.
- Understand significance of community if multiple individuals in same community are treated for latent tuberculosis infection. Make all attempts to place on some treatment plan to increase compliance through social support.

EVALUATION

■ Evaluate the effectiveness of the antitubercular drugs. Sputum specimen for acid-fast bacilli should be negative after taking antitubercular drugs for several weeks or months.

Antifungal Drugs

Antifungal drugs, also called **antimycotic drugs,** are used to treat two types of fungal infections: (1) *superficial fungal infections* of the skin or mucous membrane and (2) *systemic fungal infections* of the lung or central nervous system. Fungal infections may be mild, such as tinea pedis (athlete's foot), or severe, such as in pulmonary conditions or meningitis. Fungi, such as *Candida* spp. (yeast), are part of the normal flora of the mouth, skin, intestine, and vagina. Candidiasis might occur as an **opportunistic infection** when the body's defense mechanisms are impaired, allowing overgrowth of the fungus. Drugs such as antibiotics, oral contraceptives, and immunosuppressives may alter the body's defense mechanisms. Opportunistic fungal infections can be mild (e.g., yeast infection in the vagina) or severe (e.g., systemic fungal infection).

The antifungal drugs are classified into the following groups (Table 31–3):
- Polyenes (e.g., amphotericin B and nystatin)
- Azoles (e.g., ketoconazole)
- Antimetabolites (e.g., flucytosine)
- Antiprotozoals (e.g., atovaquone)
- Echinocandins (e.g., caspofungin)

Table 31-2

Antitubercular Drugs

Generic (Brand)	Route and Dosage	Uses and Considerations
First-Line Drugs		
ethambutol HCl (Myambutol)	A: PO: 15 mg/kg as a single dose *Retreatment:* A: PO: 25 mg/kg as a single dose for 2 mo; then decrease to 15 mg/kg/d C: >12 y: same as adult	Used as a combination drug for active TB. Decrease dose if renal insufficiency is present. *Pregnancy category:* C; PB: 10%-20%; $t^{1}/_{2}$: 3-4 h (8 h with renal dysfunction)
isoniazid (INH, Nydrazid)	See Prototype Drug Chart 31-1.	
pyrazinamide (🍁 Tebrazid)	A: PO: 20-35 mg/kg/d in 3-4 divided doses; *max:* 3 g/d	Used in combination with other antitubercular drugs for short-term and initial phase of therapy. Promote fluid intake. *Pregnancy category:* C; PB: 10%-20%; $t^{1}/_{2}$: 9.5 h
rifabutin (Mycobutin)	A: PO: 300 mg/d in 1 or 2 divided doses C: PO: 75 mg d	To treat *Mycobacterium tuberculosis* infection; to prevent disseminated *Mycobacterium avium* complex disease in clients with advanced HIV infection. *Pregnancy category:* B; PB: 85%; $t^{1}/_{2}$: 16-69 h
rifampin (Rifadin, Rimactane)	A: PO: 600 mg/d as a single dose C: PO: 10-20 mg/kg/d as a single dose; *max:* 600 mg/d	Used as a combination drug for active TB. For selective gram-positive and gram-negative bacteria, including *Neisseria meningitidis.* Liver enzymes should be monitored. *Pregnancy category:* C; PB: 85%-90%; $t^{1}/_{2}$: 3 h
rifapentine (Priftin)	A: PO: 600 mg × 2 wk for 2 mo, then 600 mg once per wk for 4 mo	To treat TB. Intervals between dose should be at least 72 h. Monitor for toxicity if drug is taken with an anticoagulant, anticonvulsant, or digoxin. It is contraindicated with oral contraceptives. *Pregnancy category:* C; PB: 97.7%; $t^{1}/_{2}$: 13.3 h
streptomycin SO$_4$	A: IM: 1 g daily or 7-15 mg/kg/d for 2-3 mo, then 2-3 times per wk C: IM: 20-40 mg/kg/d in divided doses	Used against TB as the third drug with isoniazid and rifampin or with isoniazid and ethambutol. First drug used to treat TB. *Pregnancy category:* C; PB: 30%; $t^{1}/_{2}$: 2-3 h
Second-Line Drugs		
aminosalicylate sodium, P.A.S. sodium	A: PO: 14-16 g/d in 2-3 divided doses C: PO: 275-420 mg/kg/d in 3-4 divided doses; take with food	Second-line antitubercular drug. To treat pulmonary and extrapulmonary TB. Used in combination with other antitubercular drugs. Take after meals to reduce gastric irritation. *Pregnancy category:* C; PB: 15%; $t^{1}/_{2}$: 1 h
capreomycin (Capastat)	A: IM: 1 g/d for 2-4 mo, then 1 g, 2-3 times per wk C: IM: 15 mg/kg/d	It is sensitive to the bacillus *Mycobacterium tuberculosis.* It should be used in combination with other antitubercular drugs; it is not effective when used alone. It is useful when the first-line drug is resistant to the bacilli. Hearing loss is an adverse reaction. Client should take pyridoxine (vitamin B$_6$) to avoid peripheral neuropathy. *Pregnancy category:* C; PB: UK; $t^{1}/_{2}$: 3-6 h
cycloserine (Seromycin)	A: PO: 250 mg q12h for 2 wk; may increase to 500 mg, q12h; *max:* 1 g/d C: PO: 10-20 mg/kg/d in divided doses	Broad-spectrum antimycobacterial drug for the treatment of TB. It is a second-line drug and is used when first-line drugs fail. Cycloserine should be used in combination with other antitubercular drugs. *Pregnancy category:* C; PB: UK; $t^{1}/_{2}$: 10 h
ethionamide (Trecator-SC)	A: PO: 250 mg, q8-12h C: PO: 4-5 mg/kg/q8h; *max:* 1 g/d	Like isoniazid, it is effective against the tubercle bacilli. It is used when first-line drugs fail. Client should take pyridoxine (vitamin B$_6$) to avoid peripheral neuropathy. Side effects include GI discomfort. **Caution:** Use with caution in persons with diabetes mellitus, alcoholism, and hepatic disorder. *Pregnancy category:* D; PB: UK; $t^{1}/_{2}$: 2-3 h

Other Second-Line Drugs

Kanamycin, amikacin, ciprofloxacin, and ofloxacin are effective against the tubercle bacilli in combination with antitubercular drugs. See Chapter 29, Antibacterials: Macrolides, Tetracyclines, Aminoglycosides, Fluoroquinolones.

A, Adult; *C,* child; *d,* day; *GI,* gastrointestinal; *h,* hour; *HIV,* human immunodeficiency virus; *IM,* intramuscular; *max,* maximum; *mo,* month; *PB,* protein-binding; *PO,* by mouth; $t^{1}/_{2}$, half-life; *TB,* tuberculosis; *UK,* unknown; *wk,* week; *y,* year; >, greater than, 🍁, Canadian drug.

Table 31–3

Antifungal Drugs

Generic (Brand)	Route and Dosage	Uses and Considerations
Polyenes		
amphotericin B (Fungizone)	*Test dose:* A: IV: 0.25-1 mg in 20 ml of D_5W infused over 20-30 min A: IV: 0.25-1 mg/kg/d in D_5W or 1.5 mg/kg every other day; *max:* 1.5 mg/kg/d C: IV: Same as adult, except dilution and infuse time differ	For treatment of a variety of systemic fungal (mycotic) infections, such as aspergillosis, blastomycosis, coccidioidomycosis, cryptococcosis, histoplasmosis. Nephrotoxicity may occur when given in high doses. Hypokalemia might occur. *Pregnancy category:* B; PB: 95%; $t^1/_2$: 24 h
nystatin (Mycostatin)	*Intestinal infections:* A: PO: 500,000-1,000,000 units 3 times/day or q8h *Oral candidiasis:* A: PO: 400,000-600,000 units q6-8h C: PO: 250,000-500,000 units q6h Neonate (<7 d): PO: 100,000 units q6h	To treat *Candida* infections. *Pregnancy category:* C; PB: $t^1/_2$: UK
Azoles		
fluconazole (Diflucan)	See Prototype Drug Chart 31–2.	
itraconazole (Sporanox)	A: PO: Loading dose: 200 mg q8h × 3 d; *maint:* 200 mg/d; *max:* 400 mg/d in two divided doses	Effective against various systemic fungal infections, particularly blastomycosis and histoplasmosis. *Pregnancy category:* C; PB: 99%; $t^1/_2$: 21-42 h
ketoconazole (Nizoral)	A: PO: 200-400 mg/d as a single dose C: >2 y: PO: 3.3-6.6 mg/kg/d as single dose C: <20 kg: PO: 50 mg/d	For infections by *Candida* spp., histoplasmosis, blastomycosis, and others. Treatment could last 1-6 mo for systemic infections. Take with food to avoid GI discomfort. *Pregnancy category:* C; PB: 95%; $t^1/_2$: 2-8 h
miconazole nitrate (Monistat, Micatin)	A: IV: 200-3600 mg/d in D_5W in three divided doses; infuse IV over 30-60 min C: IV: 20-40 mg/kg/d in divided doses; *max:* 15 mg/kg per inf A: Supp: 100 mg vaginal at bedtime for 7 d Available: Vaginal cream 2%; lotion	For fungal meningitis and fungal bladder infections. Also for vaginal fungal infections. *Pregnancy category:* B; PB: 92%; $t^1/_2$: 2-24 h
voriconazole (Vfend)	PO: >40 kg: 400 mg q12h on day 1, then 200 mg q12h, may increase to 300 mg q12h PO: <40 kg: 400 mg q12h on day 1 then 100 mg q12h, may increase to 150 mg q12h A/Elderly: IV: 6 mg/kg q12h day 1 then 4 mg/kg q12h	For treatment of *Aspergillosis* infection. *Pregnancy category:* D; PB: UK; $t^1/_2$: 6h-6 d
Antimetabolites		
flucytosine (Ancobon)	A: PO: 50-150 mg/kg/d in four divided doses C: >50 kg: PO: 50-150 mg/kg/d in 4 divided doses C: <50 kg: PO: 1.5-4.5 g/m^2/d in four divided doses Neonate: PO: 50-100 mg/kg/d in 1-2 divided doses	Use with amphotericin B may increase therapeutic action as well as toxicity. Fungal resistance occurs if the drug is given alone. *Pregnancy category:* C; PB: UK; $t^1/_2$: 3-6 h
Antiprotozoal		
atovaquone (Mepron)	A: PO: 750 mg b.i.d. with food × 21 d	For treatment of mild to moderate *Pneumocystis carinii* pneumonia. *Pregnancy category:* C; PB: 99%; $t^1/_2$: 2-3 d
Echinocandins		
caspofungin (Cancidas)	*Loading dose:* A: IV: 70 mg *Maintenance dose:* A: IV: 50 mg/d	For treatment of *Aspergillosis* infection. *Pregnancy category:* C; PB: UK $t^1/_2$: 9-11 h

A, Adult; *b.i.d.*, twice a day; *C*, child; *d*, day; *D_5W*, dextrose 5% in water; *GI*, gastrointestinal; *h*, hour; *inf*, infusion; *IV*, intravenous; *maint*, maintenance; *max*, maximum; *min*, minute; *mo*, month; *PB*, protein-binding; *PO*, by mouth; *supp*, suppository; *$t^1/_2$*, half-life; *t.i.d.*, three times a day; *UK*, unknown; *y*, year; >, greater than; <, less than.

Polyenes

Amphotericin B

The polyene antifungal drug of choice for treating severe systemic infection is amphotericin B. Introduced in 1956 and used currently with close supervision because of its toxicity, amphotericin B is effective against numerous fungal diseases, including histoplasmosis, cryptococcosis, coccidioidomycosis, aspergillosis, blastomycosis, and candidiasis (systemic infection).

Pharmacokinetics

Amphotericin B is highly protein bound and has a long half-life. Only 5% of the drug is excreted in the urine. Renal disease does not affect the excretion of amphotericin B.

Pharmacodynamics

Amphotericin B is not absorbed from the GI tract; therefore it is administered IV in low doses for treating systemic fungal infections. Peak effect occurs 1 to 2 hours after IV infusion, and the duration is 20 hours.

Side Effects and Adverse Reactions

Side effects and adverse reactions for amphotericin B include flush, fever, chills, nausea, vomiting, hypotension, paresthesias, and thrombophlebitis. Amphotericin B is considered *highly toxic* and can cause nephrotoxicity and electrolyte imbalance, especially hypokalemia and hypomagnesemia (low serum potassium and magnesium levels). Urinary output, blood urea nitrogen, and serum creatinine levels need to be closely monitored.

Nystatin

Nystatin (Mycostatin), another polyene antifungal drug, is administered orally or topically to treat candidal infection. It is available in suspensions, cream, ointment, and vaginal tablets. Nystatin is poorly absorbed via the GI tract; however, the oral tablet form is used for intestinal candidiasis. The more common use of nystatin is in oral suspension for candidal infection in the mouth. The client is instructed to swish the liquid within the mouth, making contact with the mucous membrane, and then to swallow the liquid after a few minutes. If the throat area is involved, instruct the client to gargle with nystatin after swishing and before swallowing.

Pharmacokinetics

Nystatin is poorly absorbed. Its protein-binding power and half-life are unknown. The drug is excreted unchanged in feces.

Pharmacodynamics

Nystatin increases permeability of the fungal cell membrane, thus causing the fungal cell to become unstable and to discharge the content. This drug has a fungistatic and fungicidal action. The onset of action for both suspension and tablet is rapid. The onset of action for vaginal tablet or cream is approximately 24 or more hours.

Azole Group

The azole group is effective against candidiasis (superficial and systemic), coccidioidomycosis, cryptococcosis, histoplasmosis, and paracoccidioidomycosis. Ketoconazole was the first effective antifungal drug that was orally absorbed.

Fluconazole and itraconazole are also azole drugs used to treat systemic fungal infection. These three antifungals can be taken orally, unlike amphotericin B, caspofungin, and voriconazole, which are only administered IV. Fluconazole, a systemic azole antifungal agent, is described in Prototype Drug Chart 31–2.

Numerous azoles are used to treat candidiasis and the tinea infections in topical preparations. These drugs are available in forms of vaginal tablet, cream, ointment, and solution. Topical antifungal agents (azoles and others) are presented in Table 31–4.

Antimetabolite

The antimetabolite flucytosine has antifungal action. It is well absorbed from the GI tract. Flucytosine is used in combination with other antifungal drugs, such as amphotericin B (see Table 31–3).

Antiprotozoal

Atovaquone (Mepron), an antiprotozoal agent, is used to treat mild to moderate *Pneumocystis carinii* pneumonia.

Echinocandins

Caspofungin (Cancidas) is used to treat *Candida* and *Aspergillosis* infections. This drug is only administered IV because it is not absorbed in the GI tract. Phlebitis at the IV site and increased AST and ALT are common adverse effects.

Nursing Process

Antifungals

ASSESSMENT

■ Obtain a medical history from client of any serious renal or hepatic disorder. Antifungal agents such as amphotericin B, fluconazole (Diflucan), flucytosine (Ancobon), and ketoconazole (Nizoral) are contraindicated if client has a serious renal or liver disease.
■ Check laboratory tests for liver enzyme values (alkaline phosphatase [ALP], alanine aminotransferase [ALT], aspartate aminotransferase [AST], gamma-glutamyl transferase [GGT]), blood urea nitrogen (BUN), bilirubin, and serum creatinine. Elevated levels can indicate liver or renal dysfunction. These test results may be used for future comparisons.
■ Record baseline vital signs for future comparison.

NURSING DIAGNOSES

■ Risk for infection
■ Risk for impaired tissue integrity

PLANNING

■ Client's fungal infection will be resolved.

NURSING INTERVENTIONS

■ Obtain a culture to determine the fungus (e.g., *Candida*).
■ Monitor client's urinary output; many of the antifungal drugs may cause nephrotoxicity.
■ Check the laboratory results and compare with baseline findings (i.e., BUN, serum creatinine, ALP, ALT, AST, bilirubin, and electrolytes). Certain antifungals could cause hepatotoxicity as well as nephrotoxicity when taking high doses over a prolonged period.
■ Record vital signs. Compare with baseline findings.
■ Observe for side effects and adverse reactions to antifungal drugs (antimycotics), such as nausea, vomiting, headache, phlebitis, and signs and symptoms of electrolyte imbalance (hypokalemia with amphotericin B).

Client Teaching

General

• Instruct client to take the drug as prescribed. Compliance is of utmost importance because discontinuing the drug too soon may result in a relapse.

• Advise client to obtain laboratory testing as indicated. Serum liver enzymes, BUN, creatinine, and electrolytes should be monitored.
• Inform client taking ketoconazole not to consume alcohol.

Self-Administration

• Educate client on the administration of nystatin (Mycostatin) suspension. Place the nystatin dose, usually 1 to 2 teaspoons, in the mouth. Swish the solution in the mouth and swallow (swish and swallow), or after swishing, have client expectorate the solution (check with health care provider).

Side Effects

• Teach client to avoid operating hazardous equipment or a motor vehicle when taking amphotericin B, ketoconazole, or flucytosine because these drugs may cause visual changes, sleepiness, dizziness, or lethargy.
• Encourage client to report side effects, such as nausea, vomiting, diarrhea, dermatitis, rash, dizziness, tinnitus, edema, and flatulence. These symptoms may occur when taking certain antifungal drugs.

PROTOTYPE DRUG CHART 31–2

FLUCONAZOLE

Drug Class
Antifungal: fluconazole
Trade Name: Diflucan
Pregnancy Category: C

Dosage
Systemic candidiasis:
A: PO/IV: 400 mg/d 1 then 200 mg/d for 4 wk
C: PO/IV: 3-6 mg/kg/d
Vaginal candidiasis:
A: PO: 150 mg times 1 dose

Contraindications
Hypersensitivity
Caution: Pregnancy

Drug-Lab-Food Interactions
Drug: Increases PT when taking warfarin; increases hypoglycemia when taken with oral sulfonylureas; increases phenytoin, cyclosporine, and haloperidol levels; decreases fluconazole level with cimetidine and rifampin

Pharmacokinetics
Absorption: PO: Well absorbed in GI tract
Distribution: PB: 12%
Metabolism: t½: 20-50 h
Excretion: In urine

Pharmacodynamics
PO: Onset: UK
Peak: 1-2 h
Duration: UK
Vag: Onset: UK
Peak: UK
Duration: UK

Therapeutic Effects/Uses
To treat *Candida* infections and cryptococcal meningitis
Mode of Action: Increase permeability of the fungal cell membrane

Side Effects
PO: Anorexia, nausea, vomiting, diarrhea (large doses), stomach cramps, rash, headache
Vaginal: Rash, burning sensation

Adverse Reactions
None known

A, Adult; *C,* child; *d,* day; *GI,* gastrointestinal; *h,* hour; *IV,* intravenous; *PB,* protein-binding; *PO,* by mouth; *PT,* prothrombin time; *t½,* half-life; *UK,* unknown; *wk,* week.

Cultural Considerations ⊕

- Recognize that clients from various cultures may not understand the purpose and procedure for the use of vaginal tablets or creams. A detailed explanation may be needed.
- Respect client's apprehensions and fear concerning the use of the topical antifungal drugs and the desire to use alternative methods. Evaluate client's method of topical administration in regard to safe practice. If the method is considered unsafe, explain why and suggest modifications. If appropriate, involve other persons for clarification.

EVALUATION

■ Evaluate the effectiveness of the antifungal (antimycotic) drug by noting the absence of the fungal infection (e.g., decreased itching, redness, and rawness).

Peptides

The two groups of **peptides** used as antibiotics are the polymyxins and bacitracin. The peptides are derived from cultures of *Bacillus subtilis*, and this group appears to interfere with bacterial cell membrane function.

Polymyxins

Polymyxins were one of the early groups of antibacterials, but many of the early drugs were discontinued because they caused nephrotoxicity. Polymyxin B is approved for pharmaceutical use. Polymyxins produce a bactericidal effect by interfering with the cellular membrane of the bacterium, thereby causing cell death. They affect most gram-negative bacteria, such as *Pseudomonas aeruginosa*, *Escherichia coli*, *Klebsiella* spp., and *Shigella* spp.

Except for colistin, which exerts action on the colon and is excreted in the feces, the polymyxins are not absorbed through the oral route. IM injection of polymyxins produces marked pain at the injection site; therefore IV administration of polymyxins at a slow infusion rate is the suggested method. Table 31–5 lists the polymyxins with their dosage and uses.

Severe Adverse Effects

High serum levels of polymyxins can cause nephrotoxicity and neurotoxicity. With nephrotoxicity, the blood urea nitrogen and serum creatinine levels are elevated; however, when the serum drug level decreases, renal toxicity is usually reversed. Signs and symptoms of **neurotoxicity** are numbness and tingling of the extremities, **paresthesias**

Table 31–4

Topical Antifungal Agents for Fungal Infections

Tinea Infections

Drug	Drug Form	Candidiasis	Tinea Pedis	Tinea Cruris	Tinea Corporis
Azoles					
butoconazole nitrate (Femstat)	2% vaginal cream	X			
clotrimazole (Femcare, Mycelex, Gyne-Lotrimin)	1% topical cream; vaginal tablet; PO: 1 troche (lozenge)	X	X	X	X
econazole (Spectazole)	1% topical cream	X	X	X	X
miconazole nitrate (Monistat, Micatin)	Vaginal suppository, 2% vaginal cream	X			
oxiconazole (Oxistat)	Cream		X	X	X
sulconazole (Exelderm)	Cream; solution		X	X	X
terconazole (Terazol-3)	Vaginal suppository; 0.4% and 0.8% vaginal cream	X			
tioconazole (Vagistat)	Vaginal suppository; 0.5% vaginal ointment	X			
Other Topical Antifungals					
ciclopirox olamine (Loprox)	Cream; lotion	X Cutaneous	X	X	X
haloprogin (Halotex)	1% cream; solution		X	X	X
naftifine (Naftin)	1% cream or gel		X	X	X
terbinafine HCl (Lamisil)	1% cream		X	X	X
tolnaftate (Aftate)	1% cream, gel, solution		X	X	X

PO, By mouth.

(abnormal sensation), and dizziness. Neurotoxicity is usually reversible when the drug is discontinued.

Bacitracin

Bacitracin has a polypeptide structure and acts by inhibiting bacterial cell-wall synthesis and damaging the cell-wall membrane. The drug action can be bacteriostatic or bactericidal. Bacitracin is not absorbed by the GI tract and, if given orally, is excreted in the feces. It is therefore given IV or IM. It crosses the blood-brain barrier and thus is effective in treating meningitis. Bacitracin is effective against most gram-positive bacteria and some gram-negative bacteria. Over-the-counter (OTC) bacitracin ointment is available for application to the skin.

Side Effects and Adverse Reactions

The side effects of bacitracin include nausea and vomiting. Severe adverse reactions are renal damage, respiratory paralysis, blood dyscrasias (life-threatening anemias), and mild to severe allergic reactions, ranging from hives to anaphylaxis.

Metronidazole

Metronidazole (Flagyl) is used primarily to treat various disorders associated with organisms in the GI tract. It is prescribed to treat intestinal amebiasis, trichomoniasis, inflammatory bowel disease, anaerobic infections, and bacterial vaginosis and is used as perioperative **prophylaxis** in colorectal surgery. Metronidazole is commonly used with other agents to treat *Helicobacter pylori*, which is associated with frequent recurrent peptic ulcers. Table 31–5 includes data related to metronidazole.

WEBSITES

For further information on *Antitubercular Drugs, Antifungal Drugs, Peptides,* and *Metronidazole,* visit these Internet resources:

Information on fluconazole:
www.hivdent.org/drugs/FLUCONAZOLE.htm
www.diseasesdatabase.com/sieve/item1.asp?glngUserChoice=4855

Information on amphotericin B:
www.nlm.nih.gov/medlineplus/druginfo/uspdi/202032.html

Further information on amphotericin B:
www.uphs.upenn.edu/bugdrug/antibiotic_manual/ampho.htm

Information on isoniazid:
www.nlm.nih.gov/medlineplus/druginfo/medmaster/a682401.html

Table 31–5

Antibacterials: Peptides

Generic (Brand)	Route and Dosage	Uses and Considerations
bacitracin (Bactrin USP)	C: <2.5 kg: IM: <900 units/kg/d in 2-3 divided doses C: >2.5 kg: IM: <1000 units/kg/d in 2-3 divided doses. Available in topical and ophthalmic ointment.	It is seldom used parenterally except for children. Topical ointment for skin infection and ophthalmic ointment for infections of the eye. *Pregnancy category:* C; PB: <20%; $t^{1}/_{2}$: UK
colistimethate sodium (IM/IV) (Coly-Mycin M)	A & C: IM/IV: 2.5-5 mg/kg/d in divided doses	For treating *Pseudomonas aeruginosa* infection. *Pregnancy category:* C; PB: UK; $t^{1}/_{2}$: 2-3 h
polymyxin B SO₄ (Aerosporin)	A: IM: 25,000 units/kg/d in 4-6 divided doses IV: 15,000-25,000 units/kg/d in 2 divided doses (q12h) C: >2 y: Same as adult	For systemic use; also available in ointment form. May cause nephrotoxicity if given with aminoglycosides or amphotericin. *Pregnancy category:* B; PB: UK; $t^{1}/_{2}$: 4.5-6 h

Additional Antibacterial Agent

metronidazole (Flagyl, Flagyl-ER, MetroGel, Protostat)	*Amebiasis:* A: PO: 500-750 mg t.i.d. for 5-10 d C: PO: 35-50 mg/kg/d in 3 divided doses *Anaerobic infections:* A: PO: 7.5 mg/kg q6h; *max:* 4 g/d A: IV: 15 mg/kg loading dose, then 7.5 mg/kg q6h *Bacterial vaginosis:* A: PO: ER preparation: 750 mg/d × 7 d *Perioperative prophylaxis:* A: IV: 1 g, 1 h before surgery; 500 mg, 6 and 12 h after first dose *Rosacea:* Thin application twice per day to affected areas Available in vaginal and topical gel	For treatment of intestinal amebiasis, trichomoniasis, inflammatory bowel disease, *H. pylori* infection causing peptic ulcers, bacterial vaginosis, and anaerobic infections and perioperative prophylaxis in colorectal surgery. Side effects may include GI discomfort, headache, depression, although not common. Not recommended during the first trimester of pregnancy. *Pregnancy category:* B; PB: UK; $t^{1}/_{2}$: 6-8 h

A, Adult; *C,* child; *d,* day; *h,* hour; *IM,* intramuscular; *IV,* intravenous; *PB,* protein-binding; $t^{1}/_{2}$, half-life; *UK,* unknown; *y,* year; >, greater than; <, less than.

Critical Thinking Case Study

C.J., age 41, has had a constant cough and night sweats for several months. He consumes 1 pint of whiskey per day. Sputum is positive for acid-fast (tubercle) bacillus. The health care provider orders a 6- to 9-month antitubercular drug regimen (time of therapy to be determined according to sputum and radiograph test results). For 2 months, C.J. takes isoniazid, rifampin, and pyrazinamide daily. The next 4 to 7 months, C.J. takes isoniazid and rifampin biweekly.

1. What could be contributing causes for C.J.'s contracting tuberculosis? Give other contributing causes for contracting tuberculosis.

2. C.J. received first-line antitubercular drugs for treatment of tuberculosis. How can the health professional determine whether the drugs are effective in eradicating the tubercle bacilli? Explain.

3. What is the nurse's role in client teaching concerning the drug regimen?

4. Name at least two serious adverse reactions that can occur when antitubercular drugs are given over an extended period.

5. What laboratory tests should be monitored while C.J. takes isoniazid and rifampin? Why?

The health care provider ordered pyridoxine to be given daily.

6. Give your rationale for the use of pyridoxine. What type of drug is it? What is its purpose, and when should it be administered?

7. What health agencies may the nurse suggest that could be helpful to C.J. during and after therapy?

Study Questions

1. What is the purpose of combination drug therapy in the treatment of tuberculosis?

2. What is a common side effect of isoniazid? Why should some clients receive pyridoxine (vitamin B_6) while taking isoniazid? What are the signs and symptoms of peripheral neuropathy?

3. What is a potential adverse reaction to the use of isoniazid and rifampin? Would the problem be intensified if the drugs were taken by an alcoholic or a client with a liver disorder? Explain.

4. Your client is to receive nystatin for an oral fungal infection. How would you instruct the client to use the oral suspension of nystatin?

5. What type of electrolyte imbalance is associated with the use of amphotericin B? What other adverse effect might result from its use?

6. What are the three oral antifungal drugs that may be taken for systemic fungal infections? How do these drugs differ from one another according to their protein-binding and half-life? What are the advantages of these drugs over amphotericin B?

7. How do the topical antifungal imidazoles clotrimazole and econazole differ from miconazole, oxiconazole, and sulconazole?

8. Why should kidney function be assessed with polymyxin administration? Against what bacteria are polymyxins and colistin effective?

32 Antiviral, Antimalarial, and Anthelmintic Drugs

ELECTRONIC RESOURCES

Additional information can be found on the companion website at *http://evolve.elsevier.com/KeeHayes/pharmacology/* or on the companion CD-ROM, which includes:

- *NCLEX-style examination review questions*
- *Pharmacology animations*
- *Medication error and (IV) therapy checklists*
- *Medication calculation problems*
- *Electronic calculators*

OBJECTIVES

- Name several antiviral and antimalarial drugs and explain their uses.
- Identify the various helminths and the human body sites used for their infestation.
- Describe the action of anthelmintics.
- Explain the side effects and adverse reactions to antiviral, antimalarial, and anthelmintic drugs.
- Identify several nursing interventions, including client teaching, for antiviral, antimalarial, and anthelmintic drug therapy.

TERMS

acquired immunodeficiency syndrome (AIDS)
anthelmintic drugs
antimalarial drugs

antiviral drugs
erythrocytic phase
helminthiasis
helminths

prophylaxis
tissue phase
trichinosis
virus

Viruses

Viruses are more difficult to eradicate than most types of bacteria. A **virus** is an obligate intracellular organism that uses the cell to reproduce. Viruses enter healthy cells and use their deoxyribonucleic acid (DNA) and ribonucleic acid (RNA) to generate more viruses. The growth cycle of viruses depends on the host cell enzymes and cell substrates for viral replication. Viruses live and reproduce when they are within living cells.

A viral infection usually can be detected only after the virus has replicated itself. Viruses can cause mild to severe infections. The influenza virus is passed primarily during sneezing and coughing. This virus enters through droplets into the respiratory tract of the unaffected person and begins replicating 24 hours before symptoms appear. General signs and symptoms of an acute viral infection include headache, low-grade fever (with a mild viral infection), nausea, vomiting, diarrhea, muscular pain, fatigue, and cough.

Vaccines

Vaccines have been developed to prevent diseases such as smallpox, chickenpox, mumps, rabies, and influenza (see Chapter 35, Vaccines). The influenza virus vaccine may change annually because influenza (flu) virus changes its genetic structure each year. However, the influenza vaccine still promotes the production of antibodies by the immune system, despite the viruses' varying genetic structures. Eggs are used to produce the flu vaccine; therefore any allergies to eggs should be determined before administration to the client. The success rate of vaccine use to prevent influenza in healthy children and adults is 65% to 90%. In older adults, vaccines are effective 60% of the time and less than 60% if an older adult has multiple health problems.

Diagnostic Tests for Influenza

Several office laboratory tests can be used to diagnose influenza. The diagnostic test Directigen Flu A has been available for many years to detect influenza A; however, it does not detect influenza B. Flu OIA (Thermo BioStar, Boulder, Colo.), QuickVue Influenza Test (Quidel, San Diego), and Zstatflu (ZymeTx, Oklahoma City) are new diagnostic tests that identify influenza A and B. These tests use throat swabs, nasal swabs, or nasal aspiration. Results are available within 10 to 20 minutes. QuickVue tends to be easy and fast for a rapid diagnosis of influenza A and B. The Food and Drug Administration (FDA) has approved two new drugs, zanamivir (Relenza) and oseltamivir phosphate (Tamiflu), that inhibit the replication and spread of the influenza virus if given within 48 hours of symptoms; thus early diagnosis of influenza is important.

Antiviral Non-HIV Drugs

Antiviral drugs are used to prevent or delay the spread of a viral infection. They inhibit viral replication by interfering with viral nucleic acid synthesis in the cell. There are groups of antiviral drugs effective against various viruses such as influenza A and B, herpes species, cytomegalovirus (CMV), and human immunodeficiency virus (HIV). Drugs for HIV are discussed in Chapter 34, HIV and AIDS-Related Agents. The antiviral non-HIV drugs are listed in Table 32–1. Interferon alfa-2a and 2b are used to treat hepatitis B and C viruses (see Chapter 37, Biologic Response Modifiers).

Nonclassified Antivirals

The first two related antivirals, amantidine hydrochloride (Symmetrel) and rimantadine hydrochloride (Flumadine), were used to treat type A influenza. Both these antivirals are nonclassified antivirals. Originally, amantidine was used to treat parkinsonism but later was found to be effective against influenza A. Neither amantidine nor rimantadine are effective against type B influenza. Three other nonclassified antivirals are (1) cidofovir, which is used to treat CMV retinitis; (2) foscarnet (Foscavir), which is used to treat HIV retinitis and herpes simplex infection in clients with **acquired immunodeficiency syndrome (AIDS);** and (3) vidarabine (Vira-A), which is used to treat herpesvirus.

Vidarabine was first introduced as an antineoplastic drug for the treatment of leukemia. In 1964 it was discovered that vidarabine exerts an antiviral effect against HSV-1, herpes zoster, varicella zoster, and CMV. Although it is not effective against herpes simplex virus type 2 (HSV-2; genital herpes), vidarabine has been used effectively to treat herpes simplex viral encephalitis.

Side Effects and Adverse Reactions

Amantadine and Rimantadine. The side effects and adverse reactions to amantadine include central nervous system (CNS) effects, such as insomnia, depression, anxiety, confusion, and ataxia; orthostatic hypotension; neurologic problems, such as weakness, dizziness, and slurred speech; and gastrointestinal (GI) disturbances, such as anorexia, nausea, vomiting, and diarrhea. The CNS side effects of rimantadine occur less often than with amantadine.

Topical Antivirals

There are three topical antiviral drugs: idoxuridine (Herplex Liquifilm), penciclovir (Denavir), and trifluridine (Viroptic). These topical agents are used to treat herpes simplex viruses.

Neuraminidase Inhibitors

A new group of antivirals, neuraminidase inhibitors, decrease the release of the virus from infected cells, thus decreasing viral spread and shortening the duration of flu symptoms. Zanamivir (Relenza) and oseltamivir phos-

Table 32–1

Non-HIV Antivirals

Generic (Brand)	Route and Dosage	Uses and Considerations
Systemic Non-HIV Antivirals		
Nonclassified Antivirals		
amantadine HCl (Symmetrel)	*Influenza A:* A: PO: 200 mg/d in 1-2 divided doses C: 1-8 y: PO: 4.4-8.8 mg/kg/d in 2-3 divided doses C: 9-12 y: PO: 100-200 mg/d in 1-2 divided doses	Primary use is prophylaxis against influenza A. Well absorbed by the GI tract. *Pregnancy category:* C; PB: UK; t½: 24 h
cidofovir (Vistide)	A: IV: 5 mg/kg once wk for 2 wk, then 5 mg/kg every other week. Take probenecid 2 g, 3 h before infusion and 1 g, 8 h after infusion.	For treatment of CMV retinitis, especially in clients with AIDS. Kidney damage may occur; monitor kidney function. *Pregnancy category:* C; PB: UK; t½: 17-65 h
foscarnet (Foscavir)	*CMV retinitis:* A: IV: Induction: 60 mg/kg infused over 1 h, q8h, for 2 to 3 wk; *maint:* 90-120 mg/kg/d infused over 2 h *Herpes simplex infections/AIDS:* A: IV: 40-60 mg/kg q8h for 2-3 wk; may include: 50 mg/kg/d for 5 to 7 d/wk up to 15 wk	For treatment of herpesviruses (HSV-1 and HSV-2, VZV) and CMV retinitis. It is expensive. It does not cause granulocytopenia or thrombocytopenia. It can cause kidney damage and hyperphosphatemia. Monitor kidney function closely. *Pregnancy category:* C; PB: UK; t½: 3-4 h
rimantadine HCl (Flumadine)	A: PO: 200 mg/d in 1 or 2 divided doses C: <10 y: PO: 5 mg/kg/d; *max:* 150 mg/d C: >10 y: PO: same as adult	For prophylaxis and treatment against influenza A virus. Drug dose is usually reduced for clients with severe hepatic or renal impairment. *Pregnancy category:* C; PB: 40%; t½: 33 h
vidarabine monohydrate (Vira-A)	A & C: IV: 10-15 mg/kg/d infused over 12-24 h	Effective against serious HSV-1, herpes zoster, and varicella zoster. *Pregnancy category:* C; PB; 20%-30%, t½: 1.5-3 h
Purine Nucleoside		
acyclovir (Zovirax)	See Prototype Drug Chart 32–1.	
famciclovir (Famvir)	*Herpes zoster:* A: PO: 500 mg q8h × 7 d	For treatment of herpes zoster. *Pregnancy category:* C; PB: UK; t½: 2-3 h
ganciclovir sodium (Cytovene)	A & C: IV: Initially: 5 mg/kg over 1 h q12h × 14-21 d; *maint:* 5 mg/kg/d over 1 h × 7 d or 6 mg/kg/d over 1 h × 5 d	For treatment of CMV systemic infection in immunocompromised clients. *Pregnancy category:* C; PB: 1%-2%; t½: 2.5-6 h
ribavirin (Virazole)	A & C: By aerosol inhalation administration	For respiratory syncytial viral infection in infants and children. *Pregnancy category:* X; PB: NA; t½: 24 h

A, Adult; *AIDS,* acquired immunodeficiency syndrome; *b.i.d.,* twice a day; *C,* child; *CMV,* cytomegalovirus; *d,* day; *DNA,* deoxyribonucleic acid; *GI,* gastrointestinal; *gt,* drop; *gtt,* drops; *h,* hour; *HIV,* human immunodeficiency virus; *HSV,* herpes simplex virus; *IV,* intravenous; *maint,* maintenance; *max,* maximum; *PB,* protein-binding; *PO,* by mouth; *t½,* half-life; *t.i.d.,* three times a day; *UK,* unknown; *VZV,* varicella-zoster virus; *wk,* week; *y,* year; >, greater than; <, less than.

phate (Tamiflu) are two neuraminidase inhibitors recently approved by the FDA. They should be taken within 48 hours of flu symptoms. These drugs inhibit the activity of neuraminidase, a viral glycoprotein, and are effective against type A and B influenza viruses. Zanamivir and oseltamivir phosphate are *not* substitutes for the "flu shot."

Gamma Globulin (Immune Globulin)

Gamma globulin (IgG) is rich in antibodies found in the blood. It provides a passive form of immunity to a virus by blocking the penetration of a virus into the host cell. It is administered during the early infectious stage to prevent a viral invasion in the body.

The human immune globulin (Gamastan) is administered intramuscularly (IM). A single-dose injection protects for approximately 2 to 3 weeks; it then may be repeated in 2 to 3 weeks. For clients who need an immediate

increase in immune globulin levels, intravenous (IV) immune globulin (Gamimune N) may be administered.

Purine Nucleosides

The synthetic purine nucleoside antiviral group is effective in interfering with the steps of viral nucleic acid (DNA) synthesis. Drugs in this group of nucleoside analogs include ribavirin (Virazole), acyclovir (Zovirax), famciclovir (Famvir), ganciclovir sodium (Cytovene), and valacyclovir (Valtrex). These drugs are effective in combating herpes simplex viruses (HSV-1, HSV-2), herpes zoster (shingles), varicella-zoster virus (chicken pox), and CMV. A new drug, valganciclovir (Valcyte), a prodrug of ganciclovir, is effective for treating CMV retinitis in clients with AIDS.

The antiviral drug ribavirin was first marketed in 1986. It is used to treat respiratory syncytial virus (RSV) in children and respiratory infections caused by the influenza A

Table 32–1

Non-HIV Antivirals—cont'd

Generic (Brand)	Route and Dosage	Uses and Considerations
Systemic Non-HIV Antivirals—cont'd		
Purine Nucleoside—cont'd		
valacyclovir HCl (Valtrex)	*Herpes zoster:* A: PO: 1 g t.i.d. × 7 d *Recurrent genital herpes:* A: PO: 500 mg b.i.d. 5 d *Reduce dosage:* Clients with decreased renal function	It is converted to acyclovir during intestinal and liver metabolism. It is effective against VZV causing herpes zoster (shingles) and recurrent genital herpes. Monitor kidney function. GI disturbances and headaches are common side effects. *Pregnancy category:* B; PB: 14%-18%; $t^1/_2$: 2.5-3.5 h
valganciclovir (Valcyte)	A: PO: Induction 900 mg b.i.d. with food for 21 d; *maint:* 900 mg/d with food	To treat CMV infected cells of retinitis in AIDS clients. It inhibits the viral DNA synthesis. It may cause leukopenia, thrombocytopenia, bone marrow depression, and aplastic anemia. *Pregnancy category:* UK; PB: UK; $t^1/_2$: UK
Neuraminidase Inhibitors		
oseltamivir phosphate (Tamiflu)	A: PO: 75 mg b.i.d. × 5 d C: 15-23 kg: PO: 45 mg b.i.d. C: >40 kg: 75 mg/d	For treatment of uncomplicated acute influenza A and B. Treatment should begin within 2 days of flu symptoms. May be taken with or without food. Side effects include transient nausea and vomiting. Dose should be reduced with renal insufficiency. *Pregnancy category:* C; PB: UK, $t^1/_2$: 6-10 h
zanamivir (Relenza)	A: Inhaler: 10 mg b.i.d. × 5 d	For treatment of influenza A and B. Treatment should begin within 2 days of flu symptoms. The inhaled drug is deposited in the oropharynx and throat. Less than 20% is absorbed systemically. *Pregnancy category:* C; PB: UK; $t^1/_2$: 2.5-5 h
Topical Non-HIV Antivirals		
idoxuridine (Herplex Liquifilm, Stoxil)	0.5% ointment: q4h during day *Solution:* Instill 1 gt during day and q2h at night; time interval can be decreased	Used primarily for HSV-1 keratitis. *Pregnancy category:* C; PB: UK; $t^1/_2$: UK
penciclovir (Denavir)	1% cream: apply q2h during the day for 4 d	For treatment of recurrent herpes labialis (cold sores) of lips. *Pregnancy category:* B; PB: UK; $t^1/_2$: UK
trifluridine (Viroptic)	1% ophthalmic solution: 1 gt q2h during the day; *max:* 9 gtt/d	Used primarily for keratoconjunctivitis because of herpes simplex virus. *Pregnancy category:* C; PB: UK; $t^1/_2$: UK

and B viruses in older adults. Ribavirin is administered by aerosol.

Acyclovir

Acyclovir was introduced as an antineoplastic drug and was later found to be effective against herpesvirus, especially HSV-2, but also against HSV-1, herpes zoster (shingles), and CMV (which can cause congenital defects). There has been reported resistance to acyclovir as a result of the lack of viral-producing enzyme (thymidine kinase) needed to convert the drug to an effective antiviral compound. Prototype Drug Chart 32–1 lists the drug data for acyclovir.

Pharmacokinetics

Acyclovir is slowly absorbed, depending on the dose, and is widely distributed to body and organ tissues. Half of the drug passes into the cerebrospinal fluid. The drug is 10% to 30% protein bound. Its half-life is 2 to 3 hours with normal renal function. Acyclovir is excreted unchanged in the urine.

Pharmacodynamics

Acyclovir interferes with the viral synthesis of DNA, thereby short-circuiting its replication. The onset of action for the oral preparation is unknown; for the intravenous (IV) route, the onset is rapid. The peak con-

centration time is within 2 hours for both routes of administration, and the duration of action for both is similar.

Probenecid can increase the effect of acyclovir. If aminoglycoside or amphotericin B are taken with acyclovir, the incidence of nephrotoxicity is increased.

Valacyclovir (Valtrex) is converted to acyclovir, which has inhibitory activity against HSV-1, HSV-2, and varicella-zoster virus or herpes zoster. With herpes zoster, valacyclovir has a greater decrease in pain and an increase in healing time (40 to 43 days) than with acyclovir (59 days).

Famciclovir (Famvir), an antiviral drug developed before valacyclovir, is equally effective as acyclovir for treating acute herpes zoster.

Ganciclovir (Cytovene, Vitrasert) is effective in treating the herpesviruses and CMV. Its primary use is to treat CMV infections. It has serious adverse reactions.

Side Effects and Adverse Reactions

Vidarabine, Acyclovir, and Ganciclovir. The side effects and adverse reactions to vidarabine, acyclovir, and ganciclovir include GI disturbances (e.g., nausea, vomiting, di-

PROTOTYPE DRUG CHART 32–1

ACYCLOVIR SODIUM

Drug Class	**Dosage**
Antiviral Trade Name: Zovirax *Pregnancy Category:* C	*Herpes simplex virus:* A: PO: 200 mg q4h, 5 × d; 400 mg t.i.d. for 7-10 d IV: 5 mg/kg 5 × d (diluted in D_5W) *Herpes zoster virus:* A: PO: 800 mg q4h 5 × d for 5-7 d C: PO: 80 mg/kg/d in 5 divided doses *Herpes simplex encephalitis:* A: IV: 10-15 mg/kg q8h × 14-21 d C: IV: 500 mg/m² q8h × 7d
Contraindications	**Drug-Lab-Food Interactions**
Hypersensitivity, severe renal or hepatic disease *Caution:* Electrolyte imbalance, nursing mothers, young children	*Drug:* Increase nephro-neurotoxicity with aminoglycosides, probenecid, interferon *Lab:* May *increase* AST, ALT, BUN
Pharmacokinetics	**Pharmacodynamics**

Absorption: PO: Slowly absorbed
Distribution: PB: 10%-30%
Metabolism: t½: PO: 2-3 h
Excretion: 95% unchanged in urine
	PO: Onset: UK
	  Peak: 1.5-2 h
	  Duration: 4-8 h
	IV: Onset: Rapid
	  Peak: 1-2 h
	  Duration: 4-8 h

Therapeutic Effects/Uses

To treat HSV-1, HSV-2 (genital)
Mode of Action: Interference with viral synthesis of DNA

Side Effects	**Adverse Reactions**
Nausea, vomiting, diarrhea, headache, tremors, lethargy, rash, pruritus, increased bleeding time, phlebitis at IV site	Urticaria, anemia, gingival hyperplasia **Life-threatening:** Nephrotoxicity (large doses), neuropathy, bone marrow depression, granulocytopenia, thrombocytopenia, leukopenia, seizure, acute renal failure

A, Adult; *ALT*, alanine aminotransferase; *AST*, aspartate aminotransferase; *BUN*, blood urea nitrogen; *C*, child; *d*, day; *DNA*, deoxyribonucleic acid; *h*, hour; *HSV*, herpes simplex virus; *IV*, intravenous; *PB*, protein-binding; *PO*, by mouth; *t½*, half-life; *t.i.d.*, three times a day; *UK*, unknown.

---

arrhea). With vidarabine, there might be CNS disturbances, such as weakness, malaise, tremors, and confusion. Adverse reactions can include a decrease in hemoglobin, white blood cells, and platelets; liver involvement (transient); and thrombophlebitis.

With acyclovir, there might be headache, dizziness, and hematuria. Insomnia, depression, and hypotension, although infrequent, can also occur. Elevated blood urea nitrogen (BUN) and serum creatinine levels can result from renal involvement; such involvement is usually transient.

Ganciclovir can cause thrombocytopenia and granulocytopenia. Because of the possible serious adverse reactions, this drug should be prescribed primarily for severe systemic CMV infections for immunocompromised clients.

Nursing Process

Antivirals

ASSESSMENT

■ Obtain a medical history from client of any serious renal or hepatic disease.

■ Determine baseline vital signs and a complete blood count (CBC). Use these findings for comparison with future results.

■ Assess baseline laboratory results, particularly blood urea nitrogen (BUN), serum creatinine, liver enzymes, bilirubin, and electrolytes. Use these results for future comparisons.

■ Evaluate baseline vital signs and urine output. Report abnormal findings.

NURSING DIAGNOSES

■ Risk for infection
■ Risk for impaired tissue integrity

PLANNING

■ Symptoms of viral infections will be eliminated or diminished.

NURSING INTERVENTIONS

■ Check client's CBC. Report abnormal results, such as leukopenia, thrombocytopenia, and low hemoglobin and hematocrit.
■ Monitor other laboratory tests, such as BUN, serum creatinine, and liver enzymes, and compare with baseline values.
■ Record client's urinary output. An antiviral drug such as acyclovir can affect renal function.
■ Note vital signs, especially blood pressure. Acyclovir and amantadine may cause orthostatic hypotension.
■ Observe for signs and symptoms of side effects. Most antiviral drugs have many side effects; see Prototype Drug Chart 32–1.
■ Check for superimposed infection (superinfection) caused by high dose and prolonged use of an antiviral drug such as acyclovir.
■ Administer oral acyclovir as prescribed. Oral dose can be taken at mealtime.
■ For IV use, dilute the antiviral drug in an appropriate amount of solution as indicated in the drug circular. Administer the IV drug over 60 minutes. *Never* give acyclovir as a bolus (IV push).

Client Teaching

General

• Advise client to maintain an adequate fluid intake to ensure sufficient hydration for drug therapy and to increase urine output.
• Instruct client with genital herpes to avoid spreading the infection by practicing sexual abstinence or by using condoms. Teach women with genital herpes to have a Pap test done every 6 months or as indicated by the health care provider. Cervical cancer is more prevalent in women with genital herpes simplex.
• Direct clients taking zidovudine to have blood cell count monitored.

Side Effects

• Encourage client to perform oral hygiene several times a day. Gingival hyperplasia (red, swollen gums) can occur with prolonged use of antiviral drugs.
• Guide client to report adverse reactions, including decrease in urine output and central nervous system changes such as dizziness, anxiety, or confusion.

• Warn client with dizziness resulting from orthostatic hypotension to arise slowly from a sitting to a standing position.
• Tell client to report any side effects associated with the antiviral drug, such as nausea, vomiting, diarrhea, increased bleeding time, rash, urticaria, or menstrual abnormalities.

Cultural Considerations

• Teach the non–English-speaking client and family members how to use ophthalmic preparations. Pictures may be helpful.

EVALUATION

■ Evaluate the effectiveness of the antiviral drug in eliminating the virus or in decreasing symptoms.
■ Determine whether side effects are absent.

Antiviral HIV Drugs

The microbe of the human immunodeficiency virus (HIV) is the cause of AIDS. HIV is a retrovirus. There are two classes of antiretroviral drugs: (1) reverse transcriptase inhibitors and (2) protease inhibitors. Antiviral drugs classified as reverse transcriptase inhibitors include delavirdine (Rescriptor), didanosine (Videx), lamivudine (Epivir), nevirapine (Viramune), stavudine (Zerit), zalcitabine (Hivid), and zidovudine (Retrovir, AZT). These drugs aid in inhibiting viral replication. Zidovudine was one of the first retroviral drugs approved by the FDA. It inhibits the action of viral reverse transcriptase, thus preventing the synthesis of DNA and allowing the T_4 lymphocytes to increase initially.

The protease inhibitor group includes indinavir (Crixivan), nelfinavir (Viracept), ritonavir (Norvir), and saquinavir (Invirase). This group of antivirals inhibits the replication of retroviruses (HIV-1 and -2). When a protease inhibitor is used in combination with a reverse transcriptase inhibitor, these drugs may greatly reduce the viral level to the point that it is undetectable. The combination of drugs helps to decrease HIV drug resistance. The antiviral drugs for suppressing HIV are discussed in Chapter 34, HIV and AIDS-related Disorders.

Antimalarial Drugs

Malaria, caused by the protozoan parasites *Plasmodium* spp. that are carried by an infected *Anopheles* mosquito, is still one of the most prevalent protozoan diseases. After the mosquito infects the human, the protozoan parasite passes through two phases: the tissue phase and the erythrocytic phase. The **tissue phase** produces no clinical symptoms in the human, but the **erythrocytic phase** (invasion of the red blood cells) causes symptoms of chills, fever, and sweating. The incubation period is 10 to 35 days, followed by flulike symptoms.

PROTOTYPE DRUG CHART 32–2

CHLOROQUINE HCl

Drug Class

Antimalarial
Trade Name: Aralen HCl
Pregnancy Category: C

Dosage

Acute malaria:
A: PO: 600 mg base/dose; then 6 h later: 300 mg/dose;
    then at 24 and 48 h: 300 mg/dose
IM: 200 mg/base q6h, PRN; *max:* 800 mg/d
C: PO: 10 mg base/kg/dose, then 6 h later: 5 mg
    base/kg/dose; then 5 mg base/kg/d for 2 d
IM: 5 mg base/kg q12h
Prophylaxis:
2 wk before and 6-8 wk after exposure
A & C: PO: 5 mg/kg/wk; *max:* 300 mg base/wk

Contraindications

Hypersensitivity to 4-aminoquinolones, renal disease,
    psoriasis, retinal changes
Caution: Alcoholism; liver dysfunction; G-6-PD deficiency;
    GI, neurologic, and hematologic disorders

Drug-Lab-Food Interactions

Drug: Increase effects of digoxin, anticoagulants,
    neuromuscular blocker; *decrease* absorption with
    antacids and laxatives
Lab: Decrease red blood cell count, hemoglobin,
    hematocrit

Pharmacokinetics

Absorption: Well absorbed from GI tract
Distribution: PB: 50%-65%
Metabolism: t½: 1.5-2 d
Excretion: Excreted slowly in urine

Pharmacodynamics

PO: Onset: Rapid
    Peak: 3.5 h
    Duration: Days to weeks
IM: Onset: Rapid
    Peak: 0.5 h
    Duration: Days to weeks

Therapeutic Effects/Uses

To treat acute malaria; prophylaxis for malaria
Mode of Action: Increased pH in the malaria parasite inhibits parasitic growth

Side Effects

Anorexia, nausea, vomiting, diarrhea, abdominal cramps,
    fatigue, pruritus, nervousness, visual disturbances
    (blurred vision)

Adverse Reactions

ECG changes, hypotension, psychosis
Life-threatening: Agranulocytosis, aplastic anemia,
    thrombocytopenia, ototoxicity, cardiovascular collapse

A, Adult; *C,* child; *d,* day; *ECG,* electrocardiogram; *G-6-PD,* glucose-6-phosphate dehydrogenase; *GI,* gastrointestinal; *h,* hour; *IM,* intramuscular; *IV,* intravenous; *max,* maximum; *PB,* protein-binding; *PO,* by mouth; *PRN,* as needed; *t½,* half-life; *wk,* week.

There are approximately 50 species of *Plasmodium;* 4 types of the species cause malaria: *P. malariae, P. ovale, P. vivax,* and *P. falciparum. P. vivax* is the most prevalent; *P. falciparum* is the most severe. Throughout the world there are about 200 million cases of malaria, but in the United States malaria is confined mainly to persons who enter the country from elsewhere. Malaria has increased since 1960 because of travel to endemic regions in the world and because of antimalarial-resistant therapy.

Treatment of malaria depends on the type of *Plasmodium* and the organism's life cycle. Quinine was the only antimalarial drug available from 1820 until the early 1940s. Synthetic **antimalarial drugs** have since been developed that are as effective as quinine and cause fewer toxic effects. When drug-resistant malaria occurs, combinations of antimalarials are used to facilitate effective treatment. Chloroquine is a commonly prescribed drug

for malaria. If drug resistance to chloroquine occurs, another antimalarial, mefloquine HCl (Lariam), or combinations of antimalarials with or without antibiotics (e.g., tetracycline, doxycycline, clindamycin) may be prescribed.

Three methods used to eradicate malaria are **prophylaxis** for the prevention of malaria, treatment for the acute attack, and prevention of relapse. Many of the synthetic antimalarials, such as chloroquine, primaquine, and pyrimethamine-sulfadoxine, are used prophylactically. Chloroquine and mefloquine are frequently used to treat an acute malarial attack. Mefloquine HCl and the combination drug atovaquone/proguanil (Malarone) are used to treat chloroquine-resistant *P. falciparum.* Chloroquine and hydroxychloroquine can be toxic to children and may even cause death; therefore the drug dose should be closely monitored. Prototype Drug Chart 32–2 lists the drug data for chloroquine HCl.

Table 32–2

Antimalarials

Generic (Brand)	Route and Dosage	Uses and Considerations
chloroquine HCl (Aralen HCl) hydroxychloroquine SO₄ (Plaquenil SO₄)	See Prototype Drug Chart 32–2. *Acute malaria:* A: PO: 620 mg base or 800 mg, then 310 mg base or 400 mg at 6, 18, and 24 h C: PO: 10 mg base/kg/dose, 6 h: 5 mg base/kg; 5 mg base/kg/d for 2 d *Prophylaxis:* 1 wk before and 6-8 wk after exposure A & C: PO: 5 mg base/kg/wk; *max:* 300 mg base/wk	Alternative to chloroquine. Dosage varies for treating malaria. Can be used adjunctively with primaquine. Give drug with meals to reduce the occurrence of GI distress. *Pregnancy category:* C; PB: 55% t¹/₂: 1.5-2 d
mefloquine HCl (Lariam)	A: PO: Single dose: 1250 mg; then 250 mg q wk × 4 wk; take with plenty of water	New antimalarial drug. Action is similar to chloroquine HCl. *Pregnancy category:* C; PB: 98%; t¹/₂: 10-21 d
primaquine phosphate	*Malaria prophylaxis:* A: PO: 15 mg/d for 14 d (single doses) C: PO: 0.3 mg/kg/d for 14 d (single doses)	Prophylaxis against certain *Plasmodium* spp. (*P. vivax* and *P. ovale*) and for relapse. Can affect white blood cell production (granulocytopenia) and acute hemolytic anemia in clients with G-6-PD deficiency. *Pregnancy category:* C; PB: UK; t¹/₂: 3.7-9.6 h
pyrimethamine (Daraprim)	*Malaria prophylaxis:* A & C: >10 y: PO: 25 mg/wk C: <4 y: PO: 6.25 mg/wk C: 4-10 y: PO: 12.5 mg/wk	Prophylaxis use for malaria. For treatment of chloroquine-resistant *Plasmodium falciparum* infections. May be used with quinacrine, quinine, or chloroquine. *Pregnancy category:* C; PB: 80%; t¹/₂: 1.5-2 d
quinacrine HCl (Atabrine HCl)	*Malaria suppression:* A: PO: 100 mg/d C: PO: 50 mg/d	For treating *Plasmodium malariae* and *Plasmodium vivax* infections. *Pregnancy category:* C; PB: UK; t¹/₂: UK
quinine SO₄ (Quinamm, Quiphile)	*Acute malaria:* A: PO: 650 mg q8h for 3-7 d C: PO: 25 mg/kg/d in 3 divided doses (q8h) for 3-7 d	Used in combination drug therapy or for chloroquine-resistant malaria. Used to treat nocturnal leg cramps. *Pregnancy category:* X; PB: 70%-95%; t¹/₂: 6-14 h
Combination of Antimalarial Drug		
atovaquone/proguanil (Malarone)	A: C >40 kg: PO: 250/100 mg = 1 tab/d C: <40 kg: 62.5/25 mg/d to 187.5/75 mg/d; based on kilograms of weight	For oral prophylaxis and treatment of malaria. It is effective for chloroquine-resistant strains. It is considered to have a greater cure rate (treatment) than mefloquine.

A, Adult; *C*, child; *d*, day; *G-6-PD*, glucose-6-phosphate dehydrogenase; *GI*, gastrointestinal; *h*, hour; *max*, maximum; *PB*, protein-binding; *PO*, by mouth; *t¹/₂*, half-life; *tab*, tablet; *UK*, unknown; *wk*, week; *y*, year; >, greater than; <, less than.

The antimalarial drug halofantrine is not available in the United States but is used in countries where acute malaria is prevalent. This drug is effective for treating chloroquine-resistant *P. falciparum*. Clients who have cardiac dysrhythmias should not take it.

Pharmacokinetics

Chloroquine HCl is well absorbed from the GI tract. It is moderately protein binding, and the drug has a long half-life. The first two doses have a loading dose effect. Because of its long half-life, the next dose is given on the second day, and the fourth dose is given on the third day. Chloroquine is metabolized in the liver to active metabolites and excreted in the urine.

Pharmacodynamics

Chloroquine HCl inhibits the malaria parasite's growth by interfering with its protein synthesis. Whether the drug is given orally or IM, the onset of action is rapid. The peak effect is slower when given orally. The duration of effect of the drug is very long—days to weeks.

Side Effects and Adverse Reactions

General side effects and adverse reactions to antimalarials include GI upset, cranial nerve VIII involvement (quinine and chloroquine), renal impairment (quinine), and cardiovascular effects (quinine).

Table 32–2 lists commonly ordered antimalarial drugs and their dosage, uses, and considerations. Quinine is an antimalarial drug, and quinidine is an antidysrhythmic drug.

PREVENTING MEDICATION ERRORS

Do not confuse...

- **quinine** (antimalarial) with **quinidine** (antidysrhythmic). These two drugs look alike, but the actions and pharmacology are very different.

A medication guideline that was developed by the FDA accompanies mefloquine (Lariam) each time it is dispensed. This type of guideline is used only for drugs that require monitoring for serious adverse effects. Adverse effects that may occur after mefloquine use include severe anxiety, restlessness, disorientation, depression, hallucinations, paranoia, and suicidal thoughts.

Nursing Process

Antimalarials

ASSESSMENT

■ Assess client's hearing, especially if he or she takes quinine or chloroquine. These drugs may affect cranial nerve VIII.
■ Check the client for visual changes. Clients who take chloroquine and hydroxychloroquine should have frequent ophthalmic examinations.

NURSING DIAGNOSES

■ Risk for infection
■ Risk for impaired tissue integrity

PLANNING

■ Client will be free of malarial symptoms.

NURSING INTERVENTIONS

■ Monitor client's urinary output and liver function by checking the urine output (>600 ml/d) and the liver enzymes. Antimalarial drugs concentrate first in the liver; serum liver enzyme levels should be checked especially if the person drinks considerable amounts of alcohol or has a liver disorder.
■ Report if client's serum liver enzymes are elevated.

Client Teaching
General
• Advise clients traveling to malaria-infested countries to receive prophylactic doses of antimalarial drug before leaving, during the visit, and upon return.
• Instruct client to take oral antimalarial drugs with food or at mealtime if GI upset occurs.
• Monitor client returning from a malaria-infested area for malarial symptoms.
• Inform client who takes chloroquine or hydroxychloroquine to report vision changes immediately.
• Warn client to avoid consuming large quantities of alcohol.

Side Effects
• Direct client to report signs and symptoms of anorexia, nausea, vomiting, diarrhea, abdominal cramps, pruritus, visual disturbances, and dizziness.

Cultural Considerations

• If client from a malaria-infested country complains of chills, high fever, and profuse sweating, client's serum should be tested for malaria. Client may receive an antimalarial drug as a prophylactic measure or for treatment of an acute attack. Explanation is necessary so client complies with the drug regimen.

EVALUATION

■ Evaluate the effectiveness of the antimalarial drug by determining that client is free of symptoms.

Anthelmintic Drugs

Helminths are large organisms (parasitic worms) that feed on host tissue. The most common site for **helminthiasis** (worm infestation) is the intestine. Other sites for parasitic infestation are the lymphatic system, blood vessels, and liver.

There are four groups of helminths: (1) cestodes (tapeworms), (2) trematodes (flukes), (3) intestinal nematodes (roundworms), and (4) tissue-invading nematodes (tissue roundworms and filariae). The cestodes (tapeworms) are segmented and enter the intestine via contaminated food. There are four species of cestodes: *Taenia solium* (pork tapeworm), *Taenia saginata* (beef tapeworm), *Diphyllobothrium latum* (fish tapeworm), and *Hymenolepis nana* (dwarf tapeworm). The segmented cestodes have heads and hooks or suckers that attach to the tissue.

The trematodes (flukes) are flat, nonsegmented parasites that feed on the host. Four types of trematodes exist: *Fasciola hepatica* (liver fluke), *Fasciolopsis buski* (intestinal fluke), *Paragonimus westermani* (lung fluke), and *Schistosoma* species (blood fluke).

Five types of nematodes may feed on the intestinal tissue: *Ascaris lumbricoides* (giant roundworm), *Necator americanus* (hookworm), *Enterobius vermicularis* (pinworm), *Strongyloides stercoralis* (threadworm), and *Trichuris trichiura* (whipworm).

Two types of nematodes are tissue invading: *Trichinella spiralis* (pork roundworm) and *Wuchereria bancrofti* (filariae). The pork roundworm or *T. spiralis* can cause **trichinosis,** which can be diagnosed by a muscle biopsy. By thoroughly cooking pork, the roundworm, if present, is destroyed.

Side Effects and Adverse Reactions
The common side effects of **anthelmintic drugs** include GI upset such as anorexia, nausea, vomiting, and occasionally diarrhea and stomach cramps. The neurologic problems associated with anthelmintics are dizziness, weakness, headache, and drowsiness. Adverse reactions do not occur frequently because the drugs usually are given only for a short period (1 to 3 days), except for niclosamide for treatment of dwarf tapeworms, piperazine for treatment of pinworms, and thiabendazole for treatment of threadworms and pork worms. Thiabendazole should be avoided if the client has liver disease.

Table 32–3

Anthelmintic Drugs

Generic (Brand)	Route and Dosage	Uses and Considerations
bithionol (Actamer)	UK	Effective against flukes. Treatment of *Paragonimus westermani* (lung fluke)
diethylcarbamazine (Hetrazan)	A: PO: 2-3 mg/kg/t.i.d.	Treatment for nematode-filariae
ivermectin (Stromectol)	A & C: >15 kg: PO: 200 mcg/kg/1 dose	A broad-spectrum antiparasitic drug. Causes paralysis to the parasite. Highly active against various mites. *Pregnancy category:* C; PB: UK; t½: 12-16 h
mebendazole (Vermox)	A: PO: 100 mg b.i.d. × 3 d Repeat in 2-3 wk if necessary C: >2y: PO: same as adult	Treatment for giant roundworm, hookworm, pinworm, whipworm. *Pregnancy category:* C
niclosamide (Niclocide)	A: PO: 2 g, single dose C: >34 kg: PO: 1.5 g, single dose C: 11-34 kg: PO: 1 g, single dose	Treatment for beef and fish tapeworms. *Pregnancy category:* B
oxamniquine (Vansil)	A: PO: 15 mg/kg/ d for 1-2 d C: PO: 10-15 mg/kg/d for 1-2 d	Treatment against mature and immature worms. *Pregnancy category:* C; PB: UK; t½: 1-2.5 h
piperazine citrate (Antepar)	*Roundworm:* A: PO: 3.5 g/d × 2 d C: PO: 75 mg/kg/d × 2 d; *max:* 3.5 g/d *Pinworms:* A & C: 65 mg/kg/d × 7 d *max:* 2.5 g/d	Treatment of roundworms and pinworms. *Pregnancy category:* B; PB: UK; t½: UK
praziquantel (Biltricide)	A & C: PO: 10-20 mg/kg single dose A & C: PO: 20 mg/kg t.i.d. × 1 d A & C: 25 mg/kg t.i.d. 1-2 d	Treatment for beef, pork, and fish tapeworms Treatment for blood flukes Treatment for liver, lung, and intestinal flukes. *Pregnancy category:* B; PB: UK; t½: 0.8-1.5 h
pyrantel pamoate (Antiminth)	A & C: PO: 11 mg/kg single dose; *max:* 1 g	Treatment of giant roundworm, hookworm, and pinworm. *Pregnancy category:* C; PB: UK; t½: UK
thiabendazole (Mintezol)	Repeat in 2 wk PRN A: <70 kg: PO: 25 mg/kg 1-2 ×/d for 2 d; repeat in 2 d PRN C: 14-70 kg: PO: 25 mg/kg 1-2 ×/d for 2 d	Treatment of threadworm and pork worm. *Pregnancy category:* C; PB: UK; t½: UK

A, Adult; *b.i.d.*, two times a day; *C*, child; *d*, day; *h*, hour; *max*, maximum; *PB*, protein-binding; *PO*, by mouth; *PRN*, as needed; *t½*, half-life; *t.i.d.*, three times a day; *UK*, unknown; *wk*, week; *y*, year; >, greater than; <, less than.

Table 32–3 lists ten anthelmintic drugs prescribed to treat various types of parasitic worms.

Nursing Process

Anthelmintics

ASSESSMENT

■ Obtain a history of foods client has eaten, especially meat and fish, and how the food was prepared.
■ Note if any other person in the household has been checked for helminths (worms).
■ Assess baseline vital signs and collect a stool specimen.

NURSING DIAGNOSES

■ Defensive coping related to the helminth and treatment regimen
■ Activity intolerance related to dizziness, headache, drowsiness

PLANNING

■ Client will be free of helminths.
■ Client will understand how to prepare foods properly to avoid recurrence.

NURSING INTERVENTIONS

■ Collect a stool specimen in a clean container. Avoid having the stool come in contact with water, urine, or chemicals, which could destroy parasitic worms.
■ Administer the prescribed anthelmintics after meals to prevent or minimize the occurrence of GI distress.
■ Report to the health care provider if client has any side effects.

Client Teaching

• Explain to the client the importance of washing hands before eating and after going to the toilet. The parasite can be transferred within the family if proper hygiene is not used.
• Instruct client to take daily showers and *not* baths.

- Advise client to change sheets, bedclothes, towels, and underwear daily.
- Tell client that, if the problem persists after therapy, a second course of anthelmintics may be necessary.
- Emphasize the importance of taking the prescribed drug at designated times and to keep health care appointments.
- Alert client that drowsiness may occur and that he or she should avoid operating a car or machinery if drowsiness occurs.
- Educate client to report any side effects to the health care provider.

Cultural Considerations

- Obtain an interpreter when necessary; do not rely on family members, who may not fully disclose because of honor and shame.

EVALUATION

- Evaluate the effect of the anthelmintics and the absence of side effects.
- Determine whether client is using proper hygiene to avoid spread of parasitic worms.

WEBSITES

For further information on *Antiviral*, *Antimalarial*, and *Anthelmintic Drugs*, visit these Internet resources:

Information on acyclovir:
www.nlm.nih.gov/medlineplus/druginfo/medmaster/a681045.html

Critical Thinking Case Study

T.P., age 75, has shingles. She complains of pain and blisters (vesicular eruptions), which partially surround her waist. The health care provider prescribed acyclovir, 800 mg, every 4 hours, five times a day for 7 days.

1. When taking the health history, what should the nurse ask T.P.?

2. How does herpes zoster differ from varicella-zoster virus (VZV)? Explain who would be more susceptible to contracting herpes zoster virus infection.

3. How is acyclovir effective for relieving T.P.'s symptoms?

4. Is the prescribed acyclovir dose correct? If so, why?

5. How does acyclovir differ from famciclovir and amantadine?

6. What comfort measures would you suggest to T.P.?

7. What should the nurse inform T.P. about being around other people?

Study Questions

1. Amantadine is an antiviral drug. For what other disease is this drug used? What are some side effects and adverse reactions to amantadine?

2. Vidarabine and acyclovir are antiviral antimetabolites. How are these drugs similar, and how do they differ in their uses?

3. What three antiviral drugs may be prescribed for advanced HIV infection?

4. Your client is to receive chloroquine as a prophylactic against malaria. How does chloroquine act to prevent malaria? What is the schedule for administration when it is used prophylactically? Discuss the significance of protein binding and the half-life of chloroquine HCl.

5. Why should the client's hematology tests be monitored while the client takes chloroquine HCl?

6. What should be included in client teaching regarding the use of antimalarials?

7. What are helminths? Most types of helminths are concentrated in what part of the body?

8. Trichinosis is caused by what organism? How can this health problem be prevented? How is it diagnosed?

9. What client teaching instructions should be included for a client diagnosed with helminths?

33 Drugs for Urinary Tract Disorders

ELECTRONIC RESOURCES

Additional information can be found on the companion website at *http://evolve.elsevier.com/KeeHayes/pharmacology/* or on the companion CD-ROM, which includes:
- *NCLEX-style examination review questions*
- *Pharmacology animations*
- *Medication error and IV therapy checklists*
- *Medication calculation problems*
- *Electronic calculators*

OUTLINE

Objectives

Terms

Introduction

Urinary Antiseptics/Antiinfectives and Antibiotics
Nitrofurantoin
Nursing Process: Urinary Antiinfective: Nitrofurantoin
Methenamine
Trimethoprim and Trimethoprim-Sulfamethoxazole

Fluoroquinolones (Quinolones)
Drug-Drug Interactions

Urinary Analgesics
Phenazopyridine

Urinary Stimulants

Urinary Antispasmodics/Antimuscarinics

Websites

Critical Thinking Case Study

Study Questions

OBJECTIVES

- Identify the groups of drugs that are urinary antiseptics and antiinfectives.
- Describe the side effects and adverse reactions to urinary antiseptics and antiinfectives.
- Give uses for a urinary analgesic, a urinary stimulant, and a urinary antispasmodic.
- Describe the nursing process, including client teaching, regarding urinary antiseptic/antiinfective drugs.

TERMS

acute cystitis
acute pyelonephritis
antimuscarinics
antispasmodics
bactericidal

bacteriostatic
micturition
urinary analgesic
urinary antiseptics/antiinfectives

urinary stimulant
urinary tract infections (UTIs)

Introduction

The largest number of urinary tract disorders are caused by **urinary tract infections (UTIs)**. UTIs may result from an upper UTI, such as pyelonephritis, or a lower UTI, such as cystitis, urethritis, or prostatitis. A group of drugs called **urinary antiseptics/antiinfectives** prevents bacterial growth in the kidneys and bladder but is not effective for systemic infections. Urinary antiseptics/antiinfectives have a **bacteriostatic** effect when given in lower dosages. They also have a **bactericidal** effect when given in higher dosages.

Urinary antiseptics/antiinfectives, urinary analgesics, urinary stimulants, and urinary antispasmodics/antimuscarinics are presented in this chapter. See Chapters 28 (Antibacterials and Their Effects: Penicillins and Cephalosporins), 29 (Antibacterials: Macrolides, Tetracyclines, Aminoglycosides, and Fluoroquinolones), and 30 (Antibacterials: Sulfonamides) for further explanation of antibiotics, fluoroquinolones, and sulfonamides that are used to treat UTIs. Diuretics are discussed in Chapter 41, Diuretics.

Acute cystitis, a lower UTI, frequently occurs in female clients because of their shorter urethra. It is more common in women of childbearing age, older women, and young girls. Acute cystitis is commonly caused by *Escherichia coli*. Other bacterial causes include the gram-positive *Staphylococcus saprophyticus* and gram-negative *Klebsiella, Proteus,* and *Pseudomonas*. Symptoms of cystitis include pain and burning on urination and urinary frequency and urgency. A urine culture is obtained before the start of any antiinfective/antibiotic drug therapy. In male clients, a lower UTI is most likely prostatitis with symptoms similar to cystitis.

Acute pyelonephritis, an upper UTI, is commonly seen in women of childbearing age, older women, and young girls. *E. coli* is the most common organism causing pyelonephritis. Symptoms include chills, high fever, flank pain, pain during urination, urinary frequency and urgency, and pyuria. The bacterial count in the urine is greater than 100,000 bacteria/ml. In severe cases, the client may be hospitalized and receive intravenous (IV) antibiotics such as an aminoglycoside, ticarcillin/clavulanic acid, or piperacillin/tazobactam.

The most commonly used agents for treating UTIs are nitrofurantoin (Furalan, Furadantin, Macrodantin), trimethoprim-sulfamethoxazole (co-trimoxazole, Bactrim, Septra), and fluoroquinolones such as cinoxacin (Cinobac), nalidixic acid (NegGram), and norfloxacin (Noroxin), and ciprofloxacin (Cipro). Treatment may consist of a single double-strength dose of the chosen drug, a short-term 3-day course, or the traditional method of 7 to 14 days of drug dosing. Fosfomycin tromethamine (Monurol), a nitrofurantoin prototype drug, is effective for UTIs as a single-dose treatment. Other agents used to treat UTIs include oral amoxicillin/clavulanic acid (Augmentin) and oral third-generation cephalosporins (cefixime, cefpodoxime proxetil, or ceftibuten). With severe UTIs, IV drug therapy followed by oral drug therapy is usually recommended.

Urinary Antiseptics/Antiinfectives and Antibiotics

Urinary antiseptics/antiinfectives are limited to the treatment of UTIs. The drug action occurs in the renal tubule and bladder and thus is effective in reducing bacterial growth. A urinalysis and culture and sensitivity test are usually performed before the initiation of drug therapy. The groups of urinary antiseptics/antiinfectives are nitrofurantoin, methenamine, trimethoprim, and the fluoroquinolones.

Nitrofurantoin

Nitrofurantoin (Furalan, Macrodantin) was first prescribed to treat UTIs in 1953. Nitrofurantoin is bacteriostatic or bactericidal, depending on the drug dosage, and is effective against many gram-positive and gram-negative organisms, especially *E. coli*. It is used to treat acute and chronic UTIs. The drug data for nitrofurantoin are given in Prototype Drug Chart 33–1.

Pharmacokinetics

Nitrofurantoin is well absorbed from the gastrointestinal (GI) tract. The drug is usually taken with food to decrease GI distress. Decreased absorption occurs when the drug is taken with antacids. Nitrofurantoin is moderately protein bound. With normal renal function, the drug is rapidly eliminated because of its short half-life of 20 minutes; however, it accumulates in the serum with urinary dysfunction.

Pharmacodynamics

When nitrofurantoin is given in low doses for prophylactic use, the drug has a bacteriostatic effect. High concentration of nitrofurantoin causes a bactericidal effect. Nitrofurantoin is effective against many gram-positive and gram-negative organisms such as *E. coli, Neisseria,* streptococci, *Staphylococcus aureus,* and others. It is not as effective against *Pseudomonas aeruginosa, Proteus* species, and some species of *Klebsiella*. The onset and duration of action are unknown. Peak action occurs 30 minutes after absorption. If sudden onset of dyspnea, chest pain, cough, fever, and chills develops, the client should contact the health care provider. Symptoms resolve after discontinuing the drug.

The nursing process for nitrofurantoin is applicable for the other urinary antiseptics/antiinfectives.

Nursing Process

Urinary Antiinfective: Nitrofurantoin

ASSESSMENT

- Obtain a history from client of clinical problems with urinary tract infection (UTI) or other urinary tract disorders.
- Check client for signs and symptoms of UTI, such as pain or burning sensation on urination and frequency and urgency of urination.
- Evaluate complete blood count (CBC) on clients with long-term therapy; monitor regularly.
- Assess renal and hepatic function.
- Determine urine pH; 5.5 is desired. However, alkalinization of the urine is *not* recommended.

NURSING DIAGNOSES

- Acute pain
- Risk for infection

PLANNING

- Client will be free of signs and symptoms of UTI within 10 days.

NURSING INTERVENTIONS

- Monitor client's output. Careful attention to output is required when administering urinary antiseptics to clients with anuria and oliguria. Report promptly any decrease in urine output.

- Before the start of drug therapy, obtain a urine culture to determine the organism causing the UTI.
- Observe client for side effects and adverse reactions to urinary antiseptic drugs. Peripheral neuropathy (tingling, numbness of extremities) may result from renal insufficiency (inability to excrete drug) or long-term use of nitrofurantoin. Peripheral neuropathy may be irreversible.
- Dilute IV nitrofurantoin in 500 ml of IV solution before administering; reconstitute in sterile water without preservative.

Client Teaching

General
- Teach client not to crush tablets or open capsules.

PROTOTYPE DRUG CHART 33–1

NITROFURANTOIN

Drug Class	**Dosage**
Urinary antiinfective Trade Name: Furalan, Furadantin, Macrodantin, ♣ Apo-nitrofurantoin, Novofuran *Pregnancy Category:* B	*Initial/recurrent UTI:* **A: PO:** 50-100 mg q.i.d. with meals and at bedtime; take with food **C: 1 mo-12 y: PO:** 5-7 mg/kg in 4 divided doses *Long-term prophylaxis:* **A: PO:** 50-100 mg at bedtime **C: 1 mo-12 y: PO:** 1 mg/kg in 1-2 divided doses
Contraindications	**Drug-Lab-Food Interactions**
Hypersensitivity, moderate to severe renal impairment, oliguria, anuria, Cl_{cr} <40 ml/min, infants <1 mo, term pregnancy, lactation with infant suspected of having G-6-PD deficiency *Caution:* Vitamin B deficiency, electrolyte imbalance, diabetes mellitus	*Drug:* *Decrease* effect with probenecid; decrease absorption with antacids
Pharmacokinetics	**Pharmacodynamics**
Absorption: Well absorbed from GI tract; enhanced with food **Distribution:** PB: 60%, crosses placenta and enters breast milk **Metabolism:** $t\frac{1}{2}$: 20-60 min **Excretion:** In urine; small amounts in bile	**PO:** Onset: UK Peak: 30 min Duration: UK

Therapeutic Effects/Uses

To treat acute and chronic UTIs
Mode of Action: Inhibits bacterial enzymes and metabolism

Side Effects	**Adverse Reactions**
Anorexia, nausea, vomiting, rust/brown discoloration of urine, diarrhea, rash, pruritus, dizziness, headache, drowsiness	Superinfection, peripheral neuropathy, hemolytic anemia, agranulocytosis **Life-threatening:** Anaphylaxis, hepatotoxicity, Stevens-Johnson syndrome

A, Adult; *C,* child; *Cl$_{cr}$,* creatinine clearance; *G-6-PD,* glucose-6-phosphate dehydrogenase; *GI,* gastrointestinal; *min,* minute; *mo,* month; *PB,* protein-binding; *PO,* by mouth; *q.i.d.,* four times a day; *t$\frac{1}{2}$,* half-life; *UK,* unknown; *UTI,* urinary tract infection; *y,* year; <, less than; ♣, Canadian drug names.

- Advise client to rinse the mouth thoroughly after taking oral nitrofurantoin. This drug can stain the teeth.
- Avoid antacids because they interfere with drug absorption.
- Instruct client to shake suspension well before taking and protect it from freezing.
- Warn client not to drive a motor vehicle or operate dangerous machinery because this drug may cause drowsiness.
- Direct clients with diabetes *not* to use Clinitest for glucose testing because a false-positive result may occur.

Diet
- Inform client to increase fluids and take the drug with food; this minimizes GI upset.

Side Effects
- Alert client that urine may turn a harmless brown.
- Encourage client to report any signs of secondary fungal or bacterial infection (superinfection), such as stomatitis or anogenital discharge or itching.

Methenamine
- Educate client to drink cranberry juice or take vitamin C with approval of the health care provider to keep the urine acidic. Foods that are alkaline, such as milk and some vegetables, may increase the urine pH. The urine pH should be less than 5.5 for the antiseptic to be effective.

Fluoroquinolones
- Warn client to avoid operating hazardous machinery or driving a car while taking the drug, especially if dizziness is present.
- Encourage client to take the drug with food and to avoid antacids because they interfere with drug absorption.
- Alert client that the urine may turn a harmless brown because of the drug.
- Direct client to report any signs of superinfection or a secondary fungal or bacterial infection.
- Tell client to avoid excessive exposure to sunlight.

Cultural Considerations ⊕
- Alleviate the fear or concerns client from a different cultural background has by explaining the treatment regimen for a UTI. An interpreter may be necessary. The use of pamphlets could help client understand the urinary tract problem.
- A detailed explanation of preventive measures of UTIs could be helpful. Proper use of toilet paper after defecation should be emphasized.

EVALUATION

■ Evaluate the effectiveness of the urinary antiinfectives in alleviating the UTI. Client is free of side effects and adverse reactions to drug.

Methenamine

Methenamine (Hiprex, Mandelamine) produces a bactericidal effect when the urine pH is less than 5.5. Methenamine is available as mandelate salt (short-acting) and as hippurate salt. It is effective against gram-positive and gram-negative organisms, especially *E. coli* and *P. aeruginosa*. It is used for chronic UTIs. Methenamine should not be taken with sulfonamides because crystalluria is likely to occur. It is absorbed readily from the GI tract, and approximately 90% of the drug is excreted in the urine unchanged. Methenamine forms ammonia and formaldehyde in acid urine; therefore the urine needs to be acidified to exert a bactericidal action. Cranberry juice (several 8-ounce glasses per day), ascorbic acid, and ammonium chloride can be taken to decrease the urine pH.

Trimethoprim and Trimethoprim-Sulfamethoxazole

Trimethoprim (Proloprim, Trimpex) can be used alone (although frequently it is not) for the treatment of UTIs or in combination with a sulfonamide, sulfamethoxazole (the combined preparation is generically called *co-trimoxazole*, or *TMP/SMZ*), to prevent the occurrence of trimethoprim-resistant organisms. It produces slow-acting bactericidal effects against most gram-positive and gram-negative organisms. Co-trimoxazole (Bactrim, Septra) is discussed in detail in Chapter 29, Antibacterials: Macrolides, Tetracyclines, Aminoglycosides, and Fluoroquinolones. Trimethoprim is used in the treatment and prevention of acute and chronic UTIs. The amount of trimethoprim in the prostatic fluid is about two to three times greater than the amount in the vascular fluid. The half-life of trimethoprim is normally 9 to 11 hours; however it is longer in clients with renal dysfunction.

Fluoroquinolones (Quinolones)

Fluoroquinolones are one of the groups of urinary antibacterials that are effective against lower UTIs. Nalidixic acid (NegGram) was developed in 1964, and cinoxacin (Cinobac), norfloxacin (Noroxin), and ciprofloxacin hydrochloride (Cipro) were marketed in the 1980s. Enoxacin was marketed in 1989, ofloxacin in 1990, and lomefloxacin in 1992. The newer fluoroquinolones (norfloxacin, ciprofloxacin, enoxacin, ofloxacin, and lomefloxacin) are effective against a wide variety of UTIs. The drug dosage should be decreased when renal dysfunction is present. The half-lives of these drugs are 2 to 4 hours but are prolonged in clients with renal dysfunction. Table 33–1 lists the urinary antiseptics/antiinfectives and their dosages, uses, and considerations.

Side Effects and Adverse Reactions

The side effects and adverse reactions to urinary antiseptics are listed herein by category.

Nitrofurantoin. Side effects of nitrofurantoin use include GI disturbances such as anorexia, nausea, vomiting, diarrhea, and abdominal pain and pulmonary reactions such as dyspnea, chest pain, fever, and cough.

Table 33–1

Antiseptics and Urinary Antiinfectives

Generic (Brand)	Route and Dosage	Uses and Considerations
fosfomycin tromethamine (Monurol)	A & C: >12 y: PO: 1-3 g packet dissolved in 4 oz water, as a single dose	To treat uncomplicated UTIs in women. Has a bactericidal effect against most gram-negative and gram-positive bacteria. Side effects include headaches and diarrhea. *Pregnancy category:* B; PB: 0; t½: 5.7 h
methenamine mandelate (Mandelamine, Mandameth)	A: PO: 1 g q.i.d. p.c. C: 6-12 y: PO: 0.5 g q.i.d. p.c. or 50 mg/kg in 4 divided doses p.c. C: <6 y: PO: 18.4 mg/kg q.i.d.	For chronic UTIs. Urine pH should be acidic (<5.5). It should not be used with sulfonamides. May cause crystalluria, so push fluids. It can cause GI irritation, so take with meals. *Pregnancy category:* C; PB: UK; t½: 3-6 h
methenamine hippurate (Hiprex, Urex)	A: PO: 1 g b.i.d. C: 6-12 y: PO: 0.5-1 g b.i.d.	Same as above
nitrofurantoin (Furalan, Furadantin, Macrodantin)	See Prototype Drug Chart 33–1.	
trimethoprim (Proloprim, Trimpex)	A: PO: 100 mg q12h or 200 mg q24h; if Cl$_{cr}$ (CrCl) is 15-30 ml/min: 50 mg q12h; if Cl$_{cr}$ <15 ml/min: do not use	For prevention and treatment of acute and chronic UTIs in both men and women. High doses can cause GI upset. Drug can be combined with sulfamethoxazole (Bactrim). *Pregnancy category:* C; PB: UK; t½: 8-11 h
ertapenem (Invanz)	A: IM/IV: 1 g every day for 10-14 days	To treat complicated UTIs. Effective against gram-positive and gram-negative bacteria. Commonly causes diarrhea, nausea, and headache. *Pregnancy category:* B; PB: 85%-95%; t½: 2-4 h
Sulfonamides		
trimethoprim-sulfamethoxazole (TMP-SMZ, Co-trimoxazole, Bactrim, Septra)	See Prototype Drug Chart 30–1.	Effective for serious UTIs and for otitis media. *Pregnancy category:* C; PB: 60%-70%; t½: 9 h
Quinolones (Fluoroquinolones)		
cinoxacin (Cinobac)	A: PO: 1 g/d in 2-4 doses for 1-2 wk *Renal dysfunction:* Initially: 500 mg; if Cl$_{cr}$ is >80 ml/min: 500 mg b.i.d.; 80-50 ml/min: 250 mg t.i.d.; 50-20 ml/min: 250 mg b.i.d.; <20 ml/min: 250 mg daily Not recommended for infants or prepubertal children.	For acute and chronic UTIs. More effective than nalidixic acid. Absorbed in prostatic tissue. Can cause dizziness and photosensitivity. Avoid excessive exposure to sunlight. *Pregnancy category:* C; PB: 60%-80%; t½: 1.5 h
ciprofloxacin (Cipro)	A: PO: mild to moderate: 250 mg q12h A: PO: severe/complicated: 500-750 mg q12h A: IV: 200-400 mg q12h; dilute and infuse over 1 h *Renal dysfunction:* Decrease dosage *Hemo or peritoneal dialysis:* 250-500 mg q24h after dialysis	Has a broad-spectrum antibacterial effect. For UTI, skin and soft tissue infections, and bone and joint infections and anthrax infection. Antacid inhibits drug absorption. Use with caution in clients with seizure disorders. Can be taken without food. Photosensitivity can occur. Avoid excessive exposure to sunlight. *Pregnancy category:* C; PB: 20%-40%; t½: 4-6 h
enoxacin (Penetrex)	*Uncomplicated UTI:* A: PO: 200 mg q12h for 7 d *Complicated or severe UTI:* A: PO: 400 mg q12h for 14 d If Cl$_{cr}$ <30 ml/min, reduce dose by 50%.	Effective against complicated and uncomplicated UTIs. Fluid intake should be increased. Take before or after meals. Phototoxicity may occur. *Pregnancy category:* C (pregnant: X); PB: UK; t½: 3-6 h
lomefloxacin (Maxaquin)	A: PO: 400 mg/d × 10 d	For UTIs and transurethral surgery prophylaxis. *Pregnancy category:* C; PB: UK; t½: 6.25-7.75 h
nalidixic acid (NegGram)	A: PO: 1 g q.i.d. for 1-2 wk; 1 g b.i.d. for long-term use C: PO: 55 mg/kg/d in 4 divided doses for 1-2 wk; 33 mg/kg/d for long-term use C: <3 mo: *Do not use*	For acute and chronic UTIs. Resistance to drug may occur. Highly protein bound. Not distributed in prostatic fluid. Take with food to avoid GI upset. Photosensitivity can occur. Contact health care provider if seizures or severe headaches occur. *Pregnancy category:* B; PB: 93%; t½: 1-2 h (elderly: 12 h)

A, Adult; *b.i.d.,* twice a day; *BUN,* blood urea nitrogen; *C,* child; *Cl$_{cr}$,* creatinine clearance; *d,* day; *GI,* gastrointestinal; *h,* hour; *IM,* intramuscular; *IV,* intravenous; *min,* minute; *mo,* month; *PB,* protein-binding; *p.c.,* after meals; *PO,* by mouth; *q.i.d.,* four times a day; *t½,* half-life; *t.i.d.,* three times a day; *UK,* unknown; *UTI,* urinary tract infection; *wk,* week; *y,* year; *>,* greater than; *<,* less than.   *Continued*

Table 33–1

Antiseptics and Urinary Antiinfectives—cont'd

Generic (Brand)	Route and Dosage	Uses and Considerations
Quinolones (Fluoroquinolones)—cont'd		
norfloxacin (Noroxin)	A: PO: 400 mg b.i.d. for 1-2 wk on empty stomach *Uncomplicated cystitis caused by E. coli, K. pneumoniae, P. mirabilis:* 400 mg b.i.d. × 3 d *Uncomplicated caused by any other organism:* 400 mg b.i.d. × 7-10 d *Complicated:* 400 mg b.i.d. × 10-21 d *Renal impairment (Cl_{cr} <50 ml/min):* 400 mg daily	For acute and chronic UTIs. Most potent drug of the quinolone group. Food may inhibit drug absorption. *Pregnancy category:* C; PB: 10%-15%; $t\frac{1}{2}$: 3-4 h
ofloxacin (Floxin)	A: PO: IV: 200 mg q12h × 10 d	For UTIs, respiratory tract and skin infections. May cause headaches, dizziness, insomnia. *Pregnancy category:* C; PB: 20%-32%; $t\frac{1}{2}$: 5-7.5 h
Other		
aztreonam (Azactam)	A: IM/IV: 500 mg-1 g q8-12h	Treatment of UTIs caused by gram-negative organisms. Also useful for low respiratory infection and septicemia. *Pregnancy category:* B; PB: 56%-60%; $t\frac{1}{2}$: 1.5-2 h
imipenem/cilastatin sodium (Primaxin)	A: IV: 250 mg-1 g q6h; *max:* 4 g/d or 50 mg/kg/d, whichever is the lesser amount C: Safety and efficacy not established Adjust dosing in clients with renal impairment.	Treatment of serious UTIs. Also useful for lower respiratory, bone, and joint infections; and septicemia and endocarditis. *Pregnancy category:* C; PB: 20%-40%; $t\frac{1}{2}$: 1 h
polymyxin B SO_4 (Aerosporin)	A & C: IV: 15,000-25,000 units/kg/d in divided doses q12h	Effective for UTIs and to prevent bacteriuria occurring from indwelling catheter. Can cause nephrotoxicity. Monitor renal function (BUN, serum creatinine). *Pregnancy category:* B; PB: UK; $t\frac{1}{2}$: 4-6 h

Methenamine. Methenamine use also has GI side effects, including nausea, vomiting, and diarrhea. There are some allergic reactions to the dye in Hiprex. Bladder irritation and crystalluria (when taken in large doses) may occur.

Trimethoprim. GI symptoms, including nausea and vomiting, and skin problems, such as rash and pruritus, can accompany trimethoprim use.

Fluoroquinolones. Nalidixic acid use can have the following side effects: headaches, dizziness, syncope (fainting), peripheral neuritis, visual disturbances, and rash. Nausea, vomiting, diarrhea, headaches, and visual disturbances can occur with cinoxacin and norfloxacin use. Photosensitivity is a common side effect associated with fluoroquinolones.

Drug-Drug Interactions

The following drug-drug interactions can occur with the use of urinary antiseptics/antiinfectives:

* Antacids decrease nitrofurantoin absorption.
* Sodium bicarbonate inhibits the action of methenamine.
* Methenamine taken with sulfonamides increases the risk of crystalluria.
* Nalidixic acid enhances the effects of warfarin (Coumadin).

* Most urinary antiseptics cause false-positive Clinitest results.

Urinary Analgesics

Phenazopyridine

Phenazopyridine hydrochloride (Pyridium), an azo dye, is a **urinary analgesic** that has been available for almost 40 years. It is used to relieve pain, burning sensation, and the frequency and urgency of urination that are symptomatic of lower UTIs. The drug can cause GI disturbances, hemolytic anemia, nephrotoxicity, and hepatotoxicity. The urine becomes a harmless reddish orange because of the dye. Phenazopyridine can alter the glucose urine test (Clinitest); therefore a blood test should be used to monitor glucose levels.

Urinary Stimulants

When bladder function is decreased or lost as a result of (1) a neurogenic bladder (a dysfunction caused by a lesion of the nervous system), (2) a spinal cord injury (paraplegia, hemiplegia), or (3) a severe head injury, a parasympathomimetic may be used to stimulate **micturition** (urination).

The drug of choice, bethanechol chloride (Urecholine), is a **urinary stimulant,** also known as a *direct-acting parasympathomimetic* (cholinomimetic). The drug action is to increase bladder tone by increasing tone of the detrusor urinal muscle, which produces a contraction strong enough to stimulate urination. Bethanechol is discussed in detail in Chapter 18, Cholinergics and Anticholinergics.

Urinary Antispasmodics/Antimuscarinics

Urinary tract spasms resulting from infection or injury can be relieved with **antispasmodics** that have a direct action on the smooth muscles of the urinary tract. This group of drugs (dimethyl sulfoxide [also called DMSO], oxybutynin [Ditropan], and flavoxate [Urispas]) is contraindicated for use if urinary or GI obstruction is present or if the client has glaucoma. Antispasmodics have the same effects as **antimuscarinics,** parasympatholytics, and anticholinergics (see Chapter 18, Cholinergics and Anticholinergics). Side effects include dry mouth, increased heart rate, dizziness, intestinal distention, and constipation. Tolterodine tartrate (Detrol) is an antimuscarinic/anticholinergic drug used to control an overactive bladder, which causes frequency in urination. This drug also decreases urge urinary incontinence. It has the same side effects as antispasmodics/anticholinergics. Table 32–2 lists drugs that are urinary analgesics, stimulants, and antispasmodics/antimuscarinics.

Table 33–2
Urinary Analgesic, Stimulant, and Antispasmodics

Generic (Brand)	Route and Dosage	Uses and Considerations
Urinary Analgesic		
phenazopyridine HCl (Pyridium, Urodine)	A: PO: 100-200 mg t.i.d. p.c. × 2 d C: PO: 12 mg/kg in 3 divided doses	For chronic cystitis to alleviate pain and burning sensation during urination. Urine will be reddish orange. Can be taken concurrently with an antibiotic. It treats only symptoms, not the underlying cause of the pain; therefore do not use long term for undiagnosed urinary tract pain. *Pregnancy category:* B; PB: UK; t½: UK
Urinary Stimulant		
bethanechol Cl (Urecholine, Duvoid, Urebeth)	A: PO: 10-50 mg t.i.d./q.i.d. 1 h a.c. or 2 h p.c.; *max:* 120 mg/d subQ: 2.5-5 mg t.i.d./q.i.d. PRN C: PO: 0.2 mg/kg t.i.d. or 0.6 mg/m² t.i.d.	For hypotonic or atonic bladder. Should not be taken if peptic ulcer is present. Can cause epigastric distress, abdominal cramps, nausea, vomiting, diarrhea, and flatulence. Can cause dizziness, lightheadedness, and fainting, especially when standing up from lying or sitting position. *Pregnancy category:* C; PB: UK; t½: UK
Urinary Antispasmodics		
dimethyl sulfoxide (DMSO, Rimso-50)	*Bladder instillation:* 50 ml of 50% sol retained for 15 min; repeat q2wk until relief	For cystitis. Administered into the bladder to remain for 15 minutes. Additional effects are antiinflammatory, anesthetic, and bacteriostatic. Can cause a garliclike taste and odor on breath and skin for up to 72 h. *Pregnancy category:* C; PB: UK; t½: UK
flavoxate HCl (Urispas)	A: PO: 100-200 mg t.i.d. or q.i.d.	For urinary tract spasms. To be avoided by persons with glaucoma. Cautious use by older adults. Side effects include nausea, vomiting, dry mouth, drowsiness, blurred vision. *Pregnancy category:* B; PB: UK; t½: UK
oxybutynin Cl (Ditropan)	A: PO: 5 mg b.i.d. or t.i.d. Elderly: PO: 2.5-5 mg b.i.d. C: >5 y: PO: 5 mg b.i.d. C: 1-5 y: PO: 0.2 mg/kg b.i.d.–q.i.d.	For urinary tract spasms and overactive bladder. Contraindicated for persons with cardiac, renal, hepatic, and prostate problems. Side effects include drowsiness, blurred vision, and dry mouth. *Pregnancy category:* B; PB: UK; t½: 1-3 h
Antimuscarinic/Anticholinergic		
tolterodine tartrate (Detrol)	A: PO: 2 mg b.i.d. Decrease to 1 mg b.i.d. with liver or kidney dysfunction.	To control overactive bladder by decreasing urinary frequency and urgency. Client with narrow-angle glaucoma should not take this drug. Dry mouth is common. *Pregnancy category:* C; PB: 96%; t½: 2-3.5 h
trospium chloride (Sanctura)	A: PO: 20 mg twice daily	To treat overactive bladder by action of a muscarinic-receptor antagonist. *Pregnancy category:* UK; PB: UK; t½: 18 h

A, Adult; *a.c.,* before meals; *b.i.d.,* twice a day; *C,* child; *d,* daily; *h,* hour; *max,* maximum; *min,* minute; *PB,* protein-binding; *p.c.,* after meals; *PO,* by mouth; *PRN,* as needed; *q.i.d.,* four times a day; *subQ,* subcutaneous; *sol,* solution; *t½,* half-life; *t.i.d.,* three times a day; *UK,* unknown; *wk,* week; *y,* year; *>,* greater than.

WEBSITES

For further information on *Drugs for Urinary Tract Disorders,* visit these Internet resources:

Information on nitrofurantoin:

www.nlm.nih.gov/medlineplus/druginfo/medmaster/a682291.html

Information on Bactrim:

www.healthsquare.com/newrx/BAC1046.HTM

Critical Thinking Case Study

F.L., age 29, is married and has a 3-year-old child. F.L. complained to her health care provider of painful urinary frequency and urgency. The client has an elevated temperature. The urine specimen indicated that the client had a urinary tract infection (UTI). Co-trimoxazole D.S. (double-strength, T-160 mg/S-800 mg) tablet twice a day for 14 days is prescribed (see Chapter 30, Antibacterials: Sulfonamides, as needed).

1. What other information should the health care provider obtain from the client?

2. What other dose of co-trimoxazole (TMP-SMZ) could be prescribed? Explain.

3. Explain what the health care provider should discuss with the client in regard to taking the drug and its possible side effects. What other information should F.L. receive?

4. What preventive measures should be discussed with the client to prevent future occurrences of UTIs?

5. What is the recommended follow-up care for F.L.?

6. What other drugs might be used instead of co-trimoxazole (TMP-SMZ)? Would one urinary antiinfective drug be more effective than another antiinfective drug? Explain.

Study Questions

1. What are the symptoms of UTIs? What group of drugs is used to alleviate these symptoms?

2. What is the major group of side effects associated with most urinary antiseptics/antiinfectives? How can they be prevented?

3. What type of drug is phenazopyridine and what is its purpose? What are two nursing interventions related to this drug?

4. What are the side effects of urinary antispasmodics? Why? Why should a person with glaucoma avoid taking a drug from this group?

5. What type of drug is tolterodine tartrate (Detrol) and for what purpose is it prescribed?

Nine

Immunologic Agents

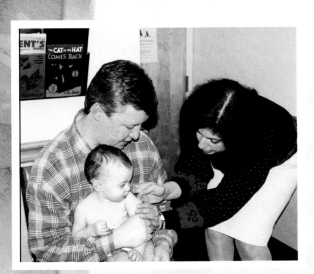

Immunity comprises functions that protect people from the effects of invasion of the body by microscopic organisms such as bacteria, viruses, molds, spores, pollens, protozoa, and cells from other persons or animals. A person remains in harmony with these organisms as long as the organisms do not enter the body's internal environment. The body has various defenses (e.g., skin) that prevent microorganisms from gaining access to its internal environment. However, these defenses are not infallible, and invasion of the body's internal environment by microorganisms occurs often. A properly functioning immune system neutralizes, eliminates, or destroys the invading microorganisms. To do this without harming the body, immune system cells use defensive actions against only *nonself* proteins and cells. This means that the immune system cells can differentiate between the body's own healthy self cells and other nonself proteins and cells.

Nonself proteins and cells include (1) all foreign cells and microorganisms, (2) infected or debilitated body cells, and (3) self cells that have undergone malignant transformation into cancer cells. This ability to recognize self versus nonself, necessary to prevent healthy body cells from being destroyed along with the invaders, is called *self-tolerance*. The immune system cells are the only body cells capable of recognizing self from nonself.

Unique proteins on the surface of all body cells of each individual serve as a personal identification code for that person. The cell-surface proteins of one person are recognized as "foreign" by the immune system of another person. These are antigens, proteins capable of stimulating an immune response.

Immune function is generally most efficient when people are in their 20s and 30s; it slowly declines with increasing age. Older adults have marginal immune function, causing increased susceptibility to a variety of pathologic conditions.

Immune System Structure

The immune system is not confined to any one organ or body area. Instead, immune system cells originate in the bone marrow. Some of these cells mature in the bone marrow; while others leave the bone marrow and mature in different body sites. After maturation, most immune system cells are released into the blood where they circulate throughout the body and exert specific effects.

Immune System Function

The three processes necessary for immunity and the cells involved in these responses can be categorized as inflammation, antibody-mediated immunity (humoral immunity), and cell-mediated immunity. Inflammation is discussed in the introduction to Unit VIII. Full immunity, or immunocompetence, requires the adequate function and interaction of all three processes, although some functions of each overlap. Long-lasting immune actions are those generated by antibody-mediated immunity and cell-mediated immunity.

Antibody-Mediated Immunity

Antibody-mediated immunity (AMI), also called *humoral immunity*, involves antigen-antibody interactions that neutralize, eliminate, or destroy foreign proteins. Antibodies for these interactions are produced by populations of B lymphocytes.

Antigen-Antibody Interactions

Antigen-antibody interactions occur in the body's internal environment. To make an antibody that can exert its effects on a specific antigen, the body must first be exposed to that antigen to the degree that the antigen enters the body. Even when exposure includes penetration, not all exposures result in the stimulation of antibody production. Invasion by the antigen must occur in such large numbers that some of the antigen either evades detection by the normal nonspecific defenses or overwhelms the abilities of the inflammatory response to neutralize, eliminate, or destroy the invader.

Acquiring Antibody-Mediated Immunity

The two broad categories of immunity are innate immunity and acquired immunity. Innate immunity is a genetically determined characteristic of an individual, group, or species. A person either has or does not have innate immunity. For example, people have many innate immunities to viruses and other microorganisms that cause specific diseases in animals. As a result, humans are not susceptible to such diseases as mange, distemper, hog cholera, or any of a variety of animal afflictions. This type of immunity cannot be developed or transferred from one person to another and is not an adaptive response to exposure or invasion by foreign proteins.

Acquired immunity is the immunity that every person's body makes (or can receive) as an adaptive response to invasion by foreign proteins. Antibody-mediated immunity is an acquired immunity. Acquired immunity occurs either naturally or artificially and can be either active or passive. Active immunity occurs when antigens enter the body and the body responds by making specific antibodies against the antigen. This type of immunity is active because the body takes an active part in making the antibodies. Active immunity can occur under conditions that are either natural or artificial. Natural active immunity occurs when an antigen enters the body without human assistance, and the body responds by actively making antibodies against that antigen (e.g., chickenpox virus). Most of the time, the first invasion of the body by this antigen results in the person manifesting signs and symptoms of the disease. However, processes occurring in the body at the same time allow the person to acquire immunity to that antigen so that he or she will not become ill after a second exposure to the same antigen. This type of immunity is the most effective and the longest lasting.

Artificial active immunity is a type of protection developed against illnesses that produce such serious side effects that total avoidance of the disease is most desirable. Small amounts of specific antigens are deliberately placed (as a vaccination) in the body so that the body responds by actively making antibodies against the antigen. Because antigens used for this procedure have been specially processed to make them less likely to proliferate within the body, this exposure does not in itself cause the disease.

Examples of diseases for which artificially acquired active immunity can be obtained include tetanus, diphtheria, measles, smallpox, mumps, and rubella. This type of immunity lasts many years, although repeated but smaller doses of the original antigen are required as a "booster" to maintain complete protection against the antigen.

Passive immunity occurs when antibodies against a specific antigen are in a person's body but the person did not actively generate these antibodies. Instead, these antibodies are made in the body of another person or animal and then transferred to the body of a specific individual. Because these antibodies are foreign to the individual, the body recognizes the antibodies as nonself and takes steps to eliminate them relatively quickly. For this reason, passive immunity can provide only immediate, short-term protection against a specific antigen.

Cell-Mediated Immunity

Cell-mediated immunity (CMI), or cellular immunity, involves many leukocyte actions, reactions, and interactions that range from the simple to the complex. This type of immunity is provided by committed lymphocyte stem cells that mature in the secondary lymphoid tissues of the thymus and pericortical areas of lymph nodes. Certain CMI responses influence and regulate the activities of antibody-mediated immunity and inflammation by producing and releasing cytokines; therefore total immunocompetence relies on optimal CMI function.

The leukocytes playing the most important roles in CMI include several specific T-lymphocyte subsets along with a special population of cells known as *natural killer cells* (NK cells). T lymphocytes further differentiate into a variety of subsets, each of which has a specific function. The three T-lymphocyte subsets crucial to the development and continuation of CMI are helper/inducer T cells, suppressor T cells, and cytotoxic/cytolytic T cells.

Protection Provided By Cell-Mediated Immunity

Specific components of CMI assist in providing protection to the body by their highly developed abilities to differentiate self from nonself. The nonself cells most easily recognized by CMI are those self cells infected by organisms that live within host cells and those self cells mutated at the DNA level and thus abnormal. CMI provides a surveillance system that rids the body of self cells that might potentially harm the body. CMI is critically important in preventing development of cancer and metastasis after exposure to carcinogens.

34 HIV and AIDS-Related Agents

LISA A. PLOWFIELD AND ROBERT KIZIOR

ELECTRONIC RESOURCES

Additional information can be found on the companion website at *http://evolve.elsevier.com/KeeHayes/pharmacology/* or on the companion CD-ROM, which includes:

- *NCLEX-style examination review questions*
- *Pharmacology animations*
- *Medication error and (IV) therapy checklists*
- *Medication calculation problems*
- *Electronic calculators*

OUTLINE

OBJECTIVES

- Describe the life cycle of the human immunodeficiency virus (HIV).
- Define antiretroviral therapy.
- List the four classifications of antiretroviral therapy, and give examples of medications in each group.
- Describe specific factors related to adherence/compliance with the medication regimen.
- Explain prophylactic treatment for opportunistic infections.

- Identify implications of the related drugs for pregnancy.

- Describe postexposure prophylaxis for health care workers.

- Describe the nursing process, including client teaching, to care for clients who take antiretroviral therapy.

TERMS

adherence/compliance
antiretroviral
CD4⁺ T cells
fusion inhibitors
highly active antiretroviral therapy (HAART)

immune response
immune system
integrase
nonnucleoside analogues
nucleoside analogues

postexposure prophylaxis (PEP)
protease
protease inhibitors
resistance

reverse transcriptase (RT)
reverse transcriptase inhibitors
viral load (VL)

Introduction

In 1981 a group of young predominantly homosexual men were diagnosed with a syndrome that was later named *acquired immunodeficiency syndrome (AIDS)*. Worldwide, approximately 42 million people are infected with human immunodeficiency virus (HIV). Approximately 20 million deaths have been attributed to HIV/AIDS.

In the United States, about 784,000 people have had AIDS, with death occurring in about 60% of these. Currently, more than 340,000 people are living with AIDS and more than 900,000 are living with HIV.

Pathology

In 1983, HIV was identified as the causative agent of AIDS. HIV is a retrovirus that causes a gradual deterioration of immune function. AIDS is characterized by profound immunologic deficits, opportunistic infection, secondary infections, and malignant neoplasms.

Once a person is infected with HIV, crucial immune cells called **CD4⁺ T cells** are disabled and killed. During the course of infection, the numbers of CD4⁺ T cells progressively decline. CD4⁺ T cells play a crucial role in the **immune response**, signaling other cells in the **immune system** to perform their special function.

Three modes of transmission of HIV infection are injection of infected blood or blood products, sexual contact, and maternal-fetal transmission. Occupational exposure accounts for a small number of infected individuals, most from needlestick injury.

Laboratory and Diagnostic Tests

A healthy, uninfected person usually has 800 to 1200 CD4⁺ T cells per cubic millimeter (mm³) of blood. When severe damage from HIV infection causes the CD4⁺ T-cell count to decrease to 200 mm³ or equal to or less than 14%, the person is particularly vulnerable to opportunistic infections and cancers and is then classified as having AIDS. Table 34–1, *A* and *B,* lists the HIV classification system. In addition to the T-cell count, another test used to evaluate the status of the client's immune system is the **viral load (VL).** HIV ribonucleic acid (RNA) (viral particles) is counted; the higher the number, the higher the viral burden.

HIV is a retrovirus. It uses three different enzymes to genetically encode, replicate, and assemble new virus within the cells (HIV can replicate only inside cells). These three enzymes are reverse transcriptase, integrase, and protease.

The virus enters the cell through the CD4 molecule on the cell surface. The virus uncoats with the help of the **reverse transcriptase (RT)** enzyme, and a single-stranded viral RNA is converted into deoxyribonucleic acid (DNA), the form in which the cell carries its genes. The viral DNA migrates to the nucleus of the cell, where it is spliced into the host DNA with the help of the second enzyme, **integrase**. Once incorporated, HIV DNA is called the *provirus* and is duplicated together with the cell genes every time the cell divides. **Protease,** the third enzyme, assists in the assembly of newly formed viral particles (Figure 34–1).

As of 1995, monotherapy with any antiretroviral agent is no longer recommended. Combination therapy known as **highly active antiretroviral therapy (HAART)** is the current treatment recommendation. Medications designed to slow or inhibit these three enzymes are called **antiretroviral** medications. In 1987 the Food and Drug Administration (FDA) approved the first RT inhibitor and in 1995 approved the first protease inhibitor. To date, no integrase inhibitors have been approved.

The goals of HAART include decreasing the VL to undetectable levels, preserving and increasing the number of CD4⁺ T cells, preventing resistance, having the client in good clinical condition, and preventing secondary infections and cancers. HIV VL testing can be performed by polymerase chain reaction or branch-chain DNA. These tests can produce differing results, so the same test should be used in clients consistently. Newer ultrasensitive VL tests will soon become the standard of care; these tests have a lower threshold of detection of 50 copies per milliliter. To obtain and maintain the goals of HAART therapy, the client must have excellent **adherence/compliance** skills. Failure to take combination therapy as directed can lead to **resistance** to or failure of antiretroviral agents. Ad-

Table 34–1A

Classification System for HIV Infection*

CD4+ T-Cell Categories	Clinical Categories for Adults		
	(A) Asymptomatic, Acute (Primary) HIV or Persistent Generalized Lymphadenopathy	(B) Symptomatic, not (A) or (C) Conditions	(C) AIDS-Indicator Conditions
(1) 500/mcL	A1	B1	C1
(2) 200-499/mcL	A2	B2	C2
(3) <200/mcL AIDS-indicator T-cell count	A3	B3	C3

From Department of Health and Human Services, Henry J. Kaiser Family Foundation: *Panel on practices for treatment of HIV infection: guidelines for the use of antiretroviral agents in HIV-infected adults and adolescents,* Dec 1, 1998.
*The revised Centers for Disease Control and Prevention classification system for HIV-infected adolescents and adults categorizes persons on the basis of CD4+ T-lymphocyte counts and clinical conditions associated with HIV infection. The system is based on three ranges of CD4+ T-lymphocyte counts and three clinical categories, represented by a matrix of nine mutually exclusive categories.

CD4+ T-Lymphocyte Categories
HIV-infected persons should be classified based on existing guidelines for the medical management of HIV-infected persons; thus the lowest accurate CD4+ T-lymphocyte count should be used (but not necessarily the most recent) for classification purposes.

Clinical Categories
Category A
Category A consists of one or more of the following conditions in an adolescent or adult (13 years of age or older) with documented HIV infection. Conditions listed in categories B and C must not have occurred.
• Asymptomatic HIV infection
• Persistent generalized lymphadenopathy
• Acute (primary) HIV infection with accompanying illness or history of acute HIV infection

Category B
Category B consists of symptomatic conditions in an HIV-infected adolescent or adult that are not included in category C and are attributed to HIV infection or are considered to have a clinical course complicated by HIV infection. Examples of conditions in category B include, but are not limited to, the following:
• Bacillary angiomatosis
• Candidiasis, oropharyngeal (thrush)
• Candidiasis, vulvovaginal; persistent, frequent, or poorly responsive to therapy
• Cervical dysplasia (moderate or severe)/cervical carcinoma in situ
• Constitutional symptoms, such as fever (38.5°C) or diarrhea lasting >1 month
• Hairy leukoplakia, oral
• Herpes zoster (shingles), involving at least two distinct episodes or more than one dermatome
• Idiopathic thrombocytopenic purpura
• Listeriosis
• Pelvic inflammatory disease, particularly if complicated by tubo-ovarian abscess
• Peripheral neuropathy
For classification purposes, category B conditions take precedence over category A conditions.

Category C
Category C includes the clinical conditions listed in the AIDS surveillance case definition. For classification purposes, once a category C condition occurs, the person remains in category C.

Table 34–1B

Pediatric HIV Classification*

Immunologic Categories	Clinical Categories			
	N: No Signs/ Symptoms	A: Mild Signs/ Symptoms	B: Moderate Signs/ Symptoms†	C: Severe Signs/ Symptoms†
1. No evidence of suppression	N1	A1	B1	C1
2. Evidence of moderate suppression	N2	A2	B2	C2
3. Severe suppression	N3	A3	B3	C3

From Department of Health and Human Services, Henry J. Kaiser Family Foundation: *Panel on practices for treatment of HIV infection: guidelines for the use of antiretroviral agents in HIV-infected adults and adolescents,* March 2004.
*Children whose HIV infection status is not confirmed are classified by using the above grid with a letter E (for perinatally exposed) placed before the appropriate classification code (e.g., EN2).
†Both category C and lymphoid interstitial pneumonitis in category B are reportable to state and local health departments as acquired immunodeficiency syndrome.

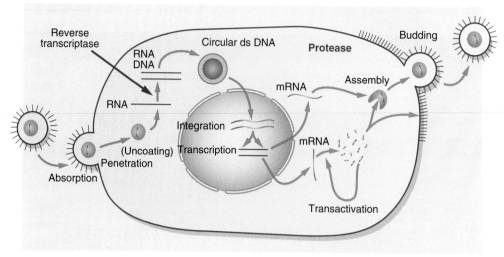

FIGURE 34–1 The life cycle of the human immunodeficiency virus.

ditionally, the clinical management of the HIV/AIDS client must include measures to minimize associated opportunistic infections and malignancies. Aggressive prophylaxis and treatment of opportunistic infections are suggested. Nutritional therapy, complementary therapy, and supportive care are also necessary.

It is recommended that antiretroviral therapy be offered to all clients with symptoms of clinical AIDS (e.g., opportunistic infection) or immunologic AIDS (e.g., CD4$^+$ cell count of <200 cells/mm^3). All asymptomatic clients with a CD4$^+$ cell count >200 but less than 350 cells/mm^3 should be offered therapy. If a client has a CD4$^+$ cell count >350 cell/mm^3, the decision to initiate therapy would depend on the client's viral load. If the viral load is >55,000 copies per milliliter, therapy is recommended. In addition, treatment should be based on the willingness and readiness of the individual, the degree of existing immunodeficiency, the risk of disease progression, and the likelihood of adherence to the prescribed treatment regimen. Recommendations for offering antiretroviral therapy in asymptomatic clients require analysis of many real and potential risks and benefits. The risks and benefits of early initiation of antiretroviral therapy in the asymptomatic HIV-infected client are listed in Box 34–1.

Management of HIV is evolving rapidly. The most current information is found on the HIV/AIDS Treatment Information Service website at www.hivatis.org/index.html or the Center for Disease Control and Prevention's Division of HIV/AIDS Prevention website at www.cdc.gov/hiv/treatment. htm. Recommendations are updated regularly.

Antiretroviral Therapy

The goals of antiretroviral therapy are to do the following:
- Suppress viral replication to slow the decline in the number of CD4$^+$ cells
- Suppress viral replication to undetectable levels
- Reduce the incidence and severity of opportunistic infections

---

BOX 34–1

Risks and Benefits of Early or Delayed Initiation of Antiretroviral Therapy in the Asymptomatic HIV-Infected Client

Potential Benefits of Early Therapy
- Control of viral replication and mutation; reduction of viral burden
- Prevention of progressive immunodeficiency; potential maintenance or reconstruction of a normal immune system
- Delayed progression to acquired immunodeficiency syndrome and prolongation of life
- Decreased risk of selection of resistant virus
- Decreased risk of drug toxicity
- Possible decreased risk of viral transmission

Potential Risks of Early Therapy
- Reduction in quality of life from adverse drug effects and inconvenience of current maximally suppressive regimens
- Earlier development of drug resistance
- Transmission of drug-resistant virus
- Limitation in future choices of antiretroviral agents as a result of development of resistance
- Unknown long-term toxicity of antiretroviral drugs
- Unknown duration of effectiveness of current antiretroviral therapies

Potential Benefits of Delayed Therapy
- Avoid negative effects of therapy including quality of life and drug-related adverse effects
- Maintain treatment options
- Delay the development of drug resistance

Potential Risks of Delayed Therapy
- Irreversibly damaging the immune system
- Increased difficulty in suppressing viral replication at a later stage of the disease
- Transmitting HIV during a longer untreated period

From Department of Health and Human Services, Henry J. Kaiser Family Foundation: *Panel on practices for treatment of HIV infection: guidelines for the use of antiretroviral agents in HIV-infected adults and adolescents,* March 23, 2004.

- Minimize adverse effects of antiretroviral therapy
- Improve quality of life
- Improve survival and reduce morbidity

Currently, **reverse transcriptase inhibitors**, **protease inhibitors**, and **fusion inhibitors** make up the classification of drugs known as *antiretroviral therapy*. RT inhibitors are further divided into **nucleoside analogues** and **nonnucleoside analogues**. As of January 2004, the FDA has approved 20 different antiretroviral agents. Protease inhibitors have changed the prognosis for millions of clients infected with HIV. Protease inhibitors combined with RT inhibitors can reduce viral plasma levels to undetectable levels, thus offering significant clinical benefit.

Antiretroviral Agents

Four classes of agents are used to treat HIV infection: nucleoside analogues, nonnucleoside analogues, protease inhibitors, and fusion inhibitors. Nucleoside and nonnucleoside analogues act by inhibiting HIV reverse transcriptase (HIV-RT), which is responsible for viral replication early in the virus life cycle. These agents prevent HIV infection of new cells but cannot prevent the production of new infections by already infected cells. Thus these agents have limited effects. The protease inhibitors block protease, an enzyme required for viral replication late in the virus life cycle. They suppress production of infectious virions in infected cell populations. The emergence of protease inhibitors has changed the prognosis for millions of persons infected with HIV. When combined with nucleoside or nonnucleoside agents, protease inhibitors can reduce viral plasma levels to undetectable levels, thus offering significant clinical benefit. Fusion inhibitors bind to viral particles and prevent adhesion to CD4+ cells. At present, fusion inhibitors should be reserved for clients for whom other therapies have failed and whose treatment options have been exhausted. Several different combinations are currently used, but the most effective combination is not yet established.

Currently, the use of HAART is the standard of care in the treatment of HIV infection. Usually HAART combines two nucleoside reverse transcriptase inhibitors (NRTIs) with either one nonnucleoside reverse transcriptase inhibitor (NNRTI) or one or two protease inhibitors.

Drug Class–Related Adverse Effects

Several class-related adverse effects have been recognized with antiretroviral drugs during the postmarketing period. For NRTIs, lactic acidosis with hepatomegaly and hepatic steatosis has been reported. For NNRTIs, rash, which occurs most commonly with nevirapine, is often mild and does not necessitate discontinuation of therapy. For protease inhibitors, reports of hyperglycemia/diabetes mellitus, increased bleeding episodes in clients with hemophilia, and fat redistribution with and without serum lipid abnormalities have been received. Because these effects were identified from spontaneous reports and other uncontrolled data, their actual incidence and the causal association with these drugs have not been definitively established. Controlled or population-based epidemiologic studies evaluating these potential class-related adverse effects are warranted. Currently, only one fusion inhibitor is available.

Nucleoside Reverse Transcriptase Inhibitors

Zidovudine (AZT, ZDV, Retrovir), approved in 1987, was the first NRTI. Zidovudine improves CD4+ counts, improves survival rates and survival times, and decreases disease progression. Zidovudine penetrates the central nervous system (CNS) and may be useful in the treatment of HIV dementia and thrombocytopenia. Additionally, it is effective in preventing infection of infants both in utero and during delivery from HIV-infected women.

Pharmacokinetics

Zidovudine is absorbed rapidly and well from the gastrointestinal (GI) tract, peaking in 30 to 90 minutes. Absorption shows considerable inter-client variation, with ranges from 42% to 95%. It is widely distributed, crossing the blood-brain barrier with good levels in cerebrospinal fluid (CSF). Tablets are best taken on an empty stomach and swallowed whole with plenty of water. Capsules may be taken with or without food (taking with food decreases nausea, but high-fat meals impair absorption). Intravenous (IV) administration should last at least 60 minutes. Zidovudine is excreted primarily in the urine.

Pharmacodynamics

Zidovudine, like other nucleoside analogues, inhibits viral enzyme reverse transcriptase, an enzyme necessary for viral HIV replication early in the viral life cycle. Zidovudine must be converted intracellularly to be active. It slows HIV replication, thus reducing the progression of HIV infection.

Prototype Drug Chart 34–1 presents the pharmacologic data for zidovudine.

Nonnucleoside Reverse Transcriptase Inhibitors (NNRTIs)

Efavirenz (Sustiva), an NNRTI, was approved by the FDA in September 1998. Efavirenz improves CD4+ counts and reduces VL. Resistance is problematic with NNRTIs; therefore, efavirenz should be used only in combination with at least one other nucleoside analogue.

Pharmacokinetics

Efavirenz is readily absorbed following oral administration. Absorption is increased with fatty meals. Peak concentration occurs within 3 to 8 hours. This drug is best taken on an empty stomach. It is widely distributed with levels in the CSF, metabolized in the liver, and excreted in the feces unchanged and in the urine as metabolite.

Pharmacodynamics

Efavirenz inhibits catalytic reaction of reverse transcriptase (enzyme necessary for viral HIV replication) independent of nucleotide binding. Its action occurs early in the viral life cycle. Efavirenz slows HIV replication, reducing progression of HIV infection. It must be used in combination therapy.

Prototype Drug Chart 34–2 presents the pharmacologic data for efavirenz.

Protease Inhibitors

Lopinavir/ritonavir (Kaletra) represents the second FDA-approved combination of two drugs from the same class. Lopinavir is used primarily for its antiretroviral activity; ritonavir is used at a reduced dosage to inhibit metabolism of lopinavir.

PROTOTYPE DRUG CHART 34–1

ZIDOVUDINE

Drug Class

Nucleoside reverse transcriptase inhibitor
Trade Name: ZDV, AZT, Retrovir
Pregnancy Category: C
FDA approved: 1987
Estimated annual cost: $4650*

Dosage

Prophylaxis vertical transmission HIV:
Maternal therapy: PO: 100 mg 5×/d Initiated at 14-34 wk
   of gestation through pregnancy
Intrapartum: IV: 2 mg/kg loading dose over 30-60 min
   followed by continuous infusion of 1 mg/kg/h until
   the cord is clamped
Newborn (syrup): PO: 2 mg/kg q6h; IV: 1.5 mg/kg over
   30 min q6h
Treatment:
A: PO: 200 mg q8h or 300 mg q12h; IV: 1 mg/kg q4h
C: PO: premature birth to 2 wk: 1.5 mg/kg q12h, increasing
   to 2 mg/kg q8h after 2 wk of age; neonatal: 2 mg/kg
   q6h; <12 y: 160 mg/m² q8h; >12 y: adult dose
C: IV: neonatal: 1.5 mg/kg q6h; <12 y: intermittent infusion: 120 mg/m² q6h; *max:* 160 mg/m² per dose; continuous infusion: 20 mg/m²/h

Contraindications

Life-threatening allergies to zidovudine or components
   of preparation
Caution: Bone marrow compromise, renal and hepatic
   dysfunction, decreased hepatic blood flow

Drug-Lab-Food Interactions

Drug: Ganciclovir and trimethoprim/sulfamethoxazole
   may *increase* risk of neutropenia; probenecid may increase concentration, risk of toxicity
Lab: May *increase* mean corpuscular volume

Pharmacokinetics

Absorption: PO: 66%-70%
Distribution: PB: 25%-38%, crosses blood-brain barrier,
   crosses placenta, peak serum levels: 30-90 min
Metabolism: t½: 60 min; extensive first-pass effect in liver
Excretion: 63%-95% in urine

Pharmacodynamics

Not applicable

Therapeutic Effects/Uses

Management of clients with HIV infection; prevention of maternal-fetal HIV transmission
Mode of Action: Inhibits viral enzyme reverse transcriptase, an enzyme necessary for viral HIV replication

Side Effects

Numbness, tingling, burning and pain in lower
   extremities, abdominal pain, rash, GI intolerance,
   fever, sore throat, headache, pruritus, muscle pain,
   difficulty swallowing, arthralgia, insomnia, confusion,
   mental changes, bluish brown bands on fingernails

Adverse Reactions

Nausea, vomiting, anemia (pale skin, unusual fatigue or
   weakness), neutropenia (fever, chills, sore throat),
   seizures

A, Adult; *C,* child; *d,* day; *FDA,* Food and Drug Administration; *GI,* gastrointestinal; *h,* hour; *HIV,* human immunodeficiency virus;
IV, intravenous; *max,* maximum; *min,* minute; *PB,* protein-binding; *PO,* by mouth; *t½,* half-life; *wk,* week; *y,* year; >, greater than;
<, less than.
*Estimated average cost as of April 2004.

PROTOTYPE DRUG CHART 34–2

EFAVIRENZ

Drug Class

Nonnucleoside reverse transcriptase inhibitor
Trade Name: Sustiva
Pregnancy Category: C
FDA approved: 1998
Estimated annual cost: $5820*

Dosage

Note: Dose given at bedtime to minimize CNS adverse
effects
A: PO: 600 mg once daily
C: PO: 10 to <15 kg: 200 mg daily; 15 to <20 kg: 250 mg
daily; 20 to <25 kg: 300 mg daily; 25 to <32.5 kg: 350
mg daily; 32.5 kg to <40 kg: 400 mg daily; ≥40 kg:
600 mg daily

Contraindications

Life-threatening allergies to efavirenz or components
of preparation; concurrent use of midazolam,
triazolam, ergot alkaloids
Caution: History of mental illness/drug abuse; liver
impairment

Drug-Lab-Food Interactions

Drug: See contraindications; carbamazepine, nevirapine,
phenobarbital, phenytoin, rifampin, St John's wort
may *decrease* effect; may decrease effect of
lopinavir/irtonavir, saquinavir, amprenavir, clarithromycin, methadone, sertraline
Lab: May *increase* HDL, total cholesterol
Food: Avoid alcohol due to liver/CNS adverse effects;
high-fat meals *increase* absorption

Pharmacokinetics

Absorption: PO: Increased following high fat meal
Distribution: PB: >99%, widely distributed (found in CSF)
Metabolism: t½: 40-55 h; metabolized in liver
Excretion: Feces primarily as unchanged drug (16%-41%);
urine primarily as metabolite (14%-34%)

Pharmacodynamics

Not applicable

Therapeutic Effects/Uses

Treatment of HIV-1 infections in combination with at least two other anti-retroviral agents.
Mode of Action: Binds to reverse transcriptase, blocking RNA dependent and DNA dependent DNA polymerase
activity including HIV-1 replication.

Side Effects

Rash; CNS effects including dizziness, insomnia, abnormal
dreams/thinking, impaired concentration, amnesia,
agitation, hallucinations, euphoria, anxiety; nausea,
diarrhea

Adverse Reactions

Aggressive reaction, allergic reaction, convulsion, liver
failure, neuropathy, suicide, abnormal vision

A, Adult; *C*, child; *CNS*, central nervous system; *CSF*, cerebrospinal fluid; *DNA*, deoxyribonucleic acid; *FDA*, Food and Drug Administration;
h, hour; *HDL*, high-density lipoprotein; *HIV-1*, human immunodeficiency virus-1; *PB*, protein-binding; *PO*, by mouth; *RNA*, ribonucleic
acid; *t½*, half-life; >, greater than; ≥, greater than or equal to; <, less than.
*Estimated annual cost as of April 2004.

Pharmacokinetics

Lopinavir/ritonavir is best taken with food. If the client is also taking didanosine, it should be taken either 1 hour before or 2 hours after lopinavir. Lopinavir is metabolized in the liver and is excreted primarily in the feces (and only minimally in the urine).

Pharmacodynamics

Lopinavir blocks protease, an enzyme required for viral replication late in the virus life cycle. Lopinavir reduces viral plasma levels, slows HIV replication, and reduces the progression of HIV infection. It must be used in combination therapy.

Prototype Drug Chart 34-3 presents the pharmacologic data for lopinavir.

Drugs that should not be used with protease inhibitors are listed in Table 34-2. Drug interactions between protease inhibitors and other drugs (requiring dose modifications) are listed in Table 34-3. Table 34-4 presents drug interactions of protease inhibitors and NNRTIs.

Antiretroviral Combinations

Recently, two fixed combination products have become available. Both products are fixed combinations of existing NRTIs. The first is Combivir (lamivudine and zidovudine); the second is Trizivir (abacavir, lamivudine, and zidovudine). See Table 34-5 for further information about these products.

Summary of Antiretroviral Agents

A list of the antiretroviral agents (nucleoside analogues, nonnucleoside analogues, protease inhibitors, and fusion inhibitors) are presented in Table 34–5 with their respective routes, dosages, and considerations. See Herbal Alert 34–1 for a list of potential herbal-antiretroviral interactions. A

HERBAL ALERT 34-1

Antiretroviral Agents and Herbal Interactions

Nucleoside Analogues
- Lentinan may enhance increases in CD4$^+$ levels when taken with didanonsine.
- Laurelwood in combination with lamivudine or zidovudine may have a synergistic effect.
- Riboflavin may reduce lactic acidosis when taken with lamivudine, zidovudine, or stavudine.

Nonnucleoside Analogues
- Bitter orange juice may inhibit metabolism of nonnucleoside analogues, increasing drug levels and the risk of adverse effects.
- Garlic or St. John's wort may decrease drug levels and therapeutic effect of nonnucleoside analogues.
- Laurelwood may have a synergistic effect when taken with nevirapine.
- Kava kava in combination with nevirapine may increase the risk of developing liver damage.

Protease Inhibitors
- Bitter orange juice may inhibit the metabolism, increase drug levels, and increase the risk of adverse effects when taken with protease inhibitors.
- Garlic or St. John's wort may decrease drug levels and therapeutic effect of protease inhibitors.
- Laurelwood may have a synergistic effect in combination with nelfinavir.
- Kava kava in combination with ritonavir may increase the risk of developing liver damage.
- Grapefruit in combination with saquinavir may increase drug absorption/drug levels and the risk of adverse effects.

Table 34–2

Drugs That Should not Be Used with Protease Inhibitors

Protease Inhibitor	Calcium Blocker	Cardiac	Lipid-Lowering Agent	Anti-mycobacterial	Neuroleptic	Psychotropic	Ergot Alkaloids
Indinavir			Simvastatin Lovastatin	Rifampin Rifapentine	Pimozide	Midazolam Triazolam	Dihydroergotamine Ergotamine‡
Ritonavir*	Bepridil	Amiodarone Flecainide Propafenone Quinidine	Simvastatin Lovastatin	Rifapentine	Pimozide	Midazolam Triazolam	Dihydroergotamine Ergotamine‡
Saquinavir			Simvastatin Lovastatin	Rifampin Rifabutin† Rifapentine	Pimozide	Midazolam Triazolam	Dihydroergotamine Ergotamine‡
Nelfinavir			Simvastatin Lovastatin	Rifampin Rifapentine	Pimozide	Midazolam Triazolam	Dihydroergotamine Ergotamine
Amprenavir	Bepridil		Simvastatin Lovastatin	Rifampin Rifapentine	Pimozide	Midazolam Triazolam	Dihydroergotamine Ergotamine‡
Lopinavir/ ritonavir*		Flecainide Propafenone	Simvastatin Lovastatin	Rifampin Rifapentine	Pimozide	Midazolam Triazolam	Dihydroergotamine Ergotamine
Atazanavir	Bepridil		Simvastatin Lovastatin	Rifampin Rifapentine	Pimozide	Midazolam Triazolam	Dihydroergotamine Ergotamine‡

From Department of Health and Human Services, Henry J. Kaiser Family Foundation: *Panel on practices for treatment of HIV infection: guidelines for the use of antiretroviral agents in HIV-infected adults and adolescents,* March 2004.

*The contraindicated drugs listed are based on theoretical considerations. Thus drugs with low therapeutic indices yet with suspected major metabolic contribution from cytochrome P450 3A, CYP2D6, or unknown pathways are included in this table. Actual interactions may or may not occur in clients.
†Reduce rifabutin dose to one fourth of the standard dose.
‡This is likely a class effect.

PROTOTYPE DRUG CHART 34–3

LOPINAVIR/RITONAVIR

Drug Class

Protease inhibitor
Trade Name: Kaletra
Pregnancy Category: C
FDA approved: 2000
Estimated annual cost: $8450

Dosage

Note: Based on mg lopinavir
A & C >12 y: PO: 400 mg b.i.d.
C: 6 mo-12 y: 7 to <15 kg: 12 mg/kg b.i.d.; 15-40 kg:
 10 mg/kg b.i.d.; >40 kg: Same as adult
Dosage when taken with **amprenavir, efavirenz,
 nelfinavir,** or **nevirapine:**
A & C >12 y: 533 mg b.i.d.
C: 6 mo-12 y: 7 to <15 kg: 13 mg/kg b.i.d.; 15-45 kg:
 11 mg/kg b.i.d.; >45 kg: Same as adult

Contraindications

Life-threatening allergies to lopinavir/ritonavir or components of preparations. Ritonavir is contraindicated
 with concurrent use of ergot alkaloids, midazolam,
 triazolam, or pimozide.
Cautions: History of pancreatitis, liver impairment

Drug-Lab-Food Interactions

Drug: See contraindications; azole antifungals, lovastatin, rifampin, simvastatin, St. John's wort
Lab: May *increase* liver function tests, cholesterol,
 triglycerides
Food: Take with food. If concurrent didanosine, take
 didanosine 1 h before or 2 h after lopinavir/ritonavir

Pharmacokinetics

Absorption: PO: Well absorbed following oral administration
Distribution: PB: 98%-99%
Metabolism: t½: 5-6 h. Metabolized in liver
Excretion: Primarily fecal elimination (83%)

Pharmacodynamics

Not applicable

Therapeutic Effects/Uses

Treatment of HIV-1 infection in combination with other antiretroviral agents.
Mode of Action: Inhibits HIV protease, allowing the enzyme incapable of processing polyprotease precursors leading
 to production of noninfectious immature HIV particles

Side Effects

Nausea, vomiting, diarrhea, asthenia

Adverse Reactions

Hyperglycemia, diabetes mellitus

A, Adult; *b.i.d.,* twice a day; *C,* child; *FDA,* Food and Drug Administration; *h,* hour; *HIV,* human immunodeficiency virus; *mo,* month;
PB, protein-binding; *PO,* by mouth; *t½,* half-life; *y,* year; >, greater than; <, less than.

guide for drug interactions, in the form of multiple charts, is presented at *www.projinf.org/fs/drugin.html,* a website dedicated solely to the treatment of HIV infection.

Nursing Process

Antiretroviral Therapy

ASSESSMENT

■ Assess whether client needs HIV testing.
■ Refer as appropriate for anonymous or confidential testing.
■ Assess for renal and hepatic disorders; use of oral contraceptives.
■ Assess for signs and symptoms related to clinical progression toward a depressed immune system including profound involuntary weight loss, chronic diarrhea, chronic weight loss, intermittent or constant fever.

■ Assess use of other prescription and OTC medications.
■ Refer high-risk clients who test negative to counseling.
■ Assess physiologic and psychosocial needs and refer to medical care and psychologic support as indicated.
■ Obtain client history for clients who test positive for HIV.
■ Obtain a medical drug, diet, and herbal history; report probable drug-drug, drug-food, or drug-herb interactions.

NURSING DIAGNOSES

■ Ineffective health maintenance related to knowledge deficit about HIV/AIDS
■ Fear related to potential outcome of HIV screening, powerlessness, and/or threat to well-being
■ Imbalanced nutrition; less than body requirements
■ Ineffective individual and/or compromised family coping related to situational crises (positive HIV screening outcome)
■ Risk for infection

Text continued on p. 507

Table 34-3

Drug Interactions Between Protease Inhibitors and Other Drugs

	Drug Interactions Requiring Dose Modifications					
	Indinavir	**Ritonavir**	**Saquinavir***	**Nelfinavir**	**Amprenavir (APR)**	**Lopinavir/ ritonavir (LPV)**
fluconazole	No dosage change	No dosage change	No data	No dosage change	No dosage change	No dosage change
ketoconazole and itraconazole	Decrease dose to 600 mg q8h	Increases ketoconazole > threefold; dose adjustment required	Increases saquinavir levels threefold; no dose change†	No dosage change	APR, ketoconazole levels increased, no dosage change	Ketoconazole levels increased, do not exceed 200 mg ketoconazole daily
rifabutin	Reduce rifabutin to half dose: 150 mg/d	Consider alternative drug or reduce rifabutin dose to one fourth	Not recommended with either Invirase or Fortovase	Reduce rifabutin to half dose: 150 mg/d	Reduce rifabutin to half dose: 150 mg/d	Reduce rifabutin to 150 mg every other day or 3 ×/wk
rifampin	Contraindicated	Unknown‡	Not recommended with either Invirase or Fortovase	Contraindicated	APR levels decreased; should not co-administer	LPV levels decreased should not co-administer
Oral contraceptives	Modest increase in Ortho-Novum levels; no dose change	Ethinyl estradiol levels decreased; use alternative or additional contraceptive method	No data	Ethinyl estradiol and norethindrone levels decreased; use alternative or additional contraceptive method	Ethinyl estradiol and norethindrone levels increased, APV levels decreased. Use alternative method of contraception	Ethinyl estradiol and norethindrone levels increased, LPV levels decreased. Use alternative method of contraception
Miscellaneous	Grapefruit juice reduces indinavir levels by 26%	Desipramine increased 145%: reduce dose Theophylline levels decreased: increase dose	Grapefruit juice increases saquinavir levels†		None	None

From Department of Health and Human Services, Henry J. Kaiser Family Foundation: *Panel on practices for treatment of HIV infection: guidelines for the use of antiretroviral agents in HIV-infected adults and adolescents,* March 2004.
d, Day; *h,* hour; *wk,* week; >, greater than.
*Several drug interaction studies have been completed with saquinavir given as Invirase or Fortovase. Results from studies conducted with Invirase may not be applicable to Fortovase.
†Conducted with Invirase.
‡Rifampin reduces ritonavir 35%. Increased ritonavir dose or use of ritonavir in combination therapy is strongly recommended. The effect of ritonavir on rifampin is unknown. Used concurrently, there may be increased liver toxicity; therefore clients on ritonavir and rifampin should be monitored closely.

Table 34–4

Protease Inhibitors and Nonnucleoside Reverse Transcriptase Inhibitors: Effect of Drug on Levels/Dose

Drug Affected	Indinavir	Ritonavir	Saquinavir*	Nelfinavir	Nevirapine	Delavirdine	Efavirenz
indinavir (IDV)	—	No data	Levels: IDV no effect SQV↑ 4-7×‡ Dose: No data	Levels: IDV↑ 50% NFV↑ 80% Dose: No data	Levels: IDV↓ 28% Dose: Standard	Levels: IDV↑ 40% Dose: IDV 600 mg q8h	Levels: IDV↓ 31% Dose: IDV 1000 mg q8h
ritonavir (RTV)	No data	—	Levels: RTV no effect SQV↑ 20×†‡ Dose: Invirase or Fortovase 400 mg b.i.d. + RTV: 400 mg b.i.d.	Levels: RTV no effect NFV↑ 1.5× Dose: No data	Levels: RTV↓ 11% Dose: Standard	Levels: RTV↑ 70% Dose: No data	Levels: RTV↑ 18% Dose: RTV 600 mg b.i.d. (500 mg b.i.d. for intolerance)
saquinavir (SQV)	Levels: SQV↑ 4-7 × IDV no effect‡ Dose: No data	Levels: SQV↑ 20×†‡ RTV no effect Dose: Invirase or Fortovase 400 mg b.i.d. + RTV: 400 mg b.i.d.	—	Levels: SQV↑ 3-5× NFV↓ 20%‡ Dose: Standard NFV Fortovase 800 mg t.i.d.	Levels: SQV↓ 25% Dose: No data	Levels: SQV↑ 5× Dose: Standard for Invirase (monitor transaminase levels)	Levels: SQV↓ 62%† Coadministration not recommended
nelfinavir (NFV)	Levels: NFV↑ 80% IDV↑ 50% Dose: No data	Levels: NFV↑ 1.5× RTV no effect Dose: No data	Levels: NFV↑ 20% SQV↑ 3-5×‡ Dose: Standard NFV Fortovase 800 mg t.i.d.	—	Levels: NFV↑ 10% Dose: Standard	Levels: NFV↑ 2× DLV↓ 50% Dose: Standard (monitor for neutropenic complications)	Levels: NFV↑ 20% Dose: Standard
nevirapine (NVP)	Levels: IDV↓ 28% Dose: Standard	Levels: RTV↓ 11% Dose: Standard	Levels: SQV↓ 25%† Dose: No data	Levels: NFV↑ 10% Dose: Standard	—	Do not use together	Coadministration not recommended
delavirdine (DLV)	Levels: IDV↑ 40% Dose: IDV 600 q8h	Levels: RTV↑ 70% Dose: No data	Levels: SQV↑ 5×† Dose: Standard for Invirase. Monitor transaminase levels	Levels: NFV↑ 2× DLV↓ 50% Dose: Standard (monitor for neutropenic complications)	Do not use together	—	Coadministration not recommended
efavirenz (EFV)	Levels: EFV no effect Dose: Standard	Level: EFV↑ 21% Dose: Standard	Levels: EFV↓ 12%‡ Coadministration not recommended	Levels: EFV no effect Dose: Standard	Coadministration not recommended	Coadministration not recommended	—

From Department of Health and Human Services, Henry J. Kaiser Family Foundation: *Panel on practices for treatment of HIV infection: guidelines for the use of antiretroviral agents in HIV-infected adults and adolescents*, March 2004.

b.i.d., Twice a day, h, hour; t.i.d., three times a day.

* Several drug interaction studies have been completed with saquinavir given as Invirase or Fortovase. Results from studies conducted with Invirase may not be applicable to Fortovase.

† Conducted with Invirase.

‡ Conducted with Fortovase.

Table 34–5

Antiretroviral Agents

Generic (Brand)	Route and Dosage	Uses and Considerations
Nucleoside Reverse Transcriptase Inhibitors		
Nucleoside Analogues		
abacavir (Ziagen) FDA approved: 1998 Estimated annual cost: $5350*	A: PO: 300 mg b.i.d.	No dietary restrictions. Hypersensitivity reaction in 3%-5% of clients on this drug (fever, GI symptoms, malaise, occasionally rash). Symptoms resolve when drug is stopped. However, if given drug again, more severe symptoms occur more rapidly, including hypotension and respiratory distress. FDA mandates that clients receive detailed description of these symptoms and carry a wallet-sized card with a description of hypersensitivity reaction with them at all times. No reports of adverse reactions with other drugs. *Pregnancy category:* UK; PB: UK; t½: UK
didanosine (ddI) (Videx) FDA approved: 1991 Estimated annual cost: $4000 enteric coated $3800 chewable	A: PO: (>60 kg): tablets: 200 mg q12h; powder: 250 mg q12h; (<60 kg): tablets: 125 mg q12h; powder: 167 mg q12h C: PO: (<90 d): 50 mg/m² q12h; (>90 d): 90–150 mg/m² q12h	Give on empty stomach. Tablets chewed, crushed, or dispersed in water (when dispersed, use within 1 h); powder should be mixed in drinking water only. Pediatric powder mixed by pharmacist and is stable for 30 days refrigerated. Avoid within 2 h of dapsone. Give in combination, never as monotherapy. *Pregnancy category:* B; PB: <5%; t½: 1.6 h
emtricitabine (Emtriva) FDA approved: 2003 Estimated annual cost: $3650	A: PO: 200 mg once daily	Give in combination, never as monotherapy. Take with or without food. *Pregnancy category:* B; PB: <4%; t½: 10 h
lamivudine (3TC, Epivir) FDA approved 1995 Estimated annual cost: $3800	A: PO: (>50 kg): 150 mg b.i.d.; (<50 kg): 2 mg/kg b.i.d. C: PO: (<30 d): 2 mg/kg q12h; (>30 d): 4 mg/kg q12h	Give in combination; never as monotherapy. May take without regard to food. Avoid alcohol. Report persistent, severe abdominal pain; nausea; vomiting; numbness; or tingling. *Pregnancy category:* C; PB: <36%; t½: 5-7 h
stavudine (Zerit) FDA approved: 1992 Estimated annual cost: $4500	A: PO: (>60 kg): 40 mg q12h; (<60 kg): 30 mg q12h C: PO: 1 mg/kg q12h (up to 30 kg)	Compounded with lactose; lactose intolerant clients can take LactAid tablets before stavudine. May take without regard to food. Avoid alcohol. Report tingling, burning, pain, or numbness of hands or feet. *Pregnancy category:* C; PB: negligible; ½: 1.44 h
tenofovir (Viread) FDA approved: 2001 Estimated annual cost: $5,700	A: PO: 300 mg once daily	Give in combination, never as monotherapy. Take with food. *Pregnancy category:* B; PB: Minimal; t½: UK
zalcitabine (ddC, Hivid) FDA approved: 1992 Estimated annual cost: $3100	A: PO: 0.75 mg q8h C: PO: 0.005-0.01 mg/kg q8h	Best given on empty stomach. Swallow tablets whole with plenty of water. *Pregnancy category:* C; PB: <4%; t½: 1-3 h
zidovudine (ZDV, AZT, Retrovir) FDA approved: 1986 Estimated annual cost: $4650	*Prophylaxis vertical transmission HIV:* Maternal therapy: PO: 100 mg 5×/d Intrapartum: IV: 2 mg/kg loading dose over 30-60 min followed by continuous infusion of 1 mg/kg/h until the cord is clamped Newborn (syrup): PO: 2 mg/kg q6h; IV: 1.5 mg/kg over 30 min q6h *Treatment:* A: PO: 200 mg q8h or 300 mg q12h; IV: 1 mg/kg q4h C: PO: premature birth to 2 wk: 1.5 mg/kg q12h, increasing to 2 mg/kg q8h after 2 wk of age; neonatal: 2 mg/kg q6h; <12 y: 160 mg/m² q8h; >12 y: adult dose C: IV: neonatal: 1.5 mg/kg q6h; <12 y: intermittent infusion: 120 mg/m² q6h; *max:* 160 mg/m² per dose; continuous infusion: 20 mg/m²/h	Protect from light. May take without regard to food. Take with food to decrease nausea; avoid high-fat meal, which decreases absorption. Infusion given over at least 60 minutes. *Pregnancy category:* C; PB: 34%-38%; t½: 1 h

A, Adult; *b.i.d.*, two times a day; *C*, child; *CNS*, central nervous system; *CPK*, creatine phosphokinase; *CSF*, cerebrospinal fluid; *d*, day; *FDA*, Food and Drug Administration; *GI*, gastrointestinal; *h*, hour; *IV*, intravenous; *LFT*, liver function test; *max*, maximum; *min*, minute; *mo*, month; *PB*, protein-binding; *PI*, protease inhibitor; *PO*, by mouth; *subQ*, subcutaneous; *t½*, half-life; *t.i.d.*, three times a day; *UK*, unknown; *wk*, week; *y*, year; *>*, greater than; *<*, less than.

*Estimated annual cost as of March 2004.

Table 34–5

Antiretroviral Agents—cont'd

Generic (Brand)	Route and Dosage	Uses and Considerations
Nucleoside Reverse Transcriptase Inhibitors—cont'd		
Fixed Combinations of Nucleosides		
lamivudine/zidovudine (Combivir) FDA approved: 2001 Estimated annual cost: $7900	A & C (>12 y): One tablet 2×/d	Give in combination, never as monotherapy. May take with or without food. This combination contains two nucleoside reverse transcriptase inhibitors exhibiting synergistic antiretroviral activity. Each tablet contains 150 mg lamivudine, 300 mg zidovudine. Not to be used in those requiring dosage adjustment such as those with reduced renal function. Zidovudine use may result in hematologic toxicity, prolonged use has been associated with symptomatic myopathy. *Pregnancy category:* C *lamivudine:* PB: <38%; t½: 5-7 h *zidovudine:* PB: 30%-38%; t½: 0.5-3 h
abacavir/lamivudine/ zidovudine (Trizivir) FDA approved: 2001 Estimated annual cost: $12,800	A & C: PO: >40 kg: 1 tablet 2×/d	May be used alone or in combination with other antiretroviral agents. This combination contains three nucleoside reverse transcriptase inhibitors. Each tablet contains 300 mg abacavir, 150 mg lamivudine, 300 mg zidovudine. Not to be used in clients requiring dosage adjustment such as those with reduced renal function or those weighing <40 kg. Zidovudine use may result in hematologic toxicity; prolonged use has been associated with symptomatic myopathy. Abacavir has been associated with fatal hypersensitivity reactions. *Pregnancy category:* C; PB: 50%; t½: 1-3 h
Nonnucleoside Analogues		
delavirdine (Rescriptor) FDA approved: 1997 Estimated annual cost: $3800	A: PO: Initially 200 mg t.i.d. for 14 d; then 400 mg t.i.d.	May take without regard to food. *Pregnancy category:* C; PB: 98%; t½: 2-11 h
nevirapine (Viramune) FDA approved: 1996 Estimated annual cost: $5100	A: PO: Initially 200 mg/d for 14 d; then 200 mg 2×/d C: PO: <3 mo: start with 5 mg/kg once daily for 14 d, followed by 120 mg/m² q12h for 14 d, followed by 200 mg/m² q12h; >3 mo: start with 120 mg/m² once daily for 14 d, increasing to 120-200 mg/m² q12h if there is no rash or other untoward effects	Give in combination, never as monotherapy. May take without regard to food. *Pregnancy category:* C; PB: 60%; t½: 25-30 h
efavirenz (EFV) (Sustiva) FDA approved: 1998 Estimated annual cost: $5820	A: PO: 600 mg/d usually at bedtime	Take with or without food. Avoid high-fat meal, which may increase drug absorption, resulting in increased side effects. About 40% of clients have problems with CNS effects: dizziness, insomnia, trouble concentrating, vivid dreams, nightmares. Usually these side effects disappear within 2 wk. Rash is not serious. *Contraindicated in pregnancy.* PB: UK; t½: 40-52 h
Protease Inhibitors		
amprenavir (Agenerase) FDA approved: 2000 Estimated annual cost: $9200	A & C (>17 y), C (13-16 y, >50 kg): PO: 1200 mg 2×/d C (4-13 y; 13–16 y, <50 kg): PO: 20 mg/kg 2×/d or 15 mg/kg 3×/d; *max:* 2400 mg/d	Give in combination, never as monotherapy. May take with or without food (avoid high-fat meal). Store at room temperature. Do not refrigerate. Capsules and oral solution are not interchangeable on a mg for mg basis. Review other medications; there are many drug interactions. *Pregnancy category:* C; PB: 90%; t½: 7.1-10.6 h

Continued

Table 34–5

Antiretroviral Agents—cont'd

Generic (Brand)	Route and Dosage	Uses and Considerations
Nucleoside Reverse Transcriptase Inhibitors—cont'd		
Protease Inhibitors—cont'd		
atazanavir (Reyataz) FDA approved: 2003 Estimated annual cost: $10,400	A: PO: 400 mg once daily	Give in combination, never as monotherapy. Take with food. *Pregnancy category:* B; PB: 86%; t$\frac{1}{2}$: 7 h
fosamprenavir (Lexiva) FDA approved: 2003 Estimated annual cost: $7600	A: 1400 mg twice daily (700 mg twice daily with ritonavir)	Give in combination, never as monotherapy. Rapidly converted to amprenavir. *Pregnancy category:* C; PB: 90% (amprenavir); t$\frac{1}{2}$: 7.7 h (amprenavir)
indinavir (Crixivan) FDA approved: 1996 Estimated annual cost: $6850	A: PO: 800 mg q8h or 1200 mg q12h C: PO: 500 mg/m² q8h	Give in combination, never as monotherapy. May take with a light meal (avoid high-fat, high-calorie, high-protein meal). If given with didanosine, give at least 1 hour before or after didanosine. Drink at least 1500 ml water daily. Compounded with lactose; lactose intolerant clients can take LactAid tablets before taking indinavir. Extremely moisture sensitive; keep in original container with desiccants; do not keep in bathroom. Monitor blood glucose. *Pregnancy category:* C; PB: 60%; t$\frac{1}{2}$: 1.8 h
lopinavir/ritonavir (Kaletra) FDA approved: 2000 Estimated annual cost: $8450	NOTE: Each capsule contains 133.3 mg lopinavir/33.3 mg ritonavir. Oral solution contains 80 mg lopinavir/20 mg ritonavir per ml. Dosing based on lopinavir component. A: PO: 400 mg (3 capsules or 5 ml) 2×/d. With concomitant therapy with efavirenz or nevirapine: 533 mg (4 capsules or 6.5 ml) 2×/d. C (6 mo-12 y): PO: 7 to <15 kg: 12 mg/kg 2×/d; 15-40 kg: 10 mg/kg 2×/d. With concomitant therapy with efavirenz or nevirapine: 7 to <15 kg: 13 mg/kg 2×/d; 15-50 kg: 11 mg/kg ×/d.	Give in combination, never as monotherapy. Take with food to enhance absorption. Capsules and oral solution to be used within 2 months when stored at room temperature. Under refrigeration, stable until expiration date printed on label. Review other medications; there are many drug interactions. *Pregnancy category:* C; PB: 98%-99%; t$\frac{1}{2}$: 5-6 h
nelfinavir (Viracept) FDA approved: 1997 Estimated annual cost: $9000	A: PO: 750 mg t.i.d. or 1250 mg b.i.d. C: PO: (2-13 y): 20-30 mg/kg q8h	Give in combination, never as monotherapy. Oral powder may be mixed with small amount of water, milk, or dietary supplement and used within 6 hours. Give with food for optimal absorption. Monitor blood glucose. *Pregnancy category:* B; PB: >98%; t: 3.5-5 h
ritonavir (Norvir) FDA approved: 1996 Estimated annual cost: $9250	A: PO: Initially 300 mg q12h, increasing by 100 mg q12h to maximum of 600 mg q12h (when given with saquinavir, ritonavir dosage is 400 mg q12h) C: PO: Initially 250 mg/m² q12h, increasing by 50 mg/m² q12h over 5 d to maximum of 400 mg/m² q12h	Store capsules, solution in refrigerator; protect from light. Refrigeration of solution not necessary if used within 30 days of reconstitution, but store below 77° F. Take with food. Review other medications before initiating them; there are many drug interactions. Give in combination, never as monotherapy. Monitor blood glucose. *Pregnancy category:* B; PB: 98%-99%; t$\frac{1}{2}$: 3 h
saquinavir (Invirase, Fortovase) FDA approved: 1997 Estimated annual cost: $8650	A: PO: Invirase: 600 mg t.i.d.; Fortovase: 1200 mg t.i.d.	First FDA-approved PI. Should be taken with a full meal. Grapefruit juice increases its bioavailability. Many drug interactions. May increase LFTs, decrease glucose levels, and alter CPK. *Pregnancy category:* B; PB: 98% with poor CSF penetration; t$\frac{1}{2}$: 13 h
Fusion Inhibitors		
enfuvirtide (Fuzeon) FDA approved: 2003 Estimated annual cost: $25,000	A: SubQ: 90 mg twice daily	Reserved for use in highly motivated clients for whom prior regimens failed and who have limited treatment options. Injection site reactions are most common. *Pregnancy category:* B; PB: 92%; t$\frac{1}{2}$: 3.2-4.4 h

■ Disturbed body image
■ Deficient knowledge
■ Disturbed sleep pattern
■ Impaired memory

PLANNING

■ Client's viral load will be undetectable.
■ Client's CD4$^+$ count will be as high as possible.
■ Client will not experience secondary infections.
■ Client will participate in medical treatment and in spiritual and psychologic support.
■ Client will promptly report new onset of symptoms and side effects.
■ Client will adhere to medication regimen and/or report difficulties related to adherence.

NURSING INTERVENTIONS

■ Promote adherence/compliance to the therapeutic regimen.
■ Promote meticulous hand washing; apply standard precautions.
■ Administer increased fluids, up to 2400 ml/d unless contraindicated.
■ Monitor laboratory reports for indications of decreasing CD4$^+$ T-lymphocyte cell counts; inform health care provider.
■ Refer client for preventive care measures including annual PAP, eye, and dental examinations.
■ Refer client for nutritional counseling.
■ Refer client for spiritual support.

Client Teaching

General

• Explain how the virus may cause severe damage to the immune system.
• Describe the modes of transmission of the virus.
• Explain common emotional responses.
• Explain the need for monitoring of health practices.
• Emphasize protective precautions to decrease risk of exposure and infection as necessary.
• Advise client not to visit anyone with any type of respiratory infection.
• Provide personal drug therapy plan in writing.
• Inform client that certain foods and herbal products may interact with antiretrovirals. (See Herbal Alert 34–1.)
• Establish client/family partnership in the plan.

Self-Administration

• Assist client to develop a system for taking the correct dose of the correct medications at the correct time. A medication organizer is a practical help to many clients.
• Instruct client of importance of having an adequate supply of medication so there is no interruption in the schedule. Omission of drugs may result in deterioration of client's condition.

Side Effects

• Advise client about what symptoms to report promptly to the health care provider.
• Discuss possible side effects and strategies to manage them.
• Provide suggestions for managing diarrhea.

Diet

• Advise client to eat a variety of foods.
• Advise client how to minimize side effects (e.g., take specific drug with food).
• Discuss BRAT diet (banana, rice, applesauce, and tea) for management of diarrhea.

Cultural Considerations

• Know that there is an oral history that the drug AZT may be harmful to certain groups of people.
• Some cultures pressure women to reproduce regardless of health status and the implications for future generations.
• AIDS is a highly stigmatized disease.
• Some religious and ethnic mores prohibit use of contraception, especially male condom use.
• Ethnic minorities may distrust health care providers and refuse treatment regimens that include research.
• Issues related to adherence and culture for women with HIV is available at *http://hab.hrsa.gov/publications/womencare.htm*.

EVALUATION

■ Evaluate the effectiveness of the antiretroviral therapy.
■ Determine whether the viral load is undetectable or as low as possible.
■ Evaluate medication adherence.

Antiretroviral Therapy: The Nurse's Role

The nurse's role with clients taking complex regimens of antiretroviral medications includes ongoing assessment, analysis, and education. Thorough assessment of the client's physiologic and psychosocial health needs is required initially. Follow-up assessment after therapy begins should include medication side effects, adherence to one's regimen, and issues affecting medication adherence. Clients may confuse medication side effects with a new onset of symptoms. Careful follow-up assessment can detect the need for additional medical care or medication regulation.

Issues of adherence are common with antiretroviral therapy. Individual assessment of adherence issues with an analysis of the client's lifestyle is essential. Multiple strategies for adherence are available and should be discussed with clients. Medication organizers are commonly used. A written schedule, medication diary, chalkboard, scheduled pager or cellular telephone messaging systems can be used to help clients maintain accurate administration. Friends, family members, and personal support systems can assist clients in adherence to medications. A client information sheet that explains the importance of adherence with HIV disease is available at *http://www.aids.org/factSheets/4-5-Adherence.html.*

Nurses can facilitate adherence by allowing sufficient time to educate clients about medications, developing a trusting relationship, and building a partnership with the client. Excellent information and strategies for adherence are available at *http://hivinsite.ucsf.edu/InSite?page=kbr-03-02-09.* When simpler regimens are available, nurses can advocate with medical providers for their clients. Therefore the nurse must maintain current knowledge of available regimens and clinical trials.

In addition to client assessment, education, and advocacy, nurses should identify problems that require additional investigation and research. Because the individual and lifestyle needs of the diverse HIV/AIDS population, research on strategies to promote adherence will continue to be needed. Best practices for adherence need to be identified.

The nurse's role with research is also needed with clinical trials. Accurate data collection, record keeping, and attention to detail are needed. Whenever medication regimens change, nurses should contribute to the ongoing evaluation of medication/regimen side effects and adverse event reporting. Adverse events can be reported at *http://www.fda.gov/medwatch/.*

Other Drugs For HIV

A welcome and unexpected new drug in the treatment of HIV infection and AIDS is Hydrea. Currently, Hydrea is not FDA approved for the treatment of AIDS. Table 34–6 presents additional data on Hydrea.

Adefovir dipivoxil (Preveon) is an NRTI that is available to clients in whom at least two NRTIs and one protease inhibitor have failed. This availability is only through an

expanded-access protocol. The primary adverse effect of adefovir has been mild to moderate nephrotoxicity. Side effects include nausea, diarrhea, asthenia, and aminotransferase activity. There are no reports of interactions with other drugs. This drug awaits FDA approval.

Trizivir, approved in 2000, is a fixed dosage combination of the nucleoside analogs abacavir, lamivudine, and zidovudine for the treatment of HIV infection. This product may be used alone or in combination with other antiretroviral agents. Each tablet contains 300 mg abacavir, 150 mg lamivudine, and 300 mg zidovudine. The recommended dosage is one tablet twice a day. It is not recommended for clients who weigh less than 40 kg, for those who require dosage adjustments because of renal impairment, or for children.

Tenofovir (Viread) is a potent inhibitor of HIV replication. It was approved by the FDA in December 2001 for combination therapy in clients for whom other regimens have failed. Tenofovir is administered daily, is well tolerated, and appears to be effective against HIV strains that are resistant to other antiretroviral agents. The most common side effects of tenofovir are nausea, vomiting, and diarrhea.

In 2003, new antiretroviral drugs were added. A key component is their simplified dosing schedule relative to many older antiretroviral agents.

Enfuvirtide (Fuzeon) is the first in a class of anti-HIV therapies called *fusion inhibitors.* Fusion inhibitors bind to viral particles and prevent adhesion to $CD4^+$ cells. Enfuvirtide is administered twice daily as a subcutaneous injection. A major adverse effect is injection site reaction, occurring in nearly all clients (98%). Presently, enfuvirtide is reserved for clients for whom other therapies have failed and whose treatment options have been exhausted.

Atazanavir (Reyataz) is a once-a-day protease inhibitor. An advantage over other protease inhibitors is that it does not increase triglyceride or low-density lipoprotein (LDL) cholesterol levels. A disadvantage is that its most common adverse effect is hyperbilirubinemia. Also, the drug may prolong the PR interval, leading to first-degree atrioventricular block.

Emtricitabine (Emtriva) is a once-a-day NRTI and is similar to lamivudine. Similar to other NRTIs, emtricitabine has the possibility of causing lactic acidosis with hepatic steatosis. The most common adverse effect (6%) is hyperpigmentation of the soles of the feet and the palms of the hands.

Fosamprenavir (Lexiva) is a phosphate ester pro-drug of amprenavir. Fosamprenavir is quickly hydrolyzed to amprenavir and is distributed in the blood as amprenavir. Side effects and drug interactions are similar to amprenavir. Food does not affect its absorption.

Adherence To Drug Regimen

Adherence to the therapeutic regimen is a major concern and issue with clients receiving antiretroviral therapy. Relative to this, the nurse must be knowledgeable about ways to promote adherence to the regimen. Nonadherence will re-

Table 34–6

Hydrea

Trade name	Hydrea
Generic name	hydroxyurea
Form	500 mg capsules
Dose	500 mg b.i.d.
Classification	Hydroxyurea is used for sickle cell disease and is not FDA approved for HIV. It is currently thought of as a possible drug or salvage therapy. In vitro studies show synergistic activity when combined with didanosine (ddI).
Oral bioavailability	Well absorbed
Major toxicity	Dose-dependent bone marrow suppression with leukopenia, anemia, and thrombocytopenia. Gastrointestinal intolerance may be severe, including stomatitis, nausea, vomiting, anorexia, diarrhea, and constipation.

b.i.d., Twice a day, *FDA,* Food and Drug Administration.

sult in HIV viral replication, increased VLs, and deterioration of the immune system. Development of resistant viral strains, enhanced with subtherapeutic levels of antiretroviral agents, is a serious current and long-term threat for clients with AIDS. Reasons commonly identified by clients for missing medications include forgetting to take them, feeling too sick, or not having the medicine with them. In addition, there are public health implications of nonadherence related to the expanding pool of drug-resistant viruses.

The following suggestions are offered to promote client adherence to the therapeutic regimen. Clients' understanding of their drug regimen is crucial to adherence, including the purpose of each medication, dosage schedule, food and fluid restrictions, recommended food choices, and storage of medications (e.g., refrigeration). Pictorial representation of the medications and a pillbox designed for medications to be taken four times a day may be helpful. Additional helpful hints to promote adherence are associating taking medications with a daily routine, such as brushing the teeth or feeding the pet; having a friend remind the client to take the medication; using a medications calendar to check off medications taken; and using the pharmacist as a resource.

Clients need the telephone number of a contact person to whom they can address questions. Discussion of anticipated side effects of the medications and how to manage their occurrence is necessary. A trusting client-provider relationship is essential. Long-term adherence to the regimen remains a major challenge and requires an interdisciplinary team approach.

Opportunistic Infections and Kaposi's Sarcoma

Once the CD4+ count decreases to less than 200/mm³, many opportunistic infections are more likely to develop. The lower the CD4+ count, the greater the risk and number of infections. In most instances, with all the microorganisms, breakthrough and progression occur. There are no cures, and lifelong treatment is required to prevent recurrence.

Candidiasis

Fungal infection. *Symptoms:* patches of inflammation with or without ulceration. May cause difficulty swallowing, nausea, sternal pain. Women may have thick vaginal discharge and pruritus. Diagnosis by KOH-scraping from mucous membranes.

Cryptococcus

Fungal infection. *Symptoms:* fever, malaise, headache, cough, GI disturbances. May localize in CNS (meningitis, encephalitis), memory loss, confusion. Diagnosis by culture of CSF.

Cytomegalovirus

Viral infection. *Symptoms:* painless, progressive loss of vision, sometimes complicated by retinal detachment. In the GI tract, causes nausea, vomiting, weight loss. Diagnosis by funduscopic examination. Primarily treated with valganciclovir. See Chapter 32, Antiviral, Antimalarial, and Anthelmintic Drugs, Table 32-1.

Herpes Simplex Virus (HSV)

Viral infection (HSV-1 and HSV-2). *Symptoms:* orolabial, genital, anorectal (pain, itching, painful defecation), mucocutaneous lesions, esophagitis, encephalitis (less common). Diagnosis by viral culture.

Histoplasmosis

Fungal infection. *Symptoms:* often asymptomatic, may cause flulike symptoms, high fever, weight loss, liver and spleen enlargement. Diagnosis by fungal cultures.

Mycobacterium avium Complex

Bacterial infection. *Symptoms:* high spiking fevers, diarrhea, night sweats, malaise, weight loss, anemia, neutropenia. Diagnosis by blood cultures or biopsy of liver, bone marrow, and lymph nodes.

Pneumocystis carinii Pneumonia

Protozoal/fungal infection. *Symptoms:* fever, dyspnea, tachypnea with or without rales or rhonchi, and nonproductive or mildly productive cough, chills, sweats. Diagnosis by bronchial washings or open lung biopsy.

Salmonella

Bacterial infection. *Symptoms:* fever, chills, night sweats. Diagnosis by blood cultures.

Toxoplasma gondii

Parasite infection. Primarily infects the brain and eye. *Symptoms:* fever, headache, seizures, focal neurologic abnormalities, and mental status changes. Diagnosis presumptive or based on computed tomography or magnetic resonance imaging.

Tuberculosis

Bacterial infection. *Symptoms:* cough, fever, sweating, malaise, fatigue, weight loss, nonpleuritic chest pain, dyspnea. Diagnosis by tuberculosis smear, culture.

Kaposi's Sarcoma

Cancer. *Symptoms:* red-blue blotches or nodules ranging in size from a few millimeters to several centimeters in diameter. The lesion may bleed. Nodules may appear in the mouth or in the viscera. Rarely seen in women. Diagnosis made by biopsy.

Therapies for common opportunistic infections, and Kaposi's sarcoma are presented in Table 34-7.

End-Stage AIDS

The era of HAART has shown that HIV-infected/AIDS clients are living longer. The increased survival time of HIV clients has shown an increase of end-stage AIDS condi-

Table 34–7

Therapies for Common Opportunistic Infections and Conditions

Clinical Disease	Prophylactic Agent	Agents—Acute Infection
Esophageal candidiasis		Fluconazole
		Itraconazole
		Amphotericin B
Cryptococcal meningitis		Amphotericin B
		Flucytosine
		Fluconazole
Cytomegaloviral retinitis	Ganciclovir	Foscarnet
		Ganciclovir
		Valganciclovir
		Cidofovir
Mycobacterium avium complex	Clarithromycin	Clarithromycin
	Azithromycin	Ethambutol
	Rifabutin	Azithromycin
		Amikacin
		Ciprofloxacin
Pneumocystis carinii pneumonia	Trimethoprim-sulfamethoxazole	Trimethoprim-sulfamethoxazole
	Dapsone	Dapsone
	Pyrimethamine	Pentamidine
	Pentamidine	Clindamycin
	Atovaquone	Primaquine
		Atovaquone
		Trimetrexate and folinic acid
Toxoplasmic encephalitis	Trimethoprim-sulfamethoxazole	Sulfadiazine
	Dapsone	Pyrimethamine
	Pyrimethamine	Folinic acid
	Atovaquone	Clindamycin
		Azithromycin
		Clarithromycin
		atovaquone
Tuberculosis	Isoniazid	Isoniazid
	Pyridoxine	Firampin
	Rifampin	Pyrazinamide
	Pyrazinamide	Ethambutol
		Streptomycin
Kaposi's sarcoma		Vinblastine
		Doxorubicin
		Daunorubicin
		Interferon alfa 2b

tions. Additionally, causes of death have changed from sepsis and opportunistic infections to liver and kidney failure, malignancies, pneumonias, and end-stage AIDS. End-stage AIDS can be manifested by pain, general weight loss, anorexia, neuropathies, dementia, constipation, diarrhea, depression, nausea, and vomiting.

Antiretroviral Therapy in Pregnancy

One of the most significant research studies in the history of HIV and AIDS was the ACTG 076 study (AIDS Clinical Trials Group Protocol, the 76th study), a phase III, randomized, double-blind, placebo-controlled clinical trial. The goal of the trial was to evaluate whether AZT (zidovudine, ZDV) administered to HIV-infected pregnant women and their infants could reduce the rate of transmission from mother to infant. Approximately 7000 infants are born to HIV-infected women in the United States each year. The study was halted

in February 1994 when the review board found a 67.5% reduction in HIV maternal-fetal transmission.

The protocol for HIV-infected pregnant women/newborns from this study (MMWR, 43 RR-11, 1994) is as follows:

• *Pregnant women:* Oral administration of 100 mg of ZDV five times daily, initiated at 14 to 34 weeks of gestation and continued throughout the pregnancy. During labor, IV administration of ZDV in a 1-hour loading dose of 2 mg/kg of body weight, followed by a continuous infusion of 1 mg/kg of body weight per hour until delivery.

• *Newborns:* Oral administration of ZDV to the newborn (ZDV syrup at 2 mg/kg of body weight per dose every 6 hours) for the first 6 weeks of life, beginning 8 to 12 hours after birth.

Consider referring all pregnant clients to the national Antiretroviral Therapy registry. The telephone number is (800) 258-4263; FAX (800) 800-1052; and website *www.APRegistry.com.*

Table 34–8

Basic and Expanded Postexposure Prophylaxis Regimens

Regimen Category	Application	Drug Regimen
Basic	Occupational HIV exposures for which there is a recognized transmission risk	4 wk (28 d) of both zidovudine 600 mg every day in divided doses (i.e., 300 mg 2×/d, 200 mg 3×/d, or 100 mg q4h) *and* lamivudine 150 mg 2×/d
Expanded	Occupational HIV exposures that pose an increased risk for transmission (e.g., larger volume of blood and/or higher virus titer in blood)	Basic regimen plus *either* indinavir 800 mg q8h *or* nelfinavir 750 mg 3×/d*

From Department of Health and Human Services, Henry J. Kaiser Family Foundation: *Panel on practices for treatment of HIV infection: guidelines for the use of antiretroviral agents in HIV-infected adults and adolescents,* March, 2004.
d, Day; h, hour; wk, week.
*Indinavir should be taken on an empty stomach (i.e., without food or with a light meal) and with increased fluid consumption (i.e., drinking six 8-oz glasses of water throughout the day); nelfinavir should be taken with meals.

The U.S. Public Health Service Task Force recommendations for use of antiretroviral agents during pregnancy for maternal health and reduction of perinatal transmission of HIV (*MMWR*, 47 RR-2, 1998) include the use of combination antiretroviral therapy. There are some early reports of increased numbers of premature births with HIV-infected pregnant women receiving combination therapy.

Postexposure Prophylaxis for Health Care Workers

As of December 1999, a total of 56 health care workers in the United States had acquired HIV infection from occupational exposure. Needlestick injuries carried a 0.33% chance of transmission; mucosal surface exposure carried a 0.09% chance of transmission. There were no transmissions from skin exposures. Of the 52 confirmed cases, nurses and laboratory technicians made up the majority of the cases; all cases involved blood or bloody body fluids (three were laboratory workers exposed to HIV viral cultures). To date, there are no confirmed cases in surgeons and no transmissions attributed to exposure to a suture needle.

The policy for **postexposure prophylaxis (PEP)** needs to be institution specific and available to all employees. The basic and expanded postexposure regimens are described in Table 34–8. HIV PEP resources and registries are presented in Table 34–9.

A comprehensive reference for PEP is the U.S. Public Health Service Statement on the Management of Occupational Exposures to HIV and Recommendations for Postexposure Prophylaxis, *MMWR* 50(RR-11): June 29, 2001.

The Future of HIV/AIDS-Related Agents

HIV/AIDS is a prime area of clinical investigations. Multiple vaccines have been tested; however, only one has been approved for large clinical trials. Vaccines are showing little that is promising for the near future. New compounds are 5 to 10 years away from reaching advanced clinical studies. Efforts are now directed to finding new treatment

options for clients who have few options left and to optimizing current treatments. Clients need to be dosed as few times a day as possible, reducing to as few pills as possible, and reducing side effects.

Fusion inhibitors represent a new class of HIV medications, and the new additions to existing antiretroviral agents are well tolerated and provide once daily dosing.

Table 34–9

National Resources

Resource or Registry	Contact Information
Centers for Disease Control and Prevention (CDC) National AIDS Clearinghouse	800-458-5231 *www.cdc.gov*
HIV/AIDS Treatment Information Service	800-HIV-0440 (448-0440)
National AIDS Hotline	800-342-AIDS (342-2437)
National Clinical Hotline	888-TRIALS-A (874-2572)
National Prevention Information Network	800-458-5231

WEBSITES

For further information on *HIV and AIDS-Related Agents,* visit these Internet resources:

AIDS Fact Sheet: Adherence:
www.aids.org/factSheets/4-5-Adherence.html

Drug Adherence in HIV/AIDS:
http://hivinsite.ucsf.edu/InSite?page=kbr-03-02-09

MedWatch:
www.fda.gov/medwatch/

HIV/AIDS Bureau—A Guide to the Clinical Care of Women with HIV/AIDS:
http://hab.hrsa.gov/publications/womencare.htm

Department of Health and Human Services (DHHS):
www.aidsinfo.nih.gov

Critical Thinking Case Study

R.S. was diagnosed with HIV infection in 1994 and began zidovudine (AZT) therapy that same year. In 1995, 3TC (Epivir, Lamivudine) was added to the zidovudine.

In early 1996, the laboratory reported R.S.'s viral load (VL) at 120,000. At that time, ritonavir was added. The VL decreased to 3500, and the CD4⁺ T cells increased from 06 mm³ to 96 mm³.

R.S. reports that it is hard to "always be taking medicine" and states, "Now that I'm back to work and going out again, I sometimes forget my pills." Additionally, there is a complaint of increased fatigue. VL increased to 8500, and CD4⁺ T cells decreased to 70 mm³.

It is believed that R.S. has become resistant to RT inhibitors and is started on dual protease inhibitors. In 6 weeks, the VL is undetectable and the CD4⁺ T cells are 85 mm³.

1. Missing doses of protease inhibitors can be very harmful to the client. Given the client's history, what can the nurse do to assist R.S. with issues related to adherence/compliance?

2. What is the rationale for including 3TC in R.S.'s therapeutic plan?

3. What action should the nurse take to facilitate R.S.'s understanding of the consequences of her nonadherence to the drug regimen?

4. What are the dangers of missing doses of protease inhibitors?

Study Questions

1. What are at least two side effects of NRTIs?

2. What are the two modes of action of nevirapine (Viramune)?

3. What is the major problem with NRTIs that requires they be used only in combination with a nucleoside analogue?

4. NNRTIs affect the concentration of oral contraceptives. True or false?

5. What was the first protease inhibitor approved by the FDA?

6. What is a toxic effect of efavirenz (EFV) that affects about 40% of clients who take this drug?

7. What are at least eight general factors to be included in client teaching about antiretroviral therapy?

8. What suggestions related to diet would you share with a client newly diagnosed with AIDS and beginning a therapeutic plan?

9. What are three nursing interventions to promote client adherence to the complex medical regimen?

10. What factors are likely to lead to problems with medication adherence?

11. What are at least three aspects of the nurse's research role related to antiretroviral therapy?

12. What are at least two cultural considerations related to clients on antiretroviral therapy?

35 Vaccines

LYNETTE M. WACHHOLZ

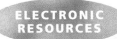 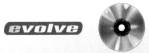

Additional information can be found on the companion website at *http://evolve.elsevier.com/KeeHayes/pharmacology/* or on the companion CD-ROM, which includes:
- *NCLEX-style examination review questions*
- *Pharmacology animations*
- *Medication error and (IV) therapy checklists*
- *Medication calculation problems*
- *Electronic calculators*

OUTLINE

OBJECTIVES

- Describe the differences between active and passive immunity.
- Describe the differences between active natural and active acquired immunity.
- Identify infectious diseases for which vaccines are currently available.
- Outline the currently recommended childhood immunization schedule.
- Identify vaccines routinely administered to adults.
- Discuss contraindications to the administration of varicella vaccine.
- Explain the nursing interventions, including client teaching, related to the administration of vaccines.

TERMS

acquired immunity
active immunity
anaphylaxis
antibodies
antigen

attenuated viruses
conjugate vaccines
immunizations
natural immunity
passive immunity

pathogen
recombinant subunit
    vaccines
seroconversion
toxoids

Introduction

Timely **immunizations** protect individuals from illness. They can also ultimately lead to the eradication of disease, as was the case with smallpox in 1977. Therefore universal immunization is a national goal. However, in the United States more than one child in three is not current with the recommended immunizations by the age of 2 years.

A recent study suggested that factors such as absence of a two-parent household, large family size, Medicaid enrollment, absence of a usual health care provider, no insurance coverage, or lack of a telephone in the home significantly increased the odds of a child experiencing vaccination delay.

Other studies have looked at racial disparities in immunization rates. One such study noted an increasing gap in coverage rates between white and black children, as well as between white and Hispanic children.

Active Immunity

Active immunity occurs as a part of the human immune response, which is activated when a **pathogen** such as a bacterium or virus invades the body. The body recognizes this pathogen as a foreign substance and promptly begins producing **antibodies** and other infection-fighting cells whose responsibility is to rid the body of this foreign substance. On the first exposure to the pathogen, the immune response is relatively slow and is typically accompanied by signs and symptoms of disease. However, the immune system retains memory of this pathogen. If this same pathogen invades the body again, the immune response, including the increased production of pathogen-specific antibodies, occurs much more rapidly and generally prevents disease. This active **natural immunity** may be present for the remaining life of the individual.

Active protection against disease may also be provoked by immunization. Vaccination involves the administration of a small amount of **antigen,** which, although capable of stimulating an immune response, does not typically produce disease. The antigen in vaccines may be produced in several ways. Traditional vaccines contain the whole or components of an inactivated (killed) microorganism. Other vaccines are **attenuated viruses** that are composed of live, attenuated (weakened) microorganisms. **Toxoids** are inactivated toxins, the harmful disease-causing substance produced by some microorganisms.

Some newer vaccines are called **conjugate vaccines.** Such vaccines require a protein or toxoid from an unrelated organism to link to the outer coat of the disease-causing microorganism. This linking creates a substance that can be recognized by the immature immune system of young infants. *Haemophilus influenzae* type B is an example of a conjugate vaccine.

Recombinant subunit vaccines involve the insertion of some of the genetic material (e.g., deoxyribonucleic acid [DNA]) of a pathogen into another cell or organism, where the antigen is then produced in massive quantities. These antigens are then used as a vaccine in place of the whole pathogen. Hepatitis B is an example of this type of vaccine.

Regardless of the composition of the vaccine, each vaccine is designed to stimulate an immune response against a specific pathogen. Booster doses are sometimes required to maintain sufficient immunity. Because the immune system retains memory, a vaccinated individual who is later exposed to the actual pathogen mounts a rapid immune response, thus preventing disease. This active artificially **acquired immunity** is the focus of this chapter.

Passive Immunity

Passive immunity occurs when an individual receives antibodies against a particular pathogen from another source. Newborn infants naturally receive passive immunity via the transfer of maternal antibodies across the placenta. Passive immunity may also be acquired via the administration of antibodies pooled from several human or animal sources that have been exposed to disease-causing pathogens. Alternatively, antibodies may be produced using recombinant DNA technology.

Whether natural or acquired, passive immunity is transient, lasting no more than several weeks to a few months. The recipient does not mount his or her own immune response. However, passive immunity is important. It helps young infants who, because of their immature immune systems, are poorly equipped to protect themselves against disease. Acquired passive immunity is important (1) when time does not permit active vaccination alone, (2) when the exposed individual is at high risk for complications of the disease, or (3) when the person suffers from an immune system deficiency that renders that person unable to produce an effective immune response.

Vaccine-Preventable Diseases

In the United States there are more than 20 infectious diseases that may be prevented by active vaccination. Many of these vaccines are routinely administered to healthy children and adults. Others are reserved for special populations, such as military personnel, travelers to certain foreign countries, or the chronically ill. Table 35–1 provides an overview of the disease manifestations and vaccine information, including route of administration and storage temperature. Vaccine-preventable diseases include anthrax, diphtheria, *Haemophilus influenzae* type B (Hib), hepatitis A, hepatitis B, influenza, Japanese encephalitis, measles, meningococcal disease, mumps, pertussis, pneumococcal disease, poliomyelitis, rabies, rubella, tetanus, tuberculosis, typhoid, varicella, and yellow fever.

Figure 35–1 summarizes the latest recommendations for childhood immunizations. Note that these recommendations change regularly; for the most current information, check the Centers for Disease Control and Prevention (CDC) website at *www.cdc.gov/nip*.

Table 35–1

Vaccine-Preventable Diseases

Disease/Route of Administration and Storage Temperature	Manifestations	Vaccine
Anthrax/subQ	• Spectrum involves three types of infection: *Cutaneous* (malignant pustule): a painless sore that develops at the site of a cut *Inhalational* (wool sorter's disease): severe dyspnea, cyanosis, fever, and death *Gastrointestinal:* abdominal pain, vomiting, bloody diarrhea, toxemia, shock, possibly death • Inhalational form associated with use of bacteria in biologic warfare	• Inactivated bacteria • Administration limited to military personnel
Diphtheria/IM	• Respiratory infection • May result in heart failure or paralysis if left untreated	• Toxoid • Contained in DTaP, DT, Td, and DTaP-hepatitis B-polio vaccines
Haemophilus influenzae type B/(Hib)/IM 35°-46° F (2°-8° C)	• Causes meningitis, pneumonia, sepsis, arthritis, and skin and throat infections • Most serious in children younger than 1 y	• Bacterial conjugate • Contained in Hib, Hib-DTaP, and Hib-hepatitis B vaccines
Hepatitis A/IM 35°-46° F (2°-8° C)	• Fever, malaise, jaundice, anorexia, and nausea • Acute, self-limited illness	• Inactivated virus • Contained in hepatitis A and hepatitis A-hepatitis B vaccines • Administered to high-risk populations and persons traveling to certain foreign countries • Also recommended for routine immunization of children in states, countries, and communities with elevated rates of hepatitis A virus infection
Hepatitis B/IM 35°-46° F (2°-8° C)	• Malaise, anorexia, arthralgias, arthritis, jaundice • Chronic infection can occur leading to liver cirrhosis, liver cancer, and death	• Recombinant viral antigen • Contained in hepatitis B, hepatitis B-Hib, hepatitis B-DTaP-polio, and hepatitis B-hepatitis A vaccines
Influenza/IM; intranasal 35°-46° F (2°-8° C)	• Fever, chills, headaches, malaise, myalgias, nasal congestion, and cough • Occasionally causes croup and pneumonia	• Inactivated viral components or live virus
Japanese encephalitis/subQ	• Headache, fever, myalgias, encephalitis	• Inactivated virus • Administered to some foreign travelers
Measles/subQ 35°-46° F (2°-8° C)	• Rash, fever, cough, nasal congestion, conjunctivitis, pneumonia • Occasionally results in encephalitis	• Live virus • Contained in measles, measles-mumps, and MMR vaccines
Meningococcal disease/subQ	• Fever, sepsis, rash, meningitis	• Old vaccine: portions of inactivated bacterial capsule; new vaccine: bacterial conjugate
Mumps/subQ 35°-46° F (2°-8° C)	• Swelling of salivary glands, fever, and headache • Rarely causes encephalitis, inflamed testicles, or permanent hearing loss	• Live virus • Contained in mumps, measles-mumps, and MMR vaccines
Pertussis ("whooping cough")/IM	• Severe coughing spasms • Rarely causes pneumonia, seizures, encephalitis, and death • Symptoms more severe in infants and young children	• Antigenic components of inactivated bacteria (acellular) • Contained in DTaP, and DTaP-Hib, and DTaP-hepatitis B-polio vaccines

BCG, Bacille Calmette-Guérin; *B-Hib*, *Haemophilus influenzae* type B; *DT*, diphtheria-tetanus; *DTaP*, diphtheria-tetanus-pertussis; *ID*, intradermal; *IM*, intramuscular; *MMR*, measles-mumps-rubella; *PO*, by mouth; *subQ*, subcutaneous; *Td*, tetanus-diphtheria; *y*, year; >, greater than; ≥, greater than or equal to; <, less than.

Continued

Table 35–1

Vaccine-Preventable Diseases—cont'd

Disease/Route of Administration and Storage Temperature	Manifestations	Vaccine
Pneumococcal disease/IM, subQ 35°-46° F (2°-8° C)	• Ear infections, sinus infections, pneumonia • Occasionally causes sepsis and meningitis	Two different types of vaccines: • Older polysaccharide vaccine contains portions of 23 serotypes of pneumococcal bacterial capsules (PPV23); administered to elderly and certain other high risk populations as long as ≥2 y of age • Newer vaccine is a protein conjugate vaccine containing portions of seven serotypes of pneumococcal bacterial capsules (PCV7); recommended for routine administration to children <2 y of age and certain other older high-risk children
Poliomyelitis subQ, IM 35°-46° F (2°-8° C)	• Mild form causes fever, sore throat, nausea, and headaches • Severe form causes paralysis and death	
Rabies IM	• Anxiety, difficulty swallowing, seizures, and invariably progresses to death	• Inactivated virus • Inactivated virus • Administered to high-risk groups (e.g., veterinarians, animal handlers) and persons traveling to areas where rabies is common
Rubella ("German measles") subQ 35°-46° F (2°-8° C)	• Rash, fever • Birth defects if acquired by pregnant women	• Live virus • Contained in rubella and MMR vaccines
Smallpox Skin prick	• High fever, severe headache, backache, abdominal pain, and lethargy lasting 2-5 days • Then extensive rash which begins as macules that progress to papules, then firm vesicles, and finally, deep-seated, hard pustules which cause significant scarring	• Live virus • Natural disease eradicated worldwide in 1980 • May be used as a weapon of bioterrorism • Limited immunization program to include military personnel, civilian health care workers, and emergency personnel began in 2002
Tetanus ("lock jaw") IM 35°-46° F (2°-8° C)	• Headache, irritability, muscle spasms (jaw, neck, arms, legs, back, and abdomen)	• Toxoid • Contained in tetanus, DTaP, DTaP-Hib, DT, DTaP-hepatitis B-polio, and Td vaccines
Tuberculosis ("TB") ID, subQ	• Highly contagious respiratory infection • May also cause meningitis and bone, joint, and skin infections	• Live bacteria • Referred to as BCG vaccine • Not routinely administered in the United States • Prevents severe disease but does not prevent infection with the bacterium
Typhoid/subQ, PO	• Fever, headache, anorexia, abdominal pain, enlarged liver and spleen, constipation, and later, diarrhea	• Available as live bacteria, inactivated, or components of typhoid bacterial capsule • Recommended only for travelers to certain countries
Varicella ("chickenpox")/subQ 5° F (−15° C) or colder	• Fever and rash, consisting of a few to hundreds of itchy, blisterlike lesions • Symptoms more severe in older children and adults • Complications may include encephalitis, bacterial skin infections, pneumonia, Reye syndrome, and death	• Live virus
Yellow fever/subQ	• Fever, jaundice, and gastrointestinal hemorrhage	• Live virus • Recommended for travelers to foreign countries with high yellow fever rates • Required by international regulations for travel to and from certain countries

Recommended Childhood and Adolescent Immunization Schedule
United States · July–December 2004

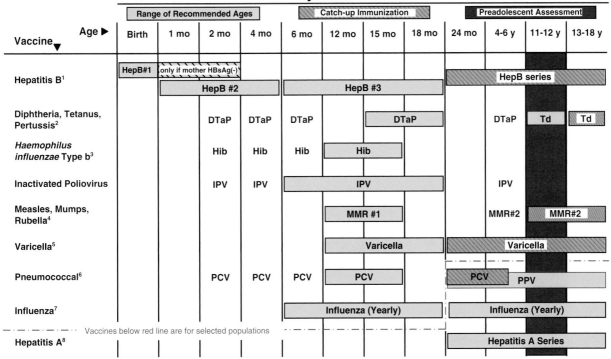

This schedule indicates the recommended ages for routine administration of currently licensed childhood vaccines, as of April 1, 2004, for children through age 18 years. Any dose not given at the recommended age should be given at any subsequent visit when indicated and feasible. ▉ Indicates age groups that warrant special effort to administer those vaccines not previously given. Additional vaccines may be licensed and recommended during the year. Licensed combination vaccines may be used whenever any components of the combination are indicated and the vaccine's other components are not contraindicated. Providers should consult the manufacturers' package inserts for detailed recommendations. Clinically significant adverse events that follow immunization should be reported to the Vaccine Adverse Event Reporting System (VAERS). Guidance about how to obtain and complete a VAERS form can be found on the Internet: www.vaers.org or by calling 800-822-7967.

1. Hepatitis B (HepB) vaccine. All infants should receive the first dose of hepatitis B vaccine soon after birth and before hospital discharge; the first dose may also be given by age 2 months if the infant's mother is hepatitis B surface antigen (HBsAg) negative. Only monovalent HepB can be used for the birth dose. Monovalent or combination vaccine containing HepB may be used to complete the series. Four doses of vaccine may be administered when a birth dose is given. The second dose should be given at least 4 weeks after the first dose, except for combination vaccines which cannot be administered before age 6 weeks. The third dose should be given at least 16 weeks after the first dose and at least 8 weeks after the second dose. The last dose in the vaccination series (third or fourth dose) should not be administered before age 24 weeks.

Infants born to HBsAg-positive mothers should receive Hep B and 0.5 mL of Hepatitis B Immune Globulin (HBIG) within 12 hours of birth at separate sites. The second dose is recommended at age 1–2 months. The last dose in the immunization series should not be administered before age 24 weeks. These infants should be tested for HBsAg and antibody to HBsAg (anti-HBs) at age 9–15 months.

Infants born to mothers whose HBsAg status is unknown should receive the first dose of the HepB series within 12 hours of birth. Maternal blood should be drawn as soon as possible to determine the mother's HBsAg status; if the HBsAg test is positive, the infant should receive HBIG as soon as possible (no later than age 1 week). The second dose is recommended at age 1–2 months. The last dose in the immunization series should not be administered before age 24 weeks.

2. Diphtheria and tetanus toxoids and acellular pertussis (DTaP) vaccine. The fourth dose of DTaP may be administered as early as age 12 months, provided 6 months have elapsed since the third dose and the child is unlikely to return at age 15–18 months. The final dose in the series should be given at age ≥4 years. **Tetanus and diphtheria toxoids (Td)** is recommended at age 11–12 years if at least 5 years have elapsed since the last dose of tetanus and diphtheria toxoid-containing vaccine. Subsequent routine Td boosters are recommended every 10 years.

3. Haemophilus influenzae type b (Hib) conjugate vaccine. Three Hib conjugate vaccines are licensed for infant use. If PRP-OMP (PedvaxHIB or ComVax [Merck]) is administered at ages 2 and 4 months, a dose at age 6 months is not required. DTaP/Hib combination products should not be used for primary immunization in infants at ages 2, 4, or 6 months but can be used as boosters following any Hib vaccine. The final dose in the series should be given at age ≥12 months.

4. Measles, mumps, and rubella vaccine (MMR). The second dose of MMR is recommended routinely at age 4–6 years but may be administered during any visit, provided at least 4 weeks have elapsed since the first dose and both doses are administered beginning at or after age 12 months. Those who have not previously received the second dose should complete the schedule by the visit at age 11–12 years.

5. Varicella vaccine. Varicella vaccine is recommended at any visit at or after age 12 months for susceptible children (i.e., those who lack a reliable history of chickenpox). Susceptible persons age ≥13 years should receive 2 doses, given at least 4 weeks apart.

6. Pneumococcal vaccine. The heptavalent **pneumococcal conjugate vaccine (PCV)** is recommended for all children age 2–23 months. It is also recommended for certain children age 24–59 months. The final dose in the series should be given at age >12 months. **Pneumococcal polysaccharide vaccine (PPV)** is recommended in addition to PCV for certain high-risk groups. See MMWR 2000;49(RR-9):1-35.

7. Influenza vaccine. Influenza vaccine is recommended annually for children aged ≥6 months with certain risk factors (including but not limited to asthma, cardiac disease, sickle cell disease, HIV, and diabetes), healthcare workers, and other persons (including household members) in close contact with persons in groups at high risk (see MMWR 2004;53[RR-6]:1-40) and can be administered to all others wishing to obtain immunity. In addition, healthy children aged 6–23 months and close contacts of healthy children aged 0–23 months are recommended to receive influenza vaccine, because children in this age group are at substantially increased risk for influenza-related hospitalizations. For healthy persons aged 5–49 years, the intranasally administered live, attenuated influenza vaccine (LAIV) is an acceptable alternative to the intramuscular trivalent inactivated influenza vaccine (TIV). See MMWR 2004;53(RR-6):1-40. Children receiving TIV should be administered a dosage appropriate for their age (0.25 mL if 6–35 months or 0.5 mL if ≥3 years). Children aged ≤8 years who are receiving influenza vaccine for the first time should receive 2 doses (separated by at least 4 weeks for TIV and at least 6 weeks for LAIV).

8. Hepatitis A vaccine. Hepatitis A vaccine is recommended for children and adolescents in selected states and regions and for certain high-risk groups; consult your local public health authority. Children and adolescents in these states, regions, and high-risk groups who have not been immunized against hepatitis A can begin the hepatitis A immunization series during any visit. The 2 doses in the series should be administered at least 6 months apart. See MMWR 1999;48(RR-12):1-37.

For additional information about vaccines, including precautions and contraindications for immunization and vaccine shortages, please visit the National Immunization Program Website at (www.cdc.gov/nip/acip/) or call the National Immunization Information Hotline at 800-232-2522 (English) or 800-232-0233 (Spanish).

Approved by the Advisory Committee on Immunization Practices (www.cdc.gov/nip/acip), the American Academy of Pediatrics (www.aap.org), and the American Academy of Family Physicians (www.aafp.org).

FIGURE 35-1 Recommended childhood and adolescent immunizations.

HERBAL ALERT 35–1

Vaccines

There are no known interactions between vaccinations and herbal preparations.

PREVENTING MEDICATION ERRORS

Do not confuse...

- Hepatitis B vaccine **Engerix-B** and **Recombivax**. These drugs have different doses.

- Hepatitis B vaccines and hepatitis B immunoglobulin (HBIG).

Childhood Immunizations

A summary of rules for childhood immunizations is also located at the Immunization Action Coalition's website at *www.immunize.org/catg.d/rules1.pdf*. Helpful information about each vaccine includes route of administration, recommended age of vaccine administration, minimum dosing intervals, and contraindications to use. The recommended vaccines are diphtheria-tetanus-pertussis (DTaP), tetanus-diphtheria (Td), polio, varicella, measles-mumps-rubella (MMR), *H. influenzae* type B, hepatitis B, pneumococcal conjugate, influenza, and in some populations hepatitis A. Children and their caregivers should be questioned regarding their use of prescription and over-the-counter medications as well as herbal preparations before immunizations are administered. See Herbal Alert 35–1.

Adult Immunizations

Whereas much emphasis is placed on regularly immunizing infants and children, adult immunizations are frequently overlooked. However, they are equally important to the health and well-being of this population. Vaccines for adults may include Td, influenza, pneumococcal polysaccharide, hepatitis B, hepatitis A, MMR, varicella, and in certain instances meningococcal polysaccharide. The recommended adult immunization schedule by age group and medical conditions is found in Figure 35–2. A summary of recommendations for adult immunization is also located at the Immunization Action Coalition's website at *www.immunize.org/catg.d/p2011b.pdf*. Helpful information for each vaccine includes route of transmission, recommended populations, routine and "catch-up" schedules, and contraindications. The CDC suggests review of adult immunization records on decade birthdays (e.g., ages 30, 40, 50).

Immunization Before Foreign Travel

Foreign travel warrants the administration of all routine vaccines indicated based on age or immunization history. Foreign travel also requires consideration of additional vaccines, depending on the client's travel destinations.

Many travelers may need to consider vaccination against typhoid and yellow fever. Typhoid is caused by a bacterium, *Salmonella enterica* typhi, which is generally spread via contaminated food and water (refer to Table 35–1 for disease manifestations). Risk of contracting this infection is greatest for travelers to India, Pakistan, Mexico, Bangladesh, the Philippines, and Haiti. Even stays of less than 2 weeks pose significant risk. Two vaccines are available for use in the United States. The live oral vaccine can be administered to persons 6 years of age and older and consists of four capsules, one taken every 48 hours, with the series completed one week before potential exposure. A booster consisting of the same four-capsule regimen is recommended every 5 years. The polysaccharide vaccine may be administered to travelers 2 years of age and older. It is administered at least 2 weeks before expected exposure as a single, intramuscular (IM) injection. A booster dose is recommended every 2 years.

Yellow fever is a mosquito-borne viral illness. The disease occurs only in sub-Saharan Africa and tropical South America. The vaccine is administered as a single injection; a booster every 10 years is recommended. In the United States, the vaccine is administered only at authorized vaccine centers throughout the country (*www2.ncid.cdc.gov/travel/yellowfever*).

Other vaccines needed for travel may include meningococcal, rabies, and Japanese encephalitis vaccines. A country-specific review of vaccinations is beyond the scope of this chapter. However, current vaccine recommendations and related travel information are available from the CDC at (888) 232-3299 or *www.cdc.gov/travel*.

Reporting of Diseases and Adverse Reactions

Health care providers are responsible for reporting cases of vaccine-preventable diseases to public health officials, who then make weekly reports to the CDC. These data identify whether an outbreak is occurring and the impact of immunization policies and procedures.

Vaccines are generally safe. Common mild reactions include swelling at the injection site and fever. Awareness of the contraindications for use of vaccines decreases the incidence of serious adverse reactions. Absolute contraindications include anaphylactic reaction to a specific vaccine or component of another vaccine or moderate or severe illness. In general, vaccines may be given if the client has the following: mild acute illness or convalescent phase of illness, antimicrobial therapy, exposure to infectious disease, and prematurity.

Health care providers must report adverse reactions to the Vaccine Adverse Events Reporting System (VAERS).

Recommended Adult Immunization Schedule by Vaccine and Age Group
UNITED STATES • OCTOBER 2004–SEPTEMBER 2005

Age group (yrs) ▶ Vaccine ▼	19–49	50–64	≥65
Tetanus, Diphtheria (Td)*	1 dose booster every 10 years[1]		
Influenza	1 dose annually[2]	1 dose annually	
Pneumococcal (polysaccharide)	1 dose[3,4]	1 dose[3,4]	
Hepatitis B*	3 doses (0, 1–2, 4–6 months)[5]		
Hepatitis A*	2 doses (0, 6–12 months)[6]		
Measles, Mumps, Rubella (MMR)*	1 or 2 doses[7]		
Varicella*	2 doses (0, 4–8 weeks)[8]		
Meningococcal (polysaccharide)	1 dose[9]		

Legend:
- For all persons in this group
- For persons lacking documentation of vaccination or evidence of disease
- For persons at risk (i.e., with medical/exposure indications)

The Recommended Adult Immunization Schedule is Approved by the Advisory Committee on Immunization Practices (ACIP), the American College of Obstetricians and Gynecologists (ACOG), and the American Academy of Family Physicians (AFFP)

* Covered by the Vaccine Injury Compensation Program.
See Footnotes for Recommended Adult Immunization Schedule on back cover.

This schedule indicates the recommended age groups for routine administration of currently licensed vaccines for persons aged ≥19 years. Licensed combination vaccines may be used whenever any components of the combination are indicated and when the vaccine's other components are not contraindicated. Providers should consult manufacturers' package inserts for detailed recommendations.

Report all clinically significant postvaccination reactions to the Vaccine Adverse Event Reporting System (VAERS). Reporting forms and instructions on filing a VAERS report are available by telephone, 800-822-7967, or from the VAERS website at http://www.vaers.org.

Information on how to file a Vaccine Injury Compensation Program claim is available at http://www.hrsa.gov/osp/vicp or by telephone, 800-338-2382. To file a claim for vaccine injury, contact the U.S. Court of Federal Claims, 717 Madison Place, N.W., Washington, DC 20005, telephone 202-219-9657.

Additional information about the vaccines listed above and contraindications for immunization is available at http://www.cdc.gov/nip or from the National Immunization Hotline, 800-232-2522 (English) or 800-232-0233 (Spanish).

Continued

FIGURE 35–2 Recommended adult immunizations by age group and by medical conditions.

Recommended Adult Immunization Schedule by Vaccine and Medical and Other Indications

UNITED STATES • OCTOBER 2004–SEPTEMBER 2005

Vaccine ▼ / Indication ▶	Pregnancy	Diabetes, heart disease, chronic pulmonary disease, chronic liver disease (including chronic alcoholism)	Congenital immunodeficiency, cochlear implants, leukemia, lymphoma, generalized malignancy, therapy with alkylating agents, antimetabolites, CSF** leaks, radiation or large amounts of corticosteroids	Renal failure /end stage renal disease, recipients of hemodialysis or clotting factor concentrates	Asplenia (including elective splenectomy and terminal complement component deficiencies)	HIV*** infection	Health-care workers
Tetanus, Diphtheria (Td)*,1	■	■	■	■	■	■	■
Influenza2	■	A, B	C	■	C	■	■
Pneumococcal (polysaccharide)3,4		B	D	D	D, E, F	D, G	
Hepatitis B*,5	■	■	■	H	■	■	■
Hepatitis A*,6	■	I	■	■	■	■	L
Measles, Mumps, Rubella (MMR)*,7	■	■	■ (Contraindicated)	■	■	J	■
Varicella*,8	■	■	K (Contraindicated)	■	■	J	■

Legend: For all persons in this group · For persons lacking documentation of vaccination or evidence of disease · For persons at risk (i.e., with medical/exposure indications) · ■ Contraindicated

* Covered by the Vaccine Injury Compensation Program.
** Cerebrospinal fluid.
*** Human immunodeficiency virus.
See Special Notes for Medical and Other Indications below. Also see Footnotes for Recommended Adult Immunization Schedule on back cover.

Special Notes for Medical and Other Indications

A. Although chronic liver disease and alcoholism are not indications for influenza vaccination, administer 1 dose annually if the patient is aged ≥50 years, has other indications for influenza vaccine, or requests vaccination.

B. Asthma is an indication for influenza vaccination but not for pneumococcal vaccination.

C. No data exist specifically on the risk for severe or complicated influenza infections among persons with asplenia. However, influenza is a risk factor for secondary bacterial infections that can cause severe disease among persons with asplenia.

D. For persons aged < 65 years, revaccinate once after ≥5 years have elapsed since initial vaccination.

E. Administer meningococcal vaccine and consider Haemophilus influenzae type b vaccine.

F. For persons undergoing elective splenectomy, vaccinate ≥2 weeks before surgery.

G. Vaccinate as soon after diagnosis as possible.

H. For hemodialysis patients, use special formulation of vaccine (40 μg/mL) or two 20 μg/mL doses administered at one body site. Vaccinate early in the course of renal disease. Assess antibody titers to hepatitis B surface antigen (anti-HB) levels annually. Administer additional doses if anti-HB levels decline to < 10 mIU/mL.

I. For all persons with chronic liver disease.

J. Withhold MMR or other measles-containing vaccines from HIV-infected persons with evidence of severe immunosuppression (see MMWR 1998;47 [No. RR-8];21–2 and MMWR 2002;51 [No. RR-2];22–4).

K. Persons with impaired humoral immunity but intact cellular immunity may be vaccinated (see MMWR 1999;48[No. RR-6]).

L. No data to support a recommendation.

FIGURE 35–2, cont'd   Recommended adult immunizations by age group and by medical conditions.

Footnotes

Recommended Adult Immunization Schedule • UNITED STATES • OCTOBER 2004–SEPTEMBER 2005

1. **Tetanus and diphtheria (Td).** Adults, including pregnant women with uncertain history of a complete primary vaccination series, should receive a primary series of Td. A primary series for adults is 3 doses; administer the first 2 doses at least 4 weeks apart and the 3rd dose 6–12 months after the second. Administer 1 dose if the person received the primary series and if the last vaccination was received ≥ 10 years previously. Consult recommendations for administering Td as prophylaxis in wound management (see *MMWR* 1991;40[No. RR-10]). The American College of Physicians Task Force on Adult Immunization supports a second option for Td use in adults: a single Td booster at age 50 years for persons who have completed the full pediatric series, including the teenage/young adult booster.

2. **Influenza vaccination.** The Advisory Committee on Immunization Practices (ACIP) recommends inactivated influenza vaccination for the following indications, when vaccine is available. *Medical indications:* chronic disorders of the cardiovascular or pulmonary systems, including asthma; chronic metabolic diseases, including diabetes mellitus, renal dysfunction, hemoglobinopathies, or immunosuppression (including immunosuppression caused by medications or by human immunodeficiency virus [HIV]; and pregnancy during the influenza season. *Occupational indications:* health-care workers and employees of long-term-care and assisted living facilities. *Other indications:* residents of nursing homes and other long-term-care facilities; persons likely to transmit influenza to persons at high risk (i.e. in-home caregivers to persons with medical indications, household/close contacts and out-of-home caregivers of children aged 0–23 months; household members and caregivers of elderly persons and adults with high-risk conditions); and anyone who wishes to be vaccinated. For healthy persons aged 5–49 years without high-risk conditions who are not contacts of severely immunocompromised persons in special care units, either the inactivated vaccine or the intranasally administered influenza vaccine (FluMist®) may be administered (see *MMWR* 2004;53[No. RR-6]).
   Note: Because of the vaccine shortage for the 2004–05 influenza season, CDC has recommended that vaccination be restricted to the following priority groups, which are considered to be of equal importance: all children aged 6–23 months; adults aged ≥65 years; persons aged 2–64 years with underlying chronic medical conditions; all women who will be pregnant during the influenza season; residents of nursing homes and long-term-care facilities; children aged 6 months–18 years on chronic aspirin therapy; health-care workers involved in direct patient care; and out-of-home caregivers and household contacts of children aged < 6 months. For the 2004–05 season, intranasally administered, live, attenuated influenza vaccine, if available, should be encouraged for healthy persons who are aged 5–49 years and are not pregnant, including health-care workers (except those who care for severely immunocompromised patients in special care units) and persons caring for children aged < 6 months (see *MMWR* 2004;53:923–4).

3. **Pneumococcal polysaccharide vaccination.** *Medical indications:* chronic disorders of the pulmonary system (excluding asthma); cardiovascular diseases; diabetes mellitus; chronic liver diseases, including liver disease as a result of alcohol abuse (e.g., cirrhosis); chronic renal failure or nephrotic syndrome; functional or anatomic asplenia (e.g., sickle cell disease or splenectomy); immunosuppressive conditions (e.g., congenital immunodeficiency, HIV infection, leukemia, lymphoma, multiple myeloma, Hodgkins disease, generalized malignancy, or organ or bone marrow transplantation); chemotherapy with alkylating agents, antimetabolites, or long-term systemic corticosteroids; or cochlear implants. *Geographic/other indications:* Alaska Natives and certain American Indian populations. *Other indications:* residents of nursing homes and other long-term-care facilities (see *MMWR* 1997;46[No. RR-8] and *MMWR* 2003;52:739–40).

4. **Revaccination with pneumococcal polysaccharide vaccine.** One-time revaccination after 5 years for persons with chronic renal failure or nephrotic syndrome; functional or anatomic asplenia (e.g., sickle cell disease or splenectomy); immunosuppressive conditions (e.g., congenital immunodeficiency, HIV infection, leukemia, lymphoma, multiple myeloma, Hodgkins disease, generalized malignancy, or organ or bone marrow transplantation); or chemotherapy with alkylating agents, antimetabolites, or long-term systemic corticosteroids. For persons aged ≥65 years, one-time revaccination if they were vaccinated ≥5 years previously and were aged < 65 years at the time of primary vaccination (see *MMWR* 1997;46[No. RR-8]).

5. **Hepatitis B vaccination.** *Medical indications:* hemodialysis patients or patients who receive clotting factor concentrates. *Occupational indications:* health-care workers and public-safety workers who have exposure to blood in the workplace; and persons in training in schools of medicine, dentistry, nursing, laboratory technology, and other allied health professions. *Behavioral indications:* injection-drug users; persons with more than one sex partner during the previous 6 months; persons with a recently acquired sexually transmitted disease (STD); all clients in STD clinics; and men who have sex with men. *Other indications:* household contacts and sex partners of persons with chronic hepatitis B virus (HBV) infection; clients and staff members of institutions for the developmentally disabled; inmates of correctional facilities; or international travelers who will be in countries with high or intermediate prevalence of chronic HBV infection for > 6 months (http://www.cdc.gov/travel/diseases/hbv.htm) (see *MMWR* 1991;40[No. RR-13]).

6. **Hepatitis A vaccination.** *Medical indications:* persons with clotting factor disorders or chronic liver disease. *Behavioral indications:* men who have sex with men or users of illegal drugs. *Occupational indications:* persons working with hepatitis A virus (HAV)-infected primates or with HAV in a research laboratory setting. *Other indications:* persons traveling to or working in countries that have high or intermediate endemicity of hepatitis A. If the combined Hepatitis A and Hepatitis B vaccine is used, administer 3 doses at 0, 1, and 6 months (http://www.cdc.gov/travel/diseases/hav.htm) (see *MMWR* 1999;48[No. RR-12]).

7. **Measles, mumps, rubella (MMR) vaccination.** *Measles component:* adults born before 1957 can be considered immune to measles. Adults born during or after 1957 should receive ≥1 dose of MMR unless they have a medical contraindication, documentation of ≥1 dose, or other acceptable evidence of immunity. A second dose of MMR is recommended for adults who 1) were recently exposed to measles or in an outbreak setting, 2) were previously vaccinated with killed measles vaccine, 3) were vaccinated with an unknown vaccine during 1963–1967, 4) are students in postsecondary educational institutions, 5) work in health-care facilities, or 6) plan to travel internationally. *Mumps component:* 1 dose of MMR vaccine should be adequate for protection. *Rubella component:* Administer 1 dose of MMR vaccine to women whose rubella vaccination history is unreliable and counsel women to avoid becoming pregnant for 4 weeks after vaccination. For women of childbearing age, regardless of birth year, routinely determine rubella immunity and counsel women regarding congenital rubella syndrome. Do not vaccinate pregnant women or those planning to become pregnant during the next 4 weeks. For women who are pregnant and susceptible, vaccinate as early in the postpartum period as possible (see *MMWR* 1998;47[No. RR-8] and *MMWR* 2001;50:1117).

8. **Varicella vaccination.** Recommended for all persons lacking a reliable clinical history of varicella infection or serologic evidence of varicella zoster virus (VZV) infection who might be at high risk for exposure or transmission. This includes health-care workers and family contacts of immuno-compromised persons; persons who live or work in environments where transmission is likely (e.g., teachers of young children, child care employees, and residents and staff members in institutional settings); persons who live or work in environments where VZV transmission can occur (e.g., college students, inmates, and staff members of correctional institutions, and military personnel); adolescents aged 11–18 years and adults living in households with children; women who are not pregnant but who might become pregnant; and international travelers who are not immune to infection.
   Note: Approximately 95% of U.S.-born adults are immune to VZV. Do not vaccinate pregnant women or those planning to become pregnant during the next 4 weeks. For women who are pregnant and susceptible, vaccinate as early in the postpartum period as possible (see *MMWR* 1999;48[No. RR-6]).

9. **Meningococcal vaccine (quadrivalent polysaccharide for serogroups A, C, Y, and W 135).** *Medical indications:* adults with terminal complement component deficiencies or those with anatomic or functional asplenia. *Other indications:* travelers to countries in which meningococcal disease is hyperendemic or epidemic (e.g., the "meningitis belt" of sub-Saharan Africa and Mecca, Saudi Arabia). Revaccination after 3–5 years might be indicated for persons at high risk for infection (e.g., persons residing in areas where disease is epidemic). Counsel college freshmen, especially those who live in dormitories, regarding meningococcal disease and availability of the vaccine to enable them to make an educated decision about receiving the vaccination (see *MMWR* 2000;49[No. RR-7]). The American Academy of Family Physicians recommends that colleges should take the lead on providing education on meningococcal infection and availability of vaccination and offer it to students who are interested. Physicians need not initiate discussion of meningococcal quadrivalent polysaccharide vaccine as part of routine medical care.

FIGURE 35–2, cont'd Recommended adult immunizations by age group and by medical conditions.

PROTOTYPE DRUG CHART 35–1

VARICELLA

Drug Class	**Dosage**
Vaccines Trade Name: Varivax *Pregnancy Category:* C	**C: 12 mo–12 y: subQ:** 0.5 ml × 1 dose **Persons ≥13 y: subQ:** 0.5 ml × 2 doses given 4-8 wk apart
Contraindications	**Drug-Lab-Food Interactions**
Previous anaphylaxis to this vaccine or to any of its components; pregnancy or possibility of pregnancy within 1 mo; immunocompromised vaccine recipient; presence of moderate to severe acute illness; active untreated tuberculosis	*Drug:* Separate from MMR vaccine by 4 wk, if not given on same day; delay VV for at least 5 mo after blood transfusion or Ig; delay Ig for 2 mo after VV; high dose immunosuppressant medications; avoid salicylates for 6 wk after VV
Pharmacokinetics	**Pharmacodynamics**
Not applicable	*Seroconversion rates:* 12 mo–12 y: >95% at 4-6 wk after vaccination ≥13 y: 78%-85% 4 wk after first dose and 99% 4 wk after second dose No booster indicated at this time.

Therapeutic Effects/Uses

Prevention of chickenpox. When administered to susceptible individuals, vaccine results in complete protection from chickenpox for the majority. For the minority in whom breakthrough chickenpox develops after vaccination, the disease is typically very mild. The vaccine also provides prophylaxis protection if administered within 3 to 5 d of exposure to chickenpox.
Mode of Action: Stimulates active immunity against natural disease

Side Effects	**Adverse Reactions**
Pain and redness at injection site, fever, chickenpox-like rash (generalized or confined to area surrounding injection site)	Anaphylaxis, thrombocytopenia, encephalitis, Stevens-Johnson syndrome

C, Child; *d,* day; *Ig,* immune globulin; *MMR,* measles-mumps-rubella; *mo,* month; *subQ,* subcutaneous; *VV,* varicella vaccine; *wk,* week; *y,* year; >, greater than; ≥, greater than or equal to.

Information and forms are available at (800) 822-7967 or www.vaers.org. The National Childhood Vaccine Injury Act of 1986 set forth the National Vaccine Injury Compensation Program (NVICP). This program provides compensation for injury or death caused by a vaccination. The NVICP does not require proof of negligence on the part of a health care provider. For more information, call the NVICP at (800) 338-2382.

Varicella Vaccine

Prototype Drug Chart 35–1 provides the pharmacologic data for varicella vaccine.

Pharmacokinetics

Biologic products such as vaccines do not undergo the pharmacokinetic processes associated with other drug therapy.

Pharmacodynamics

Seroconversion is the acquisition of detectable levels of antibodies in the bloodstream. In the case of varicella vaccine, seroconversion occurs in more than 95% of 12-month to 12-year-old recipients at approximately 4 to 6 weeks after vaccination. Susceptible clients 13 years of age and older who receive two doses of varicella vaccine 4 to 8 weeks apart show a seroconversion rate of 78% to 82% at 4 weeks after the first dose and 99% at 4 weeks after the second dose. The immune response appears to persist indefinitely after vaccination. No booster is currently indicated.

Contraindications

Varicella vaccine should be avoided in clients with a history of previous **anaphylaxis** to this vaccine or to any of its components, including gelatin and neomycin. It is also contraindicated in the presence of moderate to severe acute illness or active untreated tuberculosis.

The possible effects of the vaccine on fetal development are currently unknown; therefore varicella vaccine is contraindicated during pregnancy. However, chickenpox can sometimes cause fetal harm. Pregnancy should also be avoided for at least 1 month after each dose of the vaccine. NOTE: This recommendation differs from the product package insert, which suggests a 3-month delay in pregnancy.

Clients who are immunocompromised because of malignancies or high dose systemic steroid therapy should avoid varicella vaccine. Likewise, the vaccine is contraindicated in the presence of primary or acquired immunodeficiencies, including human immunodeficiency virus (HIV).

Drug Interactions

Frequently, a client is eligible for several immunizations at any given visit. A client receiving varicella vaccine may receive all other vaccines concurrently as long as each is administered at a separate site. If the MMR vaccine is not given the same day as the varicella vaccine, administration of the two vaccines should be spaced at least 4 weeks apart.

If a client has received a transfusion of blood or blood products, including immune globulin, administration of the varicella vaccine should be deferred at least 5 months. Likewise, such blood products should be avoided for at least 2 months after vaccination, if possible. Blood products and immune globulin interfere with the body's production of antibodies specific to chickenpox, thereby decreasing the likelihood that active immunity will develop.

Reye syndrome has occasionally occurred in children following natural chickenpox infection. The majority of these children were also receiving salicylate medications (e.g., aspirin). Therefore it is generally recommended that clients avoid salicylates for 6 weeks after vaccination.

Nursing Process

Vaccines

ASSESSMENT

- Identify barriers to timely and complete immunization (e.g., belief that vaccine-preventable diseases no longer exist, misunderstanding of *true* contraindications to immunization, concerns regarding vaccine safety and efficacy, fear of multiple injections, cost).
- Obtain medical history including history of malignancy or other immune deficiency.
- Determine history of pregnancy or possible pregnancy within the next month. Do not administer vaccines to pregnant women.
- Obtain drug history, including high-dose immunosuppressants, blood transfusions, and immune globulin.
- Obtain a list of herbal products used by client and/or primary caregiver (in case of breastfed infant).
- Determine complete allergy history, including drugs, vaccines, food, and environmental allergies.
- Assess for adverse reactions (other than allergic) to previous doses of vaccine or any vaccine component.
- Assess for symptoms of moderate to severe acute illness with or without fever.
- Screen for unvaccinated or immunodeficient household contacts.
- Obtain immunization history to determine current vaccine needs.

NURSING DIAGNOSES

- Deficient knowledge: vaccine-preventable diseases, risks and benefits of vaccination
- Ineffective health maintenance

PLANNING

- Client will adhere to recommended immunization schedule for vaccine-preventable diseases.
- Client will be free of adverse reactions.

NURSING INTERVENTIONS

- Strictly adhere to individual vaccine storage requirements to ensure potency of the product.
- Upon preparation, including reconstitution of a given vaccine, administer within time limits stated in package insert to ensure potency.
- At time of visit, administer at separate sites all vaccines for which client is eligible. Do *not* mix vaccines in the same syringe.
- Document in client's record the following data: vaccination date, route, and site; vaccine type, manufacturer, lot number, and expiration date; name, business address, and title of individual administering vaccine.
- Observe clients for signs and symptoms of adverse reactions to vaccines.
- Keep epinephrine readily available for immediate use in case of anaphylactic reaction.
- Provide client with a record of immunizations administered.

Client Teaching

General

- Discuss with client and/or client's family the manifestations of and risk of contracting vaccine-preventable diseases.
- Answer all questions regarding vaccine safety and efficacy.
- Inform female clients of childbearing age to avoid pregnancy for 1 month depending on the vaccines to be administered.
- Instruct clients to avoid contact with immunocompromised persons depending on vaccines to be administered.
- In accordance with federal law, provide client or client's family with current Vaccine Information Statements (VISs), available from the CDC, for each vaccine administered. The following data must be documented in the client's record: vaccination date, route, and site; vaccine type, manufacturer, lot number, and expiration date; name, business address, and title of individual administering vaccine.
- Remind client or client's family to bring immunization record to all visits.

- Provide client or client's family with date upon which to return for next vaccination.

Side Effects
- Discuss common side effects of vaccines such as injection site soreness, fever, and side effects specific to individual vaccines.
- Offer suggestions for management of common side effects (e.g., cold compresses for injection site soreness, acetaminophen for soreness and/or fever).
- Instruct client or client's family to contact the health care provider if signs of a serious reaction are noted.

Cultural Considerations

- Modify communications to meet cultural needs of client/family.
- Do not assume that a positive response means a definite yes.
- Use an interpreter when necessary.
- VISs are available in multiple languages and can be downloaded from the Immunization Action Coalition's website at *www.immunize.org*.

EVALUATION

- Evaluate client's or client's family's understanding of rationale for immunizations.
- Evaluate client adherence to recommended immunization schedule.

Recent Developments and the Future of Vaccines

Currently new vaccines are being brought to market and new delivery systems developed.

A small outbreak of anthrax cases in the United States in 2001 increased the level of awareness of the vaccine for anthrax. As a biological weapon, anthrax is highly lethal. It is easily produced, stored, and spread over large areas. Proper vaccination is an essential part of protection against this disease. Approved by the FDA in 1970, anthrax vaccine has been routinely and safely administered to laboratory personnel, livestock farmers, veterinarians, and utility personnel deployed during the Gulf War. The vaccine requires six injections: three given 2 weeks apart followed by three additional doses at 6, 12, and 18 months. No serious side effects have been reported, but the vaccination is contraindicated during pregnancy. An oral anthrax vaccine is on the horizon. The vaccine is derived from a genetically modified plant virus. The virus is introduced into a plant, where it then stimulates the plant to produce new proteins. These proteins are extracted and used to produce a vaccine. When the vaccine is administered to a human, the person's body reacts as if infected with anthrax and creates antibodies against the bacterium. In the event of a bioterrorism attack,

large numbers of individuals can be rapidly immunized with an oral vaccine. Additional information is available at www.anthrax.osd.mil.

Menactra, a new vaccine approved by the Food and Drug Administration (FDA) in early 2005, is a quadrivalent conjugate vaccine (MCV-4) designed to prevent meningococcal disease. It offers several advantages over the older polysaccharide vaccine (MPSV-4), including inducing longer immune memory, ensuring booster effects, and reducing nasopharyngeal carriage. In addition, the conjugate vaccine is more immunogenic in younger children than the polysaccharide vaccine. The Advisory Committee on Immunization Practices recommends this newly licensed vaccine be administered as a single dose to children 11 to 12 years old, to adolescents entering high school (15 years old), to college freshmen living in dormitories, and to certain other high-risk populations.

Smallpox was eradicated worldwide by 1980. The United States discontinued routine childhood immunization against smallpox in 1971. However, since the events of September 2001, concern has arisen that the smallpox (or variola) virus could be used as a bioterrorist weapon. Unlike anthrax, smallpox virus is not airborne and is transmitted through human bodily fluids or contaminated materials. A smallpox immunization plan has been implemented in the United States *(www.bt.cdc.gov)*. However, there has been some resistance to vaccination because of a lack of perceived threat and because of the risk of significant side effects from the vaccine. The currently available vaccine is a live virus preparation. It is administered using a bifurcated needle to deliver the vaccine into the epidermis. A skin reaction occurs at the immunization site 3 to 5 days later and eventually leaves a scar. Boosters may be recommended every 10 years.

FluMist, a live, intranasal influenza vaccine, was licensed by the FDA in 2003. Because it is a live vaccine, recipients may develop symptoms of influenza (usually mild) and theoretically may spread the disease to unprotected contacts. Therefore its use is limited to healthy individuals 5 through 49 years of age. The older, inactivated vaccine is still preferred over FluMist for health care workers and others who have close contact with immunocompromised individuals.

Work continues on new combination vaccines that reduce the number of injections as well as vaccines against infectious agents such as *Campylobacter jejuni*, human papilloma virus (HPV), parainfluenza virus, respiratory syncytial virus (RSV), *Helicobacter pylori*, rotavirus, and HIV.

New delivery systems for vaccines are currently in development to replace the "needle." Timed-release pills have the potential to offer lifetime immunity to a specific disease in a one-time dose. With this, the need for a booster vaccination is eliminated. In addition, skin patches may one day be used to administer tetanus and influenza vaccines.

WEBSITES

For further information on *Vaccines,* visit these Internet resources:

General immunization information:

Allied Vaccine Group:
www.vaccine.org

CDC's National Immunization Program:
www.cdc.gov/nip

Childhood Immunization Support Program:
www.cispimmunize.org

Children's Vaccine Program:
www.childrensvaccine.org

Food and Drug Administration:
www.fda.gov/oc/opacom/kidshtml/vaccines.htm

Immunization Action Coalition:
www.immunize.org and *www.vaccineinformation.org*

Institute for Vaccine Safety:
www.vaccinesafety.edu

National Association of Pediatric Nurse Practitioners:
www.pertussis.com and *www.hibdisease.com*

National Network for Immunization Information:
www.immunizationinfo.org

National Vaccine Program Office:
www.hhs.gov/nvpo

Parents of Kids with Infectious Diseases:
www.pkids.org

Vaccine Education Center at Children's Hospital of Philadelphia:
www.vaccine.chop.edu

The Vaccine Page:
www.vaccines.com

Travel immunization information:

CDC's Travel Health:
www.cdc.gov/travel

Travel Health Online:
www.tripprep.com

Critical Thinking Case Study

J.W., a 29-year-old woman, is seen at the immunization clinic with her 2-month-old daughter and her son, who just turned 5 years old last month. She reports they all need shots.

1. J.W. will soon be returning to work at a long-term care facility for developmentally disabled adults. She reports that her new employer is encouraging her to be immunized against hepatitis B. She wonders how long it will take her to complete the vaccine series. What is your response?

2. You administer J.W.'s first dose of hepatitis B vaccine today. When should she return for the next dose?

3. You ask J.W. about her vaccine history. She says she does not have an immunization card but remembers last receiving a "booster when I stepped on a nail at my high school graduation picnic." What "booster" did she likely receive? At what point is another booster due?

4. J.W. says her daughter needs her "regular baby shots." The infant received her first hepatitis B vaccine while in the newborn nursery. Against what vaccine-preventable illnesses will you plan to vaccinate this infant today?

5. When would this infant be due for another series of immunizations?

6. J.W. asks you about chickenpox vaccine. She would like her daughter to be vaccinated against chickenpox as soon as possible because she does not want her to suffer through chickenpox as her brother did. What is the earliest age at which her daughter can receive varicella vaccine?

7. J.W. says she has heard that you can get chickenpox from the vaccination shot. How would you respond to this comment?

8. J.W. has brought her son's immunization card. It shows he received hepatitis B vaccine at birth, 2 months, and 9 months. He received DTaP, Hib, polio (IPV), and pneumococcal (PCV) vaccines at 2 months, 4 months, and 6 months. She is worried that he will need to start his immunizations over because "he's so far behind." How would you respond to her concern?

9. For what vaccines is he due today?

Study Questions

1. What is the difference between active natural and active acquired immunity?

2. What is the difference between active and passive immunity?

3. What vaccines are typically indicated for children up to 16 years of age?

4. What are the two types of pneumococcal vaccines and for what age groups are they typically indicated?

5. If a 2-month-old infant experiences redness and tenderness at the DTaP injection site associated with a fever of 100.8° F, what vaccine should be administered at the next visit in 6 to 8 weeks?

6. What are contraindications to the use of varicella vaccine?

7. Describe the smallpox vaccination, and give reasons for resistance to vaccination.

8. What are the commonly administered immunizations before foreign travel?

9. Discuss the reasons FluMist is limited to healthy individuals 5 to 49 years of age.

10. What are the nursing interventions related to vaccine administration?

Ten

Cancer Agents

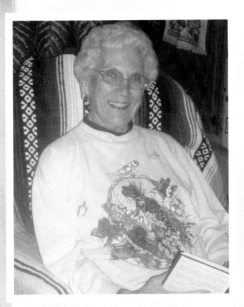

Cancer is a major health problem in our society. The causes of cancer vary and include those attributed to environment (e.g., chemicals, asbestos, radiation), genetic influence (e.g., BRAC $\frac{1}{2}$ mutation), lifestyle (e.g., smoking, alcohol use), diet (e.g., high fat), infection (e.g., Epstein-Barr, *Helicobacter pylori*), and immune suppression (e.g., HIV infection, immunosuppressive medications). Cancer (malignant, neoplastic) cells are characterized by (1) unregulated growth, (2) lack of differentiation, and (3) spread (metastasis) to other body cells and organs. Cancer cells that divide rapidly respond more effectively to anticancer therapy than do slow-growing malignant cells.

Cell Cycle

The cell cycles of normal and cancer cells are similar. The cell cycle has four phases that are directed toward cell replication, and a fifth, the resting phase. The first phase of the cell cycle is G_1, the presynthesis phase that prepares for deoxyribonucleic acid (DNA) synthesis. The second phase is the S phase, whereby DNA synthesis occurs. Next is the G_2 postsynthesis phase in which the cell is prepared for mitosis. Cell division (cytokinesis) occurs in the fourth, or M (mitosis), phase. The cells may immediately enter the G_1 phase or enter the G_0 or resting phase. Most cells in the human body are in the G_0 stage. Exceptions include metabolically active cells such as the granulocytes and epithelial cells found in the gastrointestinal tract. The cell cycle is demonstrated in Figure X–1, and the phases are described in Box X–1.

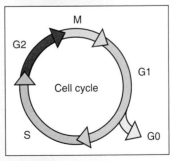

FIGURE X–1   Cell cycle. *G_1 phase (postmitotic gap):* Production of enzyme for DNA synthesis. The G_1 phase lasts 15 to 18 hours. *S phase (synthesis):* The DNA doubles. The S phase lasts 10 to 20 hours. *G_2 phase (premitotic gap):* RNA synthesis for later mitosis. The G_2 phase lasts approximately 3 hours. *M phase (mitosis):* Cell division produces two identical cells. The M phase lasts approximately 1 hour. *G_0 phase (resting):* Cells remain in this phase or return to the cell cycle for cell replication. Cells in this phase are not as sensitive to many antineoplastic drugs.

Cell Cycle and Phases

1. G_1: enzyme production needed for deoxyribonucleic acid (DNA)
2. S, or synthesis: DNA synthesis and replication
3. G_2: ribonucleic acid (RNA) and protein synthesis
4. M, or mitosis: cell division
5. G_0: resting phase

Growth Rate

Growth rate *(doubling time)* is defined as the time it takes for a cancerous tumor to double in size. Growth fraction decreases and doubling time increases as the tumor enlarges. Growth rate depends on several factors, including the cell-cycle activity of the proliferating cells in the tumor mass, the number of cells proliferating within the tumor *(growth fraction)* and the rate of cell loss from the tumor. In general, anticancer drugs are more effective against cancer cells that have a high growth fraction. Malignant tumors that have prolonged cell-cycles and a slower growth rate are more likely to be locally confined and therefore more amendable to surgical excison.

Anticancer Therapy

In the past 3 decades, significant advances have been made in the treatment of malignancies. *Chemotherapy* (chemical treatment) is the use of chemicals to kill cancer cells. Research has led to the use of new anticancer drugs and the development of standard treatment protocols (drug, dose, and schedule) for anticancer drugs to guide therapy. Nurses play a vital role in managing the treatment of people with cancer. This includes the administration of chemotherapy in health care facilities and in the homes of clients. To provide the best possible care, nurses should understand the chemotherapy regimen, contraindications, drug interactions, therapeutic effects, side effects, and adverse reactions of the chemotherapy that clients receive.

Chapter 36, Anticancer Drugs, discusses how selected anticancer drugs inhibit or prevent cell reproduction. The anticancer drugs are divided into major classes which include alkylating agents, antimetabolites, antitumor antibiotics, mitotic inhibitors, targeted therapies, and hormonal agents.

Some chemotherapy agents negatively affect cancer cells when they are actively dividing. These are called *cell-cycle specific (CCS) agents*. *Cell-cycle non-specific (CCNS) drugs* work best in the G_0 (resting) stage to disrupt cancer cells. Chemotherapy usually targets ribonucleic acid (RNA) or deoxyribonucleic acid (DNA) in cancer cells to prevent mitosis or induce apoptosis (self-death). The specific drugs selected are administered based on the type of tumor cells, the rate at which they divide, and the time that the drugs will be most effective. In general, chemotherapy is most effective in destroying cells that are rapidly dividing.

Chapter 37, Biologic Response Modifiers, describes the evolving state of biologic response modifiers, which work to (1) enhance host immunologic function, (2) destroy or interfere with tumor activities, and (3) promote differentiation of stem cells.

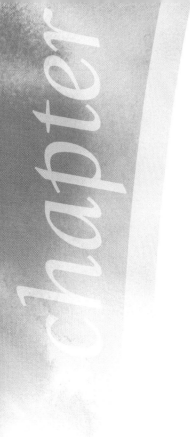

36 Anticancer Drugs

PAULA KLEMM

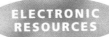 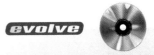

Additional information can be found on the companion website
at *http://evolve.elsevier.com/KeeHayes/pharmacology/*
or on the companion CD-ROM, which includes:
- *NCLEX-style examination review questions*
- *Pharmacology animations*
- *Medication error and (IV) therapy checklists*
- *Medication calculation problems*
- *Electronic calculators*

OUTLINE

OBJECTIVES

- Differentiate between cell-cycle specific and cell-cycle nonspecific drugs.
- Identify general side effects and adverse reactions to anticancer drugs.
- Describe the uses and considerations for alkylating compounds, antimetabolites, antitumor antibiotics, mitotic inhibitors, targeted therapy, and hormones.
- Describe client education guidelines for administering chemotherapy in the home.
- State three ways the nurse can avoid absorption of chemotherapeutic agents.
- Describe the nursing process, including client teaching, related to anticancer drugs.

TERMS

adjuvant therapy
alkylating agents
angiogenesis inhibitors
antimetabolites
antitumor antibiotics
cell-cycle nonspecific (CCNS) drugs

cell-cycle specific (CCS) drugs
combination chemotherapy
cytoprotectant (chemoprotectant)
doubling time
growth fraction

hormones
leucovorin rescue
mitotic inhibitors
monoclonal antibodies
multidrug resistance
palliative
proteasome inhibitors

protein tyrosine kinases
protocol
targeted cancer therapies
vesicant
vesication
vinca alkaloids

Introduction

In the United States, the mortality rate of cancer is second only to heart disease. Cancer is the leading cause of death in women and the second leading cause of death in children between the ages of 1 and 15 years (accidents are first). One in three women and one in two men will develop cancer over the course of their lifetime. Excluding skin cancers, the highest incidence rates in men are prostate, lung, and colorectal cancer; in women, breast, lung, and colorectal cancers have the highest incidence.

Cancer results from damage to the deoxyribonucleic acid (DNA) within the cell. DNA is the genetic substance in the body cells and transfers information necessary for the production of enzymes and protein synthesis. Cancer develops when some of the genes in a normal cell become damaged or lost (mutation). Several mutations are required before cancer can develop.

Anticancer drugs are also called *cancer chemotherapeutic agents* or *antineoplastic drugs*. Nitrogen mustard (a derivative of mustard gas that was used in warfare) was first used in the 1940s to treat clients with high white blood counts caused by leukemia and lymphoma. Soon after, methotrexate, cyclophosphamide, and fluorouracil were introduced and are still used today to treat malignancies. In the 1970s, using two or more chemotherapy agents to treat cancer was adopted and led to better response rates and increased survival time. Over the years, researchers have developed strict guidelines for the administration of anticancer drugs. Chemotherapy may be used as the sole treatment of cancer or in conjunction with other modalities (e.g., radiation, surgery, biologic response modifiers, targeted therapy). Combination chemotherapy has proven effective in curing some cancers (e.g., leukemia, Hodgkin's disease, Wilm's tumor). When cancer cannot be cured, anticancer drugs may be given to control the disease for a period of months to years. If the cancer can no longer be controlled, chemotherapy may be used to relieve symptoms associated with the disease.

Genetic, Infective, Environmental, and Dietary Influences

Cancers that have a genetic influence include breast, ovarian, endometrial, colon, and lung cancers, retinoblastoma and malignant melanoma. Many more genetic influences are expected to be found. Environment, lifestyle, viruses, and diet can influence the development of these and other types of cancers. Table 36–1 gives examples of

Table 36–1

Environmental, Infective, and Dietary Influences on Cancer Development

Environmental

Tobacco
Cancer of the lung, larynx, bladder, kidney, colon, cervix, stomach, pancreas, or breast

Asbestos
Lung cancer

Benzene
Acute myelogenous leukemia

Vinyl chloride
Sarcoma

Arsenic
Cancer of the lung, skin, sarcoma

Ionizing Radiation
Leukemia, cancer of the thyroid, breast

Ultraviolet Rays
Skin cancer

Aflatoxin
Liver cancer

Infective

Herpes Simplex 2 Virus (Genital Herpes)
Cancer of the cervix

Hepatitis B and Hepatitis C Viruses
Cancer of the liver

Epstein-Barr Virus (a cause of infectious mononucleosis)
Burkitt's lymphoma, nasopharyngeal cancers

Human papilloma Virus (HPV)
Cancer of the cervix

Human T-Cell Lymphotrophic Virus
T-cell leukemia

Helicobacter pylori
Cancer of the stomach

Diet

Animal Fat
Cancer of the colon, rectum, breast, uterus, prostate, ovary

Heterocyclic Amines (found in some smoked meats)
Cancer of the stomach, colon, rectum, pancreas, breast

Alcohol
Cancer of the mouth, throat, esophagus, liver, breast

types of environmental products, viruses, and foods that have a carcinogenic effect on cancer development in humans.

Genes can cause cells to become cancerous in three ways. *Proto-oncogenes* are normal genes that are involved in the controlled growth and division of cells. An oncogene is a mutation in a proto-oncogene. This abnormal oncogene overproduces cellular growth-control proteins and triggers unregulated cell division. Tumor-suppressor genes (antioncogenes) signal a cell to cease multiplying and act to stop the action of oncogenes. If tumor-suppressor genes become lost or dysfunctional, cells could reproduce uncontrollably. Other genes repair damage to DNA. If these DNA-repair genes are damaged, mutations are not mended and subsequently are passed on to the next generation of daughter cells. It may take a long time before enough cell mutations take place and cause cancer to develop. As a result, cancers more commonly occur in older individuals.

A number of viruses are associated with the development of cancer. The human papillomavirus (HPV) has been found in most women who have invasive cervical cancer. Individuals with human immunodeficiency virus (HIV) may develop lymphomas, anal, or genital cancers. The Epstein-Barr virus is found in almost all people with Burkitt's lymphoma in central Africa. Hepatocellular carcinoma (liver cancer) is linked to the hepatitis B virus. Other viruses that have a link to the development of cancer include human T-cell lymphotropic virus, type 1 (HTLV-1), human T-cell lyphotropic virus, type 2 (HTLV-2), and Kaposi's sarcoma-associated herpes virus.

Bacteria play a role in the development of cancer. The presence of *Helicobacter pylori* in the stomach is associated with an increased risk of developing gastric cancer. Recent research suggests that listeria monocytogenes, in combination with diet and other host factors, may increase motility and the invasion of colon cancer cells.

Environmental factors associated with the development of cancer include smoking, diet, infectious diseases, chemicals, and radiation. According to the American Cancer Society (ACS), the use of tobacco, an unhealthy diet, and inadequate physical activity account for 75% of cancer cases in the United States.

Cell-Cycle Nonspecific and Specific Drugs

In Unit X the cell cycle for normal and cancer cells, **growth fraction**, and **doubling time** are discussed (see Figure X–1). Refer to the discussion at the beginning of Unit Ten for clarification of the cell cycle and definitions.

Anticancer drugs cause cancer death by interfering with cell replication (see Figure X–1 in the Unit Ten opener). **Cell-cycle nonspecific (CCNS) drugs** act during any phase of the cell cycle, and **cell-cycle specific (CCS) drugs** exert their influence during a specific phase of the cell cycle. CCNS drugs (also called *cell-cycle independent*) kill cells during the M and G₀ phases. CCS drugs (also called *cell-cycle dependent*) are most effective against rapidly growing cancer cells. In general, the CCNS drugs include the alkylating drugs (although some alkylating agents are CCS), antitumor antibiotics, and hormones. The CCS drugs include the antimetabolites and the mitotic inhibitors. Table 36–2 and Figure 36–1 identify the types and group of drugs and the phase of the cell cycle that they affect.

Growth fraction and **doubling time** are two factors that play a major role in the response of cancer cells to anticancer drugs. Anticancer drugs are more effective against neoplastic cells that have a high growth fraction. Leukemias and some lymphomas have high growth fractions and thus respond well to anticancer drug therapy. Small and early forming cancer cells and fast-growing tumors respond well to chemotherapy and have a higher cure rate than slow-growing tumors in the advanced stages. When the tumor is 1 cm³ it is clinically detectable and con-

Table 36–2

Cell-Cycle Nonspecific (CCNS) and Cell-Cycle Specific (CCS) Agents

Type	Drug Group	Cell-Cycle Effect
CCNS	Alkylating drugs	All phases of cell division / Most effective in G₁ and S phases
CCNS	Nitrosoureas	All phases of cell division
CCS	Antimetabolites	S phase
CCNS	Antitumor antibiotics	All phases
CCS	Vinca alkaloids	M phase
CCS	Taxanes	M phase
CCS	Topoisomerase inhibitors	G₂, S phases

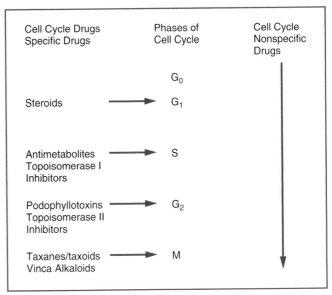

FIGURE 36–1 Cell-cycle nonspecific (CCNS) and cell-cycle specific (CCS) agents.

tains approximately one billion cancer cells and represents 30 doubling times from the initial cancer cell. At that time, symptoms may appear.

Solid tumors have a large percentage of their cell mass in the G_0 phase, so they generally have a low growth fraction and are less sensitive to anticancer drugs. High-dose chemotherapy results in better tumoricidal (tumor-killing) effects. Depending on the type of cancer, malignant cell growth is usually faster in the earlier stages of tumor development. As the tumor grows, the blood supply decreases, thereby slowing the growth rate. Anticancer agents are more effective against small tumors with sufficient blood supply. As the tumor enlarges, its growth fraction decreases and its doubling time increases, thus reducing the effectiveness of anticancer therapy.

Cancer Chemotherapy

Anticancer drugs are not selective, so both cancer cells and normal cells are affected. The side effects of chemotherapy are largely related to the toxic effects on normal cells. Antineoplastic agents are effective because normal cells are able to repair themselves and continue to grow, whereas cancer cells are less able to do so. Thus the side effects of chemotherapy are most often temporary. Chemotherapy is usually administered systemically for cancer that has spread to other parts of the body, for tumors in multiple sites, or for tumors that are too large to be removed via other means (e.g., surgery).

Some types of cancer can be cured with chemotherapy (e.g., Hodgkin's disease, Burkitt's lymphoma, Wilm's tumor, testicular cancer). Other types of cancer may be treated with surgery first, followed by chemotherapy to kill any cancer cells that may remain in the body (e.g., breast cancer, colon cancer). This is referred to as **adjuvant therapy.** Neoadjuvant chemotherapy may be given to help shrink a large tumor so that it can be surgically removed. **Palliative** chemotherapy is used to relieve symptoms associated with advanced disease (e.g., pain) and to improve the quality of life.

Chemotherapy administration is guided by specific **protocols** that were developed as a result of controlled research studies. The length of treatment is determined by the type and extent of the malignancy, kind of chemotherapy that is given, expected side effects of these drugs, and the amount of time that normal cells need to recover. Chemotherapy is usually given in cycles to improve the likelihood that cancer cells will be destroyed and that normal cells can recover. The duration, frequency, and number of cycles of chemotherapy are based on the type and size of the tumor, whether the disease has spread to other areas of the body (metastasis), and the condition of the client. Chemotherapy treatment may consist of one agent or a combination of agents. Combination chemotherapy may be administered on one day or spread out over several days. The duration of each treatment varies from minutes to days and may be repeated weekly, biweekly, or monthly, based on the protocol being followed.

Anticancer/antineoplastic drugs are listed in Box 36–1 according to their classification.

Drug Resistance

Malignant tumors often develop resistance to chemotherapeutic agents. This is termed **multidrug resistance** (MDR) and may occur for several reasons. Chemotherapy may not kill all neoplastic cells, and these cells may mutate and become resistant to the drug. Some tumor cells have a natural resistance to certain chemotherapy agents, thus making the drugs ineffective. Tumor resistance can occur as a result of *gene amplification,* in which a gene produces many copies of itself. This leads to an over production of protein that makes the chemotherapy drug less effective. Some cancer cells develop the ability to repair DNA damage caused by the antineoplastic therapy; others overproduce a P-glycoprotein (P-gp) in the cell membrane that pumps the chemotherapy out of the cells before it can be effective. Strategies for reversing the effects of MDR are being evaluated.

Combination Chemotherapy

Single-agent drug therapy is not usually used to treat cancer. Rather, combinations of drugs are employed to enhance tumoricidal effects. Chemotherapy is most effective when it is able to kill cells in all phases of the cell cycle. Combining chemotherapy (**combination chemotherapy**) drugs makes this possible.

CCS and CCNS drugs are often combined to maximize cell death. Each individual chemotherapy drug used in combination therapy should have proven activity. Using the drugs together may have a synergistic effect. In addition, each drug should have different modes of action and different dose-limiting toxicities. Using a combination of antineoplastic drugs has the advantage decreasing drug resistance and increasing destruction of cancer cells. Some of the combinations of anticancer drugs used in cancer treatment are presented in Table 36–3.

General Side Effects and Adverse Reactions

Anticancer drugs cause adverse reactions on rapidly growing normal cells (e.g., skin, hair). These drugs can also affect cells in the gastrointestinal (GI) tract, the mucous membranes, and the reproductive system. Table 36–4 lists the general adverse reactions to anticancer drugs on the fast-growing cells of the body. Selected nursing measures and considerations are included.

Anticancer Therapy in Outpatient Clinics and in the Home

The administration of anticancer drugs in outpatient clinics is common and has proven to be cost-effective and convenient. Although chemotherapy regimens have become increasingly aggressive, most clients will not be hospitalized unless they require close monitoring or are very ill. Some chemotherapy agents are administered in the home. Clients receiving highly potent drugs may need to be

BOX 36–1

Anticancer Drugs by Classifications

Alkylating Agents

nitrogen mustard (mechlorethamine hydrochloride)
chlorambucil (Leukeran)
cyclophosphamide (Cytoxan)
estramustine (Emcyt)
ifosfamide (Ifex)
mechlorethamine HCl (Mustargen)
melphalan (Alkeran)
uracil mustard
chlorambucil (Leukeran)

Nitrosoureas

carmustine (BiCNU, BCNU)
carmustine with polifeprosan 20 implant (Giliadel Wafer)
lomustine (CeeNU, CCNU)
streptozocin (Zanosar)

Alkylating-Like Agents

altretamine (Hexalen)
carboplatin (Paraplatin)
cisplatin (Platinol)
dacarbazine (DTIC)
eloxatin (Oxaliplatin)
pipobroman (Vercyte)
triethylenethiophosphoramide (Thiotepa)

Alkyl Sulfonates

busulfan (Myleran)

Antimetabolites

folic acid antagonist
methotrexate (MTX, amethopterin, Folex, Mexate)

Pyrimidine Analogues

capecitabine (Xeloda)
cytarabine HCl (Cytosar-U, ARA-C)
floxuridine (FUDR)
5-fluorouracil (5-FU, Adrucil)
gemcitabine HCl (Gemzar)
procarbazine HCl (Matulane)

Purine Analogues

cladribine (Leustatin)
fludarabine (Fludara)
6-mercaptopurine (6-MP, Purinethol)
thioguanine (Lanvis)

Ribonucleotide Reductase Inhibitors

hydroxyurea (Hydrea)
trimetrexate glucuronate (Neutrexin)
2-deoxycoformycin (Pentostatin, Nipent, DCF)

Enzyme Inhibitors

pentostatin (Nipent)

Mitotic Inhibitors

vinca alkaloids
vinblastine sulfate (Velban, Oncovin, Vincasar)
vincristine (liposomal) (Marqibo)
vinorelbine (Navelbine)

Antimicrotubules or Taxanes

docetaxel (Taxotere)
paclitaxel (Taxol)

Antitumor Antibiotics

bleomycin sulfate (Blenoxane)
dactinomycin (Actinomycin D, Cosmegen)
daunorubicin HCl (Cerubidine)
daunorubicin (liposomal) (DaunoXome)
doxorubicin (Adriamycin, Rubex)
doxorubicin HCL (liposomal) (Doxil, Caelyx, Myocet)
epirubicin (Ellence)
idarubicin (Idamycin)
mitomycin (Mutamycin)
mitoxantrone (Novantrone)
plicamycin (Mithracin, Mithracin)
valrubicin (Valstar)

Targeted Therapies

Topoisomerase I Inhibitors (Camptothecins)

irinotecan HCl (Camptosar, CPT-11)
topotecan HCl (Hycamtin)

Topoisomerase II Inhibitors (epipodophyllotoxins)

etoposide (VePesid, VP-16, Etopophos)
teniposide (Vumon, VM-26)

Tyrosine Kinase Inhibitors

gefitinib (Iressa)
imatinib mesylate (Gleevec)

Proteasome Inhibitors

bortezomib (Velcade)

Monoclonal Antibodies

cetuximab (Erbitux)
gemtuzumab-ozogamicin (Mylotarg)
rituximab (Rituxan)
trastuzumab (Herceptin)
alemtuzumab (Campath)

Angiogenesis Inhibitors

bevacizumab (Avastin)

Retinoids

bexarotene (Targretin)

Hormones, Hormonal Antagonists, and Enzymes

Androgens

testolactone (Teslac)
progesterone (Gesterol 50)

Hormonal Antagonists and Enzymes

aminoglutethimide (Cytadren)
anastrozole (Arimidex)
bicalutamide (Casodex)
exemestane (Aromasin)
flutamide (Eulexin)
fulvestant (Faslodex)
goserelin acetate (Zoladex)
letrozole (Femara)
leuprolide acetate (Lupron)
megestrol acetate (Megace)
mitotane (Lysodren)
nilutamide (Nilandron)
polyestradiol phosphate (Estradurin)
raloxifene hydrochloride (Evista)
tamoxifen citrate (Nolvadex) (nonsteroidal antiestrogen)
toremifene (Fareston)

Miscellaneous Enzymes

L-asparaginase (Elspar)
pegaspargase (Oncaspar)

Table 36–3

Selected Combinations of Anticancer Drugs

Drug	Name	Selected Uses
vinblastine, bleomycin, cisplatin (Platinol)	VBP	Testicular cancer
mechlorethamine, vincristine (Oncovin), procarbazine, prednisone	MOPP	Hodgkin's disease
cyclophosphamide, doxorubicin (Adriamycin), fluorouracil	CAF	Breast cancer, prostate cancer
taxotere, doxorubicin (Adriamycin), cyclophosphamide (Cytoxan)	TAC	Breast cancer
cyclophosphamide, epirubicin, fluorouracil	CEF	Breast cancer
cyclophosphamide, doxorubicin (Adriamycin), methotrexate	CAM	Prostate cancer
oxaliplatin, fluorouracil (5-FU), leucovorin	FOLFOX	Colorectal cancer
mitomycin C, vinblastine, cisplatin	MVP	Small cell lung cancer
mechlorethamine, vincristine, procarbazine, prednisone	MOPP	Hodgkin's lymphoma
paclitaxel, carboplatin	PC	Non-small cell lung cancer

NOTE: Doses of chemotherapy agents vary based on the drug protocol, type and stage of cancer, age, weight functional status, and comorbid conditions (e.g., heart disease, diabetes, respiratory problems, liver disease, etc.).

closely monitored for severe adverse reactions or to provide adequate hydration.

When a chemotherapy drug is given in the home, a health care provider qualified to administer anticancer agents follows the policies provided by the oncologist and the home health care agency. Client education guidelines are usually available and may include the following:

- Assess the learning needs of the client and family members.
- Provide printed information on the chemotherapeutic agents that are written at an appropriate educational level for the client/family (an eighth-grade level or lower is recommended).
- Discuss with the client/family the anticancer drug(s) that will be administered, the desired effects, and length of time per administration.
- Discuss the treatment process (i.e., intravenous access, administration of chemotherapy, duration of chemotherapy administration, monitoring side effects, follow-up).
- Discuss potential side effects of chemotherapy and how these will be handled. Include specific information on what is normal and what is not. Be sure that the client knows how to take his or her temperature.
- Give written instructions regarding diet, medications (e.g., antiemetics), and hydration as indicated.
- Emphasize self-care strategies (e.g., mouth care regimen, personal hygiene, exercise).
- Provide written guidelines for calling the physician (e.g., temperature elevation, uncontrolled vomiting, diarrhea).
- Teach the client/family that chemotherapy usually remains in the body for 48 to 72 hours after it is administered and is excreted in the urine, stool, emesis, semen, and vaginal secretions.
- Teach caregivers (including pregnant caregivers) to wear gloves (latex, nitrile, polyurethane, neoprene) when emptying a bedpan, urinal, or emesis basin or when changing soiled bed linens or clothing. Soiled linens should be washed as soon as possible.

- Provide information on the safe storage of chemotherapy medications that are kept in the home (e.g., keep in a safe place away from children and pets).
- Provide written information on safe handling of chemotherapy waste.

To reduce the nurse's exposure to chemotherapy drugs during intravenous (IV) administration, the following precautions should be followed:

- Use powder-free gloves (nitrile, polyurethane, neoprene) when handling chemotherapy.
- A mask is not needed if the drug was prepared by a pharmacist.
- Gowns (disposable, impermeable, lint-free) should be worn during the administration of IV chemotherapy.
- Gloves should be worn when disposing of body fluids (urine, feces, emesis) of clients who have received chemotherapy in the previous 48 hours.
- A face shield should be used if there is a danger of splashing when administering chemotherapy or disposing of body fluids.
- Change gloves after chemotherapy administration and if they become contaminated or punctured.
- Cytotoxic drugs can be accidentally absorbed by inhalation, contact with the skin or mucous membranes, and ingestion. The following guidelines should be followed:
  - Prepare chemotherapy in a separate work area. Use a plastic-backed absorbent pad to contain spills during preparation.
  - Wash hands before and after administration of chemotherapy.
  - Avoid hand-to-mouth or hand-to-eye contact while working with chemotherapy.
- Refer to the agency's policies for priming IV tubing and disconnecting tubing after administration.
- Refer to the agency's policies for disposal of used equipment.
- Refer to the agency's policies for chemotherapy spills or exposure.

Table 36–4

General Adverse Reactions to Anticancer Drugs

Adverse Reactions	Nursing Measures and Considerations
Bone Marrow Suppression	
Low RBC count (anemia)	Assess for fatigue, shortness of breath, low blood pressure, increased heart rate, increased respiratory rate, oliguria, and mental status changes. Anemia may be treated with ferrous sulfate or infusions of RBCs. Assess for cyanosis. Plan rest periods for the client. Administer oxygen as prescribed. Elevate the head of the bed to facilitate breathing. Provide pain mediation if pain is increasing oxygen consumption. Provide assistance to bathroom. Monitor for mental status changes. Erythropoietin may be administered to stimulate production of RBCs.
Low WBC count (neutropenia)	Susceptibility to infections increases as WBCs decrease. Visitors with colds or infections should take precautions (i.e., wear mask) or avoid visiting the client. Fever, chills, upper respiratory infections, or sore throat should be reported to the HCP. Health care professionals and visitors should wash hands before and after contact with the client. Neutrophils are the primary WBCs that fight infections. The usual signs of infection (pain, swelling, redness, warmth, pus) may be absent or greatly reduced in neutropenic clients. Monitor for an increase (or decrease) in body temperature. An elevated temperature should be considered as a sign of infection. Temperatures of 38.3°C or above should be reported to the physician immediately. Appropriate cultures (e.g., blood, urine, sputum) will be collected and an antibiotic regimen will be initiated. Assess for localized infections. Auscultate breath sounds. Monitor WBC. Colony-stimulating factors (e.g., Filgrastim) may be administered to stimulate the production of WBCs.
Low platelet count (thrombocytopenia)	Petechiae, bruising, bleeding of gums, and nosebleeds are signs of a low platelet count and should be reported to the HCP. Assess for bleeding, petechiae, ecchymoses. Assess for occult bleeding in urine, feces, and emesis. Monitor platelet counts and bleeding time. Apply pressure to injection sites. Platelet transfusions may be needed. Avoid medications that may promote bleeding (e.g., aspirin). Avoid invasive procedures (e.g., injections, indwelling catheters, rectal temperature).
GI Disturbances	
Anorexia	Loss of appetite may be related to anemia, pain, fatigue, or a bitter taste in the mouth caused by some chemotherapy agents. Provide small frequent meals high in calories and protein. Plan for rest periods. Address issues of pain control. Provide hard candy or ice chips to help relieve bitter taste.
Nausea and vomiting	Antineoplasic drugs often stimulate the chemoreceptor trigger zone (CTZ) leading to nausea and vomiting. Nausea and vomiting may be caused by irritation of the GI tract; the effects of radiation to the chest, abdomen, or brain; anxiety; constipation; pain; electrolyte imbalances; or other medications. Provide antiemetics before, during, and after chemotherapy. Assess for GI upset and medicate appropriately. Minimize noise, stimulation, odors. Frequent mouth care is needed.
Diarrhea	Diarrhea may be one of three types: osmotic (absorption defects), secretory (bacterial infection, neoplasm), or exudative (secondary to chemotherapy). The chemotherapeutic agents that are commonly associated with diarrhea are the alkylating agents, antitumor antibiotics and antimetabolites. Treatment (medications, diet changes) will depend on the cause. Diarrhea may be caused by other medications (e.g., antibiotics); comorbid conditions (e.g., Crohn's disease) or enteral feedings (e.g., tube feeding). Assess normal bowel habits, monitor for electrolyte imbalances and dehydration. Administer appropriate antidiarrheal medications (e.g., antibiotics, anticholinergics, antispasmodics, psyllium, kaolin and pectin, octreotide acetate, etc.). Teach client to eat small frequent meals; follow a low residue diet; limit spicy, fatty foods; salty foods; intake of whole grains; fresh fruits and vegetables; caffeine; and carbonated drinks. Client should avoid very hot or very cold foods (may stimulate peristalsis). Monitor intake and output.
Mucositis (stomatitis)	Many antineoplastic agents can cause changes in the oral mucosa. These changes generally occur 2 to 14 days after initiation of therapy. Assess for taste changes, tissue swelling, redness, pain, dry mouth, white patches, or a white coating on the oral mucosa. Mucositis ranges from mild to severe. Symptomatic treatment is provided. This may include frequent mouth rinses, topical anesthetics, antibiotics, antifungal medication, saliva substitutes, and pain medication. Client should avoid commercial mouthwash that contains alcohol. A soft toothbrush is recommended. Offer ice chips or ice pops; these may help relieve pain. Assess intake and output. Evaluate caloric needs.

GI, Gastrointestinal; HCP, health care provider; RBC, red blood cell; WBC, white blood cell.

Continued

Table 36–4

General Adverse Reactions to Anticancer Drugs—cont'd

Adverse Reactions	Nursing Measures and Considerations
Alopecia	Not all chemotherapeutic agents cause hair loss. Hair thinning, patchy baldness, or complete alopecia may occur, depending on the drug. Hair on all areas of the body is affected. Hair loss may be gradual (progressing with each cycle of chemotherapy), or it may be rapid. Hair regrowth usually occurs once chemotherapy is completed, although the texture may be somewhat changed. Discuss potential hair loss with the client before therapy. Discuss ways to address loss of hair (wigs, scarves, hats, turbans). Assess for body image changes.
Fatigue	Fatigue may be caused by chemotherapy, sleep disturbances, emotional distress, depression, bone marrow depression, infection, pain, or electrolyte imbalances. Assess fatigue using a visual analogue scale (0 = no fatigue; 10 = worst fatigue). Address conditions that might be contributing to fatigue (e.g., lack of sleep, pain, depression). Plan ways to help client conserve energy. Plan a well-balanced diet. Clients should be encouraged to participate in regular (but not strenuous) exercise. Encourage stress reduction measures (e.g., relaxation, guided imagery).
Infertility	If infertility occurs, it may be permanent. Pretreatment counseling is advised.

Alkylating Drugs

One of the largest groups of anticancer drugs is the alkylating compounds. **Alkylating agents** cause cross-linking of DNA strands, abnormal base pairing, or DNA strand breaks, thus preventing the cell from dividing. Drugs in this group belong to the CCNS category and kill cells in various and multiple phases of the cell cycle. However, they are most effective against cells in the G_0 phase. They are effective against many types of cancer, including acute and chronic leukemias, lymphomas, multiple myeloma, and solid tumors (e.g., breast, ovary, uterus, lung, bladder, and stomach). Drugs in this category are classified into several groups: mustard gas derivatives (e.g., cyclophosphamide [Cytoxan]), ethylenimines (e.g., triethylenotheophosphoramide [Thiotepa]), alkylsulfonates (e.g., busulfan [Myleran]), hydrazines and triazines (e.g., dacarbazine [DTIC]), nitrosoureas (e.g., carmustine [BiCNU]), and metal salts (e.g., cisplatin [Platinol]). Nitrosoureas are unique because they can cross the blood-brain barrier, making them useful in the treatment of brain cancer. Adverse reactions to these drugs are the same as those listed in Table 36–4.

Cyclophosphamide

Mechlorethamine (nitrogen mustard, Mustargen), the first alkylating drug introduced for cancer treatment, became available for clinical use during World War II. Mechlorethamine is commonly administered as part of a chemotherapy regimen to treat Hodgkin's disease. This drug is a severe **vesicant** that can cause tissue necrosis if it infiltrates into the tissues. Cyclophosphamide (Cytoxan), an analogue of nitrogen mustard, may be prescribed orally or IV. The client should be well hydrated while taking this drug to prevent hemorrhagic cystitis (bleeding as a result of severe bladder inflammation). MESNA (2-mercaptoethane sulphonate sodium) is a **cytoprotectant (chemoprotectant)** drug that is often given with high-dose cyclophosphamide to inactivate urotoxic metabolites in the bladder and minimize damage to this organ. Bone marrow suppression and alopecia are common side effects. ***Do not confuse cyclophosphamide (Cytoxan) with Cytotec.*** Prototype Drug Chart 36–1 details the pharmacologic behavior of cyclophosphamide.

Pharmacokinetics

Cyclophosphamide is well absorbed from the GI tract. Its half-life is moderate, and it is moderately protein bound. The drug is metabolized by the liver, and less than 50% is excreted unchanged in the urine.

Pharmacodynamics

Cyclophosphamide was one of the early antineoplastic drugs and is still prevalent in chemotherapy protocols to treat breast cancer, leukemia, lymphoma, multiple myeloma, ovarian cancer, retinoblastoma neuroblastoma, and sarcoma. The onset of action begins in 2 to 3 hours; however, therapeutic effect may take several days. It is one of the anticancer drugs that can be administered orally.

Several drug interactions may occur with cyclophosphamide. The client should report all medications that he or she is taking, including over-the-counter (OTC) medicines and herbal supplements. Serious drug interactions can occur when taking cyclophosphamide and the gout medication allopurinol, phenobarbital, warfarin, thiazide diuretics, and some psychiatric medications. See Herbal Alert 36–1 for cyclophosphamide.

Table 36–5 lists the alkylating drugs, uses, and considerations.

Nursing Process

Alkylating Drugs: Cyclophosphamide

ASSESSMENT

- Assess complete blood count (CBC), differential, and platelet count weekly. Drug may be withheld if red blood cell, white blood cell, and platelet counts drop below pre-determined levels.
- Conduct thorough physical assessment and document findings.
- Assess results of pulmonary function tests, chest radiographs, renal and liver function studies during therapy.
- Assess temperature; fever may be early sign of infection.

NURSING DIAGNOSES

■ Risk for infection (secondary to bone marrow depression)
■ Risk for alteration in nutrition; less than body requirement (secondary to GI side effects chemotherapy)
■ Risk for altered urinary elimination (secondary to hemorrhagic cystitis related to chemotherapy)
■ Risk for abnormal bleeding (secondary to effects of chemotherapy on the lining of the bladder and/or bone marrow depression)
■ Knowledge deficit (patient/family: related to chemotherapeutic protocol)

PLANNING

■ Client will have blood counts in the desired range
■ Client will maintain nutritional status (adequate fluid intake and output, sufficient caloric intake, stable weight)
■ Client will maintain adequate urinary output
■ Client will remain free of symptoms of hemorrhagic cystitis
■ Client will demonstrate understanding of chemotherapeutic protocol (e.g., dose, administration, side effects, adverse reactions)

NURSING INTERVENTIONS

■ Monitor blood counts and laboratory values.
■ Handle drug with care during preparation; avoid direct skin contact with anticancer drugs. Follow protocols.
■ Monitor IV site frequently for irritation and phlebitis.
■ Administer antiemetic 30 to 60 minutes before giving drug.
■ Hydrate client with IV and/or oral fluids before chemotherapy starts.
■ Monitor blood, urea, nitrogen (BUN) and creatinine prior to administration.
■ Assess for signs and symptoms of hematuria, urinary frequency, or dysuria. Teach client to empty bladder every 2 to 3 hours.
■ Increase fluids to 2 to 3 L/day to reduce the risk of hemorrhagic cystitis, urate deposition, or calculus formation.
■ Monitor fluid intake and output and nutritional intake.
■ Maintain strict medical asepsis.

Client Teaching

General
• Emphasize protective precautions, as necessary.
• Teach client to take cyclophosphamide early in the day to prevent accumulation of the drug in the bladder during the night.
• Remind client to consult with a health care provider before administration of any vaccines.
• Advise client that cyclophosphamide is excreted in breast milk. Testicular atrophy and reversible oligospermia/azospermia in males.

• Teach importance of using birth control measures as appropriate. Discuss sperm-banking with male clients as appropriate.
• Teach client that pregnancy should be avoided for 3 to 4 months after completing antineoplastic therapy in most situations. Some sources recommend that both men and women avoid conception for 2 years after completion of treatment.
• Emphasize protective isolation precautions. Advise client not to visit anyone who has a respiratory infection. A decreased WBC count puts client at high risk for acquiring an infection.
• Instruct client to promptly report signs of infection (e.g., fever, sore throat), bleeding (e.g., bleeding gums, petechiae, bruises, hematuria, blood in the stool), and anemia (e.g., increased fatigue, dyspnea, orthostatic hypotension).

Side Effects
• Instruct client about good oral hygiene with a soft toothbrush for stomatitis; use a soft toothbrush when the platelet count is <50,000 cells/mm^3.
• Remind premenopausal females that they may experience amenorrhea, menstrual irregularities, or sterility; instruct male client that he may experience impotence.
• Advise client of possible hair loss; recommend a wig, hairpiece, scarf, or turban.
• Assess for use of alternative/complementary therapy that may interact with chemotherapy agent.

Diet
• Advise client to follow a diet low in purines (e.g., organ meats, beans, peas) to alkalize urine.
• Advise client to avoid citric acid.
• Offer client food and fluids that may decrease nausea, such as cola, crackers, or ginger ale.
• Plan small, frequent meals.

Cultural Considerations ⊕
• In some non-Western cultural groups, health care decisions are made by consensus and the family plays a key role in filtering information that is given to the clients. Issues related to informed consent and full disclosure of medical information may cause distress in cultural groups who place the needs of the family above the needs of the individual. Interactions should be modified based on family structure, religious values and beliefs, time orientation, cultural health practices, and verbal and nonverbal communication.
• Hyperpigmentation of the tongue and oral mucosa after administration has been reported in African Americans.

EVALUATION

■ Client is free of infection.
■ Client will maintain target weight.
■ Client will maintain nutritional status.
■ Client will not experience hemorrhagic cystitis.
■ Client and family education needs have been met.

PROTOTYPE DRUG CHART 36–1

CYCLOPHOSPHAMIDE

Drug Class

Alkylating drug
Trade Name: Cytoxan, Procytox, Endoxan, Neosar
Pregnancy Category: D

Dosage

A: PO: Initially: 1-5 mg/kg over 2-5 d; maint: 1-5 mg/kg/d
IV: Initially: 40-50 mg/kg in divided doses over 2-5 d;
  max: 100 mg/d; *maint:* 10-15 mg/kg every 7-10 d
C: PO/IV: Initially: 1-5 mg/kg in divided doses or
  50-150 mg/m²
If bone marrow depression occurs, dosage adjustment is
  necessary.

Contraindications

Hypersensitivity, severe bone marrow depression
Caution: Pregnancy, liver or kidney disease

Drug-Lab-Food Interactions

Drug: Decreases digoxin level. Increases drug action of
  barbiturates, chloramphenicol half-life, duration of
  leukopenia if given with thiazide diuretics, effects of
  anticoagulant drugs. Potentiates doxorubicin (Adriamycin) cardiomyopathy. Actions and toxicities of allopurinol, phenothiazines, potassium iodide, imipramine,
  warfarin, succinylcholine, and thiazide diuretics are altered if any of these is given with cyclophosphamide.
Herb: Use cautiously with garlic, ginkgo, echinacea, ginseng, St. John's wort, kava, grape seed. Toxicity and actions of both cyclophosphamide and vitamin A are altered if given together. Do not use with mistletoe.
Lab: Suppresses positive reaction to uric acid, purified
  protein derivative, mumps, Candida; Papanicolaou test
  (Pap smear) may cause a false-positive result.

Pharmacokinetics

Absorption: PO: Well absorbed
Distribution: PB: 50%
Metabolism: t½: 3-12 h
Excretion: 25%-40% in urine unchanged; 5%-20% in feces
Nadir: 7-14 d

Pharmacodynamics

Effects on blood count:
PO/IV: Onset: 7 d
  Peak: 10-14 d
  Duration: 21 d

Therapeutic Effects/Uses

Breast, lung, ovarian cancers; Hodgkin's disease; leukemias; and lymphomas; an immunosuppressant agent
Mode of Action: Inhibition of protein synthesis through interference with DNA replication by alkylation of DNA

Side Effects

Nausea, vomiting, diarrhea, weight loss, hematuria,
  alopecia, impotence, sterility, ovarian fibrosis,
  headache, dizziness, dermatitis

Adverse Reactions

Hemorrhagic cystitis, secondary neoplasm, bone marrow
  depression
Life-threatening: Leukopenia, thrombocytopenia,
  cardiotoxicity (very high doses), hepatotoxicity
  (long term)

A, Adult; *C,* child; *d,* day; *DNA,* deoxyribonucleic acid; *h,* hour; *IV,* intravenous; *maint,* maintenance; *max,* maximum; *PB,* protein-
binding; *PO,* by mouth; *t½,* half-life.
NOTE: Chemotherapy drug doses are based on body weight and prescribed either as milligrams per kilogram (mg/kg) or milligrams
per meter squared (mg/m²). Doses will also vary based on the drug protocol, type and stage of cancer, age, functional status, and comorbid conditions (e.g., heart disease).

HERBAL ALERT 36–1

Cyclophosphamide

🍃 Use cautiously with garlic, ginkgo, echinacea, ginseng,
St. John's wort, kava, and grape seed. Toxicity and actions
of both cyclophosphamide and vitamin A are altered if
given together. Do not use with mistletoe.

Antimetabolites

Antimetabolites resemble natural metabolites. Thus they
disrupt the metabolic processes, and some of the agents inhibit enzyme synthesis. They are classified as CCS and affect the S phase (DNA synthesis and metabolism) of the
cell cycle. Fluorouracil (5-FU) and floxuridine (FUDR) can
be classified as CCNS as well as CCS. This group is classi-

Table 36–5

Antineoplastics: Alkylating Drugs

Generic (Brand)	Uses and Considerations
Nitrogen Mustards	
chlorambucil (Leukeran)	Lymphocytic leukemia, lymphomas, and cancer of the breast and ovaries. Side effects include nausea, vomiting, anorexia, diarrhea, abdominal upset, and leukopenia. *Pregnancy category:* D; PB: 99%; $t^{1/2}$: 1.5 h
cyclophosphamide (Cytoxan)	See Prototype Drug Chart 36–1.
estramustine phosphate sodium (Emcyt)	Progressive carcinoma of prostate. Consists of estrogen and nitrogen mustard. Common side effects include nausea, peripheral edema, thrombophlebitis, and breast tenderness. *Pregnancy category:* X; PB: UK; $t^{1/2}$: 20 h
ifosfamide (Ifex)	Testicular cancer, lymphoma, lung cancer, and sarcomas. Mesna, a uroprotective agent, is added to prevent hemorrhagic cystitis. *Pregnancy category:* D; PB: UK; $t^{1/2}$: 7-15 h (high dose)
mechlorethamine HCl (Mustargen)	Hodgkin's disease, solid tumors, and pleural effusion caused by cancer of the lung. Similar side effects as chlorambucil. *Pregnancy category:* D; PB: UK; $t^{1/2}$: <1 min
melphalan (Alkeran)	Multiple myeloma, melanoma, and cancer of the breast, ovary, and testes. *Pregnancy category:* D; PB: <30%; $t^{1/2}$: 1.5 h
temozolomide (Temodar)	Refractory anaplastic astrocytoma. *Pregnancy category:* UK, PB: UK, $t^{1/2}$: UK
uracil mustard	Chronic lymphocytic and myelocytic leukemia; non-Hodgkin's; cervix, ovary, and lung cancers. GI distress may occur. *Pregnancy category:* X; PB: UK; $t^{1/2}$: UK
Nitrosoureas	
carmustine (BiCNU)	Hodgkin's disease, multiple myeloma, melanoma, and brain tumors. May be used for cancer of the breast and lung. Nausea, vomiting, and stomatitis may occur. *Pregnancy category:* D; PB: UK; $t^{1/2}$: 15-30 min
Carmustine with Polifeprosan 20 implant (Giliadel wafer)	Chemotherapeutic wafer implant used in addition to surgery for recurrent glioblastoma multiform to improve survival. Approved by FDA in February 2003.
lomustine (CeeNu)	Advanced Hodgkin's disease and brain tumors. *Pregnancy category:* D; PB: 50%; $t^{1/2}$: 1-2 d
streptozocin (Zanosar)	Pancreatic islet cell tumor and cancer of the lung. May also be used for Hodgkin's disease and colorectal cancer. Nausea, vomiting, diarrhea, and leukopenia may occur. *Pregnancy category:* C; PB: UK; $t^{1/2}$: 30-45 min
Alkyl Sulfonates	
busulfan (Myleran)	Myelocytic leukemia. WBC should be closely monitored. May be used as preparation agent in bone marrow transplant. *Pregnancy category:* D; PB: UK; $t^{1/2}$: UK
Alkylating-Like Drugs	
altretamine (Hexalen)	Ovarian cancer. Also used for breast, cervix, colon, endometrium, head/neck, and lung cancers; lymphomas. Nausea and vomiting and peripheral neuropathy may occur. *Pregnancy category:* D; PB: 6%; $t^{1/2}$: 13 h
carboplatin (Paraplatin)	Recurrent ovarian cancer. May be used as preparation agent in bone marrow transplant. *Pregnancy category:* D; PB: 0%; $t^{1/2}$: 2-6 h
cisplatin (Platinol, CDDP)	Ovarian and testicular cancer. Used as adjunctive treatment. Has been used for cancer of the bladder, head and neck, and endometrium. Nausea, vomiting, peripheral neuropathy, stomatitis, tinnitus, and blurred vision may occur. Ototoxicity occurs in 30% of clients. *Pregnancy category:* D; PB: >90%; $t^{1/2}$: 58-75 h
oxaliplatin (Eloxatine)	Metastatic colorectal cancer. Used with 5-FU and leucovorin. Ovarian cancer, head and neck cancer, and malignant melanoma. *Pregnancy category:* D; $t^{1/2}$: 20-40 d; >90%.
dacarbazine (DTIC)	Metastatic malignant melanoma, sarcomas, neuroblastoma, and refractory Hodgkin's disease. May be given as an IV bolus (push) injection or by infusion. Common side effects are anorexia, nausea, and vomiting. *Pregnancy category:* C; PB: 5%-10%; $t^{1/2}$: 5 h
pipobroman (Vercyte)	Polycythemia and chronic myelocytic leukemia. *Pregnancy category:* D; PB: UK; $t^{1/2}$: UK
triethylenethiophosphoramide (Thiotepa)	Palliative therapy, especially breast and ovarian cancer. *Pregnancy category:* D; PB: UK; $t^{1/2}$: 1.5-2 h

NOTE: Chemotherapeutic doses and schedules will vary depending on the protocol, body surface area (m^2), age, functional status, and comorbid conditions. For a full discussion of body surface area in dosage calculation, see Chapter 4B, Methods for Calculation.

5-FU, Fluorouracil; *d*, day; *FDA*, Food and Drug Administration; *GI*, gastrointestinal; *h*, hour; *IV*, intravenous; *min*, minute; *PB*, protein-binding; $t^{1/2}$, half-life; *UK*, unknown; *WBC*, white blood cell; >, greater than; <, less than.

fied according to the substances with which they interfere and include folic acid (folate) antagonists (e.g., methotrexate [MTX]), pyrimidine antagonists (e.g., 5-FU), purine antagonists (e.g., 6-mercaptopurine [Purinethol]), and adenosine deaminase inhibitors (e.g., fludarabine [Fludara]). Antimetabolites are used to treat acute leukemia, breast cancer, head and neck cancer, lung cancer, osteosarcoma, and non-Hodgkin's lymphoma.

Methotrexate (MTX), a folic acid antagonist, was discovered in 1948 and is used for the treatment of both cancerous and noncancerous (e.g. rheumatoid arthritis) conditions. MTX acts as a substitute for folic acid, which is needed for the synthesis of proteins and DNA. Cancer clients receiving high doses of MTX must be given leucovorin calcium to "rescue" **(leucovorin rescue)** normal cells from the adverse effects of the drug.

Pharmacokinetics

MTX is metabolized in the liver and excreted in the urine. Eighty to ninety percent is excreted unchanged in the urine within 24 hours.

Pharmacodynamics

MTX is absorbed from the GI tract and peaks in 1 hour, with peak concentration in 3 to 12 hours. It is one of the anticancer drugs that can be administered orally, IV, or by injection.

Numerous drug interactions may occur with MTX. Protein-bound drugs (e.g., aspirin, phenytoin) increase the toxicity of MTX. Nonsteroidal anti-inflammatory drugs (NSAIDs) increase and prolong MTX levels. Cotrimoxazole and pyrimethamine increase MTX levels. Clients who are taking penicillins, cyclo-oxygenase 2 (COX-2) inhibitors, and OTC herbs should share this information with their physician because these products interact with MTX as well.

HERBAL ALERT 36–2

5-Fluorouracil

🍃 Use cautiously with ginseng and St. John's Wort. Do not use with mistletoe.

Table 36–6

Antineoplastics: Antimetabolites

Generic (Brand)	Uses and Considerations
Folic Acid Antagonist	
methotrexate (Amethopterin, MTX)	Solid tumors, sarcomas, choriocarcinoma, leukemia. At higher doses, clients should be well hydrated; keep urine pH 7.0 for drug solubility for excretion. Higher doses require use of leucovorin as a rescue for normal cells. *Pregnancy category:* D; PB: 50%; $t^{1/2}$: 8-16 h
Pyrimidine Analogues	
capecitabine (Xeloda)	Metastatic breast cancer and metastatic colorectal cancer. Capecitabine is converted by the body to 5-FU. Effective when cancer is resistant to paclitaxel. Reduces tumor size. Food decreases absorption rate. *Pregnancy category:* UK; PB: UK; $t^{1/2}$: 45 min
cytarabine HCl (Cytosar-U, ARA-C)	Acute leukemias and lymphomas. Also used as an immunosuppressive drug after organ transplant. May be used in combination with other anticancer drugs. Nausea, vomiting, leukopenia, and thrombocytopenia are common side effects. *Pregnancy category:* D; PB: 15% $t^{1/2}$: 1-3 h
floxuridine (FUDR)	Metastatic colon cancer and hepatomas. *Pregnancy category:* D; PB: UK; $t^{1/2}$: 20 h
5-Fluorouracil (Adrucil, 5-FU)	See Prototype Drug Chart 36–2.
gemcitabine HCl (Gemzar)	Advanced or metastatic adenocarcinoma of the pancreas, non–small-cell lung cancer and bladder cancer. Acts at the S phase of cell cycle. Monitor leukocytes and platelet count; reduce dose if these values are extremely low. *Pregnancy category:* D; PB: UK; $t^{1/2}$: 1-1.5 h
procarbazine HCl (Matulane)	Palliative treatment of advanced Hodgkin's disease and for solid tumors. May be used with other anticancer drugs. *Pregnancy category:* D; PB: UK; $t^{1/2}$: 10 min
Purine Analogues	
cladribine (Leustatin)	For treatment of hairy cell leukemia and chronic lymphocytic leukemia. Adverse reactions: bone marrow suppression, fever, nausea, vomiting, diaphoresis. *Pregnancy category:* D; PB: 20%; $t^{1/2}$: 5.4 h
fludarabine (Fludara)	Chronic lymphocytic leukemia in clients who have not responded to other alkylating drugs; low-grade non-Hodgkin's lymphoma. Anorexia, nausea, diarrhea, fever, and peripheral edema may occur. *Pregnancy category:* D; PB: UK; $t^{1/2}$: 9 h
6-Mercaptopurine (Purinethol)	First used in 1952 for treating acute lymphatic leukemia. Also used as an immunosuppressive drug. Adverse reactions may include hepatoxicity, bone marrow depression, hyperuricemia. *Pregnancy category:* D; PB: 19%; $t^{1/2}$: 45 min
thioguanine (Lanvis)	Acute and chronic myelogenous leukemia. Long duration of action. *Pregnancy category:* D; PB: UK; $t^{1/2}$: 2-11 h
Ribonucleotide Reductase Inhibitor	
hydroxyurea (Hydrea)	Melanoma, resistant chronic myelocytic leukemia, and ovarian cancer. Has a long duration of action. *Pregnancy category:* D; PB: UK; $t^{1/2}$: 3-4 h
trimetrexate glucuronate (Neutrexin)	Alternative drug therapy for *Pneumocystis carinii* pneumonia; treatment for clients with AIDS. May be used for colorectal cancer. CBC should be monitored. *Pregnancy category:* D; PB: 86%-94%; $t^{1/2}$: 11-13 h
Enzyme Inhibitor	
pentostatin (Nipent)	Hairy cell leukemia refractory to alpha-interferon. Has a very long duration of action. *Pregnancy category:* D; PB: UK; $t^{1/2}$: 6 h

NOTE: Chemotherapeutic doses and schedules will vary depending on the protocol, body surface area (m^2), age, functional status, and co-morbid conditions. For a full discussion of body surface area in dosage calculation, see Chapter 4B, Methods for Calculation.
5-FU, Fluorouracil; *AIDS,* acquired immunodeficiency syndrome; *CBC,* complete blood cell count; *h,* hour; *min,* minute; *PB,* protein-binding; $t^{1/2}$, half-life; *UK,* unknown.

PREVENTING MEDICATION ERRORS

Do not confuse...

- **fluorouracil (Efudex)** and **Efidac.**

Fluorouracil

Pharmacokinetics

Fluorouracil (5-FU) is administered IV for solid tumors and topically for superficial basal cell carcinoma. Less than 10% is bound to protein, and the half-life for the IV route is 10 to 20 minutes. A small amount of the drug is excreted in the urine, and up to 80% is excreted by the lungs as carbon dioxide.

Pharmacodynamics

Fluorouracil, a CCS drug, blocks the enzyme action necessary for DNA and ribonucleic acid (RNA) synthesis. The drug has a low therapeutic index and is used alone or in combination with other anticancer drugs. Fluorouracil can cross the blood-brain barrier. Its duration of action is 30 days.

Side Effects and Adverse Reactions

The side effects of 5-FU are similar to other anticancer drugs. These include anorexia, nausea, vomiting, diarrhea, stomatitis, alopecia, photosensitivity, increased pigmentation, rash, and erythema. Stomatitis is an early sign of toxicity and should be reported to the physician. Bone marrow depression may occur 4 to 8 days after the beginning of drug therapy. See Herbal Alert 36–2 for fluorouracil.

The general side effects for antimetabolite drugs include bone marrow suppression (leukopenia, thrombocytopenia), stomatitis (inflammation of the oral mucosa), and alopecia. Table 36–6 lists the antimetabolite drugs, uses, and considerations.

Prototype Drug Chart 36–2 on p. 543 presents the pharmacologic data for 5-FU.

Nursing Process

Antimetabolites: Fluorouracil (5-FU)

ASSESSMENT

- Assess complete blood count (CBC), differential, and platelet count weekly. Chemotherapy may be held if red cell, white cell, and platelet counts drop below predetermined levels.
- Conduct thorough physical assessment and document findings.
- Assess renal function studies before and during drug therapy.
- Assess temperature; fever may be an early sign of infection.

NURSING DIAGNOSES

- Risk for infection (secondary to bone marrow depression)

- Risk for altered nutrition; less than body requirements (secondary to GI side effects of chemotherapy)
- Risk for pain (mucositis/stomatitis) (secondary to GI side effects of chemotherapy)
- Risk for impaired perianal skin integrity (secondary to diarrhea caused by chemotherapy)
- Knowledge deficit (client/family: related to chemotherapeutic protocol)

PLANNING

- Client will have blood counts in the desired range.
- Client will maintain nutritional status (adequate fluid intake and output, adequate caloric intake, stable weight).
- Client will experience adequate pain control.
- Client will limit exposure to sunlight.
- Client will demonstrate understanding of chemotherapeutic protocol (dose, administration, side effects and adverse reactions).

NURSING INTERVENTIONS

- Monitor blood counts and laboratory values.
- Handle drug with care during preparation; avoid direct skin contact with anticancer drugs. Follow protocols.
- Monitor IV site frequently. Extravasation produces severe pain. If this occurs, apply ice pack and notify health care provider.
- Administer antiemetic 30 to 60 minutes before drug to prevent vomiting.
- Assess for hyperpigmentation along the vein in which 5-FU was administered.
- Offer client food and fluids that may decrease nausea, such as cola, crackers, or ginger ale.
- Plan small, frequent meals.
- Maintain strict medical asepsis.
- Support good oral hygiene; brush teeth with soft toothbrush and use waxed dental floss.
- Encourage mouth rinses every two hours with normal saline.
- Monitor fluid intake and output and nutritional intake. GI effects are common on the fourth day of treatment.

Client Teaching

General

- Emphasize protective precautions as necessary.
- Teach client to examine mouth daily and report signs of stomatitis (soreness, ulcerations, white patches in mouth). Oral hygiene several times a day is essential. If stomatitis occurs, rinse mouth with baking soda or normal saline. Use a soft toothbrush.
- Instruct client to take pain medication as prescribed to relieve mouth pain related to mucositis/stomatitis.
- Advise client to take year-round photosensitivity precautions. Use sunscreen when outdoors.
- Advise client not to visit anyone who has a respiratory infection. A decreased white blood cell (WBC) count puts client at risk for acquiring an infection.

- Teach importance of using birth control measures as appropriate. Discuss sperm-banking with male clients as appropriate.
- Teach client that pregnancy should be avoided for 3 to 4 months after completing antineoplastic therapy in most situations. Some sources recommend that both men and women avoid conception for 2 years after completion of treatment.
- Emphasize protective isolation precautions. Advise client not to visit anyone who has a respiratory infection. A decreased WBC count puts client at high risk for acquiring an infection.
- Instruct client to promptly report signs of infection (e.g., fever, sore throat), bleeding (e.g., bleeding gums, petechiae, bruises, hematuria, blood in the stool), and anemia (e.g., increased fatigue, dyspnea, orthostatic hypotension).

Side Effects
- Instruct client about good oral hygiene with a soft toothbrush for mucositis/stomatitis; use a soft toothbrush when the platelet count is <50,000 cells/mm^3. Rinse mouth every two hours with normal saline. Avoid the use of commercial mouthwashes that contain alcohol.
- Remind premenopausal females that they may experience amenorrhea, menstrual irregularities, or sterility; Instruct male client that he may experience impotence.
- Advise client of possible hair loss; recommend a wig, hairpiece, scarf, or turban.
- Assess for use of alternative/complementary therapy that may interact with chemotherapy agent.

Diet
- Encourage small frequent meals.
- Encourage the use of cool bland foods.
- Offer ice chips or ice pops to help relieve mouth pain.

Cultural Considerations ⊕
- In some non-Western cultural groups, health care decisions are made by consensus and the family plays a key role in filtering information that is given to the clients. Issues related to informed consent and full disclosure of medical information may cause distress in cultural groups who place the needs of the family above the needs of the individual. Interactions should be modified based on family structure, religious values and beliefs, time orientation, cultural health practices, and verbal and nonverbal communication.
- An increased incidence of hyperpigmentation has been reported in dark-skinned people. Hyperpigmentation may be seen on the skin, nails, hair, and oral mucosa. This usually disappears over time.

EVALUATION

- Client is free of infection.
- Oral mucosa is free of pain, erythema, and swelling.

- Pain is controlled.
- Skin integrity is intact.
- Client and family education needs have been met.

Antitumor Antibiotics

Antitumor antibiotics (bleomycin [Blenoxane], dactinomycin [Actinomycin D], daunorubicin [Cerubidine], doxorubicin [Adriamycin], mitomycin [Mutamycin], and plicamycin [Mithracin]) inhibit protein and RNA synthesis and bind DNA, causing fragmentation. There are several types of antitumor antibiotics, including the anthracyclines (e.g., doxorubicin, daunorubicin), chromomycins (e.g., dactinomycin, plicamycin), and miscellaneous drugs (e.g., mitomycin, bleomycin). Except for bleomycin, which has its major effect on the G_2 phase, they are classified as CCNS drugs. Dactinomycin was the first antibiotic used in the treatment of tumors in animals in the early 1940s. Bleomycin and plicamycin were introduced in 1962. These antitumor antibiotics differ from one another and are used for various cancers.

Prototype Drug Chart 36–3 presents the pharmacologic data for doxorubicin.

Doxorubicin and Plicamycin
Pharmacokinetics
Doxorubicin and plicamycin are administered IV. Doxorubicin is metabolized in the liver to active and inactive metabolites. The various metabolites affect the half-life; the initial phase of doxorubicin is 12 minutes, the intermediate phase is 3.5 hours, and the final phase is 30 hours.

Pharmacodynamics
The primary effects of doxorubicin and plicamycin differ, although they are classified as antitumor antibiotics. Doxorubicin is prescribed in combination with other anticancer agents for the treatment of cancer of the breast, ovaries, lung, and bladder and leukemias and lymphomas. Doxorubicin can cause cardiac toxicity and recipients of this drug are limited to a maximum lifetime dose of 550 mg/m^2 (See Herbal Alert 36–3 for doxorubicin). Dexrazoxane (Zinecard) is a cytoprotective (chemoprotective) agent that may be given to help prevent cardiac toxicities associated with doxorubicin administration. Plicamycin may be used in combination with other anticancer agents for the treatment of testicular carcinoma. Its primary use is for correction of hypercalcemia.

Because plicamycin affects bleeding time, use of aspirin, anticoagulants, and thrombolytic agents should be avoided. The use of cyclophosphamide with doxorubicin can increase the likelihood of hemorrhagic cystitis.

Side Effects and Adverse Reactions
The adverse reactions to the antitumor antibiotics are similar to other antineoplastics and include alopecia, nausea, vomiting, stomatitis, leukopenia, and thrombocytopenia. The anti-

HERBAL ALERT 36–3

Doxorubicin
🍃 Green tea may enhance antitumor effects, so report use to the health care provider. Use cautiously with grape seed, garlic, and St. John's Wort.

PROTOTYPE DRUG CHART 36–2

5-FLUOROURACIL

Drug Class

Antimetabolite
Trade Name: Adrucil, 5-FU, Efudex (topical)
Pregnancy Category: D

Dosage

A: IV: 12 mg/kg/d × 4 d; *max:* 800 mg/d; repeat with
  6 mg/kg on days 6, 8, 10, and 12 or as indicated
Maintenance dose: 10-15 mg/kg/wk as single dose; *max:*
  1 g/wk
Topical: 1%-2% sol/cream b.i.d. to head/neck lesions; 5%
  to other body areas
Refer to specific protocol.

Contraindications

Hypersensitivity, pregnancy, severe infection, myelosuppression, marginal nutritional status. Reduce dose
  in clients with impaired hepatic, renal function
  or malnutrition.

Drug-Lab-Herb Interactions

Drug: Bone marrow depressants *increase* chances of toxicity. Avoid live virus vaccines, which may potentiate virus
  replication. *Increased* 5-FU toxicity with concomitant use
  of leucovorin calcium. Metronidazole may *increase* 5-FU
  toxicity (clearance of 5-FU decreased). *Increased* pharmacologic effects of 5-FU when given with cimetidine
  (Tagamet). Thiazide diuretics *increase* myelosuppression.
Lab: May *decrease* albumin; may *increase* excretion
  of 5-HIAA in urine
Herb: Use cautiously with ginseng, St. John's wort. Do
  not use with mistletoe.

Pharmacokinetics

Absorption: IV and topical: 5%-10%
Distribution: PB: UK
Metabolism: t½: 10-20 min
Excretion: In urine and expired carbon dioxide
Nadir: 10-14 d

Pharmacodynamics

Effects on blood count:
IV: Onset: 1-9 d
  Peak: 9-21 d
  Duration: 30 d
Topical: Onset: 2-3 d
  Peak: 2-6 wk
  Duration: 4-8 wk

Therapeutic Effects/Uses

Cancer of breast, cervix, colon, liver, ovary, pancreas, stomach, and rectum. Given in combination with levamisole after
  surgical resection in clients with Duke's stage C colon cancer
Mode of Action: Prevention of thymidine synthetase production, thereby inhibiting DNA and RNA synthesis; not phase
  specific

Side Effects

Stomatitis, nausea, vomiting, diarrhea, alopecia, rash,
  photosensitivity. Diarrhea may be severe.

Adverse Reactions

Bone marrow depression
Life-threatening: Thrombocytopenia, myelosuppression,
  hemorrhage, renal failure

5-FU, Fluorouracil; *5-HIAA,* 5-hydroxyindoleacetic acid; *A,* adult; *b.i.d.,* two times a day; *d,* day; *DNA,* deoxyribonucleic acid; *IV,* intravenous; *max,* maximum; *min,* minute; *PB,* protein-binding; *RNA,* ribonucleic acid; *sol,* solution; *t½,* half-life; *UK,* unknown; *wk,* week.

PROTOTYPE DRUG CHART 36–3

DOXORUBICIN

Drug Class

Antitumor antibiotic
Trade Name: Adriamycin
Pregnancy Category: D

Dosage

60-75 mg/m² as a single dose every 21 days or 30 mg/m²
IV for 3 days every 4 wk. When used in combination
therapy: 40-50 mg/m² as a single IV injection every 21
to 28 days. Safety and efficacy have not been established for children.
Reduce dose with renal impairment.

Contraindications

Pregnancy, severe cardiac disease. Cardiac status and
cardiac ejection fraction should be tested before
starting doxorubicin therapy. Do not exceed a lifetime
cumulative dose of 550 mg/m² (450 mg/m² if the
client has had prior chest irradiation or is receiving
cyclophosphamide). Dexrazoxane (Zinecard) is used
to help prevent or lessen cardiac damage.
Caution: Hepatic and renal impairment

Drug-Lab-Herb Interactions

Drug: Calcium channel blockers, paclitaxol (Taxol), and
mitomycin *increase* the risk of the cardiac toxicity if
given with doxorubicin. Doxorubicin may *decrease*
digoxin levels. Doxorubicin *decreases* levels of phenytoin. Cyclophosphamide *increases* the risk of cardiac
toxicity and hemorrhage. *Increased* risk of hepatotoxicity when given with mercaptopurine. *Increased*
plasma clearance of doxorubicin when given with barbiturates. Precipitate will form when doxorubicin is
combined with heparin or 5-FU. *Decreased* metabolic
clearance of 5-FU and *increased* cytotoxicity when
given with Alfa interferon. Prolonged hemotoxic effects may occur if doxorubicin and cyclosporine are
given together.
Lab: ECG changes. *Increases* uric acid.
Herb: Green tea may enhance antitumor effects. Report
use to health care provider. Use cautiously with grape
seed, garlic, St. John's wort.

Pharmacokinetics

Absorption: IV
Distribution: PB: 80%-90%
Metabolism: t½: 3-30 h
Excretion: 50% in bile and 5% in urine
Nadir: 10-14 d (doxorubicin)

Pharmacodynamics

IV: Onset: 7-10 d
   Peak: 14 d
   Duration: 21 d

Therapeutic Effects/Uses

Breast, bladder, ovarian, and lung cancers; leukemias; lymphomas, soft tissue and bone sarcoma
Mode of Action: Inhibits DNA and RNA synthesis; has immunosuppressant activity

Side Effects

Stomatitis, anorexia, nausea, vomiting, diarrhea, rash,
alopecia. Doxorubicin is a potent vesicant. May cause
a flare reaction. Nausea and vomiting are dose related
and may begin 1-3 h after administration. Causes
discolored urine (pink to red) for up to 48 h. May
cause "radiation recall" to previously irradiated skin.

Adverse Reactions

Esophagitis; anemia; hyperpigmentation of nails, tongue,
and oral mucosa, especially in African Americans. Drug
is teratogenic, mutagenic, and carcinogenic.
Life-threatening: Thrombocytopenia, leukopenia, cardiotoxicity, congestive heart failure, electrocardiogram
changes, severe myelosuppression, anaphylaxis

5-FU, Fluorouracil; *d,* day; *DNA,* deoxyribonucleic acid; *ECG,* electrocardiogram; *h,* hour; *IV,* intravenous; *PB,* protein-binding; *RNA,* ribonucleic acid; *t½,* half-life; *wk,* week.

PREVENTING MEDICATION ERRORS

Do not confuse...

• doxorubicin (Adriamicin) with Idamycin or
  Idarubicin.

tumor antibiotics are capable of causing **vesication** (blistering of tissue). Exceptions to this are bleomycin and plicamycin. Some antitumor antibiotics can cause organ toxicities. Bleomycin causes pulmonary toxicity, and daunorubicin,
doxorubicin, and idarubicin cause cardiac toxicity.

Table 36–7 lists the antitumor antibiotics, uses, and
considerations.

Table 36-7

Antineoplastics: Antitumor Antibiotics

Generic (Brand)	Uses and Considerations
Antitumor Antibiotics	
bleomycin SO₄ (Blenoxane)	Squamous cell carcinomas, testicular tumor (when used with vinblastine and cisplatin), and lymphomas. Low incidence of bone marrow suppression. Lifetime dose is 400 units/m². A serious adverse reaction is anaphylaxis. Has a long duration of action. *Pregnancy category:* D; PB: 1%; t½: 2 h
dactinomycin (Actinomycin D, Cosmegen)	Testicular tumors, Wilms' tumor, choriocarcinoma, and rhabdomyosarcoma. Nausea and vomiting may occur during the first 24 h. Has a long duration of action. *Pregnancy category:* C; PB: 80%-90%; t½: 36 h
daunorubicin HCl (Cerubidine)	Leukemia, Ewing's sarcoma, Wilms' tumor, neuroblastoma, and non-Hodgkin's lymphoma. Has a long duration of action. *Pregnancy category:* D; PB: 80%; t½: 19 h
doxorubicin (Adriamycin)	See Prototype Drug Chart 36-3.
epirubicin (Ellence)	Cancers of breast; lung; lymph system; stomach; and ovaries. Metastatic node-positive breast cancer; adjuvant with anticancer therapy. May be used in combination therapy with cyclophosphamide and fluorouracil (CEF) for breast cancer; improved survival rate over cyclophosphamide, methotrexate, and fluorouracil (CMF). Adverse effects include bone marrow depression, cardiotoxicity (less than doxorubicin), and extravasation necrosis. Less cardiotoxic than doxorubicin with similar efficacy. *Pregnancy category:* D to X; PB: UK; t½: 33 h
idarubicin (Idamycin)	Acute monocytic leukemia and solid tumors. More potent than daunorubicin or doxorubicin. Vesicant, monitor CBC. Urine may be red. *Pregnancy category:* D; PB: 97%; t½: 22 h
mitomycin (Mutamycin)	Disseminated adenocarcinoma of breast, stomach, and pancreas. Also used for cancer of the head, neck, cervix, and lung. Monitor temperature and CBC. *Pregnancy category:* D; PB: UK; t½: 12 min
mitoxantrone (Novantrone)	Acute nonlymphocytic leukemia; may be used for breast cancer. Rash, dyspnea, hypotension, facial swelling, blue urine, sclera, skin hue change may occur. Severe hepatic dysfunction with decreased total body clearance. *Pregnancy category:* D; PB: 95%; t½: 1.5-13 d
plicamycin (Mithracin)	Testicular cancer. May be used to treat hypercalcemia. *Pregnancy category:* X; PB: UK; t½: 2-8 h
valrubicin (Valstar)	Bladder cancer. May cause urinary frequency and urgency, dysuria, hematuria, and bladder pain. *Pregnancy category:* UK; PB: UK; t½: UK

NOTE: Chemotherapeutic doses and schedules will vary depending on the protocol, body surface area (*m²*), age, functional status, and co-morbid conditions. For a full discussion of body surface area in dosage calculation, see Chapter 4B, Methods for Calculation.
CBC, Complete blood cell count; *d,* day; *h,* hour; *min,* minute; *PB,* protein-binding; *t½,* half-life; *UK,* unknown.

Nursing Process

Antitumor Antibiotics: Doxorubicin (Adriamycin)

ASSESSMENT

■ Assess complete blood count (CBC), differential, and platelet count weekly. Drug may be withheld if red blood cell, white blood cell (WBC), and platelet counts drop below predetermined levels.
■ Conduct thorough physical assessment and document findings.
■ Assess temperature; fever may be early sign of infection.
■ Assess plans for pregnancy (if appropriate).

NURSING DIAGNOSES

■ Risk for infection (secondary to bone marrow depression)
■ Risk for alternation in cardiac output (secondary to cardiotoxic effects of chemotherapy)
■ Risk for altered skin integrity (secondary to vesicant properties of chemotherapy)
■ Knowledge deficit related to antineoplastic therapy

PLANNING

■ Client will have blood cell values in the desired range.
■ Client will be free of cardiac dysfunction
■ Client's skin integrity will remain intact
■ Client will demonstrate understanding of the chemotherapy regimen, including side effects.
■ Assess client/family knowledge related to chemotherapeutic protocol.

NURSING INTERVENTIONS

■ Monitor blood counts and laboratory values.
■ Handle drug with care during preparation; avoid direct skin contact with drug.
■ Monitor IV site frequently. Doxorubicin is a severe vesicant whose effects are not immediately apparent. Give drug through a large bore, quickly running IV.

Tissue necrosis may occur 3 to 4 weeks after infiltration into tissue. Extravasation produces severe pain. If this occurs, apply ice pack and notify health care provider.
■ Administer antiemetic 30 to 60 minutes before chemotherapy.
■ Monitor for changes in urine color (pink to red). Drug is red and is excreted in the urine.
■ Offer client food and fluids that may decrease nausea, such as cola, crackers, or ginger ale.
■ Plan small frequent meals.
■ Administer prophylactic antibiotics to prevent infection.
■ Offer analgesics for pain as prescribed.
■ Maintain strict medical asepsis.
■ Support good oral hygiene. Use soft toothbrush. Use waxed dental floss.
■ Monitor fluid intake and output and nutritional intake.

Client Teaching
General
• Emphasize protective precautions (e.g., hand washing, personal hygiene), as necessary.
• Teach client the signs and symptoms of cardiac dysfunction (shortness of breath, palpitations, edema in extremities) and to report these to his health care provider.
• Teach client that complete alopecia occurs with doses >50 mg/m². Teach that hair will begin to regrow within several months after therapy is completed.
• Teach client about "radiation recall" on previously irradiated skin.
• Advise client not to visit anyone who has a respiratory infection. A decreased WBC count puts client at risk for acquiring an infection.
• Teach importance of using birth control measures as appropriate. Discuss sperm-banking with male clients as appropriate.
• Teach client that pregnancy should be avoided for 3 to 4 months after completing antineoplastic therapy in most situations. Some sources recommend that both men and women avoid conception for 2 years after completion of treatment.
• Emphasize protective isolation precautions. Advise client not to visit anyone who has a respiratory infection. A decreased WBC count puts client at high risk for acquiring an infection.
• Instruct client to promptly report signs of infection (e.g., fever, sore throat), bleeding (e.g., bleeding gums, petechiae, bruises, hematuria, blood in the stool), and anemia (e.g., increased fatigue, dyspnea, orthostatic hypotension).

Side Effects
• Assess for nausea, vomiting, and administer antiemetics as prescribed.
• Teach importance of birth control measures. Discuss sperm banking if appropriate.

• Remind premenopausal females that they may experience amenorrhea, menstrual irregularities, or sterility; instruct male client that he may experience impotence.
• Advise client of possible hair loss; recommend a wig, hairpiece, scarf, or turban.
• Assess for use of alternative/complementary therapy that may interact with chemotherapy agent.

Diet
• Encourage small frequent meals.
• Encourage eating bland foods.

Cultural Considerations
• In some non-Western cultural groups, health care decisions are made by consensus and the family plays a key role in filtering information that is given to clients. Issues related to informed consent and full disclosure of medical information may cause distress in cultural groups that place the needs of the family above the needs of the individual. Interactions should be modified based on family structure, religious values and beliefs, time orientation, cultural health practices, and verbal and nonverbal communication.
• Hyperpigmentation of the tongue and oral mucosa has been seen after the administration of doxorubicin in African Americans.

EVALUATION
■ Client is free of infection.
■ Cardiac function is maintained.
■ Client and family education needs have been met.
■ Side effects of therapy are controlled.
■ Client and family education needs have been met.

Mitotic Inhibitors

Mitotic inhibitors are plant alkaloids and other compounds that are derived from natural products that block cell division at the M phase of the cell cycle. Thus they are CCS. The vinca alkaloids (e.g., vinblastine [Velban], vincristine [Oncovin], and vinorelbine [Navelbine]) are obtained from the periwinkle plant. The antimicrotubules or taxanes group (e.g., docetaxel [Taxotere] and paclitaxel [Taxol]) are procured from the needles and bark of the yew tree.

Adverse reactions to **vinca alkaloids** include leukopenia, partial to complete alopecia, stomatitis, nausea, and vomiting. Vincristine and vinblastine may cause reversible or irreversible neurotoxicity. Signs and symptoms of neurotoxicity might include a decrease in muscular strength (numbness, tingling of fingers and toes), constipation, ptosis (drooping of the upper eyelid), hoarseness, and motor instability. Common adverse effects of the taxanes are alopecia, diarrhea, nausea, vomiting, peripheral neuropathy, stomatitis, and fever. Docetaxel may cause fluid retention. Table 36–8 lists the mitotic inhibitors and taxanes, uses and considerations.

Table 36-8

Antineoplastics: Mitotic Inhibitors

Generic (Brand)	Uses and Considerations
Mitotic Inhibitors	
vinblastine SO$_4$ (Velban)	Cancer of the testes, breast, and kidney and for treatment of lymphomas, lymphosarcomas, and neuroblastomas. Nausea, vomiting, and alopecia are common side effects. Check CBC before dosing. *Pregnancy category:* D; PB: 75%; t$^{1}/_{2}$: 25 h
vincristine SO$_4$ (Oncovin)	Cancer of the breast, lungs, and cervix; multiple myelomas, sarcomas, lymphomas, Wilms' tumor. Neurologic difficulties should be assessed. Used for treating Hodgkin's disease in combination therapy, MOPP (mechlorethamine, vincristine, procarbazine, and prednisone). *Never* should be given intrathecally. *Pregnancy category:* D; PB: 75%; t$^{1}/_{2}$: triphasic 2-85 h
vinorelbine (Navelbine)	First-line treatment for ambulatory clients with advanced, unresectable non-small cell lung cancer (NSCLC). May be used alone or in combination with cisplatin for stage IV NSCLC and in combination with cisplatin for stage III NSCLC. *Pregnancy category:* D; PB: UK; t$^{1}/_{2}$: UK
Antimicrotubule/Taxanes	
docetaxel (Taxotere)	Advanced or metastatic breast cancer. Inhibits mitosis in the cells. Has a greater antitumor activity with lower toxicity effect than paclitaxel (Taxol). Monitor WBC and platelet count; if low, dose may need to be decreased. *Pregnancy category:* D; PB: UK; t$^{1}/_{2}$: 11.1 h
paclitaxel (Taxol)	Metastatic ovarian and breast cancer. Monitor vital signs and electrocardiogram. Has a long duration of action (3 wk). Peak action is 11 d. *Pregnancy category:* D; PB: 80%-90%; t$^{1}/_{2}$: 5-17 h

NOTE: Chemotherapeutic doses and schedules will vary depending on the protocol, body surface area (m^2), age, functional status, and comorbid conditions. For a full discussion of body surface area in dosage calculation, see Chapter 4B, Methods for Calculation.
CBC, Complete blood cell count; *d*, day; *h*, hour; *PB*, protein-binding; *t$^{1}/_{2}$*, half-life; *UK*, unknown; *WBC*, white blood cell; *wk*, week.

Targeted Therapies (Topoisomerase Inhibitors, Tyrosine Kinase Inhibitors, Proteosome Inhibitors, Monoclonal Antibodies, Angiogenesis Inhibitors)

Targeted cancer therapies are a new approach in cancer treatment. They work by interfering with cancer cell growth and division in different ways and at various points in the development, growth, and spread of cancer. These therapies may interfere with proteins or enzymes in cancer cells, leading to *apoptosis* (cell death). By blocking the signals that tell cancer cells to grow and divide uncontrollably, targeted cancer therapies can help to stop the growth and division of cancer cells.

Topoisomerase I inhibitors or camptothecins (irinotecan [Camptosar], topotecan [Hycamtin]) work in the S phase and topoisomerase II inhibitors or epipodophyllotoxins (etoposide [VePesid, VP-16], teniposide [Vumon, VM-26]) work in the G$_2$ phase to interfere with the action of topoisomerase enzymes (topoisomerase I and II) to destroy the structure of DNA that is needed for replication. The adverse effects of topoisomerase I inhibitors include alopecia, constipation, nausea and vomiting, and peripheral neuropathy. Topotecan (Hycamtin) also can cause stomatitis, abdominal pain, and headache. Irinotecan (Camptosar)-associated diarrhea may occur. The side effects associated with etoposide (VP-16) administration include alopecia, anorexia, and nausea and vomiting. Nausea, vomiting, diarrhea, and mu-

cositis may result after the administration of teniposide (VM-26). Table 36–9 lists the mitotic and topoisomerase inhibitors, uses, and considerations.

Protein tyrosine kinases (PTKs) are enzymes that regulate signaling pathways in cells and regulate cell proliferation, differentiation, and antiapoptotic signals. Antiapoptotic signals allow cells to avoid programmed death. Unregulated activation of these enzymes can lead to cancer. Tyrosine kinase inhibitors (e.g., gefitinib [Iressa], imatinib mesylate [Gleevec]) interfere with receptor tyrosine kinase activity and disrupt cell signaling pathways that regulate cell proliferation. Side effects include nausea and vomiting, diarrhea, and skin rash. Gleevec may also cause indigestion, swelling around the eyes or lower legs, and muscle cramps.

The proteasome is an enzyme complex found within the cytoplasm of cells. It acts to dispose damaged cellular proteins and degrade short-lived proteins that regulate cell cycle, cell growth, and differentiation. Cancer may develop when these processes become abnormal. **Proteasome inhibitors** (e.g., bortezomib [Velcade]) prevent the breakdown of certain proteins and transcription factors and inactivate genes and proteins that help cancer cells survive antineoplastic therapy, thereby causing cancer cell death. Side effects include fatigue, malaise, nausea, vomiting, diarrhea, anorexia, constipation, thrombocytopenia, peripheral neuropathy, fever, and anemia.

Monoclonal antibodies (Moabs, mAbs) (e.g., trastuzumab [Herceptin]) recognize proteins on specific cancer cells (e.g., breast cancer). They can be used alone, or they can

Table 36–9

Antineoplastics: Targeted Therapies

Generic (Brand)	Uses and Considerations
Topoisomerase I Inhibitors	
irinotecan HCl (Camptosar)	Advanced and metastatic carcinoma of the colon and rectum. Inhibits the topoisomerase enzyme that is needed for DNA and RNA synthesis. Increased fluid intake is necessary. Monitor WBC count. *Pregnancy category:* D; PB: UK; t$\frac{1}{2}$: 6-10 h
topotecan HCl (Hycamtin)	Advanced and metastatic carcinoma of ovary. Used when other anticancer therapy fails. Inhibits topoisomerase I enzyme required for DNA replication. Monitor WBCs. *Pregnancy category:* D; PB: 35%; t$\frac{1}{2}$: 2-3 h
Topoisomerase II Derivatives	
etoposide (VePesid, VP-16)	Refractory testicular tumors, small cell lung carcinoma, Hodgkin's and non-Hodgkin's lymphomas, and acute myelogenous leukemia. Has standard chemotherapy side effects. Has a long duration of action. Transient hypotension with rapid IV infusion. *Pregnancy category:* D; PB: 97%; t$\frac{1}{2}$: 4-11 h
teniposide (Vumon, VM-26)	Acute lymphoblastic leukemia (ALL) in children. Used in combination with other anticancer drugs. Severe adverse reactions include bone marrow depression and anaphylaxis. *Pregnancy category:* D; PB: 99%; t$\frac{1}{2}$: 5 h
Tyrosine Kinase Inhibitors	
Gefitinib (Iressa)*	Approved by the FDA in May 2003. For use as a single agent in clients with locally advanced or metastatic non-small cell lung cancer who have failed to respond to platinum-based and docetaxel (Taxotere) chemotherapy. *Pregnancy category:* D; PB: UK; t$\frac{1}{2}$: 48 h
Imatinib mesylate (Gleevec)	Approved in 2001 to treat chronic myeloid leukemia (CML) and approved in February 2002 for metastatic malignant gastrointestinal stromal tumors (GIST). *Pregnancy category:* D; PB: 95%; t$\frac{1}{2}$: 18-40 h
Proteasome Inhibitors	
Bortezomib (Velcade)	Approved by the FDA in May 2003 for the treatment of multiple myeloma. Bortzezomab (Velcade) is a drug in a new class of anticancer agents known as proteasome inhibitors and is indicated for clients whose disease has relapsed after two previous treatments and have shown resistance to the last treatment. *Pregnancy category:* D; PB: 80%; t$\frac{1}{2}$: 9-15 h
Monoclonal Antibodies	
alemtuzumab (Campath)	Approved by the FDA May 7, 2001, to treat B-cell chronic lymphocytic leukemia (B-CLL). Binds to CD52 surface antigen resulting in cell lysis. *Pregnancy category:* C; t$\frac{1}{2}$: 12 d
cetuximab (Erbitux)	Metastatic colorectal cancer. Approved by FDA in February 2004. Binds to human epidermal growth factor (EGFR) and blocks activation of receptor-associated kinases. Used alone or in combination with irinotecan (Camptosar). *Pregnancy category:* C; t$\frac{1}{2}$: 114 h
gemtuzumab-ozogamicin (Mylotarg)	Relapsed acute myeloid leukemia (AML) for selected clients age 60 and older. *Pregnancy category:* D; PB: UK; t$\frac{1}{2}$: 72 h
rituximab (Rituxan)	Approved by the FDA in 2001 for the treatment of low-grade non-Hodgkin's lymphoma. Used to treat CLL (chronic lymphocytic leukemia). *Pregnancy category:* C; t$\frac{1}{2}$: 11-104 h
trastuzumab (Herceptin)	Metastatic breast cancer with tumors that over express the HER2 (human epidermal growth factor receptor 2) protein. Used in combination with paclitaxel for first line therapy, or as a single agent in second and third line therapy. Clinical trials are under way to determine the usefulness of trastuzumab in the treatment of osteosarcoma, and cancers of the lung, pancreas, salivary gland, colon, prostate, endometrium and bladder. *Pregnancy category:* B; t$\frac{1}{2}$: 1.7-12 d
Angiogenesis Inhibitors	
bevacizumab (Avastin)	Approved by the FDA in February 2004 for the treatment of metastatic colorectal cancer used in combination with 5-FU. Treatment of breast cancer and mesothelioma. *Pregnancy category:* C; t$\frac{1}{2}$: 11-50 d
Retinoids	
bexarotene (Targretin)	Bexarotene is a retinoid used in molecular targeted therapy to treat early or advanced-stage refractory cutaneous T-cell lymphoma. There have been relapses following prescribed dosing; with larger dosing, less relapse. Could cause hypoglycemia to clients with diabetes who take insulin or oral hypoglycemics. *Pregnancy category:* X; PB: UK, t$\frac{1}{2}$: 7 h

NOTE: Chemotherapeutic doses and schedules will vary depending on the protocol, body surface area (*m²*), age, functional status, and comorbid conditions. For a full discussion of body surface area in dosage calculation, see Chapter 4B, Methods for Calculation.
*Withdrawn for use with clients with newly diagnosed lung cancer because it provides no survival advantage over other chemotherapeutic agents. It is suggested that this agent only be used in clients who are already taking it and have seen some benefit. In addition, this drug may be used in studies that were approved before 2005.
5-FU, Fluorouracil; *d,* day; *DNA,* deoxyribonucleic acid; *FDA,* Food and Drug Administration; *h,* hour; *IV,* intravenous; *PB,* protein-binding; *RNA,* ribonucleic acid; *t¹/₂,* half-life; *UK,* unknown; *WBC,* white blood cell.

be used as vehicles to deliver drugs, toxins, or radioactive material to tumor sites. Trastuzumab is used in the treatment of breast cancer and blocks the effects of the growth factor protein human epidermal growth factor 2 (HER2), which transmits growth signals to the cancer cells. Side effects usually occur during the initial treatment with Herceptin and include fever, chills, pain, weakness, nausea, vomiting, diarrhea, headaches, difficulty breathing, and rashes. These side effects generally subside after the first treatment.

Another category of antineoplastic drugs, the **angiogenesis inhibitors**, acts to prevent angiogenesis (the growth of new blood vessels) to cancerous tumors (e.g., bevacizumab [Avastin]). Clinical trials are underway to evaluate the efficacy of these drugs in the treatment of cancer. Severe side effects include asthenia, pain, hypertension, diarrhea, and leukopenia. Other adverse effects may include pain, headache, hypertension, diarrhea, nausea, vomiting, anorexia, stomatitis, constipation, upper respiratory infection, nose bleed, dyspnea, exfoliative dermatitis, and proteinuria.

Liposomal Chemotherapy

A new approach to delivering chemotherapy involves the use of anticancer drugs that have been packaged inside synthetic fat globules called *liposomes*. The fatty coating helps the chemotherapy drug remain in the system longer and helps decrease side effects (e.g., hair loss, nausea, vomiting). Encapsulated forms doxorubicin (Doxil, Caelyx, Myocet), daunorubicin (DaunoXome), and vincristine (Marqibo) are being tested and other drugs are under development.

Hormonal Agents

Although **hormones** are not considered true chemotherapeutic agents, several classes of hormonal agents are used in the treatment of cancer. These include corticosteroids, sex hormones, antiestrogens, aromatase inhibitors, gonadotropin-releasing hormone analogues, and antiandrogens.

Corticosteroids

Corticosteroids (glucocorticoids) are anti-inflammatory agents that suppress the inflammatory process that occurs as a result of tumor growth. Although the exact mechanism of action is unknown, these agents may block steroid-specific receptors on the surface of cells. This blocking action slows the growth fraction of the tumor, thus retarding its growth. Prednisone, dexamethasone, and hydrocortisone can help decrease cerebral edema caused by a malignant brain tumor. Cortisone drugs give the client a sense of well-being and varying degrees of euphoria. Cortisone derivatives that are taken internally produce many side effects, such as fluid retention, potassium loss, increased risk of infection, increase in blood sugar, increase in fat distribution, muscle weakness, increased bleeding tendency, and euphoria.

Sex Hormones

The sex hormones (estrogen, androgens) or hormone-like agents are used to slow the growth of hormone dependent tumors (e.g., prostate cancer, breast cancer). Estrogen therapy is a palliative treatment used to decrease the progression of prostatic cancer in men and to slow the growth of hormone-dependent breast cancer in women. Estrogen preparations suppress tumor growth, and the drug promotes remission of the cancer for up to a year. Examples of this group of drugs are diethylstilbestrol (DES, Stilbestrol), ethinyl estradiol (Estinyl), chlorotrianisene (TACE), and conjugated estrogens (Premarin).

Progestins may be prescribed to treat breast cancer, endometrial carcinoma, and renal cancer. These drugs (e.g., hydroxyprogesterone caproate [Duralutin]), medroxyprogesterone acetate [Depo-Provera], and megestrol acetate [Megace]) act by shrinking the cancer tissues. Adverse reactions include fluid retention and thrombotic (clot) disorders.

Androgens are given to treat advanced breast cancer in premenopausal women. This male hormone promotes regression of the tumor. If androgen therapy is used for a long time, masculine secondary sexual characteristics, such as body hair growth, lowering of the voice, and muscle growth, will occur.

Antiestrogens (e.g., tamoxifen [Nolvadex]) are used to treat breast cancer tumors that are estrogen receptor positive. A newer drug, raloxifene (Evista) is a selective estrogen receptor modulator (SERM) that acts like an antiestrogen to slow tumor growth, but it has fewer side effects than tamoxifen. Both tamoxifen and raloxifene have been found to decrease the risk of breast cancer in postmenopausal women.

Gonadotropin-Releasing Hormone Analogues

Luteinizing hormone-releasing hormone (LH-RH) agonists (e.g., leuprolide [Lupron], goserelin [Zoladex]) suppress the secretion of follicle-stimulating hormone and luteinizing hormone from the pituitary gland. Initially, an increase in testosterone levels is seen. However, with continued use, the pituitary becomes insensitive to this stimulation which leads to a reduction in the production of androgens and estrogens.

Antiandrogens

Antiandrogens (e.g., flutamide [Eulexin], nilutamide [Nilandron], bicalutamide [Casodex]) are useful in treating men with hormone-responsive prostate cancer that has metastasized. These agents work by binding to androgen receptors and blocking the effects of dihydrotestosterone on the prostate cancer cells.

Aromatase Inhibitors

In postmenopausal females, the ovaries no longer produce estrogen, but androgen is converted to estrogen in this group of women. The aromatase inhibitors block the peripheral conversion of androgens to estrogens, thus suppressing the

Table 36–10

Antineoplastics: Hormones, Hormone Antagonists, and Enzymes

Generic (Brand)	Uses and Considerations
Androgens	
testolactone (Teslac)	Palliative treatment of breast carcinoma in postmenopausal women. Serum calcium levels should periodically be checked. Voice may deepen and facial hair may increase. *Pregnancy category:* D; PB: UK; t½: UK
progesterone (Gesterol 50)	Palliative treatment of endometrial and breast carcinoma. *Pregnancy category:* X; PB: UK; t½: 5 min
Hormonal Antagonists	
aminoglutethimide (Cytadren)	Adrenal carcinoma, ectopic adrenocorticotropic hormone (ACTH)-producing tumors. Drug suppresses adrenal activity. May be used in breast cancer therapy. Treatment usually used for 3 months. *Pregnancy category:* D; PB: 20%-25%; t½: 7-15 h
anastrozole (Arimidex) bicalutamide (Casodex)	Advanced breast cancer in postmenopausal women. Diarrhea, headache, hot flashes, pain, hypertension, and dyspnea might occur. *Pregnancy category:* D; PB: 40%; t½: 50 h
exemestane (Aromasin)	Advanced metastatic prostatic carcinoma. *Pregnancy category:* X; PB: UK; t½: 5.8 d
flutamide (Eulexin)	Advanced breast cancer in postmenopausal women. Prostatic cancer. *Pregnancy category:* D; PB: UK; t½: 24 h
fulvestrant (Faslodex)	Metastatic prostatic carcinoma, usually in combination with other anticancer drugs. *Pregnancy category:* D; PB: 95%; t½: 5–10 h
goserelin acetate (Zoladex)	Treatment of hormone-receptor positive metastatic breast cancer in postmenopausal women whose disease has progressed after antiestrogen therapy. *Pregnancy category:* D; PB: 99%; t½: 40 d
letrozole (Femara)	Metastatic prostatic carcinoma. It is a synthetic luteinizing hormone-releasing analogue. May also be used in breast cancer and endometriosis. Gynecomastia, breast swelling, and hot flashes may occur. *Pregnancy category:* X; PB: UK; t½: 4-6 h
leuprolide (Lupron)	Advanced breast cancer in postmenopausal women. Decreases estrogen biosynthesis. May be more effective than megestrol acetate and aminoglutethimide. *Pregnancy category:* UK; PB: UK; t½: 2 d
	Used to slow the growth of prostate cancer. Can be given daily (Lupron) or at 3- or 4-month intervals (Lupron Depot). May be used to treat endometriosis. Hypersensitivity reactions may occur in people with allergy to benzyl alcohol. Pregnant women should not take this drug (high risk of fetal damage). *Pregnancy category:* X; PB: 49%; t½: 3 h
megestrol acetate (Megace)	Palliative treatment of advanced carcinoma of the breast and endometrium. May promote weight gain by increasing appetite. *Pregnancy category:* X; PB: UK; t½: 15-20 h
mitotane (Lysodren)	Palliative treatment of inoperable adrenal cortical carcinoma. Adverse reactions include hemorrhagic cystitis, hypouricemia, and hypercholesterolemia. Monitor vital signs. *Pregnancy category:* C; PB: UK; t½: 20-160 d
nilutamide (Nilandron)	Prostatic carcinoma. Loss of libido and sexual potency may occur. Monitor liver function. *Pregnancy category:* C; PB: UK; t½: 24-72 h
polyestradiol PO4 (Estradurin)	Palliative treatment of inoperable prostatic carcinoma. Estrogen derivative. Side effects may include fluid retention, nausea, vomiting, hypertension, weight change, and thromboembolic disorders. *Pregnancy category:* X; PB: UK; t½: UK
tamoxifen citrate (Nolvadex)	Palliative treatment of advanced breast carcinoma with positive lymph nodes in postmenopausal women. Competes with estradiol at estrogen receptor sites. Decreases DNA synthesis. Reduces risk of breast cancer in postmenopausal women. *Pregnancy category:* D; PB: UK; t½: 7 d
raloxifene (Evista)	A selective estrogen receptor modulator (SERM) originally approved to fight osteoporosis in postmenopausal women. Reduces risk of breast cancer with fewer side effects than tamoxifen. *Pregnancy category:* X; PB: 95%; t½: 27 h
toremifene citrate (Fareston)	Advanced breast cancer in postmenopausal women. An antiestrogen drug. *Pregnancy category:* D; PB: >99%; t½: 5 d
Miscellaneous Enzymes	
L-asparaginase (Elspar)	Acute lymphocytic leukemia. Used in combination with another anticancer drug. Common side effects include nausea, vomiting, anorexia, leukopenia, and impaired pancreatic function. *Pregnancy category:* C; PB: 30%; t½: 8–30 h (IV)
pegaspargase (Oncaspar)	Acute lymphoblastic leukemia. A CCS agent affecting G_1 phase of the cell cycle. It interferes with DNA, RNA, and protein synthesis. *Pregnancy category:* C; PB: UK; t½: 1.4 to 5.2 d

NOTE: Chemotherapeutic doses and schedules will vary depending on the protocol, body surface area (m^2), age, functional status, and comorbid conditions. For a full discussion of body surface area in dosage calculation, see Chapter 4B, Methods for Calculation.

CCS, Cell-cycle specific; *d,* day; *DNA,* deoxyribonucleic acid; *h,* hour; *IV,* intravenous; *min,* minute; *PB,* protein-binding; *RNA,* ribonucleic acid; *t½,* half-life; *UK,* unknown; *>,* greater than.

postmenopausal synthesis of estrogen and slowing tumor growth. Aromatase inhibitors are used in the treatment of hormonally sensitive breast cancer in postmenopausal women or premenopausal women who have had their ovaries removed. Anastrozole (Arimidex), letrozole (Femara), and exemestane (Aromasin) are examples of aromatase inhibitors currently in use. Increasingly, these agents are being used before tamoxifen in postmenopausal women with hormonally responsive metastatic breast cancer. Table 36–10 lists hormonal agents, uses, and considerations.

Miscellaneous Agents

This category includes a number of antineoplastic agents in which the mechanism of action is unclear (see Table 36–10).

Summary

Many antineoplastic drugs act to disrupt cancer cells in one (CCS) or more than one (CCNS) phase of the cell cycle. These include the alkylating compounds, antimetabolites, antitumor antibiotics, mitotic inhibitors, targeted therapy, hormones, and hormone antagonists. Newer chemotherapy agents, designed to target specific enzymes or proteins in cancer cells, continue to be developed and evaluated for clinical efficacy (e.g., topoisomerase inhibitors, tyrosine kinase inhibitors, proteosome inhibitors). Other drugs designed to block growth factors on the surface of cancer cells, deliver toxic therapy directly to tumors, or block the growth of blood vessels that supply tumors are in use or being tested in clinical trials (e.g., monoclonal antibodies, angiogenesis inhibitors).

Nurses play an important role in helping people understand the procedures related to chemotherapy administration. Client/family education is critical. Nurses may need to explain the treatment protocol to clients and provide verbal and written information on the chemotherapeutic agents that will be administered. Clients require information about what side effects can be expected, how these will be addressed, and when to call their health care provider. Chemotherapy drugs are highly toxic. Nurses should provide information to clients about the safe handling and disposal of these agents if they are to be taken in the home environment.

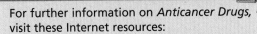

WEBSITES

For further information on *Anticancer Drugs,* visit these Internet resources:

Agency for Healthcare Research and Quality:
http://www.ahcpr.gov/

Oncolink:
http://www.oncolink.org/

PubMed National Library of Medicine:
http://www.ncbi.nlm.nih.gov/entrez/query.fcgi

U.S. Food and Drug Administration:
http://www.fda.gov/

Medline Plus:
http://www.nlm.nih.gov/medlineplus/

National Cancer Institute:
http://www.nci.nih.gov/cancertopics/chemotherapy-and-you

Critical Thinking Case Study

Your client, a 60-year-old African American woman, was recently diagnosed with breast cancer. She received combination chemotherapy consisting of oral (PO) cyclophosphamide and IV doxorubicin and fluorouracil (CAF).

Her regimen consisted of the following:

Cyclophosphamide	100 mg/m²	PO	Days 1-14
Doxorubicin	50 mg/m²	IV	Days 1, 8
Fluorouracil	500 mg/m²	IV	Day 1

1. Differentiate the drug actions of cyclophosphamide, fluorouracil, and doxorubicin.

2. What side effects and adverse reactions should the nurse assess for during therapy? Why would assessment of the cardiac, GI, and genitourinary systems be important with this drug regimen?

3. What is the maximum lifetime dose for doxorubicin? Why is this so important?

4. Describe the early signs of cardiac toxicity that you might see days to months after the administration of doxorubicin.

5. Briefly explain why hydration would be important during this drug regimen.

6. What nursing interventions would be appropriate when caring for this client?

7. Describe the teaching you would provide to the client and her family.

8. After two cycles of chemotherapy, the client complains that her mouth feels sore and it hurts to eat. Which chemotherapy agent is most likely responsible for this finding? What nursing interventions would you initiate to address this problem?

9. Analyze protective measures necessary to avoid accidental exposure to chemotherapy agents during administration.

10. The client calls you at the clinic and tells you that she has a temperature of 38.3° C. What actions would you take?

Study Questions

1. Name the five phases of the cell cycle. List the groups of drugs that are cell-cycle specific and cell-cycle nonspecific.

2. Your client is receiving cyclophosphamide, methotrexate, and fluorouracil (CMF) for the treatment of breast cancer. What information would you include in your client teaching about self-care activities related to these drugs?

3. List the common adverse reactions associated with most antineoplastic drugs.

4. What are the advantages of combination therapy for the client with cancer?

5. List the therapeutic actions of corticosteroids, such as prednisone, in the treatment of cancer.

6. What is the definition of vesicant? List the anti-cancer drugs with vesicant properties. What precautions should be taken when a client is receiving a vesicant?

7. Briefly explain how targeted therapies work in the treatment of cancer.

8. Briefly explain how angiogenesis inhibitors work in limiting tumor growth.

9. Describe nursing interventions for the client with a low platelet count.

10. Your client is receiving a chemotherapy agent that is likely to cause alopecia. What teaching would you provide for this individual?

37 Biologic Response Modifiers

ANNE E. LARA

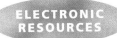

Additional information can be found on the companion website at *http://evolve.elsevier.com/KeeHayes/pharmacology/* or on the companion CD-ROM, which includes:
- *NCLEX-style examination review questions*
- *Pharmacology animations*
- *Medication error and IV therapy checklists*
- *Medication calculation problems*
- *Electronic calculators*

OUTLINE

OBJECTIVES

- Discuss the actions of the biologic response modifiers.
- Identify two client populations that may benefit from biologic response modifiers.
- List three common side effects of interferons, colony-stimulating factors, and interleukin-2.
- Describe the nursing process, including client teaching, to care for clients who receive biologic response modifiers.

TERMS

Introduction

Biologic response modifiers (BRMs) are a class of agents used to enhance the body's immune system. Advances in biochemical technology have led to the discovery of BRMs and to the identification of their clinical activities. **Recombinant DNA** (genetic engineering process that produces mass quantities of human proteins) and **hybridoma technology** (process that uses mice to mass produce monoclonal antibodies) are two advances that have led to commercial mass production of BRMs (Figures 37–1 and 37–2).

Interferons (α, β, γ), colony-stimulating factors, interleukins, tumor necrosis factor, and monoclonal antibodies are some currently known BRMs. With the exception of the monoclonal antibodies, BRMs are complex proteins produced by the cells of the immune system (Figure 37–3).

Individuals taking BRMs are immune compromised and should be counseled on concurrent drug and herb use (see Herbal Alert 37–1).

The following three BRM functions have been identified:

1. Enhance host immunologic function (immunomodulation)
2. Destroy or interfere with tumor activities (cytotoxic/cytostatic effects)
3. Promote differentiation of stem cells (other biologic effects) (Table 37–1)

The indications for BRMs are currently undergoing investigation in clinical trials. Erythropoietin, granulocyte colony-stimulating factors, granulocyte macrophage colony-stimulating factor, Neumega (oprelvekin), and interferon alpha are approved by the Food and Drug Administration (FDA) and commercially available. The interleukins, tumor necrosis factor, and some monoclonal antibodies continue to be studied in clinical trials. Only one monoclonal antibody—trastuzumab (Herceptin)—has been approved by the FDA. Interferons, interleukins, colony-stimulating factors, and trastuzumab are discussed in this chapter.

HERBAL ALERT 37–1

Biologic Response Modifiers and Herbs

🌿 Herbal preparations are generally not recommended for clients receiving biologic response modifiers (BRMs). Several herbs (echinacea, ginseng, goldenseal) act to stimulate the immune system. However, clients taking BRMs are immunocompromised and taking these preparations in combination is not recommended.

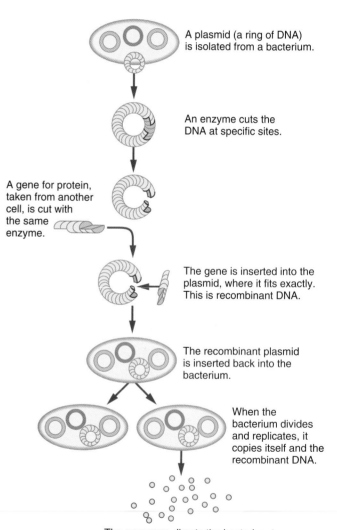

A plasmid (a ring of DNA) is isolated from a bacterium.

An enzyme cuts the DNA at specific sites.

A gene for protein, taken from another cell, is cut with the same enzyme.

The gene is inserted into the plasmid, where it fits exactly. This is recombinant DNA.

The recombinant plasmid is inserted back into the bacterium.

When the bacterium divides and replicates, it copies itself and the recombinant DNA.

The new gene directs the bacterium to make a new protein product, such as interferon.

FIGURE 37–1 Recombinant DNA. (Redrawn from *Understanding the immune system*, NIH Pub No 88-529, Bethesda, MD, 1991, National Institutes of Health, p. 29.)

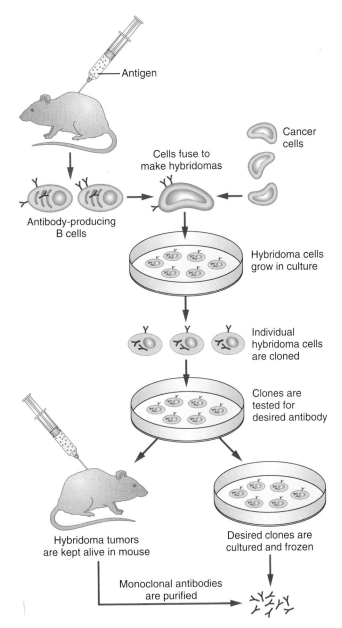

FIGURE 37–2   Hybridoma therapy. (Redrawn from *Understanding the immune system*, NIH Pub No 88-529, Bethesda, MD, 1991, National Institutes of Health, p. 28.)

Interferons

Interferons (IFNs) are a family of naturally occurring proteins that were first discovered in the 1950s. Three major types of IFNs have been identified: alpha (α) IFN, beta (β) IFN, and gamma (γ) IFN. Each type is produced by a different cell within the immune system. All three types can be manufactured using recombinant DNA technology; however, only IFN-α is FDA approved for commercial use.

Interferon-α

IFN-α is produced by B cells, T cells, **macrophages,** and null cells in response to the presence of viruses or tumor cells. IFN-α has been shown to have antiviral, antiproliferative, and immunomodulatory effects, which means that it inhibits intracellular replication of viral DNA, interferes

with tumor cell growth, and enhances natural killer cell (antitumor) activity. Recombinant IFN-α is manufactured as Roferon-A and Intron A.

In 1986, IFN-α was approved by the FDA for use in treating hairy cell leukemia; in 1989 it was approved for use in acquired immunodeficiency syndrome (AIDS)-related Kaposi's sarcoma. Clinically, IFN-α has been used to treat non-Hodgkin's lymphoma, multiple myeloma, chronic myelogenous leukemia, renal cell carcinoma, malignant melanoma, bladder cancer, and carcinoid (type of cancerlike disease). Intravesical administration of IFN-α has proved successful for low-grade bladder tumors; intraperitoneal administration of IFN-α has been used to treat ovarian cancer; and intralesional application of IFN-α has been used to treat melanoma and basal cell carcinoma. Benign conditions such as laryn-

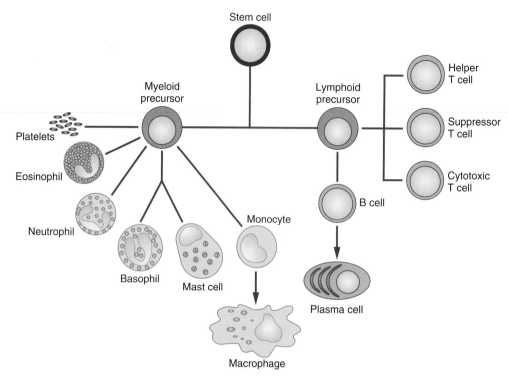

FIGURE 37–3   Cells of the immune system. (Redrawn from *Understanding the immune system*, NIH Pub No 88-529, Bethesda, MD, 1991, National Institutes of Health, p. 5.)

Table 37–1

Action of Biologic Response Modifiers

Biologic Response Modifier	Action
Interleukins	I
Interferons	I, C
Monoclonal antibodies	C
Tumor necrosis factor	C
Colony-stimulating factors	O

C, Cytotoxic/cytostatic; I, immunomodulation; O, other biologic activity.

geal papillomata and condyloma acuminatum have also been treated with IFN-α.

Pharmacokinetics

IFN-α is metabolized by the liver and filtered by the kidney. The body, however, absorbs approximately 80% of the dose. Peak serum concentrations are reached 4 to 8 hours after administration. IFN-α can be administered subcutaneously (subQ), intramuscularly (IM), and intravenously (IV), although subQ or IM administration is preferred. SubQ administration is recommended for clients with platelet counts below 50,000.

Side Effects and Adverse Reactions

The major side effect of IFN-α is a flulike syndrome. Other effects occur in the gastrointestinal (GI), neurologic, cardiopulmonary, renal, hepatic, hematologic, and dermatologic systems.

The flulike syndrome is characterized by chills, fever, fatigue, malaise, and myalgias. Chills can occur 3 to 6 hours after IFN-α administration and may progress to rigors. A fever as high as 101° F to 104° F (39° C to 40° C) may occur within 30 to 90 minutes after the onset of chills and

last 24 hours. Fatigue, malaise, and myalgias are cumulative side effects; fatigue is the dose-limiting toxicity (i.e., the side effect that necessitates a decrease in dose or discontinuation of the drug).

GI side effects include nausea, diarrhea, vomiting, anorexia, taste alterations, and xerostomia (dry mouth). These side effects are mild; anorexia is considered the dose-limiting toxicity for this system.

Neurologic side effects are reversible (after the drug is stopped) and occur in 70% of clients who receive IFN-α. These effects are manifested by mild confusion, somnolence (sleepiness), irritability, poor concentration, seizures, transient aphasia (temporary loss of ability to speak), hallucinations, paranoia, and psychoses.

Cardiopulmonary side effects are dose related and occur more frequently in older adults and clients with an underlying cardiac disease. The effects include tachycardia, pallor, cyanosis, tachypnea, nonspecific electrocardiographic changes, rare myocardial infarction, and orthostatic hypotension.

Renal and hepatic effects are dose dependent and usually result in few or no symptoms. The effects are manifested by increased blood urea nitrogen (BUN) and creatinine levels, proteinuria, and elevated transaminases.

Hematologic effects are reversible and dose limiting. Neutropenia (decreased number of neutrophils in the blood) and thrombocytopenia are manifestations of such effects. Neutropenia is usually rare and does not predispose the client to infection. **Thrombocytopenia** is more common in clients with hematopoietic (affecting the formation of blood cells) diseases than in those with solid tumors.

Table 37–2

Biologic Response Modifiers: Interferons

Generic (Brand)	Route and Dosage	Uses and Considerations
Interferon alfa-2a (Roferon-A)	*Hairy-cell leukemia, condylomata acuminata:* A: subQ/IM: 3 million international units daily for 16-24 wk	For treating hairy-cell leukemia, condyloma acuminata, and AIDS-related Kaposi's sarcoma. Flulike symptoms such as fatigue, aches, pain, fever, chills, headaches may occur. *Pregnancy category:* C; PB: UK; $t\frac{1}{2}$: 2-3 h
Interferon alfa-2b (Intron A)	A: subQ: 2 million international units/ $m^2 \times 3$ wk *Kaposi's sarcoma:* A: IM/subQ/IV: Initially: 36 million international units daily for 10-12 wk; *maint:* 36 million international units 3 × wk	For treating hairy-cell leukemia, condyloma acuminata, AIDS-related Kaposi's sarcoma, and chronic hepatitis B and non-A hepatitis. Flulike symptoms may occur. Monitor CBC, AST, ALT, ALP, LDH. *Pregnancy category:* C; PB: UK; $t\frac{1}{2}$: 2 h
Interferon gamma-1b (Actimmune)	*Body surface area >0.5 m^2:* A: subQ: 50 mcg/m^2 3 × wk *Body surface area <0.5 m^2:* A & C: >1 y: subQ: 1.5 mcg/kg 3 × wk	For treating chronic granulomatous disease. Flulike symptoms may occur. *Pregnancy category:* C; PB: UK; $t\frac{1}{2}$: 0.5-6 h
Interferon alfa-n3 (Alferon N)	*Condylomata acuminata:* A: Inject into wart: 250,000 units (0.05 ml) twice weekly; *max:* 8 wk Do *not* repeat for >3 mo after end of therapy	For treating recurring condylomata acuminata (genital venereal warts). Flulike symptoms may occur. Monitor CBC, AST, ALT, ALP, LDH. *Pregnancy category:* C; PB: UK; $t\frac{1}{2}$: 6-8 h
Interferon beta-1b (Betaseron)	*Reduce number of clinical exacerbations of multiple sclerosis:* A: >18 y: subQ: 8 million units every other day C: Not recommended	For treating multiple sclerosis (MS). Flulike symptoms may occur. *Pregnancy category:* C; PB: UK; $t\frac{1}{2}$: 8 min-4.3 h

A, Adult; *AIDS,* acquired immunodeficiency syndrome; *ALT,* alanine aminotransferase; *ALP,* alkaline phosphatase; *AST,* aspartate aminotransferase; *C,* child; *CBC,* complete blood count; *h,* hour; *IM,* intramuscular; *IV,* intravenous; *LDH,* lactate dehydrogenase; *maint,* maintenance; *max,* maximum; *min,* minute; *mo,* month; *PB,* protein-binding; *subQ,* subcutaneous; $t\frac{1}{2}$, half-life; *UK,* unknown; *wk,* week; *y,* year; *>,* greater than; *<,* less than.

Maculopapular rashes of the trunk and extremities, pruritus, irritation at the injection site, desquamation (shedding of epithelial cells of the skin), and alopecia are dermatologic effects of IFN-α. Alopecia can occur after more than 4 months of therapy.

Dosing and Preparation

Roferon-A is available in liquid and powder forms. The liquid is supplied in 3 million or 18 million international units/mL vials. The powder is available as 18 million international units/vial at a concentration of 3 million international units/0.5 ml. When mixed with 3 ml of bacteriostatic water diluent, the vial concentration is 6 million international units/milliliter, or 3 million international units/0.5 ml. Both the liquid and powder should be refrigerated at 36° F to 46° F (2° C to 8° C) and used within 1 month. The vials should not be frozen or shaken.

Intron A is supplied as a lyophilized powder in 3, 5, and 25 million international units. The powder is reconstituted with bacteriostatic water diluent. Final vial concentrations are 3 million international units/vial (3 million international units/vial with 1 ml of diluent), 5 million international units/ml (5 million international units/vial with 2 ml of diluent), and 5 million international units/ml (25 million international units/vial with 5 ml of diluent). The vials can be shaken to hasten powder dissolution. The final solution is stable for 30 days when stored at 36° F to 46° F (2° C to 8° C). The IFN alphas are listed in Table 37–2 with their dosages, uses, and considerations.

Administration

The administration of IFN-α is contraindicated in clients with known hypersensitivity to IFN-α, mouse immunoglobulin, or any component of the product. It should be used cautiously in clients with severe cardiac, renal, or hepatic disease and in those with seizure disorders or central nervous system dysfunction. Manufacturers recommend administering the agent to persons 18 years or older only under the supervision of a qualified physician. There have been no studies demonstrating the safety and effectiveness of IFN-α in pregnant women, nursing mothers, or children. Women of childbearing age should use contraceptives while receiving IFN-α because of the agent's effects on serum estradiol and progesterone concentrations. Studies have demonstrated no fertility or teratogenic effects in men.

It is recommended that baseline and periodic complete blood counts (CBCs) and liver function tests be performed during the course of IFN therapy. Manufacturers suggest that clients undergo IFN therapy for at least 6 months before a decision is made whether to continue treatment in those who respond or discontinue treatment in those who do not; optimal treatment duration has not been determined. Dose reductions of 50% or drug discontinuation should be considered if adverse reactions occur. Concurrent or prior treatment with chemotherapeutic agents or radiation therapy may increase the effectiveness and toxicity of IFN-α.

Colony-Stimulating Factors

Hematopoietic **colony-stimulating factors (CSFs)** are proteins that stimulate or regulate the growth, maturation, and differentiation of bone marrow stem cells (Figure 37–4). The CSFs are manufactured through recombinant DNA techniques.

Although CSFs are not directly tumoricidal, they are useful in cancer treatment because they do the following:

- Decrease the length of posttreatment neutropenia (the length of time the neutrophils [a type of white blood cell] are decreased secondary to chemotherapy), thereby reducing the incidence and duration of infection
- Permit the delivery of higher doses of drugs. **Myelosuppression** (suppression of bone marrow activity) is often a dose-limiting toxicity of chemotherapy. Higher, possibly tumoricidal doses of drugs cannot be administered because of potentially life-threatening side effects. CSFs can minimize the myelosuppression toxicity thus allowing the delivery of higher doses of drugs.
- Reduce bone marrow recovery time after bone marrow transplantation
- Enhance macrophage or granulocyte tumor-, virus-, and fungus-destroying ability
- Prevent severe thrombocytopenia after myelosuppressive chemotherapy

CSFs have been used to treat clients with neutropenia secondary to disease or treatment and can be administered both IV and subQ. The CSFs that are FDA approved for clinical use are erythropoietin, granulocyte colony-stimulating factor (G-CSF), granulocyte macrophage colony-stimulating factor (GM-CSF), and Neumega (oprelvekin).

Erythropoietin

Erythropoietin (EPO) (Procrit) is a glycoprotein produced by the kidney that stimulates red blood cell production in response to hypoxia (decreased oxygen to body tissues). Specifically, EPO stimulates the division and differentiation of committed red blood cell progenitors (parent cells destined to become circulating red blood cells) in the bone marrow. EPO is currently FDA approved for use in clients with anemia secondary to chronic renal failure (CRF), zidovudine (AZT)-treated human immunodeficiency virus (HIV) infections, or cancer and its treatment. The use of EPO in clients with anemia may decrease the need for and frequency of red cell transfusion. EPO is marketed under the brand name Epogen.

Pharmacokinetics

Erythropoietin (EPO) can be administered IV (IV push) or subQ. According to the manufacturer, EPO administered by IV is eliminated at a rate consistent with first-order kinetics (process by which the drug is eliminated in part by hepatic and renal blood flow). It has a circulating half-life ranging from approximately 4 to 13 hours in clients with CRF. Plasma

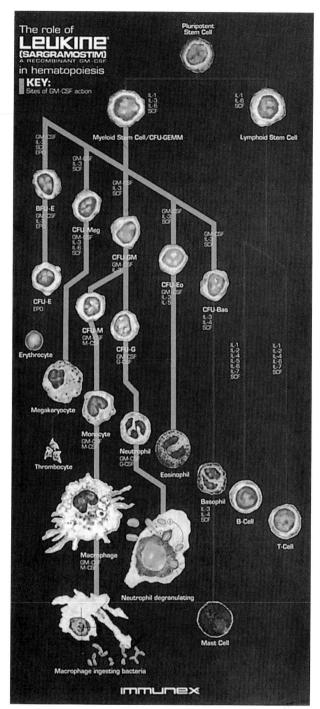

FIGURE 37–4 The role of sargramostim (Leukine) in hematopoiesis. (Courtesy Immunex Corp., San Francisco.)

levels of EPO have been detected for at least 24 hours. After subQ administration of EPO to CRF clients, peak serum levels are achieved within 5 to 24 hours. The half-life of IV-administered EPO is approximately 20% shorter in normal clients without CRF than in clients with CRF. Pharmacokinetic studies have not been done with HIV-infected clients. See Prototype Drug Chart 37–1.

Side Effects and Adverse Reactions

The side effects of EPO include hypertension, headache, arthralgias (joint pain), nausea, edema, fatigue, diarrhea, vomiting, chest pain, injection site skin reaction, asthenia

PROTOTYPE DRUG CHART 37–1

EPOEITIN ALFA (ERYTHROPOIETIN)

Drug Class

Biologic response modifier
Trade Name: Epogen, Procrit, ♣ Eprex
Pregnancy Category: C

Dosage

A: 50-100 units/kg 3 × wk
IV: Dialysis clients
IV/subQ: Nondialysis, CRF clients
IV/subQ: 100 U/kg 3 × wk for 8 wk in AZT-treated
    HIV-infected clients
Initial dose to those with EPO levels <500 mU/ml and re-
    ceiving <4200 mg of AZT/wk. Clients with EPO level
    >500 mU/ml are unlikely to respond to EPO therapy.

Contraindications

Uncontrolled hypertension, hypersensitivity to mamma-
    lian cell-derived products or human albumin
Caution: Pregnancy, lactation, porphyria; safety in chil-
    dren not known

Drug-Lab-Food Interactions

Drug: None known
Lab: Increase hematocrit, *decrease* plasma volume
Food: None known

Pharmacokinetics

Absorption: subQ, IV
Distribution: PB: UK
Metabolism: t½: 4-13 h in clients with CRF; 20% less
    in those with normal renal function
Excretion: In urine

Pharmacodynamics

IV: Onset: 7-10 d
    Peak: 2-4 wk
    Duration: UK
subQ: Onset: 7-10 d
    Peak: 5-24 h
    Duration: UK

Therapeutic Effects/Uses

To treat anemia secondary to CRF or AZT (zidovudine) treatment of HIV infections. Use in clients with anemia
    secondary to cancer or its treatment is under investigation.
Mode of Action: Increased production of RBCs, triggered by hypoxia or anemia

Side Effects

Sense of well-being, hypertension, arthralgias, nausea,
    edema, fatigue, injection site reaction, rash, diarrhea,
    shortness of breath

Adverse Reactions

Seizures, hyperkalemia
Life-threatening: Cerebrovascular accident, myocardial
    infarction

A, Adult; *CRF,* chronic renal failure; *d,* day; *EPO,* erythropoietin; *h,* hour; *HIV,* human immunodeficiency virus; *IV,* intravenous; *PB,*
protein-binding; *RBC,* red blood cell; *subQ,* subcutaneous; *t½,* half-life; *UK,* unknown; *wk,* week; <, less than; >, greater than; ♣,
Canadian drug name.

(weakness), dizziness, seizures, thrombosis (clots), and allergic reactions. Studies demonstrate that EPO administration is well tolerated with no reports of serious allergic reactions or anaphylaxis. Rare transient skin reactions have been
reported. Blood pressure may increase in clients with CRF
who receive EPO during the early phase of treatment when
the hematocrit (Hct) is increasing. About 25% of clients with
CRF who receive dialysis may require initiation of or increase
in antihypertensive therapy. It is postulated that increases in
blood pressure may relate to increases in Hct; therefore it is
recommended that the dose of EPO be decreased if the Hct
increase exceeds four points in any 2-week period. Similarly,
an increase in Hct may cause increased vascular access clotting (clots in blood vessel at connection site with artificial
kidney) in hemodialysis clients. Clients may require increased heparinization during EPO therapy to prevent clotting of the artificial kidney. Seizures occurred in clients with

CRF who received EPO during clinical trials; activity was particularly evident during the first 90 days of therapy.

Dosing

EPO should be administered at starting doses of 50 to
100 units/kg three times a week. The dose should be reduced when the Hct reaches the 30% to 33% range or increases by more than four points in any 2-week period. The
dosage must be individualized to maintain the Hct within
the target range. Dose changes should be made in the
range of 25 units/kg three times a week.

According to the manufacturer, if a client does not respond to EPO or maintain a response, the following situations must be considered and evaluated:

1. Iron deficiency
2. Underlying infections, inflammatory, or malignant
    processes

3. Occult blood loss
4. Underlying hematologic disease
5. Folic acid or vitamin B_{12} deficiency
6. Hemolysis
7. Aluminum intoxication
8. Osteitis fibrosa cystica (fibrous degeneration with formation of cysts and nodules secondary to hyperparathyroidism)

Administration

EPO administration is contraindicated in clients with (1) uncontrolled hypertension, (2) known hypersensitivity to mammalian cell-derived products, and (3) known hypersensitivity to human albumin. Evaluation of iron stores should occur during EPO therapy. Transferrin saturation should be at least 20% and ferritin should be at least 100 ng/ml. Iron supplements may be used to increase and maintain transferrin saturation to support EPO-stimulated erythropoiesis.

The safety and effectiveness of EPO therapy in pregnant women, nursing mothers, and children have not been established. There are no known EPO drug interactions.

Preparation

The following are the manufacturers' preparation and administration recommendations for EPO:
1. Do not shake because shaking may denature the glycoprotein, rendering it biologically inactive.
2. Use only one dose per vial. Do not reenter the vial. Discard any unused portion because the vial contains no preservatives.
3. Store the 2000-, 3000-, 4000-, 10,000-, or 20,000-unit vials at 36° F to 46° F (2° C to 8° C). Do not freeze.
4. Warm the vial to room temperature before subQ administration.
5. Use the smallest volume of EPO per injection (1 ml or less per injection) to decrease injection site discomfort.
6. Use ice to numb the injection site.
7. Do not use the same needle to draw medication into the syringe and to inject the medication. Use a new needle to inject medication.

Granulocyte and Pegfilgrastim (Neulasta) Colony-Stimulating Factor

Granulocyte colony-stimulating factor (G-CSF) and Pegfilgrastim **(Neulasta)**, marketed as filgrastim (Neupogen), are human **granulocyte** (type of white blood cell [WBC] responsible for fighting infection) colony-stimulating factor produced by recombinant DNA technology. G-CSF is a glycoprotein produced by monocytes (a type of WBC), fibroblasts (immature fiber-producing cells), and endothelial cells (cells that line the heart cavity and blood and lymph vessels). It regulates the production of **neutrophils** (granular leukocytes, WBCs) within the bone marrow. G-CSF is FDA approved and commercially available to decrease the incidence of infections in clients receiving myelosuppressive chemotherapeutic agents. G-CSF has been evaluated as

an adjunct to chemotherapy for both solid tumor and hematologic malignancies and in studies using a number of different chemotherapy regimens. Filgrastim and Pegfilgrastim are commercially available forms of G-CSF. Prototype Drug Chart 37–2 gives the drug data for filgrastim and pegfilgrastim.

Filgrastim

Pharmacokinetics

Filgrastim administration results in a two-phase neutrophil response. An early response is seen within 24 hours of administration. Following the chemotherapy-induced **nadir** (low point), a second peak in circulating neutrophils is observed. The proliferation-induced increase in neutrophils usually begins 4 to 5 days after administration is initiated, but timing may vary based on the type and dose of the myelosuppressive therapy and the client's underlying disease and prior treatment history. The elimination half-life of G-CSF in both normal clients and those with cancer is 3.5 hours. Clearance rates are approximately 0.5 to 0.7 ml/min/kg.

Side Effects and Adverse Reactions

The side effects of filgrastim therapy include nausea, vomiting, skeletal pain, alopecia, diarrhea, neutropenia, fever, mucositis, fatigue, anorexia, dyspnea, headache, cough, skin rash, chest pain, generalized weakness, sore throat, stomatitis, constipation, and pain of unspecified origin. Of these reactions, bone pain is the only consistently observed reaction attributed to G-CSF therapy. The bone pain was of mild to moderate severity and well controlled with nonnarcotic analgesia. It occurs more frequently in clients receiving higher (20 to 100 mcg/kg daily) IV doses than in clients receiving lower (3 to 10 mcg/kg daily) subcutaneous doses.

Dosing

G-CSF can be administered subQ and by IV infusion. The recommended starting dose of G-CSF is 5 mcg/kg daily subQ or IV infusion. The maximum tolerated dose has not been established. Doses may be increased in 5-mcg/kg increments for each chemotherapy cycle, according to the duration and severity of the absolute neutrophil count nadir. The **absolute neutrophil count (ANC)** is determined using the following equation:

$$\text{ANC} = \text{Total white blood count (WBC)} \times \text{percentage of neutrophils} + \text{percentage of bands}$$

G-CSF should not be administered 24 hours before or after the administration of therapeutic agents because of the potential sensitivity of rapidly dividing myeloid cells to chemotherapy. G-CSF may stimulate the proliferation of rapidly dividing cells, which may be destroyed by chemotherapy drugs.

G-CSF causes a transient increase in neutrophil counts 1 to 2 days after initiation of therapy. However to achieve a sustained therapeutic response, G-CSF therapy should be continued until postchemotherapy nadir ANC is 10,000/mm³. Premature discontinuation of G-CSF therapy before expected ANC recovery is not recommended.

PROTOTYPE DRUG CHART 37–2

FILGRASTIM

Drug Class	**Dosage**
Granulocyte colony-stimulating factor (G-CSF) Trade Name: Neupogen *Pregnancy Category:* C	A: IV inf/subQ: 5 mcg/kg/d C: 5-10 mcg/kg/d Refer to specific protocols.
Contraindications	**Drug-Lab-Food Interactions**
Hypersensitivity to *Escherichia coli*-derived proteins; 24 hours before or after cytotoxic chemotherapy *Caution:* Pregnancy, lactation; safety in children not known	*Drug:* None known *Lab: Increase* lactic acid, LDH, alkaline phosphatase; transient *increase* in neutrophils *Food:* None known
Pharmacokinetics	**Pharmacodynamics**
Absorption: subQ: Well absorbed **Distribution:** PB: UK **Metabolism:** t½: 2-3.5 h **Excretion:** Probably in urine	IV/subQ: Onset: 24 h Peak: 3-5 d Duration: 4-7 d

Therapeutic Effects/Uses

To decrease incidence of infection in clients receiving myelosuppressive chemotherapeutic agents; adjunct to
chemotherapy for both solid tumor and hematologic malignancies
Mode of Action: Increases production of neutrophils and enhances their phagocytosis

Side Effects	**Adverse Reactions**
Nausea, vomiting, skeletal pain, alopecia, diarrhea, fever, skin rash, anorexia, headache, cough, chest pain, sore throat, constipation	Neutropenia, dyspnea, splenomegaly, psoriasis, hematuria **Life-threatening:** Thrombocytopenia, myocardial infarc- tion, adult respiratory distress syndrome in clients with sepsis

A, Adult; *C,* child; *d,* day; *h,* hour; *IV,* intravenous; *LDH,* lactate dehydrogenase; *PB,* protein-binding; *subQ,* subcutaneous; *t½,* half-
life; *UK,* unknown.

Administration

G-CSF administration has no demonstrable effects on
fertility in male and female rats. Its carcinogenic potential is not known. Caution should be used when G-CSF
is given to pregnant women and nursing mothers. The
manufacturer recommends that the benefits justify the
potential risks.

Filgrastim's efficacy has not been demonstrated in children, although safety data indicate that it does not cause
any greater toxicity in children than in adults.

There has been no evidence of other drug interaction
with filgrastim, but its administration is contraindicated in
clients with known hypersensitivity to *Escherichia coli*-
derivant proteins.

Preparation

Neupogen is supplied as 1-ml vials containing 300 mcg of
filgrastim or as 1.6-ml vials containing 480 mcg of filgrastim. Both vials are preservative free; therefore the manufacturer recommends that the vials be used one time only
and that any vials left at room temperature for longer than
6 hours be discarded. Filgrastim should be stored in a refrigerator at 36° F to 46° F (2° C to 8° C). Do not freeze
or shake the vials.

Pegfilgrastim

Pharmacokinetics

Filgrastim is eliminated via the kidneys. Pegfilgrastim is a pegylated
(**pegylation** is the process of adding a polyethylene glycol [PEG] molecule
to another molecule) form of filgrastim. Pegfilgrastim therefore becomes
a larger substance and as a result is not as easily eliminated from the body
via the kidneys. The decreased rate of urinary excretion keeps this G-CSF
in the body longer, thereby reducing the frequency of injections. Filgrastim requires daily IV or subcutaneous injections for up to 2 weeks to be effective, whereas pegfilgrastim only requires a once per chemotherapy cycle
injection to be effective. This reduction in dosing frequency reduces daily
clinic trips for daily injections for clients and their families.

Pegfilgrastim is used to decrease the incidence of infections and
febrile neutropenia in clients receiving chemotherapy for nonmyeloid
malignancies.

Side Effects and Adverse Reactions

Side effects are similar to those of filgrastim with the most
frequently reported adverse event being bone pain. This
bone pain is effectively reduced with acetaminophen 650 mg
or 400 mg ibruprofen by mouth every 4 to 6 hours.

PROTOTYPE DRUG CHART 37-3

SARGRAMOSTIM

Drug Class

Granulocyte macrophage colony-stimulating factor (GM-CSF)
Trade Name: Leukine
Pregnancy Category: C

Contraindications

Within 24 h of chemotherapy administration or within 12 h after last dose of radiation therapy; excessive leukemia myeloid blast cells in bone marrow; hypersensitivity to GM-CSF, yeast-derived products
Caution: Pregnancy, lactation, congestive heart failure; safety in children not established; not FDA approved for children

Pharmacokinetics

Absorption: IV: Essentially complete
Distribution: PB: UK
Metabolism: t½: 2 h
Excretion: Probably in urine

Dosage

A: IV 250 mcg/m²/d as a 2-h infusion for 21 d after autologous BMT; a maximum tolerated dose has not been determined
Some protocols use subQ administration.

Drug-Lab-Food Interactions

Drug: Lithium and steroids may *increase* effect
Lab: *Increase* in WBC and platelet counts, bilirubin, creatinine, and liver enzymes
Food: None known

Pharmacodynamics

IV: Onset: 7-14 d
  Peak: UK
  Duration: Baseline WBC by 1 wk after administration

Therapeutic Effects/Uses

To accelerate growth and development of bone marrow and circulating blood cell activity in autologous BMT
Mode of Action: Increased production and functional activity of eosinophils, macrophages, monocytes, and neutrophils

Side Effects

Generally well tolerated; diarrhea, fatigue, chills, weakness, local irritation at injection site; peripheral edema, rash

Adverse Reactions

Pleural/pericardial effusion, rigors, GI hemorrhage, dyspnea

A, Adult; *BMT,* bone marrow transplant; *d,* day; *FDA,* Food and Drug Administration; *GI,* gastrointestinal; *h,* hour; *IV,* intravenous; *PB,* protein-binding; *subQ,* subcutaneous; *t½,* half-life; *UK,* unknown; *WBC,* white blood cell; *wk,* week.

Dosing and Administration

The recommended dose is 6 mg of Pegfilgrastim administered as a single, subcutaneous injection given at least 24 hours after chemotherapy once per chemotherapy cycle.

Preparation, Storage, and Handling

Pegfilgrastim is supplied in prefilled syringes containing 6 mg in 0.6 ml. This colorless, preservative-free medication should be protected from light and refrigerated at 2° C to 8° C. Only one injection is to be given by syringe. Any unused pegfilgrastim should be discarded.

Granulocyte Macrophage Colony-Stimulating Factor

Granulocyte macrophage colony-stimulating factor (GM-CSF) belongs to a group of growth factors that support survival, clonal expression, and differentiation (maturation) of hematopoietic progenitor cells. GM-CSF induces partially committed progenitor (parent) cells to divide and differentiate in the granulocyte macrophage (a type of WBC responsible for recognizing and destroying bacteria through phagocytosis) pathway. GM-CSF, unlike G-CSF, is a multilineage factor, promoting proliferation of myelomonocytic,

megakaryocytic, and erythroid progenitors. Activated T cells, endothelial cells, and fibroblasts produce GM-CSF in vivo. Commercial production of GM-CSF is accomplished through recombinant DNA technology. GM-CSF is FDA approved for commercial use to induce and support myeloid reconstitution after autologous bone marrow transplant (BMT). A GM-CSF product is commercially available as sargramostim (Leukine). Prototype Drug Chart 37–3 presents the drug data for sargramostim.

Pharmacokinetics

GM-CSF has been found to effectively accelerate myeloid engraftment (growth and development of bone marrow and subsequent circulating blood cell activity) in autologous BMT. After autologous BMT in clients with non-Hodgkin's lymphoma, acute lymphoblastic leukemia, or Hodgkin's disease, GM-CSF administration resulted in accelerated myeloid engraftment, decreased duration of antibiotic use, reduced duration of infectious episodes, and shortened hospitalizations.

Side Effects and Adverse Reactions

Side effects of GM-CSF administration include fever, mucous membrane disorder, asthenia, malaise, sepsis, nausea, diarrhea, vomiting, anorexia, liver damage, alopecia, rash, peripheral edema, dyspnea, blood dyscrasias, renal dysfunction, and central nervous system disorder. GM-CSF should be administered with caution to clients with preexisting pleural or precardial effusions because it may increase fluid retention. Sequestration of granulocytes in the pulmonary circulation has been seen with GM-CSF administration. The phenomenon has resulted in dyspnea and suggests that special attention be given to respiratory symptoms during or immediately following GM-CSF infusions, a caution that is especially important for clients with underlying pulmonary disease. If dyspnea occurs, the GM-CSF infusion should be reduced by half or discontinued.

Supraventricular dysrhythmia has been observed during GM-CSF infusion, suggesting cautious administration in clients with preexisting cardiac disease. Renal and hepatic dysfunction, as indicated by elevated serum creatinine, bilirubin, and liver function tests, have occurred with GM-CSF administration. If these values become elevated, GM-CSF dosage should be reduced or therapy interrupted.

GM-CSF therapy is contraindicated in clients with excessive leukemia myeloid blast cells in the bone marrow or peripheral blood (>10%) and in clients with known hypersensitivity to GM-CSF, yeast-derived products, or any component of the product. Because of the sensitivity of rapidly dividing hematopoietic progenitor cells to cytotoxic chemotherapy or radiologic therapy, GM-CSF should not be administered within 24 hours before or after chemotherapy or within 12 hours before or after radiation therapy.

GM-CSF should be administered to pregnant women or nursing mothers only if clearly indicated (i.e., if the benefits outweigh the risks). Efficacy in the pediatric population has not been established.

Carcinogenic, mutagenic, or fertility effects have not been determined. Full evaluation of drug interactions have not been conducted; however, drugs that may potentiate the myeloproliferative effects of GM-CSF, such as lithium and corticosteroids, should be used with caution.

Dosing

The recommended dose of GM-CSF is 250 mcg/m²/day for 21 days as a 2-hour infusion beginning 2 to 4 hours after autologous bone marrow infusion.

Administration

GM-CSF should not be administered within 24 hours of chemotherapy administration or within 12 hours before or after radiation therapy. Manufacturers recommend dose reduction or discontinuation in the presence of a severe adverse reaction, blast cell (immature, possibly malignant cell) appearance, or underlying disease progression. GM-CSF therapy should be stopped if the ANC is greater than 20,000 cells/mm³ to avoid potential complications associated with leukocytosis.

Preparation

Leukine is supplied as a sterile, white, preservative-free lyophilized powder (powder that goes into solution quickly) in vials containing 250 or 500 mcg of sargramostim. The powder is reconstituted with 1 ml of sterile water for injec-

tion. During reconstitution, the diluent should be directed at the side of the vial and the contents gently swirled but not shaken. Further dilution with 0.9% sodium chloride only is done in preparation for the 2-hour IV infusion. The final concentration of solution should be greater than 10 mcg/ml. The infusion should be completed within 6 hours of preparation to ensure stability and potency. Sargramostim powder, reconstituted vials, and diluted solution should be refrigerated at 36° F to 46° F (2° C to 8° C).

Neumega (Oprelvekin)

Neumega is recombinant human interleukin-11, which is a platelet growth factor. This product can potentially prevent recurrent severe chemotherapy-induced thrombocytopenia. The active ingredient of Neumega is oprelvekin. Oprelvekin, according to the manufacturer, stimulates megakaryocyte and thrombocyte production. This effect results in functionally and morphologically normal circulating platelets. Neumega is advertised as "a much needed option in clients who are receiving myelosuppressive chemotherapy." The reasons for this claim are twofold: (1) with use of this product, chemotherapy administration does not have to be delayed because of a low platelet count, and (2) the need for potentially risk-associated platelet transfusions is reduced. Neumega is therefore indicated to prevent severe thrombocytopenia and to reduce the need for platelet transfusions following myelosuppressive chemotherapy. Efficacy is most evident in those who experience severe thrombocytopenia following the previous chemotherapy cycle.

Pharmacokinetics

Neumega is available for subQ administration in single-use vials containing 5 mg of oprelvekin as a sterile, lyophilized powder. When reconstituted with 1 ml of sterile water for injection, the resulting solution has a pH of 7.0 and a concentration of 5 mg/ml.

Product dosing should begin 6 to 24 hours after the completion of chemotherapy. Studies have shown that daily subQ dosing for 14 days increased the platelet count in a dose-dependent way. Platelet counts begin to increase between 5 and 9 days after the start of the Neumega administration. After use of the product is stopped, platelet counts continued to increase for up to 7 days and then return to baseline within 14 days.

Animal studies have demonstrated that Neumega is rapidly cleared from the serum and distributed to highly perfused organs. The kidney is the primary route of elimination, although most of the product is metabolized before excretion. Neumega is contraindicated in clients with a history of hypersensitivity to the product or any of its components.

Side Effects and Adverse Reactions

The side effects of Neumega include fluid retention, cardiovascular events, ophthalmologic events, and allergic reactions. Mild to moderate fluid retention without weight gain has resulted from product administration. Fluid retention, reversible within several days of product discontinuation, was manifested by peripheral edema; exertional dyspnea; and worsening of preexisting pleural effusions, ascites, and pericardial effusions. Transient atrial arrhythmias (fibrillation or flutter) have occurred in approximately 10% of clients. These arrhythmias may be related to fluid retention, advanced age, or underlying cardiac disease. Papilledema and transient visual blurring have been reported in about 1.5% of clients. The only reported allergic reaction has been a transient rash at the injection site. There have been no reports of anaphylaxis or hypersensitivity reactions.

Drug interactions between Neumega and other medications have not been fully evaluated. No studies have been done to assess the carcinogenic potential of the product. In addition, no studies have determined its use in children or in pregnant women or nursing mothers; its use in these situations should be carefully evaluated.

Dosing

The recommended dose of Neumega in adults is 50 mcg/kg given once daily. It should be administered subQ as a single injection in the thigh, abdomen, hip, or upper arm. Pediatric dosing (based on a pharmacokinetic study) should be 75 to 100 mcg/kg. The first dose of Neumega should be given 6 to 24 hours after the completion of chemotherapy. Platelet counts should be monitored to determine the duration of the Neumega therapy.

Administration

Administration should continue until the postnadir count is greater than 50,000 cells/μl. Dosing beyond 21 days is not recommended. Neumega should be discontinued at least 2 days before chemotherapy is begun.

Preparation

Reconstituted Neumega is a clear, colorless, isotonic solution with a pH of 7.0. During reconstitution, excessive agitation should be avoided. The sterile water for injection USP should be directed at the side of the vial and the contents gently swirled. A single-dose vial should not be reentered or reused. The parenteral drug products should be visually inspected; if they are discolored or contain particulate matter, they should be discarded.

Neumega should be used within 3 hours of reconstitution if it has been stored at either 36° F to 46° F (2° C to 8° C) or at room temperature up to 77° F (25° C). Neumega should not be frozen, and the reconstituted product should not be shaken.

Client Information

Self-administration of Neumega should not be attempted until the client fully understands the health care provider's instructions about its preparation, correct dose, and proper method for injection. The injection site should not be rubbed. The dose should be given at the same time each day. If a dose is missed, the next scheduled dose should be taken.

NOTE: Clients can safely receive concurrent doses of EPO, G-CSF and Neumega. Different injection sites should be used for each agent.

Interleukins

Interleukins are a group of proteins produced by the body's WBCs—the lymphocytes. Because interleukins are hormonelike glycoproteins manufactured by the lympho-cytes, they are sometimes called **lymphokines.** One of the most widely studied interleukins is interleukin-2 (IL-2).

This substance, first defined in 1976, has been found to have antitumor activities. The greatest antitumor effect has been identified in those with renal cell cancer or malignant melanoma.

IL-2 is produced commercially through recombinant DNA technology. It is marketed as aldesleukin (Proleukin) for use in the treatment of metastatic renal cell carcinoma.

Pharmacokinetics

IL-2, administered either by IV infusion or subQ injection, is rapidly distributed to the extravascular, extracellular space and eliminated from the body by metabolism in the kidney. The serum half-life of IL-2 is short. Because of this rapid clearance, IL-2 is administered in frequent, short infusions.

Side Effects and Adverse Reactions

The side effects most frequently reported as a result of IL-2 use include hypotension, nausea, vomiting, diarrhea, mental status changes, oliguria/anuria, anemia, thrombocytopenia, fever, chills, sinus tachycardia, pulmonary congestion, dyspnea, pain at injection site, fatigue, weakness, malaise, and elevated liver function tests. See Table 37–3 for additional side effects. According to the manufacturer, Proleukin should be permanently discontinued if certain organ system toxicities occur (Table 37–4) and held and then restarted under specific parameters for other toxicities (Table 37–5).

Preparation

Proleukin is supplied in single-use vials, each of which contains 22×10^6 units of Proleukin. Unreconstituted vials should be stored in a refrigerator at 36° F to 46° F (2° C to 8° C). When reconstituted aseptically with 1.2 ml of sterile water for injection, each vial contains 18 million IU (1.1 mg) of Proleukin. Bacteriostatic water should not be used. Inject the sterile water into the vial. The contents should be gently swirled, not shaken. The resulting solution should be a clear, colorless to pale yellow liquid. Discard any unused portion of the liquid. The indicated dose of Proleukin should be withdrawn from the vial and diluted into a 50-ml 5% dextrose IV bag. The IV bag, if not used immediately, can be stored for 48 hours in a refrigerator. Infuse over a 15-minute period through nonfiltered IV tubing. See Table 37–6 for dosage and administration information.

Monoclonal Antibody

Monoclonal antibodies are engineered in the laboratory with the specific purpose of targeting antigens and receptors that are expressed most frequently on cancer cells. Because of the specificity of the monoclonal antibody "targets," the use of these substances has become known as **targeted therapy. Epidermal growth factor receptor (EGFR), human epidermal growth factor 2 (HER2),** and **vascular endothelial growth factor (VEGF)** are three classes of targeted therapy.

Table 37–3

Incidence of Adverse Events to Interleukin-2

Events by Body System	% of Clients	Events by Body System	% of Clients
Cardiovascular		**Gastrointestinal**	
Hypotension	85	Nausea and vomiting	87
(requiring pressors)	71	Diarrhea	76
Sinus tachycardia	70	Stomatitis	32
Arrhythmias	22	Anorexia	27
Atrial	8	Gastrointestinal bleeding	13
Supraventricular	5	(requiring surgery)	2
Ventricular	3	Dyspepsia	7
Junctional	1	Constipation	5
Bradycardia	7	Intestinal perforation/ileus	2
Premature ventricular	5	Pancreatitis	<1
contractions			
Premature atrial contractions	4		
Myocardial ischemia	3	**Neurologic**	
Myocardial infarction	2	Mental status changes	73
Cardiac arrest	2	Dizziness	17
Congestive heart failure	1	Sensory dysfunction	10
Myocarditis	1	Special sensory disorders	7
Stroke	1	(vision, speech, taste)	
Gangrene	1	Syncope	3
Pericardial effusion	1	Motor dysfunction	2
Endocarditis	1	Coma	1
Thrombosis	1	Seizure (grand mal)	1

From *Proleukin: aldesleukin for injection*, Emeryville, Calif, 2000, Cetus/Chiron Corp.
<, Less than.

Table 37–4

Organ System Toxicities with Interleukin-2

Organ System	Permanently Discontinue Treatment for the Following Toxicities
Cardiovascular	Sustained ventricular tachycardia (5 beats)
	Cardiac rhythm disturbances not controlled or unresponsive to management
	Recurrent chest pain with electrocardiographic changes, documented angina, or myocardial infarction
	Pericardial tamponade
Pulmonary	Intubation required >72 h
Renal	Renal dysfunction requiring dialysis >72 h
Central nervous system	Coma or toxic psychosis lasting >48 h
	Repetitive or difficult to control seizures
Gastrointestinal	Bowel ischemia/perforation/gastrointestinal bleeding requiring surgery

From *Proleukin: aldesleukin for injection*, Emeryville, Calif, 2000, Cetus/Chiron Corp.
h, Hour; >, greater than.

Gefiinitib (Iressa) and cetuximab (Erbitux) are monoclonal antibodies in the EGFR class, trastuzumab (Herceptin) is in the HER2 class, and Bevacizumab (Avastin) is in the VEGF class.

Trastuzumab and a nonclassified monoclonal antibody, Rituximab, will be described.

Trastuzumab

Trastuzumab (Herceptin) is a recombinant humanized monoclonal antibody approved by the FDA for solo treatment of metastatic breast cancer in clients whose condition is refractory to chemotherapy or in combination with paclitaxel (Taxol) for first-line treatment of metastatic breast cancer. The drug is specifically for clients with tumors that overexpress the HER2 protein found in 25% to 30% of those with metastatic breast cancer. HER2 is structurally similar to the epidermal growth factor receptor.

Pharmacokinetics

The metabolism and elimination of trastuzumab are unknown. Following IV infusion, the half-life is dose dependent; the half-life is about 6 days with a weekly maintenance dose of 2 mg/kg. The initial dose is 4 mg/kg IV over 1.5 hours, followed by weekly maintenance doses of 2 mg/kg over half an hour. The estimated cost for 23 weeks of treatment for a 120-pound woman is about $14,000.

Table 37–5

Interleukin-2 Dose Held and Given

Organ System	Hold Dose For:	Subsequent Doses May be Given If:
Cardiovascular	Atrial fibrillation, supraventricular tachycardia, or bradycardia that requires treatment or is recurrent or persistent	Client is asymptomatic with full recovery to normal sinus rhythm
	Systolic BP <90 mm Hg with increasing requirements for pressors	Systolic BP 90 mm Hg and stable or improving requirements for pressors
	Any ECG change consistent with MI or ischemia with or without chest pain; suspicion of cardiac ischemia	Client is asymptomatic, MI has been ruled out, clinical suspicion of angina is low
Pulmonary	O_2 saturation <94% on room air or <90% with 2 L O_2 by nasal prongs	O_2 saturation 94% on room air or 90% with 2 L O_2 by nasal prongs
Central nervous system	Mental status changes, including moderate confusion or agitation	Mental status changes completely resolved
Systemic	Sepsis syndrome, client is clinically unstable	Sepsis syndrome has resolved, client is clinically stable, infection is under treatment
Renal	Serum creatinine 4.5 mg/dL or a serum creatinine of 4 mg/dL in the presence of severe volume overload, acidosis, or hyperkalemia	Serum creatinine <4 mg/dL and fluid and electrolyte status is stable
	Persistent oliguria, urine output of 10 ml/h for 16 to 24 h with rising serum creatinine	Urine output >10 ml/h with a decrease of serum creatinine 1.5 mg/dl or normalization of serum creatinine
Hepatic	Signs of hepatic failure including encephalopathy, increasing ascites, liver pain, hypoglycemia	All signs of hepatic failure have resolved*
Gastrointestinal	Stool guaiac repeatedly >3-4+	Stool guaiac negative
Skin	Bullous dermatitis or marked worsening of preexisting skin condition (avoid topical steroid therapy)	Resolution of all signs of bullous dermatitis

From *Proleukin: aldesleukin for injection,* Emeryville, Calif, 2000, Cetus/Chiron Corp.
BP, Blood pressure; *ECG,* electrocardiographic; *h,* hour; *MI,* myocardial infarction; O_2, oxygen; >, greater than; <, less than.
*Discontinue all further treatment for that course. Consider starting a new course of treatment at least 7 weeks after cessation of adverse event and hospital discharge.

Table 37–6

Interleukin*

Generic (Brand)	Route and Dosage	Uses and Considerations
interleukin-2 (Proleukin)	*Metastatic renal cancer:* A: IV: 600,000 international units/kg (0.037 mg/kg) by a 15-min IV infusion q8h for a total of 14 doses. Following 9 days of rest, the schedule is repeated for another 14 doses, for a maximum of 28 doses per course *Renal cancer studies:* 18 million international units/m²/d for 5 d, followed by 2 d rest, then 9 million or 18 million international units/m²/d, 5 d/wk, for 5 wk	For treating metastatic renal cancer. This dosage schedule and route have also been used in renal cancer studies.

A, Adult; *d,* day; *h,* hour; *IV,* intravenous; *min,* minute; *wk,* week.
*Clients receiving IL-2 by any route, in any dose, and in any setting—inpatient or outpatient—should be monitored closely for signs of toxicity.

Side Effects and Adverse Reactions

Trastuzumab can be cardiotoxic; this risk is increased in older adults, in those with previous cardiac disease, and in those with previous exposure to an anthracycline. A flulike symptom complex (fever, chills, nausea, vomiting, headache, asthenia, and pain) occurs in about 40% of clients after first and sometimes later infusions. However, trastuzumab does not cause myelosuppression or alopecia.

Rituximab

Rituximab (Rituxan) is a monoclonal antibody used to treat clients with relapsed or refractory low-grade or follicular, CD20-positive, B-cell non-Hodgkin's lymphoma. The mechanism of action of this genetically engineered chimeric murine/human monoclonal antibody is directed against the CD20 antigen found on the surface of normal and malignant B lymphocytes. The antibody is an IgGI kappa immunoglobulin, which binds specifically to the antigen CD20.

Table 37–7

Additional Monoclonal Antibodies (Targeted Therapies)

Drug	Indications	Adverse Reactions
gemtuzumab ogogamicin (Mylotarg)	Humanized MAb conjugated with antitumor antibiotic calicheamicin. Treatment of CD33 positive AML in clients over 60 y in first relapse or not eligible for other chemo; 30% remission rate.	Severe bone marrow suppression in all clients due to CD33 antigen on normal cells. Other serious events are hypersensitivity reactions (anaphylaxis, hepatotoxicity, tumor lysis syndrome). Give acetaminophen and diphenhydramine before infusion to reduce infusion reactions that usually occur within 24 h. Corticosteroids and meperidine may also be needed. Monitor electrolytes, CBC, platelets, and liver enzymes.
alemtuzumab (Campath)	Humanized MAb for treatment of B-cell CLL for those treated with alkylating agents and refractory to fludarabine.	Hematologic toxicity, opportunistic infections, infusion reactions. Premedicate and titrate the dose slowly. Prophylaxis for *Pneumocystis carinii* and herpes is recommended. Monitor CBC and CD4 counts.
ibritumomab tiuxetan (Zevalin)	Radiolabeled MAb for B-cell non-Hodgkin's lymphoma as part of regimen after administration of rituximab (follow premed guidelines)	Severe, prolonged, and delayed bone marrow suppression. Monitor CBC and platelet count.
tositumomab and iodine-131 tositumomab (Bexxar)	Mouse derived MAb for CD20-positive, follicular non-Hodgkin's lymphomas refractory to rituximab with relapse.	Severe and prolonged neutropenia, thrombocytopenia, and anemia. Need thyroid protective medications (start 1 d before and continue for 14 d after). Monitor CBC and serum creatinine. Iodine-131 contraindicated in pregnancy.
cetuximab (Erbitux)	Chimeric MAb, binds to EGRF, for advanced metastatic colon cancer in combination with irinotecan (Camptosar).	May get infusion reactions, usually with first treatment, mild to severe. Pretreat with diphenhydramine. Test for EGRF before use.
bevacizumab (Avastin)	Humanized MAb, angiogenesis inhibitor. First-line treatment for metastatic colorectal cancer in combination with 5-FU.	GI perforation, hemorrhage, impaired wound healing. Also kidney damage and CHF, HTN. Monitor BP, serial urinalysis (hold drug if 24-h urine protein is >2 g).

AML, Acute monocytic leukemia; *BP,* blood pressure; *CBC,* complete blood cell count; *CHF,* chronic heart failure; *CLL,* chronic lymphocytic leukemia; *d,* day; *EGRF,* epidermal growth factor receptor; *5-FU,* fluorouracil; *g,* gram; *GI,* gastrointestinal; *h,* hour; *HTN,* hypertension; *MAb,* monoclonal antibody; *y,* year; >, greater than.

Pharmacokinetics and Pharmacodynamics

Following IV infusion, rituximab shows immediate results in a rapid and sustained depletion or circulating and tissue-based B cells. The half-life is 60 hours after the first infusion and 174 hours after the fourth infusion. Rituximab is detectable in clients 3 to 6 months after completion of treatment; B-cell recovery begins about 6 months after completion of treatment.

Side Effects and Adverse Reactions

Adverse reactions in greater than 10% of clients include headache, fever, chills, nausea, leukopenia, asthenia, and angioedema.

Dosing

IV push of bolus should not be administered to avoid hypersensitivity reactions. Premedication of acetaminophen and diphenhydramine should be considered before infusion of rituximab to attenuate infusion-related events. Withholding antihypertensive medications should be considered 12 hours before infusion of rituximab to avoid transient hypotension during infusion.

The recommended adult dose of rituximab is 375 mg/m² IV once weekly × 4 doses (days 1, 8, 15, and 22). The initial rate is 50 mg per hour every 30 minutes to a maximum of 400 mg per hour.

Refer to Table 37–7 for information on additional monoclonal antibodies (targeted therapies). See the Preventing Medication Errors box for a safety alert related to BRMs.

PREVENTING MEDICATION ERRORS

Do not confuse these BRMs:

- **Epoietin alfa (Epogen, Procrit)** with **Neupogen**
- **Filgrastim (Neupogen)** with **Epogen, Nutramigen**
- **Sargramostim (Leukine)** with **Leukeran**
- **Interferon alfa-2a (Roferon-A)** with **Interferon alfa 2b**
- **Interferon alfa-2b (Intron-A)** with **Interferon alfa-2a**
- **Interferon beta-1a (Avonex, Rebif)** with **Avelox, interferon beta-1b**
- **Interferon beta-1b (Betaseron)** with **Interferon beta-1a**
- **Interleukin-2 (Il-2, Proleukin)** with **Interferon 2**

Nursing Process

Biologic Response Modifiers

ASSESSMENT

■ Obtain a drug and herb history from client.

■ Obtain baseline information about client's physical status. This should include height, weight, vital signs, laboratory values (complete blood count [CBC], uric acid, electrolytes, blood urea nitrogen [BUN], creatinine, and liver function tests), cardiopulmonary assessment, intake and output, skin assessment, daily activities status (i.e., ability to perform activities of daily living, sleep-rest cycle), nutritional status, presence or absence of underlying symptoms of disease, and the use of current or past medication and treatment.

■ Assess CBC (with filgrastim, sargramostim, and Neumega) before therapy and biweekly throughout therapy to avoid leukocytosis and thrombocytosis. Assess renal and hepatic function tests in clients with dysfunction (liver enzymes, BUN, serum creatinine). With erythropoietin, assess blood pressure before start of and especially early in therapy. Most clients will need supplemental iron. Desired levels are >100 ng/ml for serum ferritin and >20% for serum iron transferrin saturation.

■ Obtain baseline data regarding client's psychosocial status, including educational level, ability and desire to learn, support systems, past coping strategies, presence or absence of emotional difficulties, and self-care abilities.

■ Assess client for signs and symptoms of biologic response modifiers (BRMs), such as fatigue, chills, diarrhea, and weakness. With filgrastim, be alert to changes in clients with preexisting cardiac conditions.

■ Assess client's and family's ability to administer subcutaneous BRMs.

■ Determine client's and family's understanding of BRMs and related side effects.

NURSING DIAGNOSES

■ Altered nutrition; less than body requirements
■ Risk for infection
■ Risk for deficient fluid volume
■ Impaired oral mucous membrane
■ Fatigue
■ Disturbed body image
■ Anxiety
■ Fear
■ Risk for caregiver role strain

PLANNING

■ Client and family will verbalize an understanding of the importance of reporting BRM-related side effects.

■ Client and family will demonstrate correct and safe BRM administration.

■ Client and family will identify strategies to deal with BRM-related side effects.

■ Client will remain free of infection (filgrastim and sargramostim).

■ Client will remain free of hemorrhage.

NURSING INTERVENTIONS

■ Monitor client's temperature at the onset of chills.

■ Administer prescribed meperidine 25 to 50 mg intravenously to decrease rigors.

■ Premedicate client with acetaminophen to reduce chills and fever and with diphenhydramine to reduce nausea.

■ Cover client with blankets to promote warmth during chills.

■ Encourage client to rest when tired and to notify health care provider if profound fatigue or anorexia occurs.

■ Encourage client to drink at least 2 L of fluid a day to promote excretion of cellular breakdown products.

■ Administer an antiemetic as necessary. Premedicate client with antiemetic and administer antiemetic around the clock for 24 hours after BRM administration to further delay nausea or vomiting.

■ Consult dietitian, social worker, and physical or occupational therapist as necessary.

■ Provide client and family the opportunity to discuss the effect of BRM therapy on the quality of life.

■ Refer client and family to a financial counselor if reimbursement of BRM therapy is problematic.

■ Administer BRM at bedtime to decrease the consequences of fatigue.

■ Continue with the same brand of BRM, and notify the health care provider if considering changing the brand.

■ Remember, with sargramostim, use only one dose per vial; be alert for expiration date. Avoid shaking vial. Reconstituted solutions are clear; use within 6 hours and discard unused portion. Recall that albumin may be added, depending on drug concentration, to prevent adsorption of drug to components of the drug delivery system.

■ Remember, with filgrastim, drug vials are for one-time use; any vial left at room temperature for more than 6 hours should be discarded. Drug vials are preservative free. Store in refrigerator at 2° C to 8° C. Avoid shaking vials.

■ Remember, with Neumega, avoid excessive agitation during preparation. Use only one dose per vial. Inspect the parenteral product and discard if it is discolored or has particulate matter. Use within 3 hours of reconstitution if stored at 36° F to 46° F (2° C to 8° C). Avoid freezing or shaking the drug.

Client Teaching

General

- Explain to client and family the rationale for BRM therapy.
- Explain the frequency and rationale for studies and procedures during BRM therapy.
- Inform client and family that most BRM side effects disappear within 72 to 96 hours after discontinuation of therapy.
- Instruct clients of childbearing age to use contraceptives during BRM therapy and for 2 years after completion of therapy.
- Provide client with information regarding the effect of BRM-related fatigue on sexuality.
- Explain to client that herb use concurrent with BRM therapy is not recommended. See Herbal Alert 37–1.

Side Effects

- Advise client to report episodes of difficulty in concentration, confusion, or somnolence.
- Report weight loss.
- Report dyspnea, palpitations, and signs of infection or bleeding.

Self-Administration

- Demonstrate correct drug administration techniques.
- Provide client and family with written or video instructions regarding BRM self-administration.

Cultural Considerations ⊕

- Obtain an interpreter when necessary; do not rely on family members, who may not fully disclose because of honor or shame.

EVALUATION

- Evaluate client's and family's education strategies by asking them to discuss the potential effect of BRM therapy on the quality of life.
- Evaluate client's and family's BRM self-administration technique.
- Evaluate periodically client's and family's management of BRM-related side effects.
- There will be a decreased incidence of infection in clients after autologous bone marrow transplantation.
- There will be a decreased incidence of thrombocytopenia in clients after chemotherapy administration.

Summary

BRM therapy is growing rapidly. As clinical trial results yield more information about BRM activity and clinical efficacy, the indications for the use of BRMs will expand. As more is learned about the effect of BRMs on the quality of client life, attention will be directed toward side effect management and symptom prevention. Nurses play a key role in both the identification and management of BRM-related toxicities. Through assessment of clients receiving BRMs and a knowledge of BRM activity, nurses can develop a plan of care that will result in clients receiving BRM therapy in a safe and comfortable manner.

WEBSITES

For further information on *Biologic Response Modifiers,* visit these Internet resources:

Side effects of biologic response modifiers:
http://cancer-symptoms.org/cancer-treatments/Biological-Response-Modifiers.htm

Cancer treatment: Immunotherapy and biological response modifiers:
http://www.bccancer.bc.ca/PPI/CancerTreatment/ImmunotherapyBiologicalResponseModifiers.htm

Critical Thinking Case Study

J.W., age 55, has metastatic non–small cell cancer of the lung. His past treatment regimen included external-beam chest irradiation and combination chemotherapy. Two weeks before hospitalization, J.W. received a course of carboplatin, vinblastine (Velban), and methotrexate as an outpatient. He was admitted to the hospital with neutropenia, thrombocytopenia, and anemia. Upon assessment, J.W. was cachectic, weak, and able to perform activities of daily living only with assistance. Admitting laboratory data were Hgb (hemoglobin) 6.9, Hct (hematocrit) 20.6, platelets 16,000, and WBC 600 with ANC of 96. J.W. was started on Neupogen 480 mcg subQ daily; EPO 10,000 U subQ every other day; and Neumega 50 mcg/kg subQ daily. Parenteral antibiotic therapy was also initiated. Nursing diagnoses for J.W. included a potential for infection related to neutropenia, fatigue related to anemia, and anxiety related to hospitalization.

Nursing interventions included the following:

1. Maintaining good hand washing before and after client contact

2. Allowing no one with cold or infection to enter client's room

3. Obtaining vital signs and pulmonary assessment every 4 hours

4. Inspecting all sites associated with a risk for infection (e.g., venipuncture sites, oral cavity, perirectal area) every shift

5. Applying no suppositories, enemas, or urinary catheters and obtaining no rectal temperatures

6. Monitoring laboratory values daily

7. Wearing masks at all times during client contact

8. Providing bedside physical therapy

9. Giving emotional support to client and family

10. Instructing client and family in giving subQ injections and about the signs and symptoms of infection

J.W. continued therapy with filgrastim (Neupogen), oprelvekin (Neumega), and erythropoietin (EPO). The following laboratory data were obtained:

LAB TESTS	DAY 1	DAY 2	DAY 3	DAY 4	DAY 5
Hgb	6.9	6.5	7.1	7.8	7.9
Hct	20.6	19.4	21.6	22.9	22.9
Platelets	16,000	15,000	16,000	20,000	30,000
WBC/ANC	600/96	1000/0	1200/168	9400/4700	31,500/18,270

Neupogen was discontinued on day 5 and antibiotics were discontinued on day 4, but EPO and Neumega were continued. J.W.'s physical therapy was continued in the physical therapy department. Because J.W. refused red blood cell transfusion on the basis of religious beliefs, he was discharged to home (day 5) on EPO 10,000 units subQ every other day and Neumega 50 mcg/kg subQ daily for 7 days.

1. Why were Neupogen, Neumega, and EPO indicated?

2. What is an often overlooked side effect of EPO? Based on this side effect, what should be closely monitored in a client receiving this agent?

3. On days 1 to 4, for what is a client receiving this agent at high risk?

M.J., age 38, has stage IV breast cancer that was diagnosed 3 years ago. When first diagnosed, she underwent lumpectomy, axillary node dissection, and breast irradiation. She recently was seen by her medical oncologist with complaints of lower back pain and dyspnea at rest. Magnetic resonance imaging (MRI) identified bone metastasis in the thoracic and lumbar spine, and chest radiographs revealed a large left-sided pleural effusion. M.J. has a history of atrial fibrillation. She takes MS Contin and MSIR (morphine sulfate) for back pain. She receives radiation to her lower thoracic and lumbar spine. She has also received two courses of chemotherapy. She tolerated the first course without incident. Ten days after the second course, however, she was seen at the emergency department with shortness of breath, fever, chills, weakness, and a 2-day history of epistaxis and bruising. Laboratory results are Hb 9.5, WBC 1000 with 30% neutrophils, 50% lymphocytes, 5% bands, platelet count 9000. She is admitted to the oncology unit with orders for IV fluid, empiric antibiotics, Neupogen, and Neumega. M.J. is a single mother who lives at home with her two children, a 10-year-old son and a 6-year-old daughter.

Critical Thinking Case Study—cont'd

1. Why are Neupogen and Neumega indicated? What is the client's ANC?

2. How would the products be ordered?

3. What are the expected side effects of these agents?

4. What are the nursing interventions for the client's hospital stay and postdischarge?

5. How long should Neupogen and Neumega be administered?

6. Discuss the use of trastuzumab (Herceptin) in this client's situation.

Study Questions

1. Identify the three functions of BRMs.

2. Describe how colony-stimulating factors exert their effect in the body.

3. List the side effects of interferon-α, G-CSF, GM-CSF, Neumega, interleukin-2, and trastuzumab (Herceptin).

4. Discuss client and family teaching strategies for clients receiving EPO.

5. Explain how to administer EPO, G-CSF, GM-CSF, and Neumega.

6. Describe the nursing assessment for clients receiving interleukin-2. The discussion should include preadministration, administration, and postadministration assessments.

7. Identify at least six monoclonal antibodies.

8. Mrs. A. lives 120 miles from her medical oncologist office and relies on her working daughter for transportation to and from the doctor's office. Which GCSF would be most appropriate for her and why?

9. Identify nursing interventions for clients receiving monoclonal antibodies.

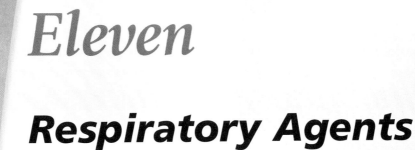

Eleven

Respiratory Agents

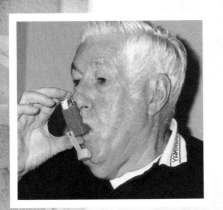

The respiratory tract is divided into two major parts: (1) the upper respiratory tract, which consists of the nares, nasal cavity, pharynx, and larynx, and (2) the lower respiratory tract, which consists of the trachea, bronchi, bronchioles, alveoli, and alveolar-capillary membrane. Air enters through the upper respiratory tract and travels to the lower respiratory tract where gas exchanges occur. Figure XI–1 illustrates these components.

Ventilation and *respiration* are distinct terms and should not be used interchangeably. *Ventilation* is the movement of air from the atmosphere through the upper and lower airways to the alveoli. *Respiration* is the process whereby gas exchange occurs at the alveolar-capillary membrane. Respiration has the following three phases:

1. Ventilation, in which oxygen passes through the airways
2. Perfusion, in which blood from the pulmonary circulation is adequate at the alveolar-capillary bed
3. Diffusion (molecules move from higher concentration to lower concentration) of gases, in which oxygen passes into the capillary bed to be circulated and carbon dioxide leaves the capillary bed and diffuses into the alveoli for ventilatory excretion

Perfusion is influenced by alveolar pressure. For gas exchange, the perfusion of each alveolus must be matched by adequate ventilation. Factors such as mucosal edema, secretions, and bronchospasm increase the resistance to airflow and decrease ventilation and diffusion of gases.

The chest cavity is a closed compartment bounded by 12 ribs, the diaphragm, thoracic vertebrae, sternum, neck muscles, and intercostal muscles between the ribs. The pleura are membranes that encase the lungs. The lungs are divided into lobes: the right lung has three lobes and the left lung has two lobes. The heart, which is not attached to the lungs, lies on the midleft side in the chest cavity.

Lung Compliance

Lung compliance (lung volume based on the unit of pressure in the alveoli) determines the lung's ability to stretch (i.e., tissue elasticity). Lung compliance is determined by (1) connective tissue (collagen and elastin) and (2) surface tension in the alveoli that is controlled by surfactant. Surfactant lowers the surface tension in the alveoli and prevents interstitial fluid from entering. Increased (high) lung compliance is present with chronic obstructive pulmonary disease (COPD), and decreased (low) lung compliance occurs with restrictive pulmonary disease. With low compliance, there is decreased lung volume, resulting from increased connective tissue or increased surface tension; the lungs become "stiff," and it takes greater than normal pressure to expand lung tissue.

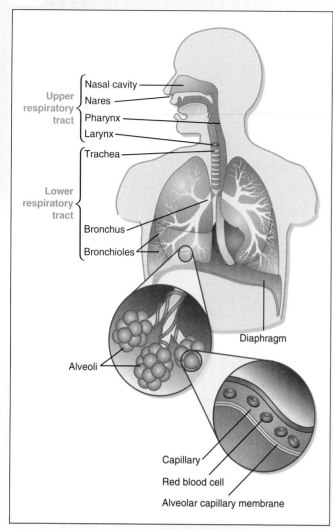

FIGURE XI–1   Basic structures of the respiratory tract.

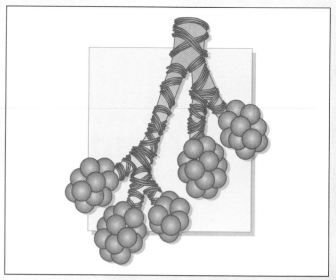

FIGURE XI–2   The bronchial smooth muscle fibers become more closely spaced as they near the alveoli.

Control Of Respiration

Oxygen (O_2), carbon dioxide (CO_2), and hydrogen (H^+) ion concentration in the blood influence respiration. Chemoreceptors are sensors that are stimulated by changes in these gases and ion. The central chemoreceptors, located in the medulla near the respiratory center and cerebrospinal fluid, respond to an increase in carbon dioxide and a decrease in pH by increasing ventilation. However, if the carbon dioxide level remains elevated, the stimulus to increase ventilation is lost.

Peripheral chemoreceptors, located in the carotid and aortic bodies, respond to changes in oxygen (PO_2) levels. A low blood oxygen level ($PO_2 < 60$ mm Hg) stimulates the peripheral chemoreceptors, which in turn stimulate the respiratory center in the medulla, and ventilation is increased. If oxygen therapy increases the oxygen level in the blood, the PO_2 may be too high to stimulate the peripheral chemoreceptors, and ventilation will be depressed.

Bronchial Smooth Muscle

The tracheobronchial tube is composed of smooth muscle whose fibers spiral around the tracheobronchial tube, becoming more closely spaced as they near the terminal bronchioles (Figure XI–2). Contraction of these muscles constricts the airway. The sympathetic and parasympathetic nervous systems affect the bronchial smooth muscle in opposite ways. The vagus nerve (parasympathetic nervous system) releases acetylcholine, which causes bronchoconstriction. The sympathetic nervous system releases epinephrine, which stimulates the beta$_2$ receptor in the bronchial smooth muscle, resulting in bronchodilation. These two nervous systems counterbalance each other to maintain homeostasis.

Cyclic adenosine monophosphate (cyclic AMP) in the cytoplasm of bronchial cells increases bronchodilation by relaxing the bronchial smooth muscles. The pulmonary enzyme phosphodiesterase can inactivate cyclic AMP. Drugs of the methylxanthine group (theophylline) inactivate phosphodiesterase thus permitting cyclic AMP to function.

This unit includes Chapter 38, Drugs for Common Upper Respiratory Disorders, and Chapter 39, Drugs for Acute and Chronic Lower Respiratory Disorders. Chapter 38 discusses drugs used to relieve cold symptoms, such as antihistamines, decongestants, antitussives, and expectorants. Drugs used to alleviate and control airway obstruction are presented in Chapter 39. These include the sympathomimetics (adrenergics), particularly the beta$_2$ adrenergics; the methylxanthines, such as theophylline; leukotriene receptor antagonists; glucocorticoids; cromolyn sodium; and mucolytics.

38 Drugs for Common Upper Respiratory Disorders

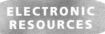

Additional information can be found on the companion website at *http://evolve.elsevier.com/KeeHayes/pharmacology/* or on the companion CD-ROM, which includes:

* *NCLEX-style examination review questions*
* *Pharmacology animations*
* *Medication error and IV therapy checklists*
* *Medication calculation problems*
* *Electronic calculators*

OUTLINE

OBJECTIVES

* Compare *antihistamine, decongestant, antitussive,* and *expectorant drug groups.*
* Differentiate between *rhinitis, sinusitis,* and *pharyngitis.*
* Identify the side effects of nasal decongestants and explain how they can be avoided.
* Describe the nursing process, including client teaching, for drugs used to treat the common cold.

TERMS

acute pharyngitis
acute rhinitis
allergic rhinitis
antihistamines

antitussives
common cold
decongestants
expectorants

rebound nasal congestion
rhinorrhea
sinusitis

Introduction

Upper respiratory infections (URIs) include the common cold, acute rhinitis, sinusitis, and acute pharyngitis. The common cold is the most prevalent type of URI. Adults have an average of two to four colds per year, and children have an average of 4 to 12 colds per year. Incidence is seasonally variable, with approximately 50% of the population experiencing a winter cold and 25% experiencing a summer cold. Normally, a cold is not considered a life-threatening illness; however, it causes physical and mental discomfort and loss of time at work and school. The common cold is an expensive illness in the United States—more than $500 million is spent each year on over-the-counter (OTC) cold and cough preparations.

Common Cold, Acute Rhinitis, and Allergic Rhinitis

The **common cold** is caused by the rhinovirus and affects primarily the nasopharyngeal tract. **Acute rhinitis** (acute inflammation of the mucous membranes of the nose) usually accompanies the common cold. Acute rhinitis is not the same as **allergic rhinitis,** often called *hay fever,* which is caused by pollen or a foreign substance (e.g., animal dander). Nasal secretions increase in both acute rhinitis and allergic rhinitis.

A cold is most contagious 1 to 4 days before the onset of symptoms (the incubation period) and during the first 3 days of the cold. Transmission occurs more frequently from touching contaminated surfaces and then touching the nose or mouth than it does from viral droplets released by sneezing.

There is an old saying, "Curing a cold takes 1 week with treatment or 7 days without treatment." Home remedies include rest, chicken noodle soup, hot toddy (sugar, alcohol, and tea), vitamin C (which is debatable), and megadoses of vitamins (which is controversial). The four groups of drugs used to manage cold symptoms are antihistamines (H_1 blocker), decongestants (sympathomimetic amines), antitussives, and expectorants. These drugs can be used singly or in combination preparations.

Symptoms of the common cold include **rhinorrhea** (watery nasal discharge), nasal congestion, cough, and increased mucosal secretions. If a bacterial infection secondary to the cold occurs, infectious rhinitis may result and the nasal discharge becomes tenacious, mucoid, and yellow or yellow-green. The nasal secretions are discolored by white blood cells and cellular debris that are byproducts of the fight against the bacterial infection. Antibiotics used to treat bacterial respiratory infections are discussed in Chapters 28 (Antibacterials: Penicillins and Cephalosporins), 29 (Antibacterials: Macrolides, Tetracyclines, Aminoglycosides, and Fluoroquinolones), and 30 (Antibacterials: Sulfonamides).

Antihistamines

Antihistamines, H_1 blockers or H_1 antagonists, compete with histamine for receptor sites, thus preventing a histamine response. The two types of histamine receptors, H_1 and H_2, cause different responses. When the H_1 receptor is stimulated, the extravascular smooth muscles, including those lining the nasal cavity, are constricted. With stimulation of the H_2 receptor, an increase in gastric secretions occurs, which is a cause of peptic ulcer (see Chapter 46, Antiulcer Drugs). These two types of histamine receptors should not be confused. Antihistamines decrease nasopharyngeal secretions by blocking the H_1 receptor.

Although antihistamines are commonly used as cold remedies, these agents can also treat allergic rhinitis. However, the antihistamines are not useful in an emergency situation such as anaphylaxis. Most antihistamines are rapidly absorbed in 15 minutes, but they are not potent enough to combat anaphylaxis.

First-Generation Antihistamines

The antihistamine group can be divided into first and second generations. Most first-generation antihistamines cause drowsiness, dry mouth, and other anticholinergic symptoms, whereas second-generation antihistamines have fewer anticholinergic effects and a lower incidence of drowsiness. Many OTC cold remedies contain a first-generation antihistamine, which can cause drowsiness; therefore clients should be alerted not to drive or operate dangerous machinery when taking such medications. The anticholinergic properties of most antihistamines cause dryness of the mouth and decreased secretions, making them useful in treating rhinitis caused by the common cold. Antihistamines also decrease the nasal itching and tickling that cause sneezing.

The first-generation antihistamine diphenhydramine (Benadryl) has been available for years and is frequently combined with other ingredients in cold remedy preparations. Its primary use is to treat rhinitis. Prototype Drug Chart 38–1 lists the pharmacologic behavior of diphenhydramine.

Second-Generation Antihistamines

The second-generation antihistamines are frequently called *nonsedating antihistamines* because they have little to no effect on sedation. In addition, these antihistamines cause fewer anticholinergic symptoms. Although a moderate amount of alcohol and other central nervous system (CNS) depressants may be taken with second-generation antihistamines, many clinicians advise against such use.

The second-generation antihistamines, cetirizine (Zyrtec), fexofenadine (Allegra), and loratadine (Claritin), have half-lives between 7 to 15 hours. Azelastine (Astelin, Optivar) is a second-generation antihistamine that has a half-life of 22

PROTOTYPE DRUG CHART 38–1

DIPHENHYDRAMINE

Drug Class	**Dosage**
Antihistamine	**A: PO:** 25-50 mg q6-8h
Trade Name: Benadryl, ❦ Allerdryl	**A: IM/IV:** 10-50 mg as single dose, q4-6h; *max:* 400 mg/d
Pregnancy Category: B	**C: PO/IM/IV:** 5 mg/kg/d in 4 divided doses; *max:* 300 mg/d
Contraindications	**Drug-Lab-Food Interactions**
Acute asthmatic attack, severe liver disease, lower respiratory disease, neonate; MAOIs	*Drug: Increase* CNS depression with alcohol, narcotics, hypnotics, barbiturates; avoid use of MAOIs
Caution: Narrow-angle glaucoma, benign prostatic hypertrophy, pregnancy, newborn or premature infant, breastfeeding, urinary retention	

Pharmacokinetics	**Pharmacodynamics**
Absorption: PO: Well absorbed	**PO:** Onset: 15-45 min
Distribution: PB: 98%	Peak: 1-4 h
Metabolism: t½: 2-7 h	Duration: 4-8 h
Excretion: In urine as metabolites	**IM:** Onset: 15-30 min
	Peak: 1-4 h
	Duration: 4-7 h
	IV: Onset: Immediate
	Peak: 0.5-1 h
	Duration: 4-7 h

Therapeutic Effects/Uses

To treat allergic rhinitis, itching; to prevent motion sickness; sleep aid; antitussive
Mode of Action: Blocks histamine₁ thereby decreasing allergic response; affects respiratory system, blood vessels, and GI system

Side Effects	**Adverse Reactions**
Drowsiness, dizziness, fatigue, nausea, vomiting, urinary retention, constipation, blurred vision, dry mouth and throat, reduced secretions, hypotension, epigastric distress, hearing disturbances; excitation in children; photosensitivity	**Life-threatening:** Agranulocytosis, hemolytic anemia, thrombocytopenia

A, Adult; *C,* child; *CNS,* central nervous system; *d,* day; *GI,* gastrointestinal; *h,* hour; *IM,* intramuscular; *IV,* intravenous; *MAOIs,* monoamine oxidase inhibitors; *max,* maximum; *min,* minute; *PB,* protein-binding; *PO,* by mouth; *t¹/₂,* half-life; ❦, Canadian drug name.

---

hours and is administered by nasal spray. Table 38–1 lists the first- and second-generation antihistamines used to treat rhinitis.

Pharmacokinetics

Diphenhydramine can be administered orally, intramuscularly (IM), or intravenously (IV). It is well absorbed from the gastrointestinal (GI) tract, but systemic absorption from topical use is minimal. It is highly protein bound (98%) and has an average half-life of 2 to 7 hours. Diphenhydramine is metabolized by the liver and excreted as metabolites in the urine.

Pharmacodynamics

Diphenhydramine blocks the effects of histamine by competing for and occupying H₁-receptor sites. It has anticholinergic effects and should not be used by clients with narrow-angle glaucoma. Drowsiness is a major

side effect of the drug; in fact, it is sometimes used in sleep-aid products. Diphenhydramine is also used as an antitussive (i.e., it alleviates cough). Its onset of action can occur in as few as 15 minutes when taken orally and IM. IV administration results in an immediate onset of action. The duration of action is 4 to 8 hours.

Diphenhydramine can cause CNS depression if taken with alcohol, narcotics, hypnotics, or barbiturates.

Side Effects of Most First-Generation Antihistamines

The most common side effects of first-generation antihistamines are drowsiness, dizziness, fatigue, and disturbed coordination. Skin rashes and anticholinergic symptoms (e.g., dry mouth, urine retention, blurred vision, wheezing) may also occur.

Table 38-1

Antihistamines for Treatment of Allergic Rhinitis

Generic (Brand)	Route and Dosage	Uses and Considerations
First-Generation Antihistamines		
Alkylamine Derivatives		
brompheniramine maleate (Bromphen, Dimetane)	A: PO: 4 mg q4-6h or SR: 8 mg q8-12h; *max:* 24 mg/d IM/IV/subQ: 10 mg q8-12h; *max:* 40 mg/d C: 6-12 y: PO: 2 mg q4-6h; *max:* 12 mg/d	For allergies. Also present in various cough and decongestant formulas. *Pregnancy category:* C; PB: UK; t½: 25-36 h
chlorpheniramine maleate (Chlor-Trimeton, Kloromin, Phenetron, Telechlor, Teldrin)	A: PO: 2-4 mg q4-6h; *max:* 24 mg/24 h SR: 8-12 mg q8-12 h C: 6-12 y: PO: 2 mg q4-6h; *max:* 12 mg/d	For allergies including allergic rhinitis. May be used in combination with nasal decongestant. *Pregnancy category:* C; PB: 72%; t½: 20-24 h
dexchlorpheniramine maleate (Dexchlor, Poladex, Polaramine)	A: PO: 2 mg q4-6h or SR: 4-6 mg q8-12h or at bedtime C: >6 y: PO: 1 mg q4-6h or SR: 4 mg at bedtime	Relief of allergic rhinitis. May be used with epinephrine to treat anaphylactic reaction. *Pregnancy category:* B; PB: UK; t½: UK
Ethanolamine Derivatives		
clemastine fumarate (Tavist)	A: PO: 1.34-2.68 mg b.i.d./t.i.d.; *max:* 8 mg/d C: <12 y: PO: 0.67-1.34 mg b.i.d.	For relief of allergic rhinitis and urticaria. *Pregnancy category:* C; PB: UK; t½: UK
diphenhydramine (Benadryl)	See Prototype Drug Chart 38-1.	
Ethylenediamines		
tripelennamine (PBZ)	A: PO: 25-50 mg q4-6h or 100 mg sustained release q8-12h, *max:* 600 mg/d C: PO: 5 mg/kg/d in 4-6 divided doses, *max:* 300 mg/d	For relief of symptoms of allergic conditions. *Pregnancy category:* B; PB: UK; t½: UK
Piperidine Derivatives		
azatadine maleate (Optimine)	A: PO: 1-2 mg b.i.d./t.i.d. C: <12 y: PO: not recommended	Relief of allergic rhinitis and chronic urticaria. Drowsiness, dizziness, and hypotension may occur. *Pregnancy category:* B; PB: UK; t½: 9-12 h
cyproheptadine HCl (Periactin)	A: PO: 4-20 mg/d in divided doses; *max:* 0.5 mg/kg/d C: >6 y: PO: 4 mg q8-12h; *max:* 16 mg/d C: 2-6 y: PO: 2 mg q8-12 h	For allergies (rhinitis, conjunctivitis, pruritus). Common side effects include drowsiness, dry mouth, dizziness, and epigastric distress. *Pregnancy category:* B; PB: UK; t½: UK

A, Adult; *b.i.d.*, twice a day; *C*, child; *d*, day; *h*, hour; *IM*, intramuscular; *IV*, intravenous; *max*, maximum; *mo*, month; *PB*, protein-binding; *PO*, by mouth; *q.i.d.*, four times a day; *subQ*, subcutaneous; *SR*, sustained-release; *t½*, half-life; *tab*, tablet; *t.i.d.*, three times a day; *UK*, unknown; *y*, year; >, greater than; <, less than.

Nursing Process

Antihistamine: Diphenhydramine

ASSESSMENT

- Determine baseline vital signs.
- Obtain drug history; report if drug-drug interaction is probable.
- Assess for signs and symptoms of urinary dysfunction, including retention, dysuria, and frequency.
- Note complete blood count (CBC) during drug therapy.
- Assess cardiac and respiratory status.
- If allergic reaction, obtain history of environmental exposures, drugs, recent foods eaten, and stress.

NURSING DIAGNOSES

- Impaired tissue integrity
- Risk for imbalanced fluid volume
- Disturbed sleep pattern

PLANNING

- Client will have decreased nasal congestion, mucosal secretions, and cough.
- Client will sleep 6 to 8 hours per night.

NURSING INTERVENTIONS

- Give with food to decrease gastric distress.
- Administer IM in large muscle. Avoid subQ injection.

Table 38–1

Antihistamines for Treatment of Allergic Rhinitis—cont'd

Generic (Brand)	Route and Dosage	Uses and Considerations
First-Generation Antihistamines—cont'd		
Piperidine Derivatives—cont'd		
phenindamine (Nolahist)	A, C: >12 y: PO: 25 mg q4-6h, *max:* 150 mg/d C: <12 y: 12.5 mg q4-6h, *max:* 75 mg/d	For temporary relief of allergic rhinitis. *Pregnancy category:* B; PB: UK; $t\frac{1}{2}$: UK
Other Antihistamines		
triprolidine and pseudoephedrine (Actifed)	A: PO: 1 tab q4-6h; *max:* 4 tab/d C: >6 y: PO: ½ tab q6-8h; *max:* 2 tab/d	For rhinitis. A combination of an antihistamine and decongestant. *Pregnancy category:* B; PB: UK; $t\frac{1}{2}$: 3 h
triprolidine HCl (Zymine, Myidil)	A: PO: 2.5 mg b.i.d., t.i.d.; *max:* 10 mg/d C: 6-12 y: PO: 1.25 mg b.i.d., t.i.d.; *max:* 5 mg/d C: 2-5 y: PO: 0.6 mg t.i.d./q.i.d.; *max:* 2.5 mg/d C: 4 mo-2 y: PO: 0.3 mg t.i.d./q.i.d.; *max:* 1.25 mg/d	For allergies. Similar effects as other antihistamines. It has a low incidence of drowsiness. *Pregnancy category:* C; PB: UK; $t\frac{1}{2}$: UK
Second-Generation Antihistamines		
azelastine (Astelin)	*Nasal Spray* A, C: >12 y, and elderly: 1-2 sprays to each nostril q12h	For allergic rhinitis. May cause headaches, mild sedation, and bitter taste. *Pregnancy category:* UK; PB: UK; $t\frac{1}{2}$: UK
cetirizine (Zyrtec)	A: 5-10 mg/d	For allergic rhinitis and urticaria. Has few anticholinergic effects. *Pregnancy category:* C; PB: 93%; $t\frac{1}{2}$: 8 h
fexofenadine (Allegra) with pseudoephedrine (Allegra-D)	A, C: >12 y, and elderly: PO: 60 mg q12h	To treat allergic rhinitis and rhinorrhea. Has less sedative effect. *Pregnancy category:* C; PB: UK; $t\frac{1}{2}$: 14.4 h
loratadine (Claritin)	A, C: >6 y: PO: 10 mg/d	Relief of allergic rhinitis and urticaria. Long-acting H_1 blocking effect. *Pregnancy category:* B; PB: UK; $t\frac{1}{2}$: 3-20 h; *metabolite:* 28h
desloratadine (Clarinex)	A: PO: 5 mg daily	For relief of allergic rhinitis. *Pregnancy category:* C; PB: 85%-89%; $t\frac{1}{2}$: 27 h

Client Teaching

General

- Encourage client to avoid driving a motor vehicle and performing other dangerous activities if drowsiness occurs or until stabilized on drug.
- Avoid alcohol and other central nervous system depressants.
- Instruct client to take drug as prescribed. Notify health care provider if confusion or hypotension occurs.
- For prophylaxis of motion sickness, take drug at least 30 minutes before offending event and also before meals and at bedtime during the event.
- Inform the breastfeeding mother that small amounts of drug pass into the breast milk. Because children are more susceptible to the side effects of antihistamines (e.g., unusual excitement or irritability), breastfeeding is not recommended while using these drugs.

Side Effects

- Advise family members or parents that children are more sensitive to the effects of antihistamines. Nightmares, nervousness, and irritability are more likely to occur in children.
- Inform older adults that they are more sensitive to the effects of antihistamines. Confusion; difficult or painful urination; dizziness; drowsiness; feeling faint; and dryness of the mouth, nose, or throat are more likely to occur in older clients.
- For temporary relief of mouth dryness, suggest using sugarless candy or gum, ice chips, or a saliva substitute.

Cultural Considerations

- Decrease language barriers by decoding the jargon of health care environment for those with language difficulties and for those who are not in the health care field.

EVALUATION

■ Evaluate effectiveness of drug in relieving allergic symptoms or as a sleep aid.

Nasal and Systemic Decongestants

Nasal congestion results from dilation of nasal blood vessels caused by infection, inflammation, or allergy. With this dilation, there is a transudation of fluid into the tissue spaces, resulting in swelling of the nasal cavity. Nasal **decongestants** (sympathomimetic amines) stimulate the alpha-adrenergic receptors, thus producing vascular constriction (vasoconstriction) of the capillaries within the nasal mucosa. The result is shrinking of the nasal mucous membranes and a reduction in fluid secretion (runny nose).

Nasal decongestants are administered by nasal spray or drops or in tablet, capsule, or liquid form. Frequent use of decongestants, especially nasal spray or drops, can result in tolerance and **rebound nasal congestion** (rebound va-

sodilation instead of vasoconstriction). Rebound nasal congestion is caused by irritation of the nasal mucosa.

Systemic decongestants (alpha-adrenergic agonists) are available in tablet, capsule, and liquid form and are used primarily for allergic rhinitis, including hay fever and acute coryza (profuse nasal discharge). Examples of systemic decongestants are ephedrine (Ephedrine), phenylephrine (Neo-Synephrine), and pseudoephedrine (Sudafed). In the past, phenylpropanolamine was used in many cold remedies; however, the Food and Drug Administration (FDA) ordered its removal from OTC cold remedies and weight-loss aids because of reports that suggested the drug might cause stroke, hypertension, renal failure, and cardiac dysrhythmias. These other agents are frequently combined with an antihistamine, analgesic, or antitussive in oral cold remedies. The advantage of systemic decongestants is that they relieve nasal congestion for a longer period than nasal decongestants; however, currently there are long-acting nasal decongestants. Nasal decongestants usually act promptly and cause fewer side effects than systemic decongestants. Table 38–2 lists

Table 38–2

Systemic and Nasal Decongestants (Sympathomimetic Amines)

Generic (Brand)	Route and Dosage	Uses and Considerations
ephedrine SO₄ (Efedron)	A: PO: 25-50 mg t.i.d./q.i.d. PRN; *max:* 150 mg/d subQ/IM/IV: 12.5-25 mg; may repeat; *max:* 150 mg/24 h C: 6-12 y: 6.25-12.5 mg q4h; *max:* 75 mg/d	Relief of allergic rhinitis, nasal congestion, sinusitis, mild acute and chronic asthma; improves narcotic-impaired respiration; corrects hypotension. It is an alpha- and beta-adrenergic agonist. OTC drug used alone or in combination. *Pregnancy category:* C; PB: UK; t½: 3-6 h
naphazoline HCl (Allerest, Privine)	A & C: >12 y: 2 gtt or 0.05% spray in each nostril; q3-6h, 5 d C: 6-12 y: 0.025%, 1-2 gtt in each nostril	Relief of nasal congestion, allergic rhinitis. Can cause rebound congestion, transient hypertension, bradycardia, and cardiac dysrhthmias. Use only 3-5 d. *Pregnancy category:* C; PB: UK; t½: UK
oxymetazoline HCl (Afrin)	A & C: >6 y: 0.05% gtt or spray; 2-3 gtt or 1-2 sprays in each nostril b.i.d. C: 2-5 y (0.025% gtt only): 2-3 gtt b.i.d. (q10-12h)	Long-acting decongestant. Taken twice a day, morning and evening. Can cause rebound congestion. Use only 3-5 d. *Pregnancy category:* C; PB: UK; t½: UK
phenylephrine HCl (Neo-Synephrine, Sinex)	A: Sol (0.25%-1%): 2-3 gtt or 1-2 sprays in each nostril q4h C: 6-12 y: Sol (0.25%): 1-2 gtt or sprays in each nostril q4th C: 6 mo-5 y: Sol (0.125%-0.16%): 1-2 gtt in each nostril q4h	For rhinitis. Less potent than epinephrine. Can cause transient hypertension and headaches. Do not use for longer than 3-5 d. *Pregnancy category:* C; PB: UK; t½: 2.5 d
pseudoephedrine (Novafed, Sudafed)	A: PO: 60 mg q4-6h; 120 mg SR q12h; *max:* 240 mg/d C: 6-12 y: 30 mg q4-6h; *max:* 120 mg/d C: 2-5 y: 15 mg q4-6h; *max:* 60 mg/d	For rhinitis. Less CNS stimulation and hypertension than ephedrine. *Pregnancy category:* C; PB: UK; t½: 9-15 h
tetrahydrozoline (Tyzine)	A & C: >6 y: Nasal: 2-4 drops of 0.1% sol or spray in each nostril q3h PRN C: 2-6 y: Nasal: 2-4 drops of 0.5% sol or spray in each nostril q3h PRN	For relief of nasopharyngeal congestion. *Pregnancy category:* C; PB: UK; t½: UK
xylometazoline (Otrivin, Neo-Synephrine II)	A: Nasal: 1-2 sprays or 1-2 drops of 0.1% sol in each nostril q8-10h, *max:* 3 doses/d C: 6-12 y: Nasal: 1 spray or 2-3 drops of 0.05% sol in each nostril q8-10h, *max:* 3 doses/d C: <6 mo: Nasal: 1 drop of 0.05% sol in each nostril q6h, *max:* 3 doses/d	For temporary relief of nasal congestion associated with the common cold, sinusitis, acute and chronic rhinitis, hay fever, and other allergies. *Pregnancy category:* C; PB: UK; t½: UK

A, Adult; *b.i.d.,* twice a day; *C,* child; *CNS,* central nervous system; *d,* day; *gtt,* drops; *h,* hour; *IM,* intramuscular; *IV,* intravenous; *max,* maximum; *OTC,* over-the-counter; *PB,* protein-binding; *PO,* by mouth; *PRN,* as necessary; *q.i.d.,* four times a day; *subQ,* subcutaneous; *sol,* solution; *SR,* sustained release; *t½,* half-life; *t.i.d.,* three times a day; *UK,* unknown; *y,* year; *>,* greater than; *<,* less than.

nasal and systemic decongestants and their dosages, uses, and considerations.

Side Effects and Adverse Reactions

The incidence of side effects is low with topical preparations such as nose drops. Decongestants can make a client jittery, nervous, or restless. These side effects decrease or disappear as the body adjusts to the drug.

Usage of nasal decongestants longer than 5 days could result in rebound nasal congestion. Instead of the nasal membranes constricting, vasodilation occurs, causing increased stuffy nose and nasal congestion. The nurse should emphasize the importance of limiting the use of nasal sprays and drops.

As with any alpha-adrenergic drug (e.g., decongestants), blood pressure and blood glucose levels can increase. These drugs are contraindicated or to be used with extreme caution in clients with hypertension, cardiac disease, hyperthyroidism, and diabetes mellitus.

Drug Interactions

When using decongestants with other drugs, drug interactions can occur. Pseudoephedrine may decrease the effect of beta-blockers. Taking monoamine oxidase (MAO) inhibitors may increase the possibility of hypertension or cardiac dysrhythmias. The client should also avoid large amounts of caffeine (coffee, tea) because it can increase restlessness and palpitations caused by decongestants.

Intranasal Glucocorticoids

Intranasal glucocorticoids or steroids are effective for treating allergic rhinitis. Because these agents are steroids, they have an antiinflammatory action, thus decreasing the allergic

rhinitis symptoms of rhinorrhea, sneezing, and congestion. The following are six examples of intranasal steroids:

- beclomethasone (Beconase, Vancenase, Vanceril)
- budesonide (Rhinocort)
- dexamethasone (Decadron)
- flunisolide (Nasalide)
- fluticasone (Flonase)
- triamcinolone (Nasacort)

These drugs may be used alone or in combination with H_1 antihistamine. With continuous use, dryness of the nasal mucosa may occur.

It is rare for systemic effects of the steroids to occur; however, it is more likely for systemic effects to result with the use of intranasal dexamethasone, which should not be used for longer than 30 days. The other intranasal glucocorticoids undergo rapid deactivation after absorption. Most allergic rhinitis is seasonal; therefore the drugs are for short-term use unless otherwise indicated by the health care provider. Table 38–3 lists the intranasal glucocorticoids and their dosages, uses, and considerations.

Antitussives

Antitussives act on the cough-control center in the medulla to suppress the cough reflex. The cough is a protective way to clear the airway of secretions or any collected material. A sore throat may cause coughing that increases throat irritation. If the cough is nonproductive and irritating, an anti-

Table 38–3

Intranasal Glucocorticoids

Generic (Brand)	Route and Dosage	Uses and Considerations
beclomethasone (Beconase, Vancenase, Vanceril)	A: 1-2 puffs/sprays, b.i.d. to q.i.d. C: 6-12 y: 1-2 sprays b.i.d. to q.i.d.	To treat seasonal allergic rhinitis and bronchial asthma. Not for acute asthma. *Pregnancy category:* C; PB: UK; $t\frac{1}{2}$: 3-15 h
budesonide (Pulmicort, Rhinocort)	A & C: >6 y: 2 sprays b.i.d. or 4 sprays in the morning	For seasonal rhinitis in adults and children. May be used in maintenance therapy for asthma. *Pregnancy category:* C; PB: UK; $t\frac{1}{2}$: 2.5-3 h
dexamethasone (Decadron)	A: 2 sprays b.i.d. or t.i.d. C: 6-12 y: 1-2 sprays b.i.d.	Administered orally, intravenously, ophthalmically, topically, and intranasally. A potent steroid used for short-term therapy. May have a systemic effect. *Pregnancy category:* C; PB: UK; $t\frac{1}{2}$: 3-4.5 h
flunisolide (AeroBid, Nasalide)	A: 2 sprays b.i.d. to t.i.d. C: 6-14 y: 1 spray t.i.d. or 2 sprays b.i.d.	For seasonal rhinitis for adults and children. May be used for steroid-dependent asthma. *Pregnancy category:* C; PB: UK; $t\frac{1}{2}$: 1-2 h
fluticasone (Flonase, Flovent)	A: 2 sprays daily or 1 spray b.i.d. C: >6 y: 1 spray daily	For seasonal allergic rhinitis. When symptoms have decreased, reduce dose to 1 spray daily. *Pregnancy category:* C; PB: UK; $t\frac{1}{2}$: 3.1 h
mometasone furoate (Nasonex)	A: 2 sprays daily	For seasonal allergic rhinitis. *Pregnancy category:* C; PB: UK; $t\frac{1}{2}$: UK Note: Direct spray away from nose septum; gently sniff.
triamcinolone (Nasacort)	A: 1-2 sprays daily	For allergic rhinitis. Has many uses, such as an immunosuppressant. *Pregnancy category:* C; PB: UK; $t\frac{1}{2}$: 2-5 h

A, Adult; *b.i.d.*, twice a day; *C*, child; *h*, hour; *PB*, protein-binding; *q.i.d.*, four times a day; *t\frac{1}{2}*, half-life; *t.i.d.*, three times a day; *UK*, unknown; *y*, year; >, greater than.

PROTOTYPE DRUG CHART 38–2

DEXTROMETHORPHAN HYDROBROMIDE

Drug Class	**Dosage**
Antitussive	**A: PO:** 10-20 mg q4-8h; *max:* 120 mg/24 h
Trade Name: Robitussin DM, Romilar, Sucrets Cough Control, PediaCare, Benylin DM, and others; 🍁 Balminil DM, Neo-DM, Ornex DM	**C: 6-12 y: PO:** 5-10 mg q4-6h; *max:* 60 mg/d
	C: 2-5 y: PO: 2.5-5.0 mg q4-8h; *max:* 30 mg/d
	Sustained Action Liquid (Delsym):
Pregnancy Category: C	**A:** 60 mg q12h
	C: 6-12 y: 30 mg q12h
	C: 2-5 y: 15 mg q12h

Contraindications	**Drug-Lab-Food Interactions**
Chronic obstructive pulmonary disease, chronic productive cough, hypersensitivity; MAOIs	*Drug:* Increase effect/toxicity with MAOIs, narcotics, sedative-hypnotics, barbiturates, antidepressants, alcohol

Pharmacokinetics	**Pharmacodynamics**
Absorption: PO: Rapidly absorbed	**PO:** Onset: 15-30 min
Distribution: PB: UK	Peak: UK
Metabolism: t½: UK	Duration: 3-6 h
Excretion: In urine	

Therapeutic Effects/Uses

To provide temporary suppression of a nonproductive cough; to reduce viscosity of tenacious secretions
Mode of Action: Inhibition of the cough center in the medulla

Side Effects	**Adverse Reactions**
Nausea, dizziness, drowsiness, sedation	Hallucinations at high doses
	Life-threatening: None known

A, Adult; *C,* child; *d,* day; *h,* hour; *MAOIs,* monoamine oxidase inhibitors; *max,* maximum; *min,* minute; *PB,* protein-binding; *PO,* by mouth; *t½,* half-life; *UK,* unknown; *y,* year; 🍁, Canadian drug names.

tussive may be taken. Hard candy may decrease the constant, irritating cough. Dextromethorphan, a nonnarcotic antitussive, is widely used in OTC cold remedies. Prototype Drug Chart 38–2 lists the drug data related to dextromethorphan (Benylin).

The three types of antitussives are nonnarcotic, narcotic, or combination preparations. Antitussives are usually used in combination with other agents (Table 38–4).

Pharmacokinetics

Dextromethorphan is available in syrup or liquid form, chewable capsules, and lozenges in numerous cold and cough remedy preparations. Brand name formulations include Robitussin DM, Romilar, PediaCare, Contac Cold Formula, Sucrets cough formulas, and many others. The drug is rapidly absorbed and exerts its effects 15 to 30 minutes after oral administration. Its protein-binding percentage and half-life are unknown. Dextromethorphan is metabolized by the liver and excreted in the urine.

Pharmacodynamics

Dextromethorphan, a nonnarcotic antitussive, suppresses the cough center in the medulla; however, it does not depress respiration. In addition, it causes neither physical dependence nor tolerance. If the cough lasts longer than 1 week and a fever or rash is present, medical care should be sought. Clients with underlying medical conditions should seek prompt medical attention.

The onset of action for dextromethorphan is relatively fast and its duration is 3 to 6 hours. Usually, preparations containing dextromethorphan can

be used several times a day. CNS depression may occur if the drug is used with alcohol, narcotics, sedative-hypnotics, barbiturates, or antidepressants.

Expectorants

Expectorants loosen bronchial secretions so they can be eliminated by coughing. They can be used with or without other pharmacologic agents. Expectorants are found in many OTC cold remedies along with analgesics, antihistamines, decongestants, and antitussives. The most common expectorant in such preparations is guaifenesin. Hydration is the best expectorant. Table 38–4 lists the drug data for antitussives and expectorants.

Nursing Process

Common Cold

ASSESSMENT

■ Determine whether there is a history of hypertension, especially if a decongestant is an ingredient in the cold remedy.

■ Note baseline vital signs. An elevated temperature of 99° F (37.2° C) to 101° F (38.3° C) may indicate a viral infection caused by a cold.

■ Obtain drug history; report if drug-drug interaction is probable. Dextromethorphan HCl given with MAOIs, narcotics, sedative-hypnotics, barbiturates, antidepressants, and alcohol may increase toxicity.

■ Assess cardiac and respiratory status.

NURSING DIAGNOSES

■ Fatigue

■ Sleep deprivation resulting from chronic coughing

■ Risk for infection

PLANNING

■ Client will be free of nonproductive cough. A secondary bacterial infection does not occur.

■ Client will be free of a secondary bacterial infection.

NURSING INTERVENTIONS

■ Monitor vital signs. Blood pressure can become elevated when a decongestant is taken. Dysrhythmias can also occur.

■ Observe color of bronchial secretions. Yellow or green mucus is indicative of a bronchial infection. Antibiotics may be needed.

■ Be aware that codeine preparations for cough suppression can lead to tolerance and physical dependence.

Client Teaching

General

• Tell client that hypotension and hyperpyrexia may occur when dextromethorphan is taken with MAOIs.

• Instruct client on proper use of a nasal spray and proper use of puff or squeeze products. Instruct client not to use more than one or two puffs, four to six times a day, for 5 to 7 days. Rebound congestion can occur with overuse.

• Advise client to read the label on OTC drugs and to check with the health care provider before taking cold remedies. This is especially important when taking other drugs or when client has a major health problem such as hypertension or hyperthyroidism.

• Inform client that antibiotics are not helpful in treating common cold viruses. However, they may be prescribed if a secondary infection occurs.

• Encourage older client with heart disease, asthma, emphysema, diabetes mellitus, or hypertension to contact the health care provider concerning the selection of drug, including OTC drugs.

• Direct client not to drive during initial use of a cold remedy containing an antihistamine because drowsiness is common.

• Instruct client to maintain adequate fluid intake. Fluids liquify bronchial secretions to ease elimination by coughing.

• Teach client not to take a cold remedy before or at bedtime. Insomnia may occur if it contains a decongestant.

• Encourage client to get adequate rest.

• Inform client that common cold and flu viruses are transmitted frequently by hand-to-hand contact or touching a contaminated surface. Cold viruses can live on the skin for several hours and on hard surfaces for several days.

• Instruct client to avoid environmental pollutants, fumes, smoking, and dust to lessen unnecessary cough.

• Teach client to perform three effective coughs before bedtime to promote uninterrupted sleep.

• Direct client and parents to store the drug out of reach of small children; request childproof caps.

• Advise client to contact the health care provider if cough persists for more than 1 week or is accompanied with chest pain, fever, or headache.

Self-Administration

• Instruct client about self-administration of medications such as nose drops and inhalants.

• Encourage client to cough effectively, to take deep breaths before coughing, and to be in the upright position.

Cultural Considerations ⊕

• Accept client's remedies to treat the common cold, which may be the result of cultural practices. Discuss practices that could cause body harm.

• Present ways to care for the common cold for clients from various cultural backgrounds, such as increasing fluid intake and rest and using tissues to remove nasal and bronchial secretions. Advise client to contact a health professional if the cold persists and if the body temperature is greater than 101° F (38.3° C).

EVALUATION

■ Evaluate the effectiveness of the drug therapy. Determine that client is free of a nonproductive cough, has adequate fluid intake and rest, and is afebrile.

Sinusitis

Sinusitis is an inflammation of the mucous membranes of one or more of the maxillary, frontal, ethmoid, or sphenoid sinuses. A systemic or nasal decongestant may be indicated. Acetaminophen, fluids, and rest may also be helpful. For acute or severe sinusitis, an antibiotic may be prescribed.

Table 38–4

Antitussives and Expectorants

Generic (Brand)	Route and Dosage	Uses and Considerations
Narcotic Antitussives		
codeine CSS II	A: PO: 10-20 mg q4-6h; *max:* 120 mg/d C: 6-12 y: PO: 5-10 mg q4-6h; *max:* 60 mg/d C: 2-5 y: PO: 2.5-4.5 mg q4-6h; *max:* 18 mg/d	Schedule II drug. Can be a Schedule V drug when combined in cough syrup. Usually mixed with an antihistamine, decongestant, and/or expectorant. Can cause drowsiness, dizziness, nausea, constipation, and respiratory depression. *Pregnancy category:* C; PB: 7%; $t^1/_2$: 2.5-4 h
guaifenesin and codeine (Cheracol, Robitussin A-C) CSS V	*Temporary relief of cough caused by minor irritation:* A: PO: 5-10 ml q6-8h C: 2-6 y: PO: 2.5 ml q6-8h PRN	An expectorant that is combined with a narcotic antitussive. Also to control a cough caused by the common cold or bronchitis. *Pregnancy category:* C; PB: UK; $t^1/_2$: UK
hydrocodone bitartrate (Hycodan) CSS III	A: PO: 5-10 mg q4-6h; *max:* 15 mg/d C: PO: 1.25 mg q4-6h; 0.6 mg/kg/d in 3-4 divided doses, not to exceed 10 mg/single dose	Relief of cough and pain. Has similar side effects as codeine. *Pregnancy category:* C; PB: UK; $t^1/_2$: 3-4 h
Nonnarcotic Antitussives		
benzonatate (Tessalon)	*Relief of nonproductive cough:* A: PO: 100 mg t.i.d. or q4h; *max:* 600 mg/d C: <10 y: PO: 8 mg/kg/d in 3-6 divided doses	Relief of cough. It does not decrease the respiratory center. Has few side effects. *Pregnancy category:* C; PB: UK; $t^1/_2$: UK
dextromethorphan hydrobromide (Benylin)	See Prototype Drug Chart 38–2.	
promethazine with dextromethorphan	A: PO: 5 ml q4-6h; *max:* 30 ml/d C: 6-12 y: PO: 2.5-5 ml q4-6h; *max:* 20 ml/d C: 2-6 y: PO: 1.25-5 ml, q4-6h	For cough. A combination of a phenothiazine and a nonnarcotic antitussive. *Pregnancy category:* C; PB: UK; $t^1/_2$: UK
Expectorants		
guaifenesin (Robitussin, Anti-Tuss, Glycotuss)	A: PO: 200-400 mg q4h; *max:* 2.4 g/d C: 6-12 y: PO: 100-200 mg q4h; *max:* 1.2 g/d C: 2-5 y: PO: 50-100 mg q4h; *max:* 600 mg/d	For dry, unproductive cough. Can cause nausea and vomiting. Can be combined with other cold remedies. Take with glass of water to loosen mucus. *Pregnancy category:* C; PB: UK; $t^1/_2$: UK
Antitussive/Expectorant		
guaifenesin and dextromethorphan (Robitussin-DM)	A: PO: 10 ml q6-8h C: 6-12 y: PO: 5 ml q6-8h C: 2-5 y: PO: 2.5 ml q6-8h	For nonproductive cough. *Pregnancy category:* C; PB: UK; $t^1/_2$: UK

A, Adult; *C,* child; *CSS,* Controlled Substance Schedule; *d,* day; *h,* hour; *max,* maximum; *PB,* protein-binding; *PO,* by mouth; *PRN,* as necessary; $t^1/_2$, half-life; *t.i.d.,* three times a day; *UK,* unknown; *y,* year; <, less than.

Acute Pharyngitis

Acute pharyngitis (inflammation of the throat, or "sore throat") can be caused by a virus, beta-hemolytic streptococci (strep throat), or other bacteria. It can occur alone or with the common cold and rhinitis or acute sinusitis. Symptoms include elevated temperature and cough. A throat culture should be obtained to rule out beta-hemolytic streptococcal infection. If the culture is positive for beta-hemolytic streptococci, a 10-day course of antibiotics is often prescribed. Saline gargles, lozenges, and increased fluid intake are usually indicated. Acetaminophen may be taken to decrease an elevated temperature. Antibiotics are not effective for viral pharyngitis.

WEBSITES

For further information on *Drugs for Common Upper Respiratory Disorders,* visit these Internet resources:

Information on cetirizine:
www.nlm.nih.gov/medlineplus/druginfo/medmaster/a698026.html

Information on loratadine:
www.health-net.info/loratadine.html

Critical Thinking Case Study

G.H., age 35, has allergic rhinitis. Her prescriptions include loratadine (Claritin), 5 mg per day, and fluticasone, two nasal inhalations per day. Previously she had taken OTC drugs and asked whether she should continue to take the OTC drug with her prescriptions. She has never used a nasal inhaler.

1. What additional information is needed from G.H. concerning her health problem?

2. What is your response to G.H. concerning the use of OTC drugs with her prescriptive drugs?

3. How would you instruct G.H. to use a nasal inhaler? Explain. (See Chapter 3, Principles of Drug Administration.)

4. What are the similarities and differences between loratadine and diphenhydramine? Could one of these antihistamines be more effective than the other? Explain.

5. Design a client teaching plan for G.H. in regard to medications and environmental allergens.

6. What could you suggest to decrease allergens (e.g., dust mites) in the home?

Study Questions

1. Antihistamines can be used for the common cold. What are the desired and undesired effects of antihistamines?

2. How do first-generation and second-generation antihistamines differ? Give examples.

3. What are antitussives and expectorants? How are they administered?

4. A client has a cold and complains of nasal congestion. He has been using a nasal decongestant every 3 hours for several days. He says the nasal congestion is as bad as before he started the medication. What nursing interventions, including client teaching, should be given?

5. A client complains of a sore throat. The pharynx appears red. What nursing action should be taken?

6. T.S. says that she was with a friend the day before her friend got a "head cold." She asks whether she can avoid getting the cold by staying away from her friend. What would your response be? What client teaching is recommended?

39 Drugs for Acute and Chronic Lower Respiratory Disorders

ELECTRONIC RESOURCES

Additional information can be found on the companion website at *http://evolve.elsevier.com/KeeHayes/pharmacology/* or on the companion CD-ROM, which includes:
- *NCLEX-style examination review questions*
- *Pharmacology animations*
- *Medication error and IV therapy checklists*
- *Medication calculation problems*
- *Electronic calculators*

OUTLINE

OBJECTIVES

- Contrast chronic obstructive pulmonary disease (COPD) and restrictive lung disease.
- Differentiate the drug groups used to treat COPD and asthma and the desired effects of each.
- Describe the side effects of beta₂-adrenergic agonists and methylxanthines.
- Compare the therapeutic serum or plasma theophylline level and the toxic level.
- Contrast the therapeutic effects of leukotriene antagonists, glucocorticoids, cromolyn, antihistamines, and mucolytics for COPD and asthma.
- Describe the nursing process, including client teaching, related to drugs commonly used for COPD, including asthma, and restrictive lung disease.

TERMS

asthma	bronchodilators	chronic obstructive pul-	glucocorticoids
bronchial asthma	bronchospasm	monary disease (COPD)	mucolytics
bronchiectasis	chronic bronchitis	emphysema	restrictive lung disease

Introduction

Chronic obstructive pulmonary disease (COPD) and re-strictive pulmonary disease are the two major categories of lower respiratory tract disorders. COPD is caused by airway obstruction with increased airway resistance of airflow to lung tissues. Four major pulmonary disorders cause COPD: chronic bronchitis, bronchiectasis, emphysema, and asthma. Chronic bronchitis, bronchiectasis, and emphy-sema frequently result in irreversible lung tissue damage. The lung tissue changes resulting from an acute asthmatic attack are normally reversible; however, if the asthma attacks are frequent and asthma becomes chronic, irreversible changes in the lung tissue may result. Clients with COPD usually have a decrease in forced expiratory volume in 1 sec-ond (FEV_1) as measured by pulmonary function tests.

Restrictive lung disease is a decrease in total lung capac-ity as a result of fluid accumulation or loss of elasticity of the lung. Pulmonary edema, pulmonary fibrosis, pneumonitis, lung tumors, thoracic deformities (scoliosis), and disorders affecting the thoracic muscular wall (e.g., myasthenia gravis) are among the types and causes of restrictive pulmonary disease.

Drugs discussed in this chapter are primarily used to treat COPD, particularly asthma. These drugs include bron-chodilators (sympathomimetics [primarily beta$_2$-adrenergic agonists], methylxanthines [xanthines]), leukotriene antago-nists, glucocorticoids, cromolyn, anticholinergics, and mu-colytics. Some of these drugs may also be used to treat re-strictive pulmonary diseases.

Chronic Obstructive Pulmonary Disease

Asthma is an inflammatory disorder that involves a hyper-responsiveness of the airways with varying amount of air-way obstruction. This disorder is triggered by stimuli such as stress, allergens, and pollutants.

Bronchial asthma, one of the COPD lung diseases, is char-acterized by bronchospasm (constricted bronchioles), wheezing, mucus secretions, and dyspnea. There is resistance to airflow caused by obstruction of the airway. In acute and chronic asthma, minimal to no changes are seen in the struc-ture and function of lung tissues when the disease process is in remission. In chronic bronchitis, emphysema, and bron-chiectasis, there is permanent, irreversible damage to the physical structure of the lung tissue. Symptoms are similar in these three pulmonary disorders to those of asthma, except wheezing does not occur. Figure 39–1 displays the overlap-

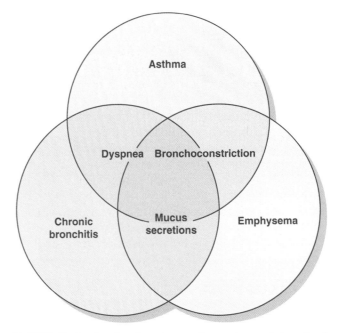

FIGURE 39–1 Overlapping signs and symptoms of chronic ob-structive pulmonary disease (COPD) conditions.

ping symptoms of COPD conditions. Frequently, there is a steady deterioration over a period of years.

Chronic bronchitis is a progressive lung disease caused by smoking or chronic lung infections. Bronchial inflamma-tion and excessive mucous secretion result in airway ob-struction. Productive coughing is a response to excess mucus production and chronic bronchial irritation. Inspiratory and expiratory rhonchi may be heard on auscultation. Hypercap-nia (increased carbon dioxide retention) and hypoxemia (decreased blood oxygen) lead to respiratory acidosis.

In **bronchiectasis**, there is abnormal dilation of the bronchi and bronchioles secondary to frequent infection and inflammation. The bronchioles become obstructed by the breakdown of the epithelium of the bronchial mucosa. Tissue fibrosis may result.

Emphysema is a progressive lung disease caused by ciga-rette smoking, atmospheric contaminants, or lack of the alpha$_1$-antitrypsin protein that inhibits proteolytic enzymes that destroy alveoli (air sacs). The proteolytic enzymes are re-leased in the lung by bacteria or phagocytic cells. The termi-nal bronchioles become plugged with mucus, causing a loss in the fiber and elastin network in the alveoli. The alveoli en-large as many of the alveolar walls are destroyed. Air be-comes trapped in the overexpanded alveoli, leading to inad-equate gas (oxygen and carbon dioxide) exchange.

Cigarette smoking is the most common risk factor for COPD, especially with chronic bronchitis and emphysema. There is no cure for COPD at this time; however, it remains preventable in most cases. Because cigarette smoking is the most directly related cause, not smoking significantly prevents COPD from developing. Quitting smoking will slow the disease process.

Medications frequently prescribed for COPD include the following:

- Bronchodilators, such as sympathomimetics (adrenergics), parasympatholytics (anticholinergic drug, Atrovent), and methylxanthines (caffeine, theophylline), are used to assist in opening narrowed airways.
- Glucocorticoids (steroids) are used to decrease inflammation.
- Leukotriene modifiers reduce inflammation in the lung tissue, and cromolyn and nedocromil act as antiinflammatory agents by suppressing the release of histamine and other mediators from the mast cells.
- Expectorants are used to assist in loosening the mucus from the airways.
- Antibiotics may be prescribed to prevent serious complications from bacterial infections.

A table listing suggested pharmacotherapy for smoking cessation, from the *Nurse Practitioners Prescribing Reference (NPPR)*, Fall issue, 2004, is presented on the **evolve** website. The table includes behavior modification, transdermal and chewing gum products, and prescribed agents such as Nicotrol nasal spray, Nicotrol inhaler, and buproprion oral medication.

Bronchial Asthma

Bronchial asthma is a COPD characterized by periods of bronchospasm resulting in wheezing and difficulty in breathing. **Bronchospasm**, or bronchoconstriction, results when the lung tissue is exposed to extrinsic or intrinsic factors that stimulate a bronchoconstrictive response. Factors that can trigger an asthmatic attack (bronchospasm) include humidity; air pressure changes; temperature changes; smoke; fumes (exhaust, perfume); stress; emotional upset; exercise; and allergies to animal dander, dust mites, food, and drugs (e.g., aspirin, indomethacin, ibuprofen). Reactive airway disease (RAD) is a cause of asthma resulting from sensitivity stimulation from allergens, dust, temperature changes, and cigarette smoking.

Pathophysiology

Mast cells, found in connective tissue throughout the body, are directly involved in the asthmatic response, particularly to extrinsic factors. Allergens attach themselves to mast cells and basophils, resulting in an antigen-antibody reaction on the mast cells in the lung; thus the mast cells stimulate the release of chemical mediators such as histamines, cytokines, serotonin, eosinophil chemotactic factor of anaphylaxis (ECF-A), and leukotrienes. Eosinophil counts are usually elevated during an allergic reaction, which indicates that an inflammatory process is occurring.

These chemical mediators stimulate bronchial constriction, mucous secretions, inflammation, and pulmonary congestion. Histamine and ECF-A are strong bronchoconstrictors. Bronchial smooth muscles are wrapped spirally around the bronchioles, and the bronchioles contract as they are stimulated by these mediators.

Figure 39–2 shows the factors contributing to bronchoconstriction. Cyclic adenosine monophosphate (cyclic AMP, or cAMP), a cellular signaling molecule, is involved in many cellular activities and is responsible for maintaining bronchodilation. When histamine, ECF-A, and leukotrienes inhibit the action of cAMP, bronchoconstriction results. The sympathomimetic (adrenergic) **bronchodilators** and methylxanthines increase the amount of cAMP in bronchial tissue cells.

In an acute asthmatic attack, the short-acting sympathomimetics (beta$_2$-adrenergic agonists) are the first line of defense. They promote cAMP production and enhance bronchodilation. Long-acting sympathomimetics are used for maintenance. Sympathomimetics (adrenergics) are also discussed in Chapter 17, Adrenergics and Adrenergic Blockers.

Sympathomimetics: Alpha- and Beta$_2$-Adrenergic Agonists

Sympathomimetics increase cAMP, causing dilation of the bronchioles. In an acute bronchospasm caused by anaphylaxis from an allergic reaction, the nonselective sympathomimetic epinephrine (Adrenalin), which is an alpha$_1$, beta$_1$, and beta$_2$ agonist, is given subcutaneously to promote bronchodilation and elevate the blood pressure. Epinephrine is administered in emergency situations to restore circulation and increase airway patency (see Chapter 57, Adult and Pediatric Emergency Drugs).

For bronchospasm associated with chronic asthma or COPD, selective beta$_2$-adrenergic agonists are given by aerosol or as a tablet. These drugs act primarily on the beta$_2$ receptors; therefore the side effects are *less severe* than those of epinephrine, which acts on alpha$_1$, beta$_1$, and beta$_2$ receptors.

Albuterol

The newer beta-adrenergic drugs for asthma are more selective for beta$_2$ receptors. High doses or overuse of the beta$_2$-adrenergic agents for asthma may cause some degree of beta$_1$ response such as nervousness, tremor, and in-

PREVENTING MEDICATION ERRORS

Do not confuse...

- **albuterol** (beta$_2$-adrenergic) with **Accupril** (cardiovascular agent). Both names look alike, but the class and action are very different.

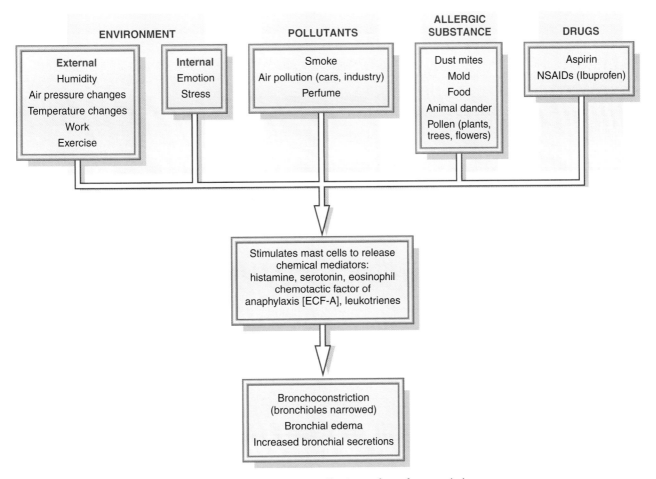

FIGURE 39–2 Factors contributing to bronchoconstriction.

creased pulse rate. The ideal beta$_2$ agonist is one that has a rapid onset of action, longer duration of action, and few side effects. Albuterol (Proventil, Ventolin) is a selective beta$_2$ drug that is effective for treatment and control of asthma by causing bronchodilation with long duration of action. See Prototype Drug Chart 17–2 for drug data related to albuterol.

Metaproterenol

The second beta-adrenergic agent is metaproterenol (Alupent, Metaprel), which was first marketed in 1961. It has some beta$_1$ effect but is primarily used as a beta$_2$ agent. It can be administered orally or by inhalation with a metered-dose inhaler or a nebulizer.

PREVENTING MEDICATION ERRORS

Do not confuse...

- **Alupent** (beta-adrenergic) with **Atrovent** (another beta-adrenergic bronchodilator). Both these beta-adrenergic drugs look alike, but their pharmacology (e.g., interactions, side effects, adverse effects) is different.

For long-term asthma treatment, beta$_2$-adrenergic agonists are frequently administered by inhalation. This route of administration usually delivers more drug directly to the constricted bronchial site. The effective inhalation drug dose is less than it would be by the oral route; there are also fewer side effects in using this route. The onset of action of the drug is more rapid (1 minute) by inhalation than orally (15 minutes). Prototype Drug Chart 39–1 lists the pharmacologic behavior of metaproterenol.

Pharmacokinetics

Metaproterenol is well absorbed from the GI tract. Its protein-binding percentage and half-life are unknown. It is metabolized by the liver and excreted in the urine.

Pharmacodynamics

Metaproterenol reverses bronchospasm by relaxing the bronchial smooth muscle. The drug acts on the beta$_2$ receptor, promoting bronchodilation, and increases cAMP.

The onset of action for oral and inhalational metaproterenol is fast and its duration is short. Excessive use of the drug by inhalation may cause tolerance and paradoxic bronchoconstriction. Because it has some beta$_1$ properties, it can cause tremor, nervousness, heart palpitations, and increased heart rate when taken in large doses. A few drug interactions need to be considered. When metaproterenol is taken with a beta-adrenergic blocker, its effects are decreased. Other sympathomimetic agents increase the effects of metaproterenol.

PROTOTYPE DRUG CHART 39–1

METAPROTERENOL

Drug Class	**Dosage**
Bronchodilator: adrenergic beta$_2$ and some beta$_1$ Trade Name: Alupent, Metaprel *Pregnancy Category: C*	**A & C >9 y and >27 kg:** PO: 20 mg q6-8h **C 6-9 y or <27 kg:** PO: 10 mg q6-8h **A & C >12 y:** MDI 2-3 inhalations as single dose; wait 2 min before second dose, if necessary; use only q3-4h to maximum of 12 inhalations/d

Contraindications	**Drug-Lab-Food Interactions**
Hypersensitivity, cardiac dysrhythmias *Caution:* Narrow-angle glaucoma, cardiac disease, hypertension	*Drug: Increase* action with sympathomimetics; *decrease* with beta blockers *Lab: Decreased* serum potassium

Pharmacokinetics	**Pharmacodynamics**
Absorption: PO: Well absorbed **Distribution:** PB: UK **Metabolism:** t½: UK **Excretion:** In urine as metabolites	**PO:** Onset: 15-30 min Peak: 1 h Duration: 4 h **subQ:** Onset: 1-5 min Peak: 1 h Duration: 3-4 h

Therapeutic Effects/Uses

To treat bronchospasm, asthma; to promote bronchodilation
Mode of Action: Relaxation of smooth muscle of bronchi

Side Effects	**Adverse Reactions**
Nervousness, tremors, restlessness, insomnia, headache, nausea, vomiting, hyperglycemia, muscle cramping in extremities	Tachycardia, palpitations, hypertension **Life-threatening:** Cardiac dysrhythmias, cardiac arrest, paradoxical bronchoconstriction

A, Adult; *C*, child; *h*, hour; *MDI*, metered-dose inhaler; *min*, minute; *PB*, protein-binding; *PO*, by mouth; *subQ*, subcutaneous; *t½*, half-life; *UK*, unknown; *y*, year; >, greater than; <, less than.

Isoproterenol

The first beta-adrenergic agent used for bronchospasm was isoproterenol (Isuprel), introduced in 1941. It has no alpha-agonist properties, but it is considered a non-selective beta agonist because it stimulates both beta$_1$ and beta$_2$ receptors. Because the beta$_1$ receptors are stimulated, the heart rate increases and tachycardia may result. Beta$_2$ stimulation promotes bronchodilation. Isoproterenol is administered by inhalation using an aerosol inhaler or nebulizer, or intravenously (IV) for severe asthmatic attacks. Its duration of action is short. Because of its severe side effects from beta$_1$ response, it is seldom prescribed.

 PREVENTING MEDICATION ERRORS

Do not confuse...

- **Isuprel** (beta-adrenergic) with **Isordil** (nitrate vasodilator). Both names look alike, but the class and action are very different.

Use of an Aerosol Inhaler

If the beta$_2$ agonist is given by a metered-dose inhaler (MDI) or dry powdered inhaler (DPI), correct use of the inhaler and dosage intervals need to be explained to the client. If the client does not receive effective relief from the inhaler, either the client's technique is faulty or the canister is empty (see Chapter 3, Principles of Drug Administration, Figure 3–16, to determine the amount of drug left in the canister). A spacer device may be attached to the inhaler to improve drug delivery to the lung with less deposition in the mouth (see Chapter 3, Principles of Drug Administration, Figure 3–15). If the client does not use the inhaler properly to deliver the drug dose, the medication may be trapped in the upper airways. Because of drug inhalation, mouth dryness and throat irritation could result. The correct method of using the inhaler is described in the Nursing Process: Bronchodilator: Adrenergic box. See Chapter 3, Principles of Drug Administration, for a detailed discussion of aerosol inhalers' use.

Excessive use of the aerosol drug can lead to tolerance and loss of drug effectiveness. Occasionally, severe paradoxical airway resistance (bronchoconstriction) develops with repeated, excessive use of sympathomimetic oral inhalation. Frequent dosing can cause tremors, nervousness, and increased heart rate. Table 39–1 lists the sympathomimetics used as bronchodilators.

Side Effects and Adverse Reactions
Epinephrine

The side effects and adverse reactions of epinephrine include tremors, dizziness, hypertension, tachycardia, heart palpitations, cardiac dysrhythmias, and angina. The client needs to be closely monitored when epinephrine is administered.

Beta$_2$-Adrenergics

The side effects associated with beta$_2$ drugs (e.g., albuterol, terbutaline) include tremors, headaches, nervousness, increased pulse rate, and palpitations (high doses). The beta$_2$ agonists may increase blood glucose levels; therefore clients with diabetes should be taught to monitor their serum glucose levels closely. Side effects of beta$_2$ agonists may diminish after a week or longer. The bronchodilating effects may decrease with continued use. It is believed that tolerance to these drugs can develop; if this occurs, the dose may need to be increased. Failure to respond to a previously effective dose may indicate worsening asthma that requires reevaluation before increasing the dose.

Anticholinergics

Recently, a new anticholinergic drug, ipratropium bromide (Atrovent), was introduced to treat asthmatic conditions by dilating the bronchioles. Unlike other anticholinergics,

---

Table 39–1

Adrenergic Bronchodilators and Anticholinergics

Generic (Brand)	Route and Dosage	Uses and Considerations
Alpha- and Beta-Adrenergic		
ephedrine SO$_4$ (Ephedsol) Alpha$_1$, beta$_1$, beta$_2$	A: PO: 25-50 mg q3-4h; *max:* 150 mg/d PRN; subQ/IM/IV: 12.5-25 mg PRN C: >2 y: PO: 2-3 mg/kg/d in 4-6 divided doses C: 6-12 y: PO: 6.25-12.5 mg q4h; *max:* 75 mg	Relief of allergic rhinitis and sinusitis; improves respiration caused by narcotic excess; corrects hypotensive state. Nervousness, tachycardia, and insomnia could occur. *Pregnancy category:* C; PB: UK; t^1/$_2$: 3-6 h
epinephrine (Adrenalin, Primatene Mist, Bronkaid Mist) Alpha$_1$, beta$_1$, beta$_2$	A: subQ: 0.1-0.5 mg or ml of 1:1000 sol; may repeat q10-15 min PRN C: subQ: 0.01 mg or ml of 1:1000 sol; may repeat q20min-4h PRN Inhal: 1-2 puffs of 1:100 q15 min × 2 doses, then q3h	For relief of acute bronchoconstriction and to combat anaphylactic reaction. It is a nonselective (alpha, beta$_1$, and beta$_2$) adrenergic drug. Used frequently by nebulizer. Side effects include nervousness, tremors, dizziness, palpitations, tachycardia, and other cardiac dysrhythmias. *Pregnancy category:* C; PB: UK; t^1/$_2$: UK
Beta-Adrenergic		
albuterol (Proventil, Ventolin) Beta$_2$	A & C: >6 y: Inhal MDI: 1-2 puffs q4-6h or 2 puffs 15 min before exercise A: PO: 2-4 mg t.i.d. or q.i.d.; *max:* 8 mg q.i.d. SR: 4-8 mg q12h C: 6-12 y: PO: 2 mg t.i.d./q.i.d. C: 2-6 y: PO: 0.1 mg/kg t.i.d.; *max:* 4 mg/dose	Treatment of acute and chronic asthma, bronchitis, and exercise-induced bronchospasm. Onset of action orally is 30 minutes and duration of action is 4-6 hours; SR: 8-12 hours. *Pregnancy category:* C; PB: UK; t^1/$_2$:4-5 h
bitolterol mesylate (Tornalate) Beta$_1$ (some), beta$_2$	A: Inhal MDI: 2 puffs (1-3 min apart), q4-6h; *max:* 12 inhal/d	Treatment of asthma and acute bronchitis. It can be used as a single-treatment therapy or in combination with theophylline or corticosteroid. Tremors and nervousness may occur. Has a longer duration of action than many other adrenergics (5-8 hours) by inhalation. *Pregnancy category:* C; PB: UK; t^1/$_2$: 3 h
isoetharine HCl (Bronkosol) Beta$_1$ (some), beta$_2$	Inhal: 1-2 puffs A: IPPB: 0.5-1.0 ml of 5% sol or 0.5 ml of 1% sol diluted in 3 ml of NSS	For bronchoconstriction and reversible obstructive pulmonary disease. Rapid onset (1-5 min); short duration of action (1-4 hours). *Pregnancy category:* C; PB: UK; t^1/$_2$: UK
isoproterenol (Isuprel) Beta$_1$ and beta$_2$	A & C: Inhal: 1-2 puffs q4-6h	For bronchoconstriction. Nonselective (beta$_1$ and beta$_2$). Beta$_1$ effect causes heart rate to increase. Monitor heart rate and blood pressure. The absorption of the sublingual drug can be variable and unpredictable. *Pregnancy category:* C; PB: UK; t^1/$_2$: 2-5 min

A, Adult; *C,* child; *COPD,* chronic obstructive pulmonary disease; *d,* day; *h,* hour; *IM,* intramuscular; *inhal,* inhalation; *IPPB,* intermittent positive-pressure breathing; *IV,* intravenous; *max,* maximum; *MDI,* metered dose inhaler; *min,* minute; *NSS,* normal saline solution; *PB,* protein-binding; *PO,* by mouth; *PRN,* as needed; *q.i.d.,* four times a day; *subQ,* subcutaneous; *sol,* solution; *SR,* sustained-release; *t^1/$_2$,* half-life; *t.i.d.,* three times a day; *UK,* unknown; *y,* year; *>,* greater than.

Continued

Table 39–1

Adrenergic Bronchodilators and Anticholinergics—cont'd

Generic (Brand)	Route and Dosage	Uses and Considerations
Beta-Adrenergic—cont'd		
levalbuterol (Xopenex) Beta₂	A & C: >12 y: Nebulizer 0.63-1.25 mg/ 3 ml q6-8h PRN	Treatment of acute bronchospasm and prevention of exercise-induced asthma. Product from albuterol derivative. Expensive. Rapid absorption and short acting. Side effects are nervousness and tremors. *Pregnancy category:* UK; PB: UK; t½: UK
metaproterenol sulfate (Alupent, Metaprel) Beta₁ (some) and beta₂	See Prototype Drug Chart 39–1.	
pirbuterol acetate (Maxair) Beta₂	*Prevention:* A & C: >12 y: Inhal MDI: 2 puffs q4-6h *Bronchospasm:* A & C: >12 y: Inhal MDI: 2 puffs (1-3 min apart) followed by 1 puff; not to exceed 12 inhal/d	Treatment of asthma. Moderate duration of action (5 hours). *Pregnancy category:* C; PB: UK; t½: 2-3 h
formoterol fumarate (Foradil Aerolizer)	A & C: >5 y: Inhal: Inhale contents of 1 capsule q12h	Treatment of asthma and prevention of exercise-induced asthma. *Pregnancy category:* C; PB: UK; t½: 10 h
tiotropium (Spiriva)	A: Inhal: Inhale contents of 1 capsule daily	Treatment of bronchospasm associated with chronic obstructive pulmonary disease (COPD). It is first long-acting inhaled anticholinergic drug for treatment of COPD. *Pregnancy category:* UK; PB: UK; t½: 5-6 days
salmeterol (Serevent) Beta₂	*Maintenance bronchodilation:* A & C: >12 y: Inhal MDI: 2 puffs q12h *Prevention of exercise-induced bronchospasm:* A & C: >12 y: Inhal MDI: 2 puffs 30-60 min before exercise	Treatment for chronic asthma and exercise-induced bronchospasm. Not effective for treating acute bronchospasms. Has a long duration of action (12 h). *Pregnancy category:* C; PB: 94%-98%; t½: 5.5 h
terbutaline SO₄ (Brethine, Bricanyl) Beta₂	Inhal MDI: 1-2 puffs q4-6h A: PO: 2.5-5 mg t.i.d. subQ: 0.25-0.5 mg q8h IV: 10 mcg/min, gradually increase; *max:* 80 mcg/min C: >12 y: PO: 2.5 mg t.i.d.	To treat reversible airway obstruction caused by asthma, bronchitis, and emphysema. May cause nervousness, tremors, lightheadedness, palpitations, or tachycardia if taken in excess. Slow to moderate onset (15-30 min); long oral duration (4-8 h) and moderate inhaled duration (3-6 h). *Pregnancy category:* B; PB: 25%; t½: 3-11 h
Anticholinergics		
ipratropium bromide (Atrovent)	*COPD:* A: Inhal MDI: 2 puffs t.i.d., q.i.d. >4h intervals; *max:* 12 inhal/d	To treat bronchospasm associated with COPD, including asthma. Use with caution in clients with narrow-angle glaucoma. *Pregnancy category:* B; PB: UK; t½: 1.5-2 h
ipratropium with albuterol (Combivent)	A: Inhal MDI: 2 puffs t.i.d., q.i.d.	Anticholinergic agent combines with beta₂-adrenergic agonist to increase bronchodilation. With the use of this combination of drugs, the duration of action is prolonged. *Pregnancy category:* UK; PB: UK; t½: UK

ipratropium has few systemic effects. It is administered by aerosol.

Clients who use a beta-agonist inhalant should administer it 5 minutes before using ipratropium. When using the anticholinergic agent in conjunction with an inhaled glucocorticoid (steroid) or cromolyn, the ipratropium should be used 5 minutes before the steroid or cromolyn. This causes the bronchioles to dilate so the steroid or cromolyn can be deposited in the bronchioles.

The combination of ipratropium bromide with albuterol sulfate (Combivent) is used to treat chronic bronchitis. The combination is more effective and has a longer duration of action than if either agent is used alone. These two agents combined increase the FEV₁, which is the parameter used to evaluate asthmatics and

obstructive lung disease and the response to bronchodilator therapy. Table 39–2 lists the inhalants for asthma control.

Methylxanthine (Xanthine) Derivatives

The second major group of bronchodilators used to treat asthma are the methylxanthine (xanthine) derivatives, which include aminophylline, theophylline, and caffeine. Xanthines also stimulate the central nervous system (CNS) and respiration, dilate coronary and pulmonary vessels, and cause diuresis. Because of their effect on respiration and pulmonary vessels, xanthines are used in the treatment of asthma.

Table 39-2

Inhalants for Asthma Control

Categories	Inhalant Agents
Adrenergics	
Beta₁ and beta₂	isoproterenol (Isuprel)
Beta₂ and some beta₁	bitolterol mesylate (Tornalate)
	isoetharine HCl (Bronkosol)
	metaproterenol sulfate (Alupent, Metaprel)
Beta₂	albuterol (Proventil, Ventolin)
	pirbuterol acetate (Maxair)
	salmeterol (Serevent)
	terbutaline sulfate (Brethine, Brethaire)
Anticholinergics	ipratropium bromide (Atrovent)
	ipratropium and albuterol (Combivent)
Antiinflammatory Drugs	
cromolyn and nedocromil	cromolyn (Intal)
	nedocromil (Tilade)
glucocorticoids (corticosteroids)	beclomethasone (Beclovent, Vanceril)
	budesonide (Rhinocort)
	dexamethasone (Decadron)
	flunisolide (Nasalide)
	fluticasone (Flonase)
	mometasone furoate (Nasonex)
	triamcinolone (Nasacort)

Theophylline

The first theophylline preparation, aminophylline, was produced in 1936. Theophylline relaxes the smooth muscles of the bronchi, bronchioles, and pulmonary blood vessels by inhibiting the enzyme phosphodiesterase, resulting in an increase in cAMP, which promotes bronchodilation.

Theophylline has a low therapeutic index and a narrow therapeutic range of 10 to 20 mcg/ml. The serum or plasma theophylline concentration level should be monitored frequently to avoid severe adverse effects. Toxicity is likely to occur when the serum level is greater than 20 mcg/ml. Certain theophylline preparations can be given with sympathomimetic (adrenergic) drug agents, but the dose may need to be adjusted.

Theophylline was once used as the first-line drug for treating clients with chronic asthma and other COPDs. However, theophylline use has declined sharply because there is a potential danger of serious adverse effects (e.g., dysrhythmias, convulsions, cardiorespiratory collapse) and efficacy has not been found to be greater than beta agonists or glucocorticoids. Because of its numerous adverse reactions, drug-drug interactions, and narrow therapeutic drug range, it is prescribed for maintenance therapy for clients with chronic stable asthma and other COPDs. Theophylline drugs are NOT prescribed for clients with seizure disorders or cardiac, renal, or liver disease. Clients who receive theophylline preparations need to be closely monitored for serious side effects and drug interactions.

Table 39-3 lists the theophylline preparations and their dosages, uses, and considerations.

Pharmacokinetics

Theophylline is usually well absorbed after oral administration, but absorption may vary according to the specific dosage form. Theophylline is also well absorbed from oral liquids and uncoated plain tablets. Sustained-release dosage forms are slowly absorbed. Food and antacids may decrease the rate, but not the extent, of absorption; large volumes of fluid and high-protein meals may increase the rate of absorption. The dose size can also affect the rate of absorption: larger doses are absorbed more slowly. Theophylline can also be administered in IV fluids.

The theophylline drugs are metabolized by liver enzymes, and 90% of the drug is excreted by the kidneys. Tobacco smoking increases metabolism of theophylline drugs, thereby decreasing the half-life of the drug. The half-life is also shorter in children. With a short half-life, theophylline is readily excreted by the kidneys; therefore the drug dose may need to be increased to maintain the therapeutic serum/plasma range. In nonsmokers and older adults, the average half-life of theophylline is 7 to 9 hours, and the dose requirements may be decreased. However, in smokers and children, the half-life is 4 to 5 hours, and the dose requirement may be increased. In premature infants, the half-life is 15 to 55 hours. In clients with congestive heart failure (CHF), cor pulmonale, COPD, or liver disease, the half-life is 12 hours. Kidney function may be decreased in older adults, so to avoid drug toxicity, caution should be used regarding the theophylline dosage.

Pharmacodynamics

Theophylline increases the level of cAMP, resulting in bronchodilation. The average onset of action for oral theophylline preparations is 30 minutes; for sustained-release capsules, it is 1 to 2 hours. The duration of action for the sustained-release form is 8 to 24 hours and approximately 6 hours for other oral and IV theophylline preparations.

Side Effects and Adverse Reactions

Side effects and adverse reactions to theophylline include anorexia, nausea and vomiting, gastric pain caused by increased gastric acid secretion, intestinal bleeding, nervousness, dizziness, headache, irritability, cardiac dysrhythmias, tachycardia, palpitations, marked hypotension, hyperreflexia, and seizures. Adverse CNS reactions (e.g., headaches, irritability, restlessness, nervousness, insomnia, dizziness, seizures) are often more severe in children than in adults. To decrease the potential for side effects, clients should not take other xanthines while taking theophylline.

Theophylline toxicity is most likely to occur when serum concentrations exceed 20 mcg/ml. Theophylline can cause hyperglycemia, decreased clotting time, and, rarely, increased white blood cell count (leukocytosis). Because of the diuretic effect of xanthines, including theophylline, clients should avoid caffeinated products (e.g., coffee, tea, colas, chocolate) and increase their fluid intake.

Rapid IV administration of aminophylline (a theophylline product) can cause dizziness, flushing, hypotension, severe bradycardia, and palpitations. To avoid severe adverse effects, IV theophylline preparations MUST be administered slowly via an infusion pump.

Drug Interactions

Beta-blockers, cimetidine (Tagamet), propranolol (Inderal), and erythromycin decrease the liver metabolism rate and increase the half-life and effects of theophylline; barbiturate

Table 39–3

Theophylline Preparations

Generic (Brand)	Route and Dosage	Uses and Considerations
aminophylline—theophylline ethylenediamine (Somophyllin)	A: PO: LD 400 mg; then increase dose according to body weight; *max:* 24 mg/kg/d IV: LD: 6 mg/kg over 30 min; then 0.2-0.9 mg/kg/h C: PO: LD: 7.5 mg/kg; then 3-6 mg/kg q6-8h IV: LD 6 mg/kg then 1 mg/kg/h **Caution:** Individual titration is based on serum theophylline levels.	IV for acute asthmatic attack. For IV use, drug must be diluted. Oral preparations are tablets or elixirs. For oral use, give with food to avoid GI distress. Side effects include restlessness, syncope, palpitation, tachycardia, hyperventilation, and cardiac dysrhythmias. *Pregnancy category:* C; PB: UK; t$^1/_2$: 4-9 h
dyphylline—dihydroxypropyl theophylline-like (Dilor, Lufyllin)	A: PO: 15 mg/kg q.i.d. A: IM: 250-500 mg q6h C: >6 y: PO: 4-7 mg/kg/d in 4 divided doses Therapeutic serum theophylline range: 10-20 mcg/ml	Treatment of asthma, chronic bronchitis, and emphysema. One tenth as potent as theophylline. Structure is similar to that of theophylline, but it does not convert to theophylline in the body. *Pregnancy category:* C; PB: UK; t$^1/_2$: 2 h
oxtriphylline—choline theophyllinate (Choledyl)	A: PO: 200 mg q8h C: 2-12 y: PO: 4 mg/kg q6h Therapeutic serum theophylline range: 10-20 mcg/ml	Relief of asthma and COPD. Useful for long-term therapy. Drug tolerance is infrequent. Contains 64% theophylline. *Pregnancy category:* C; PB: UK; t$^1/_2$: 3-13 h
theophylline (Theo-Dur and others)	Dose individualized according to serum theophylline levels *Initially:* A: PO: 16 mg/kg/d; *max:* 300 mg/d C: >45 kg: PO: 300 mg/d divided q8-12h C: <45 kg: PO: 12-14 mg/kg/d Premature neonates: >24 h postnatal age: 1.5 mg/kg q12h; Premature neonates: <24 h postnatal age: 1.0 mg/kg q12h; May increase in 25% increments after 3 days as tolerated until dose effective	To promote bronchodilation and to treat asthma and chronic obstructive pulmonary disease

A, Adult; *C,* child; *COPD,* chronic obstructive pulmonary disease; *d,* day; *GI,* gastrointestinal; *h,* hour; *IM,* intramuscular; *IV,* intravenous; *LD,* loading dose; *max,* maximum; *min,* minute; *PB,* protein-binding; *PO,* by mouth; *q.i.d.,* four times a day; *t$^1/_2$,* half-life; *UK,* unknown; *y,* year; *>,* greater than; *<,* less than.

and carbamazepine decrease its effects. In both situations, the theophylline dosage would need adjustment. Theophylline increases the risk of digitalis toxicity, decreases the effects of lithium, and decreases theophylline levels with phenytoin. If theophylline and a beta-adrenergic agonist are given together, a synergistic effect can occur; cardiac dysrhythmias may result.

Nursing Process

Bronchodilator: Leukotriene Receptor Antagonist

ASSESSMENT

■ Obtain a medical and drug history; report probable drug-drug interactions.
■ Note baseline vital signs for abnormalities and for future comparisons.
■ Assess for wheezing, decreased breath sounds, cough, and sputum production.

■ Assess sensorium levels for confusion and restlessness caused by hypoxia and hypercapnia.
■ Determine hydration; diuresis may result in dehydration in children and older adults.

NURSING DIAGNOSES

■ Ineffective breathing pattern
■ Impaired gas exchange
■ Ineffective airway clearance
■ Noncompliance with drug therapy
■ Activity intolerance

PLANNING

■ Client will be free of wheezing and lung fields will be clear within 2 to 5 days.
■ Client is taking oral drugs and using inhaler as prescribed.

NURSING INTERVENTIONS

■ Monitor vital signs. Blood pressure and heart rate can increase greatly. Check for cardiac dysrhythmias.

■ Provide adequate hydration. Fluids aid in loosening secretions. Monitor drug therapy. Observe for side effects.
■ Administer medication after meals to decrease gastrointestinal distress.

Client Teaching

General

- Teach client to monitor pulse rate.
- Encourage client to monitor amount of medication remaining in the canister.
- Advise client not to take OTC preparations without first checking with the health care provider. Some OTC products may have an additive effect.
- Instruct client to avoid smoking. Smoking increases drug elimination.
- Discuss ways to alleviate anxiety such as relaxation techniques and music.
- Advise client having asthma attacks to wear an ID bracelet or MedicAlert tag.

Self-Administration

- Teach client to correctly use the inhaler or nebulizer. Caution against overuse because side effects and tolerance may result.

Correct use of metered-dose inhaler to deliver beta$_2$ agonist

1. Insert the medication canister into the plastic holder.
2. Shake the inhaler well *before* using. Remove cap from mouthpiece.
3. Breathe *out* through the mouth. Open mouth wide and hold mouthpiece 1 to 2 inches from mouth or place inhaler mouthpiece in mouth. A spacer may be used. Discuss technique with health care provider.
4. With mouth open, take *slow deep* breath through mouth and at same time push the top of the medication canister once.
5. Hold breath for a few seconds; exhale slowly through pursed lips.
6. If a second dose is required, wait 2 minutes and repeat the procedure by first shaking the canister in the plastic holder with the cap in place.
7. Before using a new inhaler or if the inhaler has not been used recently, do a "test spray" before administering the metered dose.
8. If a glucocorticoid inhalant is to be used with a bronchodilator, wait 5 minutes before using the inhaler containing the steroid for the bronchodilator effect.

Cultural Considerations ⊕

- Respect the cultural beliefs of client concerning alternative ways to treat asthma or other chronic obstructive pulmonary disease. Client should be told if these ways are unsafe and explained in terms that can be understood.
- If client from a different cultural background does not comply with the drug regimen, the health care provider might consult a health care provider of a similar background and provide a written plan.

EVALUATION

■ Evaluate the effectiveness of the bronchodilator. Client is breathing without wheezing and without side effects of the drug.

Leukotriene Receptor Antagonists and Synthesis Inhibitors

Leukotriene (LT) is a chemical mediator that can cause inflammatory changes in the lung. The cysteinyl leukotrienes promote an increase in eosinophil migration, mucus production, and airway wall edema, which result in bronchoconstriction. LT receptor antagonists and LT synthesis inhibitors, called *leukotriene modifiers*, are effective in reducing the inflammatory symptoms of asthma triggered by allergic and environmental stimuli. These drug groups are not recommended for the treatment of an acute asthma attack. They are used for exercise-induced asthma. Three leukotriene modifiers—zafirlukast (Accolate), zileuton (Zyflo), and montelukast sodium (Singulair)—are available in the United States. These drugs are listed in Table 39-4.

Zafirlukast (Accolate) was the first drug in the class of leukotriene modifiers. It acts as an LT receptor antagonist, thus reducing the inflammatory process and decreasing bronchoconstriction. It is administered orally and absorbed rapidly. It has a moderate to moderately long half-life and is given twice a day. Zileuton (Zyflo) is an LT synthesis inhibitor. It decreases the inflammatory process and bronchoconstriction. Zileuton has a short half-life and is given four times a day. Zafirlukast and zileuton are for adults and children older than 12 years. Montelukast (Singulair) is a new LT receptor antagonist. It has a short half-life of 2.5 to 5.5 hours and is considered safe for use in children 6 years and older.

This category of drugs is the newest group used to control asthma. Again, LT receptor antagonists and synthesis inhibitors should not be used during an acute asthmatic attack. They are only for prophylactic and maintenance drug therapy for chronic asthma.

Nursing Process

Bronchodilator: Montelukast

ASSESSMENT

■ Obtain a medical, drug, and herbal history; report probable drug-drug or drug-herb interactions.
■ Note baseline vital signs for identifying abnormalities and for future comparisons.
■ Assess for wheezing, decreased breath sounds, cough, and sputum production.
■ Assess sensorium levels for confusion and restlessness caused by hypoxia and hypercapnia.

■ Assess theophylline blood levels. Toxicity occurs at a higher frequency with levels greater than 20 mcg/ml.
■ Determine hydration; diuresis may result in dehydration in children and older adults.

NURSING DIAGNOSES

■ Ineffective airway clearance
■ Activity intolerance
■ Knowledge deficit related to OTC drugs

PLANNING

■ Client will be free of wheezing or significantly improved; lung fields will be clear within 2 to 5 days.
■ Client is taking oral drugs and using inhaler as prescribed.

NURSING INTERVENTIONS

■ Monitor vital signs. Blood pressure may decrease and heart rate may increase. Check for cardiac dysrhythmias.
■ Provide adequate hydration. Fluids aid in loosening secretions. Monitor drug therapy. Observe for side effects.
■ Check serum plasma theophylline levels (normal level is 10 to 20 mcg/ml).
■ Administer medication at regular intervals around the clock to have a sustained therapeutic level.
■ Administer medication after meals to decrease GI distress.
■ Do *not* crush enteric-coated or sustained-release (SR) tablets or capsules.
■ Provide pulmonary therapy by chest clapping and postural drainage, as appropriate.

Client Teaching

General

• Advise client that if allergic reaction occurs (e.g., rash, urticaria), drug should be discontinued and a health care provider should be notified.
• Direct client not to take OTC preparations without first checking with the health care provider. Some OTC products may have an additive effect.
• Encourage client to stop smoking while under medical supervision. Avoid marked sudden changes in smoking amounts, which could affect theophylline blood levels. Smoking increases drug elimination, which may require an increased drug dose.
• Discuss ways to alleviate anxiety such as relaxation techniques and music.
• Advise client having frequent or severe asthma attacks to wear an ID bracelet or MedicAlert tag.
• Encourage client contemplating pregnancy to seek medical advice before taking a theophylline preparation.
• Advise client to keep the drug stored out of the reach of small children; request childproof caps.

✍ Inform client that certain herbal products may interact with theophylline. (See Herbal Alert 39–1.)

Self-Administration

• Instruct client to correctly use the nebulizer in conjunction with theophylline.
• Teach client to monitor pulse rate and report to health care provider any irregularities in comparison with baseline.

Diet

• Advise client that a high-protein, low-carbohydrate diet increases theophylline elimination. Conversely, a low-protein, high-carbohydrate diet prolongs the half-life; dosage may need adjustment.

Cultural Considerations ⊕

• When offering a prescription, instructions, or pamphlets to Asian and Pacific Islanders, use both hands to show respect.

EVALUATION

■ Evaluate the effectiveness of the bronchodilators. Client is breathing without wheezing and without side effects of the drug.
■ Determine serum theophylline levels to make sure they are within the accepted range.
■ Evaluate tolerance to activity.

Glucocorticoids (Steroids)

Glucocorticoids, members of the corticosteroid family, are used to treat respiratory disorders, particularly asthma. These drugs have an antiinflammatory action and are indicated if the asthma is unresponsive to bronchodilator therapy or if the client has an asthma attack while on maximum doses of a theophylline or an adrenergic drug. It is thought that glucocorticoids have a synergistic effect when given with a beta$_2$ agonist.

Glucocorticoids can be given using the following methods:
• **MDI inhaler:** beclomethasone (Vanceril, Beclovent)
• **Tablet:** triamcinolone (Amcort, Aristocort, Azmacort), dexamethasone (Decadron), prednisone, prednisolone, and methylprednisolone
• **Intravenous:** dexamethasone (Decadron), hydrocortisone

Inhaled glucocorticoids are *not* helpful in treating a severe asthmatic attack, because it may take 1 to 4 weeks for an inhaled steroid to reach its full effect. Clients with acute COPD are usually given IV glucocorticoids for rapid effectiveness and later gradually weaned off to oral or inhaled

---

HERBAL ALERT 39–1

Lower Respiratory Disorders

🌿 *Ephedra* may increase the effect of the theophylline group and may cause theophylline toxicity.

Table 39–4

Antiinflammatory Drugs for Chronic Obstructive Pulmonary Disease

Generic (Brand)	Route and Dosage	Uses and Considerations
Leukotriene Modifiers (Do *Not* Administer for Acute Asthmatic Attack)		
Leukotriene Receptor Antagonists		
zafirlukast (Accolate)	A: PO: 20 mg b.i.d. 1 h before or 2 h after meals C: >12 y: PO: same as adults C: 7-12 y: PO: 10 mg b.i.d.	For prophylaxis and maintenance therapy for chronic asthma. Reduces inflammation within the bronchial tubes and airways. *Pregnancy category:* B; PB: >99%, $t^{1/2}$: 10 h
montelukast (Singulair)	See Prototype Drug Chart 39–2.	
Leukotriene Synthesis Inhibitors		
zileuton (Zyflo)	A: PO: 600 mg q.i.d. C: >12 y: PO: 600 mg q.i.d.	For prophylaxis and maintenance therapy for chronic asthma. Reduces inflammation in the airways and decreases bronchoconstriction. Hepatotoxicity may result; liver enzymes should be closely monitored. *Pregnancy category:* C; PB: 93%; $t^{1/2}$: 2.5 h
Glucocorticoids (Corticosteroids)		
Intranasal Spray (see Chapter 38, Table 38–3)		
beclomethasone (Beconase, Vancenase)		
budesonide (Pulmicort, Rhinocort)		
dexamethasone (Decadron)		
flunisolide (AeroBid, Nasalide)		
fluticasone (Flonase, Flovent)		
mometasone furoate (Elocon, Nasonex)		
triamcinolone (Nasacort)		
Aerosol Inhalation (see Chapter 49, Table 49–5)		
beclomethasone (Beconase, Vanceril)		
dexamethasone (Decadron)		
flunisolide (AeroBid, Nasalide)		
triamcinolone (Azmacort, Kenalog, Nasacort)		
Oral and Intravenous Administration (see Chapter 49, Table 49–5)		
betamethasone (Celestone)		
cortisone acetate (Cortone acetate, Cortistan)		
dexamethasone (Decadron)		
fludrocortisone acetate (Florinef acetate)		
hydrocortisone (Cortef, Hydrocortone)		
methylprednisolone (Medrol, Solu-Medrol, Depo-Medrol)		
paramethasone acetate (Haldrone)		
prednisolone (Delta-Cortef, Hydeltrasol)		
prednisone		
triamcinolone (Aristocort, Kenacort, Azmacort)		
Combination Drug: Glucocorticoid and Beta₂ Agonist		
fluticasone propionate (Flonase) and salmeterol (Serevent) (Advair Combination— 100 mcg/50 mcg)	A & C: >12 y: DPI diskus inhal: 1 puff b.i.d.	For asthma; not to treat acute asthmatic attacks. If insufficient response, fluticonase dose may be increased.
Cromolyn and Nedocromil (Do Not Use for Acute Asthmatic Attack)		
cromolyn sodium (Intal)	A & C: >6 y: Inhal MDI: 1 puff q.i.d.; available: oral solution and powder, intranasal	For chronic asthma and prophylactic use. Suppresses inflammation in the bronchial tube; does not have bronchodilating effects. Prevents the release of histamine. *Pregnancy category:* B; PB: UK; $t^{1/2}$: 80 min
nedocromil sodium (Tilade)	A & C: >6 y: Inhal MDI: 2 puffs, q.i.d.; may decrease to b.i.d. to t.i.d.	For maintenance therapy for mild to moderate asthma. Has antiinflammatory effect. Suppresses the release of histamine. *Pregnancy category:* B; PB: UK; $t^{1/2}$: 1.5-3 h

A, Adult; *b.i.d.*, twice a day; *C*, child; *DPI*, dry powdered inhaler; *h*, hour; *inhal*, inhalation; *MDI*, metered dose inhaler; *min*, minute; *PB*, protein-binding; *PO*, by mouth; *q.i.d.*, four times a day; $t^{1/2}$, half-life; *t.i.d.*, three times a day; *UK*, unknown; *y*, year; >, greater than.

PROTOTYPE DRUG CHART 39–2

MONTELUKAST

Drug Class	**Dosage**
Bronchodilator: Leukotriene receptor Antagonist Trade Name: Singulair *Pregnancy Category:* B	A: PO: 10 mg daily at bedtime C: 6-14 y: PO: 5 mg daily at bedtime C: 2-5y: 4 mg daily at bedtime
	Drug-Lab-Food Interactions
Contraindications	*Lab:* Abnormal liver function tests (ALT, AST)
Hypersensitivity, severe asthma attack, status asthmaticus *Caution:* Severe liver disease	
Pharmacokinetics	**Pharmacodynamics**
Absorption: Well absorbed **Distribution:** PB: 99% **Metabolism:** t½: 2.7-5.5 h **Excretion:** Feces	PO: Onset: UK Peak: 3-4 h Duration: UK

Therapeutic Effects/Uses

For the prevention and maintenance treatment of asthma
Mode of Action: Binds with leukotriene receptors to inhibit smooth muscle contraction and bronchoconstriction

Side Effects	**Adverse Effects**
Fever, headache, dizziness, fatigue, nasal congestion cough, sore throat, dental pain, influenza, dyspepsia, abdominal pain, rash	None known **Life-threatening:** None known

A, Adult; *ALT,* alanine aminotransferase; *AST,* aspartate aminotransferase; *C,* child; *h,* hour; *PB,* protein-binding; *PO,* by mouth; *t½,* half-life; *UK,* unknown; *y,* year.

---

preparations. Glucocorticoid preparations are discussed in detail in Chapter 49, Endocrine Pharmacology: Pituitary, Thyroid, Parathyroids, and Adrenals.

Glucocorticoids can irritate the gastric mucosa and should be taken with food to avoid ulceration. When discontinuing glucocorticoids, taper the dosage slowly to prevent adrenal insufficiency. A single dose usually does not cause adrenal suppression. The use of an oral inhaler minimizes the risk of adrenal suppression associated with oral systemic glucocorticoid therapy. Inhaled glucocorticoids are preferred to oral preparations unless they fail to control the asthma.

A new combination drug containing the glucocorticoid fluticasone propionate 100 mcg and salmeterol 50 mcg, known as Advair diskus (DPI), is effective in keeping the asthma in check. Advair is used every day, with only one inhalation in the morning and one at night. This drug does not replace fast-acting inhalers for sudden symptoms. The purpose of Advair is to alleviate airway constriction and inflammation.

Side Effects and Adverse Reactions

Side effects associated with the orally inhaled glucocorticoids are generally local (e.g., throat irritation, hoarseness, dry mouth, coughing) rather than systemic. Oral, laryn-

geal, and pharyngeal fungal infections have occurred but can be reversed with discontinuation and antifungal treatment. *Candida albicans* infections may be prevented by the use of a spacer with the inhaler, rinsing the mouth with water after each dose, and washing the apparatus (cap and plastic nose or mouthpiece) daily with warm water.

Oral and injectable glucocorticoids have many side effects. Short-term use causes no significant side effects. Most adverse reactions are seen within 2 weeks of glucocorticoid therapy.

When oral and IV steroids are used for prolonged periods, fluid retention (puffy eyelids, edema in the lower extremities, moon face, weight gain), thinning of the skin, purpura, abnormal subcutaneous (fat) distribution, increased blood sugar, and impaired immune response are likely to occur. With long-term oral use, side effects are significant and include fluid retention, hyperglycemia, and impaired immune response.

Cromolyn and Nedocromil

Cromolyn sodium (Intal) is used for prophylactic treatment of bronchial asthma and therefore must be taken daily. It is *not* used for acute asthmatic attacks. Cromolyn does not have bronchodilator properties but instead acts by inhibiting the release of histamine, which can cause an asthma reaction. Its most common side effects are cough and a bad taste. These effects can be decreased by drinking water before and after the inhalation.

Cromolyn is administered by inhalation. It can be used with beta adrenergics and xanthine derivatives. Rebound bronchospasm is a serious side effect of cromolyn. The drug should not be discontinued abruptly because a rebound asthmatic attack can result.

Action and uses of nedocromil sodium are similar to those of cromolyn sodium. It has an antiinflammatory effect and suppresses the release of histamine, leukotrienes, and other mediators from the mast cells. Like cromolyn, it should not be used for an acute asthmatic attack but instead is used to prevent bronchospasm and an acute asthmatic attack. The inhalation may cause an unpleasant taste. Nedocromil is believed to be more effective than cromolyn.

Table 39–4 lists the antiinflammatory drugs for COPD, which include LT receptor antagonists, LT synthesis inhibitors, glucocorticoids (intranasal spray, aerosol, inhalation, oral, intramuscular, and intravenous), and cromolyn sodium and nedocromil sodium.

Drug Therapy for Asthma According to Severity

Chronic asthma may be controlled through a long-term drug treatment program and by a quick-relief program during an acute phase. A list of four steps for controlling and treating chronic asthma according to the severity of the asthma is presented in Table 39–5. This treatment regimen was developed by the National Asthma Education and Prevention Program of the National Heart, Lung, and Blood Institute in Bethesda, Maryland, in 1997. The long-term drug treatment program may vary according to the symptoms of the asthma and its severity. The quick-relief drug therapy is the same for all classes of asthma.

Drug Therapy for Asthma According to Age

Young Children

Cromolyn and nedocromil are drugs used to treat the inflammatory effects of asthma in children. Oral glucocorticoids may be prescribed for the young child to control a moderate to severe asthmatic state. An inhalation dose of a glucocorticoid should be about 400 to 800 mcg/daily. If the condition is severe, selected young children may be ordered an oral beta$_2$-adrenergic agonist.

Older Adults

Drug selection and dosage need to be considered for the older adult with an asthmatic condition. Beta$_2$-adrenergic agonists and methylxanthines (e.g., theophylline) can cause tachycardia, nervousness, and tremors in older adults, espe-

cially those with cardiac conditions. Frequent use of glucocorticoids can increase the risk of the client developing cataracts, osteoporosis, and diabetes mellitus. If a theophylline drug is ordered, dosages of glucocorticoids are normally decreased.

Mucolytics

Mucolytics act like detergents by liquefying and loosening thick mucous secretions so they can be expectorated. Acetylcysteine (Mucomyst) is administered by nebulization. The drug should not be mixed with other drugs. The medication may be administered with a bronchodilator (not mixed together) for clients with asthma or hyperactive airway disease because the increased secretions may obstruct the bronchial airways. The bronchodilator should be given 5 minutes before the mucolytic. Side effects include nausea and vomiting, stomatitis (oral ulcers), and "runny nose."

Acetylcysteine (Mucomyst) can be used as an antidote for acetaminophen overdose if given within 12 to 24 hours after the overdose ingestion. It can be given orally diluted in juice or soft drinks.

Dornase alfa (Pulmozyme) is an enzyme that digests the deoxyribonucleic acid (DNA) in thick sputum secretions of clients with cystic fibrosis (CF). This agent helps reduce respiratory infections and improves pulmonary function. Improvement usually occurs in 3 to 7 days with its use. Side effects include chest pain, sore throat, laryngitis, and hoarseness.

Antimicrobials

Antibiotics are used only if an infection results from retained mucus secretions.

WEBSITES

For further information on *Drugs for Acute and Chronic Lower Respiratory Disorders*, visit these Internet resources:

Guidelines for the diagnosis and management of asthma:
http://www.nhlbi.nih.gov/guidelines/asthma/asthsumm.htm

beclomethasone dipropionate [Qvar]:
www.centerwatch.com/cgi-bin/cl.pl?p=patient/drugs/dru779.html

Information on alpha$_1$-proteinase inhibitor–human [Zemaira]:
www.zemaira.com

Information on combination drug, albuterol sulfate and ipratropium bromide [DuoNeb]:
www.centerwatch.com/cgi-bin/cl.pl?p=patient/drugs/dru688.html

Table 39-5

Stepwise Approach for Managing Asthma in Adults and Children Older Than 5 Years of Age: Treatment

Classify Severity: Clinical Features Before Treatment or Adequate Control		Medications Required to Maintain Long-Term Control
Symptoms/Day **Symptoms/Night**	**PEF or FEV$_1$** **PEF Variability**	**Daily Medications**
Step 4 Severe persistent Continual Frequent	$\leq$60% >30%	• Preferred treatment: — High-dose inhaled corticosteroids AND — Long-acting inhaled beta$_2$-agonists — AND, if needed, — Corticosteroid tablets or syrup long term (2 mg/kg/day, generally do not exceed 60 mg per day). (Make repeat attempts to reduce systemic corticosteroids and maintain control with high-dose inhaled corticosteroids.)
Step 3 Moderate persistent Daily >1 night/wk	>60% to <80% >30%	• Preferred treatment: — Low-to-medium dose inhaled corticosteroids and long-acting inhaled beta$_2$-agonists. • Alternative treatment (listed alphabetically): — Increase inhaled corticosteroids within medium-dose range OR — Low-to-medium dose inhaled corticosteroids and either leukotriene modifier or theophylline. If needed (particularly in patients with recurring severe exacerbations): • Preferred treatment: — Increase inhaled corticosteroids within medium-dose range and add long-acting inhaled beta$_2$-agonists. • Alternative treatment (listed alphabetically): — Increase inhaled corticosteroids within medium-dose range and add either leukotriene modifier or theophylline.
Step 2 Mild persistent >2/wk but <1 × /day >2 nights/mo	$\geq$80% 20-30%	• Preferred treatment: — Low-dose inhaled corticosteroids. • Alternative treatment (listed alphabetically): cromolyn, leukotriene modifier, nedocromil, OR sustained-release theophylline to serum concentration of 5-15 mcg/ml.
Step 1 Mild intermittent $\leq$2 days/wk $\leq$2 nights/mo	$\geq$80% <20%	• No daily medication needed. • Severe exacerbations may occur, separated by long periods of normal lung function and no symptoms. A course of systemic corticosteroids is recommended.
Quick Relief All patients		• Short-acting bronchodilator: 2-4 puffs short-acting inhaled beta$_2$-agonists as needed for symptoms. • Intensity of treatment will depend on severity of exacerbation; up to 3 treatments at 20-min intervals or a single nebulizer treatment as needed. (Course of systemic corticosteroids may be needed.) • Use of short-acting beta$_2$-agonists >2 times/wk in intermittent asthma (daily, or increasing use in persistent asthma) may indicate the need to initiate (increase) long-term-control therapy.

Step down
Review treatment every 1 to 6 months; a gradual stepwise reduction in treatment may be possible.

Step up
If control is not maintained, consider step up. First, review patient medication technique, adherence, and environmental control.

Goals of Therapy: Asthma Control
• Minimal or no chronic symptoms day or night
• Minimal or no exacerbations
• No limitations on activities; no school/work missed
• Maintain (near) normal pulmonary function
• Minimal use of short-acting inhaled beta$_2$-agonist
• Minimal or no adverse effects from medications

Note
• The stepwise approach is meant to assist, not replace, the clinical decisonmaking required to meet individual patient needs.
• Classify severity: assign patient to most severe step in which any feature occurs (PEF is % of personal best; FEV$_1$ is % predicted).
• Gain control as quickly as possible (consider a short course of systemic corticosteroids); then step down to the least medication necessary to maintain control.
• Minimize use of short-acting inhaled beta$_2$-agonists. Overreliance on short-acting inhaled beta$_2$-agonists (e.g., use of approximately one canister a month even if not using it every day) indicates inadequate control of asthma and the need to initiate or intensify long-term control therapy.
• Provide education on self-management and controlling environmental factors that make asthma worse (e.g., allergens and irritants).
• Refer to an asthma specialist if there are difficulties controlling asthma or if step 4 care is required. Referral may be considered if step 3 care is required.

FEV$_1$, Forced expiratory volume in 1 second; *min*, minute; *mo*, month; *PEF*, peak expiratory flow; *wk*, week; >, greater than; $\geq$, greater than or equal to; <, less than; $\leq$, less than or equal to.
The National Asthma Education and Prevention Program (NAEPP) Expert Panel Report: *Guidelines for the diagnosis and management of asthma—update on selected topics 2002.* http://www.nhlbi.nih.gov/guidelines/asthma/asthsumm.htm.

Critical Thinking Case Study

M.A., age 55, was recently diagnosed with bronchial asthma. Her mother and three brothers also have asthma. In the past year, M.A. has had three asthmatic attacks that were treated with prednisone and albuterol (Proventil) inhaler. Prednisone 10 mg was prescribed for 5 days as follows: day 1, one tablet four times that day; day 2, one tablet three times that day; day 3, one tablet two times that day; day 4, one tablet in the morning; day 5, one-half tablet in the morning.

1. Explain the purpose for the use of prednisone during an asthmatic attack. Explain why the dosage is decreased (tapered) over a period of 5 days.

2. Can cromolyn sodium be substituted for prednisone during an asthmatic attack? Explain.

3. M.A. is prescribed albuterol. What effect does albuterol have on controlling asthma?

4. Albuterol is administered by an inhaler. For each drug dose, M.A. is to take two puffs. What instructions should she be given concerning the use of the inhaler?

To minimize the frequency of M.A.'s asthmatic attacks, the health care provider prescribed Theo-Dur 200 mg b.i.d. The albuterol inhalation is to be taken as needed. Nursing interventions include client history of asthmatic attacks and physical assessment.

5. What should the nurse include when taking the client's history concerning asthmatic attacks? What physical assessment would suggest an asthmatic attack?

6. What type of drug is Theo-Dur? Why should the nurse ask M.A. whether she smokes?

7. What are the side effects and adverse reactions and drug interactions related to Theo-Dur?

8. What nonpharmacologic measures can the nurse suggest that may decrease the frequency of asthmatic attacks?

Study Questions

1. A client uses an albuterol aerosol inhaler four times a day to prevent an asthmatic attack. What type of drug is albuterol? What is its action? What client teaching should be included concerning dose administration and side effects?

2. Theophylline drugs are administered in tablets to prevent asthmatic attacks and in intravenous fluids as aminophylline to prevent acute asthmatic attacks. What is the effect of theophylline? What is its serum therapeutic range? Why is the serum level monitored?

3. When is cromolyn sodium used to treat asthma? Why should cromolyn *not* be abruptly discontinued?

4. A client is instructed to use two aerosol inhalers: a bronchodilator (Proventil) and a glucocorticoid

(Vanceril). What client teaching should be included on administering these drugs together?

5. A client was having a mild asthmatic attack. The health care provider ordered methylprednisolone 4 mg for six days with decreasing dosages over the six days (i.e., six tablets the first day, five tablets the second day, four tablets the third day, and so forth). The client asks the following: What is the purpose of this drug for treating my asthma? Why should I take fewer tablets each day? Why should I take it with food or after a meal? What are appropriate responses?

6. What is the action of leukotriene antagonists?

7. What are mucolytics? When are they used?

Twelve

Cardiovascular Agents

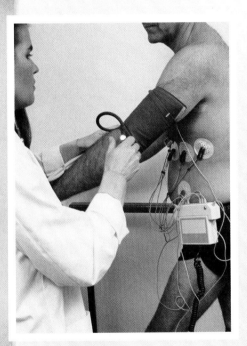

The cardiovascular system includes the heart, blood vessels (arteries and veins), and blood. Blood rich in oxygen (O_2), nutrients, and hormones moves through vessels called *arteries*, which narrow to arterioles. Capillaries transport rich nourished blood to body cells and absorb waste products such as carbon dioxide (CO_2), urea, creatinine, and ammonia. The deoxygenated blood returns to the circulation by the venules and veins to be eliminated by the lungs and kidneys with other waste products (Figure XII–1).

The heart's pumping action serves as the energy source that circulates blood to body cells. Blockage of vessels can inhibit blood flow.

Heart

The heart is composed of four chambers: the right and left atria and the right and left ventricles (Figure XII–2). The right atrium receives deoxygenated blood from the circulation, and the right ventricle pumps blood through the pulmonary artery to the lungs for gas exchange (carbon dioxide for oxygen). The left atrium receives oxygenated blood, and the left ventricle pumps the blood into the aorta for systemic circulation.

The heart muscle, called the *myocardium*, surrounds the ventricles and atria. The ventricles are thick walled, especially the left ventricle, to achieve the muscular force needed to pump blood to the pulmonary and systemic circulations. The atria are thin walled, have less pumping action and serve as receptacles for blood from the circulation and lungs.

The heart has a fibrous covering called the *pericardium*, which protects it from injury and infection. The *endocardium* is a three-layered membrane that lines the inner part of the heart chambers. Four valves—two atrioventricular (tricuspid and mitral) and two semilunar (pulmonic and aortic)—control blood flow between the atria and ventricles and between the ventricles and the pulmonary artery and the aorta. There are two coronary arteries. The right coronary artery supplies blood to the right atrium and ventricle of the heart, and the left coronary artery supplies blood to the left atrium and ventricle of the heart. The left coronary artery divides near its origin to form the left circumflex artery and the anterior descending artery. Blockage to one of these arteries can result in a myocardial infarction (MI), or heart attack.

Conduction of Electrical Impulses

The myocardium is capable of generating and conducting its own electrical impulses. The cardiac impulse usually originates in the *sinoatrial (SA) node* located in the posterior wall of the right atrium. The SA node is frequently called the *pacemaker*, because it regulates the heartbeat

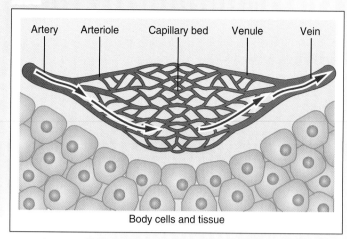

FIGURE XII–1 Basic structures of the vascular system.

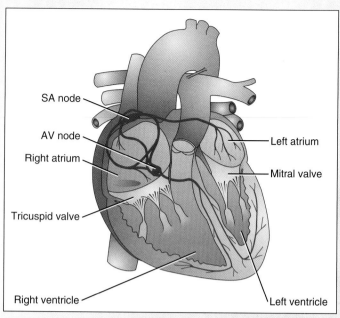

FIGURE XII–2 Anatomy of the heart. *AV node,* Atrioventricular node; *SA node,* sinoatrial node.

(firing of cardiac impulses), which is approximately 60 to 80 beats/min. The *atrioventricular (AV) node,* located in the posterior right side of the interatrial septum, has a continuous tract of fibers called the *bundle of His,* or the AV bundle. The AV node is called the *functional pacemaker,* having a rate of 40 to 60 beats/min. If the SA node fails, the AV node takes over, thus causing a slower heart rate. The AV node sends impulses to the ventricles. These two conducting systems (SA node and AV node) can act independently of each other. The ventricle can contract independently 30 to 40 times per minute.

Drugs that affect cardiac contraction include calcium, digitalis preparations, and quinidine and its related preparations. The autonomic nervous system (ANS) and the drugs that stimulate or inhibit it influence heart contractions. The sympathetic nervous system and the drugs that stimulate it *increase* heart rate; the parasympathetic nervous system and the drugs that stimulate it *decrease* heart rate.

Regulation of Heart Rate and Blood Flow

The heart beats approximately 60 to 80 times per minute in an adult, pumping blood into the systemic circulation. As blood travels, resistance to blood flow develops and arterial pressure increases. The average systemic arterial pressure, known as blood pressure, is 120/80 mmHg. Arterial blood pressure is determined by peripheral resistance and *cardiac output,* the volume of blood expelled from the heart in 1 minute, which is calculated by multiplying the heart rate by the stroke volume. The average cardiac output is 4 to 8 L/min. *Stroke volume,* the amount of blood ejected from the left ventricle with each heart beat, is approximately 70 ml/beat.

Three factors—preload, contractility, and afterload—determine the stroke volume (Figure XII–3). *Preload* refers to the blood flow force that stretches the ventricle. *Contractil-*

ity is the force of ventricular contraction, and *afterload* is the resistance to ventricular ejection of blood caused by opposing pressures in the aorta and systemic circulation.

Specific drugs can increase or decrease preload and afterload, affecting both stroke volume and cardiac output. Most vasodilators decrease preload and afterload thus decreasing arterial pressure and cardiac output.

Circulation

There are two types of circulation—pulmonary, and systemic or peripheral. With pulmonary circulation, the heart pumps deoxygenated blood from the right ventricle through the pulmonary artery to the lungs. In this situation, the artery carries blood that has a high concentration of carbon dioxide. Oxygenated blood returns to the left atrium by the pulmonary vein.

With systemic or peripheral circulation, the heart pumps blood from the left ventricle to the aorta and into the general circulation. Arteries and arterioles carry the blood to capillary beds. Nutrients in the capillary blood are transferred to cells in exchange for waste products. Blood returns to the heart through venules and veins.

Blood

Blood is composed of plasma, red blood cells (erythrocytes), white blood cells (leukocytes), and platelets. Plasma, made up of 90% water and 10% solutes, constitutes 55% of the total blood volume. The solutes in plasma include glucose, protein, lipids, amino acids, electrolytes,

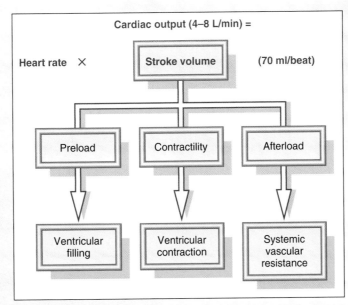

FIGURE XII-3   Cardiac output and stroke volume.

minerals, lactic and pyruvic acids, hormones, enzymes, oxygen, and carbon dioxide.

The major function of blood is to provide nutrients, including oxygen, to body cells. Most of the oxygen is carried in the hemoglobin of red blood cells (RBCs). The white blood cells (WBCs) are the major defense mechanism of the body and act by engulfing microorganisms. They also produce antibodies. The platelets are large cells that cause blood to coagulate. RBCs have a life span of approximately 120 days, whereas the life span of WBCs is only 2 to 24 hours.

Unit XII, Cardiovascular Agents, is composed of five chapters dealing with drugs for cardiac disorders, diuretics and antihypertensive drugs, and drugs for circulatory disorders. Cardiac glycosides, antianginals, and antidysrhythmics are described in Chapter 40. Chapter 41 discusses the five categories of diuretics. Five major categories of antihypertensive agents are presented in Chapter 42. The five groups of drugs covered in Chapter 43 and 44 are the anticoagulants, antiplatelets, thrombolytics, antilipidemics, and peripheral vasodilators.

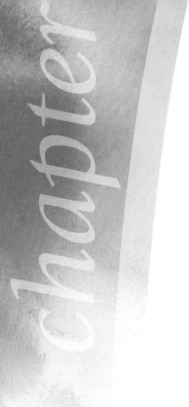

40 Cardiac Glycosides, Antianginals, and Antidysrhythmics

ELECTRONIC RESOURCES   *evolve*

Additional information can be found on the companion website at *http://evolve.elsevier.com/KeeHayes/pharmacology/* or on the companion CD-ROM, which includes:
- *NCLEX-style examination review questions*
- *Pharmacology animations*
- *Medication error and (IV) therapy checklists*
- *Medication calculation problems*
- *Electronic calculators*

OBJECTIVES

- Explain the actions related to cardiac glycosides, antianginal drugs, and antidysrhythmic drugs.
- Describe the signs and symptoms of digitalis toxicity.
- Identify the side effects and adverse reactions of nitrates, beta-blockers, calcium channel blockers, quinidine, and procainamide.
- Explain the nursing process, including client teaching, related to cardiac glycosides, antianginal drugs, and antidysrhythmic drugs.

Introduction

Three groups of drugs—cardiac glycosides, antianginals, and antidysrhythmics—are discussed in this chapter. Drugs in these groups regulate heart contraction, heart rate and rhythm, and blood flow to the myocardium (heart muscle).

Cardiac Glycosides

Digitalis began being used as early as 1200 AD, making it one of the oldest drugs. It is still used in a purified form. Digitalis is obtained from the purple and white foxglove plant, and it can be poisonous. In 1785 William Withering of England used digitalis to alleviate "dropsy," edema of the extremities caused by kidney and cardiac insufficiency. Digitalis preparations are effective in treating **congestive heart failure (CHF)**, also known as congestive cardiac failure (CCF). (Withering did not realize that "dropsy" was the result of heart failure.) When the heart muscle (*myocardium*) weakens and enlarges, it loses its ability to pump blood through the heart and into the systemic circulation. This is called **heart failure,** or pump failure. When compensatory mechanisms fail and the peripheral and lung tissues are congested, the condition is CHF. Heart failure can be left sided or right sided. The client has left-sided heart failure when the left ventricle does not contract sufficiently to pump the blood returned from the left atrium and lungs into the aorta, causing excessive amounts of blood to remain in the lung tissue. Usually the client has shortness of breath (SOB) and dyspnea. Right-sided heart failure occurs when the heart does not sufficiently pump the blood returned into the right atrium from the systemic circulation. As a result, the blood and its constituents are backed into peripheral tissues causing peripheral edema. One type of heart failure can lead to the other. Myocardial hypertropy resulting in *cardiomegaly* (increased heart size) can be a major problem associated with progressive heart failure.

With heart failure, there is an increase in preload and afterload. An increase in preload results from an increase in blood in the ventricle at the end of diastole. This occurs because of a pathologic increase in the elasticity of the ventricular walls that is associated with a weakened heart. With an increased afterload, there is an increased pressure or force in the ventricular wall caused by increased resistance in the aorta, which must be overcome to open the aortic valve so blood can be injected into the circulation. The American College of Cardiology (ACC) and the American Heart Association (AHA) in 2001 has classified heart failure in stages according to its severity. Table 40–1 lists the stages of heart failure according to ACC/AHA. Detailed information related to the staging process of heart failure can be found on the internet at *www.acc.org/clinical/guidelines/failure/hf_index.htm* and *www.americanheart.org/presenter.jhtml?identifier=11841.*

Cardiac glycosides, also called *digitalis glycosides,* are a group of drugs that inhibit the sodium-potassium pump; thus they increase intracellular calcium, which causes the cardiac muscle fibers to contract more efficiently. Digitalis preparations have four effects on the heart muscle: (1) a positive **inotropic** action (increases myocardial contraction stroke volume), (2) a negative **chronotropic** action (decreases heart rate), and (3) a negative **dromotropic** action (decreases conduction of the heart cells). The increase in myocardial contractility increases cardiac, peripheral, and kidney function by increasing cardiac output, decreasing preload, improving blood flow to the periphery and kidneys, decreasing edema, and increasing fluid excretion. As a result, fluid retention in the lung and extremities is decreased.

Cardiac glycosides are also used to correct **atrial fibrillation** (cardiac dysrhythmia with rapid uncoordinated contractions of atrial myocardium) and **atrial flutter** (cardiac dysrhythmia with rapid contractions of 200 to 300 beats per minute [bpm]). This is accomplished by the negative

Table 40–1

ACC/AHA *Stages of Heart Failure (HF)*

Stage	Characteristics According to Stages
1	High risk for HF without symptoms or structural heart disease
2	Structural heart disease without symptoms of HF
3	Structural heart disease with symptoms of HF
4	Severe structural heart disease and marked symptoms of HF

ACC, American College of Cardiology; *AHA,* American Heart Association.

chronotropic effects (decreases heart rate) and negative dromotropic effects (decreases conduction through the atrioventricular [AV] node).

Nonpharmacologic Measures to Treat Heart Failure

Nondrug therapy is an integral part of the regimen for controlling heart failure. The nondrug component of the regimen should be tailored to meet the needs of each client; however, the following are some general recommendations. The client should limit salt intake to 2 g daily, which is approximately 1 teaspoon. Alcohol intake should be either decreased to one drink per day or completely avoided. Excessive alcohol use can lead to cardiomyopathy. Smoking should be avoided because it deprives the heart of oxygen (O_2). Obesity increases cardiovascular problems; thus obese clients should decrease fat and caloric intake. Mild exercise such as walking or bicycling is recommended.

Laboratory Tests

Atrial natriuretic hormone or peptide

Reference value: 20-77 pg/ml; 20-77 ng/l (SI units). An elevated atrial natriuretic hormone (ANH) or peptide (ANP) may confirm CHF. ANH is secreted from the atria of the heart and acts as an antagonist to renin and aldosterone. It is released during expansion of the atrium, produces vasodilation, and increases glomerular filtration rate.

Brain natriuretic peptide

Reference values: Desired value: <100 pg/ml; positive value: >100 pg/ml. The brain natriuretic peptide (BNP) test aids in the diagnoses of heart failure. Diagnosing heart failure is difficult in persons with lung disease who are experiencing dyspnea and in those who are obese or elderly. Frequently the BNP is higher than 100 pg/ml in women who are 65 years old or older. An 80-year-old woman's BNP may be 160 pg/ml; however, with heart failure, the BNP is markedly higher, as high as 400 pg/ml. BNP is considered a more sensitive test than ANP for diagnosing heart failure. Today, there is a bedside/emergency department machine to measure BNP.

Digoxin

Prototype Drug Chart 40–1 gives the pharmacologic data for digoxin, a cardiac glycoside.

Pharmacokinetics

The absorption rate of digoxin in oral tablet form is greater than 70%. The rate is 90% in liquid form and 90% to 100% in capsule form. The protein-binding power for digoxin is low; however, its half-life is 36 hours. Because of its long half-life, drug accumulation can occur. Side effects should be closely monitored to detect digitalis toxicity. Clients should be made aware of side effects that need to be reported to the health care provider. Serum digoxin levels are most commonly drawn when actual digitoxicity is suspected. This allows the health care provider to ascertain the extent of such toxicity and to confirm elimination of the drug after it is stopped or decreased in dosage (see Digitalis Toxicity).

Thirty percent of digoxin is metabolized by the liver, and 70% is excreted by the kidneys mostly unchanged. Kidney dysfunction can affect the excretion of digoxin. Thyroid dysfunction can alter the metabolism of cardiac glycosides. For clients with hypothyroidism, the dose of digoxin should be decreased; in hyperthyroidism, the dose may need to be increased.

Digitoxin is a potent cardiac glycoside that has a very long half-life and is highly protein bound. This drug is seldom prescribed. The names *digoxin* and *digitoxin* are very similar; therefore the nurse must be extremely careful to administer the correct drug. The client should consistently take the same brand of digoxin to avoid unnecessary side effects or adverse reactions.

Pharmacodynamics

In clients with a failing heart, cardiac glycosides increase myocardial contraction, which increases cardiac output and improves circulation and tissue perfusion. Because these drugs decrease conduction through the AV node, the heart rate decreases.

The onset and peak actions of oral and intravenous (IV) digoxin vary. The **therapeutic serum level** is 0.5 to 2.0 ng/ml for digoxin and 10 to 35 ng/ml for digitoxin. To treat CHF, the lower serum therapeutic levels should be obtained, and for atrial flutter or fibrillation, the higher therapeutic serum levels are required.

Of these two drugs, digoxin is more frequently used. It can be administered orally or IV. Table 40–2 lists the drug data for digitalis preparations.

Digitalis Toxicity

Overdose or accumulation of digoxin causes digitalis toxicity. Signs and symptoms include anorexia, diarrhea, nausea and vomiting, **bradycardia** (pulse rate below 60 bpm), premature ventricular contractions, cardiac dysrhythmias, headaches, malaise, blurred vision, visual illusions (white, green, yellow halos around objects), confusion, and delirium. Older adults are more prone to toxicity.

Cardiotoxicity is a serious adverse reaction to digoxin; ventricular dysrhythmias result. Three cardiac-altered functions can contribute to digoxin-induced ventricular dys-

PREVENTING MEDICATION ERRORS

Do not confuse...

- **digitoxin with digoxin.** Both drugs are cardiac glycosides. Digoxin (lanoxin) is usually the choice drug because its half-life is 36 hours, whereas the half-life of digitoxin is 4 to 9 days.

Right Drug:

Maintenance dose for digoxin is 0.125 to 0.5 mg/dl. With the older adult, dose is usually 0.125 mg/dl.

Right Assessment:

Check for digoxin or digitalis toxicity. Pulse rate (heart rate) should be above 60 bpm. For other signs and symptoms, see Digitalis Toxicity, above. Monitor the therapeutic serum level of digoxin, 0.5 to 2.0 ng/ml. Digoxin can have an accumulative effect.

PROTOTYPE DRUG CHART 40–1

DIGOXIN (LANOXIN)

Drug Class

Cardiac glycoside
Trade Name: Lanoxin
Pregnancy Category: C

Dosage

A: PO: 0.5-1 mg initially in 2 divided doses (digitaliza-
tion); *maint*: 0.125-0.5 mg/daily
IV: Same as PO dose given over 5 min
Elderly: 0.125 mg/daily
C: PO: 1 mo-2 y: 0.01–0.02 mg/kg in 3 divided doses;
maint: 0.012 mg/kg/daily in 2 divided doses
IV: Dosage varies
C: PO: 2-10 y: 0.012-0.04 mg/kg in divided doses
Pediatric doses are usually ordered in mcg in elixir form.

Contraindications

Ventricular dysrhythmias, second- or third-degree heart
  block
Caution: AMI, renal disease, hypothyroidism, hypokalemia

Drug-Lab-Food Interactions

Drug: Increase digoxin serum level with quinidine,
  flecainide, verapamil; *decrease* digoxin absorption
  with antacids, colestipol; *increase* risk for digoxin toxicity with thiazide diuretics, loop diuretics
Lab: Hypokalemia, hypomagnesemia, hypercalcemia

Pharmacokinetics

Absorption: PO tablet: 60%-70%; PO liquid: 90%;
  PO capsule: 90%-100%
Distribution: PB: 25%
Metabolism: t½: 30-45 h
Excretion: 70% in urine; 30% by liver metabolism

Pharmacodynamics

PO: Onset: 1-5 h
  Peak: 6-8 h
  Duration: 2-4 d
IV: Onset: 5-30 min
  Peak: 1-5 h
  Duration: 2-4 d

Therapeutic Effects/Uses

To treat CHF, atrial tachycardia, flutter, or fibrillation
Mode of Action: Inhibits the sodium-potassium ATPase thus promoting increased force of cardiac contraction, cardiac
  output, and tissue perfusion; decreases ventricular rate

Side Effects

Anorexia, nausea, vomiting, headache, blurred vision
  (yellow-green halos), diplopia, photophobia, drowsiness,
  fatigue, confusion

Adverse Reactions

Bradycardia, visual disturbances
Life-threatening: Atrioventricular block, cardiac
  dysrhythmias

A, Adult; *AMI,* acute myocardial infarction; *ATPase,* adenosine triphosphatase; *C,* child; *CHF,* congestive heart failure; *d,* day; *h,* hour;
IV, intravenous; *maint,* maintenance; *min,* minute; *mo,* month; *PB,* protein-binding; *PO,* by mouth; *t½,* half-life; *y,* year.

rhythmias: (1) suppression of AV conduction, (2) increased automaticity, and (3) a decreased refractory period
in ventricular muscle. The antidysrhythmics phenytoin
and lidocaine are effective in treating digoxin-induced ventricular dysrhythmias.

Antidote for Cardiac/Digitalis Glycosides

Digoxin immune Fab (ovine, Digibind) may be given to
treat severe digitalis toxicity. This agent binds with digoxin
to form complex molecules that can be excreted in the
urine; thus digoxin is unable to bind at the cellular site of
action. Signs and symptoms of digoxin toxicity should be
reported promptly to the health care provider. Serum
digoxin levels should be closely monitored. Digitalis tox-

icity may result in first-degree, second-degree, or complete
heart block.

Drug Interactions

Drug interaction with digitalis preparations can cause digitalis toxicity. Many of the potent diuretics, such as
furosemide (Lasix) and hydrochlorothiazide (Hydro-
Diuril), promote the loss of potassium from the body. The
resultant **hypokalemia** (low serum potassium level) increases the effect of the digitalis preparation at its myocardial cell site of action, resulting in digitalis toxicity. Cortisone preparations taken systemically promote sodium
retention and potassium excretion or loss and can also
cause hypokalemia. Clients who take digoxin along with a

potassium-wasting diuretic or a cortisone drug should consume foods rich in potassium or take potassium supplements to avoid hypokalemia and digitalis toxicity. Antacids can decrease digitalis absorption if taken at the same time. To prevent this problem, doses should be staggered.

Nursing Process

Cardiac Glycosides: Digoxin

ASSESSMENT

■ Obtain a drug and herbal history. Report if a drug-drug or drug-herb interaction is probable. If client is taking digoxin and a potassium-wasting diuretic or cortisone drug, hypokalemia might result, causing digitalis toxicity. A low serum potassium level enhances the action of digoxin. A client taking a thiazide and/or cortisone with digoxin should take a potassium supplement.

■ Obtain a baseline pulse rate for future comparisons. Apical pulse should be taken for a full minute and should be >60 bpm.

■ Assess for signs and symptoms of digitalis toxicity. Common symptoms include anorexia, nausea, vomiting, bradycardia, cardiac dysrhythmias, and visual disturbances. Report symptoms immediately to the health care provider.

NURSING DIAGNOSES

■ Decreased cardiac output
■ Ineffective tissue perfusion (cardiopulmonary, cerebral)
■ Anxiety related to cardiac problem

PLANNING

■ Client checks pulse rate daily before taking digoxin. Client will report pulse rate of <60 bpm or a marked decline in pulse rate.

■ Client eats foods rich in potassium to maintain a desired serum potassium level (see Client Teaching, Diet).

NURSING INTERVENTIONS

■ Do *not* confuse *digoxin* with *digitoxin*. Read the drug labels carefully. Digoxin has a long half-life but has a shorter half-life than digitoxin.

■ Check the apical pulse rate before administering digoxin. Do *not* administer if pulse rate is <60 bpm.

■ Determine the signs of peripheral and pulmonary edema, which indicate congestive heart failure is present.

■ Check the serum digoxin level. The normal therapeutic drug range for digoxin is 0.5 to 2 ng/ml. A serum digoxin level of >2.0 ng/ml is indicative of digitalis toxicity. Check serum potassium level (normal range, 3.5 to 5.3 mEq/L) and report if hypokalemia (<3.5 mEq/L) is present.

Client Teaching

General

• Explain to client the importance of compliance with the drug therapy. A visiting nurse may ensure that the medications are properly taken.

• Advise client not to take OTC drugs without first consulting the health care provider to avoid adverse drug interactions.

• Keep drugs out of reach of small children. Request childproof bottles.

• Instruct client or parent of child to check pulse rate before administering the drug.

• Inform client of possible herb-drug interactions. (See Herbal Alert 40–1.)

Self-Administration

• Instruct client how to check the pulse rate before taking digoxin and to call the health care provider for pulse rate <60 bpm or irregular pulse.

Side Effects

• Instruct client to report side effects such as a pulse rate of <60 bpm, nausea, vomiting, headache, and visual disturbances, including diplopia.

Diet

• Advise client to eat foods rich in potassium such as fresh and dried fruits, fruit juices, and vegetables, including potatoes.

Cultural Considerations ⊕

• It is essential that clients from various cultural backgrounds taking digoxin, diuretics, and potassium supplements for heart failure do not miss drug doses of their medication. Client should be fully aware of adverse effects and readily report them to the health care provider.

• Speak clearly and slowly; allow time for client to respond.

• Be certain that client understands the purposes for taking these drugs. The Amish people respect authority and usually follow orders without question.

EVALUATION

■ Evaluate the effectiveness of digoxin by noting client's response to the drug (decreased heart rate, decreased chest rales) and the absence of side effects. Continue monitoring the pulse rate.

Table 40-2

Cardiac Glycosides and Inotropic Agents

Generic (Brand)	Route and Dosage	Uses and Considerations
Rapid-Acting Digitalis		
digoxin (Lanoxin)	See Prototype Drug Chart 40-1.	
Long-Acting Digitalis		
digitoxin (Crystodigin)	A: PO/IV: LD: 0.8-1.2 mg; *maint:* PO: 0.05-3 mg/d	For CHF. Serum therapeutic level is 15-30 ng/ml. Because of its long half-life, this drug is seldom given. *Pregnancy category:* C; PB: 97%; $t^{1}/_{2}$: 7-8 h
Phosphodiesterase Inhibitors (Positive Inotropic Bipyridines)		
amrinone lactate (Inocor)	A: IV: LD: 0.75 mg/kg bolus over 2-3 min; *maint:* IV inf: 5-10 mcg/kg/min; *max:* 10 mcg/kg/d	For CHF, amrinone may be prescribed when digoxin and diuretics have not been effective. It may be used in conjunction with diuretic; however, it is incompatible with furosemide. Drug is for short-term use. *Pregnancy category:* C; PB: 10%-50%; $t^{1}/_{2}$: 3.5-7h
milrinone lactate (Primacor)	A: IV: Initially: 50 mcg/kg/over 10 min *Continuous infusion:* 0.375-0.75 mcg/kg/min with 0.45%-0.9% saline	For short-term treatment of CHF. May be given before heart transplantation. Heart rate and blood pressure should be monitored. *Pregnancy category:* C; PB: 70%; $t^{1}/_{2}$: 1.5-2.5 h
Atrial Natriuretic Peptide Hormone		
nesiritide (Natrecor)	A: IV bolus: 2 mcg/kg, followed by 0.01 mcg/kg/min, by IV infusion	To treat acute CHF by increasing sodium loss. It is useful in managing dyspnea at rest. It causes vasodilation. Contraindication includes clients with a systolic BP less than 90 mm Hg. *Pregnancy category:* C; PB: UK; $t^{1}/_{2}$: 18-22 min
Antidote for Digitalis Toxicity		
digoxin immune Fab (ovine, Digibind)	Dose varies. Use manufacturer's dosing guidelines. Approx 760 mg, IV diluted in 50 ml of NSS. Infuse over 30 min.	To correct serious digitalis toxicity. This agent binds with digoxin to form complex molecules. A serum digoxin level >2.0 ng is indicative of digitalis toxicity. Onset of action is 30 min and duration of action can be 3-4 days. *Pregnancy category:* C; PB: UK; $t^{1}/_{2}$: 15-20 h

A, Adult; *BP,* blood pressure; *CHF,* congestive heart failure; *d,* day; *h,* hour; *inf,* infusion; *IV,* intravenous; *LD,* loading dose; *maint,* maintenance; *min,* minute; *NSS,* normal saline solution; *PB,* protein-binding; *PO,* by mouth; *$t^{1}/_{2}$,* half-life; *UK,* unknown; >, greater than.

HERBAL ALERT 40-1

Cardiac Glycosides: Digoxin

🍃 *Ginseng* may falsely elevate digoxin levels.

🍃 *St. John's wort* decreases the absorption of digoxin and thus decreases the serum digoxin level.

🍃 *Psyllium* (Metamucil) may decrease digoxin absorption.

🍃 *Hawthorn* may increase the effect of digoxin.

🍃 *Licorice* can potentiate the effect of digoxin. It promotes potassium loss (hypokalemia), which increases the effect of digoxin. It may cause digitalis toxicity.

🍃 *Aloe* may increase the risk of digitalis toxicity. It increases potassium loss, which increases the effect of digoxin.

🍃 *Ma-huang* or ephedra increases the risk of digitalis toxicity.

🍃 *Goldenseal* may decrease the effects of cardiac glycosides and increase the effects of antidysrhythmics.

Phosphodiesterase Inhibitors

The phosphodiesterase inhibitors are another positive inotropic group of drugs given to treat acute CHF or when there is no response to the use of other agents. This drug group inhibits the enzyme phosphodiesterase, thus promoting a positive inotropic response and vasodilation. The two drugs in this group are amrinone lactate (Inocor) and milrinone lactate (Primacor). These drugs increase stroke volume and cardiac output and promote vasodilation. They are administered IV for no longer than 48 to 72 hours. Severe cardiac dysrhythmias might result from the use of phosphodiesterase inhibitors; therefore the client's electrocardiogram (ECG) and cardiac status should be closely monitored.

Other Agents Used to Treat Heart Failure

Vasodilators, angiotensin-converting enzyme (ACE) inhibitors, angiotensin II receptor antagonists (blockers), diuretics (thiazides, furosemide), spironolactone (Aldactone), and some beta-blockers are other drug groups prescribed to treat heart failure.

Vasodilators can be used to treat heart failure. The vasodilators decrease venous blood return to the heart; thus there is a decrease in cardiac filling, ventricular stretching (preload), and oxygen demand on the heart. The arteriolar dilators act in three ways: (1) to reduce cardiac afterload, which increases cardiac output; (2) to dilate the arterioles of the kidneys, which improves renal perfusion and increases fluid loss; and (3) to improve circulation to the skeletal muscles.

ACE inhibitors are usually prescribed for heart failure. ACE inhibitors dilate venules and arterioles, which improves renal blood flow and decreases blood fluid volume. They also moderately decrease the release of aldosterone; thus sodium and fluid retention are reduced. Also, the angiotensin II receptor antagonists (blocker), such as valsartan (Diovan), were recently approved for CHF in clients who cannot tolerate an ACE inhibitor.

Diuretics are the first-line drug treatment for reducing fluid volume and are frequently prescribed with digoxin or other agents.

Spironolactone (Aldactone), a potassium-sparing diuretic, is used in treating moderate to severe CHF. Aldosterone secretions are increased in CHF; this promotes body loss of potassium and magnesium needed by the heart and increases sodium and water retention. Spironolactone blocks the production of aldosterone. This drug improves heart rate variability and decreases myocardial fibrosis. The recommended dose is 12.5 to 25 mg per day. Occurrence of hyperkalemia (excess serum potassium) is rare unless the client is receiving 50 mg daily and has renal insufficiency. However, the serum potassium level should be closely monitored.

Certain beta-blockers are usually contraindicated for clients with heart failure because this drug class reduces cardiac contractility. However, in some cases, beta-blockers, such as carvedilol (Coreg) and metoprolol tartrate (Toprol-XL), have been shown to improve cardiac performance. Nonetheless, beta-blockers are not recommended for clients with class IV heart failure.

Nesiritide (Natrecor) is a atrial natriuretic peptide hormone that inhibits antidiuretic hormone (ADH) by increasing urine sodium loss. It is used in correcting CHF by promoting vasodilation, natriuresis, and diuresis. It is useful for treating clients who have acute decompensated CHF with dyspnea at rest or who have dyspnea with little physical movement.

BiDil, a combination of hydralazine (for blood pressure) and isosorbide dinitrate (a dilator to relieve heart pain) has received FDA panel approval for treating heart failure, especially in African Americans. African Americans have more than twice the rate of heart failure as whites, and a research study has shown this drug to be effective in treating heart failure in the African-American population.

Antianginal Drugs

Antianginal drugs are used to treat **angina pectoris.** This is a condition of acute cardiac pain caused by inadequate blood flow to the myocardium resulting from either plaque occlusions within or spasms of the coronary arteries. With decreased blood flow, there is a decrease in O_2 to the myocardium, which results in pain. Anginal pain is frequently described by the client as tightness, pressure in the center of the chest, and pain radiating down the left arm. Referred pain felt in the neck and left arm commonly occurs with severe angina pectoris. Anginal attacks may lead to myocardial infarction (MI) or heart attack. Anginal pain usually lasts for only a few minutes. Stress tests, cardiac profile laboratory tests, and cardiac catheterization may be needed to determine the degree of blockage in the coronary arteries.

Types of Angina Pectoris

The frequency of anginal pain depends on many factors, including the type of angina. There are three types of angina.

- *Classic (stable):* Occurs with stress or exertion
- *Unstable (preinfarction):* Occurs frequently over the course of a day with progressive severity
- *Variant (Prinzmetal, vasospastic):* Occurs during rest

The first two types are caused by a narrowing or partial occlusion of the coronary arteries; variant angina is caused by vessel spasm (vasospasm). It is common for a client to have both classic and variant angina. Unstable angina often indicates an impending MI. This is an emergency that needs immediate medical intervention.

Nonpharmacologic Measures to Control Angina

A combination of pharmacologic and nonpharmacologic measures is usually necessary to control and prevent anginal attacks. Nonpharmacologic ways of decreasing anginal attacks are to avoid heavy meals, smoking, extremes in weather changes, strenuous exercise, and emotional upset. Proper nutrition, moderate exercise (only after consulting with a health care provider if the client already has angina), adequate rest, and relaxation techniques should be used as preventive measures.

Types of Antianginal Drugs

Antianginal drugs increase blood flow either by increasing oxygen supply or by decreasing oxygen demand by the myocardium. Three types of antianginals are nitrates, beta-blockers, and calcium channel blockers. The major systemic effect of nitrates is a reduction of venous tone,

Table 40–3

Effects of Antianginal Drug Groups on Angina

Drug Group	Variant (Vasospastic) Angina	Classic (Stable) Angina
Nitrates	Relaxation of coronary arteries, which decreases vasospasms and increases O₂ supply	Dilation of veins, which decreases preload and decreases O₂ demand
Beta-blockers	Not effective	Decreases heart rate and contractility, which decreases O₂ demand
Calcium channel blockers	Relaxation of coronary arteries, which decreases vasospasms and increases O₂ supply	Dilation of arterioles, which decreases afterload and decreases O₂ demand. Verapamil and diltiazem decrease heart rate and contractility.

Modified from Lehne RA: *Pharmacology for nursing care,* ed 4, Philadelphia, 2001, Saunders, p. 493.
O_2, Oxygen.

which decreases the workload of the heart and promotes vasodilation. Beta-blockers and calcium channel blockers decrease the workload of the heart and decrease oxygen demands.

Nitrates and calcium channel blockers are effective in treating variant (vasospastic) angina pectoris. Beta-blockers are not effective for this type of angina. With stable angina, beta-blockers can effectively be used to prevent angina attacks. Table 40–3 lists the effects of antianginal drug groups on angina.

Nitrates

Nitrates, developed in the 1840s, were the first agents used to relieve angina. The nitrates affect the blood vessels in the venous circulation and coronary arteries. They cause generalized vascular and coronary vasodilation, thus increasing blood flow through the coronary arteries to the myocardial cells. This group of drugs reduces myocardial ischemia but can cause hypotension.

The sublingual (SL) tablet, absorbed under the tongue, comes in various dosages, but the average dose prescribed is 0.4 mg or gr $^1/_{150}$ following cardiac pain, repeated every 5 minutes for a total of three doses. The effects of SL nitroglycerin last for 10 minutes. The SL tablets decompose when exposed to heat and light. For this reason, they should be kept in their original airtight glass containers. The tablets themselves are normally dispensed in these original glass containers, which have screw-cap tops that are not childproof. This facilitates emergency use by older adults who may have reduced manual dexterity and are experiencing an anginal attack. The client may experience dizziness, faintness, or headache as a result of the peripheral vasodilation. If pain persists, the client should immediately call for medical assistance.

Sublingual (SL) nitroglycerin is the most commonly used nitrate. It is not swallowed because it undergoes first-pass metabolism by the liver, which decreases its effectiveness. Instead, it is given SL and is readily absorbed into the circulation through the SL vessels. Nitroglycerin is also available in topical (ointment, transdermal patch), buccal extended-release tablet, oral extended-release capsule and tablet, aerosol spray (inhalation), and IV forms. Prototype Drug Chart 40–2 summarizes the action of nitroglycerin (nitrates).

There are various types of organic nitrates. Isosorbide dinitrate (Isordil, Sorbitrate) can be administered SL by tablets and orally by chewable tablets, immediate-release tablets, and sustained-release tablets and capsules. Isosorbide mononitrate (Monoket, Imdur) can be given orally by immediate-release and sustained-release tablets.

Pharmacokinetics

Nitroglycerin, taken SL, is absorbed rapidly and directly into the internal jugular vein and the right atrium. Approximately 40% to 50% of nitrates absorbed through the gastrointestinal (GI) tract are inactivated by liver metabolism (first-pass metabolism in the liver). The nitroglycerin in Nitro-Bid ointment and in the Transderm-Nitro patch is absorbed slowly through the skin. It is excreted primarily in the urine.

Pharmacodynamics

Nitroglycerin acts directly on the smooth muscle of blood vessels, causing relaxation and dilation. It decreases cardiac **preload** (the amount of blood in the ventricle at the end of diastole) and **afterload** (peripheral vascular resistance) and reduces myocardial O₂ demand. With dilation of the veins, there is less blood return to the heart, and with dilation of the arteries, there is less vasoconstriction and resistance.

The onset of action of nitroglycerin depends on the method of administration. With SL and IV use, the onset of action is rapid (1 to 3 minutes); it is slower with the transdermal method (30 to 60 minutes). The duration of action of the transdermal nitroglycerin patch is approximately 24 hours. Because Nitro-Bid ointment is effective for only 6 to 8 hours, it must be reapplied three to four times a day. The use of Nitro-Bid ointment has declined since the advent of the transdermal nitroglycerin patch, which is applied only once a day. It is important to note that the patch should be removed nightly to allow for an 8- to 12-hour nitrate-free interval. This is also true for most other forms of nitroglycerin. This is necessary to avoid tolerance associated with uninterrupted use or continued dosage increases of nitrate preparations. Table 40–4 lists the drug data for the nitrates.

Side Effects and Adverse Reactions

Headaches are one of the most common side effects of nitroglycerin, but they may become less frequent with continued use. Otherwise, acetaminophen may provide some relief. Other side effects include hypotension, dizziness, weakness, and faintness. When nitroglycerin ointment or transdermal patches are discontinued, the dose should be tapered over several weeks to prevent the rebound effect of

PROTOTYPE DRUG CHART 40–2

NITROGLYCERIN

Drug Class

Antianginal
Trade Name: Nitrostat, Nitro-Bid, Transderm-Nitro
patch, NTG, 🍁 Nitrogard SR, Nitrol Nitrate
Pregnancy Category: C

Dosage

A: PO/SL: 0.3, 0.4, 0.6 mg; repeat q5min × 3 as needed;
SR: 2.5-26 mg, 2-4 × d
IV: Initially: 5 mcg/min; dose may be increased
Oint: 2% 1-2 inch to chest or thigh area
Patch: 2.5-15 mg/d to chest or thigh area

Contraindications

Marked hypotension, AMI, increased intracranial pressure,
severe anemia
Caution: Severe renal or hepatic disease, early MI

Drug-Lab-Food Interactions

Drug: Increase effect with alcohol, beta-blockers, calcium channel blockers, antihypertensives; *decrease*
effects of heparin

Pharmacokinetics

Absorption: SL: >75% absorbed; oint and patch: slow
absorption
Distribution: PB: 60%
Metabolism: t½: 1-4 min
Excretion: Liver and urine

Pharmacodynamics

SL: Onset: 1-3 min
Peak: 4 min
Duration: 20-30 min
SR Cap: Onset: 20-45 min
Duration: 3-8 h
Oint: Onset: 20-60 min
Peak: 1-2 hours
Duration: 2-12 h
Patch: Onset: 30-60 min
Peak: 1-2 h
Duration: 20-24 h
IV: Onset: 1-3 min
Duration: 3-5 min

Therapeutic Effects/Uses

To control angina pectoris (anginal pain)
Mode of Action: Decrease myocardial demand for oxygen; decrease preload by dilating veins thus indirectly
decreasing afterload

Side Effects

Nausea, vomiting, headache, dizziness, syncope, weakness,
flush, confusion, pallor, rash, dry mouth

Adverse Reactions

Hypotension, reflex tachycardia, paradoxical bradycardia
Life-threatening: Circulatory collapse

A, Adult; *AMI*, acute myocardial infarction; *cap*, capsule; *d*, day; *h*, hour; *IV*, intravenous; *MI*, myocardial infarction; *min*, minute; *NTG*,
nitroglycerin; *PB*, protein-binding; *PO*, by mouth; *SL*, sublingual; *SR*, sustained-release; *t½*, half-life; 🍁, Canadian drug names; >,
greater than.

severe pain caused by **myocardial ischemia** (lack of blood supply to the heart muscle). In addition, *reflex tachycardia* may occur if the nitrate is given too rapidly; the heart rate increases greatly because of overcompensation of the cardiovascular system.

PREVENTING MEDICATION ERRORS

Do not confuse...

• **Nitrostat** and **Nystatin.** Nitrostat is a nitroglycerin drug that promotes coronary vasodilation and thus increases blood flow to the coronary arteries. Nystatin is an antifungal antibiotic that has fungistatic and fungicidal activity against yeasts and fungi.

Drug Interactions

Beta-blockers, calcium channel blockers, vasodilators, and alcohol can enhance the hypotensive effect of nitrates. IV nitroglycerin may antagonize the effects of heparin.

Beta-Blockers

Beta-adrenergic blockers block the beta₁- and beta₂-receptor sites. **Beta-blockers** decrease the effects of the sympathetic nervous system by blocking the action of the catecholamines epinephrine and norepinephrine, thereby decreasing the heart rate and blood pressure. They are used as antianginal, antidysrhythmic, and antihypertensive drugs. Beta-blockers are effective as antianginals because, by decreasing the heart rate and myocardial contractility, they reduce the need for oxygen consumption and, consequently, they reduce anginal pain. These drugs are most useful for classic (stable) angina.

Table 40–4

Antianginals

Generic (Brand)	Route and Dosage	Uses and Considerations
Nitrates		
Short Acting		
nitroglycerin (Nitrostat, Nitro-Bid, Transderm-Nitro)	See Prototype Drug Chart 40–2.	
Long Acting		
isosorbide dinitrate (Isordil, Sorbitrate)	A: SL: 2.5-10 mg q.i.d. Chewable: 5-10 mg PRN PO: 2.5-30 mg q.i.d. a.c. and bedtime SR: 40 mg q6-12h	To prevent anginal attacks. Drug can lower blood pressure. Tolerance builds up over time. Headaches, dizziness, light-headedness, and flush may occur. *Pregnancy category:* B; PB: UK; t½: 1-4 h
isosorbide mononitrate (Imdur)	A: PO: SR: 30-60 mg q morning; *max:* 240 mg/d	To prevent anginal attacks. Sustained-release form provides controlled delivery and a 6-hour drug-free period. By allowing a drug-free period, tolerance to nitrates is reduced; effectiveness is increased. *Pregnancy category:* C; PB: 5%; t½: 6.6 h
Beta-Adrenergic Blockers		
atenolol (Tenormin) (Beta₁)	A: PO: 25-100 mg/d; *max:* 200 mg/d	To control angina pectoris. Also effective in managing hypertension. Blood pressure and heart rate should be monitored. Cardioselective drug, blocking beta₁. Can be used by clients with asthma. *Pregnancy category:* C; PB: 5%-15%; t½: 6-7 h
metoprolol tartrate (Lopressor) Toprol XL (Beta₁)	A: PO: 50-100 mg in 2 divided doses; May increase to 100-400 mg/daily Elderly: PO 25 mg/daily. May increase dose A: IV: 5 mg q 2 min	Similar to atenolol by blocking beta₁. High doses of metoprolol can effect beta₂ and could cause bronchoconstriction. It can reduce cardiac oxygen demand, which decreases heart rate and contractility. *Pregnancy category:* C; PB: 12%; t½: 3-7 h
nadolol (Corgard) (Beta₁ and beta₂)	A: PO: 40 mg/d; dose may be increased; *max:* 240-320 mg/d in divided doses	To treat angina pectoris and hypertension. *Pregnancy category:* C; PB: 28%; t½: 10-24 h (renal disease: 45 h)
propranolol HCl (Inderal) (Beta₁ and beta₂)	A: PO: Initially: 10-20 mg t.i.d.-q.i.d.; *maint:* 20-60 mg t.i.d.-q.i.d.; *max:* 320 mg/d SR: 80-160 mg/d	First beta-blocker, blocking beta₁ and beta₂. It is no longer the drug of choice to prevent angina because of the risk of bronchospasm. Heart rate, blood pressure, and respiratory status should be monitored. *Pregnancy category:* C; PB: 90%; t½: 3-6 h
Calcium Channel Blockers		
amlodipine (Norvasc)	A: PO: Initially: 10 mg; *maint:* 2.5-10 mg/d Elderly: Initially: 2.5 mg/d	Management of angina pectoris and hypertension. May be given with another antianginal or antihypertensive drug. *Pregnancy category:* C; PB: 95%; t½: 30-50 h
bepridil HCl (Vascor)	A: PO: Initially 200 mg/d × 10 d; *maint:* 300 mg/d; *max:* 400 mg/d	Treatment of angina pectoris. May be used as single drug or in combination with nitrates. Given as a single dose. *Pregnancy category:* C; PB: 99%; t½: 2-24 h
diltiazem HCl (Cardizem)	A: PO: 30-60 mg q.i.d.; may increase to 360 mg/d in 4 divided doses SR: 60 mg q12h; *max:* 360 mg/daily CD: 120-180 mg/d; *max:* 360 mg/daily	For angina pectoris. Hypotensive effect is not as severe as with nifedipine. Kidney function should be monitored. *Pregnancy category:* C; PB: 70%-85%; t½: 3.5-9 h
felodipine (Plendil)	A: PO: Initially: 5 mg/d single dose; *maint:* 2.5-10 mg/d Elderly: Initially: 2.5 mg/daily	To treat chronic angina pectoris and manage hypertension. Reduces O₂ demand by the heart. A potent peripheral vasodilator thus increasing heart rate and myocardial contractility. *Pregnancy category:* C; PB: >99%; t½: 10-16 h
isradipine (DynaCirc)	A: PO: 2.5-7.5 mg t.i.d.	Primary use is to treat hypertension. Also can be given for angina pectoris. *Pregnancy category:* C; PB: 99%; t½: 5-11 h

A, Adult; *a.c.,* before meals; *b.i.d.,* twice a day; *CD,* controlled delivery; *CHF,* congestive heart failure; *d,* day; *h,* hour; *IV,* intravenous; *maint,* maintenance; *max,* maximum; *MI,* myocardial infarction; *min,* minute; *O₂,* oxygen; *PB,* protein-binding; *PO,* by mouth; *PRN,* as necessary; *q.i.d.,* four times a day; *SL,* sublingual; *SR,* sustained-release; *t.i.d.,* three times a day; *t½,* half-life; *UK,* unknown; *>,* greater than.   *Continued*

Table 40–4

Antianginals—cont'd

Generic (Brand)	Route and Dosage	Uses and Considerations
Calcium Channel Blockers—cont'd		
nicardipine HCl (Cardene, Cardene SR)	A: PO: 20 mg t.i.d.; *maint:* 20-40 mg t.i.d. SR: 30 mg b.i.d.; *maint:* 30-60 mg b.i.d.	Used for angina pectoris. May be used alone or in combination with other antianginals. Used also for hypertension. Peripheral edema, headache, dizziness, and light-headedness may occur. *Pregnancy category:* C; PB: 95%; t$\frac{1}{2}$: 5 h
nifedipine (Procardia, Adalat)	A: PO: 10-30 mg q6-8h; *max:* 180 mg/daily	For angina pectoris. Blood pressure should be closely monitored, especially if client is taking nitrates or beta-blockers. Is a potent calcium blocker. *Pregnancy category:* C; PB: 92%-98%; t$\frac{1}{2}$: 2-5 h
nisoldipine (Sular, Nisocor)	A: PO: Initially: 20 mg/d; *maint:* 10-40 mg/d in 2 divided doses Elderly: A: PO: 10-20 mg/daily	To treat angina pectoris and hypertension. Suppresses contraction of cardiac and vascular smooth muscle. Increases heart rate and cardiac output. Decreases blood pressure. *Caution:* Clients with heart disease are prone to MI and CHF. *Pregnancy category:* C; PB: >99%; t$\frac{1}{2}$: 7-12 h
verapamil HCl (Calan, Isoptin, Verelan)	A: PO: 40-120 mg t.i.d.; *max:* 480 mg/daily IV: 5-10 mg over 2 min; may repeat if needed in 15-30 min	Treatment of angina pectoris, cardiac dysrhythmias, and hypertension. Peripheral edema, constipation, dizziness, headache, and hypotension may occur. *Pregnancy category:* C; PB: 90%; t$\frac{1}{2}$: 3-8 h

Beta-blockers, which are discussed in detail in Chapter 17, Adrenergics and Adrenergic Blockers, are subdivided into nonselective beta-blockers (blocking beta$_1$ and beta$_2$) and selective (cardiac) beta-blockers (blocking beta$_1$).

Examples of nonselective beta-blockers are propranolol (Inderal), nadolol (Corgard), and pindolol (Visken). These drugs decrease the pulse rate and can cause bronchoconstriction. The cardioselective beta-blockers act more strongly on the beta$_1$ receptor, thus decreasing the pulse rate and avoiding bronchoconstriction because of their relative lack of activity at the beta$_2$ receptor. Examples of selective beta-blockers are atenolol (Tenormin) and metoprolol (Lopressor, Toprol-XL). Selective beta-blockers are the group of choice for controlling angina pectoris. Table 40–4 lists the beta-blockers most frequently used for angina.

Pharmacokinetics

Beta-blockers are well-absorbed orally. Absorption of sustained-release capsules is slow. The half-life of propranolol (Inderal) is 3 to 6 hours. Of the selective beta-blockers, atenolol (Tenormin) has a half-life of 6 to 7 hours, and the half-life of metoprolol (Lopressor) is 3 to 7 hours. Propranolol and metoprolol are metabolized and excreted by the liver. Half of atenolol is excreted unchanged by the kidneys, and half is excreted unabsorbed in the feces.

Pharmacodynamics

Because beta-blockers decrease the force of myocardial contraction, the oxygen demand by the myocardium is reduced, and the client can tolerate increased exercise with less oxygen needed. Beta-blockers tend to be more effective for classic (stable) angina than for variant (vasospastic) angina.

The onset of action of the nonselective beta-blocker propranolol is 30 minutes, its peak action is reached in 1 to 1.5 hours, and its duration is 4 to 12 hours. For the cardioselective beta-blockers, the onset of action of atenolol is 60 minutes, its peak action occurs in 2 to 4 hours, and its du-

ration of action is 24 hours; the onset of action of metoprolol is reached in 15 minutes and the duration of action is 6 to 12 hours.

Side Effects and Adverse Reactions

Both nonselective and selective beta-blockers cause a decrease in pulse rate and blood pressure. For the nonselective beta-blockers, bronchospasm, behavioral or psychotic response, and impotence (with use of Inderal) are potential adverse reactions.

Vital signs need to be closely monitored in the early stages of beta-blocker therapy. When discontinuing use, the dosage should be tapered for 1 or 2 weeks to prevent a rebound effect, such as reflex tachycardia or life-threatening cardiac dysrhythmias.

Calcium Channel Blockers

Calcium channel blockers, or *calcium blockers,* were introduced in 1982 for the treatment of angina pectoris, certain dysrhythmias, and hypertension. Calcium activates myocardial contraction, increasing the workload of the heart and the need for more oxygen. Calcium blockers decrease cardiac contractility (negative inotropic effect that relaxes smooth muscle), decrease afterload, decrease peripheral resistance, and reduce the workload of the heart, thus decreasing the need for oxygen. They are effective in controlling variant (vasospastic) angina by relaxing coronary arteries and in classic (stable) angina by decreasing oxygen demand. Figure 40–1 shows the suggested steps for treating classic and variant angina pectoris. Table 40–4 presents the drug data for the calcium blockers used to treat angina.

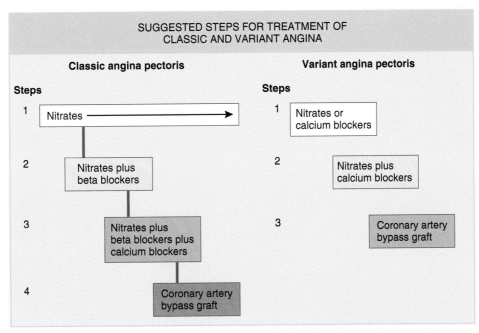

FIGURE 40–1 Suggested steps for treating classic and variant angina pectoris.

Pharmacokinetics

Three calcium blockers—verapamil (Calan), nifedipine (Procardia), and diltiazem (Cardizem)—have been effectively used for the long-term treatment of angina. Eighty to ninety percent of calcium channel blockers are absorbed through the GI mucosa. However, the first-pass metabolism by the liver decreases the availability of free circulating drug, and only 20% of verapamil, 45% to 65% of diltiazem, and 35% to 40% of nifedipine are bioavailable. All three drugs are highly protein-bound (80%-90%), and their half-life is 2 to 6 hours.

Several other calcium blockers are available: nicardipine HCl (Cardene), amlodipine (Norvasc), bepridal HCl (Vascor), felodipine (Plendil), and nislodipine (Sular). All are highly protein-bound (>95%). Nicardipine has the shortest half-life at 5 hours. Bepridil is used for angina pectoris.

Pharmacodynamics

Bradycardia is a common problem with the use of verapamil, the first calcium blocker. Nifedipine, the most potent of the calcium blockers, promotes vasodilation of the coronary and peripheral vessels, and hypotension can result. The onset of action is 10 minutes for verapamil and 30 minutes for nifedipine and diltiazem. Verapamil's duration of action is 3 to 7 hours when given orally and 2 hours when given IV; for nifedipine and diltiazem, the duration of action is 6 to 8 hours.

Side Effects and Adverse Reactions

The side effects of calcium blockers include headache, hypotension (more common with nifedipine and less common with diltiazem), dizziness, and flushing of the skin. Reflex tachycardia can occur as a result of hypotension. Calcium blockers can cause changes in liver and kidney function, and serum liver enzymes should be checked periodically. Calcium blockers are frequently given with other antianginal drugs such as nitrates to prevent angina.

Nifedipine, in its immediate-release form (10- and 20-mg capsules), has been associated with an increased incidence of sudden cardiac death, especially when prescribed in high doses for outpatients. This is not true of the sustained-release preparations (Procardia XL, Adalat CC). For this reason, immediate-release nifedipine is usually prescribed only as needed in the hospital setting for acute rises in blood pressure.

Nursing Process

Antianginals

ASSESSMENT

- Obtain baseline vital signs for future comparisons.
- Obtain health and drug histories. Nitroglycerin is contraindicated for marked hypotension or acute myocardial infarction (AMI).

NURSING DIAGNOSES

- Decreased cardiac output
- Anxiety related to cardiac problems
- Acute pain
- Activity intolerance

PLANNING

- Client takes nitroglycerin or other antianginals and angina pain is controlled.

NURSING INTERVENTIONS

- Monitor vital signs. Hypotension is associated with most antianginal drugs.

■ Have client sit or lie down when taking a nitrate for the first time. After administration, check the vital signs while client is lying down and then sitting up. Have client rise slowly to a standing position.

■ Offer sips of water before giving sublingual (SL) nitrates; dryness may inhibit drug absorption.

■ Monitor effects of IV nitroglycerin. Report angina that persists.

■ Apply Nitro-Bid ointment to the designated mark on paper. Do *not* use fingers because the drug can be absorbed; use a tongue blade or gloves. For the Transderm-Nitro patch, do not touch the medication portion.

■ Do *not* apply the Nitro-Bid ointment or the Transderm-Nitro patch in any area on the chest in the vicinity of defibrillator-cardioverter paddle placement. Explosion and skin burns may result.

Client Teaching

General

• A SL nitroglycerin tablet is used if chest pain occurs. Repeat in 5 minutes if the pain has not subsided and again in another 5 minutes if it persists. Do *not* give more than three tablets. If the chest pain persists >15 minutes, immediate medical help is necessary. *Call 911.*

• Instruct client not to ingest alcohol while taking nitroglycerin to avoid hypotension, weakness, and faintness.

• Tolerance to nitroglycerin can occur. If client's chest pain is not completely alleviated, client should notify the health care provider.

Beta-Blockers and Calcium Blockers

• Inform client not to discontinue these drugs without the health care provider's approval. Withdrawal symptoms, such as reflex tachycardia and pain, may be severe.

Self-Administration

• Demonstrate to client how (SL) nitroglycerin tablets are taken. The tablet is placed under the tongue for quick absorption. A stinging or biting sensation may indicate the tablet is fresh. With the newer SL nitroglycerin, the biting sensation may not be present. The bottle is stored away from light and kept dry. Keep in original screw-cap, amber glass bottle. The amber color of the glass provides light protection and the screw-cap closure protects from moisture in the air, which can easily reduce the potency of the tablets.

• Instruct client about the Transderm-Nitro patch. Apply once a day, usually in the morning. Rotation of skin sites is necessary. Usually the patch is applied to the chest wall; however, the thighs and arms are used. Avoid hairy areas.

Side Effects

• Headaches commonly occur when first taking nitroglycerin products and last about 30 minutes. Acetaminophen is suggested for relief.

• If hypotension results from SL nitroglycerin, place client in supine position with legs elevated.

Beta-Blockers and Calcium Blockers

• Instruct client how to take a pulse rate. Advise the client to call the health care provider if dizziness or faintness occurs; this may indicate hypotension.

Cultural Considerations ⊕

• Ascertain from African-American, Hispanic, and obese clients their understanding of foods common to people from their culture that may contribute to cardiac conditions. Speak clearly and slowly.

• Discuss with clients from various cultures the importance of the drug regimen. An interpreter may be necessary to ensure the client's compliance with drug and diet regimens.

EVALUATION

■ Evaluate client's response to nitrate product for relieving anginal pain. Note headache, dizziness, or faintness.

Antidysrhythmic Drugs

Cardiac Dysrhythmias

A **cardiac dysrhythmia (arrhythmia)** is defined as any deviation from the normal rate or pattern of the heartbeat; this includes heart rates that are too slow (bradycardia), too fast **(tachycardia)**, or irregular. The terms *dysrhythmia* (disturbed heart rhythm) and *arrhythmia* (absence of rhythm) are used interchangeably, despite the slight difference in meaning.

The ECG identifies the type of dysrhythmia. The P wave of the ECG reflects atrial activation, the QRS complex indicates the ventricular depolarization, and the T wave reflects ventricular **repolarization** (return of cell membrane potential to resting after depolarization). The PR interval indicates AV conduction time, and the QT interval reflects the ventricular action potential duration. Atrial dysrhythmias prevent proper filling of the ventricles and decrease the cardiac output by one third. Ventricular dysrhythmias are life threatening because ineffective filling of the ventricle results in decreased or absent cardiac output. With ventricular tachycardia, ventricular fibrillation is likely to occur, followed by death. Cardiopulmonary resuscitation (CPR) is necessary to treat these clients.

Cardiac dysrhythmias frequently follow an MI (heart attack) or can result from **hypoxia** (lack of oxygen to body tissues), **hypercapnia** (increased carbon dioxide in the blood), excess catecholamines, or electrolyte imbalance.

Cardiac Action Potentials

Electrolyte transfer occurs through the cardiac cell membrane. When sodium and calcium enter a cardiac cell, **depolarization** (myocardial contraction) occurs. Sodium enters

Table 40–5

Classes and Actions of Antidysrhythmic Drugs

Classes	Actions	Indications
Class I		
Fast (Sodium) Channel Blockers		
IA	Slows conduction and prolongs repolarization	Atrial and ventricular dysrhythmias, paroxysmal atrial tachycardia (PAT), supraventricular dysrhythmias
IB	Slows conduction and shortens repolarization	Acute ventricular dysrhythmias
IC	Prolongs conduction with little to no effect on repolarization	Life-threatening ventricular dysrhythmias
Class II		
Beta-blockers	Reduces calcium entry; decreases conduction velocity, automaticity, and recovery time (refractory period)	Atrial flutter and fibrillation, tachydysrhythmias, ventricular and supraventricular dysrhythmias
Class III		
Prolong repolarization	Prolongs repolarization during ventricular dysrhythmias; prolongs action potential duration	Life-threatening atrial and ventricular dysrhythmias; resistant to other drugs
Class IV		
Calcium channel blockers	Blocks calcium influx; slows conduction velocity, decreases myocardial contractility (negative inotropic), and increases refraction in the AV node	Supraventricular tachydysrhythmias; prevention of paroxysmal supraventricular tachycardia (PSVT)

AV, Atrioventricular.

rapidly to start the depolarization, and calcium enters later to maintain it. This influx of calcium leads to an increased release of intracellular calcium from the sacroplasmic reticulum, resulting in cardiac contraction. In the presence of myocardial ischemia, the contraction can be irregular.

Cardiac action potentials are frequent depolarization followed by repolarization of myocardial cells. Figure 40–2 illustrates the action potential of a ventricular cardiac cell during the course of a heartbeat. There are five phases. Phase 0 is the rapid depolarization, caused by an influx of sodium ions. Phase 1 is initial repolarization, which coincides with termination of sodium ion influx. Phase 2 is the *plateau* and is characterized by the influx of calcium ion, which prolongs the action potential and promotes atrial and ventricular muscle contraction. Phase 3 is rapid repolarization caused by influx of the potassium ion. Phase 4 is the resting membrane potential between heartbeats. It is

normally flat in ventricular muscle but begins to rise in the cells of the sinoatrial (SA) node as they slowly depolarize toward the threshold potential just before depolarization occurs, initiating the next heartbeat.

Types of Antidysrhythmic Drugs

The desired action of **antidysrhythmic (antiarrhythmic) drugs** is to restore the cardiac rhythm to normal. Box 40–1 describes the various mechanisms by which this is accomplished.

The antidysrhythmics are grouped into four classes: (1) fast (sodium) channel blockers IA, IB, and IC; (2) beta-blockers; (3) drugs that prolong repolarization; and (4) slow (calcium) channel blockers. Table 40–5 lists the classes, actions, and indications for cardiac antidysrhythmic drugs. Table 40–6 lists the drug data for the commonly administered antidysrhythmics.

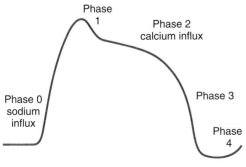

FIGURE 40–2 Cardiac action potential.

BOX 40–1

Pharmacodynamics of Antidysrhythmics

Mechanisms of Action

- Block adrenergic stimulation of the heart
- Depress myocardial excitability and contractility
- Decrease conduction velocity in cardiac tissue
- Increase recovery time (repolarization) of the myocardium
- Suppress automaticity (spontaneous depolarization to initiate beats).

Table 40-6

Antidysrhythmics

Generic (Brand)	Route and Dosage	Uses and Considerations
Class I		
Fast (Sodium) Channel Blockers IA		
disopyramide phosphate (Norpace, Napamide)	A: PO: 100-200 mg q6h CR: 300 mg q12h C: 4-12 y: PO: 10-15 mg/kg/d in divided doses 13-18 y: PO: 6-15 mg/kg/d in divided doses	Prevention and suppression of unifocal and multifocal premature ventricular contractions (PVCs). For ventricular dysrhythmias. May cause anticholinergic symptoms. Serum therapeutic level: 3-8 mcg/ml. *Pregnancy category:* C; PB: 50%-66%; t$^1/_2$: 4-10 h
procainamide HCL (Procan, Pronestyl)	A: PO: 250-500 mg q3-4h SR: 250 mg-1 g q12h or q6h IM: 50 mg/kg/day in 4 divided doses IV: Inf: 20 mg/min for 25-30 min (500-600 mg) C: PO: 40-60 mg/kg/day in 4 divided doses TDM: 4-8 mcg/ml	It controls dysrhythmias (PVC), ventricular tachycardia. It depresses myocardial excitability by slowing down conduction of cardiac tissue. *Pregnancy category:* C; PB: 20%, t$^1/_2$: 3-4 h
quinidine sulfate, polygalacturonate, gluconate (Quinidex, Cardioquin)	A: PO: 200-300 mg t.i.d.-q.i.d. C: PO: 30 mg/kg or 900 mg/m^2 in 5 divided doses	For atrial, ventricular, and supraventricular dysrhythmias. Nausea, vomiting, diarrhea, abdominal pain, or cramps are common side effects. If given with digoxin, it can increase digoxin concentration. Serum therapeutic level: 2-6 mcg/ml. *Pregnancy category:* C; PB: 80%; t$^1/_2$: 6-7 h
Fast (Sodium) Channel Blockers IB		
lidocaine (Xylocaine)	A: IV: 50-100 mg bolus in 2-3 min; then IV inf: 20-50 mcg/kg/min	For acute ventricular dysrhythmias following MI and cardiac surgery. Serum therapeutic range: 1.5-6 mcg/ml. *Pregnancy category:* B; PB: 60%-80%; t$^1/_2$: 1.5-2 h
mexiletine HCl (Mexitil)	A: PO: 200-400 mg q8h	Analogue of lidocaine. Treatment for acute and chronic ventricular dysrhythmias. Take with food to decrease GI distress. Common side effects include nausea, vomiting, heartburn, tremor, dizziness, nervousness, lightheadedness. Serum therapeutic range: 0.5-2 mcg/ml. *Pregnancy category:* C; PB: 50%-60%; t$^1/_2$: 10-12 h
tocainide HCl (Tonocard)	A: PO: LD: 600 mg. PO: 400 mg q8h; *max:* 2.4 g/d	For ventricular dysrhythmias, especially PVC. Similar to lidocaine except in oral form. Serum therapeutic level: 4-10 mcg/ml. *Pregnancy category:* C; PB: 10%-20%; t$^1/_2$: 10-17 h
Fast (Sodium) Channel Blockers IC		
flecainide (Tambocor)	A: PO: Initial: 50-100 mg q12h, increase by 50 mg q12h q4d; *maint:* 150 mg q12h; *max:* 300 mg/d	For life-threatening ventricular dysrhythmias; prevention of paroxysmal supraventricular tachycardia (PSVT) and paroxysmal atrial fibrillation or flutter (PAF). Avoid use in cardiogenic shock, second- or third-degree heart block, or right bundle branch block. *Pregnancy category:* C; PB: 40%-50%; t$^1/_2$: 12-27 h
propafenone HCl (Rythmol)	A: PO: 150-300 mg q8h; *max:* 900 mg/d	Treatment of life-threatening ventricular dysrhythmias. Avoid use if cardiogenic shock, uncontrolled CHF, heart block, severe hypotension, bradycardia, and bronchospasms occur. *Pregnancy category:* C; PB: 97%; t$^1/_2$: 5-8 h
Other Class I		
moricizine (Ethmozine)	A: PO: Initially: 200-300 mg q8h; *maint:* 300 mg q8h; decrease dose for clients with liver and kidney disease	To treat life-threatening ventricular dysrhythmias. Blocks sodium channels, decreases conduction velocity in atria and ventricles, and prolongs refractory period in the AV node. May cause bradycardia, heart block, and CHF in high doses. *Pregnancy category:* B; PB: UK; t$^1/_2$: 1.5-3.5 h

A, Adult; *AV*, atrioventricular; *b.i.d.*, two times a day; *BP*, blood pressure; *C*, child; *CHF*, congestive heart failure; *CR*, controlled release; *d*, day; *FDA*, Food and Drug Administration; *GI*, gastrointestinal; *h*, hour; *IM*, intramuscular; *inf*, infusion; *IV*, intravenous; *LD*, loading dose; *maint*, maintenance; *max*, maximum; *MI*, myocardial infarction; *min*, minute; *PAT*, paroxysmal atrial tachycardia; *PB*, protein-binding; *PO*, by mouth; *q.i.d.*, four times a day; *SR*, sustained release; *t$^1/_2$*, half-life; *t.i.d.*, three times a day; *UK*, unknown; *y*, year; *>*, greater than; *<*, less than.

Table 40–6

Antidysrhythmics—cont'd

Generic (Brand)	Route and Dosage	Uses and Considerations
Class II		
Beta-Adrenergic Blockers		
acebutolol HCl (Sectral) (Beta$_1$ blocker)	A: PO: 200 mg b.i.d.; may increase dose	Management of ventricular dysrhythmias. Also used for angina pectoris and hypertension. Primarily for PVC. New beta-blocker that affects the beta$_1$ receptor in the heart. Can cause bradycardia and decrease cardiac output. *Pregnancy category:* B; PB: 26%; t$^1/_2$: 3-13 h
esmolol (Brevibloc) (Beta$_1$ blocker)	A: IV: LD: 500 mcg; kg/over 1 min; *maint:* 50-100 mcg/kg/min; *max:* 200 mcg/kg/min	To control atrial flutter and fibrillation. For short-term use only. Mainly for clients having dysrhythmias during surgery. May cause bradycardia, heart block, and CHF. *Pregnancy category:* C; PB: 55%; t$^1/_2$: 9 min
propranolol HCl (Inderal) (Beta$_1$ and beta$_2$ blocker)	A: PO: 10-30 mg t.i.d.-q.i.d. A: IV bolus: 0.5-3 mg at 1 mg/min	For ventricular dysrhythmias, PAT, and atrial and ventricular ectopic beats. Clients with asthma should not use drug. *Pregnancy category:* C; PB: 90%; t$^1/_2$: 3-6 h
sotalol HCl (Betapace) (Beta$_1$ and beta$_2$ blocker; also Class III)	A: PO: 80 mg b.i.d.; *max:* 240-320 mg/d in divided doses Increase dose interval with renal dysfunction	For ventricular dysrhythmias. Avoid if bronchial asthma or heart block is present. *Pregnancy category:* B; PB: 0%; t$^1/_2$: 12 h
Class III		
Prolong Repolarization		
adenosine (Adenocard)	A: IV: 6 mg (bolus: 1-2 sec); repeat if necessary, 12 mg bolus × 2 doses	Treatment of PSVT, Wolff-Parkinson-White syndrome. Avoid if second- or third-degree AV block or atrial flutter or fibrillation is present. *Pregnancy category:* C; PB: UK; t$^1/_2$: <10 sec
amiodarone HCl (Cordarone)	A: PO: LD: 400-1600 mg/d in divided doses; *maint:* 200-600 mg/d; dose may be individualized	For life-threatening ventricular dysrhythmias. Initially dosage is greater and then decreases over time. Therapeutic serum level: 1-2.5 mcg/ml. *Pregnancy category:* D; PB: 96%; t$^1/_2$: 5-100 daily
bretylium tosylate (Bretylol)	A: IM: 5-10 mg/kg q6-8h IV: 5-10 mg/kg; may repeat in 15-30 min, IV drip or IV bolus	For ventricular tachycardia and fibrillation (to convert to a normal sinus rhythm). Used when lidocaine and procainamide are ineffective. *Pregnancy category:* C; PB: UK; t$^1/_2$: 4-17 h
dofetilide (Tikosyn)	PO: 250-1000 mcg/d in 2 divided doses Dose is based on calculated creatinine clearance	A selective potassium-channel blocker that prolongs repolarization. Prescribed for atrial flutter and fibrillation. Renal function should be monitored. *Pregnancy category:* C; PB: 60%-70%; t$^1/_2$: 10 h
sotalol (Betapace)	A: PO: Same as Class II *(See sotalol in Class II)*	Beta-blocker. Can be classified as Class II or III. To treat life-threatening ventricular dysrhythmias (ventricular tachycardia). Slows heart rate, decreases AV conduction, increases AV refractory period, and decreases systolic and diastolic BP. *Caution:* second- and third-degree heart block. *(See sotalol in Class II.)*
Class IV		
Calcium Channel Blockers		
verapamil HCl (Calan, Isoptin)	A: PO: 240-480 mg/d in 3-4 divided doses IV: 5-10 mg IV push	For supraventricular tachydysrhythmias, prevention of PSVT. Also used for angina pectoris and hypertension. Avoid use if cardiogenic shock, second- or third-degree AV block, severe hypotension, severe CHF occur. Serum therapeutic level 80-300 ng/ml or 0.08-0.3 mcg/ml. *Pregnancy category:* C; PB: 90%; t$^1/_2$: 3-8 h
diltiazem (Cardizem)	A: IV: 0.25 mg/kg IV bolus over 2 min, or 5-10 mg/h in IV infusion	For PSVT and atrial flutter or fibrillation. Avoid use if second- or third-degree AV block or hypotension occurs. *Pregnancy category:* C; PB: 70%-80%; t$^1/_2$: 3-8 h

Continued

Table 40–6		
Antidysrhythmics—cont'd		
Generic (Brand)	**Route and Dosage**	**Uses and Considerations**
Others		
phenytoin (Dilantin)	A: IV: 100 mg q5-10min until dysrhythmia ceases; *max:* 1000 mg	Treatment of digitalis-induced dysrhythmias. Not approved as dysrhythmic drug by FDA. Serum level <20 mcg/ml. *Pregnancy category:* D; PB: 95%; t½: 22 h
digoxin (Lanoxin)	A: IV: LD: 0.6-1 mg/d in 24 h C: >10 yr: IV: LD: 8-12 mcg/kg	For atrial flutter or fibrillation; to prevent recurrence of paroxysmal atrial tachycardia. *Pregnancy category:* C; PB: 20%-25%; t½: >36 h
ibutilide fumarate (Corvert)	A: >60 kg: IV infusion: 1 mg over 10 min; may repeat in 10 min A: IV: <60 kg: 0.01 mg/kg (0.1 ml/kg) given over 10 min	To treat atrial flutter and fibrillation. Prolongs cardiac action potential and increases atrial and ventricular refractories. *Pregnancy category:* C; PB: UK; t½: 6 h

Class I: Fast (Sodium) Channel Blockers

Fast (sodium) channel blockers decrease the fast sodium influx to the cardiac cells. The drug response is decreased conduction velocity in the cardiac tissues, suppression of the automaticity that decreases the likelihood of ectopic foci, and increased recovery time (repolarization or refractory period). There are three subgroups of fast channel blockers: IA slows conduction and prolongs repolarization (quinidine, procainamide, disopyramide); IB slows conduction and shortens repolarization (lidocaine, mexiletine HCl); and IC prolongs conduction with little to no effect on repolarization (flecainide).

Lidocaine, an IB or fast (sodium) channel blocker II, was used in the 1940s as a local anesthetic and is still used for that purpose. Later, it was determined that lidocaine had antidysrhythmic properties as well. It is still effective for treating acute ventricular dysrhythmias by some cardiologists. It slows conduction velocity and decreases action potential amplitude. Onset of action (IV) is rapid. About one third of lidocaine reaches the general circulation. A bolus of lidocaine is short lived. Other IB sodium channel blockers are mexiletine and tocainide.

Class II: Beta-Blockers

The drugs in the second class, beta-blockers, decrease conduction velocity, automaticity, and recovery time (refractory period). Examples are propranolol (Inderal) and acebutolol (Sectral). Beta-blockers are more frequently prescribed for dysrhythmias than sodium channel blockers.

Class III: Prolong Repolarization

Drugs in the third class prolong repolarization and are used in emergency treatment of ventricular dysrhythmias when other antidysrhythmics are ineffective. These drugs, bretylium (Bretylol) and amiodarone (Cordarone), increase the refractory period (recovery time) and prolong the action potential duration (cardiac cell activity).

Class IV: Calcium Channel Blockers

The fourth class consists of the calcium channel blocker verapamil (Calan, Isoptin) and diltiazem (Cardizem). Verapamil is a slow (calcium) channel blocker that blocks calcium influx, thereby decreasing the excitability and contractility (negative inotropic) of the myocardium. It increases the refractory period of the AV node, which decreases ventricular response. Verapamil is contraindicated for clients with AV block or congestive heart failure.

Prototype Drug Chart 40–3 provides information about the beta-blocker, acebutolol HCL (Sectral), which can be prescribed to treat recurrent stable ventricular dysrhythmias. Also, the pharmacokinetics and pharmacodynamics of acebutolol are given.

Pharmacokinetics

The cardioselective beta drug acebutolol (Sectral) is well absorbed in the GI tract. It is metabolized in the liver to active metabolites; 50% to 60% of the drug is eliminated in the bile via feces, and 30% to 40% is excreted in the urine. The half-life for the drug is 3 to 4 hours, but the half-life for the metabolites is 8 to 13 hours.

Pharmacodynamics

Acebutolol is prescribed for ventricular dysrhythmias as well as for angina pectoris and hypertension. As an antidyshythmic drug, the onset of action is 1 hour; peak time is 4 to 6 hours, and duration of action is 10 hours. To treat hypertension, the duration of action is 20 to 24 hours.

Side Effects and Adverse Reactions for Antidysrhythmic Drugs

Quinidine, the first drug used to treat cardiac dysrhythmias, has many side effects, such as nausea, vomiting, diarrhea, confusion, and hypotension. It can also cause heart block and neurologic and psychiatric symptoms. Procainamide causes less cardiac depression than quinidine.

High doses of lidocaine can cause cardiovascular depression, bradycardia, hypotension, seizures, blurred vision, and double vision. Less serious side effects may include dizziness, light-headedness, and confusion. The use of lidocaine is contraindicated in clients with ad-

PROTOTYPE DRUG CHART 40–3

ACEBUTOLOL HCl

Drug Class

Beta$_1$ blocker, Cardioselective beta-adrenergic antagonist
Trade Name: Sectral, Monitan
Pregnancy Category: B

Dosage

Ventricular dysrhythmias:
A: PO: 200 mg, b.i.d., q12h
May increase to 600-1200 mg in two divided doses.
Not for children <12 y

Contraindications

Second and third degree heart block, severe bradycardia, severe CHF, cardiogenic shock
Caution: Undergoing major surgery, renal and hepatic impairment, labile mellitus

Drug-Lab-Food Interactions

Drug: Increase effects with diuretics; prolong hypoglycemic effects of insulin and oral antidiabetics; antagonist effect with albuterol, metoproterenol, terbutaline.
Lab: May *increase* ALT, AST, ALP, ANA titer, BUN, lipoproteins, potassium.

Pharmacokinetics

Absorption: Well absorbed
Distribution: PB: UK
Metabolism: t½: 3-4 h; metabolites: 8-13 h
Excretion: 90%-100% in bile/feces and urine

Pharmacodynamics

For Ventricular dysrhythmias
PO: Onset: 1 h
Peak: 4-6 h
Duration: 10 h

Therapeutic Effects/Uses

To aid in the treatment for recurrent stable ventricular dysrhythmias, angina pectoris, and hypertension.
Mode of Action: Drug blocks beta$_1$-adrenergic receptors in the cardiac tissues.

Side Effects

Dizziness, nausea, headache, hypotension, diaphoresis, fatigue, constipation or diarrhea, occasionally impotence

Adverse Reactions

Palpitations with abrupt withdrawal
Life-threatening: agranulocytosis, bronchospasm with high doses

A, Adult; *ALT*, alanine aminotransferase; *AST*, aspartate aminotransferase; *ALP*, alkaline phosphatase; *ANA*, antinuclear antibodies; *b.i.d.*, twice a day; *BUN*, blood urea nitrogen; *CHF*, congestive heart failure; *h*, hour; *PB*, protein-binding; *PO*, by mouth; *UK*, unknown; *t½*, half-life; *y*, year; <, less than.

vanced AV block. It should also be used with caution in clients with liver disorder and heart failure. Mexiletine and tocainide also have side effects similar to lidocaine. They are contraindicated for use in clients with cardiogenic shock or in those with second- or third-degree heart block.

Side effects of beta-blockers are bradycardia and hypotension. Bretylium and amiodarone can cause nausea, vomiting, hypotension, and neurologic problems. Side effects of calcium blockers include nausea, vomiting, hypotension, and bradycardia.

It should be noted that *all* antidysrhythmic drugs are potentially prodysrhythmic. This is because of both the pharmacologic activity of the drug on the heart and the inherently unpredictable activity of a diseased heart, with or without the use of drugs. In some cases, life-threatening ventricular dysrhythmias can result from appropriate and skillful attempts at drug therapy to treat clients with heart disease. For these reasons, antidysrhythmic drug therapy is often initiated during continuous cardiac monitoring of the client's heart rhythm in a hospital setting.

Nursing Process

Antidysrhythmics

ASSESSMENT

■ Obtain health and drug histories. The history may include shortness of breath (SOB), heart palpitations, coughing, chest pain (type, duration, and severity), previous angina or cardiac dysrhythmias, and drugs that client currently takes.
■ Obtain baseline vital signs and electrocardiogram (ECG) for future comparisons.
■ Check early cardiac enzyme results (aspartate aminotransferase, lactate dehydrogenase, creatine phosphokinase) to compare with future laboratory results.

NURSING DIAGNOSES

■ Decreased cardiac output
■ Anxiety related to irregular heartbeat
■ Risk for activity intolerance

PLANNING

■ Client will no longer experience abnormal sinus rhythm.
■ Client will comply with the antidysrhythmic drug regimen.

NURSING INTERVENTIONS

■ Monitor vital signs. Hypotension can occur.
■ Administer drug by IV push or bolus over a period of 2 to 3 minutes or as prescribed.
■ Monitor ECG for abnormal patterns and report findings, such as premature ventricular contractions (PVCs), increased PR and QT intervals, and/or widening of the QRS complex. Increased QT interval is a risk factor for *torsades des pointes.*

Client Teaching

General

• Instruct client to take the prescribed drug as ordered. Drug compliance is essential.
• Provide specific instructions for each drug (e.g., photosensitivity for amiodarone).

Side Effects

• Instruct client to report side effects and adverse reactions to the health care provider. These can include dizziness, faintness, nausea, and vomiting.
• Advise client to avoid alcohol, caffeine, and tobacco. Alcohol can intensify the hypotensive reaction; caffeine increases the catecholamine level; and tobacco promotes vasoconstriction.

Cultural Considerations ⊕

• Ascertain from African-American, Hispanic, and obese clients their understanding of foods common to people from their culture that may contribute to cardiac conditions.

• Discuss with clients from various cultures the importance of the drug regimen. An interpreter may be necessary to ensure client's compliance with drug and diet regimens.

EVALUATION

■ Evaluate the effectiveness of the prescribed antidysrhythmic by comparing heart rates with the baseline heart rate and assessing client's response to the drug. Report side effects and adverse reactions. The drug regimen may need to be adjusted. A proarrhythmic effect may occur, which may require discontinuation of the drug.

WEBSITES

For further information on *Cardiac Glycosides, Antianginals, and Antidysrhythmics,* visit these Internet resources:

Medline Plus Medical Encyclopedia:
http://www.nlm.nih.gov/medlineplus/ency/article/000165.htm

Medline Plus Drug Information—nitroglycerin:
http://www.nlm.nih.gov/medlineplus/druginfo/medmaster/a601086.html

American Heart Association—nitroglycerin:
http://www.circ.ahajournals.org/cgi/content/full/108/11/e78?etoc

Health Net—metoprolol:
http://www.health-net.info/metoprolol.html

Health Net—acebutolol:
http://www.health-net.info/acebutolol.html

Milrinone (Primacor):
http://milrinone.com/

Heart Center Online:
http://www.heartcenteronline.com/index2.cfm

Study Questions

1. Your client takes digoxin 0.25 mg/d. What are the nursing responsibilities for client teaching in regard to pulse monitoring and side effects? What is the serum therapeutic range?

2. Drug interactions are associated with digitalis drugs. What are the effects of potassium-wasting diuretics and cortisone with digitalis?

3. What effects do electrolytes have on digitalis toxicity?

4. How are nitroglycerin products administered? Explain. What is a common, temporary side effect of

nitrates that occurs early in the course of administration? How is this side effect treated?

5. Beta-blockers are administered from which drug groups for cardiac conditions? What are two side effects of beta-blockers?

6. Calcium channel blockers are given from which drug groups for cardiac conditions? Which calcium blockers are used for dysrhythmias?

7. How do the fast (sodium) channel blockers affect the heart?

Critical Thinking Case Study

S.T., age 64, has congestive heart failure (CHF), which has been controlled with digoxin, furosemide (Lasix), and a low-sodium diet. She is taking potassium chloride (KCl) 20 mEq orally per day. Three days ago, S.T. had flulike symptoms of anorexia, lethargy, and diarrhea. Her fluid and food intake was diminished. She refused to take the KCl, stating that the drug makes her sick. She has taken the digoxin and furosemide daily.

The nurse's assessment during the home visit includes poor skin turgor, poor muscle tone, irregular pulse rate, and decreased bowel sounds. The nurse obtained a blood sample for serum electrolytes; results indicated potassium (K) 2.9 mEq/L, sodium (Na) 137 mEq/L, and chloride (Cl) 96 mEq/L.

1. List reference values for serum potassium (K), serum sodium (Na), and serum chloride (Cl)? Are S.T.'s electrolytes within normal range? Explain.

2. What physical findings of S.T. are indicative of which electrolyte imbalance?

3. What are the reasons for the electrolyte imbalance?

4. S.T. said she was not taking KCl because the drug makes her sick. What information can you give her concerning the administration of potassium?

5. What is the effect of furosemide on digoxin when there is a potassium deficit? Explain.

6. The nurse should assess S.T. for digitalis toxicity. Why? List the signs and symptoms of digitalis toxicity.

S.T. was referred to the health care provider because of her serum potassium deficit and its effect on digoxin. A repeat serum potassium determination was taken and the result was 2.8 mEq/L. A liter of dextrose 5% in water with KCl 40 mEq/L was administered over 4 hours.

7. How many milliequivalents of KCl per hour would S.T. receive? Does this amount constitute an acceptable dosage?

8. Why is it important that the nurse check the rate of intravenous fluids containing potassium, the hourly urine output, and vital signs?

9. Because of the low serum potassium level, what other electrolyte value should be checked and why?

After S.T.'s serum electrolytes returned to normal, the health care provider instructed her to continue taking the prescribed KCl dosage daily with her other medications.

10. S.T. asked why she has to continue taking these drugs. What should be your response?

11. The nurse instructs S.T. to eat foods rich in potassium. Which foods are the richest sources of potassium?

D.K., age 72, had a myocardial infarction (MI) 5 years ago. He has been having angina attacks at night and at rest while watching television. He complains of stabbing pain in the chest that lasts 5 minutes. Pain does not radiate to the arm. D.K. is prescribed propranolol (Inderal), 20 mg q.i.d. His vital signs are blood pressure, 108/58; pulse, 56 (at times irregular); respirations, 28. His clinical history indicates that he has mild asthma.

1. What other clinical information is needed in regard to D.K.'s health problem and drug?

2. Of the various types of angina, D.K.'s angina occurrence may indicate which type? Explain.

3. What assessments should the nurse make while D.K. is taking propranolol? Is propranolol an appropriate anginal drug for D.K.? Explain.

4. What client teaching should be included for D.K. in regard to his health history and drug?

D.K. notified the health care provider that he was having "dizzy spells." His blood pressure was 86/50, pulse 46, and respirations 30. His propranolol was stopped, and diltiazem (Cardizem), 30 mg q.i.d., was ordered. He is experiencing an increasing amount of wheezing.

5. What are the correlations between D.K.'s dizziness, wheezing, and vital signs to propranolol?

6. Is the diltiazem ordered for D.K. within the therapeutic dosage range? In what ways would this drug benefit D.K.?

7. List the side effects of diltiazem that should be included in client teaching. What other pertinent information should the nurse include in the teaching data for D.K.?

8. What other drug regimen might be helpful to D.K.?

41 Diuretics

OUTLINE

OBJECTIVES

- Explain the action and uses of diuretics.
- Identify the various groups of diuretics.
- Describe several side effects and adverse reactions related to thiazide, loop, and potassium-sparing diuretics.
- Explain the nursing interventions, including client teaching, related to diuretics, especially thiazide, loop, and potassium-sparing diuretics.

TERMS

antihypertensive
diuresis
diuretics
hypercalcemia
hyperglycemia
hyperkalemia
hypertension
hyperuricemia
hypokalemia
natriuresis
naturetic
oliguria
osmolality
potassium-sparing diuretics
potassium-wasting diuretics
saluretic

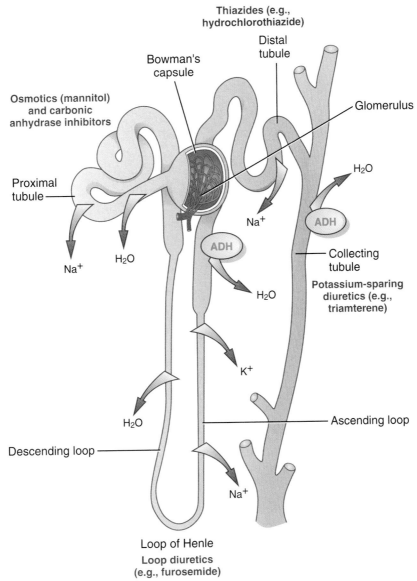

FIGURE 41–1 Diuretics act on different segments of the renal tube: osmotic, mercurial, and carbonic anhydrase inhibitor diuretics affect the proximal tubule; loop (high-ceiling) diuretics affect the loop of Henle; thiazides affect the distal tubule; and potassium-sparing diuretics act primarily on the collecting tubules.

Introduction

Diuretics are used for two main purposes: to decrease hypertension (lower blood pressure) and to decrease edema (peripheral and pulmonary) in congestive heart failure (CHF) and renal or liver disorders. **Hypertension** is an elevated blood pressure. Diuretics discussed in this chapter are used either alone or in combination to decrease blood pressure and edema.

Diuretics produce increased urine flow **(diuresis)** by inhibiting sodium and water reabsorption from the kidney tubules. Most sodium and water reabsorption occurs throughout the renal tubular segments (proximal, loop of Henle [descending loop and ascending loop], and collecting tubule). Diuretics can affect one or more segments of

the renal tubules. Figure 41–1 illustrates the renal tubule along with the normal process of water and electrolyte reabsorption and the diuretic effects on the tubules.

Every 1.5 hours, the total volume of the body's extracellular fluid (ECF) goes through the kidneys (glomeruli) for cleansing; this is the first process for urine formation. Small particles such as electrolytes, drugs, glucose, and waste products from protein metabolism are filtered in the glomeruli. Larger products such as protein and blood cells are not filtered with normal renal function, and they remain in the circulation. Sodium and water are the largest filtrate substances.

Normally, 99% of the filtered sodium that passes through the glomeruli is reabsorbed. From 50% to 55% of

Table 41–1

Diuretics: Thiazides

Generic (Brand)	Route and Dosage	Uses and Considerations
Short-Acting		
chlorothiazide (Diuril)	*Hypertension:* A: PO: 250-500 mg/d or b.i.d. *Edema:* A: PO: 500-1000 mg/d A: IV: 250-1000 mg/d in 1-2 divided doses C: >1 y: PO: 20 mg/kg/d in 2 divided doses C: <6 mo: PO: 10-30 mg/kg/d in divided doses	For hypertension and peripheral edema. Adults may be given IV chlorothiazide, but it is not recommended for infants and children. *Pregnancy category:* B; PB: 20%-80%; $t^{1/2}$: 1-2 h
hydrochlorothizide (HydroDiuril, HCTZ)	See Prototype Drug Chart 41–1.	
Intermediate-Acting		
bendroflumethiazide (Naturetin)	A: PO: 2.5-20 mg/d C: PO: *maint:* 0.05-0.1 mg/kg/d or 1.5-3 mg/m²/d or in divided doses	Treatment of hypertension and edema associated with CHF and cirrhosis. Has similar effects as the prototype drug HCTZ. Hypokalemia, hyperglycemia, and hyperuricemia may occur. *Pregnancy category:* UK; PB: 94%; $t^{1/2}$: 3-4 h
benzthiazide (Exna)	*Hypertension:* A: PO: 25-100 mg/d or 25-100 mg in divided doses *Edema:* A: PO: 25-200 mg/d C: PO: 1-4 mg/kg/d in 3 divided doses	Similar to hydrochlorothiazide. *Pregnancy category:* D; PB: UK; $t^{1/2}$: UK
hydroflumethiazide (Saluron, Diucardin)	*Hypertension:* A: PO: 50-100 mg/d *Edema:* A: PO: 25-200 mg/d C: PO: 1 mg/kg/d	Similar to hydrochlorothiazide, its effects, side effects, adverse reactions, and abnormal laboratory results. *Pregnancy category:* C; PB: 74%; $t^{1/2}$: 17 h
Long-Acting		
methyclothiazide (Aquatensen, Enduron)	*Hypertension/edema:* A: PO: 2.5-10 mg/d C: PO: 0.05-0.1 mg/kg/d	For hypertension and edema associated with CHF and renal or liver dysfunction. Side effects and drug interactions are similar to those of HCTZ. It has a long duration of action. *Pregnancy category:* C; PB: UK; $t^{1/2}$: UK

A, Adult; *b.i.d.,* twice a day; *C,* child; *CHF,* congestive heart failure; *d,* daily; *h,* hour; *IV,* intravenous; *maint,* maintenance; *max,* maximum; *mo,* month; *PO,* by mouth; *PB,* protein-binding; *$t^{1/2}$,* half-life; *UK,* unknown; *wk,* week; *y,* year; >, greater than; <, less than.

sodium reabsorption occurs in the proximal tubules, 35% to 40% in the loop of Henle, 5% to 10% in the distal tubules, and less than 3% in the collecting tubules. Diuretics that act on the tubules closest to the glomeruli have the greatest effect in causing **natriuresis** (sodium loss in the urine). A classic example is the osmotic diuretic mannitol. The diuretic effect depends on the drug reaching the kidneys and its concentration in the renal tubules.

Diuretics have an **antihypertensive** effect by promoting sodium and water loss by blocking sodium and chloride reabsorption. This causes a decrease in fluid volume and lowering of blood pressure. In addition, with fluid loss, edema (fluid retention in body tissues) should decrease. When sodium is retained, water is also retained in the body and the blood pressure increases.

Many diuretics cause the loss of other electrolytes, including potassium, magnesium, chloride, and bicarbonate. The diuretics that promote potassium excretion are classified as **potassium-wasting diuretics,** and those that promote potassium retention are called **potassium-sparing diuretics.**

The following five categories of diuretics are effective in removing water and sodium:
- Thiazide and thiazide-like
- Loop or high-ceiling
- Osmotic
- Carbonic anhydrase inhibitor
- Potassium-sparing

The thiazide, loop or high-ceiling, and potassium-sparing diuretics are the most frequently prescribed types for hypertension and for edema associated with CHF. All are potassium wasting, except those in the potassium-sparing group.

Combination diuretics have been marketed that contain both potassium-wasting and potassium-sparing drugs primarily for the treatment of hypertension. The combinations have an additive effect in reducing the blood pressure. The combination of potassium-wasting and potassium-sparing diuretic is discussed in the section on potassium-

Table 41-1

Diuretics: Thiazides—cont'd

Generic (Brand)	Route and Dosage	Uses and Considerations
Long-Acting—cont'd		
polythiazide (Renese-R)	*Hypertension:* A: PO: 2-4 mg/d *Edema:* A: PO: 1-4 mg/d C: PO: 0.02-0.08 mg/kg/d	Similar to hydrochlorothiazide. *Pregnancy category:* D; PB: 84%; $t\frac{1}{2}$: 25 h
trichlormethiazide (Diurese Metahydrin, Naqua)	*Hypertension:* A: PO: 2-4 mg/d in 1-2 divided doses *Edema:* A: PO: 1-4 mg/d or b.i.d. C: PO: 0.07 mg/kg/d in divided doses	Similar to HCTZ. It has a long duration of action (24 hours). *Pregnancy category:* B; PB: UK; $t\frac{1}{2}$: 2.5-7 h
Thiazide-Like Diuretics		
(This group has similar effects to but not exactly like HCTZ.)		
chlorthalidone (Hygroton)	*Hypertension:* A: PO: 12.5-50 mg/d *Edema:* A: PO: 25-100 mg/d; *max:* 200 mg/d C: PO: 2 mg/kg/3 × wk	For hypertension and edema associated with CHF and renal or liver dysfunction. It has a very long duration of action (24-72 h). *Pregnancy category:* C; PB: 75%; $t\frac{1}{2}$: 40-54 h
indapamide (Lozol)	*Hypertension/edema:* A: PO: 2.5 mg/d; may increase to 5 mg/d	For hypertension and edema. A long-acting diuretic. May be classified as a loop diuretic. *Pregnancy category:* B; PB: 75%; $t\frac{1}{2}$: 14-18 h
metolazone (Zaroxolyn)	*Hypertension:* A: PO: 2.5-5.0 mg/d *Edema:* A: PO: 5-20 mg/d	For hypertension and edema. Intermediate-acting diuretic. More effective than thiazides in clients with decreased renal function. *Pregnancy category:* D; PB: 33%; $t\frac{1}{2}$: 8-14 h
quinethazone (Hydromox)	A: PO: 50-100 mg/d; *max:* 200 mg/d in divided doses	For edema. Intermediate-acting diuretic. *Pregnancy category:* D; PB: UK; $t\frac{1}{2}$: UK

sparing diuretics. Chapter 42, Antihypertensive Drugs, discusses the combinations of antihypertensive agents with hydrochlorothiazide.

Thiazides and Thiazide-Like Diuretics

The first thiazide, chlorothiazide, was marketed in 1957; it was followed 1 year later by hydrochlorothiazide. There are numerous thiazide and thiazide-like preparations. Thiazides act on the distal convoluted renal tubule, beyond the loop of Henle, to promote sodium, chloride, and water excretion. Thiazides are used to treat hypertension and peripheral edema. They are not effective for immediate diuresis. Table 41-1 lists the drugs, dosages, uses, and considerations for the thiazide and thiazide-like diuretics. Drug dosages for hypertension and edema are similar.

The thiazide diuretics are used primarily for clients with normal renal function. If the client has a renal disorder and the creatinine clearance is less than 30 ml/min, the effectiveness of the thiazide diuretic is greatly decreased. Thiazides cause a loss of sodium, potassium, and magnesium, but they promote calcium reabsorption. **Hypercalcemia** (calcium excess) may result, which can be haz-

ardous to the client if he or she is digitalized or has cancer that causes hypercalcemia. Thiazides affect glucose tolerance; thus hyperglycemia can also occur. Thiazides should be used cautiously in clients with diabetes mellitus. Laboratory test results (e.g., electrolytes, glucose) need to be monitored.

The thiazide drug hydrochlorothiazide has been combined with selected angiotensin-converting enzyme (ACE) inhibitors, beta-blockers, alpha-blockers, angiotensin II blockers, and centrally acting sympatholytics to control hypertension. See Prototype Drug Chart 41-1 for the pharmacologic data for hydrochlorothiazide.

Pharmacokinetics

Thiazides are well absorbed from the gastrointestinal (GI) tract. Hydrochlorothiazide has a moderate protein-binding power. The half-life of the thiazide drugs is longer than that of the loop diuretics. For this reason, thiazides should be administered in the morning to avoid nocturia (nighttime urination) and sleep interruption.

Pharmacodynamics

Thiazides act directly on arterioles, causing vasodilation, which can lower blood pressure. Other action includes the excretion of sodium chloride and water, which causes a decrease in vascular fluid and thus decreases cardiac output and blood pressure. The onset of action of hydrochlorothiazide occurs within 2 hours. The peak concentration times are long

PROTOTYPE DRUG CHART 41–1

HYDROCHLOROTHIAZIDE

Drug Class	**Dosage**
Thiazide diuretic Trade Name: HydroDiuril, HCTZ, Esidrix, Oretic, 🍁 Apo-Hydro, Urozide *Pregnancy Category:* B	A: PO: Hypertension: 12.5-50 mg/d Edema: Initially: 25-200 mg in divided doses; *maint:* 25-100 mg/d C: PO: 1-2 mg/kg/d in divided doses C: <6 mo: PO: 1-3 mg/kg/d in divided doses

Contraindications	**Drug-Lab-Food Interactions**
Renal failure with anuria, electrolyte depletion *Caution:* Hepatic cirrhosis, renal dysfunction, diabetes mellitus, gout, systemic lupus erythematosus	*Drug:* Increase digitalis toxicity with digitalis and hy- pokalemia; *increase* potassium loss with steroids; potassium loss; *decrease* antidiabetic effect; *decrease* thiazide effect with cholestyramine and colestipol *Lab:* Increase serum calcium, glucose, uric acid; *decrease* serum potassium, sodium, magnesium

Pharmacokinetics	**Pharmacodynamics**

Absorption: Readily absorbed from the GI tract
Distribution: PB: 65%
Metabolism: t½: 6-15 h
Excretion: In urine
	PO: Onset: 2 h
	  Peak: 3-6 h
	  Duration: 6-12 h

Therapeutic Effects/Uses

To increase urine output; to treat hypertension, edema from CHF, hepatic cirrhosis, renal dysfunction
Mode of Action: Action is on the renal distal tubules by promoting sodium, potassium, and water excretion, decreasing
preload and cardiac output; also decreases edema; acts on arterioles, causing vasodilation thus decreasing blood
pressure

Side Effects	**Adverse Reactions**
Dizziness, vertigo, weakness, nausea, vomiting, diarrhea, hyperglycemia, constipation, rash, photosensitivity	Severe dehydration, hypotension **Life-threatening:** Severe potassium depletion, marked hypotension, uremia, aplastic anemia, hemolytic ane- mia, thrombocytopenia, agranulocytosis

A, Adult; *C,* child; *CHF,* congestive heart failure; *d,* day; *GI,* gastrointestinal; *h,* hour; *maint,* maintenance; *mo,* month; *PB,* protein-
binding; *PO,* by mouth; *t½,* half-life; <, less than; 🍁, Canadian drug names.

(3 to 6 hours). Thiazides are divided into three groups according to their duration of action: short-acting thiazides, with a duration time of less than 12 hours; intermediate-acting, with a duration time of 12 to 24 hours; and long-acting, with a duration time of more than 24 hours.

Side Effects and Adverse Reactions

Side effects and adverse reactions of thiazides include electrolyte imbalances (hypokalemia, hypercalcemia, hypomagnesemia, and bicarbonate loss), **hyperglycemia** (elevated blood sugar), **hyperuricemia** (elevated serum uric acid level), and hyperlipidemia (elevated blood lipid level). Signs and symptoms of hypokalemia should be assessed, and serum potassium levels must be closely monitored. Potassium supplements are frequently needed. Serum calcium and uric acid levels should be checked because thiazides block calcium and uric acid excretion. Thiazides affect the metabolism of carbohydrates, and hyperglycemia can result, especially in clients with high to high-normal

blood sugar levels. Thiazides can increase serum cholesterol, low-density lipoprotein, and triglyceride levels. A drug may be ordered to lower blood lipids. Other side effects include dizziness, headaches, nausea, vomiting, constipation, urticaria (hives) (rare), and blood dyscrasias (rare).

Table 41–2 summarizes the serum chemistry abnormalities that can occur with thiazide use.

Contraindications

Thiazides are contraindicated for use in renal failure. Symptoms of severe kidney impairment or shutdown include **oliguria** (marked decrease in urine output), elevated blood urea nitrogen (BUN), and elevated serum creatinine.

Drug Interactions

Of the numerous drug interactions, the most serious occurs with digoxin. Thiazides can cause **hypokalemia,** which enhances the action of digoxin, and digitalis toxicity can occur. Potassium supplements are frequently prescribed, and

Table 41–2

Serum Chemistry Abnormalities Associated with Thiazides

Serum Chemistry Parameter	Abnormal Results
Electrolytes	
Potassium	Hypokalemia (low serum potassium). Potassium is excreted from the distal renal tubule.
Magnesium	Hypomagnesemia (low serum magnesium). Potassium and sodium loss prompt magnesium loss.
Calcium	Hypercalcemia (elevated serum calcium). Thiazides may block calcium excretion.
Chloride	Hypochloremia (low serum chloride). Sodium and potassium losses produce chloride loss.
Bicarbonate	Minimal bicarbonate loss from proximal tubule.
Uric acid	Hyperuricemia (elevated uric acid). Thiazides can block uric acid excretion.
Blood sugar	Hyperglycemia (increased blood sugar). Thiazides increase fasting blood sugar levels and those of prediabetic state.
Blood lipids	Cholesterol, low-density lipoproteins, and triglycerides can be elevated.

serum potassium levels are monitored. Thiazides also induce hypercalcemia, which enhances the action of digoxin resulting in possible digitalis toxicity. Signs and symptoms of digitalis toxicity (bradycardia, nausea, vomiting, visual changes) should be reported. Thiazides enhance the action of lithium, and lithium toxicity can occur. Thiazides potentiate the action of other antihypertensive drugs, which may be used in combination drug therapy for hypertension.

Nursing Process

Diuretics: Thiazides

ASSESSMENT

■ Assess vital signs, weight, urine output, and serum chemistry values (electrolytes, glucose, uric acid) for baseline levels.
■ Check peripheral extremities for presence of edema. Note pitting edema.
■ Obtain a history of drugs and herbs that are taken daily. Review for drugs and herbals that may cause drug interaction, including digoxin, corticosteroids, antidiabetics, ginkgo, and licorice.

NURSING DIAGNOSES

■ Risk for deficient fluid volume
■ Impaired patterns of urinary elimination

PLANNING

■ Client's blood pressure will be decreased and/or return to normal value.
■ Client's edema will be decreased.
■ Client's serum chemistry levels remain within normal ranges.

NURSING INTERVENTIONS

■ Monitor vital signs and serum electrolytes, especially potassium, glucose, uric acid, and cholesterol levels. Report changes. If client is taking digoxin and hypokalemia occurs, digitalis toxicity frequently results.
■ Observe for signs and symptoms of hypokalemia, such as muscle weakness, leg cramps, and cardiac dysrhythmias.
■ Check client's weight daily at a specified time. A weight gain of 2.2 to 2.5 pounds is equivalent to an excess liter of body fluids.
■ Monitor urine output to determine fluid loss or retention.

Client Teaching

General
• Emphasize the need for compliance. Client may not "feel better" for some time or may not "feel worse" if treatment is missed or discontinued.
• Suggest that client take hydrochlorothiazide in early morning to avoid sleep disturbance resulting from nocturia.
• Keep drugs out of reach of small children. Request childproof bottle.
• Inform client that certain herbal products may interact with thiazide diuretics. See Herbal Alert 41–1.

Self-Administration
• Instruct client or family member how to take and record his or her blood pressure. Record daily results.

Side Effects
• Instruct client to slowly change positions from lying to standing because dizziness may occur as a result of orthostatic (postural) hypotension.
• Advise client who may be prediabetic to have blood sugar checked periodically because large doses of hydrochlorothiazide increase blood glucose levels.

- Suggest that client use sun block when in direct sunlight.

Diet

- Instruct client to eat foods rich in potassium, such as fruits, fruit juices, and vegetables. Potassium supplements may be ordered.
- Advise client to take drugs with food to avoid gastrointestinal upset.

Cultural Considerations ⊕

- Respect cultural beliefs and values. If client from a foreign background tells the health care provider that she or he only eats pasta and does not eat fruits and vegetables, the nurse may have two options: to encourage client to eat fruits and vegetables or to contact the health care provider so that an adequate potassium supplement would be prescribed to overcome potassium loss. An interpreter may be necessary.
- Emphasize the importance of client taking a potassium supplement with the potassium-wasting diuretic. In addition, advise client of consequences and dangers of not taking potassium supplements or lack of appropriate diet while taking potassium-wasting diuretics.

EVALUATION

■ Evaluate the effectiveness of drug therapy. Client's blood pressure and edema will be reduced and blood chemistry will remain within normal range.

■ Determine the absence of side effects and adverse reactions to therapy.

Loop (High-Ceiling) Diuretics

The loop, or high-ceiling, diuretics act on the ascending loop of Henle by inhibiting chloride transport of sodium into the circulation (inhibits passive reabsorption of sodium). Sodium and water are lost, together with potassium, calcium, and magnesium. Loop diuretics can affect blood sugar and increase the uric acid level. The drugs in this group are potent and cause marked depletion of water and electrolytes. The effects of loop diuretics are dose related (i.e., increasing the dose increases the effect and

---

HERBAL ALERT 41–1

Diuretics

⚘ *Aloe* can decrease the serum potassium level thereby causing hypokalemia when taken with a potassium-wasting diuretic such as thiazide diuretics.

⚘ *Uva ursi* may increase the effects of diuretics. It may cause electrolyte imbalance.

⚘ *Gingko* may increase blood pressure when taken with thiazide diuretics.

⚘ *Licorice* can increase potassium loss, leading to hypokalemia.

---

response of the drug). This response is called *high-ceiling diuretics*. Loop diuretics are more potent than thiazides as diuretics, inhibiting reabsorption of sodium two to three times more effectively, but they are less effective as antihypertensive agents.

Loop diuretics can increase renal blood flow up to 40%. It is a frequently prescribed diuretic for clients whose creatinine clearance is less than 30 ml/min and for those with end-stage renal disease. This group of diuretics causes excretion of calcium, unlike thiazides, which inhibit calcium loss.

The first loop diuretics marketed were ethacrynic acid (Edecrin) in the late 1950s and furosemide (Lasix) in 1960. Bumetanide (Bumex) is more potent than furosemide on a per milligram-for-milligram basis. Furosemide and bumetanide are derivatives of sulfonamides. Ethacrynic acid, a phenoxyacetic acid derivative, is a seldom-chosen loop diuretic. It is usually reserved for clients allergic to sulfa drugs. Prototype Drug Chart 41–2 lists the drug data for the loop diuretic furosemide.

Pharmacokinetics

Loop diuretics are rapidly absorbed by the GI tract. These drugs are highly protein bound with half-lives that vary from 30 minutes to 1.5 hours. Loop diuretics compete for protein-binding sites with other highly protein-bound drugs.

Pharmacodynamics

Loop diuretics have a great **saluretic** (sodium-chloride–losing) or **natruetic** (sodium-losing) effect and can cause rapid diuresis, thus decreasing vascular fluid volume and causing a decrease in cardiac output and blood pressure. Because furosemide is a more potent diuretic than thiazide diuretics, it causes a vasodilatory effect; thus renal blood flow increases before diuresis. Furosemide is used when other conservative measures fail, such as sodium restriction and use of less-potent diuretics. The oral dose of furosemide is usually twice that of an intravenous (IV) dose.

The onset of action of loop diuretics occurs within 30 to 60 minutes. The onset of action for IV furosemide is 5 minutes. Duration of action is shorter than that of the thiazides.

Side Effects and Adverse Reactions

The most common side effects are fluid and electrolyte imbalances, such as hypokalemia, hyponatremia, hypocalcemia, hypomagnesemia, and hypochloremia. Hypochloremic metabolic alkalosis may result, which can worsen the hypokalemia. Orthostatic hypotension can occur. Thrombocytopenia, skin disturbances, and transient deafness are rarely seen. Prolonged use of loop diuretics could cause thiamine deficiency. Table 41–3 lists the physiologic and laboratory changes associated with loop diuretics.

Drug Interaction

The major drug interaction is with digitalis preparations. If the client takes digoxin with a loop diuretic, digitalis toxicity can result. Hypokalemia enhances the action of digoxin and increases the risk of digitalis toxicity. The client needs potassium replacement with food or supplements. Table 41–4 lists the data for the four loop (high-ceiling) diuretics.

PROTOTYPE DRUG CHART 41–2

FUROSEMIDE

Drug Class

Loop (high ceiling) diuretic
Trade Name: Lasix, ✤ Fumide, Furomide
Pregnancy Category: C

Dosage

A: PO: 20-80 mg single dose/d; may increase in 6-8 h,
  20-40 mg; *max:* 600 mg/d
IM/IV: 20-40 mg single dose; over 1-2 min IV; repeat
  20 mg in 2 h
C: PO: 2 mg/kg single dose; repeat in 6-8 h; *max:* 6 mg/kg/d
IM/IV: 1 mg/kg single dose; repeat 1 mg/kg in 2 h

Contraindications

Presence of severe electrolyte imbalances, hypovolemia,
  anuria, hypersensitivity to sulfonamides, hepatic coma

Drug-Lab-Food Interactions

Drug: Increase orthostatic hypotension with alcohol; *increase* ototoxicity with aminoglycosides; *increase* bleeding with anticoagulants; *increase* potassium loss with steroids; *increase* digitalis toxicity and cardiac dysrhythmias with digoxin and hypokalemia; *increase* lithium toxicity; *increase* amphotericin B ototoxicity and nephrotoxicity
Lab: Increase BUN, blood/urine glucose, serum uric acid, ammonia; *decrease* potassium, sodium, calcium, magnesium, chloride serum levels

Pharmacokinetics

Absorption: PO: Readily absorbed from the GI tract
Distribution: PB: 95%
Metabolism: t½: 30-50 min
Excretion: In urine, some in feces; crosses placenta

Pharmacodynamics

PO: Onset: <60 min
  Peak: 1-4 h
  Duration: 6-8 h
IV: Onset: 5 min
  Peak: 20-30 min
  Duration: 2 h

Therapeutic Effects/Uses

To treat fluid retention/fluid overload caused by CHF, renal dysfunction, cirrhosis; hypertension; acute pulmonary edema
Mode of Action: Inhibition of sodium and water reabsorption from the loop of Henle and distal renal tubules;
  potassium, magnesium, and calcium also may be excreted

Side Effects

Nausea, diarrhea, electrolyte imbalances, vertigo,
  cramping, rash, headache, weakness, ECG changes,
  blurred vision, photosensitivity

Adverse Reactions

Severe dehydration; marked hypotension
Life-threatening: Renal failure, thrombocytopenia,
  agranulocytosis

A, Adult; *BUN,* blood urea nitrogen; *C,* child; *CHF,* congestive heart failure; *d,* day; *ECG,* electrocardiogram; *GI,* gastrointestinal; *h,* hour; *IM,* intramuscular; *IV,* intravenous; *max,* maximum; *min,* minute; *PB,* protein-binding; *PO,* by mouth; *t½,* half-life; <, less than; ✤, Canadian drug names.

Nursing Process

Diuretics: Loop (High-Ceiling)

ASSESSMENT

■ Obtain a history of drugs that are taken daily. Note whether client is taking a drug that may cause an interaction, such as alcohol, aminoglycosides, anticoagulants, corticosteroids, lithium, amphotericin B, or digitalis. Recognize that furosemide is highly protein-bound and can displace other protein-bound drugs such as warfarin (Coumadin).

■ Assess vital signs, serum electrolytes, weight, and urine output for baseline levels.
■ Compare client's drug dose with recommended dose and report discrepancy.
■ Note whether client is hypersensitive to sulfonamides.

NURSING DIAGNOSES

■ Risk for deficient fluid volume

PLANNING

■ Client's edema and/or hypertension will be decreased.
■ Client's serum chemistry levels will remain within normal ranges.

NURSING INTERVENTIONS

■ Check the half-life of furosemide. With a short half-life, the drug can be repeated or given more than once a day.

■ Check onset of action for furosemide, orally and IV. If the drug is given IV, the urine output should increase in 5 to 20 minutes. If urine output does not increase, notify the health care provider. Severe renal disorder may be present.

■ Monitor urinary output to determine body fluid gain or loss. Urinary output should be at least 25 ml/h or 600 ml/24 hour.

■ Check client's weight to determine fluid loss or gain. A loss of 2.2 to 2.5 pounds is equivalent to a fluid loss of 1 liter.

■ Monitor vital signs. Be alert for marked decrease in blood pressure.

■ Administer IV furosemide slowly; hearing loss may occur if rapidly injected.

■ Observe for signs and symptoms of hypokalemia (<3.5 mEq/L), such as muscle weakness, abdominal distention, leg cramps, and/or cardiac dysrhythmias.

■ Monitor serum potassium levels, especially when a client is taking digoxin. Hypokalemia enhances the action of digitalis, causing digitalis toxicity.

Client Teaching

General
• To prevent sleep disturbance and nocturia, instruct client to take furosemide in the morning and *not* in the evening.

Side Effects
• Instruct client to arise slowly to prevent dizziness resulting from fluid loss.

Diet
• Suggest taking furosemide at mealtime or with food to avoid nausea.

Cultural Considerations ⊕

• Respect cultural beliefs and values. If client from a foreign background tells the health care provider that she or he only eats pasta and does not eat fruits and vegetables, the nurse may have two options: to encourage the client to eat fruits and vegetables or to contact the health care provider so that an adequate potassium supplement would be prescribed to overcome potassium loss. An interpreter may be necessary.

• Emphasize the importance of client taking a potassium supplement with the potassium-wasting diuretic. In addition, advise client of consequences and dangers of not taking potassium supplements or lack of appropriate diet while taking potassium-wasting diuretics.

Table 41–3

Physiologic and Laboratory Changes Associated with Loop Diuretics

Physiologic/Laboratory Changes	Possible Effects of Loop (High-Ceiling) Diuretics
Physiologic Changes	
Hypotension	Postural (orthostatic) hypotension can result because of ECFV deficit.
Ototoxicity	Hearing impairment, although rare, may occur. It is more common with use of ethacrynic acid. Diuretics in other categories are not considered ototoxic. *Caution:* Avoid taking a loop diuretic with a drug that can be ototoxic, such as aminoglycoside.
Skin disturbances	Pruritus, urticaria, exfoliative dermatitis, and purpura may occur in some persons allergic to the drug or when taking the loop diuretic in high doses over a long period.
Photosensitivity	When exposed to sun or sunlamp for a prolonged time, severe sunburn could result. The client should use sun block and avoid long sun exposure.
Hypovolemia	Excess extracellular fluid is lost through increased urine excretion.
Laboratory Changes	
Hypokalemia, hypomagnesemia, hyponatremia, hypocalcemia, hypochloremia	Potassium, magnesium, sodium, calcium, and chloride are lost from the body from increased urine excretion. Chloride, an anion, is attached to the cations potassium and sodium; thus chloride is lost along with potassium and sodium.
Hyperglycemia	Increased glycogenolysis may contribute to an elevated blood sugar level. Clients with diabetes should closely monitor their blood glucose levels when taking a loop diuretic.
Hyperuricemia	Elevated uric acid levels are common in clients susceptible to gout.
Elevated BUN and creatinine	These elevations may result from ECFV loss. Hemoconcentration can cause elevated BUN and creatinine levels, which are reversible when fluid volume returns to normal levels.
Thrombocytopenia, leukopenia	A decrease in platelet and white blood cell counts is rare, but they should be closely monitored.
Elevated lipids	Loop diuretics can decrease high-density lipoproteins (HDL) and increase low-density lipoproteins (LDL). Clients with elevated cholesterol levels should have their levels of HDL and LDL checked. Regardless of the lipid effects, loop diuretics are useful for clients with serious fluid retention caused by a cardiac condition such as CHF.

BUN, Blood urea nitrogen; *CHF,* congestive heart failure; *ECFV,* extracellular fluid volume.

EVALUATION

■ Evaluate the effectiveness of drug action: decreased fluid retention or fluid overload, decreased respiratory distress, and increased cardiac output.
■ Check for side effects and increase in urine output.

Osmotic Diuretics

Osmotic diuretics increase the **osmolality** (concentration) of the plasma and fluid in the renal tubules. Sodium, chloride, potassium (to a lesser degree), and water are excreted. This group of drugs is used to prevent kidney failure, to decrease intracranial pressure (ICP) (e.g., cerebral edema), and to decrease intraocular pressure (IOP) (e.g., glaucoma). Mannitol is a potent osmotic potassium-wasting diuretic frequently used in emergency situations, such as for ICP and IOP. In addition, mannitol can be used with cisplatin and carboplatin in cancer chemotherapy to induce a frank diuresis with decreased side effects of treatment.

Mannitol is the most frequently prescribed osmotic diuretic, followed by urea. Diuresis occurs within 1 to 3 hours after IV administration. Table 41–4 describes the two osmotic diuretics.

Table 41–4

Diuretics: Loop (High-Ceiling), Osmotics, and Carbonic Anhydrase Inhibitors

Generic (Brand)	Route and Dosage	Uses and Considerations
Loop (High-Ceiling)		
bumetanide (Bumex)	A: PO: 0.5-2.0 mg/d; *max:* 10 mg/d IV: 0.5-1.0 mg/dose; repeat in 2-4 h C: PO: 0.015 mg/kg/d	Treatment of renal disease and hypertension and edema associated with CHF. Similar effects as furosemide. *Pregnancy category:* C; PB: 95%; t½: 1-1.5 h
ethacrynic acid (Edecrin)	A: PO: 50-100 mg/d or b.i.d.; *max:* 400 mg/d IV: 0.5-1.0 mg/kg/dose or 50-100 mg/d C: PO: 1 mg/kg/d	For severe edema (pulmonary and peripheral). It is a potent diuretic and has rapid action. Also used for hypercalcemia. Moderate to high doses may cause ototoxicity. *Pregnancy category:* B; PB: 95%; t½: 1-1.5 h
furosemide (Lasix)	See Prototype Drug Chart 41–2.	
torsemide (Demadex)	*Hypertension:* A: PO/IV: Initially: 5 mg/d; *maint:* PO: 5-10 mg/d; IV: in 2 min *CHF:* A: PO/IV: 10-20 mg/d; *max:* 200 mg/d	Similar to furosemide. *Pregnancy category:* C; PB: >97%; t½: 2-4 h
Osmotics	*ICP/IOP:*	
mannitol	A: IV: 1.5-2.0 mg/kg; 15%-25% sol infused over 30-60 min *Edema, ascites, or oliguria:* A: IV: 50-100 g; 10%-20% sol infused over 90 min to 6 h	For oliguria and decreasing ICP. To prevent acute renal failure. Used in narrow-angle glaucoma for reducing IOP. Client should have effective renal function. It is a potent diuretic. *Pregnancy category:* C; PB: UK; t½: 1.5 h
urea (Ureaphil)	A: IV: 1.0-1.5 g/kg of 30% sol, inf over 1-2.5 h; *max:* 120 g/d C: >2 y: IV: 0.5-1.5 g/kg of 30% sol, inf over 1-2.5 h	Same uses as mannitol. Not the drug of choice. Used during prolonged surgery to prevent acute renal failure. *Pregnancy category:* C; PB: UK; t½: 1 h
Carbonic Anhydrase Inhibitors		
acetazolamide (Diamox)	A: PO/IV: 250 mg q12h; dose may vary A: SR: 500 mg/d or b.i.d. C: PO: 10-15 mg/kg/d in divided doses C: IV: 5-10 mg/kg/d; dose may vary	For edema, treating absence (petit mal) seizures, and open-angle glaucoma. May cause hyperglycemia, hyperuricemia, and hypercalcemia. Metabolic acidosis can result. *Pregnancy category:* C; PB: 90%; t½: 2.5-5.5 h
dichlorphenamide (Daranide, Oratrol)	A: PO: 100 mg q12h; *maint:* 25-50 mg/d-t.i.d.	Treatment of open-angle glaucoma by reducing the IOP and for narrow-angle glaucoma before surgery. *Pregnancy category:* C; PB: UK; t½: UK
methazolamide (Neptazane)	A: PO: 50-100 mg b.i.d.-t.i.d.	Similar to dichlorphenamide. *Pregnancy category:* C; PB: 50%-60%; t½: 14 h

A, Adult; *b.i.d.,* twice a day; *C,* child; *CHF,* congestive heart failure; *d,* day; *h,* hour; *ICP,* intracranial pressure; *inf,* infusion; *IOP,* intraocular pressure; *IV,* intravenous; *maint,* maintenance dose; *max,* maximum; *min,* minute; *PB,* protein-binding; *PO,* by mouth; *sol,* solution; *SR,* sustained-release; *t½,* half-life; *t.i.d.,* three times a day; *UK,* unknown; *y,* year; *>,* greater than.

Side Effects and Adverse Reactions

The side effects and adverse reactions of mannitol include fluid and electrolyte imbalance, pulmonary edema from rapid shift of fluids, nausea, vomiting, tachycardia from rapid fluid loss, and acidosis. Crystallization of mannitol in the vial may occur when the drug is exposed to a low temperature. The vial should be warmed to dissolve the crystals. The mannitol solution should not be used for IV infusion if crystals are present and have not been dissolved.

Carbonic Anhydrase Inhibitors

The carbonic anhydrase inhibitors acetazolamide, dichlorphenamide, ethoxzolamide, and methazolamide block the action of the enzyme carbonic anhydrase, which is needed to maintain the acid-base balance (hydrogen and bicarbonate ion balance). Inhibition of this enzyme causes increased sodium, potassium, and bicarbonate excretion. With prolonged use, metabolic acidosis can occur.

This group of drugs is used primarily to decrease IOP in clients with open-angle (chronic) glaucoma. These drugs are not used in narrow-angle or acute glaucoma. Other uses include diuresis, management of epilepsy, and treatment of high-altitude or acute mountain sickness. Table 41–4 presents the drug data for carbonic anhydrase inhibitor diuretics. The drug may also be used for a client in metabolic alkalosis who needs a diuretic. Carbonic anhydrase inhibitors may be alternated with a loop diuretic.

Side Effects and Adverse Reactions

Acetazolamide can cause fluid and electrolyte imbalance, metabolic acidosis, nausea, vomiting, anorexia, confusion, orthostatic hypotension, and crystalluria. Hemolytic anemia and renal calculi can also occur. These drugs are contraindicated during the first trimester of pregnancy.

Potassium-Sparing Diuretics

Potassium-sparing diuretics, which are weaker than thiazides and loop diuretics, are used as mild diuretics or in combination with another diuretic (e.g., hydrochlorothiazide or antihypertensive drugs). Continuous use of potassium-wasting diuretics requires a daily oral potassium supplement because the kidneys excrete potassium, sodium, and body water. However, potassium supplements are *not* used when the client takes a potassium-sparing diuretic; in fact, serum potassium excess, called **hyperkalemia,** results when a potassium supplement is taken with a potassium-sparing diuretic. The serum potassium should be periodically monitored when the client continuously takes a potassium-sparing diuretic. If the serum potassium level is greater than 5.2 mEq/L, the client should discontinue the potassium-sparing diuretic and re-

strict foods high in potassium (see Chapter 15, Fluid and Electrolyte Replacement).

Potassium-sparing diuretics act primarily in the collecting duct renal tubules to promote sodium and water excretion and potassium retention. The drugs interfere with the sodium-potassium pump that is controlled by the mineralocorticoid hormone aldosterone (sodium retained and potassium excreted).

Spironolactone (Aldactone), an aldosterone antagonist discovered in 1958, was the first potassium-sparing diuretic. Aldosterone is a mineralocorticoid hormone that promotes sodium retention and potassium excretion. Spironolactone blocks the action of aldosterone and inhibits the sodium-potassium pump (i.e., potassium is retained and sodium is excreted). As a result of the action of spironolactone, the heart rate is more regular, and the possibility of myocardial fibrosis is decreased. The effects of spironolactone may take 48 hours.

Amiloride and triamterene are two additional potassium-sparing diuretics commonly prescribed. Amiloride (Midamor) is effective as an antihypertensive agent. Triamterene (Dyrenium) is useful in the treatment of edema caused by CHF or cirrhosis of the liver. Spironolactone (Aldactone), amiloride (Midamor), and triamterene (Dyrenium) should not be taken with ACE inhibitors because they can also increase serum potassium levels. Prototype Drug Chart 41–3 provides the pharmacologic data for triamterene.

When potassium-sparing diuretics are used alone, they are less effective than when used in combination to reduce body fluid and sodium. These drugs are usually combined with a potassium-wasting diuretic (e.g., thiazide)—primarily hydrochlorothiazide or a loop diuretic. The combination of potassium-sparing and potassium-wasting diuretics intensifies the diuretic effect and prevents potassium loss. The common combination diuretics are spironolactone (Aldactone) and hydrochlorothiazide (Aldactazide), amiloride and hydrochlorothiazide (Moduretic), and triamterene and hydrochlorothiazide (Dyazide, Maxzide). Table 41–5 lists the potassium-sparing diuretics and the combination potassium-wasting and potassium-sparing diuretics.

Side Effects and Adverse Reactions

The main side effect of these drugs is hyperkalemia. Caution must be used when giving potassium-sparing diuretics to a client with poor renal function because the kidneys excrete 80% to 90% of the potassium. Urine output should be at least 600 ml per day. Clients should *not* use potassium supplements while taking potassium-sparing diuretics unless the serum potassium level is low. If a potassium-sparing diuretic is given with the antihypertensive drug ACE inhibitor, hyperkalemia could become severe or life-threatening because both drugs retain potassium. Monitoring serum potassium levels is necessary. GI disturbances (anorexia, nausea, vomiting, diarrhea) can occur.

PROTOTYPE DRUG CHART 41–3

TRIAMTERENE

Drug Class

Potassium-sparing diuretic
Trade Name: Dyrenium
Pregnancy Category: B

Contraindications

Severe kidney or hepatic disease, severe hyperkalemia
Caution: Renal or hepatic dysfunction, diabetes mellitus

Dosage

A: PO: **Edema:** 100 mg/d in 2 divided doses, p.c.; not to exceed 300 mg/d
C: PO: 2-4 mg/kg/d in divided doses

Drug-Lab-Food Interactions

Drug: Increase serum potassium level with potassium supplements; *increase* effects of antihypertensives and lithium; life-threatening hyperkalemia if given with ACE inhibitor
Lab: Increase serum potassium level; may *increase* BUN, AST, alkaline phosphatase levels; *decrease* serum sodium, chloride

Pharmacokinetics

Absorption: PO: Rapidly absorbed from GI tract
Distribution: PB: 67%
Metabolism: $t\frac{1}{2}$: 1.5-2.5 h
Excretion: In urine, mostly as metabolites and bile

Pharmacodynamics

PO: Onset: 2-4 h
  Peak: 6-8 h
  Duration: 12-16 h

Therapeutic Effects/Uses

To increase urine output; to treat fluid retention/overload associated with CHF, hepatic cirrhosis, or nephrotic syndrome
Mode of Action: Action on the distal renal tubules to promote sodium and water excretion and potassium retention

Side Effects

Nausea, vomiting, diarrhea, rash, dizziness, headache, weakness, dry mouth, photosensitivity

Adverse Reactions

Life-threatening: Severe hyperkalemia, thrombocytopenia, megaloblastic anemia

A, Adult; *ACE,* angiotensin-converting enzyme; *AST,* aspartate aminotransferase; *BUN,* blood urea nitrogen; *C,* child; *CHF,* congestive heart failure; *d,* day; *GI,* gastrointestinal; *h,* hour; *PB,* protein-binding; *p.c.,* after meals; *PO,* by mouth; $t\frac{1}{2}$, half-life.

Nursing Process

Diuretics: Potassium-Sparing

ASSESSMENT

■ Obtain a history of drugs that are taken daily. Note whether client is taking a potassium supplement or using a salt substitute.
■ Assess vital signs, serum electrolytes, weight, and urinary output for baseline levels.
■ Compare client's drug dose with the recommended dose and report any discrepancy.

NURSING DIAGNOSES

■ Risk for deficient fluid volume

PLANNING

■ Client's fluid retention and blood pressure will be decreased.
■ Client's serum electrolytes remain within their normal values.

NURSING INTERVENTIONS

■ Check the half-life of triamterene. With a long half-life, drug dose is usually administered once a day and sometimes twice a day.
■ Monitor urinary output. Urine output should increase. Report if urine output is <30 ml/h or <600 ml/day.
■ Monitor vital signs. Report abnormal changes.
■ Observe for signs and symptoms of hyperkalemia (increased serum potassium level: >5.3 mEq/L), such as nausea, diarrhea, abdominal cramps, tachycardia and later bradycardia, peaked narrow T wave on electrocardiogram, or oliguria.
■ To avoid nocturia, administer triamterene in the morning and not in the evening.

Client Teaching

General
• Instruct client to take triamterene with or after meals to avoid nausea.
• Do not discontinue drug without consulting the health care provider.

Side Effects
- Instruct client to avoid exposure to direct sunlight because the drug can cause photosensitivity.
- Advise client to report possible side effects of the drug, such as rash, dizziness, or weakness.

Diet
- Advise clients with high average serum potassium levels to avoid foods rich in potassium when taking potassium-sparing diuretics.

EVALUATION

■ Evaluate the effectiveness of the potassium-sparing diuretic, such as triamterene. Fluid retention (edema) is decreased or absent.
■ Determine whether urine output has increased and the serum potassium level is within normal range.

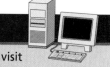

WEBSITES

For further information on *Diuretics*, visit these Internet resources:

Health Net—spironolactone:
http://www.health-net.info/spironolactone.html

Medline Plus Drug Information—spironolactone:
http://www.nlm.nih.gov/medlineplus/druginfo/medmaster/a682627.html

Medline Plus Drug Information—furosemide:
http://www.nlm.nih.gov/medlineplus/druginfo/medmaster/a682858.html

Furosemide:
http://www.marvistavet.com/html/body_furosemide.html

Table 41–5

Diuretics: Potassium-Sparing

Generic (Brand)	Route and Dosage	Uses and Considerations
Single Agents		
amiloride HCl (Midamor)	A: PO: 5 mg/d; may increase to 10-20 mg/d in 1-2 divided doses	For diuretic-induced hypokalemia; used for hypertension, CHF, and cirrhosis of the liver. Serum potassium level should be monitored to detect hyperkalemia. *Pregnancy category:* B; PB: 23%; $t_{1/2}$: 6-9 h
spironolactone (Aldactone)	*Hypertension:* A: PO: 25-100 mg/d in 1-2 divided doses *Edema:* A: PO: 25-200 mg/d in divided doses C: PO: 3.3 mg/kg/d in divided doses	For edema and hypertension. Dosage for hypertension is usually slightly lower than for edema. Has a long duration of action. *Pregnancy category:* C; PB: 98%; $t_{1/2}$: 1.5-2 h
triamterene (Dyrenium)	See Prototype Drug Chart 41-3.	
Combinations		
amiloride HCl and hydrochlorothiazide (Moduretic)	A: PO: 1-2 tab (amiloride 5 mg/hydrochlorothiazide 50 mg)	Combinations contain potassium-wasting and potassium-sparing diuretics. Drugs are to control hypertension and edema. They are used to prevent the occurrence of hypokalemia.
spironolactone and hydrochlorothiazide (Aldactazide)	A: PO: 25/25 and 50/50 mg tab	Same as Moduretic.
triamterene and hydrochlorothiazide (Dyazide, Maxzide)	A: PO: 1-2 cap b.i.d., p.c. (Dyazide: triamterene 50 mg/hydrochlorothiazide 25 mg)	Dyazide: each tablet contains triamterene 50 mg and hydrochlorothiazide 25 mg. Maxzide comes in two strengths: triamterene 37.5 mg or 75 mg and hydrochlorothiazide 50 mg or 75 mg. *Pregnancy category:* B; PB: UK; $t_{1/2}$: UK

A, Adult; *b.i.d.*, twice a day; *C*, child; *cap*, capsule; *CHF*, congestive heart failure; *d*, day; *h*, hour; *PB*, protein-binding; *p.c.*, after meals; *PO*, by mouth; $t_{1/2}$, half-life; *tab*, tablet; *UK*, unknown.

Critical Thinking Case Study

J.Q., age 58, has recently been diagnosed with hypertension. His blood pressure is 158/92. He has been prescribed hydrochlorothiazide (HydroDiuril), 50 mg daily. He has been told to eat foods rich in potassium.

1. How does hydrochlorothiazide differ from furosemide? What are their similarities and differences?

2. Why is it necessary for J.Q. to eat foods rich in potassium when taking hydrochlorothiazide? Explain.

3. What are the nursing interventions that should be considered while J.Q. takes HydroDiuril?

J.Q. became weak and complained of nausea and vomiting. His muscles were "soft." His serum potassium level was 3.3 mEq/L. J.Q.'s diuretic was changed to triamterene/hydrochlorothiazide (Dyazide). Again, he is advised to eat foods rich in potassium. Refer to Chapter 15, Fluid and Electrolyte Replacement, as needed.

4. Explain the rationale for changing J.Q.'s diuretic.

5. Should J.Q. receive a potassium supplement? Explain.

6. What nursing interventions should be followed for J.Q.?

7. What care plan should the nurse develop for J.Q. in relation to client teaching?

8. What medical follow-up care is needed for J.Q.?

Study Questions

1. The client receives hydrochlorothiazide (HydroDiuril) 50 mg daily and digoxin 0.25 mg daily. Is hydrochlorothiazide a potassium-wasting or potassium-sparing diuretic? What types of electrolyte imbalances can occur? Explain.

2. Client teaching is essential when caring for a client receiving hydrochlorothiazide and digoxin. How should the client be instructed regarding diet and vital signs? What are the signs and symptoms of digitalis toxicity?

3. What electrolyte imbalances may occur when taking hydrochlorothiazide over a prolonged period?

4. A client has diabetes mellitus and takes hydrochlorothiazide. Why should the client's blood glucose level be closely monitored?

5. What type of diuretic is furosemide (Lasix)? What electrolyte imbalances can this drug cause?

6. A client takes triamterene. What type of diuretic is triamterene? What effect can this have on the potassium level?

7. Why would a combination diuretic (triamterene and hydrochlorothiazide) be prescribed?

8. The client's blood pressure is 142/92. What non-pharmacologic measures should be suggested to lower the blood pressure?

42 Antihypertensive Drugs

OBJECTIVES

- Identify the categories of antihypertensive drugs, along with the stepped-care approach and the modified pharmacologic approach to antihypertensive drugs.
- Explain the pharmacologic action of the individual groups of antihypertensive drugs.
- Describe the side effects and adverse reactions to sympatholytics (beta-blockers, centrally acting and peripherally acting alpha-blockers, alpha- and beta-blockers), direct-acting vasodilators, and angiotensin antagonists.
- Explain the nursing interventions, including client teaching, related to antihypertensives.

TERMS

antihypertensive
essential hypertension
hypertension

secondary hypertension
stepped-care hypertension approach

sympatholytics

Hypertension

Hypertension is an increase in blood pressure such that the systolic pressure is greater than 140 mmHg and the diastolic pressure is greater than 90 mmHg. **Essential hypertension** is the most common type, affecting 90% of persons with high blood pressure. The exact origin of essential hypertension is unknown; however, contributing factors include (1) a family history of hypertension, (2) hyperlipidemia, (3) African American background, (4) diabetes, (5) obesity, (6) aging, (7) stress, and (8) excessive smoking and alcohol ingestion. Ten percent of hypertension cases are related to renal and endocrine disorders and are classified as **secondary hypertension.**

Selected Regulators of Blood Pressure

The kidneys and the blood vessels strive to regulate and maintain a "normal" blood pressure. The kidneys regulate blood pressure via the renin-angiotensin system. The process is illustrated in Figure 42–1. Renin (from the renal cells) stimulates production of angiotensin II (a potent vasoconstrictor), which causes the release of aldosterone (adrenal hormone that promotes sodium retention and thereby water retention). Retention of sodium and water causes fluid volume to increase thus elevating blood pressure. The baroreceptors in the aorta and carotid sinus and the vasomotor center in the medulla also assist in the regulation of blood pressure. Catacholamines such as norepinephrine released from the sympathetic nerve terminals and epinephrine released from the adrenal medulla increase blood pressure through vasoconstriction activity.

Other hormones that contribute to blood pressure regulation are the antidiuretic hormone (ADH) and atrial natriuretic peptide (hormone) (ANP). ADH is produced by the hypothalamus and is stored and released by the posterior pituitary gland (neurohypophysis). This hormone stimulates the kidneys to conserve and retain water when there is a fluid volume deficit; however, when there is a fluid overload, ADH secretion is inhibited, and the kidneys then excrete more water. ANP is released by the atrium of the heart and responds to fluid overload by stimulating the kidneys to increase the glomerular filtration rate, thereby increasing the elimination of sodium and water. In addition, ANP causes vasodilation and inhibits renin and aldosterone secretions. The hormone brain natriuretic peptide (BNP) is released from the atrium like ANP when volume overload occurs within the heart chambers. ANP and BNP aid in volume homeostasis and are useful for identifying heart failure.

Physiologic Risk Factors

Certain physiologic risk factors contribute to hypertension. A diet with excess fat and carbohydrates can increase blood pressure. Carbohydrate intake can affect sympathetic nervous activity. Alcohol increases renin secretions, causing the production of angiotensin II. Obesity affects the sympathetic and cardiovascular systems by increasing cardiac output, stroke volume, and left-ventricular filling. Two

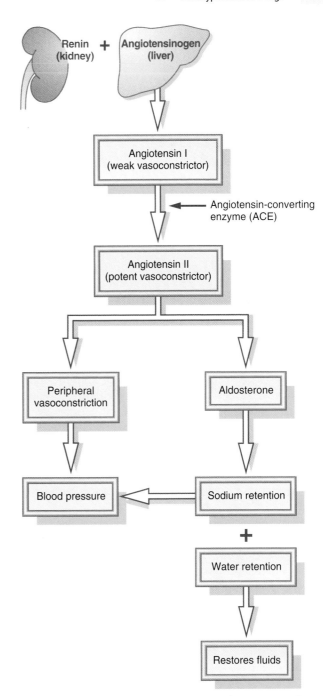

FIGURE 42–1 Renin-angiotensin system. Renin, an enzyme located in the juxtaglomerular cells of the kidney, is released when blood pressure decreases. This diagram shows how the renin-angiotensin system restores fluid balance and stabilizes blood pressure.

thirds of hypertensive persons are obese. Normally, weight loss can decrease hypertension, as can mild to moderate sodium restriction.

Cultural Responses to Antihypertensive Agents

African Americans are more likely to develop hypertension at an earlier age than white Americans. They also have a higher mortality rate from hypertension than the white population.

The use of beta-adrenergic blockers (beta-blockers) and angiotensin-converting enzyme (ACE) inhibitors is less effective for the control of hypertension in African Americans unless the drug is combined or given with a diuretic. This group is susceptible to low-renin hypertension; therefore they do not respond well to beta-blockers and ACE inhibitors. The antihypertensive drugs that are effective for African Americans are the alpha$_1$ blockers and calcium channel blockers (calcium blockers). African American clients do respond to diuretics as the *initial* monotherapy for controlling hypertension. White clients usually have high-renin hypertension and respond well to all antihypertensive agents.

The Asian population is twice as sensitive as whites to beta-blockers and other antihypertensives. A reduction in antihypertensive dosing is frequently needed. American Indians have a reduced or lower response to beta-blockers compared with whites. Monitoring blood pressure and drug dosing should be an ongoing assessment for these cultural groups.

Hypertension in Older Adults

By the age of 60 years, more than half of the older population has hypertension. Of those more than 60 years of age, most have systolic hypertension, and only 26% of these older adults have their blood pressure controlled at 140/90 mmHg or below. Both systolic and diastolic hypertension are associated with increased cardiovascular morbidity and mortality. With antihypertensive therapy, the greatest decrease in cardiovascular disorders is 34% for stroke and 19% for coronary heart disease.

One of the troublesome side effects of the use of antihypertensive agents in older adults, especially frail or institutionalized persons, is orthostatic hypotension. If orthostatic hypotension occurs, the antihypertensive drug dose may need to be decreased or another antihypertensive drug used. Older adults with hypertension should be instructed to modify their lifestyle activities. This includes restricting dietary sodium to 2.4 g daily, avoiding tobacco, and losing weight if obese.

Nonpharmacologic Control of Hypertension

A sufficient decrease in blood pressure can be accomplished by nonpharmacologic methods. There are many nonpharmacologic ways to decrease blood pressure; however, if the systolic pressure is greater than 140 mmHg, **antihypertensive** drugs are generally ordered. Nondrug methods to decrease blood pressure include (1) stress-reduction techniques, (2) exercise (increases high-density lipoproteins [HDL]), (3) salt restriction, (4) decreased alcohol ingestion, and (5) weight reduction (Figure 42–2).

When hypertension *cannot* be controlled by nonpharmacologic means, antihypertensive drugs are prescribed.

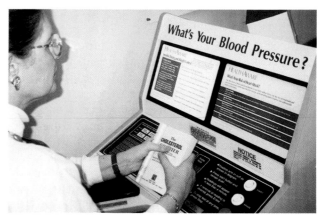

FIGURE 42–2   Blood pressure should be charted at specific intervals, especially if the client has an elevated cholesterol level or borderline hypertension.

However, nonpharmacologic methods should be combined with antihypertensive drugs to control hypertension.

New Guidelines for Hypertension

Blood pressure guidelines for determining hypertension have been revised and are contained in the Seventh Report of the Joint National Committee on Prevention, Detection, Evaluation, and Treatment of High Blood Pressure, or JNC-7. The purpose of the new guidelines is to decrease the risk of cardiovascular disease (CVD). The new guidelines for normal blood pressure is less than 120/80 mmHg. Prehypertension is the second category, with the systolic blood pressure (SBP) 120 to 139 and the diastolic blood pressure (DBP) 80 to 89. No longer is normal blood pressure equal to or less than 140/90. If the client's blood pressure was considered normal, e.g., 130/85 a year ago, it is now in the new category of prehypertension. Stage 1 hypertension is 140/90 to 159/99, and stage 2 hypertension is greater than 160/100. Table 42–1 lists the new guidelines for hypertension.

Two of three clients with hypertension have uncontrolled blood pressure or are not optimally treated. The SBP is more important than the DBP as a CVD risk for clients 50 years or older. According to the JNC-7, if the blood pressure is greater than 20/10 mmHg above goal, a

Table 42–1		
Guidelines for Determining Hypertension		
Category	**Systolic Pressure (mmHg)**	**Diastolic Pressure (mmHg)**
Normal	<120	<80
Prehypertension	120-139	80-89
Stage 1 hypertension	140-159	90-99
Stage 2 hypertension	>160	>100

>, Greater than; <, less than.

drug regimen should be started. CVD risk doubles with each increase of 20/10 mmHg starting at 115/75 mmHg.

Pharmacologic Control of Hypertension

An individualized approach to the treatment of hypertension is used by many health care providers. All drugs are considered *initial agents* when first prescribed for hypertension. Reduction of other cardiovascular risk factors and the use of fewer drugs (i.e., substituting instead of adding drugs) at the lowest effective doses are emphasized. It has been suggested that after a client has taken an antihypertensive drug for a year the drug dose and its effect on client's blood pressure should be evaluated.

In 1993, the JNC-5 classified treatment for elevated SBP, hypertension into four stages; stage 1, SBP 140 to 160; stage 2, SBP 160 to 180; stage 3, SBP 180 to 200; and stage 4, SBP greater than 200. As a result of the staging, the **stepped-care hypertension approach** for treating the four stages was developed; it included a single drug to multiple drugs. Now the JNC-7 uses three classifications for defining an elevated SBP: *prehypertension*, SBP 120 to 139; stage 1, SBP 140 to 160; and stage 2, SBP greater than 160. JNC-7 combines the previous stages 2, 3, and 4 as stage 2; it states that the drug management of the former three groups are the same as that for stage 2. Most clients may need two or more antihypertensive drugs to achieve goal blood pressure. A thiazide diuretic may be the first antihypertensive drug prescribed.

Antihypertensive drugs, used either singly or in combination with other drugs, are classified into six categories: (1) diuretics, (2) sympatholytics (sympathetic depressants), (3) direct-acting arteriolar vasodilators, (4) ACE inhibitors, (5) angiotensin II receptor antagonists (blockers), and (6) calcium channel blockers.

Diuretics

Diuretics promote sodium depletion, which decreases extracellular fluid volume (ECFV). Diuretics are effective as first-line drugs for treating mild hypertension. Hydrochlorothiazide (HydroDiuril), a thiazide, is the most frequently prescribed diuretic to control mild hypertension. It can be used alone for recently diagnosed or mild hypertension or with other antihypertensive drugs. Many antihypertensive drugs can cause fluid retention; therefore diuretics are often administered with antihypertensive agents. The various types of diuretics are discussed in Chapter 41.

Thiazide diuretics should not be used for clients with renal insufficiency (creatinine clearance level <30 ml/min). The loop (high-ceiling) diuretics such as furosemide (Lasix) are usually recommended because they do not depress renal blood flow. Diuretics are not used if hypertension is the result of renin-angiotensin-aldosterone involvement because they tend to elevate the serum renin level.

BOX 42–1

Combination of Thiazides with Antihypertensive Drugs

Thiazide with Potassium-Sparing Diuretics
- hydrochlorothiazide with spironolactone (Aldactazide)
- hydrochlorothiazide with amiloride (Moduretic)
- hydrochlorothiazide with triamterene (Dyazide, Maxzide)

Thiazide with Beta-Blockers
- hydrochlorothiazide with bisoprolol fumarate (Ziac)
- hydrochlorothiazide with metoprolol (Lopressor HCT)
- bendroflumethiazide with nadolol (Corzide)
- hydrochlorothiazide with propranolol (Inderide)
- hydrochlorothiazide with timolol (Timolide)
- chlorthalidone (thiazide-like diuretic) with atenolol (Tenoretic)

Thiazide with ACE Inhibitors
- hydrochlorothiazide with benazepril (Lotensin HCT)
- hydrochlorothiazide with captopril (Capozide)
- hydrochlorothiazide with enalapril maleate (Vaseretic)
- hydrochlorothiazide with fosinopril (Monopril HCT)
- hydrochlorothiazide with lisinopril (Prinzide, Zestoretic)
- hydrochlorothiazide with moexipril (Uniretic)
- hydrochlorothiazide with quinapril (Accuretic)

Thiazide with Angiotensin II Antagonists
- hydrochlorothiazide with candesartan (Atacand HCT)
- hydrochlorothiazide with eprosartan (Teveten HCT)
- hydrochlorothiazide with irbesartan (Avalide)
- hydrochlorothiazide with losartan (Hyzaar)
- hydrochlorothiazide with omesartan medoxomil (Benicar HCT)
- hydrochlorothiazide with telmisartan (Micardis HCT)
- hydrochlorothiazide with valsartan (Diovan HCT)

Thiazide with Centrally Acting Alpha$_2$ Agonist
- chlorthalidone with clonidine (Combipres)
- hydrochlorothiazide with methyldopa (Aldoril)

Thiazide with Alpha-Blocker
- polythiazide with prazosin (Minizide)

Combination of a Calcium-Channel Blocker with a Statin Drug
- amlodipine with atorvastatin (Caduet)

ACE, Angiotensin-converting enzyme; *HCT*, hydrochlorothiazide.

The combination of potassium-wasting and potassium-sparing diuretics may be useful instead of a single thiazide drug; less potassium excretion would occur. In addition, thiazides can be combined with other antihypertensive drugs to increase their effectiveness. Box 42–1 lists the combinations of thiazides with other drugs. Many drug products on the market include combinations of thiazide diuretics with potassium-sparing diuretics, beta-blockers, ACE inhibitors, or angiotensin II antagonists. ACE inhibitors tend to increase the serum potassium (K) level; so when they are combined with the thiazide diuretic, serum potassium loss is minimized.

Sympatholytics (Sympathetic Depressants)

The **sympatholytics** comprise five groups of drugs: (1) beta-adrenergic blockers, (2) centrally acting alpha$_2$-agonists, (3) alpha-adrenergic blockers, (4) adrenergic neuron blockers (peripherally acting sympatholytics), and (5) alpha$_1$ and beta$_1$ adrenergic blockers. The beta-adrenergic blockers block the beta receptors. The alpha-adrenergic blockers block the alpha receptors.

Beta-Adrenergic Blockers

Beta-adrenergic blockers, frequently called *beta-blockers*, are used as step I antihypertensive drugs or in combination with a diuretic in the step II approach to treating hypertension. Beta-blockers are also used as antianginals and antidysrhythmics (see Chapter 40, Cardiac Glycosides, Antianginals, and Antidysrhythmics).

Beta (B$_1$ and B$_2$)-adrenergic blockers reduce cardiac output by diminishing the sympathetic nervous system response thereby decreasing basal sympathetic tone. With continued use of beta-blockers, vascular resistance is diminished and blood pressure is lowered. Beta-blockers reduce heart rate, contractility, and renin release. There is a greater hypotensive response in clients with higher renin levels.

African American hypertensive clients do not respond well to beta-blockers for the control of hypertension. Instead, hypertension can be controlled by combining beta-blockers with diuretics.

There are numerous types of beta-blockers. The nonselective beta-blockers, such as propranolol (Inderal), inhibit beta$_1$ (heart) and beta$_2$ (bronchial) receptors. Heart rate slows (blood pressure decreases secondary to the decrease in heart rate), and bronchoconstriction occurs because of unopposed parasympathetic tone. Cardioselective beta-blockers are preferred because they act mainly on the beta$_1$ rather than the beta$_2$ receptors; as a result, bronchoconstriction is less likely to occur. Acebutolol (Sectral), atenolol (Tenormin), betaxolol (Kerlone), bisoprolol (Zebeta), and metoprolol (Lopressor) are cardioselective beta-blockers that block beta$_1$ receptors.

Cardioselectivity does not confer absolute protection from bronchoconstriction. In tests measuring forced expiratory volume in 1 second (FEV$_1$) as a measure of B$_2$ reactivity, only atenolol demonstrated true protection. Other cardioselective beta-blockers were only partially effective. Studies also show that, at the upper end of the dosage range, cardioselectivity is less effective. In clients with preexisting bronchospasms or other pulmonary disease, beta-blockers, even those considered cardioselective, should be used with caution. Some experts regard this as a relative contraindication. The real value of beta selectivity is in maintaining renal blood flow and minimizing the hypoglycemic effects of beta blockade.

The combination of beta-blockers with hydrochlorothiazides is packaged together in tablet form (see Box 42–1).

Usually, the hydrochlorothiazide dose is 12.5 to 25 mg, approximately half of the average dose.

Again, beta-blockers tend to be more effective in lowering blood pressure in clients who have an elevated serum renin level. The cardioselective prototype drug metoprolol (Lopressor) is presented in Prototype Drug Chart 42–1.

Beta-blockers should not be used by clients with second- or third-degree atrioventricular (AV) block or sinus bradycardia. A noncardioselective beta-blocker such as propranolol (Inderal) should not be given to a client with chronic obstructive pulmonary disease (COPD).

Pharmacokinetics

Metoprolol is well absorbed from the gastrointestinal (GI) tract. Its half-life is short and also its protein-binding power is low.

Pharmacodynamics

Cardioselective beta-adrenergic blockers block beta$_1$ receptors thereby decreasing heart rate and blood pressure. The nonselective beta-blockers block beta$_1$ and beta$_2$ receptors, which can result in bronchial constriction. Beta-blockers cross the placental barrier and can enter breast milk.

The onset of action of oral beta-blockers is usually 30 minutes or less, and the duration of action is 6 to 12 hours. When beta-blockers are administered intravenously (IV), the onset of action is immediate, peak time is 20 minutes (compared with 1.5 hours orally), and duration of action is 4 to 10 hours.

Side Effects and Adverse Reactions

Side effects and adverse reactions include decreased pulse rate; markedly decreased blood pressure; and, with noncardioselective beta$_1$ and beta$_2$ blockers, bronchospasm. Beta-blockers should not be abruptly discontinued because rebound hypertension, angina, dysrhythmias, and myocardial infarction can result. Beta-blockers can cause insomnia, depression, nightmares, and sexual dysfunction. Other side effects are discussed in Chapter 40. Table 42–2 presents the drug data for beta-blockers commonly used to treat hypertension.

Noncardioselective beta-blockers inhibit the liver's ability to convert glycogen to glucose in response to hypoglycemia. Because of this side effect, beta-blockers should be used with caution in clients with diabetes mellitus. In addition, the depression of heart rate masks the symptom (tachycardia) of hypotension.

Nursing Process

Antihypertensives: Beta-Blockers

ASSESSMENT

■ Obtain a medication and herbal history from client. Report if a drug-drug or drug-herbal interaction is probable.
■ Obtain vital signs. Report abnormal blood pressure. Compare vital signs with baseline finding.

■ Check laboratory values related to renal and liver function. An elevated blood urea nitrogen (BUN) and serum creatinine may be caused by metoprolol or cardiac disorder. Elevated cardiac enzymes, such as aspartate transaminase (AST) and lactate dehydrogenase (LDH), could result from use of metoprolol or from a cardiac disorder.

NURSING DIAGNOSES

■ Decreased cardiac output
■ Noncompliance with drug regimen
■ Sexual dysfunction

PLANNING

■ Client's blood pressure will be decreased or will return to normal value.
■ Client takes the medication as prescribed.

NURSING INTERVENTIONS

■ Monitor vital signs, especially blood pressure and pulse.
■ Monitor laboratory results, especially BUN, serum creatinine, AST, and LDH.

Client Teaching

General

• Instruct client to comply with drug regimen: *abrupt discontinuation of the antihypertensive drug may cause rebound hypertension.*
 Inform client that herbs can interfere with beta-blockers (see Herbal Alert 42–1).
• Suggest that client avoid OTC drugs without first checking with the health care provider. Many OTC drugs carry warnings against use in the presence of hypertension or use concurrently with antihypertensives.

PROTOTYPE DRUG CHART 42–1

METOPROLOL

Drug Class	**Dosage**
Antihypertensive: beta$_1$-blocker Trade Name: Lopressor, ♣ Betaloc, Apo-Metoprolol, Toprol SR *Pregnancy Category:* C; D (second and third trimester)	*Hypertension:* A: PO: 50-100 mg/d in 1-2 divided doses; *maint:* 100-450 mg in divided doses; *max:* 450 mg/d in divided doses; Geriatric: 25 mg/d; *maint:* 25-300 mg/d SR: 50-100 mg/d; *max:* 450 mg/d *Myocardial infarction:* A: PO: 100 mg b.i.d. IV: 5 mg q2min × 3 doses
Contraindications	**Drug-Lab-Food Interactions**
Second- and third-degree heart block, cardiogenic shock, CHF, sinus bradycardia *Caution:* Hepatic, renal, or thyroid dysfunction; asthma; peripheral vascular disease; type 1 diabetes mellitus	*Drug: Increase* bradycardia with digitalis; *increase* hypotensive effect with other antihypertensives, alcohol, anesthetics
Pharmacokinetics	**Pharmacodynamics**

Absorption: PO: 95%
Distribution: PB: 12%
Metabolism: t½: 3-7 h
Excretion: In urine
	PO: Onset: 15 min
	  Peak: 1.5 h
	  Duration: 10-19 h
	IV: Onset: Immediate
	  Peak: 20 min
	  Duration: 5-10 h

Therapeutic Effects/Uses

To control hypertension
Mode of Action: Promotion of blood pressure reduction via beta$_1$-blocking effect

Side Effects	**Adverse Reactions**
Fatigue, weakness, dizziness, nausea, vomiting, diarrhea, mental changes, nasal stuffiness, impotence, decreased libido, depression	Bradycardia, thrombocytopenia **Life-threatening:** Complete heart block, bronchospasm, agranulocytosis

A, Adult; *b.i.d.,* twice a day; *CHF,* congestive heart failure; *d,* day; *h,* hour; *IV,* intravenous; *maint,* maintenance; *max,* maximum; *min,* minute; *PB,* protein-binding; *PO,* by mouth; *SR,* sustained release; *t½,* half-life; ♣, Canadian drug names.

- Suggest that client wear a MedicAlert bracelet or carry a card indicating the health problem and prescribed drugs.
- Instruct client in a trauma situation to inform the health care provider of drugs taken daily, such as a beta-blocker. Beta-blockers block the compensatory effects of the body to the shock state. Glucagon may be needed to reverse the effects so client can be resuscitated.

Self-Administration

- Instruct client or family member how to take a radial pulse and blood pressure. Advise client to report abnormal findings to the health care provider.

Side Effects

- Advise client that antihypertensives may cause dizziness resulting from orthostatic hypotension. Instruct the client to remain in a sitting position for several minutes before standing.
- Instruct client to report dizziness, slow pulse rate, changes in blood pressure, heart palpitation, confusion, or gastrointestinal upset to the health care provider.
- Alert client with diabetes mellitus to possible hypoglycemic symptoms.
- Inform client that antihypertensives may cause sexual dysfunction (e.g., impotence).

Diet

- Teach client and family members nonpharmacologic methods to decrease blood pressure, such as a low-fat and low-salt diet, weight control, relaxation techniques, exercise, smoking cessation, and decreased alcohol ingestion (1 to 2 oz daily).
- Advise client to report constipation. Foods high in fiber, a stool softener, and increased water intake (except in clients with congestive heart failure) are usually indicated.

Cultural Considerations ⊕

- African-American clients with hypertension should avoid taking beta-blockers because these agents are not generally effective in controlling their hypertension. However, taking a diuretic with a beta-blocker increases the effectiveness for these clients.

EVALUATION

- ▪ Evaluate the effectiveness of the drug therapy (i.e., decreased blood pressure, the absence of side effects).
- ▪ Determine that client adheres to the drug regimen.

Centrally Acting Alpha$_2$ Agonists

Centrally acting alpha$_2$ agonists decrease the sympathetic response from the brainstem to the peripheral vessels. They stimulate the alpha$_2$ receptors, which in turn decreases sympathetic activity; increases vagus activity; decreases cardiac output; and decreases serum epinephrine, norepinephrine, and renin release. All these actions result

---

HERBAL ALERT 42–1

Antihypertensives

- ❧ *Ma-huang* and *ephedra* decrease or counteracts the effect of antihypertensive drugs. When taken with beta-blockers, hypertension may continue or increase.
- ❧ *Ephedra* increases hypertension when taken with beta-blockers.
- ❧ *Black cohosh* increases the hypotensive effect of antihypertensive drugs.
- ❧ *Hawthorn* may increase the effects of beta-blockers and angiotensin-converting enzyme (ACE) inhibitors.
- ❧ *Licorice* antagonizes the effects of antihypertensive drugs.
- ❧ *Goldenseal* may increase the effects of antihypertensives.
- ❧ *Parsley* may increase the cause of hypotension when taken with an antihypertensive drug.

---

in reduced peripheral vascular resistance. This group of drugs has minimal effects on cardiac output and blood flow to the kidneys. Beta-blockers are not given with centrally acting sympatholytics that can accentuate both bradycardia during therapy and rebound hypertension on discontinuing drug therapy.

Drugs in this group include methyldopa, clonidine, guanabenz, and guanfacine. Methyldopa (Aldomet) was one of the first drugs widely used to control hypertension. In high doses, methyldopa and clonidine can cause sodium and water retention. Frequently, methyldopa and clonidine are administered with diuretics. Clonidine is available in a transdermal preparation that provides a 7-day duration of action. New transdermal patches are replaced every 7 days and may be left on while bathing. Skin irritations have occurred in approximately 20% of clients. Guanabenz and guanfacine are newer centrally acting alpha$_2$ agonists with effects similar to clonidine. Guanfacine has a long half-life and usually is taken once a day. Table 42–2 lists the centrally acting alpha$_2$ agonists along with the beta-blockers.

Side Effects and Adverse Reactions

The side effects and adverse reactions include drowsiness, dry mouth, dizziness, and slow heart rate (bradycardia). Methyldopa should not be used in clients with impaired liver function, and serum liver enzymes should be monitored periodically in all clients. This group of drugs must not be abruptly discontinued because a hypertensive crisis can result. If the drug needs to be stopped immediately, another antihypertensive drug is usually prescribed to avoid rebound hypertensive symptoms (e.g., restlessness, tachycardia, tremors, headache, and increased blood pressure). Rebound hypertension is less likely to occur with guanabenz and guanfacine. The nurse should emphasize the need to take the medication as prescribed. This group of drugs can cause sodium and water retention, resulting in peripheral edema. A diuretic may be ordered with methyldopa or clonidine to decrease water and sodium retention (edema). Clients who are pregnant or contemplating preg-

Table 42–2

Antihypertensives: Beta-blockers and Central Alpha₂-Agonists

Generic (Brand)	Route and Dosage	Uses and Considerations
Beta-Adrenergic Blockers		
acebutolol HCl (Sectral) Cardioselective beta₁	A: PO: 400-800 mg/d in 1 or 2 divided doses; *max:* 1200 mg/d	For hypertension and cardiac dysrhythmia. It may be used alone or in combination with a diuretic. Side effects include dizziness, fatigue, hypotension, bradycardia, constipation/diarrhea. Vital signs should be closely monitored. *Pregnancy category:* B; PB: 26%; t½: 6-7 h
atenolol (Tenormin) Cardioselective beta₁	A: PO: 25-100 mg/d	For hypertension and angina. Similar side effects as acebutolol. *Pregnancy category:* C; PB: 6%-16%; t½: 6-7 h
betaxolol HCl (Kerlone) Cardioselective beta₁	A: PO: 10-20 mg/d. Also for ophthalmic use (glaucoma)	For hypertension and glaucoma. Ophthalmic preparation is used to decrease IOP. *Pregnancy category:* C; PB: UK; t½: 14-22 h
bisoprolol fumarate (Zebeta) Beta₁-blocker	A: PO: Initially: 5 mg/d; *maint:* 2.5-20 mg/d	For hypertension and angina pectoris. Long-acting beta₁ blocker. Heart rate and blood pressure may be decreased. *Pregnancy category:* C; PB: <30%; t½: 9-12 h
carteolol HCl (Cartrol) Nonselective beta₁ and beta₂	A: PO: 2.5-5.0 mg/d	For hypertension and glaucoma. It should be avoided for clients who have asthma because of its beta₂-blocker effect. It may be used in combination with a thiazide diuretic. *Pregnancy category:* C; PB: 23%-30%; t½: 4-6 h
carvedilol (Coreg) alpha-blocker; nonselective beta₁ and beta₂	A: PO: Initially: 3.125-6.25 mg, b.i.d. May increase after 1-2 wk; *max:* 50 mg/d Elderly: Same as adult	For treating essential hypertension. Contraindicated for decompensated cardiac failure bronchial asthma, bronchospastic conditions severe bradycardia. Food delays absorption. *Pregnancy category:* C; PB: 98%; t½: 7-10 h
metoprolol (Lopressor) Cardioselective beta₁	See Prototype Drug Chart 42–1.	
nadolol (Corgard) Nonselective beta₁ and beta₂	A: PO: 40-80 mg/d; *max:* 320 mg/d	For hypertension and angina pectoris. Similar to carteolol HCl. *Pregnancy category:* C; PB: 30%; t½: 10-24 h
penbutolol SO₄ (Levatol) Nonselective beta₁ and beta₂	A: PO: 10-20 mg/d; *max:* 80 mg/d	Treatment of stage 1 and 2 hypertension. Clients with asthma should avoid taking drug. *Pregnancy category:* C; PB: 80%- 98%; t½: 5 h
pindolol (Visken) Nonselective beta₁ and beta₂	A: PO: 5 mg b.i.d.-t.i.d.; *maint:* 10-30 mg in divided doses; *max:* 60 mg/d in divided doses	For hypertension. May be used alone or in combination with thiazide diuretic. Also may be used for angina pectoris. *Pregnancy category:* B; PB: 50%; t½: 3-4 h
propranolol (Inderal) Nonselective beta₁ and beta₂	A: PO: Initially: 40 mg b.i.d.; SR: 80 mg/d; *maint:* 120-240 mg/d in divided doses; *max:* 480 mg/d C: PO: Initially 1 mg/kg/d in 2 divided doses; *maint:* 2 mg/kg/d	For hypertension, angina, and cardiac dysrhythmias. The first beta-blocker. May cause bronchospasm because of beta₂-blocker effect. *Pregnancy category:* C; PB: 90%; t½: 3-6 h
timolol maleate (Blocadren) Nonselective beta₁ and beta₂	A: PO: Initially: 10 mg b.i.d.; *maint:* 20-40 mg/d in 2 divided doses; *max:* 60 mg/d Also for ophthalmic use (glaucoma)	For hypertension, angina pectoris, and glaucoma. It is used as step 1 antihypertensive, like most of the beta-blockers. Similar to propranolol. *Pregnancy category:* C; PB: 60%; t½: 3-4 h
Central Alpha₂ Agonists		
clonidine HCl (Catapres)	A: PO: Initially: 0.1 mg b.i.d.; *maint:* 0.2-1.2 mg/d in divided doses; *max:* 2.4 mg/d A: Transdermal patch: 100 mcg (0.1 mg)/q7d 200 mcg (0.2 mg)/q7d 300 mcg (0.3 mg)/q7d	For hypertension. Long-acting. Well absorbed from GI tract. Can be taken with a diuretic. Step 2 antihypertensive drug. Decreases sympathetic effect. Drowsiness, dizziness, and dry mouth may occur. *Pregnancy category:* C; PB: 20%-40%; t½: 6-20 h
guanabenz acetate (Wytensin)	A: PO: 4 mg b.i.d.; may increase to 4-8 mg/d; *max:* 32 mg b.i.d.	For hypertension and tachycardia. Can be taken with a thiazide diuretic. Intermediate acting. May cause drowsiness, dizziness, headache, fatigue, and dry mouth. If GI distress occurs, take with food. *Pregnancy category:* C; PB: 90%; t½: 4-14 h
guanfacine HCl (Tenex)	A: PO: 1 mg/d at bedtime; may increase to 2-3 mg/d	For hypertension. Long acting. May be taken alone or with a thiazide diuretic. *Pregnancy category:* B; PB: 70%; t½: >17 h
methyldopa (Aldomet)	A: PO: 250-500 mg b.i.d.; *max:* 3 g/d IV: 250-500 mg q6h; *max:* 1 g q6h C: PO: 10 mg/kg/d in 2-4 divided doses	For stage 1 to 3 hypertension. May be used alone or in combination with a diuretic. Long acting. Can be given IV. If GI upset occurs, take with food. *Pregnancy category:* C; PB: <15%; t½: 1.7 h

A, Adult; *b.i.d.,* twice a day; *C,* child; *d,* day; *GI,* gastrointestinal; *h,* hour; *IOP,* intraocular pressure; *IV,* intravenous; *maint,* maintenance; *max,* maximum; *PB,* protein-binding; *PO,* by mouth; *SR,* sustained release; *t½,* half-life; *t.i.d.,* three times a day; *UK,* unknown; *wk,* week; *>,* greater than; *<,* less than.

Table 42–3

Antihypertensives: Sympatholytics: Alpha-Adrenergic and Peripherally Acting Blockers and Direct-Acting Vasodilators

Generic (Brand)	Route and Dosage	Uses and Considerations
Selective Alpha-Adrenergic Blockers		
doxazosin mesylate (Cardura)	A: PO: Initially: 1 mg/d; *maint:* 2-4 mg/d; *max:* 16 mg/d	For stage 1 or 2 hypertension. May be used alone or with another antihypertensive. May cause orthostatic hypotension, headache, dizziness, and GI upset. *Pregnancy category:* B; PB: 98%; t½: 22 h
prazosin HCl (Minipress)	See Prototype Drug Chart 42–2.	
terazosin HCl (Hytrin)	A: PO: Initially: 1 mg at bedtime; *maint:* 1-5 mg/d; *max:* 20 mg/d	For stage 1 or 2 hypertension. May be used alone or with another antihypertensive drug. Dizziness and headache may occur. *Pregnancy category:* C; PB: 95%; t½: 9-12 h
Alpha-Adrenergic Blockers		
phenoxybenzamine HCl (Dibenzyline)	A: PO: Initially: 10 mg/d at bedtime; *maint:* 20-40 mg b.i.d./t.i.d. C: PO: 0.2 mg/kg/d in 1-2 divided doses; may increase dose by 0.2 mg	For hypertension related to adrenergic excess, pheochromocytoma. It lowers peripheral resistance. Has a long action. *Pregnancy category:* C; PB: UK; t½: 24 h
phentolamine (Regitine)	A: IM/IV: 2.5-5 mg; repeat q5min until controlled; then q2-3h PRN C: IM/IV: 0.05-0.1 mg/kg; repeat if needed	For hypertensive crisis caused by pheochromocytoma, MAO inhibitors, or clonidine withdrawal. It is a potent antihypertensive drug. In heart failure, it decreases afterload and increases cardiac output. For hypertension, it antagonizes the effects of epinephrine and norepinephrine causing vasodilation. *Pregnancy category:* C; PB: UK; t½: 20 min
tolazoline HCl (Priscoline HCl)	NB: IV: Initially: 1-2 mg/kg; followed by 1-2 mg/kg/h for 24-48 h; expected effect within 30 min of initial dose A: IM/IV: 10-50 mg q.i.d.	For pulmonary hypertension of newborn and for peripheral vasospastic disorders. *Pregnancy category:* C; PB: UK; t½: 3-10 h
Adrenergic Neuron Blockers (Peripherally Acting Sympatholytics)		
guanadrel sulfate (Hylorel)	A: PO: Initially: 5 mg b.i.d.; *maint:* 20-75 mg/d in divided doses	For moderate to severe hypertension. Intermediate-acting duration. Rapid onset. *Pregnancy category:* B; PB: 20%; t½: 10-12 h
guanethidine monosulfate (Ismelin)	A: PO: Initially: 10 mg/d; *maint:* 25-50 mg/d; *max:* 3 mg/kg/d C: PO: 0.2 mg/kg/d; *max:* 1-1.6 mg/kg/d	For severe hypertension. Long acting. Can be taken with a diuretic. Potent antihypertensive drug. May cause marked orthostatic hypotension, edema, weight gain, diarrhea, and bradycardia. *Pregnancy category:* C; PB: UK; t½: 5 d
reserpine (Serpasil, Serpalan)	A: PO: Initially: 0.25-0.5 mg/d for 1-2 wk; *maint:* 0.1-0.25 mg/d	One of the early antihypertensives. For hypertension. Currently, not frequently used. May cause nightmares and vivid dreams. *Pregnancy category:* C; PB: 90%; t½: 4.5-11 h

A, Adult; *b.i.d.,* twice a day; *C,* child; *d,* day; *GI,* gastrointestinal; *h,* hour; *IM,* intramuscular; *IV,* intravenous; *maint,* maintenance; *MAO,* monoamine oxidase; *max,* maximum; *min,* minute; *NB,* newborn; *PB,* protein-binding; *PO,* by mouth; *PRN,* as needed; *q.i.d.,* four times a day; *sec,* second; *t½,* half-life; *t.i.d.,* three times a day; *UK,* unknown; *wk,* week.

nancy should avoid clonidine. Methyldopa is frequently used to treat chronic or pregnancy-induced hypertension; however, it crosses the placental barrier, and small amounts may enter the breast milk of a lactating client.

Alpha-Adrenergic Blockers

This group of drugs blocks the alpha-adrenergic receptors, resulting in vasodilation and decreased blood pressure. They help maintain the renal blood flow rate. The alpha-blockers are useful in treating hypertension in clients with lipid abnormalities. They decrease the very-low-density lipoproteins (VLDL) and the low-density lipoproteins (LDL) that are responsible for the buildup of fatty plaques in the arteries (atherosclerosis). In addition, they increase high-density lipopro-

tein (HDL) levels ("friendly" lipoprotein). Alpha-blockers are safe for clients with diabetes because they do not affect glucose metabolism. They also do not affect respiratory function.

The selective alpha$_1$-adrenergic blockers—prazosin, terazosin, and doxazosin—are used mainly to reduce blood pressure and can be used to treat benign prostatic hypertrophy (BPH). Prazosin is a commonly prescribed drug. Terazosin and doxazosin have longer half-lives than prazosin, and they are normally given once a day. When prazosin is taken with alcohol or other antihypertensives, the hypotensive state can be intensified. These drugs, like the centrally acting alpha$_2$ agonists, cause sodium and water retention with edema; therefore diuretics are frequently given with them to decrease fluid accumulation in the extremities.

Table 42–3

Antihypertensives: Sympatholytics: Alpha-Adrenergic and Peripherally Acting Blockers and Direct-Acting Vasodilators—cont'd

Generic (Brand)	Route and Dosage	Uses and Considerations
Alpha₁- and Beta₁-Adrenergic Blockers		
carteolol HCl (Cartrol, Ocupress)	A: PO: Initially: 2.5 mg/d.; *maint:* 2.5-5 mg/d.; *max:* 10 mg/d	To treat hypertension. It may be used alone or in combination with other antihypertensive agents. Not for hypertensive crisis or client with open-angle glaucoma. *Pregnancy category:* C; PB: 20%-30%; t½: 4-6 h
labetalol HCl (Trandate, Normodyne)	A: PO: Initially: 100 mg b.i.d.; *maint:* 200-800 mg/d in 2 divided doses; *max:* 1200-2400 mg/d A: IV: 20 mg over 2 min; continuous infusion: 2 mg/min; *max:* 300 mg as total dose	For stage 1 or 2 hypertension. May be used alone or with a thiazide diuretic. May cause orthostatic hypotension, palpitation, and syncope. *Pregnancy category:* C; PB: 50%; t½: 4-8 h
Direct-Acting Vasodilators		
diazoxide (Hyperstat, Proglycem)	A & C: IV: 1-3 mg/kg in bolus (30 sec); repeat in 5-15 min PRN; *max:* 150 mg	For hypertensive emergency. Dose may be repeated in 5-15 min until adequate decrease in blood pressure is achieved. Oral antihypertensive drugs may follow. *Pregnancy category:* C; PB: 90%; t½: 20-45 h
hydralazine HCl (Apresoline HCl)	A: PO: Initially: 10 mg q.i.d.; *maint:* 25-50 mg q.i.d. *Severe hypertension:* IM-IV: 10-40 mg, repeat PRN C: PO: 0.1-0.2 mg/kg/dose	For hypertension. Short-acting duration. Can be taken with diuretic to decrease edema and beta-blocker to prevent tachycardia. Dizziness, tremors, headaches, tachycardia, and palpitation may occur. Vital signs should be closely monitored. *Pregnancy category:* C; PB: 87%; t½: 2-6 h
minoxidil (Loniten, Rogaine)	A: PO: Initially: 5 mg/d; *maint:* 10-40 mg/d in single or divided doses; *max:* 100 mg/d C: PO: Initially: 0.2 mg/kg/d; *max:* 5 mg/d; *maint:* 0.25-1 mg/kg/d in divided doses; *max:* 50 mg/d *Topical for alopecia:* 2% sol b.i.d.	For hypertension. Can be taken with a diuretic to reduce edema and with a beta-blocker to prevent tachycardia. Long-acting effect. When discontinuing drug, it should be slowly decreased to avoid rebound hypertension; should not be abruptly withdrawn. Vital signs should be closely monitored. *Pregnancy category:* C; PB: 0%; t½: 3.5-4 h
sodium nitroprusside (Nipride, Nitropress)	A: IV: 1-3 mcg/kg/min in D₅W; *max:* 10 mcg/kg/min	For hypertensive crisis. A potent antihypertensive drug. Drug decomposes in light; container must be wrapped in aluminum foil. Good for 24 h. Drug should be discarded if red or blue. Can cause cyanide toxicity. Measure cyanide and thiocyanate levels. May cause profound hypotension. *Pregnancy category:* C; PB: UK; t½: 10 min

The more potent alpha-blockers—phentolamine, phenoxybenzamine, and tolazoline—are used primarily for hypertensive crisis and severe hypertension resulting from catecholamine-secreting tumors of the adrenal medulla (pheochromocytomas).

Pharmacokinetics

Prazosin is absorbed through the GI tract; however, a large portion of prazosin is lost during hepatic first-pass metabolism. The half-life is short, so the drug should be administered twice a day. Prazosin is highly protein bound, and when it is given with other highly protein-bound drugs, the client should be assessed for adverse reactions.

Pharmacodynamics

The selective alpha-adrenergic blockers dilate the arterioles and venules, decreasing peripheral resistance and lowering the blood pressure. With prazosin, the heart rate is only slightly increased, whereas with nonselective alpha-blockers, such as phentolamine and tolazo-line, the blood pressure is greatly reduced and reflex tachycardia can occur. Nonselective alpha-blockers are more effective for acute hypertension; selective alpha-blockers are more useful for long-term essential hypertension.

The onset of action of prazosin occurs between 30 minutes and 2 hours. The duration of action of prazosin is 10 hours. Table 42–3 presents the drug data for selective and nonselective alpha-blockers.

Side Effects and Adverse Reactions

The side effects of prazosin, doxazosin, and terazosin include orthostatic hypotension (dizziness, faintness, lightheadedness, increased heart rate), which may occur with first dose, nausea, drowsiness, and nasal congestion caused by vasodilation, edema, and weight gain.

Side effects of phentolamine include hypotension, reflex tachycardia caused by the severe decrease in blood pressure, nasal congestion caused by vasodilation, and GI disturbances.

PROTOTYPE DRUG CHART 42–2

PRAZOSIN HCl

Drug Class	**Dosage**
Antihypertensive: alpha-adrenergic blocker Trade Name: Minipress *Pregnancy Category:* C	A: PO: 1 mg b.i.d.-t.i.d.; *maint:* 3–15 mg/d; *max:* 20 mg/d in divided doses
Contraindications	**Drug-Lab-Food Interactions**
Renal disease	*Drug: Increased* hypotensive effect with other antihy- pertensives, nitrates, alcohol
Pharmacokinetics	**Pharmacodynamics**
Absorption: GI: 60% (5% to circulation) **Distribution:** PB: 95% **Metabolism:** t½: 3 h **Excretion:** In bile and feces; 10% in urine	**PO:** Onset: 0.5-2 h Peak: 2-4 h Duration: 10 h

Therapeutic Effects/Uses

To control hypertension, refractory CHF; to treat benign prostatic hypertrophy
Mode of Action: Dilation of peripheral blood vessels via blocking the alpha-adrenergic receptors

Side Effects	**Adverse Reactions**
Dizziness, drowsiness, headache, nausea, vomiting, diarrhea, impotence, vertigo, urinary frequency, tinnitus, dry mouth, incontinence, abdominal discomfort	Orthostatic hypotension, palpitations, tachycardia, pancreatitis

A, Adult; *b.i.d.,* twice a day; *CHF,* congestive heart failure; *d,* day; *GI,* gastrointestinal; *h,* hour; *maint,* maintenance; *max,* maximum;
PB, protein-binding; *PO,* by mouth; *t½,* half-life; *t.i.d.,* three times a day.

Drug Interactions

Drug interactions occur when alpha-adrenergic blockers are taken with anti-inflammatory drugs and nitrates (e.g., nitroglycerin for angina). Peripheral edema is intensified when prazosin and an anti-inflammatory drug are taken daily. Nitroglycerin taken for angina lowers the blood pressure. If prazosin is taken with nitroglycerin, syncope (faintness) caused by a decrease in blood pressure can occur. The selective alpha-adrenergic blocker prazosin is shown in Prototype Drug Chart 42–2.

Nursing Process

Antihypertensives: Alpha-Adrenergic Blockers

ASSESSMENT

■ Obtain a medication history from client, including current drugs. Report if a drug-drug or drug-herbal interaction is probable. Prazosin is highly protein-bound and can displace other highly protein-bound drugs.
■ Obtain baseline vital signs and weight for future comparisons.
■ Check urinary output. Report if it is decreased (<600 ml/day), because drug is contraindicated if renal disease is present.

NURSING DIAGNOSES

■ Risk for activity intolerance
■ Knowledge deficit related to drug regimen
■ Impaired sexuality patterns

PLANNING

■ Client's blood pressure will decrease.
■ Client will follow proper drug regimen.

NURSING INTERVENTIONS

■ Monitor vital signs. The desired therapeutic effect of prazosin may not fully occur for 4 weeks. A sudden marked decrease in blood pressure should be reported.
■ Check daily for fluid retention in the extremities. Prazosin may cause sodium and water retention.

Client Teaching

General
• Instruct client to comply with drug regimen. *Abrupt discontinuation of the antihypertensive drug may cause rebound hypertension.*
• Inform client that orthostatic hypotension may occur. Explain that before rising, client should sit and dangle the feet.

Self-Administration

- Instruct client or family member how to take a blood pressure reading. A record for daily blood pressures should be kept.

Side Effects

- Caution client that dizziness, light-headedness, and drowsiness may occur, especially when the drug is first prescribed. If these symptoms occur, the health care provider should be notified.
- Inform male client that impotence may occur if high doses of the drug are prescribed. This problem should be reported to the health care provider.
- Instruct client to report if edema is present in the morning.
- Inform client not to take cold, cough, or allergy OTC medications without first contacting the health care provider.

Diet

- Encourage client to decrease salt intake unless otherwise indicated by the health care provider.

Cultural Considerations ⊕

- African-American clients with hypertension can take alpha-adrenergic blockers and calcium channel blockers but should avoid taking beta-blockers because these agents are not generally effective in controlling their hypertension. However, taking a diuretic with a beta-blocker increases the effectiveness for these clients.
- Asians are twice as sensitive to the effects of propranolol on the blood pressure and heart rate, so the dose should be decreased or another antihypertensive drug may be given.
- Obtain an interpreter when necessary.

EVALUATION

- Evaluate the effectiveness of the drug in controlling blood pressure and the absence of side effects.
- Evaluate client's adherence to medication schedule.

Adrenergic Neuron Blockers (Peripherally Acting Sympatholytics)

Adrenergic neuron blockers are potent antihypertensive drugs that block norepinephrine release from the sympathetic nerve endings, causing a decrease in norepinephrine release that results in a lowering of blood pressure. There is a decrease in both cardiac output and peripheral vascular resistance. Reserpine and guanethidine (the two most potent drugs) are used to control severe hypertension. Orthostatic hypotension is a common side effect, so the client should be advised to rise slowly from a reclining or sitting position. Use of reserpine may cause vivid dreams, nightmares, and suicidal intention. The drugs in this group can cause sodium and water retention. These drugs can be taken alone or with a diuretic to decrease peripheral edema.

Alpha₁- and Beta₁-Adrenergic Blockers

This group of drugs blocks both the $alpha_1$ and $beta_1$ receptors. Labetalol (Normodyne) and carteolol (Cartrol) are examples of alpha-/beta-blockers. Blocking the $alpha_1$-receptor results in dilation of the arterioles and veins occurs. The effect on the alpha-receptor is stronger than the effect on the beta-receptor; therefore blood pressure is lowered and pulse rate is moderately decreased. By blocking the cardiac $beta_1$-receptor, the heart rate and atrioventricular (AV) contractility are decreased. Large doses of alpha-/beta-blockers could block $beta_2$-adrenergic receptors, thus increasing airway resistance. Clients who have severe asthma should not take large doses of labetalol or carteolol. Table 42–3 lists these two alpha-/beta-blockers.

Common side effects of these drugs include orthostatic (postural) hypotension, GI disturbances, nervousness, dry mouth, and fatigue. Large doses of labetalol or carteolol may cause AV heart block.

Direct-Acting Arteriolar Vasodilators

Vasodilators are potent antihypertensive drugs. Direct-acting vasodilators act by relaxing the smooth muscles of the blood vessels, mainly the arteries, causing vasodilation. Vasodilators promote an increase in blood flow to the brain and kidneys. With vasodilation, the blood pressure decreases and sodium and water are retained, resulting in peripheral edema. Diuretics can be given with a direct-acting vasodilator to decrease the edema.

Reflex tachycardia is caused by the vasodilation and decrease in blood pressure. Beta-blockers are frequently prescribed with arteriolar vasodilators to decrease the heart rate; this counteracts the effect of reflex tachycardia.

Two of the direct-acting vasodilators, hydralazine and minoxidil, are used for moderate to severe hypertension; nitroprusside and diazoxide are prescribed for acute hypertensive emergency. The latter two drugs are very potent vasodilators that rapidly decrease the blood pressure. Nitroprusside acts on the arterial and venous vessels, and diazoxide acts on the arterial vessels. Table 42–3 lists direct-acting vasodilators.

Side Effects and Adverse Reactions

The effects of hydralazine are numerous and include tachycardia, palpitations, edema, nasal congestion, headache, dizziness, GI bleeding, lupuslike symptoms, and neurologic symptoms (tingling, numbness). Minoxidil has similar side effects as well as tachycardia, edema, and excess hair growth. It can precipitate an anginal attack.

Nitroprusside and diazoxide can cause reflex tachycardia, palpitations, restlessness, agitation, nausea, and confusion. Hyperglycemia can occur with diazoxide because the drug inhibits insulin release from the beta cells of the pancreas. Nitroprusside and diazoxide are discussed in greater detail in Chapter 57, Adult and Pediatric Emergency Drugs.

Angiotensin Antagonists (Angiotensin-Converting Enzyme [ACE] Inhibitors)

Drugs in this group inhibit ACE, which in turn inhibits the formation of angiotensin II (vasoconstrictor) and blocks the release of aldosterone. Aldosterone promotes sodium retention and potassium excretion. When aldosterone is blocked, sodium is excreted along with water, and potassium is retained. ACE inhibitors cause little change in cardiac output or heart rate, and they lower peripheral resistance. Figure 42–1 illustrates the renin-angiotensin system. These drugs can be used in clients who have elevated serum renin levels.

The ACE inhibitors are used primarily to treat hypertension; some of these agents are also effective in treating heart failure. The first ACE inhibitor, captopril (Capoten), became available in the early 1970s. By the mid-1990s, there were five ACE inhibitors, and in the late 1990s, there were 10. These 10 ACE inhibitors include benazepril (Lotensin), captopril (Capoten), enalapril maleate (Vasotec), fosinopril (Monopril), lisinopril (Prinivil, Zestril), moexipril (Univasc), perindopril (Aceon), quinapril (Accupril), ramipril (Altace), and trandolapril (Mavik), which are presented in Table 42–4. These drugs are not intended for first-line antihypertensive therapy.

African Americans and older adults do not respond to ACE inhibitors with the desired reduction in blood pressure, but when taken with a diuretic, the blood pressure usually will be lowered. ACE inhibitors should not be given during pregnancy because they reduce placental blood flow.

It is necessary to reduce the drug dose, except for fosinopril (Monopril), for clients with renal insufficiency.

Except for moexipril (Univasc), which should be taken on an empty stomach for maximum effectiveness, ACE inhibitors can be administered with food.

Side Effects and Adverse Reactions

The side effects of these drugs include constant or irritating cough, nausea, vomiting, diarrhea, headache, dizziness, fatigue, insomnia, serum potassium excess (hyperkalemia), and tachycardia. Because of the risk of hyperkalemia, these drugs generally should not be taken with potassium-sparing diuretics or salt substitutes that contain potassium. The major adverse effects are first-dose hypotension and hyperkalemia. Hypotension results because of the vasodilating effect. First-dose hypotension is more common in clients also taking diuretics.

Nursing Process

Antihypertensives: Angiotensin Antagonist (ACE) Inhibitors

ASSESSMENT

■ Obtain a drug and herbal history from client of current drugs that are taken. Report if a drug-drug or drug-herbal interaction is probable.

■ Obtain baseline vital signs for future comparisons.
■ Check the laboratory values for serum protein, albumin, blood urea nitrogen (BUN), creatinine, and white blood cell (WBC) count, and compare with future serum levels.

NURSING DIAGNOSES

■ Knowledge deficit related to drug regimen
■ Anxiety related to hypertensive state

PLANNING

■ Client's blood pressure will be within desired range.
■ Client is free of moderate to severe side effects.

NURSING INTERVENTIONS

■ Monitor laboratory tests related to renal function (BUN, creatinine, protein) and blood glucose levels. *Caution:* Watch for hypoglycemic reaction in clients with diabetes mellitus. Urine protein may be checked in the morning using a dipstick.
■ Report to the health care provider occurrences of bruising, petechiae, and/or bleeding. These may indicate a severe adverse reaction to an angiotensin antagonist such as captopril.

Client Teaching

General
• Instruct client not to abruptly discontinue use of captopril without notifying the health care provider. *Rebound hypertension could result.*
• Inform client not to take OTC drugs (e.g., cold or allergy medications) without first contacting the health care provider. See also Herbal Alert 42–1.

Self-Administration
• Teach client how to take and record his or her blood pressure. A blood pressure chart should be established, and blood pressure changes should be reported.

Side Effects
• Explain to client that dizziness and/or light-headedness may occur during the first week of captopril therapy. If dizziness persists, the health care provider should be notified.
• Instruct client to report any occurrence of bleeding.

Diet
• Instruct client to take captopril 20 minutes to 1 hour before a meal. Food decreases 35% of captopril absorption.
• Inform client that the taste of food may be diminished during the first month of drug therapy.

Cultural Considerations ⊕
• African Americans do not respond well to angiotensin-converting enzyme (ACE) inhibitors unless the drug is taken with a diuretic.

EVALUATION

■ Evaluate the effectiveness of the drug therapy (i.e., absence of severe side effects, blood pressure return to desired range).

Angiotensin II Receptor Antagonists (Blockers)

Angiotensin II receptor antagonists (A-II blockers or ARBs) are a new group of antihypertensive drugs. This group is similar to ACE inhibitors in that they prevent the release of

aldosterone (sodium-retaining hormone). They act on the renin-angiotensin system. The difference between ARBs and ACE inhibitors is that ARBs block the angiotensin II from the AT_1 receptors found in many tissues, whereas ACE inhibitors inhibit the angiotensin-converting enzyme in the formation of angiotensin II. The ARBs cause vasodilation and decrease peripheral resistance.

Losartan (Cozaar), valsartan (Diovan), irbesartan (Avapro), candesartan cilexetil (Atacand), eprosartan (Teveten), olmesartan medoxomil (Benicar) and telmisartan (Micardis) are examples of ARBs. These agents block the vasoconstrictor effects of angiotensin II at the receptor site.

Table 42–4

Antihypertensives: ACE Inhibitors and Angiotensin II Antagonists

Generic (Brand)	Route and Dosage	Uses and Considerations
Angiotensin Antagonists (ACE Inhibitors)		
benazepril HCl (Lotensin)	A: PO: Initially: 10 mg/d; *maint:* 20-40 mg/d in 2 divided doses	Management of stage 1 and 2 hypertension. Headache, dizziness, hypotension, nausea, diarrhea, or constipation may occur. *Pregnancy* category: C and D; PB: 97%; $t^{1/2}$: 10 h
captopril (Capoten)	A: PO: Initially: 12.5-25 mg, b.i.d.-t.i.d.; *maint:* 25-100 mg, b.i.d.-t.i.d.; *max:* 450 mg/d	To reduce blood pressure and to control CHF. Inhibits angiotensin I conversion to angiotensin II. Irritating cough is a side effect; it retains potassium. *Pregnancy category:* C and D (second and third trimester); PB: 25%-30%; $t^{1/2}$: 2-3 h with normal renal function
enalapril maleate (Vasotec)	A: PO: Initially: 5 mg/d; *maint:* 10-40 mg/d in 1-2 divided doses IV: 1.25 mg q6h infuse in 5 min *Hypertensive emergencies:* IV: 5 mg q6h as needed	For hypertension and CHF. Similar to captopril and benazepril. Has a long duration of action (orally). *Pregnancy category:* C and D (second and third trimester); PB: 50%-60%; $t^{1/2}$: 1.5-2 h
fosinopril (Monopril)	A: PO: 5-40 mg/d; *max:* 80 mg/d	To treat hypertension and heart failure. Reduces peripheral resistance (afterload) and improves cardiac output. Dose does not have to be reduced because of renal insufficiency. *Pregnancy category:* C and D (second and third trimester); PB: 97%; $t^{1/2}$: 3-4 h; 12 h active metabolite
lisinopril (Prinivil, Zestril)	A: PO: Initially: 10 mg/d; *maint:* 20-40 mg/d; *max:* 80 mg/d	For hypertension and CHF. Usually given in combination with a diuretic. Has a long duration of action (24 hours). Monitor vital signs. *Pregnancy category:* D; PB: 0%; $t^{1/2}$: 12 h
moexipril (Univasc)	A: PO: 7.5 mg/d; *max:* 30 mg/d in divided doses	For treatment of hypertension. Reduce dose with renal insufficiency; creatinine clearance <40 ml/min. May increase serum lithium levels and cause toxicity. *Pregnancy category:* C and D (second and third trimester); PB: 50%; $t^{1/2}$: 2-9 h
perindopril (Aceon)	A: PO: 2-8 mg/d	To treat mild to moderate hypertension. It reduces vasoconstriction. Common side effect of ACE inhibitors is cough. *Pregnancy category:* C and D (second and third trimester); PB: 10%-60%; $t^{1/2}$: 1.5-3 h (parent drug); 25-30 h
quinapril HCl (Accupril)	A: PO: 10-20 mg/d; *max:* 80 mg/d in divided doses Elderly: A: PO: 2.5-5 mg/d	To treat hypertension and heart failure. A potent, long-acting, second-generation ACE inhibitor. Reduces systemic vascular resistance and increases cardiac output. *Pregnancy category:* D; PB: 97%; $t^{1/2}$: 2 h
ramipril (Altace)	A: PO: 2.5-5 mg/d; *max:* 20 mg/d	Treatment of stage 1 and 2 hypertension and CHF. Similar to captopril. Has a long duration of action (24 h). *Pregnancy category:* D; PB: 97%; $t^{1/2}$: 2-3 h
trandolapril (Mavik)	A: PO: 1 mg/d; may increase weekly to 2-4 mg/d; *max:* 8 mg/d	To treat hypertension. May be used alone or combined with other antihypertensives. Diuretics should be discontinued 2 to 3 days before taking trandolapril. Reduce dose if client has renal (creatinine clearance <30 ml/min) or hepatic insufficiency. African-Americans respond to trandolapril including those with low-renin hypertension. *Pregnancy category:* C and D; PB: 80%; $t^{1/2}$: 6 h

A, Adult; *ACE*, angiotensin-converting enzyme; *b.i.d.*, two times a day; *CHF*, congestive heart failure; *d*, day; *h*, hour; *IV*, intravenous; *maint*, maintenance; *max*, maximum; *min*, minute; *PB*, protein-binding; *PO*, by mouth; *$t^{1/2}$*, half-life; *t.i.d.*, three times a day; *UK*, unknown; >, greater than; <, less than.

Continued

Table 42-4

Antihypertensives: ACE Inhibitors and Angiotensin II Antagonists—cont'd

Generic (Brand)	Route and Dosage	Uses and Considerations
Combinations with Calcium Blockers		
benazepril with amlodipine (Lotrel)		
enalapril with diltiazem (Teczem)		
enalapril with felodipine (Lexxel)		
trandolapril with verapamil (Tarka)		
Angiotensin II Receptor Antagonists		
candesartan (Atacand)	A: PO: 16 mg/d; *maint:* 8-32 mg/d	For treating hypertension. It may be used when the client does not respond or cannot tolerate ACE inhibitors. It may be combined with the calcium blocker amlodipine for a more effective response in decreasing high blood pressure. *Pregnancy category:* C and D (second and third trimester); PB: >99%; $t^{1}/_{2}$: 9 h
eprosartan (Teveten)	A: PO: Initially: 200 mg/d; 400-800 mg/d or in 2 divided doses	To treat mild to moderate hypertension. Does not cause the "cough" that ACE inhibitors do. Food can cause a slight delay in drug absorption. *Pregnancy* category: C and D (second and third trimester); PB: 98%; $t^{1}/_{2}$: 5-9 h
irbesartan (Avapro)	A: PO: 150 mg/d; *maint:* 150-300 mg/d	For treating hypertension. It may be used alone or in combination with other antihypertensive drugs. *Pregnancy category:* C and D (second and third trimester); PB: 90%; $t^{1}/_{2}$: 11-15 h
losartan potassium (Cozaar)	A: PO: 25-50 mg/d, in single dose or in 2 divided doses; *max:* 100 mg/d	For treating hypertension. It may be used alone or in combination with other antihypertensive drugs. *Pregnancy category:* C and D (second and third trimester); PB: 95%; $t^{1}/_{2}$: 1.5-2 h
olmesartan medoxomil (Benicar)	A: PO: 20 mg/d; may increase 40 mg/d Elderly: Same as adult	Inhibits binding angiotensin II to AT_1 receptors. It promotes vasodilation and decreases peripheral resistance. Not to be given if the client volume is depleted. *Pregnancy category:* C and D (second and third trimester); PB: UK; $t^{1}/_{2}$: 13 h
telmisartan (Micardis)	A: PO: 40-80 mg/d	To treat mild to moderate hypertension. Does not cause the "cough" associated with ACE inhibitors. Angioedema has been reported, though it is rare. *Pregnancy category:* C and D (second and third trimester); PB: 99.5%; $t^{1}/_{2}$: 24 h
valsartan (Diovan)	A: PO: 80 mg/d; *max:* 320 mg/d	For treating hypertension. Similar action to candesartan, irbesartan, and losartan. *Pregnancy category:* C and D (second and third trimester); PB: 99%; $t^{1}/_{2}$: 6 h
Aldosterone Receptor Antagonist		
eplerenone (Inspra)	A: PO: 50 mg/d; may increase to 50 mg b.i.d.	It binds aldosterone at the mineralocortcoid receptor. It is contraindicated if the serum potassium is >5.5 mEq/l, creatinine clearance is <50 ml/min, type 2 diabetes, and taking potassium-sparing diuretics. Drug is used to treat hypertension and CHF postmyocardial infarction. *Pregnancy category:* B; PB: UK; $t^{1}/_{2}$: UK

The Food and Drug Administration (FDA) approves them for the treatment of hypertension. The combination of losartan potassium and hydrochlorothiazide tablets and valsartan and hydrocholorothiazide tablets and others should not cause serum potassium excess or loss.

Prototype Drug Chart 42–3 gives the pharmacologic data related to losartan potassium (Cozaar).

Pharmacokinetics

Losartan potassium (Cozaar) is prescribed primarily to manage hypertension. It comes in a combination drug, losartan potassium with a low dose of hydrochlorothiazide, called Hyzaar. It is rapidly absorbed in the GI tract and undergoes first-pass metabolism in the liver to form active metabolites. It is highly protein bound and should not be given during pregnancy especially the second and third trimester. The half-life is 1.2 to 2 hours, and the half-life of the metabolite is 6 to 9 hours. The drug is excreted in the urine and feces.

Pharmacodynamics

Losartan potassium is a potent vasodilator. It blocks the binding of angiotensin II to the AT_1 receptors found in many tissues. Its peak time is 6 hours, and it has a long duration of action: 24 hours.

Like ACE inhibitors, the ARBs are less effective for treating hypertension in African Americans. In addition, ARBs, like ACE inhibitors, may cause angioedema. These agents can be taken with or without food and are suitable for clients with mild hepatic insufficiency.

PROTOTYPE DRUG CHART 42–3

LOSARTAN POTASSIUM

Drug Class

Antihypertensive: angiotensin II receptor antagonist
Trade Name: Cozaar. Also Hyzaar (hydrochlorothiazide
 with losartan potassium)
Pregnancy Category: C (first trimester); D (second and
 third trimesters)

Dosage

Hypertension:
A: PO: 25-50 mg/d in single or 2 divided doses; *max:*
 100 mg/d
C: Safety not established

Contraindications

Pregnancy, breast feeding
Caution: Renal and hepatic impairments

Drug-Lab-Food Interactions

Drug: Phenobarbital *decreases* effects of losartan and
 its metabolites.
Lab: May *increase* AST, ALT, ALP, bilirubin, BUN,
 creatinine, Hct, Hgb.

Pharmacokinetics

Absorption: Rapidly absorbed, 25-30 in blood circulation
Distribution: PB: 90-95%
Metabolism: $t\frac{1}{2}$: 1.2-2 h; metabolite: 6-9 h
Excretion: 35% in urine and 60% in bile/feces

Pharmacodynamics

PO: Onset: <1 h
 Peak: 6 h
 Duration: 24 h

Therapeutic Effects/Uses

To treat hypertension
Mode of Action: Potent vasodilator; inhibits the binding of angiotensin II

Side Effects

Dizziness, diarrhea, insomnia, and occasional cough

Adverse Reactions

Upper respiratory infection

A, Adult; *ALP,* alkaline phosphatase; *ALT,* alanine aminotransferase; *AST,* aspartate aminotransferase; *BUN,* blood urea nitrogen; *C,* child;
d, day; *h,* hour; *Hct,* hematocrit; *Hgb,* hemoglobin; *max,* maximum; *PO,* by mouth; *PB,* protein-binding; $t\frac{1}{2}$, half-life; <, less than.

Calcium Channel Blockers

Slow calcium channels are found in the myocardium
(heart muscle) and smooth muscle cells. Free calcium increases muscle contractility, peripheral resistance, and
blood pressure. Calcium channel blockers, also called *calcium antagonists* and *calcium blockers,* decrease calcium levels and promote vasodilation. The large central arteries are
not as sensitive to calcium blockers as the coronary and
cerebral arteries and the peripheral resistance vessels. Calcium blockers are highly protein bound but have a short
half-life. Slow-release preparations decrease the frequency
of administering calcium blockers. Table 42–5 lists the calcium blockers. Calcium blockers are also discussed in
Chapter 40, Cardiac Glycosides, Antianginals, and Antidysrhythmics.

Verapamil (Calan) is used to treat chronic hypertension,
angina pectoris, and cardiac dysrhythmias. Verapamil and
diltiazem act on the arterioles and the heart. The dihy-
dropyridines are the largest family group of calcium channel blockers and consist of seven drugs; six of these are
used to control hypertension. The calcium blocker ni-
modipine is used to treat subarachnoid hemorrhage.

Nifedipine (Procardia) was the first drug in this group.
Nifedipine decreases blood pressure in older adults and
in those with low serum renin values. Nifedipine and
verapamil are potent calcium blockers. Nifedipine, in its
immediate-release form (10- and 20-mg capsules), has
been associated with an increased incidence of sudden
cardiac death, especially when prescribed for outpatients
at high doses. This is not true of the sustained-release
preparations (i.e., Procardia XL, Adalat CC). For this reason, immediate-release nifedipine is usually prescribed
for acute rises in blood pressure only on an "as needed"
basis in the hospital setting.

 PREVENTING MEDICATION ERRORS

Do not confuse...

- **Diovan** and **Dioval;** they sound alike and look
 alike. Diovan (valsartan) is an angiotensin II receptor blocker, or ARB, an antihypertensive drug.
 Dioval is an estradiol, an estrogen hormone. If
 both drugs are in the home, caution must be
 taken to select the *correct* drug, especially male
 person who is supposed to receive Diovan and female person who is supposed to receive Dioval.

Table 42–5

Antihypertensives: Calcium Channel Blockers

Generic (Brand)	Route and Dosage	Uses and Considerations
Phenylalkylamines		
verapamil (Calan SR, Isoptin SR)	A: PO: 40-80 mg t.i.d. A: PO SR: 120-240 mg/d in 2 divided doses; *max:* 480 mg/d	For hypertension (sustained-release form). One of the first calcium blockers. Also used for variant angina and cardiac dysrhythmias. Common side effects include dizziness, headache, hypotension, bradycardia, and constipation. *Pregnancy category:* C; PB: 90%; t½: 3-8 h
Benzothiazepines		
diltiazem HCl (Cardizem, Cardizem CD or SR)	A: PO SR: Initially: 60-120 mg b.i.d.; *max:* 240-360 mg/d	For hypertension (sustained-release form). Also for angina pectoris; IV form for cardiac dysrhythmias (atrial fibrillation). Headache, bradycardia, and hypotension may occur. *Pregnancy category:* C; PB: 70%-80%; t½: 3.5-9 h
Dihydropyridines		
amlodipine (Norvasc)	A: PO: 5-10 mg/d. Elderly: 2.5-5.0 mg/d	To treat mild and moderate hypertension and angina pectoris. Decreases peripheral vascular resistance (vasodilation). May be used alone or with other antihypertensives. *Pregnancy category:* C; PB: >95%; t½: 30-50 h (older adults with hepatic insufficiency: 50-100 h)
felodipine (Plendil)	A: PO: Initially: 5 mg; *maint:* 5-10 mg/d; *max:* 20 mg/d	Treatment for stage 1 and 2 hypertension, CHF, and angina. Potent calcium blocker. Flush, peripheral edema, palpitations, dizziness, and headache may occur. Long duration of action. *Pregnancy category:* C; PB: 99%; t½: 10-16 h
isradipine (DynaCirc)	*Hypertension:* A: PO: 1.25-10 mg b.i.d.; *max:* 20 mg/d	Management of hypertension, CHF, and angina pectoris. For hypertension, drug may be used alone or with a diuretic. *Pregnancy category:* C; PB: 99%; t½: 5-11 h
nicardipine HCl (Cardene, Cardene SR)	A: PO: 20-40 mg t.i.d. SR: 30-60 mg b.i.d. A: IV: initially: 5 mg/h; increase dose PRN; *max:* 15 mg/h C: IV: 1-3 mcg/kg/min	To treat essential hypertension and vasospastic angina. IV therapy for short-term therapy for hypertension. Decreases systemic resistance; heart rate and cardiac output are increased. *Pregnancy category:* C; PB: 95%; t½: 2-4 h
nifedipine (Procardia)	A: PO: 10-20 mg t.i.d. A: PO SR: 30-90 mg/d; *max:* 180 mg/d	For hypertension and angina pectoris. Potent calcium channel blocker. Common side effects include dizziness, light-headedness, headache, flushing, peripheral edema, and nausea. Drug may be taken alone or with a diuretic. *Pregnancy category:* C; PB: 92%-98%; t½: 2-5 h
nisoldipine (Sular, Nisocor)	A: PO: 10-20 mg/d in 2 divided doses; *max:* 40 mg/d	To treat hypertension and angina. It can be used alone or combined with another antihypertensive drug. It is similar to nifedipine, causing vasodilation and is 10 times more potent than nifedipine. It is considered a potent coronary vasodilator. *Pregnancy category:* C; PB: 99%; t½: 2-14 h

A, Adult; *b.i.d.,* twice a day; *C,* child; *CHF,* congestive heart failure; *d,* day; *h,* hour; *IV,* intravenous; *maint,* maintenance; *max,* maximum; *min,* minute; *PB,* protein-binding; *PO,* by mouth; *PRN,* as needed; *SR,* sustained release; *t½,* half-life; *t.i.d.,* three times a day; *>,* greater than.

PROTOTYPE DRUG CHART 42–4

AMLODIPINE

Drug Class

Calcium Channel Blocker
Trade Name: Norvasc; Lotrel is a combination of
  amlodipine with benazepril
Pregnancy Category: C

Dosage

A: PO: 5-10 mg/d
Elderly: PO: 2.5-5 mg/d

Contraindications

Severe hypotension
Caution: Liver disease, CHF, aortic stenosis, pregnancy
  (category C), lactation

Drug-Lab-Food Interactions

Drug: Increase bradycardia with adenosine.
Lab: May increase amlodipine with grapefruit juice

Pharmacokinetics

Absorption: Gradual; >90% absorbed from GI tract
Distribution: PB: >95%
Metabolism: $t\frac{1}{2}$: 30-50 h; elderly $t\frac{1}{2}$: 50-100 h
Excretion: Urine and feces as inactive metabolites

Pharmacodynamics

PO: Onset: Gradual
  Peak: 6-9 h
  Duration: 24 h

Therapeutic Effects/Uses

To treat mild and moderate hypertension and angina pectoris.
Mode of Action: It decreases peripheral vascular resistance (vasodilation), thus promotes a decrease in blood pressure

Side Effects

Peripheral edema, headache, flushing, dizziness, nausea

Adverse Reactions

Reflex tachycarda, marked hypotension

A, Adult; *CHF*, congestive heart failure; *d*, day; *GI*, gastrointestinal; *h*, hour; *PB*, protein-binding; *PO*, by mouth; *t½*, half-life.

Prototype Drug Chart 42–4 gives the pharmacologic data related to amlodipine (Norvasc).

Pharmacokinetics

Amlodipine (Norvasc), like other calcium blockers, is highly protein bound. It is gradually absorbed via the GI tract. Because the half-life of amlodipine is longer than other calcium blockers, it is taken once a day.

Pharmacodynamics

Amlodipine may be used alone or with other antihypertensive drugs. Peripheral edema may occur because of its vasodilator effect, so persons with edema may need to take another type of antihypertensive drug. This drug has a long duration of action, so it is prescribed only once a day. Amlodipine may be combined with the ACE inhibitor Lotrel.

Normally, beta-blockers are not prescribed with calcium blockers because both drugs decrease myocardium contractility. Calcium blockers lower blood pressure better in African Americans than drugs in other categories.

Side Effects and Adverse Reactions

The side effects and adverse reactions of calcium channel blockers include flush, headache, dizziness, ankle edema, bradycardia, and AV block.

WEBSITES

For further information on *Antihypertensive Drugs*, visit these Internet resources:

Center Watch—enalapril (Lexxel):
http://www.centerwatch.com/patient/drugs/dru210.html

Medline Plus Drug Information—captopril:
http://www.nlm.nih.gov/medlineplus/druginfo/medmaster/a682823.html

Health Digest—captopril:
http://www.healthdigest.org/drugs/captopril.html

Novartis—diovan:
http://www.diovan.com/index.jsp?checked=y

Medline Plus Drug Information—losartan potassium:
http://www.nlm.nih.gov/medlineplus/druginfo/medmaster/a695008.html

Health Digest—doxazosin mesylate:
http://www.healthdigest.org/drugs/doxazosinmesylate.html

Critical Thinking Case Study

G.G., a 72-year-old African American, has congestive heart failure (CHF). She has diabetes. Her vital signs are blood pressure 176/94; pulse 92; respirations 30. Her medications include hydrochlorothiazide 50 mg/d, atenolol 50 mg/d, and digoxin 0.25 mg/d.

1. Why was hydrochlorothiazide prescribed for G.G.? Explain the effects of hydrochlorothiazide on blood pressure (see Chapter 41, Diuretics).

2. Abnormal electrolytes and other laboratory test results may occur when taking hydrochlorothiazide. Would the serum electrolyte and laboratory values be expected to *increase* or *decrease*?

   a. Sodium   d. Magnesium
   b. Potassium   e. Glucose
   c. Calcium   f. Uric acid

3. Why should G.G.'s blood glucose level be monitored while she is taking hydrochlorothiazide?

4. What effect may result when G.G. takes digoxin and hydrochlorothiazide? Explain.

5. Atenolol is what type of antihypertensive? Would atenolol be effective in lowering G.G.'s blood pressure if given as the only antihypertensive drug? Explain.

6. How effective is the combination of hydrochlorothiazide and atenolol for controlling G.G.'s blood pressure? Explain.

7. When using a combination drug therapy to correct hypertension, would the dosage for each drug be the same? Explain.

8. When abruptly discontinuing beta-blockers for hypertension without the client taking another antihypertensive, what might occur? Explain how adverse effects can be avoided.

G.G.'s blood glucose is 229. Her drugs for controlling hypertension are changed to prazosin 10 mg t.i.d. Her cholesterol and LDL are elevated. Her serum potassium level was 3.2 mEq/L.

9. Why were G.G.'s drugs, hydrochlorothiazide and atenolol, discontinued? Explain.

10. What type of antihypertensive is prazosin? Explain the physiologic action of prazosin for lowering the blood pressure.

11. Does prazosin have an effect on the blood glucose level? What effect could prazosin have on G.G.'s abnormal lipid levels? Explain.

G.G.'s ankles have become edematous. Hydrochlorothiazide was prescribed.

12. Why was hydrochlorothiazide added to the drug regimen? What are some of the reasons?

13. Is the daily prazosin dose within the safe therapeutic prescribed range for G.G.? Explain. (See Prototype Drug Chart 42–2.)

14. List the groups of antihypertensive drugs that can cause sodium and water retention?

Study Questions

1. What nonpharmacologic methods decrease blood pressure?

2. What is the purpose of the stepped-care approach or modified pharmacologic approach in the treatment of hypertension? Explain the function of diuretics in controlling hypertension.

3. A major side effect of sympatholytic drugs and direct-acting vasodilators is sodium and water retention. How should this problem be assessed? What drug is given with the antihypertensives to decrease this side effect? What electrolyte imbalances might occur with the use of the additional drug?

4. What are the similarities and differences between ACE inhibitors and A-II blockers?

5. What antihypertensive drug might be given for a hypertensive crisis? How is it administered?

6. What is the nursing process as it relates to administering beta-adrenergic blockers, alpha-adrenergic blockers, angiotensin antagonists, and calcium channel blockers?

43 Anticoagulants, Antiplatelets, and Thrombolytics

ELECTRONIC RESOURCES

Additional information can be found on the companion website at *http://evolve.elsevier.com/KeeHayes/pharmacology/* or on the companion CD-ROM, which includes:
- *NCLEX-style examination review questions*
- *Pharmacology animations*
- *Medication error and (IV) therapy checklists*
- *Medication calculation problems*
- *Electronic calculators*

OUTLINE

OBJECTIVES

- Describe the action for anticoagulants, antiplatelets, and thrombolytics.
- Identify the side effects and adverse reactions of anticoagulants, antiplatelets, and thrombolytics.
- Give the nursing processes, including client teaching, for anticoagulants and thrombolytics.

TERMS

activated partial thromboplastin time (aPTT)
acute myocardial infarction
  (AMI)
aggregation
anticoagulants
antiplatelets

fibrinolysis
international normalized
  ratio (INR)
ischemia
myocardial infarction
necrosis

partial thromboplastin time
  (PTT)
prothrombin time (PT)
thromboembolism
thrombolytics
thrombosis

Introduction

Various drugs are used to maintain or restore circulation. The three major groups of these drugs are (1) anticoagulants, (2) antiplatelets (antithrombotics), and (3) thrombolytics. The *anticoagulants* prevent the formation of clots that inhibit circulation. The *antiplatelets* prevent platelet **aggregation** (clumping together of platelets to form a clot). The *thrombolytics*, popularly called *clot busters*, attack and dissolve blood clots that have already formed. Each of these 3 drug groups are discussed separately.

Pathophysiology: Thrombus Formation

Thrombosis is the formation of a clot in an arterial or venous vessel. The formation of an arterial thrombus could be caused by blood stasis (because of decreased circulation), platelet aggregation on the blood vessel wall, and blood coagulation. Arterial clots are usually made up of both white and red clots with the white clots *(platelets)* initiating the process, followed by fibrin formation and the trapping of red blood cells in the fibrin mesh. Blood clots found in the veins are from platelet aggregation with fibrin that attaches to red blood cells. Both types of thrombus can be dislodged from the vessel and become an embolus (moving blood clot through the blood stream).

Platelets usually do not stick together unless there is a break in the endothelial lining of the blood vessels. When platelets adhere to the broken surface of an endothelial lining, they synthesize thromboxane A_2, which is a product of prostaglandins and also a potent stimulus for platelet aggregation (clumping of platelet cells). The platelet receptor protein that binds fibrinogen, known as *glycoprotein IIb/IIIa* or *GP IIb/IIIa*, also promotes platelet aggregation. Thromboxane A_2 and adenosine diphosphate (ADP) increase the activation of this receptor.

As the thrombus inhibits blood flow, fibrin, platelets, and red blood cells (erythrocytes) surround the clot, building the clot's size and structure. As the clot occludes the blood vessel, tissue ischemia occurs.

The venous thrombus usually develops because of slow blood flow. The venous clot can occur rapidly. Small pieces of the venous clot can detach and travel to the pulmonary artery and then to the lung. Inadequate oxygenation and gas exchange in the lungs result.

Oral and parenteral anticoagulants (warfarin and heparin) act primarily by preventing venous thrombosis, whereas antiplatelet drugs primarily act by preventing arterial thrombosis. However, both groups of drugs suppress thrombosis in general.

Anticoagulants

Anticoagulants are used to inhibit clot formation. Unlike thrombolytics, they do *not* dissolve clots that have already formed but rather act prophylactically to prevent new clots from forming. Anticoagulants are used in clients with venous and arterial vessel disorders that put them at high risk

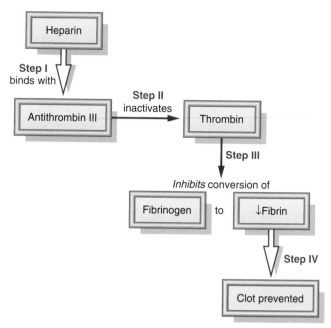

FIGURE 43–1   Action of the parenteral anticoagulant heparin.

for clot formation. The venous problems include deep vein thrombosis (DVT) and pulmonary embolism, and the arterial problems include coronary thrombosis **(myocardial infarction)**, presence of artificial heart valves, and cerebrovascular accidents (CVA, or stroke).

Heparin

Anticoagulants are administered orally or parenterally (subcutaneously [subQ] and intravenously [IV]). Heparin, introduced in 1938, is a natural substance in the liver that prevents clot formation. It was first used in blood transfusions to prevent clotting. Heparin is used in open-heart surgery to prevent blood from clotting and in the critically ill client with disseminated intravascular coagulation (DIC). Its primary use is to prevent venous thrombosis, which can lead to pulmonary embolism or stroke.

Heparin combines with antithrombin III, which accelerates the anticoagulant cascade of reactions that prevents thrombosis formation. By inhibiting the action of thrombin, conversion of fibrinogen to fibrin does not occur and the formation of a fibrin clot is prevented (Figure 43–1).

Heparin is poorly absorbed through the gastrointestinal (GI) mucosa, and much is destroyed by heparinase, a liver enzyme. Because heparin is poorly absorbed orally, it is given subQ for prophylaxis or IV to treat acute thrombosis. It can be administered as an IV bolus or in IV fluid for continuous infusion. Heparin prolongs clotting time. **Partial thromboplastin time (PTT)** and **activated partial thromboplastin time (aPTT)** are monitored during therapy. Heparin can decrease the platelet count, causing thrombocytopenia. If hemorrhage occurs, the anticoagulant antagonist protamine sulfate is given IV. Protamine can be an anticoagulant, but in the presence of heparin, it is an antagonist. Before discontinuing heparin, oral therapy with warfarin therapy is begun.

Low-Molecular-Weight Heparins

These derivatives of standard heparin were recently introduced to prevent venous thromboembolism. By extracting only the low-molecular-weight fractions of standard heparin through depolymerization, studies have shown the equivalent of anticoagulation with a lower risk of bleeding. Low-molecular-weight heparins (LMWHs) produce more stable responses at recommended doses. As a result, frequent laboratory monitoring is not required. LMWHs bind to antithrombin III, which inhibits the synthesis of factor Xa and the formation of thrombin.

There are five LMWHs: enoxaparin sodium (Lovenox), dalteparin sodium (Fragmin), ardeparin (Normiflo), danaparoid (Orgaran), and tinzaparin sodium (Innohep). Although danaparoid is considered a LMW heparin drug, it does not have heparin in its structure so it is referred to as LMW heparinoid. The uses for danaparoid are the same as other LMWHs. The synthetic anticoagulant fondaparinux (Arixtra) is administered subcutaneously, and its indirectly inhibits thrombin production. It is closely related in structure to heparin and LMW heparins, and its uses are for the same purposes as LMWHs. These agents are used to prevent DVT after hip- and knee-replacement surgery (enoxaparin, ardeparin, danaparoid) and abdominal surgery (dalteparin). They can be administered at home because aPTT monitoring is not necessary; however, heparin must be given in the hospital. The LMWH is administered subQ once or twice a day depending on the drug or the drug regimen. The drugs are available in pre-filled syringes with attached needles. The client or family member is taught how to administer the subQ injection, which is usually given in the abdomen. The average treatment is for 7 to 14 days. The LMWH is usually started in the hospital within 24 hours after surgery.

The half-life of LMWHs is two to four times longer than that of heparin. Clients should be instructed not to take antiplatelet drugs such as aspirin while taking LMWHs or heparin. Bleeding because of LMWH use is less likely to occur than when heparin is given. Heparin has a shorter half-life than LMWHs. LMWH overdose is rare; if bleeding occurs, protamine sulfate is the anticoagulant antagonist

PREVENTING MEDICATION ERRORS

Do not confuse...

- **Enoxaparin** and **enoxacin,** which are look-alike drugs. Enoxaparin is a low-molecular-weight heparin (LMWH), and enoxacin is a fluoroquinolone antibiotic. Both are generic drugs.

- **Lovenox** and **Lotronex.** Both are trade (brand) name drugs. Lovenox is a trade name for enoxaparin, a LMWH drug. Lotronex is a gastrointestinal (GI) drug.

used. The dosage for protamine sulfate is 1 mg of protamine for every 1 mg of LMWH given.

The LMWHs are contraindicated for clients with strokes, peptic ulcers, and blood anomalies. These drugs should not be given to clients having eye, brain, or spinal surgery.

Oral Anticoagulants

Three oral anticoagulants that are used today include warfarin (Coumadin), dicumarol, and anisindione (Miradon). Warfarin and dicumarol belong to the coumarin drug family, and anisindione is from the indandione group. Anisindione causes many side effects, so it is seldom ordered. Warfarin (Coumadin) is the most commonly prescribed oral anticoagulant. Warfarin is synthesized from dicumarol. Before warfarin was available for human use, it was used in rodenticides to kill rats by causing hemorrhage.

Oral anticoagulants inhibit hepatic synthesis of vitamin K, thus affecting the clotting factors II, VII, IX, and X. These drugs are used mainly to prevent thromboembolic conditions such as thrombophlebitis, pulmonary embolism, and embolism formation caused by atrial fibrillation, which can lead to a stroke (CVA). Oral anticoagulants prolong clotting time and are monitored by the **prothrombin time (PT)**. This laboratory test is usually performed before administering the next drug dose until the therapeutic level has been reached. **International normalized ratio (INR)** is a new laboratory test introduced to account for the variability in reported PTs from different laboratories. Reagents used in the PT test are compared with an international reference standard and reported as the INR. The normal INR is 1.3 to 2. Clients on warfarin therapy are maintained at an INR of 2 to 3.

There are three parenteral anticoagulants that are administered IV; argatroban (Acova), bivalirudin (Angiomax), and lepirudin (Rufludan). All three drugs directly inhibit thrombin; however, bivalirudin binds with and inhibits free-flowing thrombin. These drugs differ from heparin-like anticoagulants, which inhibit thrombin indirectly; these three intravenous anticoagulants inhibit thrombin directly.

Monitoring at regular intervals is required for the duration of drug therapy. The coumarins have long half-lives and very long durations of action (dicumarol has a longer action than warfarin); therefore drug accumulation can occur, which may cause internal bleeding. The nurse must observe for petechiae, ecchymosis, tarry stools, and hematemesis.

Parenteral and oral anticoagulants (heparin and warfarin) are presented in Prototype Drug Chart 43–1.

Pharmacokinetics

Heparin is poorly absorbed through the GI mucosa, and much is destroyed by heparinase, a liver enzyme. Heparin is given parenterally, either subcutaneously for prophylactic anticoagulant therapy or IV (bolus or continuous infusion) for an immediate response. Warfarin, an oral anticoagulant, is well absorbed through the GI mucosa; however, food will delay but not inhibit absorption.

The half-life of heparin is dose related; high doses prolong the half-life. The half-life of warfarin is 0.5 to 3 days, in contrast to 1 to 2 hours

PROTOTYPE DRUG CHART 43–1

HEPARIN AND WARFARIN SODIUM

Drug Class

Anticoagulant
Trade Names:
heparin: Lipo-Hepin, Calciparine, 🍁 Hepalean, Calcilean
Pregnancy Category: C
warfarin: Coumadin, 🍁 Warfilone
Pregnancy Category: D

Dosage

heparin:
A: subQ: 5000-7500 units q6h or 8000-10,000 units q8h
IV: Bolus: 5000 units; inf: 20,000-40,000 units over 24 h
C: IV: 50 units/kg bolus; 50-100 units/kg q4h or
20,000 units m²/24 h
warfarin:
A: PO: LD: 10 mg/d for 2-3 d; *maint:* 2-10 mg/d
Elderly: PO: 2.5 mg/d
Dose is usually titrated according to INR for adults and
the elderly.

Contraindications

heparin/warfarin: Bleeding disorder, peptic ulcer, severe
hepatic or renal disease, hemophilia, CVA
warfarin: Blood dyscrasias, eclampsia

Drug-Lab-Food Interactions

Drug: heparin: Increase effect with aspirin, NSAIDs,
thrombolytics, probenecid; *decrease* effect with nitroglycerin, protamine
warfarin: Increase effect with amiodarone, aspirin,
NSAIDs, sulfonamides, thyroid drugs, allopurinol, histamine₂ blockers, oral hypoglycemics, metronidazole,
miconazole, methyldopa, diuretics, oral antibiotics, vitamin E; *decrease* effect with barbiturates, laxatives,
phenytoin, estrogens, vitamins C and K, oral contraceptives, rifampin
Lab: May *increase* AST, ALT
Food: Decrease diet rich in vitamin K

Pharmacokinetics

Absorption: *heparin:* subQ or IV; *warfarin:* PO: Well
absorbed
Distribution: PB: *heparin:* >80%; *warfarin:* 99%
Metabolism: t½: *heparin:* 1-2 h; *warfarin:* 0.5-3 d
Excretion: *heparin:* Slowly in urine and reticuloendothelial
system; *warfarin:* in urine and bile

Pharmacodynamics

heparin
SC: Onset: 20-60 min
Peak: 2 h
Duration: 8-12 h
IV: Onset: immediate
Peak: 5-10 minutes
Duration: 2-6 h
warfarin:
PO: Onset: >2 d
Peak: 1-3 d
Duration: 2.5-5 d

Therapeutic Effects/Uses

heparin/warfarin: To prevent blood clotting
Mode of Action: *heparin:* Inhibits thrombin, which prevents the conversion of fibrinogen to fibrin
warfarin: Depression of hepatic synthesis of vitamin K clotting factors (II [prothrombin], VII, IX, and X)

Side Effects

heparin: Itching, burning
warfarin: Anorexia, nausea, vomiting, diarrhea, abdominal
cramps, rash, fever

Adverse Reactions

heparin/warfarin: Bleeding, ecchymoses
warfarin: Stomatitis
Life threatening: *heparin/warfarin:* hemorrhage

A, Adult; *ALT,* alanine aminotransferase; *AST,* aspartate aminotransferase; *C,* child; *CVA,* cerebrovascular accident; *d,* day; *h,* hour; *inf,*
infusion; *INR,* international normalized ratio; *IV,* intravenous; *LD,* loading dose; *maint,* maintenance; *NSAIDs,* nonsteroidal antiinflammatory drugs; *PB,* protein-binding; *PO,* by mouth; *subQ,* subcutaneous; *t½,* half-life; *>,* greater than; 🍁, Canadian drug names.

for heparin. Because warfarin has a long half-life and is highly protein-bound, the drug can have cumulative effects. Bleeding can occur, especially if another highly protein-bound drug is administered with warfarin. Kidney and liver disease prolong the half-life of both heparin and warfarin. Warfarin is metabolized to inactive metabolites that are excreted by the kidneys and in bile.

Pharmacodynamics

Heparin, administered for acute thromboembolic disorders, prevents thrombus formation and embolism. It has been effectively used to treat DIC, which causes multiple thrombi in small blood vessels. Warfarin is effective for long-term anticoagulant therapy. The PT level should be 1.5 to 2 times the reference value to be therapeutic, or INR should be 2.0 to

Table 43–1

Comparison of Oral and Parenteral Anticoagulants

Factors to Consider	Heparin	Warfarin (Coumadin)
Methods of administration	Subcutaneously Intravenously	Primarily orally
Drug action	Binds with antithrombin III, which inactivates thrombin and clotting factors, thus inhibiting fibrin formation	Inhibits hepatic synthesis of vitamin K, which decreases prothrombin and the clotting factors VII, IX, X
Uses	Treatment of venous thrombosis, pulmonary embolism, thromboembolic complications (e.g., heart surgery, disseminated intravascular coagulation)	Treatment of deep venous thrombosis, pulmonary embolism, transient ischemic attack, prophylactic for cardiac valves
Contraindication/caution	Hemophilia, peptic ulcer, severe (stage 3 or 4) hypertension, severe liver or renal disease, dissecting aneurysm	Hemophilia, peptic bleeding ulcer, blood dyscrasias, severe liver or kidney disease, acute myocardial infarction, alcoholism
Laboratory tests	Partial thromboplastin time (PTT): 60-70 sec Anticoagulant: 1.5-2 × control in seconds Activated partial thromboplastin time (aPTT): 20-35 sec Anticoagulant: aPTT: up to 40 sec	Prothrombin time (PT): 11-15 sec Anticoagulant: 1.25-2.5 × control in seconds International normalized ratio (INR): 1.3-2.0 Anticoagulant: INR 2.0-3.0 Prosthetic heart valves: INR up to 3.5
Side/adverse effects	Bleeding, hemorrhage, hematoma, severe hypotension	Bleeding, hemorrhage, GI bleeding, ecchymoses, hematuria
Antidote	Protamine sulfate, 1 mg per 100 units of heparin (see Table 43–2)	Vitamin K_1 PO/subQ/IM/IV: 2.5-10 mg, C: subQ/IM: 5-10 mg Infant: 1 mg Vitamin K_4: A: PO/IM/IV: 5-15 mg/d (see Table 43–2)

A, Adult; *C,* child; *d,* day; *GI,* gastrointestinal; *IM,* intramuscular; *IV,* intravenous; *PO,* by mouth; *sec,* second; *subQ,* subcutaneous.

3.0. INR has effectively replaced the use of PT, because PT can vary from laboratory to laboratory and reagent to reagent. Higher INR levels (up to 3.5) are usually required for clients with prosthetic heart valves, cardiac valvular disease, and recurrent emboli. Heparin does not cross the placental barrier, unlike warfarin; therefore warfarin use is not suggested during pregnancy.

Intravenous heparin has a rapid onset; its peak time of action is reached in minutes, and its duration of action is short. After an IV heparin dose, the client's clotting time will return to normal in 2 to 6 hours. SubQ heparin is more slowly absorbed through the blood vessels in fatty tissue. The coumarins (warfarin and dicumarol) have long onset of action, peak concentration, and duration of action times; thus drug accumulation may occur. Dicumarol has a longer action time than warfarin. Vitamin K counteracts the effect of warfarin, but it can take up to 24 hours for it to be effective.

Table 43–1 gives the comparison summary between oral and parenteral anticoagulants, according to methods of administration, drug action, uses, contraindications, laboratory tests, side effects and adverse reactions, and antidotes.

Side Effects and Adverse Reactions

Bleeding (hemorrhaging) is the major adverse effect of warfarin. Clients should be monitored closely for signs of bleeding (e.g., petechiae, ecchymosis, hematemesis). PT or INR testing should be scheduled at recommended intervals.

Drug Interactions

Because warfarin and dicumarol are highly protein bound, they are affected by drug interactions. Aspirin, nonsteroidal antiinflammatory drugs (NSAIDs), other types of antiinflammatory drugs, sulfonamides, phenytoin, cimetidine

(Tagamet), allopurinol, and oral hypoglycemic drugs for diabetes can displace warfarin or dicumarol from the protein-bound site, causing more free-circulating anticoagulant. Numerous other drugs also increase the action of warfarin, and bleeding is likely to occur. Acetaminophen (Tylenol) should be used instead of aspirin for clients taking warfarin or dicumarol. For frank bleeding resulting from excess free drug, parenteral vitamin K is given as a coagulant to decrease bleeding and promote clotting. However, caution must be used with this approach because the prothrombin can remain depressed for prolonged periods.

Table 43–2 lists the drug data for the anticoagulants, the antiplatelets, and the anticoagulant antagonists.

Exanta

Filmtabletten (Exanta) was recently developed to decrease the risk of blood clots and stroke. The reason for the use of this drug is for the clients who have bleeding problems related to warfarin (Coumadin). The benefits for the use of Exanta, according to the pharmaceutical company, are that there would not be any food or alcohol interactions, need for dose adjustment, or need for INR (PT) testing. The pharmaceutical company planned that the drug would be released in January 2005 as an anticoagulant. The Food and Drug Administration (FDA) announced that a panel of medical experts advised the FDA that more long-term studies are needed to determine the safety of the drug. Their concern is that Exanta can cause an elevation of the liver enzymes and could cause liver damage. The drug is being used in Europe. It may take several years for the final FDA approval of Exanta.

Table 43–2

Anticoagulants, Antiplatelets, and Anticoagulant Antagonists

Generic (Brand)	Route and Dosage	Uses and Considerations
Anticoagulant		
Heparins		
heparin sodium (Lipo-Hepin)	A: subQ: 5000-7500 units q6h or 8000-10,000 units q8h A: IV: Bolus: 5000 units, inf: 20,000-40,000 units over 24 h; dose varies according to aPTT level C: IV: units/kg bolus, 50-100 units/kg q4h or 20,000 units/m²/24 h	For thromboembolism as a prophylaxis against clotting. Is not given IM because of pain and hematoma. Drugs that inactivate heparin: digitalis, tetracycline, IV penicillin, phenothiazine, and quinidine; aPTT should be monitored. Protamine sulfate is the antidote for bleeding control. Dose is 1-1.5 mg for every 100 units of heparin subQ. *Pregnancy category:* C, PB: 95%; t½: 1-1.5 h
Low-molecular-weight heparins (LMWHs)		
ardeparin (Normiflo)	A: subQ: 50 units/kg, q12h	To prevent postoperative thromboembolism especially following knee replacement. Is not influenced by PT and aPTT lab tests. *Pregnancy category:* C; PB: UK; t½: 3 h
dalteparin sodium (Fragmin)	A: subQ: 2500 international units/d for 5-10 d starting 1-2 h before surgery	For prevention of DVT before surgery and for those who at risk of thromboembolism. Similar to enoxaparin. *Pregnancy category:* B; PB: UK; t½: 3-5 h
enoxaparin sodium (Lovenox)	A: subQ: 30 mg b.i.d.	For thromboembolism. Prevents and treats DVT and pulmonary embolism. Bleeding is an adverse reaction. Monitor CBC. *Pregnancy category:* B; PB: UK; t½: 4.5 h
tinzaparin sodium (Innohep)	A: subQ: 175 antiXa international units q24h	To prevent and treat DVT and thromboembolic events. Can be administered in conjunction with warfarin sodium. *Pregnancy category:* UK; PB: UK; t½: 3-4 h
LMW Heparinoid		
Danaparoid (Orgaran)	A: subQ: 750 units, q12h	Similar to LMWHs, but does not have heparin structure. It has little effect on thrombin activity and little to no effect on suppressing platelet aggregation. It is used to prevent DVT after hip surgery, *Pregnancy category:* B, PB: UK; t½: 24 h
Anticoagulants		
Coumarins		
dicumarol (Bishydroxy-coumarin)	A: PO: LD: 200-300 mg/24 h; *maint:* 25-200 mg/d based on PT	For thromboembolism as long-term prophylaxis. Has a longer duration than warfarin. INR should be monitored. Oral absorption may be erratic. *Pregnancy category:* D; PB: 99%; t½: 1-2 d
warfarin (Coumadin)	See Prototype Drug Chart 43–1.	
Indanedione Derivative		
anisindione (Miradon)	A: PO: 300 mg first d; 200 mg second d; 100 mg third d, then 25 to 250 mg/d	An indanedione derivative for anticoagulation. Urine may appear orange. *Pregnancy category:* X; PB: 98%; t½: 3-5 d
Synthetic Anticoagulant		
Fondaparinux (Arixtra)	A: subQ: 2.5 mg/d	Inhibits indirectly thrombin production and coagulation is suppressed. Closely related to heparin and LMWHs. Used to prevent DVT after hip fracture or replacement surgery and knee-replacement surgery. May cause somewhat more bleeding than LMWHs. Long duration time. *Pregnancy category:* C; PB: UK; t½: 17-21 h (longer with renal insufficiency)
Anticoagulants (Intravenous)		
argatroban (Acova)	A: IV: 2 mcg/kg/min; Dose is adjusted to maintain aPTT at 1.5-3 times the baseline	Directly inhibits thrombin (thrombin inhibitor). Same effect as lepirudin. Decreases the development of new thrombosis. *Pregnancy category:* B; PB: 54%; t½: 40-52 min
bivalirudin (Angiomax)	A: IV bolus: 1 mg/kg; following 4 h IV: 2.5 mg/kg/h; following 0.2 mg/kg/h	Bivalirudin binds with and inhibits free-flowing thrombin. Not effective if the thrombin is bound to clots. Adverse effect is bleeding. *Pregnancy category:* B; PB: 0%; t½: 25 min
lepirudin (Refludan)	A: IV bolus: 0.4 mg/kg over 15-20 sec; Followed by 0.15 mg/kg/h for 2-10 d	Directly inhibits thrombin. Used as a prophylaxic and treatment of a thrombosis due to HIT. Titrated to aPTT ratio. Liver function should be normal. Adverse effect is bleeding. *Pregnancy category:* B; PB: UK; t½: 1.3 h

A, Adult; *aPTT,* activated partial thromboplastin time; *b.i.d.,* twice a day; *C,* child; *CBC,* complete blood count; *d,* day; *DVT,* deep vein thrombosis; *h,* hour; *HIT,* heparin-induced thrombocytopenia; *IM,* intramuscular; *inf,* infusion; *INR,* international normalized ratio; *IV,* intravenous; *LD,* loading dose; *LMWH,* low-molecular-weight heparin; *maint,* maintenance; *min,* minute; *PB,* protein-binding; *PO,* by mouth; *PT,* prothrombin time; *sec,* second; *subQ,* subcutaneous; *t½,* half-life; *UK,* unknown.

Table 43-2

Anticoagulants, Antiplatelets, and Anticoagulant Antagonists—cont'd

Generic (Brand)	Route and Dosage	Uses and Considerations
Antiplatelets		
Anagrelide HCl (Agrylin)	A: PO: 1 mg, b.i.d. May be increased by 0.5 mg/wk if necessary. Maintain platelet count: >600,000 mcl.	Inhibits platelet aggregation by affecting aggregating agents; ADP, cAMP, and collagen. Adverse reactions include CHF, heart block, pulmonary hypertension, cardiomyopathy. Onset: 7-10 days after appropriate dose. *Pregnancy category:* C; PB: UK; $t^{1/2}$: 1.2-1.8 h
aspirin	A: PO: 81-325 mg/d or every other day	For prevention of thrombosis before or after CVA or MI. Client should check with health care provider before taking aspirin for antiplatelet therapy. Aspirin should be avoided with peptic ulcer or liver dysfunction. Enteric-coated preparation decreases GI upset. *Pregnancy category:* D; PB: 76%-90%; $t^{1/2}$: 10-12 h
Cilostazol (Pletal)	A: PO: 100 mg, b.i.d. 1 h before or 2 h after AM and PM meals.	Inhibits platelet aggregation and is a vasodilator. Also indicated for intermittent claudication. Smoking may decrease serum levels. Adverse reactions include CHF, tachycardia, cerebral ischemia, atrial flutter or fibrillation. *Pregnancy category:* C; PB: 95%-98%; $t^{1/2}$: 1-13 h
clopidogrel (Plavix)	See Prototype Drug Chart 43-2.	
dipyridamole (Persantine)	A: PO: 50-100 mg t.i.d.-q.i.d.	For prevention of thromboembolism post-MI and associated with prosthetic devices (heart valves and hip replacement); prevention of TIA. Monitor blood pressure. *Pregnancy category:* B; PB: >91%; $t^{1/2}$: 10-12 h
sulfinpyrazone (Anturane)	A: PO: 200-400 mg b.i.d.; *max:* 800 mg/d	Used for treating gout. Has antiplatelet function. May be used in AV shunts for hemodialysis to prevent clotting. *Pregnancy category:* C; PB: 95%-99%; $t^{1/2}$: 3 h
ticlopidine (Ticlid)	A: PO: 250 mg b.i.d.	To prevent the risk of strokes and thrombin formation. To treat intermittent claudication and sickle cell disease. Avoid if client has a hematopoietic disorder such as thrombocytopenia or bleeding peptic ulcer. *Pregnancy category:* B; PB: UK; $t^{1/2}$: 24 h-5 d
Combination of Antiplatelet Drugs		
aggrenox (dipyridamole and aspirin)	*Stroke prevention:* 1 capsule, b.i.d. (aspirin 25 mg and ER-dipyridamole 200 mg)	Combination of aspirin and ER-dipyridamole for stroke prevention with clients that had TIA.
Antiplatelets: Glycoprotein (GP) IIb/IIIa Receptor Antagonists		
abciximab (ReoPro)	A: IV bolus: 0.25 mg/kg given 10-60 min before PTCA. Inject 4.5 ml abciximab into 250 ml of NSS or D_5W. Follow with a continuous infusion of 10 mcg/min (17 ml/h) for 12 h	To prevent acute cardiac ischemia before and following PTCA and for unstable angina. *Pregnancy category:* C; PB: UK; $t^{1/2}$: 30 min
eptifibatide (Integrilin)	A: IV bolus: 180 mcg/kg, then 2 mcg/kg/min for up to 72 h	For acute cardiac syndromes (unstable angina and non-Q-wave MI). Can be used with angioplasty. *Pregnancy category:* B; PB: 25%; $t^{1/2}$: 2.5 h
tirofiban (Aggrastat)	A: IV: 0.4 mcg/kg/min for 30 min, then 0.1 mcg/kg/min for 12-24 h after angioplasty	New agent. For acute cardiac syndromes (unstable angina and non-Q-wave MI). Also may be used with angioplasty. *Pregnancy category:* B; PB: 35% unbound; $t^{1/2}$: UK
Anticoagulant Antagonists		
protamine SO_4	A: IV: Initially: 1 mg/100 units heparin administered; 10-50 mg in 3-10 min slow push; *max:* 50 mg in any 10-min period	Used to stop bleeding during heparin therapy. Binds and neutralizes heparin. *Pregnancy category:* C; PB: UK; $t^{1/2}$: UK
vitamin K_1, phytonadione (AquaMEPHYTON, Mephyton, Konakion)	A: PO/IM/IV: 2-10 mg q12-24 h as needed C: subQ/IM: 5-10 mg	For control of bleeding caused by as needed warfarin or dicumarol. If frank bleeding occurs, fresh or frozen plasma or Plasmanate may be needed. Depending on form and route, vitamin K takes effect in 1-24 h. Hemorrhage is usually controlled in 3-6 h. *Pregnancy category:* C; PB: UK; $t^{1/2}$: UK

ADP, Adenosine diphosphate; *AV,* arteriovenous; *cAMP,* cyclic adenosine monophosphate; *CHF,* congestive heart failure; *CVA,* cerebrovascular accident; *ER,* extended release; *GI,* gastrointestinal; *max,* maximum; *MI,* myocardial infarction; *NSS,* normal saline solution; *PTCA,* percutaneous transluminal coronary angioplasty; *q.i.d.,* four times a day; *TIA,* transient ischemic attack; *t.i.d.,* three times a day; *wk,* week; *>,* greater than.

Oral Anticoagulant Antagonists

Bleeding occurs in about 10% of clients taking oral anticoagulants. Vitamin K_1 (phytonadione), antagonist of warfarin, is used for warfarin overdose or uncontrollable bleeding. Usually 1 to 10 mg of vitamin K_1 is given at once if bleeding occurs. If vitamin K_1 fails to control bleeding, then fresh whole blood or fresh-frozen plasma or platelets are generally given.

Nursing Process

Anticoagulants: Warfarin (Coumadin) and Heparin

ASSESSMENT

■ Obtain a history of abnormal clotting or health problems that affect clotting, such as severe alcoholism or severe liver or renal disease. Warfarin is contraindicated for clients with blood dyscrasias, peptic ulcer, cerebrovascular accident (CVA), hemophilia, or severe hypertension. Use with caution in client with acute traumatic injury.

■ Obtain a drug and herbal history of current drugs and herbs client takes. Report if a drug-drug or drug-herbal interaction is probable. Warfarin is highly protein-bound and can displace other highly protein-bound drugs, or warfarin could be displaced, which may result in bleeding.

■ Develop a flow chart that lists prothrombin time (PT) or international normalized ratio (INR) and warfarin dosages. A baseline PT or INR should be obtained before warfarin is administered.

NURSING DIAGNOSES

■ Risk for injury (bleeding)
■ Knowledge deficit

PLANNING

■ Client's PT will be 1.25 to 2.5 times the control level or INR will be 2 to 3. For a client receiving heparin, the activated partial thromboplastin time (aPTT) should be checked.

■ Abnormal bleeding will be rapidly addressed while client is taking an anticoagulant. The PT, INR, or aPTT level(s) will be closely monitored.

NURSING INTERVENTIONS

■ Monitor vital signs. An increased pulse rate followed by a decreased systolic pressure can indicate a fluid volume deficit resulting from external or internal bleeding.

■ Monitor PT or INR for warfarin (Coumadin) and aPTT for heparin before administering the anticoagulant. The PT should be 1.25 to 2.5 times the control level or INR 2.0 to 3.0 except for prosthetic heart valves (up to INR 3.5). The platelet count should be monitored, because anticoagulants can decrease platelet count.

■ Check for bleeding from the mouth, nose (epistaxis), urine (hematuria), and skin (petechiae, purpura).

■ Check stools periodically for occult blood.

■ Monitor older adults closely for bleeding. Their skin is thin and the capillary beds are fragile.

■ Keep anticoagulant antagonists (protamine for heparin and vitamin K for warfarin) available when drug dose is increased or there are indications of frank bleeding. Fresh-frozen plasma may be needed for transfusion.

Client Teaching

General

• Instruct client to inform the dentist when taking an anticoagulant. Contacting the health care provider may be necessary.

• Explain client to use a soft toothbrush to prevent the gums from bleeding.

• Instruct client to shave with an electric razor. Bleeding from shaving cuts may be difficult to control.

• Advise client to have laboratory tests such as PT performed as ordered by the health care provider. Warfarin dose is regulated according to the INR derived from the PT.

• Suggest that client carries a medical ID card or wear jewelry (MedicAlert) that lists the person's name, telephone number, and drug name.

• Encourage client *not* to smoke. Smoking increases drug metabolism; thus the warfarin dose may need to be increased. If the person insists on smoking, notify the health care provider.

• Instruct client to check with the health care provider before taking OTC drugs. Aspirin should *not* be taken with warfarin because aspirin intensifies its action and bleeding is apt to occur. Suggest that client use acetaminophen.

• Inform client that many herbal products (see Herbal Alert 43–1) interact with anticoagulants and may increase bleeding. The international normalized ratio (INR) or prothrombin time (PT) should be closely monitored.

• Teach client to control external hemorrhage (bleeding) from accidents or injuries by applying firm, direct pressure for at least 5 to 10 minutes with a clean, dry absorbent material.

Side Effects

• Advise client to report bleeding, such as petechiae, ecchymosis, purpura, tarry stools, bleeding gums, epistaxis, or expectoration of blood.

Diet

- Advise client to avoid alcohol, which could contribute to increased bleeding, and large amounts of green leafy vegetables, fish, liver, coffee, or tea (caffeine), which are rich in vitamin K.

Cultural Considerations ⊕

- Certain cultural groups may lack understanding related to health problems, drug therapy, adverse effects, and follow-up care concerning thrombophlebitis or other conditions that cause a thrombus formation.
- Respect the cultural beliefs of client regarding his or her method for treating a vascular problem. If the method may be harmful, explanations along with a nursing plan should be initiated.

EVALUATION

- Evaluate the effectiveness of drug therapy. Client's PT or INR values are within the desired range and client is free of significant side effects.

Antiplatelet Drugs

Antiplatelets are used to prevent thrombosis in the arteries by suppressing platelet aggregation. Heparin and warfarin prevent thrombosis in the veins.

Antiplatelet drug therapy is mainly for prophylactic use such as: (1) prevention of myocardial infarction or stroke for clients with familial history, (2) prevention of a repeat myocardial infarction or stroke, and (3) prevention of a stroke for clients having transient ischemic attacks (TIAs).

For clients with familial history of stroke or myocardial infarction, the recommended aspirin dose is 81, 162, or 325 mg per day. Because aspirin has a prolonged antiplatelet activity, it should be discontinued at least 7 days before surgery.

HERBAL ALERT 43–1

Anticoagulants

- *Dong quai, feverfew, garlic, ginger, ginkgo,* and *bilberry* may increase bleeding when taken with anticoagulants such as warfarin (Coumadin). Warfarin has an additive effect and increases the international normalized ratio (INR) and prothrombin time (PT).
- Excessive doses of *anise* may interfere with anticoagulants.
- *Ginseng* may decrease the effects of warfarin thereby decreasing the INR.
- *Alfalfa* may decrease anticoagulant activity.
- *Goldenseal* may decrease the effect of heparin and oral anticoagulants.
- *Black haw* increases the action of anticoagulants.
- *Chamomile* may interfere with the actions of anticoagulants.
- *Valerian* may decrease the effects of warfarin.

Other antiplatelet drugs include dipyridamole (Persantine), ticlopidine (Ticlid), clopidogrel (Plavix), anagrelide HCl (Agrylin), abciximab (ReoPro), eptifibatide (Integrilin), and tirofiban (Aggrastat). Dipyridamole, ticlopidine, and clopidogrel have similar effects as aspirin but are more expensive. Cilostazol (Pletal) inhibits platelet aggregation and is a vasodilator that may be used for intermittent claudication. Clopidogrel (Plavix) is the antiplatelet drug that is frequently used after a myocardial infarction or stroke, prescribed singly or with aspirin. It has been stated that Plavix and aspirin are more effective in inhibiting platelet aggregation if used together than if used as separate drugs. Prototype Drug Chart 43–2 gives the pharmacologic data for clopidogrel (Plavix).

Pharmacokinetics

Clopidogrel (Plavix) is rapidly absorbed and has a highly protein-binding power. It is metabolized to active metabolite formation in which it prevents platelet aggregation. The half-life is 8 hours; it is usually prescribed once a day. The excretion of the drug metabolite is equally in the urine and feces.

Pharmacodynamics

Clopidogrel (Plavix) prevents platelet aggregation by blocking the binding of adenosine diphosphate (ADP) to the platelet ADP receptor. Plavix prolongs bleeding time; therefore it should be discontinued for 7 days preceding surgery. The onset of action of Plavix is 1 to 2 hours, and its peak time is 2 to 3 hours. The drug should not be taken if the client has a bleeding peptic ulcer, any active bleeding, or intracranial hemorrhage.

Abciximab, eptifibatide, and tirofiban are used primarily for acute coronary syndromes (unstable angina or non-Q-wave myocardial infarction) and for preventing reocclusion of coronary arteries following percutaneous transluminal coronary angioplasty (PTCA). These drugs are usually given before and after PTCA. The drug of choice for angioplasty is abciximab. Abciximab, eptifibatide, and tirofiban block the binding of fibrinogen to the glycoprotein IIb/IIIa receptor on the platelet surface. They are called *platelet glycoprotein (GP) IIb/IIIa receptor antagonists*. Following IV infusion, the antiplatelet effects for abciximab persist for 24 to 48 hours, and for eptifibatide and tirofiban, the antiplatelet effects last for 4 hours.

Herbal products can interact with antiplatelet drugs (see Herbal Alert 43–2).

Thrombolytics

Thromboembolism (occlusion of an artery or vein caused by a thrombus or embolus) results in **ischemia** (deficient blood flow) that causes **necrosis** (death) of the tissue distal to the obstructed area. It takes approximately 1 to 2 weeks for the blood clot to disintegrate by natural fibrinolytic mechanisms. If a new thrombus or embolus can be dissolved more quickly, the tissue necrosis is minimized and blood flow to the area is reestablished faster. This is the basis for thrombolytic therapy.

HERBAL ALERT 43–2

Antiplatelets

- *Dong quai, feverfew, garlic,* and *ginkgo* interfere with platelet aggregation. When one of these herbs is taken with an antiplatelet drug, such as aspirin, increased bleeding may occur.

PROTOTYPE DRUG CHART 43–2

CLOPIDOGREL BISULFATE

Drug Class	**Dosage**
Antiplatelet Trade Name: Plavix *Pregnancy Category* B	A: PO: 75 mg daily

Contraindications	**Drug-Lab-Herb Interactions**
Intracranial hemorrhage, peptic ulcer *Caution:* Liver disease, GI bleeding, surgery, bleeding from trauma	*Drug:* May *increase* bleeding when taken with NSAIDs; interferes with metabolism of phenytoin, warfarin, fluvastatin. *Lab:* Prolongs bleeding time. *Herb:* May *increase* bleeding when taken with ginger, garlic, ginkgo, feverfew

Pharmacokinetics	**Pharmacodynamics**
Absorption: Rapid **Distribution:** PB: 94%-98% **Metabolism:** t½: 8 h **Excretion:** 50% urine and 50% feces	PO: Onset: 1-2 h Peak: 2-3 h Duration: UK

Therapeutic Effects/Uses

To prevent reoccurrence of a MI, stroke, and prevent vascular death
Mode of Action: It inhibits platelet aggregation. It prevents the enzyme, ADP, from binding with the ADP platelet receptor.

Side Effects	**Adverse Reactions**
Upper RTI, flulike symptoms, dizziness, headaches, fatigue, chest pain, diarrhea	None of significance. May cause hypertension, bronchitis

A, Adult; *ADP,* adenosine diphosphate; *GI,* gastrointestinal; *h,* hour; *PB,* protein-binding; *PO,* by mouth; *MI,* myocardial infarction; *NSAIDs,* nonsteroidal antiinflammatory drugs; *RTI,* respiratory tract infection; *t½,* half-life; *UK,* unknown.

PREVENTING MEDICATION ERRORS

Do not confuse...

Right Drug

- Tenecteplase (TNKase) and tissue plasminogen activator (t-PA). These two drugs look alike, and even though they are from the same drug class—thrombolytics—the drugs are different and their administration time is different.

Right Dose and Time

- TNKase and t-PA have different dosages. Their administration time is also different. TNKase is administered as a single dose; t-PA is administered in three different doses and times. The first dose is a bolus, and the second and third doses are over 30 minutes and 60 minutes.

Thrombolytics have been used since the early 1980s to promote the fibrinolytic mechanism (converting plasminogen to plasmin, which destroys the fibrin in the blood clot). The thrombus, or blood clot, disintegrates when a thrombolytic drug is administered within 4 to 6 hours after an **acute myocardial infarction (AMI)**; necrosis resulting from the blocked artery is prevented or minimized and hospitalization time may be decreased. The need for cardiac bypass or coronary angioplasty can be evaluated soon after thrombolytic treatment. A thrombolytic drug should be administered within 3 hours of a thrombolic stroke. These drugs are also used for pulmonary embolism, DVT, noncoronary arterial occlusion from an acute thromboembolism, and thrombolic stroke.

Six commonly used thrombolytics are streptokinase, urokinase, tissue plasminogen activator (t-PA, alteplase), anisoylated plasminogen streptokinase activator complex (APSAC, anistreplase), reteplase (Retavase), and tenecteplase (TNKase). Streptokinase and urokinase are enzymes that act

PROTOTYPE DRUG CHART 43–3

TISSUE PLASMINOGEN ACTIVATOR (tPA)

Drug Class	**Dosage**
Thrombolytic Agent Trade Name tPA, Alteplase *Pregnancy Category:* C	A: IV bolus: 15 mg, then 50 mg infused over 30 min then 35 mg infused over 60 min; *max:* 100 mg

Contraindications	**Drug-Lab-Food Interactions**
Internal bleeding, bleeding disorders, recent CVA, surgery or trauma, bacterial endocarditis, severe liver dysfunction, severe uncontrolled hypertension	***Drug:*** *Increase* bleeding when taken with oral anticoagulants, NSAIDs, cefotetan, plicamycin. ***Lab:*** *Decrease* in plasminogen, fibrinogen, hematocrit, and hemoglobin

Pharmacokinetics	**Pharmacodynamics**

Absorption: Direct IV
Distribution: PB: UK
Metabolism: t½: 25-30 min
Excretion: Urine
	PO: Onset: Immediate
	  Peak: 5-10 min
	  Duration: 3 h

Therapeutic Effects/Uses

To dissolve clot following an acute MI, pulmonary embolism, acute ischemic stroke
Mode of Action: tPA promotes conversion of plasminogen to plasmin. Plasmin, an enzyme, digests the fibrin matrix of clots. tPA initiates fibrinolysis.

Side Effects	**Adverse Reactions**
bleeding	**Life threatening:** intracerebral hemorrhage, stroke, atrial or ventricular dysrhythmias.

A, Adult; *CVA,* cerebrovascular accident; *h,* hour; *IV,* intravenous; *PB,* protein-binding; *max,* maximum; *min,* minute; *NSAIDs,* nonsteroidal antiinflammatory drugs; *PO,* by mouth; *t½,* half-life; *tPA,* tissue plasminogen activator; *UK,* unknown.

systemically to promote the conversion of plasminogen to plasmin. t-PA and APSAC activate plasminogen by acting specifically on the clot. They also promote the conversion of plasminogen to plasmin. Plasmin, an enzyme, digests the fibrin in the clot. Plasmin also degrades fibrinogen, prothrombin, and other clotting factors. These six drugs induce **fibrinolysis** (fibrin breakdown).

Streptokinase may cause hypotension when first administered. Drug dosage may need to be adjusted. Reteplase (Retavase), a derivative of t-PA, is a fairly recent thrombolytic drug. Anticoagulants and antiplatelet drugs increase the risk of hemorrhage; therefore they should be avoided until the thrombolytic effect has passed. The health care provider needs to determine whether the client has taken any of these drugs before seeking treatment.

Prototype Drug Chart 43–3 gives the pharmacologic data for tPA.

Pharmacokinetics

The commercial preparation of tissue plasminogen activator (tPA) is identical to the natural human tPA, an enzyme that converts plasminogen to plasmin. It is administered as an IV bolus initially, then is infused over 30 minutes, and then 60 minutes. The half-life of tPA is 25 to 30 minutes. Tissue plasminogen activator costs about $2750 and is five times more expensive than streptokinase, but it is not as expensive as TNKase and urokinase. The client probably would not have allergic reactions to tPA as they might to steptokinase, anistreplase, and urokinase.

Pharmacodynamics

Tissue plasminogen activator promotes thrombolysis by converting plasminogen to plasmin. Plasmin degrades fibrin, fibrinogen, and factors V, VIII, and XII. Peak action of tPA is 5 to 10 minutes. The duration of action is 3 hours.

Side Effects and Adverse Reactions

Allergic reactions can complicate thrombolytic therapy. Anaphylaxis (vascular collapse) occurs more frequently with streptokinase than with the other thrombolytics. If the drugs are administered through an intracoronary catheter after myocardial infarction, reperfusion dysrhythmia or hemorrhagic infarction at the myocardial necrotic area can result. The major complication of thrombolytic drugs is hemorrhage. The antithrombolytic drug aminocaproic acid (Amicar) is used to stop bleeding by inhibiting plasminogen activation, which inhibits thrombolysis.

Table 43–3

Thrombolytics

Generic (Brand)	Route and Dosage	Uses and Considerations
Thrombolytics		
anistreplase (APSAC, Eminase)	A: IV: 30 units over 2-5 min	Treatment following an AMI, causing lysis of the thrombi. Decreases the infarction size. *Pregnancy category:* C; PB: UK; $t^{1}/_{2}$:1.5-2 h
reteplase (Retavase)	A: IV bolus: 10 units over 2 min, then repeat 10 units in 30 min (total of 20 units)	To treat coronary thrombosis by causing lysis of the thrombi; inhibits the fibrin aspect of the thrombus. A derivative of t-PA (Alteplase). Considered more effective than t-PA with less risk of hemorrhage. *Pregnancy category:* C; PB: UK; $t^{1}/_{2}$: 13-16 min
streptokinase (Streptase, Kabikinase)	*Myocardial infarction:* A: IV: 1,500,000 international units diluted in 45 ml; infuse in 53 ml; infuse over 60 min *Pulmonary embolism:* A: IV: LD: 250,000 international units/h for 24-72 h (24 h for PE; 72 h for DVT).	Dissolves blood clots caused by coronary artery thrombi, DVT, PE; converts plasminogen to plasmin for dissolving fibrin deposits. Should be given after AMI within 4 h. *Pregnancy category:* C; PB: UK; $t^{1}/_{2}$: 20-80 min
tenecteplase (TNKase)	A: IV: *Max:* 50 mg *NOTE:* Dose is based on body weight.	To reduce mortality associated with AMI. A "clot buster" that can be administered in 5 seconds in one dose. *Pregnancy category:* C; PB: UK; $t^{1}/_{2}$: 11-138 min
tissue-type plasminogen activator (t-PA, alteplase, Activase)	See Prototype Drug Chart 43–3.	
urokinase (Abbokinase)	A: IV: LD: 4400 international units/kg diluted and infuse over 10 min, then continuous infusion: 4400 international units/kg over 12 h *Occluded coronary artery:* Dose may be increased.	Same uses as streptokinase. Causes less allergic reaction and is more expensive than streptokinase. Not susceptible to antistreptokinase antibodies. May also be used for peripheral artery occlusion. *Pregnancy category:* B; PB: UK; $t^{1}/_{2}$: 10-20 min
Plasminogen Inactivator		
aminocaproic acid (Amicar)	A: PO/IV: LD: 4-5 g first hour Inf: 1-1.25 g/h for 8 h; *max:* 30 g/d	Treatment for excessive bleeding that may result from heart surgery, severe trauma, abruptio placentae, and thrombolytic drugs such as streptokinase, t-PA, and urokinase. Side effects include dizziness, headache, orthostatic, hypotension, and thrombophlebitis. *Pregnancy category:* C; PB: 0%; $t^{1}/_{2}$: 1-2 h

A, Adult; *AMI,* acute myocardial infarction; *d,* day; *DVT,* deep vein thrombosis; *h,* hour; *Inf,* infusion; *IV,* intravenous; *LD,* loading dose; *max,* maximum; *min,* minute; *PB,* protein-binding; *PE,* pulmonary embolism; $t^{1}/_{2}$, half-life; *t-PA,* tissue plasminogen activator; *UK,* unknown.

Table 43–3 lists the drug data for the thrombolytic drugs.

Nursing Process

Thrombolytics

ASSESSMENT

■ Assess baseline vital signs and compare with future values.
■ Check baseline complete blood count (CBC), prothrombin time (PT), or international normalized ratio (INR) values before administration of streptokinase.

■ Obtain a medical and drug history. Contraindications for use of streptokinase include a recent cerebrovascular accident (CVA), active bleeding, severe hypertension, and anticoagulant therapy. Reported if client takes aspirin or nonsteroidal antiinflammatory drugs (NSAIDs). Thrombolytics are contraindicated for the client with a recent history of traumatic injury, especially head injury.

NURSING DIAGNOSES

■ Decreased cardiac output
■ Anxiety related to severe health problem
■ Impaired tissue integrity
■ Risk for injury

PLANNING

■ The blood clot will be dissolved, and client will be closely monitored for active bleeding.
■ Client's vital signs will be monitored for stability during and after thrombolytic therapy.
■ Thrombolytic drug should be administered 4 hours after myocardial infarction.

NURSING INTERVENTIONS

■ Monitor vital signs. Increased pulse rate followed by decreased blood pressure usually indicates blood loss and impending shock. Record vital signs and report changes.
■ Observe for signs and symptoms of active bleeding from the mouth or rectum. Hemorrhage is a serious complication of thrombolytic treatment. Aminocaproic acid can be given as an intervention to stop the bleeding.
■ Check for active bleeding for 24 hours after thrombolytic therapy has been discontinued: q15min for the first hour, every q30min until the eighth hour, and then hourly.
■ Observe for signs of allergic reaction to streptokinase, such as itching, hives, flush, fever, dyspnea, bronchospasm, hypotension, and/or cardiovascular collapse.
■ Avoid administering aspirin or nonsteroidal antiinflammatory drugs (NSAIDs) for pain or discomfort when client is receiving a thrombolytic. Acetaminophen can be substituted.
■ Monitor the electrocardiogram (ECG) for the presence of reperfusion dysrhythmias as the blood clot is dissolving; antidysrhythmic therapy may be indicated.
■ Avoid venipuncture/arterial sticks.

Client Teaching

General
• Explain the thrombolytic treatment to client and family. Be supportive.

Side Effects
• Instruct client to report any side effects, such as lightheadedness, dizziness, palpitations, nausea, pruritus, or urticaria.

EVALUATION

■ Determine the effectiveness of drug therapy: clot has dissolved, vital signs are stable, no signs or symptoms of active bleeding, and client is pain free.

WEBSITES

For further information on *Anticoagulants, Antiplatelets, and Thrombolytics,* visit these Internet resources:

Plavix:
http://www.plavix.com

Medline Plus Drug Information—clopidogrel:
http://www.nlm.nih.gov/medlineplus/druginfo/uspdi/203403.html

Wichita MedEd Online—Antithrombotics—heparin:
http://www2.kumc.edu/wichita/meded/cvresource/antithrombotic/heparin/

Lovenox:
http://www.lovenox.com/

Medline Plus Drug Information—anticoagulants:
http://www.nlm.nih.gov/medlineplus/druginfo/uspdi/202050.html

Critical Thinking Case Study

T.M., age 57, has thrombophlebitis in the right lower leg. IV heparin, 5000 units by bolus, was given. Following the IV bolus, heparin 5000 units given subQ q6h was prescribed. Other therapeutic means to decrease pain and alleviate swelling and redness were also prescribed. An aPTT test was ordered.

1. Was T.M.'s heparin order per day within the safe daily range?

2. What are the various methods for administering heparin?

3. Why was an aPTT test ordered? How would you determine whether T.M. is within the desired range? Explain.

After 5 days of heparin therapy, T.M. was prescribed warfarin (Coumadin) 5 mg PO daily. An INR test was ordered.

4. What is the pharmacologic action of warfarin? Is the warfarin dose within the daily dosage range? Explain.

5. What is the half-life and protein-binding for warfarin? If a client takes a drug that is highly protein bound, would there be a drug interaction? Explain.

6. Why was INR ordered for T.M.? What is the desired range?

7. What serious adverse reactions could result with prolonged use or large doses of warfarin?

8. What client teaching interventions should the nurse include? List three client teaching interventions.

9. Months later, T.M. had hematemesis. What nursing action should be taken?

Study Questions

1. In what routes can heparin be administered? When? Why? Give rationales.

2. What drugs enhance the action of warfarin (drug interaction)? How is warfarin (Coumadin) therapy monitored? Explain.

3. Explain how protamine is used. What is its action?

4. What is an appropriate nursing plan of care for a client with thrombocytopenia?

5. The client had an AMI within the last 3 hours. A thrombolytic drug is given. What type of nursing assessment should be performed and for how long?

6. What are at least three client situations that contradict the use of thrombolytic therapy?

7. What are the differences between an anticoagulant and a thrombolytic?

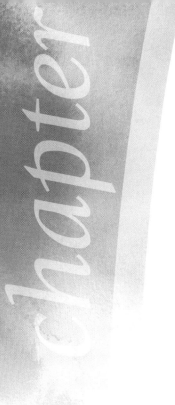

44 Antilipidemics and Peripheral Vasodilators

ELECTRONIC RESOURCES

Additional information can be found on the companion website at *http://evolve.elsevier.com/KeeHayes/pharmacology/* or on the companion CD-ROM, which includes:

- *NCLEX-style examination review questions*
- *Pharmacology animations*
- *Medication error and IV therapy checklists*
- *Medication calculation problems*
- *Electronic calculators*

OBJECTIVES

- Describe the action of the two main drug groups: antilipidemics and peripheral vasodilators.
- Identify the side effects and adverse reactions of antilipidemics and peripheral vasodilators.
- Describe the nursing process, including client teaching, for antilipidemics and peripheral vasodilators.

TERMS

antilipidemics
chylomicrons
high-density lipoproteins (HDL)

hyperlipidemia
ischemia
lipoproteins
low-density lipoproteins (LDL)

peripheral vasodilators
very low-density lipoproteins (VLDL)

Introduction

Various drugs are used to maintain or decrease blood lipid concentrations and promote dilation of vessels. Antilipidemics that lower blood lipids are also called *hypolipidemics* or *antilipidemics*. Peripheral vasodilators are drugs that dilate vessels that have been narrowed by vasospasm.

Antilipidemics

Antilipidemics lower abnormal blood lipid levels. Lipids composed of cholesterol, triglycerides, and phospholipids are transported in the body and are bound to protein in various amounts. These **lipoproteins** are classified as **chylomicrons, very low-density lipoproteins (VLDL), low-density lipoproteins (LDL),** and **high-density lipoproteins (HDL).** The HDL (friendly or "good" lipoproteins) have a higher percentage of protein and less lipids. Their function is to remove cholesterol from the bloodstream and deliver it to the liver. The other three lipoproteins are composed mainly of cholesterol and triglycerides and contribute to atherosclerotic plaque in the blood vessels; they are "bad" lipoproteins. Table 44–1 presents the composition of the lipoproteins.

Serum cholesterol and triglyceride measurements are frequently part of a regular physical examination or readmission evaluation and are used as baseline test results. If the levels are high, a 12- to 14-hour fasting lipid profile

may be ordered. When cholesterol, triglycerides, and LDL are elevated, the client is at increased risk for coronary artery disease (CAD). Table 44–2 lists the various serum lipids and their reference values (normal serum levels) according to a risk classification.

Nonpharmacologic Methods for Cholesterol Reduction

Before antilipidemics are prescribed, nondrug therapy should be initiated for decreasing blood pressure. The saturated fats and cholesterol in the diet should be reduced. Total fat intake should be 30% or less of caloric intake, and cholesterol intake should be 300 mg or less. The client should read labels on containers and buy appropriate foods. Clients should choose lean meats, especially chicken and fish.

In many cases, diet alone will not lower blood lipid levels. Because 75% to 85% of serum cholesterol is endogenously (internally) derived, dietary modification alone will typically lower total cholesterol levels by only 10% to 30%. This, and the fact that adherence to dietary restrictions is often short lived, explains why many clients do not respond to diet modification alone.

Exercise is an important aspect of the nonpharmacologic method to reduce cholesterol. For the hypertensive older adult, exercise can be walking and bicycling. If the client is obese, body-weight reduction decreases choles-

Table 44–1

Lipoprotein Groups

Lipoprotein Subgroups	Composition of the Lipoproteins			
	Protein (%)	Cholesterol (%)	Triglycerides (%)	Phospholipids (%)
Chylomicrons	1-2	1-3	80-95	3-6
Very low density (VLDL)	6-10	8-20	45-65	15-20
Low density (LDL)	18-22	45-50	4-8	18-24
High density (HDL)	45-55	15-20	2-7	26-32

Modified from Henry J: *Clinical diagnosis and management by laboratory methods,* ed 18, Philadelphia, 1991, Saunders, p. 189.

Table 44–2

Serum Lipid Values

Lipids	Desirable (mg/dl)	Level of Risk for CAD		
		Low Risk (mg/dl)	Moderate Risk (mg/dl)	High Risk (mg/dl)
Cholesterol	150-200	<200	200-240	>240
Triglycerides	40-150	Values vary with age	Values vary with age	>190
Lipoproteins				
LDL	<100	100-130	130-159	>160
HDL	45-60	>60	35-50	<35

CAD, Coronary artery disease; *HDL,* high-density lipoproteins; *LDL,* low-density lipoproteins; <, less than; >, greater than.

Table 44–3

Hyperlipidemia: Lipoprotein Phenotype

Type	Major Lipids
I	Increased chylomicrons and increased triglycerides. Uncommon.
IIA	Increased low-density lipoprotein (LDL) and increased cholesterol.
IIB	Increased very low-density lipoprotein (VLDL), increased LDL, increased cholesterol and triglycerides. Very common.
III	Moderately increased cholesterol and triglycerides. Uncommon.
IV	Increased VLDL and markedly increased triglycerides. Very common.
V	Increased chylomicrons, VLDL, and triglycerides. Uncommon.

Types II and IV are commonly associated with coronary artery disease.

terol levels and the risk of CAD. Smoking is another risk factor that should be eliminated. Smoking increases LDL cholesterol and decreases the HDL.

If nonpharmacologic methods are ineffective for reducing cholesterol and the lipoproteins LDL and VLDL and **hyperlipidemia** remains, antilipidemic drugs are prescribed. It must be emphasized to the client that dietary changes need to be made and an exercise program followed even after drug therapy has been initiated. The type of antilipidemics ordered depends on the lipoprotein phenotype (Table 44–3).

Types of Antilipidemics

Drugs that lower lipid levels include bile-acid sequestrants, fibrates (fibric acid), nicotinic acid, and hepatic 3-hydroxy-3 thylglutaryl coenzyme A (HMG-CoA) reductase inhibitors (statins). The statins have fewer adverse effects and are well tolerated.

One of the first antilipidemics was cholestyramine (Questran), introduced in 1959. It is a resin that binds with bile acids in the intestine and is effective against hyperlipidemia type II. The drug comes in a gritty powder, which is mixed thoroughly in water or juice.

Colestipol (Colestid) is a resin antilipidemic similar to cholestyramine. Both are effective in lowering cholesterol. Bile acid sequestrants should not be used as the only therapy in clients with elevated triglycerides because they typically raise triglyceride levels.

Clofibrate (Atromid-S) and gemfibrozil (Lopid) are fibric acid derivatives that are effective in reducing triglyceride and VLDL levels. They are used primarily to reduce hyperlipidemia type IV but can also be used for type II hyperlipidemia. These drugs are highly protein bound and should not be taken with anticoagulants because they compete for protein sites. The anticoagulant dose should be reduced during antilipidemic therapy, and the international normalized ratio (INR) should be closely monitored. Clofibrate,

once a popular antilipidemic, is not suggested for long-term use because of its many side effects, such as cardiac dysrhythmias, angina, thromboembolism, and gallstones.

Nicotinic acid, or niacin (vitamin B_2), reduces VLDL and LDL. Nicotinic acid is actually very effective at lowering cholesterol levels, and its effect on the lipid profile is highly desirable. Because it has numerous side effects and large doses are required, as few as 20% of clients can tolerate niacin initially. However, with proper client counseling, careful drug titration, and concomitant use of aspirin, this number can be increased to as high as 60% to 70%.

Probucol, a bisphenol, is poorly absorbed after oral dosage. It lowers the LDL and cholesterol levels in type II hyperlipidemia, but it is not as effective as other antilipidemic drugs. It is highly lipid soluble and is stored in body fat; thus it is slow to eliminate from the body. Diarrhea may result from use. Probucol is contraindicated for clients with cardiac dysrhythmias.

Statins

The statin drugs, first introduced in 1987, inhibit the enzyme HMG CoA reductase in cholesterol biosynthesis; thus the statins are called *HMG CoA reductase inhibitors*. By inhibiting cholesterol synthesis in the liver, this group of antilipidemics decreases the concentration of cholesterol and decreases the LDL and slightly increases the HDL cholesterol. Reduction of LDL cholesterol may be seen in as early as 2 weeks. The statin group has been useful in decreasing CAD and reducing mortality rates.

Numerous statins have been approved in the past few years. The present group of statins includes atorvastatin calcium (Lipitor), fluvastatin (Lescol), lovastatin (Mevacor), pravastatin sodium (Pravachol), simvastatin (Zocor), and rosuvastatin calcium (Crestor). Lovastatin was the first statin used to decrease cholesterol. It is effective in lowering LDL (hyperlipidemia type II) within several weeks; gastrointestinal (GI) disturbances, headaches, muscle cramps, and tiredness are early complaints. Serum liver enzymes should be monitored, and an annual eye examination is needed because cataract formation may result from lovastatin therapy. The other four statins have actions similar to lovastatin in decreasing serum cholesterol, LDL, VLDL, and triglycerides, and they slightly elevate HDL. Atorvastatin (Lipitor), lovastatin (Mevacor), and simvastatin (Zocor) are more effective at lowering LDL than the other statins.

If antilipidemic therapy is withdrawn, cholesterol and LDL levels return to pretreatment levels. The client taking an antilipidemic should understand that antilipidemic drug therapy is a lifetime commitment for maintaining a decrease in serum lipid levels. Abruptly stopping the statin drug could cause the client to have a threefold more rebound effect that may cause death from an AMI.

Laboratory Test

Homocysteine: Reference values: 4-17 mcmol/L (fasting). Homocysteine, an amino acid, is a by-product of protein. It is found in protein, such as eggs, chicken, beef, and cheddar

PROTOTYPE DRUG CHART 44–1

ATORVASTATIN

Drug Class	**Dosage**
Antilipidemic; HMG-CoA Reductase Inhibitor Trade Name: Lipitor *Pregnancy Category:* X	A: PO: 10 mg/daily; may increase dose up to 80 mg/daily C: Safety is not established
Contraindications	**Drug-Lab-Food Interactions**
Active liver disease, pregnancy *Caution:* History of liver disease, increase alcohol ingestion, trauma, severe metabolic endocrine disorders, uncontrolled seizures	*Drug: Decrease* effect with antacids, propranolol. May *increase* digoxin level, oral contraceptives. *Increase* effects with macrolide antibiotics, antifungals
Pharmacokinetics	**Pharmacodynamics**
Absorption: Rapid **Distribution:** PB: 98% **Metabolism:** t$\frac{1}{2}$: 14 h; metabolites: 20-30 h **Excretion:** Primarily in the bile; some via urine	PO: Onset: 2 wk for decrease in cholesterol Peak: 1-2 h; 2-4 wk to be effective Duration: 24 h

Therapeutic Effects/Uses

To decrease cholesterol levels and to decrease serum lipids especially LDL and triglycerides
Mode of Action: Inhibits HMG-CoA reductase. HMG-CoA reductase is necessary for hepatic production of cholesterol.

Side Effects	**Adverse Reactions**
Rare Headache, rash/pruritus, constipation/diarrhea, sinusitis, pharynitis	Rhabdomyolysis, myalgia, photosensitivity, cataracts

A, Adult; *C*, child; *h*, hour; *HMG-CoA*, 3-hydroxy-3 methyl-glutaryl coenzyme; *PO*, by mouth; *PB:* protein-binding; *t½:* half-life; *LDL*, low-density lipoproteins; *wk*, week.

---

cheese. A high level of homocysteine has been linked to cardiovascular disease, stroke, and the possibility of Alzheimer's disease. Also, it may promote blood clotting. It has been stated that an increase in serum homocysteine can damage the inner lining of blood vessels and promote a thickening and loss of flexibility in the blood vessel. The three vitamins that can lower the serum level of homocysteine are vitamin B$_6$ (pyridoxine), vitamin B$_{12}$ (cyanocobalamin), and folic acid.

Prototype Drug Chart 44–1 list the data of a frequently prescribed antilipidemic, atorvastatin (Lipitor). The five statins are commonly used drugs to reduce cholesterol, LDL, and triglycerides.

Pharmacokinetics

Atorvastatin (Lipitor) decreases the LDL by 25% with lower doses and 55% with higher doses. It increases the HDL, but not as high as some of the other statins, such as pravastatin and simvastatin. It decreases the triglyceride levels by 20% with lower doses and 50% with higher doses, a greater reduction than with the other statins. Atorvastatin is highly protein bound, so it is usually prescribed once a day. It has a half-life of 14 hours, which is moderately long, and the half-life for its metabolites is 20 to 30 hours.

Pharmacodynamics

The positive effect of lowering the lipids with atorvastatin is seen in about 2 weeks. The peak time after a dose of atorvastatin is 1 to 2 hours; however, it takes 2 to 4 weeks for therapeutic effect of the drug to take effect.

When the client is taking high doses of atorvastatin or any statins, myopathy and rhabdomyolysis (disintegration of striated muscle fibers) may occur. If client complains of muscle pain or tenderness, it should be reported immediately.

Side Effects and Adverse Reactions

Side effects and adverse reactions of cholestyramine include constipation and peptic ulcer. Constipation can be decreased or alleviated by increasing intake of fluids and foods high in fiber. Early signs of peptic ulcer are nausea and abdominal discomfort, followed later by abdominal pain and distention. To avoid GI discomfort, the drug must be taken with and followed by sufficient fluids.

The many side effects of nicotinic acid (e.g., GI disturbances, flushing of the skin, abnormal liver function [elevated serum liver enzymes], hyperglycemia, hyperuricemia) decrease its usefulness. However, as mentioned, aspirin and careful drug titration can reduce side effects to a manageable level in most clients.

The statin drugs can cause a dose-related increase in liver enzyme levels. Serum liver enzyme levels (alkaline phosphatase, alanine aminotransferase, gamma-glutamyl transferase) should be monitored. Baseline liver enzyme studies should be prescribed before statin drug therapy. A slight transient increase in a serum liver enzyme level may be within normal value for the client, but it should be rechecked in a week or more. Clients with acute hepatic disorder should not take a statin drug.

A serious skeletal muscle adverse effect known as *rhabdomyolysis* has been reported with the use of the statin drug class. Clients should be advised to report promptly any unexplained muscle tenderness or weakness, especially if accompanied by fever or malaise.

Table 44–4 lists the drug data for the antilipidemics.

Nursing Process

Antilipidemics (Statins)

ASSESSMENT

■ Assess vital signs and serum chemistry values (cholesterol, triglycerides, aspartate aminotransferase [AST], alanine aminotransferase [ALT], creatine phosphokinase [CPK]) for baseline values.
■ Obtain a medical history. Atorvastatin and statin drugs are contraindicated for clients with a liver disorder. Pregnancy category is X.

NURSING DIAGNOSES

■ Impaired tissue integrity
■ Anxiety related to elevated cholesterol level

PLANNING

■ Client's cholesterol level will be <200 mg/dl in 6 to 8 weeks.
■ Client will be taught to choose foods low in fat, cholesterol, and complex sugars.

NURSING INTERVENTIONS

■ Monitor client's blood lipid levels (cholesterol, triglycerides, low-density lipoprotein [LDL], and high-density lipoprotein [HDL]) every 6 to 8 weeks for the first 6 months after any statin therapy and then every 3 to 6 months. For lipid level profile, client should fast for 12 to 14 hours. Desired cholesterol value is <200 mg/dl; triglyceride value is <150 mg/dl (can vary); LDL is <100 mg/dl; and HDL is >60 mg/dl. Cholesterol levels of >240 mg/dl, LDL levels of >160 mg/dl, and HDL levels of <35 mg/dl can lead to severe cardiovascular or cerebral vascular accident (CVA).
■ Monitor laboratory tests for liver function, such as ALT, ALP, and gamma-glutamyl transferase (GGT). Antilipidemic drugs may cause liver disorder.
■ Observe for signs and symptoms of GI upset. Taking the drug with sufficient water or with meals may alleviate some of the GI discomfort.

Client Teaching

General

● Advise client that if there is a family history of hyperlipidemia, his or her children should have a baseline blood lipid level obtained and monitored. Instruct the client that children should decrease fatty foods in the diet.
● Emphasize the need to comply with the drug regimen to lower the blood lipids. Side effects should be reported to the health care provider.
● Inform client that it may take several weeks before blood lipid levels decline. Explain that laboratory tests for blood lipids (cholesterol, triglycerides, LDL, and HDL) are usually ordered every 3 to 6 months.
● Advise client to have serum liver enzymes monitored as indicated by the health care provider. Lovastatin, pravastatin, and simvastatin are contraindicated in acute hepatic disease and pregnancy.
● Instruct client to have an annual eye examination and to report changes in visual acuity.

Clofibrate, Gemfibrozil, Probucol

● Advise client taking clofibrate and probucol that decreased libido and impotence may occur and should be reported. Drug dosage can be changed or another antilipidemic may be ordered.
● Instruct clients with diabetes or those at risk for developing diabetes to monitor blood glucose levels if they take gemfibrozil. Dietary changes or insulin adjustment may be necessary.
● Advise client with cardiac dysrhythmias to tell the health care provider before starting probucol. Cardiac dysrhythmias should be monitored and reported.

Nicotinic Acid

● Instruct client to take the drug with meals to decrease GI discomfort.

Self-Administration

● For cholestyramine and cholestipol, instruct client to mix the powder well in water or juice.

Side Effects

Cholestyramine, Colestipol, and Nicotinic Acid (Niacin)

● Advise client that constipation may occur with cholestyramine and colestipol. Increasing fluid intake and food bulk should help to alleviate the problem.
● Explain to client that flush is common and should decrease with continued use of the drug. Usually, the drug is started at a low dose.
● Advise client that large doses of nicotinic acid can cause vasodilation, producing dizziness and faintness (syncope).

Statins

● Explain to client that the serum liver enzyme levels are periodically monitored.

- Encourage client to report promptly any unexplained muscle tenderness or weakness that may be caused by rhabdomyolysis.
- Instruct client not to abruptly stop the statin drug because a serious rebound effect might occur that could lead to an AMI and possible death. Before stopping a statin, client should talk to his or her health care provider.

Diet

- Explain to client that GI discomfort is a common problem with most antilipidemics. Suggest increasing fluid intake when taking the medication.
- Instruct client to maintain a low-fat diet by eating foods that are low in animal fat, cholesterol, and complex sugars. Lovastatin and other antilipidemics are not a substitute for a diet that is low in fat.

Cultural Considerations ⊕

- Respect client's belief of how to control his or her cholesterol level.
- Do not criticize folk practices; explanations and modification to plan of care may be necessary if the method client uses is not effective or is unsafe.

EVALUATION

- Evaluate the effectiveness of the antilipidemic drug. Client's cholesterol level is within desired range.
- Determine that client is on a low-fat, low-cholesterol diet.

Table 44–4

Antilipidemics

Generic (Brand)	Route and Dosage	Uses and Considerations
Bile-Acid Sequestrants		
cholestyramine resin (Questran)	A: PO: 4 g t.i.d. a.c. and at bedtime; mix powder in 120-240 ml of fluid; *max:* 24 g/d	Cholestyramine resin was the first antilipidemic produced. For type II hyperlipoproteinemia (LDL). Decrease in LDL is apparent in 1 week. Drug powder should be mixed well in fluid. It does not have any effect on VLDL and HDL but could increase triglyceride levels. GI upset and constipation can occur. Vitamin A, D, K deficiency may occur because of decreased GI absorption. *Pregnancy category:* C; PB: UK; t½: UK
colesevelem (Welchol)	A: PO: 3 tablets (625 mg/tablet) b.i.d. or 6 tablets, daily	It has a cholesterol-lowering effect by binding with bile salts in the intestines to form an insoluble complex with fecal excretions, thus, reducing circulating cholesterol including LDL. Triglycerides may be slightly increased. Contraindications with bowel obstruction. May be used in combination with a statin drug. Pregnancy B; PB: UK; t½: UK
colestipol HCl (Colestid)	A: PO: 10-30 g/d in divided doses before meals	To reduce cholesterol and LDL levels. Same as cholestyramine. *Pregnancy category:* C; PB: UK; t½: UK
Fibrates (Fibric Acid)		
clofibrate (Atromid-S)	A: PO: 500 mg q.i.d.	For lowering cholesterol, VLDL, and triglyceride. For types IIB (VLDL), IV, V hyperlipidemia. Drug is more effective for higher cholesterol levels. Therapeutic effect occurs in 2-5 days. Drug should not be taken during pregnancy. Gallstones can occur with long-term use. *Pregnancy category:* C; PB: 90%-95%; t½: 12-25 h
fenofibrate (Tricor)	A: PO: 67-201 mg/d	Treatment of type IV and V hyperlipidemia, and for hypertriglyceridemia. Specified diet should be part of drug therapy. Monitor serum creatinine levels. *Pregnancy category:* C; PB: 99%; t½: 21 h
gemfibrozil (Lopid)	A: PO: 600 mg b.i.d. before meals; *max:* 1500 mg/d	For VLDL and elevated triglycerides; LDL may decrease and HDL may increase. For types II (VLDL, LDL), III, IV, V hyperlipidemia. Do not use in combination with lovastatin because of increase in CPK. *Pregnancy category:* B; PB: >90%; t½: 1.5 h
Nicotinic Acid		
nicotinic acid (Niacin)	A: PO: Initially: 100 mg t.i.d.; *maint;* 1-3 g/d p.c. in 3 divided doses; *max:* 6 g/d	For VLDL and LDL: types II, III, IV, V hyperlipidemia. Doses are 100 times higher than for RDA to lower VLDL. See text. *Pregnancy category:* C; PB: UK; t½: 45 min

A, Adult; *a.c.,* before meals; *b.i.d.,* twice a day; *CPK,* creatine phosphokinase; *d,* day; *GI,* gastrointestinal; *h,* hour; *HDL,* high-density lipoprotein; *LDL,* low-density lipoprotein; *maint,* maintenance; *max,* maximum; *min,* minute; *PB,* protein-binding; *p.c.,* after meals; *PO,* by mouth; *q.i.d.,* four times a day; *RDA,* recommended daily allowance; *t½,* half-life; *t.i.d.,* three times a day; *UK,* unknown; *VLDL:* very low-density lipoprotein; *>,* greater than.

Peripheral Vasodilators

A common problem in older adults is peripheral arterial (vascular) disease (PAD, PVD). It is characterized by numbness and coolness of the extremities, intermittent claudication (pain and weakness of limb when walking but no symptoms at rest), and possible leg ulcers. The primary cause is arteriosclerosis and hyperlipidemia resulting in atherosclerosis. The arteries become occluded.

Peripheral vasodilators increase blood flow to the extremities. They are used in peripheral vascular disorders of venous and arterial vessels. They are more effective for disorders resulting from vasospasm (Raynaud's disease) than from vessel occlusion or arteriosclerosis (arteriosclerosis obliterans, thromboangiitis obliterans [Buerger's disease]). In Raynaud's disease, cold exposure or emotional upset can trigger vasospasm of the toes and fingers; these clients have benefited from vasodilators. Clients with diabetes mellitus are more likely to have PAD by two to four times the usual rate and are at risk of claudication.

Although the following drugs have different actions, they all promote vasodilation: tolazoline (Priscoline), isoxsuprine (Vasodilan), nicotinyl alcohol, and papaverine (Cerespan, Genabid). Nicotinyl alcohol and papaverine are direct-acting peripheral vasodilators. The alpha-blocker prazosin (Minipress) and the calcium channel blocker nifedipine (Procardia) have also been used as peripheral vasodilators.

Individuals with dyslipidemia and PAD, who are treated with HMG-CoA reductase inhibitors (statins), may get improvement for claudication symptoms as well as a decrease in serum lipids. Also, clients with PAD and who are hypertensive receive improvement for both conditions when taking the antihypertensive drug, ramipril (Altace), an ACE inhibitor. The antiplatelet drugs clopidogrel (Plavix) and aspirin have been used to decrease PAD symptoms. Another antiplatelet drug, cilostazol (Pletal), has been approved by the Food and Drug Administration (FDA) for treating intermittent claudication. It decreases arterial thrombi. The herb ginkgo biloba, taken with an an-

Table 44-4

Antilipidemics—cont'd

Generic (Brand)	Route and Dosage	Uses and Considerations
Antihyperlipidemic		
ezetimibe (Zetia)	A: PO: 10 mg, daily	It inhibits cholesterol absorption in the small intestine. Also, it reduces the total cholesterol, LDL, triglycerides, and increases HDL. Caution use should be with liver dysfunction and elevated serum transaminase levels. *Pregnancy category:* C; PB: UK, t½: UK
Vastatins and Statins (HMG-CoA Reductase Inhibitors)		
atorvastatin calcium (Lipitor)	A: PO: 10 mg/d; *max:* 80 mg/d	To reduce hyperlipidemia (LDL, cholesterol, and triglycerides). May increase digoxin levels. *Caution* in clients with history of liver disease. *Pregnancy category:* X; PB: 98%; 14 h
fluvastatin sodium (Lescol)	A: PO: Initially: 20-40 mg at bedtime; *maint:* 20-80 mg/d	Treatment of types IIA and IIB hyperlipidemia, total cholesterol, and elevated triglycerides. HDL is slightly increased. Monitor liver function (liver enzymes). *Pregnancy category:* X; PB: 98%; t½: 1.2 h
lovastatin (Mevacor)	A: PO: 20-80 mg/day in 1-2 divided doses with meals	It is given to control cholesterol by inhibiting cholesterol synthesis. Lovastatin decreases LDL and increases some HDL. Liver enzyme should be checked. *Pregnancy category:* X; PB: 95%; t½: 1-2 h
pravastatin sodium (Pravachol)	A: PO: 10-40 mg/d	Decreases serum cholesterol, LDL, VLDL, and triglycerides. HDL is slightly increased. Monitor liver enzymes. *Pregnancy category:* X; PB: 55%; t½: 1.5-2.5 h
rosuvastatin calcium (Crestor)	A: PO: 10 mg, daily	A strong new statin drug that cuts LDL in half for 52% of those taking it. Reduces total cholesterol, LDL, triglycerides, and increases HDL. Muscle pain and weakness should be reported. Liver enzyme should be checked. *Pregnancy category:* X; PB: UK, t½: UK
simvastatin (Zocor)	A: PO: Initially: 5-10 mg/d in evening; *maint:* 20-80 mg/d in the evening; *max:* 80 mg/d	Similar to lovastatin. Monitor liver enzymes. *Pregnancy category:* X; PB: 95%; t½: UK
Combination Anticholesterol Drug		
Vytorin (Eyetimibe/Simvastatin)	A: PO: 10/10 mg to 10/80 mg	A combination of ezetimibe (Zetia) and simvastatin (Zocor). Ezetimibe decreases absorption of cholesterol in the small intestines. Simvastatin (Zocor) interfers with the production of the cholesterol in the liver.

PROTOTYPE DRUG CHART 44–2

ISOXSUPRINE HCl

Drug Class	**Dosage**
Peripheral vasodilator Trade Name: Vasodilan, Vasoprine *Pregnancy Category:* C	A: PO: 10-20 mg t.i.d.-q.i.d.

Contraindications	**Drug-Lab-Food Interactions**
Arterial bleeding, severe hypotension, postpartum, tachycardia *Caution:* Bleeding disorders, tachycardia	*Drug: Decrease* blood pressure with antihypertensives

Pharmacokinetics	**Pharmacodynamics**
Absorption: PO: Readily absorbed **Distribution:** PB: UK **Metabolism:** t½: 1.251.5 h **Excretion:** In urine	PO: Onset: 0.5 h Peak: 1 h Duration: 3 h

Therapeutic Effects/Uses

To increase circulation caused by peripheral vascular disease (Raynaud's disease, arteriosclerosis obliterans) and cerebrovascular insufficiency
Mode of Action: Action is directly on vascular smooth muscle

Side Effects	**Adverse Reactions**
Nausea, vomiting, dizziness, syncope, weakness, tremors, rash, flush, abdominal distention, chest pain	Hypotension, tachycardia, palpitations

A, Adult; *h*, hour; *PB*, protein-binding; *PO*, by mouth; *q.i.d.*, four times a day; *t½*, half-life; *t.i.d.*, three times a day; *UK*, unknown.

---

tiplatelet drug, has been used to treat intermittent claudication because of its vasodilating and antioxidant effects, although this herb has not been approved by the FDA. Most of the group of drugs used for treating PAD do not cure the health problem but aid in relieving PAD symptoms.

Isoxsuprine hydrochloride, a beta-adrenergic antagonist with slight alpha-adrenergic antagonist effects, is effective for relaxing the arterial walls within skeletal muscles. Prototype Drug Chart 44–2 gives the drug data for isoxsuprine.

Isoxsuprine

Pharmacokinetics

Isoxsuprine is readily absorbed from the GI tract. It has a short half-life of 1.25 to 1.5 hours. Because of its half-life, the drug can be taken three to four times a day.

Pharmacodynamics

Isoxsuprine is a beta₂-adrenergic agonist. It causes vasodilation on arteries within the skeletal muscles. Bronchodilation may also occur. This drug has a short onset of action, peak time, and duration of action.

Side Effects and Adverse Reactions

Light-headedness, dizziness, orthostatic hypotension, tachycardia, palpitation, flush, and GI distress may occur.

The effectiveness of peripheral vasodilators in increasing blood flow by vasodilation is questionable in the presence of arteriosclerosis. These drugs may decrease some of the symptoms of cerebrovascular insufficiency. The drug data for the peripheral vasodilators are given in Table 44–5.

Pentoxifylline

Pentoxifylline (Trental), classified as an hemorrheologic agent, improves microcirculation and tissue perfusion by decreasing blood viscosity and improving the flexibility of erythrocytes thus increasing tissue oxygenation. It is not a vasodilator, although it dilates rigid arteriosclerotic blood vessels including arterioles, capillaries, and venules. It is a derivative from the xanthine group. Pentoxifylline has been approved by FDA for clients with intermittent claudication and has been prescribed for those with Buerger's disease resulting from arterial occlusions. However, in one research study, pentoxifylline was not determined to be more effective than taking a placebo.

Reactions to an overdose of pentoxifylline include flushing of the skin, faintness, sedation, and GI disturbances. The drug should be taken with food. The client should avoid smoking because nicotine increases vasocon-

Table 44–5

Vasodilators (Peripheral)

Generic (Brand)	Route and Dosage	Uses and Considerations
Alpha-Adrenergic Antagonists		
isoxsuprine HCl (Vasodilan)	See Prototype Drug Chart 44–2.	
tolazoline HCl (Priscoline HCl)	A: subQ/IM/IV: 10-50 mg q.i.d. NB: IV: Initially: 1-2 mg/kg, followed by 1-2 mg/kg/h for 24-48 h; initial dose effect: 30 min	For neonatal pulmonary hypertension and in vascular occlusive diseases in adults. Causes vasodilation and decreases peripheral resistance. Improves circulation in thromboangiitis obliterans, Raynaud's disease, frostbite, and peripheral vasospastic disorders. *Pregnancy category:* C; PB: UK; t½: A: 10 h, NB: 3-10 h
Direct-Acting Peripheral Vasodilators		
ergoloid mesylates (Hydergine)	A: PO/SL: 1 mg t.i.d.; dose may increase to 4-12 mg/d	For cerebrovascular insufficiency. To improve cognitive skills, self-care, and mood, especially in the older adult. SL tablets should be placed under the tongue. May cause GI distress, orthostatic hypotension. *Pregnancy category:* C; PB: UK; t½: 3-12 h
nicotinyl alcohol (Ronigen [Canada only])	A: PO: 150-300 mg b.i.d.	Acts as vasodilator. Can cause flush and orthostatic hypotension. *Pregnancy category:* UK; PB: UK; t½: UK
papaverine (Pavabid)	A: PO: 100-300 mg q12h or 150 mg q8h SR: 150 mg q12h; *max:* 300 mg q12h IV: 30-120 mg q3h PRN	For arterial spasms. Reduces ischemia of the brain, heart, and peripheral vessels. One of the oldest vasodilators. Side effects: flush, GI upset, headaches, increased heart rate and respiration. *Pregnancy category:* C; PB: 90%; t½: 1.5 h
Hemorrheologic		
cilostazol (Pletal)	See Table 43–2.	
pentoxifylline (Trental)	A: PO: 400 mg t.i.d. with meals	For peripheral vascular disorders. Alleviates intermittent claudication. Also improves cerebral function for those with cerebrovascular insufficiency and may decrease stroke incidence for those having recurrent TIA. *Pregnancy category:* C; PB: UK; t½: 0.5-1 h

A, Adult; *b.i.d.*, twice a day; *d*, day; *GI*, gastrointestinal; *h*, hour; *IM*, intramuscular, *IV*, intravenous; *NB*, newborn; *max*, maximum; *min*, minute; *PB*, protein-binding; *PO*, by mouth; *PRN*, as necessary; *q.i.d.*, four times a day; *subQ*, subcutaneous; *SL*, sublingual; *SR*, sustained-release tablet; *t½*, half-life; *TIA*, transient ischemic attack; *t.i.d.*, three times a day; *UK*, unknown.

striction. Clients taking an antihypertensive drug along with pentoxifylline may need to have the antihypertensive dosage decreased to avoid side effects.

Nursing Process

Vasodilators: Isoxsuprine (Vasodilan)

ASSESSMENT

■ Obtain baseline vital signs for future comparison.
■ Assess for signs of inadequate blood flow to the extremities: pallor, coldness of extremity, and pain.

NURSING DIAGNOSES

■ Impaired tissue integrity
■ Pain related to inadequate blood flow to extremity

PLANNING

■ Client's blood flow to the extremities will improve, and client's pain will be controlled.

NURSING INTERVENTIONS

■ Monitor vital signs, especially blood pressure and heart rate. Tachycardia and orthostatic hypotension can be problematic with peripheral vasodilators.

Client Teaching

General
• Inform client that a desired therapeutic response may take 1.5 to 3 months.
• Advise client not to smoke; smoking increases vasospasm.
• Instruct client to use aspirin or aspirin-like compounds only with the health care provider's approval. Salicylates help to prevent platelet aggregation.

Side Effects
• Encourage client to change position slowly but frequently to avoid orthostatic hypotension. Orthostatic hypotension is common when taking high doses of a vasodilator.
• Instruct client to report side effects of isoxsuprine, such as flush, headaches, and dizziness.

Diet

• Suggest that client with gastrointestinal disturbances take isoxsuprine with meals.

• Advise client not to ingest alcohol with a vasodilator because it may cause a hypotensive reaction.

EVALUATION

■ Evaluate the effectiveness of the isoxsuprine therapy; blood flow is increased in the extremities and pain has subsided.

■ Client experiences no side effects from the prescribed drug.

WEBSITES

For further information on *Antilipidemics and Peripheral Vasodilators,* visit these Internet resources:

Medline Plus—clopidogrel:
http://www.nlm.nih.gov/medlineplus/druginfo/uspdi/203403.html

Lipitor:
http://www.lipitor.com

Medline Plus—anticoagulants:
http://www.nlm.nih.gov/medlineplus/druginfo/uspdi/202050.html

Critical Thinking Case Study

J.H. had a myocardial infarction (MI) 3 years ago. He was prescribed gemfibrozil (Lopid) 600 mg, twice daily, before meals. His cholesterol remained between 220 to 240 mg/dl and his LDL 140 mg/dl. His anticholesterol drug was changed to simvastatin (Zocor) 20 mg/day in the evening.

1. How does simvastatin differ from gemfibrozil?

2. Why do you think that J.H.'s cholesterol drug, gemfibrozil, was changed to simvastatin?

3. While J.H. is taking simvastatin, which group of serum levels should be monitored?

4. How long after J.H. took simvastatin should his cholesterol and lipoproteins be checked?

5. What is the maximum dose for simvastatin?

6. J.H. complains of muscle pain and muscle weakness. What might this indicate?

7. Could J.H. receive both gemfibrozil and simvastatin? Explain.

8. J.H. is on vacation and does not have enough simvastatin tablets. What should he do?

Study Questions

1. The client has a serum cholesterol level of 265 mg/dl, a triglyceride level of 235 mg/dl, and an LDL level of 180 mg/dl. Do these serum levels indicate hypolipidemia, normolipidemia, or hyperlipidemia? What nonpharmacologic measure should the nurse suggest that can aid in decreasing blood lipids?

2. Explain how the statin drugs decrease cholesterol.

3. Which serum levels should be monitored when the client is taking statin drugs?

4. What severe skeletal muscle adverse reaction could occur?

5. Name the "friendly" lipoprotein. The LDL desirable value level should be _____.

6. What are the uses of peripheral vasodilators? What two common side effects can occur?

Thirteen

Gastrointestinal Agents

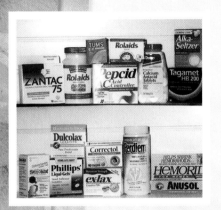

The gastrointestinal (GI) system (tract), comprising the alimentary canal and the digestive tract, begins at the oral cavity of the mouth and ends at the anus. Major structures of the GI system are (1) the oral cavity (mouth, tongue, and pharynx), (2) the esophagus, (3) the stomach, (4) the small intestine (duodenum, jejunum, and ileum), (5) the large intestine (cecum, colon, and rectum), and (6) the anus. The accessory organs and glands that contribute to the digestive process are (1) the salivary glands, (2) the pancreas, (3) the gallbladder, and (4) the liver (Figure XIII–1). The main functions of the GI system are digestion of food particles and absorption of the digestive contents (nutrients, electrolytes, minerals, and fluids) into the circulatory system for cellular use. Digestion and absorption take place in the small intestine and, to a lesser extent, in the stomach. Undigested material passes through the lower intestinal tract with the aid of peristalsis to the rectum and anus, where it is excreted as feces, or stool.

Oral Cavity

The oral cavity, or mouth, starts the digestive process by (1) breaking up food into smaller particles; (2) adding saliva, which contains the enzyme amylase for digesting starch (the beginning of the digestive process); and (3) swallowing, a voluntary movement of food that becomes involuntary (peristalsis) in the esophagus, stomach, and intestines. Swallowing occurs in the pharynx (throat), which connects the mouth and esophagus.

Esophagus

The esophagus, a tube that extends from the pharynx to the stomach, is composed of striated muscle in its upper portion and smooth muscle in its lower portion. The inner lining of the esophagus is a mucous membrane that secretes mucus. The peristaltic process of contraction begins in the esophagus and ends in the lower large intestine. There are two sphincters: the superior esophageal (hyperpharyngeal) sphincter and the lower esophageal sphincter. The lower esophageal sphincter prevents gastric reflux into the esophagus, a condition called *reflux esophagitis*.

Stomach

The stomach is a hollow organ that lies between the esophagus and the intestine. The body of the stomach has lesser and greater curvatures. It can hold 1000 to 2000 ml of gastric contents and empties in 2 to 6 hours (average is 3 to 4 hours), depending on gastric content and motility. Two sphincters, the *cardiac sphincter*, which lies at the upper opening of the stomach, and the *pyloric sphincter*, located at the lower portion of the stomach or the head of the duodenum, regulate the entrance of food into the stomach.

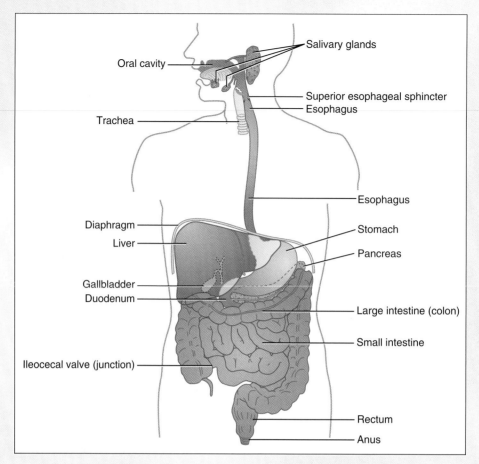

FIGURE XIII–1 The gastrointestinal system and alimentary canal.

The interior lining of the stomach has mucosal folds that contain glands that secrete gastric juices. The four types of cells in the stomach mucosa that secrete these juices are (1) *chief cells,* which secrete the proenzyme pepsinogen (pepsin); (2) *parietal cells,* which secrete hydrochloric acid (HCl); (3) *gastrin-producing cells,* which secrete gastrin, a hormone that regulates enzyme release during digestion; and (4) *mucus-producing cells* that release mucus to protect the stomach lining, which extends into the duodenum.

Small Intestine

The small intestine begins at the pyloric sphincter of the stomach and extends to the ileocecal valve at the cecum. Most drug absorption occurs in the duodenum, but lipid-soluble drugs and alcohol are absorbed from the stomach. The lower digestive process begins in the stomach, but most of the digestive contents are absorbed from the small intestine. The duodenum releases the hormone secretin, which suppresses gastric acid secretion, causing the intestinal juices to have a higher pH than the gastric juices. The intestinal cells also release the hormone cholecystokinin, which in turn stimulates the release of pancreatic enzymes and the contraction of the gallbladder to release bile into the duodenum. Hormones, bile, and pancreatic enzymes (trypsin, chymotrypsin, lipase, and amylase) complete the

digestion of carbohydrates, protein, and fat in preparation for absorption.

Large Intestine

The large intestine accepts undigested material from the small intestine, absorbs water, secretes mucus, and with peristaltic contractions moves the remaining intestinal contents to the rectum for elimination. Defecation completes the process.

Drugs For Gastrointestinal Disorders

Vomiting, diarrhea, and constipation are GI problems that frequently require drug intervention. Chapter 45, Drugs for Gastrointestinal Tract Disorders, describes the antiemetics used to control vomiting. This chapter also discusses emetics used to eliminate ingested toxins and drugs, antidiarrheal drugs, and laxatives. The nursing process is considered in relation to each of these drug groups.

Chapter 46, Antiulcer Drugs, discusses drugs used to prevent and treat peptic ulcers (gastric and duodenal). These drugs include tranquilizers, anticholinergics, antacids, histamine$_2$ blockers, proton pump inhibitors, pepsin inhibitor, and prostaglandin analogue antiulcer drug.

45 Drugs for Gastrointestinal Tract Disorders

ELECTRONIC RESOURCES

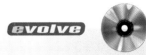

Additional information can be found on the companion website at *http://evolve.elsevier.com/KeeHayes/pharmacology/* or on the companion CD-ROM, which includes:
- *NCLEX-style examination review questions*
- *Pharmacology animations*
- *Medication error and IV therapy checklists*
- *Medication calculation problems*
- *Electronic calculators*

OUTLINE

OBJECTIVES

- Identify causes of vomiting, diarrhea, and constipation.
- Explain the action and side effects of antiemetics, emetics, antidiarrheals, and laxatives.
- Describe the nursing process, including client teaching, of antiemetics, emetics, antidiarrheals, and laxatives.
- Identify contraindications to the use of antiemetics, emetics, antidiarrheals, and laxatives.

TERMS

adsorbents	cathartics	diarrhea	opiates
antidiarrheals	chemoreceptor trigger	emetics	osmotics
antiemetics	zone (CTZ)	emollients	purgatives
cannabinoids	constipation	laxatives	vomiting center

Introduction

Drug groups used to correct or control vomiting, diarrhea, and constipation are antiemetics, emetics, antidiarrheals, and laxatives. Each of these drug groups is discussed separately. Drugs used to treat peptic ulcers are discussed in Chapter 46, Antiulcer Drugs.

Vomiting

Vomiting (emesis), the expulsion of gastric contents, has a multitude of causes, including motion sickness, viral and bacterial infection, food intolerance, surgery, pregnancy, pain, shock, effects of selected drugs (e.g., antineoplastics), radiation, and disturbances of the middle ear that affect equilibrium. Nausea, a queasy sensation, may or may not precede the expulsion. The cause of the vomiting must be identified. Antiemetics can mask the underlying cause of vomiting and should not be used until the cause has been determined unless the vomiting is so severe as to cause dehydration and electrolyte imbalance.

Two major cerebral centers—the **chemoreceptor trigger zone (CTZ)**, which lies near the medulla, and the **vomiting center** in the medulla—cause vomiting when stimulated (Figure 45–1). The CTZ receives most of the impulses from drugs, toxins, and the vestibular center in the ear and transmits them to the vomiting center. The neurotransmitter dopamine stimulates the CTZ, which in turn stimulates the vomiting center. Levodopa, a drug with dopamine-like properties, can cause vomiting by stimulating the CTZ. Some sensory impulses, such as odor, smell, taste, and gastric mucosal irritation, are transmitted directly to the vomiting center. The neurotransmitter acetylcholine is also a vomiting stimulant. When the vomiting center is stimulated, the motor neuron responds by causing contraction of the diaphragm, the anterior abdominal muscles, and the stomach. The glottis closes, the abdominal wall moves upward, and vomiting occurs.

Nonpharmacologic measures should be used first when nausea and vomiting occur. If the nonpharmacologic measures are not effective, antiemetics are combined with nonpharmacologic measures. The two major groups of antiemetics are *nonprescription* (antihistamines, bismuth subsalicylate, phosphorated carbohydrate solution) and *prescription* (antihistamines, dopamine antagonists, benzodiazepines, serotonin antagonists, glucocorticoids, cannabinoids, and miscellaneous antiemetics).

Nonpharmacologic Measures

The nonpharmacologic methods of decreasing nausea and vomiting include administration of weak tea, flattened carbonated beverage, gelatin, Gatorade, and Pedialyte (for use in children). Crackers and dry toast may be helpful. When dehydration becomes severe, intravenous (IV) fluids are needed to restore body fluid balance.

Nonprescription Antiemetics

Nonprescription **antiemetics** (antivomiting agents) can be purchased as over-the-counter (OTC) drugs. These drugs are frequently used to prevent motion sickness and have minimal effect on controlling severe vomiting resulting from anticancer agents (antineoplastics), radiation, and toxins. To prevent motion sickness, the antiemetic should be taken 30 minutes before travel. These drugs are not effective in relieving motion sickness if taken after vomiting has occurred.

Selected antihistamine antiemetics such as dimenhydrinate (Dramamine), cyclizine hydrochloride (Marezine), meclizine hydrochloride (Antivert), and diphenhydramine hydrochloride (Benadryl) can be purchased OTC to prevent nausea, vomiting, and dizziness (vertigo) caused by motion by inhibiting vestibular stimulation in the middle

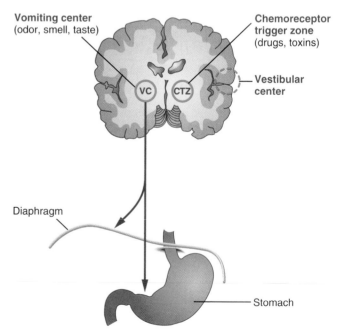

FIGURE 45–1 The chemoreceptor trigger zone and vomiting center.

ear. Benadryl is also used to prevent or alleviate allergic reactions to drugs, insects, and food by acting as an antagonist to the histamine$_1$ (H$_1$) receptors.

The side effects of antihistamine antiemetics are similar to those of anticholinergics: drowsiness, dryness of the mouth, and constipation. Table 45–1 lists the nonprescription antihistamines used for vomiting caused by motion sickness.

Several nonprescription drugs such as bismuth subsalicylate (Pepto-Bismol) act directly on the gastric mucosa to suppress vomiting. They are marketed in liquid and chewable tablet forms and can be taken for gastric discomfort or diarrhea. Phosphorated carbohydrate solution (Emetrol), a hyperosmolar carbohydrate, decreases nausea and vomiting by changing the gastric pH; it may also decrease smooth-muscle contraction of the stomach. Its effectiveness as an antiemetic has not been verified. Clients with diabetes mellitus should avoid this drug because of its high sugar content.

Antiemetics were once frequently used for the treatment of nausea and vomiting during the first trimester of pregnancy, but they are no longer recommended because they may cause harm to the fetus. Instead, nonpharmacologic methods should be used to alleviate nausea and vomiting during pregnancy, and OTC antiemetics should be avoided. If the vomiting becomes severe and threatens the well-being of the mother and fetus, an antiemetic such as trimethobenzamide (Tigan) can be administered, although this drug is classified as pregnancy category C. Other antiemetics may be prescribed cautiously.

Prescription Antiemetics

Common prescription antiemetics are classified into the following groups: (1) antihistamines, (2) anticholinergics, (3) dopamine antagonists, (4) benzodiazepines, (5) serotonin antagonists, (6) glucocorticoids, (7) cannabinoids (for clients with cancer), and (8) miscellaneous. Many of these drugs act as antagonists to dopamine, histamine, serotonin, and acetylcholine, which are associated with vomiting. Antihistamines and anticholinergics act primarily on the vomiting center; they also act by decreasing stimulation of the CTZ and vestibular pathways. The cannabinoids act on the cerebral cortex. Phenothiazines and the miscellaneous antiemetics, such as diphenidol, metoclopramide, and trimethobenzamide, act on the CTZ center. Drug combination therapy is commonly used to manage chemotherapy-induced nausea and vomiting. Lorazepam (Ativan), glucocorticoids, and serotonin (5–HT$_3$) receptor antagonists are quite effective in combination therapy. Lorazepam, haloperidol, and glucocorticoids are not approved by the Food and Drug Administration (FDA) as antiemetics but are extremely effective when combined for this unlabeled use.

Antihistamines and Anticholinergics

Only a few prescription antihistamines and anticholinergics are used in the treatment of nausea and vomiting. Table 45–2 lists these drugs and their dosages, uses, and considerations.

Table 45–1

Nonprescription Antiemetics: Antihistamine

Generic (Brand)	Route and Dosage	Uses and Considerations
Motion Sickness		
buclizine HCl (Bucladin-S Softab)	*Prophylaxis:* A: PO: 50 mg 0.5 h before travel; may repeat in 4-6 h	Prevention of motion sickness that may cause nausea and vomiting. Drowsiness and dry mouth can occur. Avoid taking alcohol and central nervous system depressants. *Pregnancy category:* C; PB: UK; t$^{1}/_2$: UK
cyclizine HCl (Marezine)	A: PO: 50 mg 0.5 h before travel; may repeat in 4-6 h; *max:* 200 mg/d IM: 50 mg q4-6h PRN C: 6-12 y: PO: 25 mg daily/ t.i.d. *Postoperative vomiting:* A: IM: 50 mg 0.5 h before surgery ends; may repeat q4-6h PRN	Similar to buclizine. Has been used for postoperative nausea and vomiting. *Pregnancy category:* B; PB: UK; t$^{1}/_2$: UK
dimenhydrinate (Calm-X, Dimetabs, Dramamine)	A: PO: 50-100 mg q4-6h; *max:* 400 mg/d; IM/IV: 50 mg PRN C: 6-12 y: PO: 25-50 mg PRN; *max:* 150 mg/d C: <2 y: Not recommended	Primarily used to prevent motion sickness. Drowsiness, dizziness, dry mouth, and hypotension may occur. *Pregnancy category:* B; PB: UK; t$^{1}/_2$: UK
meclizine HCl (Antivert, Antrizine, Bonine)	A & C >12 y: PO: 25-50 mg 1 h before travel, after meal; may repeat q24h *Vertigo:* A: PO: 25-100 mg/d in divided doses	Prevention of nausea, vomiting, and dizziness. Drowsiness and dry mouth may occur. *Pregnancy category:* B; PB: UK; t$^{1}/_2$: 6 h

A, Adult; *C,* child; *d,* day; *h,* hour; *IM,* intramuscular; *max,* maximum; *PB,* protein-binding; *PO,* by mouth; *PRN,* as needed; *t$^{1}/_2$,* half-life; *t.i.d.,* three times a day; *UK,* unknown; *y,* year; >, greater than; <, less than.

Table 45–2

Prescription Antiemetics

Generic (Brand)	Route and Dosage	Uses and Considerations
Prescription Antihistamines		
hydroxyzine (Vistaril, Atarax)	A: PO/IM: 25–100 mg t.i.d. or q.i.d. PRN	For postoperative nausea and vomiting, vertigo (dizziness). Given preoperatively with narcotics to decrease nausea. Give hydroxyzine deep IM. Drowsiness and dry mouth usually occur. *Pregnancy category*: C; PB: UK; t$\frac{1}{2}$: 3 h
promethazine (Phenergan)	See Prototype Drug Chart 45–1	
Anticholinergic		
scopolamine (Transderm-Scop)	A: transdermal patch Deliver: 0.5 mg in 3 d	For motion sickness. Has numerous anticholinergic side effects. One patch behind ear at least 4 hours before antiemetic effect is required. Patch is effective for 3 days. Alternate ears if using for longer than 3 days. Wash hands after applying patch disc. Wear no more than one disc/patch at a time. *Pregnancy category*: C; PB: <25%; t$\frac{1}{2}$: 8 h
Dopamine Antagonists		
Phenothiazines		
prochlorperazine maleate (Compazine)	A: PO/IM: 5-10 mg t.i.d.-q.i.d., PRN (give deep IM) SR: 10 mg q12h PR: 5-25 mg PRN C: PO/Rect: 2.5 mg b.i.d.-t.i.d.	Primary use is for severe nausea and vomiting. Secondary use is to reduce anxiety and tension and for psychosis. Drowsiness, dizziness, EPS, and dry mouth may occur. *Pregnancy category*: C; PB: >90%; t$\frac{1}{2}$: 23 h
promethazine (Phenergan)	See Prototype Drug Chart 45–1.	
Butyrophenones		
droperidol (Inapsine)	A: IM/IV: 2.5-10 mg, 0.5-1 h before surgery C: 2-12 y: IM/IV: 0.088-0.165 mg/kg, 0.5-1 h before surgery C: <2 y: Not recommended	Prevention of nausea and vomiting during surgical and diagnostic procedures. May cause hypotension, tachycardia, and EPS. *Pregnancy category*: C; PB: UK; t$\frac{1}{2}$: 2.5 h
Benzodiazepine		
lorazepam (Ativan)	A: PO: 2-6 mg/d in 2-3 divided doses; *max*: 10 mg/d	For prevention of nausea and vomiting resulting from cancer chemotherapy. It is usually administered with an antiemetic such as metoclopramide. *Pregnancy category*: D; PB: 85%; t$\frac{1}{2}$: 10-20 h
Serotonin (5-HT$_3$) Receptor Antagonist		
dolasetron mesylate (Anzemet)	*Cancer chemotherapy:* A: PO/IV: 100 mg, 1 h before chemotherapy C: >2 y: PO/IV: 1.8 mg/kg 1 h before chemotherapy A & C: PO/IV: *max*: 100 mg	To prevent nausea and vomiting before chemotherapy. Drug can also be used in pre- and postoperative surgery to prevent and treat nausea and vomiting. It acts on the serotonin 5-HT$_3$ receptor in the stomach and the CTZ. *Pregnancy category*: B; PB: UK; t$\frac{1}{2}$: 10 min to 7 h

A, Adult; *a.c.*, before meals; *AIDS*, acquired immunodeficiency syndrome; *b.i.d.*, two times a day; C, child; *CNS*, central nervous system; *CSS*, Controlled Substances Schedule; *CTZ*, chemoreceptor trigger zone; *d*, day; *EPS*, extrapyramidal symptoms; *h*, hour; *IM*, intramuscular; *IV*, intravenous; *max*, maximum; *min*, minute; *PB*, protein-binding; *PO*, by mouth; *PR*, per rectum; *PRN*, as needed; *q.i.d.*, four times a day; *sec*, second; *SR*, sustained release; t$\frac{1}{2}$, half-life; *t.i.d.*, three times a day; *UK*, unknown; *y*, year; >, greater than; <, less than.

Side Effects and Adverse Reactions

Side effects include drowsiness, which can be a major problem, dry mouth, blurred vision caused by pupillary dilation, tachycardia (with anticholinergic use), and constipation. These drugs should *not* be used in clients with glaucoma.

Dopamine Antagonists

These agents suppress emesis by blocking dopamine$_2$ receptors in the CTZ. The categories of dopamine antagonists include phenothiazines, butyrophenones, and

metoclopramide. Common side effects of the dopamine antagonists are extrapyramidal symptoms (EPS), which are caused by blocking the dopamine receptors, and hypotension. See Chapter 25 (Antipsychotics and Anxiolytics) for a more detailed description of EPS and phenothiazines.

Phenothiazine Antiemetics

Selected piperazine phenothiazines are used to treat nausea and vomiting resulting from surgery, anesthetics, chemotherapy, and radiation sickness. They act by in-

Table 45-2

Prescription Antiemetics—cont'd

Generic (Brand)	Route and Dosage	Uses and Considerations
Serotonin (5-HT₃) Receptor Antagonist—cont'd		
granisetron (Kytril)	A: PO: 1 mg b.i.d. (1 h before and 12 h after chemotherapy) A: IV: 10 mcg/kg/30 min before chemotherapy	Prevention of nausea and vomiting caused by cancer chemotherapy. Acts on the CTZ and vomiting center. Headache may occur. *Pregnancy category:* B; PB: 65%; t$\frac{1}{2}$: 4-10 h
ondansetron HCl (Zofran)	A: PO: 8 mg b.i.d. (first dose 30 min before, and 8 h and 16 h after chemotherapy) A: IV: 0.15 mg/kg/30 min before chemotherapy; then 4 and 8 h after (total, 3 doses)	For nausea and vomiting related to cancer chemotherapy, especially treatment with cisplatin. *Pregnancy category:* B; PB: 70%-75%; t$\frac{1}{2}$: 4 h
palonosetron (Aloxi)	A: IV: 0.25 mg over 30 sec, 30 min before chemotherapy	To prevent nausea and vomiting associated with cancer chemotherapy. Pregnancy category: B; PB: 62%; t$\frac{1}{2}$: 40 h
Cannabinoids		
dronabinol (Marinol) CSS II	*Chemotherapy-induced nausea:* A: PO: 5 mg/m² 1-3 h before chemotherapy; then q2-4h after; *max:* 15 mg/m²/dose	For nausea and vomiting caused by cancer chemotherapy. Taken before and for 24 hours after chemotherapy. It can be an appetite stimulant for clients with AIDS. Common side effects include drowsiness, dizziness, dry mouth, impaired thinking, and euphoria. *Pregnancy category:* B; PB: 98%; t$\frac{1}{2}$: 20-24 h
Miscellaneous		
diphenidol HCl (Vontrol)	*Nausea, vomiting, and vertigo:* A: PO: 25-50 mg q4h PRN; *max:* 300 mg/d C: >6 y: PO: 0.9 mg/kg; *max:* 5.5 mg/kg/d	For nausea, vomiting, and vertigo because of Ménière's disease and surgery of the middle ear. *Pregnancy category:* C; PB: UK; t$\frac{1}{2}$: 4 h
metoclopramide HCl (Reglan)	A: PO: 10 mg a.c. and at bedtime IV: 1-2 mg/kg 30 min before chemotherapy; then repeat q2h for two doses; then q3h for three doses; infuse diluted solution over not less than 15 min	For nausea and vomiting related to cancer chemotherapy treatment. It increases gastric and intestinal emptying. Avoid alcohol and CNS depressants. EPS may occur. *Pregnancy category:* B; PB: 30%; t$\frac{1}{2}$: 4-7 h
trimethobenzamide HCl (Tigan, Arrestin, Ticon)	A: PO: 250 mg t.i.d.-q.i.d. IM/PR: 200 mg t.i.d.-q.i.d. C: 15-40 kg: PO/PR: 15-20 mg/kg/d divided in three to four doses or 100-200 mg, t.i.d.-q.i.d.	For postoperative nausea and vomiting, motion sickness, and vertigo. Avoid with CNS depressants and if sensitive to benzocaine or similar local anesthetics. *Pregnancy category:* C; PB: UK; t$\frac{1}{2}$: UK
aprepitant (Emend)	A: PO: 125 mg on day 1, 80 mg on days 2 and 3	For nausea and vomiting related to cancer chemotherapy. *Pregnancy category:* B; PB: 95%; t$\frac{1}{2}$: 9-13 h

hibiting the CTZ. When used in clients with cancer, these drugs are commonly given the night before treatment, the day of the treatment, and for 24 hours after treatment. Not all phenothiazines are effective antiemetic agents. When prescribed for vomiting, the drug dosage is usually smaller than when used for psychiatric disorders.

Chlorpromazine (Thorazine) and prochlorperazine edisylate (Compazine) were the first phenothiazines used for both psychosis and vomiting. Promethazine (Phenergan), a phenothiazine introduced as an antihistamine in the 1940s, has a sedative effect and can also be used for motion sickness as well as management of nausea and vomiting. Promethazine is the most frequently prescribed antiemetic drug. Prototype Drug Chart 45-1 describes the action and effects of promethazine.

Pharmacokinetics

Promethazine is readily absorbed in the gastrointestinal (GI) tract. It has 60% to 90% protein-binding capacity. Promethazine is metabolized by the liver and excreted in the urine and feces.

Pharmacodynamics

Promethazine blocks the H₁-receptor sites on effector cells and impedes histamine-mediated responses. The onset of action of oral and intramuscular (IM) administration is 20 minutes, and the duration of action is from 2 to 8 hours. The onset of action of intravenous (IV) promethazine is 5 minutes; the duration of action is the same as the oral preparation.

Drug and Laboratory Interactions

Central nervous system (CNS) depression increases when promethazine is taken with alcohol, narcotics, sedative-hypnotics, and general anesthetics. Anticholinergic effects increase when promethazine is combined with antihista-

PROTOTYPE DRUG CHART 45–1

PROMETHAZINE HCl

Drug Class

Antiemetic: phenothiazine
Trade Name: Phenergan
Pregnancy Category: C

Dosage

A: PO/PR/IM/IV: 12.5-25 mg q4-6h PRN
C: PO/PR/IM/IV: 0.25-0.5 mg/kg q4-6h PRN

Contraindications

Hypersensitivity, narrow-angle glaucoma, severe liver
    disease, intestinal obstruction, blood dyscrasias, bone
    marrow depression
Caution: Cardiovascular disease, liver dysfunction, asthma,
    respiratory dysfunction, hypertension, elderly and
    debilitated clients

Drug-Lab-Food Interactions

Drug: Increases CNS depression and anticholinergic effects
    when taken with alcohol and other CNS depressants
Lab: False pregnancy test

Pharmacokinetics

Absorption: PO: easily absorbed from GI tract
Distribution: PB: 60%-90%
Metabolism: t½: UK
Excretion: In urine and feces

Pharmacodynamics

PO: Onset: 20 min
    Peak: UK
    Duration: 2-8 h
IM: Onset: 20 min
    Peak: UK
    Duration: 2-8 h
IV: Onset: 5 min
    Peak: UK
    Duration: 2-8 h
PR: Onset: 20 min
    Peak: UK
    Duration: 2-8 h

Therapeutic Effects/Uses

To treat and prevent motion sickness, nausea, and vomiting
Mode of Action: Blocks H, receptor sites; inhibits chemoreceptor trigger zone

Side Effects

Drowsiness, confusion, anorexia, dry mouth and eyes,
    constipation, blurred vision, photosensitivity,
    hypertension, hypotension, transient leukopenia,
    urinary retention

Adverse Reactions

Extrapyramidal syndrome (tardive dyskinesia, akathisia)
Life-threatening: Agranulocytosis, respiratory depression

A, Adult; *C,* child; *CNS,* central nervous system; *GI,* gastrointestinal; *h,* hour; *IM,* intramuscular; *IV,* intravenous; *min,* minute; *PB,* protein-binding; *PO,* by mouth; *PR,* per rectum; *PRN,* as needed; *t½,* half-life; *UK,* unknown; >, greater than; <, less than.

mines, anticholinergics such as atropine, and other phenothiazines. Promethazine may interfere with urinary pregnancy tests, producing false results.

Side Effects and Adverse Reactions

Phenothiazines have antihistamine and anticholinergic properties. The side effects of phenothiazine antiemetics are moderate sedation, hypotension, EPS, CNS effects (restlessness, weakness, dystonic reactions, agitation), and mild anticholinergic symptoms (dry mouth, urinary retention, constipation). Because the dose is lower for vomiting than for psychosis, the side effects are not so severe. Promethazine is relatively free of EPS at antiemetic doses. Table 45–2 lists the drug data for the phenothiazines along with other prescription antiemetics.

Butyrophenones

Haloperidol (Haldol) and droperidol (Inapsine), like phenothiazines, block the dopamine₂ receptors in the CTZ. They are used to treat postoperative nausea and vomiting and emesis associated with toxins, cancer chemotherapy, and radiation therapy. Antiemetic doses are smaller for haloperidol than required for antipsychotic effects. Like phenothiazines, EPSs are likely to occur if these drugs are used over an extended time. Hypotension may result; therefore blood pressure should be monitored.

Metoclopramide

Metoclopramide (Reglan) suppresses emesis by blocking the dopamine receptors in the CTZ. It is used in the treatment of postoperative emesis, cancer chemotherapy, and radiation therapy. High doses can cause sedation and diarrhea. With this agent, the occurrence of EPS is more prevalent in children than in adults. Metoclopramide should not be given if the client has GI obstruction, hemorrhage, or perforation.

Benzodiazepines

Selected benzodiazepines indirectly control nausea and vomiting that may occur with cancer chemotherapy. Lorazepam (Ativan) is the choice drug. Previously, diazepam (Valium) was the desired benzodiazepine. Lorazepam effectively provides emesis control, sedation, anxiety reduction, and amnesia in combination with a glucocorticoid and serotonin 5-HT$_3$ receptor antagonist.

Serotonin (5-HT$_3$) Receptor Antagonists

Serotonin antagonists suppress nausea and vomiting by blocking the serotonin receptors (5-HT$_3$) in the CTZ and the afferent vagal nerve terminals in the upper GI tract.

Serotonin antagonists—ondansetron (Zofran), granisetron (Kytril), dolasetron (Anzemet), and Palonosetron (Aloxi)—are the most effective of all antiemetics in suppressing nausea and vomiting caused by cancer chemotherapy-induced emesis or emetogenic anticancer drugs. Ondansetron (the first serotonin antagonist), granisetron, and dolasetron do not block the dopamine receptors; therefore, they do not cause EPS as do the phenothiazine antiemetics. These drugs can be administered orally and IV. They are also effective in preventing nausea and vomiting before and after surgery. Common side effects include headache, diarrhea, dizziness, and fatigue.

Glucocorticoids (Corticosteroids)

Dexamethasone (Decadron) and methylprednisolone (Solu-Medrol) are two agents that are effective in suppressing emesis associated with cancer chemotherapy. These drugs are administered IV. Because these glucocorticoids are administered IV and for only a short while, the side effects normally caused by glucocorticoids may be diminished. Glucocorticoids are discussed in Chapter 49, Endocrine Pharmacology: Pituitary, Thyroid, Parathyroids, and Adrenals.

Cannabinoids

Cannabinoids, the active ingredients in marijuana, were approved for clinical use in 1985 to alleviate nausea and vomiting resulting from cancer treatment. These agents may be prescribed for clients receiving chemotherapy who do not respond to or are unable to take other antiemetics. They are contraindicated for clients with psychiatric disorders. Cannabinoids can be used as an appetite stimulant for clients with acquired immunodeficiency syndrome (AIDS). The cannabinoid dronabinol (Marinol) is described in Table 45–2.

Side Effects and Adverse Reactions

Side effects occurring as a result of cannabinoid use include mood changes, euphoria, drowsiness, dizziness, headaches, depersonalization, nightmares, confusion, in-

coordination, memory lapse, dry mouth, orthostatic hypotension or hypertension, and tachycardia. Less common symptoms are depression, anxiety, and manic psychosis.

Miscellaneous Antiemetics

Diphenidol (Vontrol) and trimethobenzamide (Tigan) are miscellaneous antiemetics because they do not act strictly as antihistamines, anticholinergics, or phenothiazines. These drugs suppress the impulses to the CTZ. Diphenidol also prevents vertigo by inhibiting impulses to the vestibular area.

Side Effects and Adverse Reactions

The side effects and adverse reactions of the miscellaneous antiemetics are drowsiness and anticholinergic symptoms (dry mouth, increased heart rate, urine retention, constipation, blurred vision). Trimethobenzamide can cause hypotension, diarrhea, and EPS (abnormal involuntary movements, postural disturbances, and alteration in muscle tone).

Table 45–2 lists the drug data for the miscellaneous antiemetics along with other prescription antiemetics.

Nursing Process

Antiemetics

ASSESSMENT

- Determine a history of the onset, frequency, and amount of vomiting and contents of the vomitus. If appropriate, elicit from client possible causative factors such as food (seafood, mayonnaise).
- Obtain a history of present health problems. Clients with glaucoma should avoid many of the antiemetics.
- Record vital signs for abnormalities and for future comparison.
- Assess urinalysis before and during therapy.

NURSING DIAGNOSES

- Nutrition, imbalanced nutrition: Less than Body Requirements
- Fluid Volume, Deficient, Risk for, related to vomiting

PLANNING

- Client will adhere to nonpharmacologic methods and/or drug regimen to alleviate vomiting.
- The underlying cause of vomiting is determined and corrected.

NURSING INTERVENTIONS

- Check vital signs. If vomiting is severe, dehydration may occur, and shocklike symptoms may be present.
- Monitor bowel sounds for hypoactivity or hyperactivity.
- Provide mouth care after vomiting. Encourage client to maintain oral hygiene.

Client Teaching

General

- Instruct client to store drug in tight, light-resistant container if required.
- Teach client to avoid OTC preparations.
- Direct client not to consume alcohol while taking antiemetics. Alcohol can intensify the sedative effect.
- Advise pregnant women to avoid antiemetics during the first trimester because of possible teratogenic effects on the fetus. Encourage pregnant women to seek medical advice about OTC or prescription antiemetics.

Side Effects

- Tell client to report sore throat, fever, and mouth sores; notify health care provider and have blood drawn for a complete blood count (CBC).
- Alert client to avoid driving a motor vehicle or engaging in dangerous activities because drowsiness is common with antiemetics. If drowsiness becomes a problem, a decrease in dosage may be indicated.
- Warn client with a hepatic disorder to seek medical advice before taking phenothiazines. Instruct client to report dizziness.
- Suggest to client nonpharmacologic methods of alleviating nausea and vomiting such as flattened carbonated beverages, weak tea, crackers, and dry toast.

Cultural Considerations

- Respect clients' cultural beliefs and alternative methods for treating nausea and vomiting. Discuss with clients the safety of their methods, other nondrug methods, and the purpose of an antiemetic if prescribed.
- An interpreter may be needed to assist non–English-speaking clients to understand the drug schedule for prescribed antiemetics and their side effects.

EVALUATION

- Evaluate the effectiveness of the nonpharmacologic methods or antiemetic by noting the absence of vomiting. Identify any side effects that may result from drug.

Emetics

Emetics are drugs used to induce vomiting. When an individual has consumed certain toxic substances, induced vomiting (emesis) may be indicated to expel the substance before absorption occurs. There are many ways to induce vomiting without using drugs, such as putting the finger in the back part of the throat.

Vomiting should not be induced if caustic substances, such as ammonia, chlorine bleach, lye, toilet cleaners, or battery acid, have been ingested. Regurgitating these substances can cause additional injury to the esophagus. To prevent aspiration, vomiting should also be avoided if petroleum distillates are ingested; these include gasoline, kerosene, paint thinners, and lighter fluid. Activated charcoal is given when emesis is contraindicated.

Ipecac

Ipecac is an OTC drug. Most health care providers instruct parents to keep ipecac in the household; however, it should be kept out of the reach of children. When the client purchases ipecac, instruct the client to get ipecac *syrup* and *not* ipecac fluid extract, which is more potent. Ipecac syrup induces vomiting by stimulating the CTZ in the medulla and acting directly on the gastric mucosa. Ipecac should be taken with a glass of water or other fluid (do not give milk or carbonated beverages). If vomiting does not occur in 20 to 30 minutes, repeat the dose. The absorption of ipecac is minimal when vomiting is induced. However, when ipecac does not induce vomiting and is absorbed, cardiotoxicity may occur. When vomiting is not induced, clients should be treated with activated charcoal or gastric lavage and cardiovascular support if necessary. Individuals with bulimia and anorexia nervosa may develop cardiomyopathy and death following frequent abuse of ipecac. Prototype Drug Chart 45–2 gives the drug data for ipecac.

Pharmacokinetics

Following a dose of ipecac, eight or more ounces of tepid water or juice should be given. The absorption of ipecac is minimal. The protein-binding is unknown, and the half-life is short (Table 45–3).

Pharmacodynamics

Ipecac acts on the CTZ in the medulla and on the gastric mucosa to induce vomiting. The onset of action for ipecac is 15 to 30 minutes, and the duration of action is 20 to 25 minutes.

Nursing Process

Emetic: Ipecac Syrup

ASSESSMENT

- Determine the toxic substance ingested. Do *not* induce vomiting if caustics or petroleum products have been ingested.
- Check the time elapsed since the ingestion; lavage may be indicated.
- Record client's vital signs. Report abnormal findings.

NURSING DIAGNOSES

- Risk for absorption of toxic substance
- Risk for infection

PLANNING

- Toxic substance will be expelled before absorption.
- Client will have minimal or no adverse effects of the toxic substance.

NURSING INTERVENTIONS

- Call the poison control center to report the toxic ingestion and for instructions.
- Monitor vital signs. Report changes.

■ Offer sufficient fluids with ipecac syrup; warm clear liquids are best. Avoid carbonated beverages because they cause abdominal distention. Do *not* give milk or milk products. Position client in high Fowler's position. Fluids dilute the toxic substance and are vehicles for expelling the substance. If emetic is unsuccessful, gastric lavage may be performed or activated charcoal may be given to adsorb the toxic substance.

■ Do *not* offer ipecac syrup or fluids to a semiconscious or unconscious person because of the danger of aspiration. Gastric lavage is usually performed in such cases.

■ Do *not* induce vomiting if the toxic substance is a caustic or a petroleum distillate.

■ Prepare for forceful vomiting; have large basin ready, and move clothing to protected area.

Client Teaching

General

* Instruct the parent or other family member to have ipecac syrup on hand. Explain that ipecac syrup is an OTC drug.
* Explain to the parent that ipecac should be given with sufficient fluids. Advise that ipecac syrup is *not* given if the toxic substance is a caustic or petroleum product.

* Advise client or parents *never* to remove toxic substances from original labeled containers. Instruct parents on the use of childproof caps for future prevention.
* Inform the parent to keep readily available the telephone numbers of the poison control center and all emergency services.

Cultural Considerations ⊕

* Recognize that clients from various cultural groups may need additional guidance in regard to (1) storing drugs and chemical agents out of the reach of children, (2) giving first aid related to the substance the child ingested, and (3) knowing how to contact a poison center. A written information sheet in client's language may be beneficial.

EVALUATION

■ Evaluate the effectiveness of ipecac syrup for inducing vomiting.

■ Continue monitoring vital signs.

■ Continue monitoring for signs and symptoms related to the effect of ingested substance.

PROTOTYPE DRUG CHART 45–2

IPECAC SYRUP

Drug Class	**Dosage**
Emetic *Pregnancy Category:* C	A: PO: 15-30 ml, followed by 200-300 ml tepid water C: >1-12 y: PO: 15 ml, followed by 200-300 ml tepid water C: <1 y: PO: 5-10 ml, followed by 100-200 ml tepid water Repeat initial dose if vomiting does not occur within 30 min only if the child is older than 1 y.
Contraindications	**Drug-Lab-Food Interactions**
Hypersensitivity, depressed gag reflex, unconsciousness or semiconsciousness, poisoning with caustic or petroleum products, convulsions	*Drug: Decrease* effect with activated charcoal, carbonated beverages, or milk
Pharmacokinetics	**Pharmacodynamics**
Absorption: Minimal **Distribution:** PB: UK **Metabolism:** t½: 2 h **Excretion:** GI (vomiting)	PO: Onset: 15-30 min Peak: UK Duration: 20-25 min

Therapeutic Effects/Uses

To induce vomiting after poisoning
Mode of Action: Acts on chemoreceptor trigger zone (induces vomiting) and irritates gastric mucosa

Side Effects	**Adverse Reactions**
Diarrhea, sedation, lethargy; protracted vomiting	**Life-threatening:** Cardiotoxicity if ipecac is not vomited (hypotension, tachycardia, chest pain)

A, Adult; *C*, child; *GI*, gastrointestinal; *h*, hour; *min*, minute; *PB*, protein-binding; *PO*, by mouth; *t½*, half-life; *UK*, unknown; *y*, year; >, greater than; <, less than.

Table 45–3

Emetics and Adsorbent

Generic (Brand)	Route and Dosage	Uses and Considerations
Emetics		
ipecac syrup (OTC preparation)	See Prototype Drug Chart 45–2.	
Adsorbent		
charcoal (CharcoAid, CharcoCaps)	*For poisoning, use CharcoAid:* A: PO: 30-100 g dose in 6-8 oz of water *For flatus, use CharcoCaps:* A: PO: 520 mg, after meals; repeat PRN; *max:* 4 g/d	Promotes absorption of poison/toxic substances. Promotes absorption of intestinal gas. Both drugs are not systemically absorbed. *Pregnancy category:* C; PB: NA; t$\frac{1}{2}$: NA

A, Adult; *CNS,* central nervous system; *d,* day; *max,* maximum; *NA,* not applicable; *OTC,* over-the-counter; *PB,* protein-binding; *PO,* by mouth; *PRN,* as necessary; t$\frac{1}{2}$, half-life.

Diarrhea

Diarrhea (frequent liquid stool) is a symptom of an intestinal disorder. Causes include (1) foods (spicy, spoiled), (2) fecal impaction, (3) bacteria *(Escherichia coli, Salmonella)* or virus (parvovirus, rotavirus), (4) toxins, (5) drug reaction, (6) laxative abuse, (7) malabsorption syndrome caused by lack of digestive enzymes, (8) stress and anxiety, (9) bowel tumor, and (10) inflammatory bowel disease, such as ulcerative colitis or Crohn's disease. Diarrhea can be mild to severe. Antidiarrheals are not to be used for more than 2 days and should not be used if fever is present.

Because intestinal fluids are rich in water, sodium, potassium, and bicarbonate, diarrhea can cause minor or severe dehydration and electrolyte imbalances. The loss of bicarbonate places the client at risk for developing metabolic acidosis. Clients with diarrhea should avoid foods rich in fat and milk products. Diarrhea can develop very quickly and can be life threatening to young clients and older adults, who may not be able to compensate for the fluid and electrolyte losses.

Nonpharmacologic Measures

The cause of diarrhea should be identified. Nonpharmacologic treatment for diarrhea is recommended until the underlying cause can be determined. This includes use of clear liquids and oral solutions (Gatorade; Pedialyte or Ricolyte [both for use in children]) and IV electrolyte solutions. Antidiarrheal drugs are frequently used in combination with nonpharmacologic treatment.

Traveler's Diarrhea

Traveler's diarrhea, also called *acute diarrhea* and *Montezuma's revenge,* is usually caused by *E. coli.* It ordinarily lasts less than 2 days; however, if it becomes severe, fluoroquinolone antibiotics are usually prescribed. Loperamide (Imodium) may be used to slow peristalsis and to decrease the frequency of defecation, but it can also slow the exit of the organism from the GI tract. Traveler's diarrhea can be reduced by drinking bottled water, washing fruit, and eating cooked vegetables. Meats should be cooked until well done.

Antidiarrheals

There are various **antidiarrheals** for treating diarrhea and decreasing hypermotility (increased peristalsis). Usually there is an underlying cause of the diarrhea that needs to be corrected as well. The antidiarrheals are classified as (1) opiates and opiate-related agents, (2) somatostatin analogue, (3) adsorbents, and (4) miscellaneous antidiarrheals.

Opiates and Opiate-Related Agents

Opiates decrease intestinal motility, thereby decreasing peristalsis. Constipation is a common side effect of opium preparations. Examples are tincture of opium, paregoric (camphorated opium tincture), and codeine. Opiates are frequently combined with other antidiarrheal agents. Opium antidiarrheals can cause CNS depression when taken with alcohol, sedatives, or tranquilizers. Duration of action of opiates is approximately 2 hours.

Diphenoxylate (Lomotil, Reasec [for use in Europe]) is an opiate that has less potential for causing drug dependence than other opiates such as codeine. Difenoxin (Motofen) is an active metabolite of diphenoxylate; however, it is more potent than diphenoxylate. Both drugs are combined with atropine to decrease abdominal cramping, intestinal motility, and hypersecretion. Lomotil (diphenoxylate with atropine) is frequently prescribed for "traveler's diarrhea," and Motofen (difenoxin with atropine) is prescribed to treat nonspecific and chronic diarrhea. With prolonged use of these drugs, physical dependence may occur. Diphenoxylate product is approximately 50% atropine, which will discourage against drug abuse. The action and effects of diphenoxylate with atropine (Lomotil) are listed in Prototype Drug Chart 45–3.

Loperamide (Imodium) is structurally related to diphenoxylate but can cause less CNS depression than

PROTOTYPE DRUG CHART 45–3

DIPHENOXYLATE WITH ATROPINE

Drug Class

Antidiarrheal
Trade Name: Lomotil
Pregnancy Category: C
CSS V

Dosage

A: PO: 2.5-5 mg b.i.d.-q.i.d. PRN
C: >2 y: PO: 0.3-0.4 mg/kg/d in 4 divided doses or 2 mg
    2-4 ×/d (use liquid form only; 2.5 mg/5 ml)

Contraindications

Severe hepatic or renal disease, glaucoma, severe
    electrolyte imbalance; children <2 y

Drug-Lab-Food Interactions

Drug: Increase CNS depression with alcohol, antihista-
    mines, narcotics, sedative-hypnotics; MAOIs may en-
    hance hypertensive crisis
Lab: Increase serum liver enzymes, amylase

Pharmacokinetics

Absorption: PO: Well absorbed
Distribution: PB: UK
Metabolism: t½: 2.5 h
Excretion: In feces and urine

Pharmacodynamics

PO: Onset: 45-60 min
    Peak: 2 h
    Duration: 3-4 h

Therapeutic Effects/Uses

To treat diarrhea by slowing intestinal motility
Mode of Action: Inhibition of gastric motility

Side Effects

Drowsiness, dizziness, constipation, dry mouth, weakness,
    flush, rash, blurred vision, mydriasis, urine retention

Adverse Reactions

Angioneurotic edema
Life-threatening: Paralytic ileus, toxic megacolon, severe
    allergic reaction

A, Adult; *b.i.d.,* twice a day; *C,* child; *CNS,* central nervous system; *CSS,* Controlled Substances Schedule; *d,* day; *h,* hour; *MAOIs,*
monoamine oxidase inhibitors; *min,* minute; *PB,* protein-binding; *PO,* by mouth; *PRN,* as necessary; *q.i.d.,* four times a day; *t½,*
half-life; *UK,* unknown; *y,* year; >, greater than; <, less than.

diphenoxylate and difenoxin. It can be purchased as an OTC drug, and it protects against diarrhea, reduces fecal volume, and decreases intestinal fluid and electrolyte losses.

Clients with severe hepatic impairment should not take products containing diphenoxylate, difenoxin, and loperamide. Children and older adults who take diphenoxylate are more susceptible to respiratory depression than other age groups.

Pharmacokinetics

Diphenoxylate with atropine is well absorbed from the GI tract. The diphenoxylate is metabolized by the liver mainly as metabolites. There are two half-lives: 2.5 hours for diphenoxylate and 3 to 20 hours for the diphenoxylate metabolites. The drug is excreted in the feces and urine.

Pharmacodynamics

Diphenoxylate with atropine is an opium agonist with anticholinergic properties (atropine) that decreases GI motility (peristalsis). It has a moderate onset of action of 45 to 60 minutes, and the duration of action is 3 to 4 hours. Many side effects are caused by the anticholinergic atropine. Clients with severe glaucoma should take another antidiarrheal that does not have an anticholinergic effect. If this drug is taken with alcohol, narcotics, or sedative-hypnotics, CNS depression can occur.

Somatostatin Analog

Octreotide (Sandostatin) is a somatostatin analogue that is prescribed to inhibit gastric acid, pepsinogen, gastrin, cholecystokinin, and serotonin secretions and intestinal fluid. In addition, it decreases smooth-muscle contractility. It is frequently prescribed for severe diarrhea resulting from metastatic cancer.

Adsorbents

Adsorbents act by coating the wall of the GI tract and adsorbing the bacteria or toxins that cause the diarrhea. Adsorbent antidiarrheals include kaolin and pectin. These agents are combined in Kaopectate, a mild or moderate antidiarrheal that can be purchased OTC and used in combination with other antidiarrheals. An example is Parepectolin, which contains paregoric (an opiate) and Kaopectate (an adsorbent). Bismuth salts (Pepto-Bismol) is considered an adsorbent because it adsorbs bacterial toxins. Bismuth salts can also be used for gastric discomfort. It is an OTC drug that is used for traveler's diarrhea. Colestipol and cholestyramine (Questran) are prescriptive drugs that have been used to

Table 45–4

Antidiarrheals: Opiates and Opiate Related, Somatostatin Analogue, Adsorbents, and Miscellaneous

Generic (Brand)	Route and Dosage	Uses and Considerations
Opiates and Opiate Related		
camphorated opium tincture (paregoric) CSS III	Camphorated: 5-10 ml b.i.d.-q.i.d. C: PO: 0.25-0.5 ml/kg daily-q.i.d.	To decrease incidence of diarrhea. Decreases GI peristalsis. *Pregnancy category:* B (D at term); PB: UK; t½: 2-3 h
deodorized opium tincture CSS II	A: PO: 0.6 ml or 10 gtt q.i.d. mixed with water; *max:* 6 ml/d C: PO: 0.005-0.01 ml/kg/dose q3-4 h; *max:* 6 doses/d	For acute, nonspecific diarrhea. To treat withdrawal symptoms in neonates of mothers who are addicted to opiates. Not to be used for diarrhea caused by poison. Avoid taking alcohol and CNS depressants. *Pregnancy category:* B (D at term); PB: UK; t½: 2-3 h
difenoxin and atropine (Motofen) CSS IV	A: PO: Initially: 2 mg; then 1 mg after each loose stool; *max:* 8 mg/d for 2 d C: <2 y: Not recommended	For acute nonspecific and chronic diarrhea. Combination of a synthetic narcotic and atropine. Avoid use in narrow-angle glaucoma. Dry mouth, flush, and tachycardia may occur. *Pregnancy category:* C; PB: UK; t½: 12-24 h
diphenoxylate with atropine (Lomotil) CSS V	See Prototype Drug Chart 45–3.	
loperamide HCl (Imodium)	A: PO: Initially: 4 mg; then 2 mg after each loose stool; *max:* 16 mg/d C: 2-5 y: PO: 1 mg t.i.d. C: 6-8 y: PO: 2 mg b.i.d. C: 9-12 y: PO: 2 mg t.i.d.	For diarrhea. Newest OTC drug. Does not affect the CNS. Less than 1% reaches systemic circulation. *Pregnancy category:* B; PB: 98%; t½: 7-12 h
Somatostatin Analog		
octreotide acetate (Sandostatin)	*Diarrhea related to carcinoid tumors:* A: subQ: Initially 0.05-0.1 mg/d (50-100 mcg/d) in divided doses for 2 wk; then increase according to response; *maint:* 0.1-0.6 mg/d (100-600 mcg/d) in two to four divided doses; *max:* 0.75 mcg/d (750 mcg/d)	For severe diarrhea resulting from metastatic carcinoid tumors. It suppresses secretion of serotonin, gastrin, and pancreatic peptides. *Pregnancy category:* B; PB: 65%; t½: 1.5 h
Adsorbents		
bismuth salts (Pepto-Bismol)	*Prevention of traveler's diarrhea:* A: PO: 2 tab q.i.d. a.c. and at bedtime *Treatment:* A: PO: 2 tab or 30 ml q30-60min PRN	For diarrhea, gastric distress. OTC liquid and tablet form. *Pregnancy category:* UK; PB: UK; t½: UK
kaolin-pectin (Kapectolin, Kaopectate)	A: 60-120 ml after each loose stool C: 6-12 y: 30-60 ml after each loose stool	For diarrhea. Administered after each loose stool. OTC drug. *Pregnancy category:* B; PB: 97%; t½: 7-14 h
Miscellaneous		
furazolidone (Furoxone)	A: PO: 100 mg q.i.d.; *max:* 400 mg/d C: >1 mo: PO: 5-8 mg/kg/d in four divided doses C: >5 y: 25-50 mg q.i.d.	Management of diarrhea and enteritis caused by bacteria or protozoa. Common side effects include nausea and vomiting. *Pregnancy category:* C; PB: UK; t½: UK
parepectolin CSS V	A & C: >12 y: 15-30 ml after each loose stool; *max:* 120 ml/d C: 6-12 y: 5-10 ml after each loose stool; *max:* 40 ml/d	Contains paregoric (an opiate) and Kaopectate. OTC drug; however, must be signed for at pharmacy because it contains opium. *Pregnancy category:* D; PB: UK; t½: UK

A, Adult; *a.c.,* before meals; *b.i.d.,* twice a day; *C,* child; *CNS,* central nervous system; *CSS,* Controlled Substances Schedule; *d,* day; *GI,* gastrointestinal; *h,* hour; *max,* maximum; *min,* minute; *mo,* month; *OTC,* over-the-counter; *PB,* protein-binding; *PO,* by mouth; *PRN,* as needed; *q.i.d.,* four times a day; *subQ,* subcutaneous; *t½,* half-life; *tab,* tablet; *t.i.d.,* three times a day; *UK,* unknown; *wk,* week; *y,* year; >, greater than; <, less than.

treat diarrhea when due to excess bile acids in the colon. They are effective, although they have not been approved by the Food and Drug Administration for that purpose. Table 45–4 lists the drug data for commonly used antidiarrheals.

Miscellaneous Antidiarrheals

Various miscellaneous antidiarrheals are prescribed to control diarrhea. These drugs include furazolidone, lactobacillus, and parepectolin (paregoric, kaolin, pectin, alcohol). Table 45–4 includes these drugs.

Nursing Process

Antidiarrheals

ASSESSMENT

■ Obtain a history of any viral or bacterial infection, drugs taken, and foods ingested that could be contributing factors to diarrhea. Many of the antidiarrheals are contraindicated if the client has liver disease, narcotic dependence, ulcerative colitis, or glaucoma.

■ Check vital signs to provide baseline for future comparison and to determine body fluid and electrolyte losses.

■ Determine frequency and consistency of bowel movements.

■ Assess bowel sounds. Hyperactive sounds can indicate increased intestinal motility.

■ Report if client has a narcotic drug history. If opiate or opiate-related antidiarrheals are given, drug misuse or abuse may occur.

NURSING DIAGNOSES

■ Diarrhea

■ Nutrition, Imbalanced: Less than Body Requirements

■ Fluid Volume, Imbalanced, Risk for

PLANNING

■ Client will have bowel movements that are formed.

■ Client's body fluids will be restored.

NURSING INTERVENTIONS

■ Record vital signs. Report tachycardia or a systolic blood pressure decrease of 10 to 15 mmHg. Monitor respirations. Opiates and opiate-related drugs can cause central nervous system (CNS) depression.

■ Monitor the frequency of bowel movements and bowel sounds. Notify the health care provider if intestinal hypoactivity occurs when taking drug.

■ Check for signs and symptoms of dehydration resulting from persistent diarrhea. Fluid replacement may be necessary. With prolonged diarrhea, check serum electrolytes.

■ Administer antidiarrheals cautiously to clients with glaucoma, liver disorders, or ulcerative colitis or to pregnant women.

■ Recognize that drug may need to be withheld if diarrhea continues for more than 48 hours or acute abdominal pain develops.

Client Teaching

General

• Instruct client not to take sedatives, tranquilizers, or other narcotics with drug. CNS depression may occur.

• Inform client to avoid OTC preparations; they may contain alcohol.

• Advise client to take the drug only as prescribed. Drug may be habit forming; do not exceed recommended dose.

• Encourage client to drink clear liquids. Advise the client not to ingest fried foods or milk products until after the diarrhea has stopped.

• Teach client that constipation can result from the overuse of antidiarrheal drugs.

Cultural Considerations ⊕

• While the more traditional and older individuals in some cultures do not maintain eye contact, the acculturated and more educated usually do maintain eye contact. Do not assume that lack of eye contact means that client is not listening or does not care. It might indicate respect.

EVALUATION

■ Evaluate the effectiveness of the drug; diarrhea has stopped.

■ Monitor long-term use of opiates and opiate-related drugs for possible abuse and physical dependence.

■ Continue to monitor vital signs. Report abnormal changes.

Constipation

Constipation (accumulation of hard fecal material in the large intestine) is a relatively common complaint and a major problem for older adults. Insufficient water intake and poor dietary habits are contributing factors. Other causes include (1) fecal impaction, (2) bowel obstruction, (3) chronic laxative use, (4) neurologic disorders (paraplegia), (5) ignoring the urge to defecate, (6) lack of exercise, and (7) selected drugs, such as anticholinergics, narcotics, and certain antacids.

Nonpharmacologic Measures

Nonpharmacologic management includes a diet that contains bulk (fiber), water, exercise, and routine bowel habits. A "normal" number of bowel movements is one to three a day to three a week. What is normal varies from person to person; the nurse should determine what "normal" bowel habits are for each client. At times, a laxative may be needed, but the client should also use nonpharmacologic measures to prevent constipation.

Laxatives

Laxatives and **cathartics** are used to eliminate fecal matter. Laxatives promote a soft stool, and cathartics result in a soft to watery stool with some cramping. Frequently, the dosage determines whether the drug acts as a laxative or cathartic.* **Purgatives** are "harsh" cathartics that cause a watery stool with abdominal cramping. There are four types of laxatives: (1) osmotics (saline), (2) stimulants (contact or irritants), (3) bulk-forming, and (4) emollients (stool softeners).

Laxatives should be avoided if there is any question that the client has an intestinal obstruction; severe abdominal pain; or symptoms of appendicitis, ulcerative colitis, or diverticulitis. Most laxatives stimulate peristalsis. Laxative abuse from chronic use is a common problem, especially with older adults. Laxative dependence can be a problem; therefore client teaching is an important nursing responsibility.

Osmotic (Saline) Laxatives

Osmotics (hyperosmolar laxatives) include salts or saline products, lactulose, and glycerin. The saline products consist of sodium or magnesium, and a small amount is systemically absorbed. Serum electrolytes should be monitored to avoid electrolyte imbalance. The hyperosmolar salts pull water into the colon and increase water in the feces to increase bulk, which stimulates peristalsis. Saline cathartics cause a semiformed to watery stool according to low or high doses. Good renal function is needed to excrete any excess salts. Saline cathartics are contraindicated for clients with congestive heart failure.

Osmotic laxatives contain three types of electrolyte salts, including the (1) sodium salts (sodium phosphate or Phospho-Soda, sodium biphosphate); (2) magnesium salts (magnesium hydroxide [milk of magnesia], magnesium citrate, magnesium sulfate [Epsom salts]); and (3) potassium salts (potassium bitartrate, potassium phosphate). High doses of salt laxatives are used for bowel preparation for diagnostic and surgical procedures. Another laxative used for bowel preparation is polyethylene glycol (PEG) with electrolytes, commonly called *GoLYTELY*. With PEG, however, a large volume of solutions, approximately 3 to 4 L over 3 hours, is used. Clients may be advised to keep GoLYTELY refrigerated to make it more palatable. The positive aspect is that the solution is an isotonic, nonabsorbable osmotic substance that contains sodium salts and potassium chloride; thus it can be used by clients with renal impairment or cardiac disorder.

Lactulose, another saline laxative that is not absorbed, draws water into the intestines to form a soft stool. It decreases the serum ammonia level and is useful in liver diseases, such as cirrhosis. Glycerin acts like lactulose, increasing water in the feces in the large intestine. The bulk that results from the increased water in the feces stimulates peristalsis and defecation.

Side Effects and Adverse Reactions

Adequate renal function is needed to excrete excess magnesium. Clients who have renal insufficiency should avoid magnesium salts. Hypermagnesemia can result from con-

tinuous use of magnesium salts, causing symptoms such as drowsiness, weakness, paralysis, complete heart block, hypotension, flush, and respiratory depression.

The side effects of lactulose from excess use include flatulence, diarrhea, abdominal cramps, nausea, and vomiting. Clients who have diabetes mellitus should avoid lactulose because it contains glucose and fructose.

Stimulant (Contact) Laxatives

Stimulant (contact or irritant) laxatives increase peristalsis by irritating sensory nerve endings in the intestinal mucosa. Types include those containing phenolphthalein (Ex-Lax, Feen-A-Mint, Correctol), bisacodyl (Dulcolax), cascara sagrada, senna (Senokot), and castor oil (purgative). Bisacodyl and phenolphthalein are two of the most frequently used and abused laxatives. They can be purchased OTC. The results usually occur in 6 to 12 hours. Bisacodyl and several others of these drugs are used to empty the bowel before diagnostic tests (barium enema). Prototype Drug Chart 45-4 gives the pharmacologic data for the stimulant laxative bisacodyl.

Castor oil is a harsh laxative (purgative) that acts on the small bowel and produces a watery stool. The action is quick, within 2 to 6 hours, and the laxative should not be taken at bedtime. Castor oil is seldom used to correct constipation. It is used mainly for bowel preparation.

Pharmacokinetics

The contact laxative bisacodyl is minimally absorbed from the GI tract. It is excreted in the feces, but because of the small amount of bisacodyl absorption, a portion is excreted in the urine.

Pharmacodynamics

Bisacodyl promotes defecation. Bisacodyl irritates the colon, causing defecation, and psyllium compounds increase fecal bulk and peristalsis. The onset of action of oral bisacodyl occurs within 6 to 12 hours and within 15 to 60 minutes with the suppository (rectal administration).

Side Effects and Adverse Reactions

Side effects include nausea, abdominal cramps, weakness, and reddish brown urine caused by excretion of phenolphthalein, senna, or cascara.

With excessive and chronic use of bisacodyl, fluid and electrolyte (especially potassium and calcium) imbalances are likely to occur. Systemic effects occur infrequently because of minimal absorption of bisacodyl. Mild cramping and diarrhea are side effects of bisacodyl.

Castor oil should not be used in early pregnancy because it stimulates uterine contraction. Spontaneous abortion may result. Prolonged use of senna can damage nerves, which may result in loss of intestinal muscular tone. Table 45-5 lists the osmotic and stimulant laxatives.

Bulk-Forming Laxatives

Bulk-forming laxatives are natural fibrous substances that promote large, soft stools by absorbing water into the intestine, increasing fecal bulk and peristalsis. These agents are nonabsorbable. Defecation usually occurs within 8 to

---

*These terms are often used interchangeably. *Laxative* refers to both terms in this chapter.

PROTOTYPE DRUG CHART 45–4

BISACODYL

Drug Class

Laxative: stimulant
Trade Name: Dulcolax; ✲ Apo-Bisacodyl, Bisacolax
Pregnancy Category: C

Dosage

A: PO: 5-15 mg in AM or PM PRN; *max:* 30 mg
C: >6 y: PO: 5-10 mg; 0.3 mg/kg/d
A & C: >2 y: Rectal supp: 5-10 mg/d
C <2 y, infants: 5 mg

Contraindications

Hypersensitivity, fecal impaction, intestinal/biliary
  obstruction, appendicitis, abdominal pain, nausea,
  vomiting, rectal fissures

Drug-Lab-Food Interactions

Drug: Decrease effect with antacids, histamine$_2$ blockers, milk

Pharmacokinetics

Absorption: Minimal absorption (5%-15%)
Distribution: PB: UK
Metabolism: t½: UK
Excretion: In bile and urine

Pharmacodynamics

PO: Onset: 10-15 min
  Peak: UK
  Duration: 6-12 h
PR: Onset: 15-60 min
  Peak: UK
  Duration: 6-12 h

Therapeutic Effects/Uses

Short-term treatment for constipation; bowel preparation for diagnostic tests
Mode of Action: Increases peristalsis by direct effect on smooth muscle of intestine

Side Effects

Anorexia, nausea, vomiting, cramps, diarrhea

Adverse Reactions

Dependence, hypokalemia
Life-threatening: Tetany

A, Adult; *C,* child; *d,* day; *h,* hour; *max,* maximum; *min,* minute; *PB,* protein-binding; *PO,* by mouth; *PR,* per rectum; *PRN,* as needed;
supp, suppository; *t½,* half-life; *UK,* unknown; *y,* year; >, greater than; <, less than; ✲, Canadian drug names.

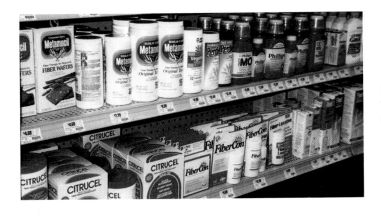

FIGURE 45–2 Various over-the-counter laxatives are available.
The bulk-forming laxatives, such as Metamucil, Perdiem, Citrucel, and FiberCon, do not cause laxative dependence.

24 hours; however, it may take up to 3 days after drug therapy is started for the stool to be soft and well formed.
Powdered bulk-forming laxatives, which sometimes come
in flavored and sugar-free forms, should be mixed in a
glass of water or juice, stirred, and drank immediately, followed by a half to a full glass of water. Insufficient fluid intake can cause the drug to solidify in the GI tract, which
can result in intestinal obstruction. This group of laxatives

does not cause laxative dependence and may be used by
clients with diverticulosis, irritable bowel syndrome, and
ileostomy and colostomy (Figure 45–2).
  Calcium polycarbophil (FiberCon), methylcellulose
(Citrucel), fiber granules (Perdiem), and psyllium hydrophilic mucilloid (Metamucil) are examples of bulk-
forming laxatives. Clients with hypercalcemia should
avoid calcium polycarbophil because of the calcium in the

Table 45–5

Laxatives: Osmotic (Saline) and Stimulant

Generic (Brand)	Route and Dosage	Uses and Considerations
Osmotics: Saline		
glycerin	A: Supp: 3 g C: <6 y: Supp: 1-1.5 g	To relieve constipation. Use with caution for clients with cardiac, renal, or liver disease and for the elderly or for those who are dehydrated. *Pregnancy category:* C; PB: UK; $t^{1}/_{2}$: 30-45 min
lactulose (Cephulac, Chronulac, Enulose)	*Chronic constipation:* A: PO: 30-60 ml/d PRN C: PO: 7.5 ml/d after breakfast	For constipation. Also used in liver disease for ammonia elimination. May be used for constipation after barium studies. Poorly absorbed. *Pregnancy category:* C; PB: UK; $t^{1}/_{2}$: UK
magnesium citrate (Citroma, Evac-Q-Mag)	A: PO: 120-240 ml C: PO: 4 ml/kg/dose or half adult dose	For constipation or to complete bowel elimination before diagnostic procedures and surgery. *Pregnancy category:* UK; PB: UK; $t^{1}/_{2}$: UK
magnesium hydroxide (milk of magnesia)	A: PO: 20-60 ml/d C: PO: 0.5 ml/kg/dose	For constipation. Take with a glass of water in morning or evening. With frequent use, good renal function is necessary. *Pregnancy category:* B; PB: UK; $t^{1}/_{2}$: UK
magnesium oxide (Maox, Mag-Ox)	A: PO: 2-4 g at bedtime with 8 oz water Do not use in client with renal failure.	Similar to magnesium hydroxide. Pregnancy category: B; PB: UK; $t^{1}/_{2}$: UK
magnesium SO$_4$ (Epsom salts)	A: PO: 10-15 g in 8 oz water C: PO: 5-10 g in water	For complete bowel elimination before surgery. Hypermagnesemia can occur if used frequently. Also used in pregnancy to control seizures with severe toxemia of pregnancy (given IV). Caution for use in renal dysfunction. *Pregnancy category:* B; PB: UK; $t^{1}/_{2}$: UK
sodium biphosphate (Fleet Phospho-Soda)	A: PO: 15-30 ml mixed in water	For constipation or bowel preparation. Contraindicated with CHF. *Pregnancy category:* UK; PB: UK; $t^{1}/_{2}$: UK
sodium phosphate with sodium biphosphate (Fleet Enema)	*Enema:* A: 60-120 ml C: 30-60 ml	For constipation or bowel preparation for diagnostic procedures. Frequent Fleet Enema may cause fluid imbalance in the elderly. *Pregnancy category:* UK; PB: UK; $t^{1}/_{2}$: UK
Stimulants		
bisacodyl (Dulcolax)	See Prototype Drug Chart 45–4.	
cascara sagrada	A: PO: Tab: 325 mg/d Fluid extract: 1 ml/d Aromatic fluid extract: 5 ml/d	For acute constipation or bowel preparation. Can be mixed with milk of magnesia. Onset: 6-12 h. *Pregnancy category:* C; PB: UK; $t^{1}/_{2}$: UK
castor oil (Neoloid, Purge)	A: PO: 15-60 ml C: 6-12 y: 5-15 ml	For bowel preparation for diagnostic tests. Harsh cathartic or purgative. Not commonly used for constipation. *Pregnancy category:* X; PB: UK; $t^{1}/_{2}$: UK
phenolphthalein (Ex-Lax, Feen-A-Mint, Correctol)	A & C: >12 y: 30-200 mg/d C: 6-12 y: 30-60 mg	For acute constipation. Onset: 6-10 h. Urine is reddish color. *Pregnancy category:* C; PB: UK; $t^{1}/_{2}$: UK
senna (Senokot)	A: PO: 2 tab or 1-2 tsp (granules) diluted in water; *max:* 4 tab/d	For constipation. Available in granules, syrup, and suppository. Prolonged use may cause fluid and electrolyte imbalances. Flatus and abdominal cramps may occur. *Pregnancy category:* C; PB: UK; $t^{1}/_{2}$: UK

A, Adult; *C,* child; *CHF,* congestive heart failure; *d,* day; *h,* hour; *IV,* intravenous; *max,* maximum; *min,* minute; *PB,* protein-binding; *PO,* by mouth; *PRN,* as needed; *supp,* suppository; *t*$^{1}/_{2}$, half-life; *tab,* tablet; *tsp,* teaspoon; *UK,* unknown; *y,* year; *>,* greater than; *<,* less than.

PROTOTYPE DRUG CHART 45–5

PSYLLIUM

Drug Class	**Dosage**
Laxative: Bulk forming Trade Name: Metamucil, Naturacil; ✤ Karacil *Pregnancy Category:* C	A: PO: 1-2 tsp in 8 oz water/d followed by 8 oz water C: >6 y: PO: 0.5-1 tsp in 4 oz water, followed by ≥4 oz water
Contraindications	**Drug-Lab-Food Interactions**
Hypersensitivity, fecal impaction, intestinal obstruction, abdominal pain	*Drug:* Decrease absorption of oral anticoagulants, aspirin, digoxin, nitrofurantoin
Pharmacokinetics	**Pharmacodynamics**
Absorption: Not absorbed **Distribution:** PB: NA **Metabolism:** t½: NA **Excretion:** In feces	PO: Onset: 10-24 h Peak: 1-3 d Duration: UK

Therapeutic Effects/Uses

To control chronic constipation
Mode of Action: Acts as bulk-forming laxative by drawing water into intestine

Side Effects	**Adverse Reactions**
Anorexia, nausea, vomiting, cramps, diarrhea	Esophageal or intestinal obstruction if not taken with adequate water **Life-threatening:** Bronchospasm, anaphylaxis

A, Adult; *C*, child; *d*, day; *h*, hour; *NA*, nonapplicable; *PB*, protein-binding; *PO*, by mouth; *t½*, half-life; *tsp*, teaspoon; *UK*, unknown; >, greater than; ≥, greater than or equal to; ✤, Canadian drug name.

---

drug. Prototype Drug Chart 45–5 presents the bulk-forming laxative psyllium (Metamucil).

Pharmacokinetics

The bulk-forming laxative Metamucil is a nondigestible and nonabsorbent substance that, when mixed with water, becomes a viscous solution. Because it is not absorbed, there is no protein-binding or half-life for the drug. Metamucil is excreted in the feces.

Pharmacodynamics

The onset of action for Metamucil is 10 to 24 hours. Peak action is 1 to 3 days. The duration of action is unknown.

Side Effects and Adverse Reactions

Bulk-forming laxatives are not systemically absorbed; therefore there is no systemic effect. If bulk-forming laxatives are excessively used, nausea, vomiting, flatus, or diarrhea may occur. Abdominal cramps may occur if the drug is used in dry form.

Emollients (Stool Softeners)

Emollients are stool softeners (surface-acting or wetting drugs) and lubricants used to prevent constipation. These drugs decrease straining during defecation. Stool softeners work by lowering surface tension and promoting water accumulation in the intestine and stool. They are frequently prescribed for clients after myocardial infarction or surgery. They are also given before administration of other laxatives in treating fecal impaction. Docusate calcium (Surfak), docusate potassium (Dialose), docusate sodium (Colace), and docusate sodium with casanthranol (Peri-Colace) are examples of stool softeners.

Lubricants such as mineral oil increase water retention in the stool. Mineral oil absorbs essential fat-soluble vitamins A, D, E, and K. Some of the minerals can be absorbed into the lymphatic system.

Side Effects and Adverse Reactions

Side effects include nausea, vomiting, diarrhea, and abdominal cramping. This drug is not indicated for children, older adults, or clients with debilitating diseases because they might aspirate the mineral oil, resulting in lipid pneumonia.

The docusate group of drugs may cause mild cramping.

Contraindications

Contraindications to the use of laxatives include inflammatory disorders of the GI tract, such as appendicitis, ulcerative colitis, undiagnosed severe pain that could be caused by an inflammation of the intestine (diverticulitis, appendicitis), pregnancy, spastic colon, or bowel obstruction. Laxatives are contraindicated when any of these conditions is suspected.

Table 45–6 presents the drug data for the laxatives.

Table 45–6

Laxatives: Bulk Forming, Emollients, and Evacuants

Generic (Brand)	Route and Dosage	Uses and Considerations
Bulk Forming		
calcium polycarbophil (FiberCon, Fiberall, Mitrolan)	A: PO: 1 g q.i.d; *max:* 6 g/d C: 6-12 y: PO: 500 mg/d t.i.d.; *max:* 3 g C: 2-5 y: PO: 500 mg/d b.i.d.; *max:* 1.5 g/d	Prevention of constipation. Also used to treat acute nonspecific diarrhea or diarrhea associated with irritable bowel syndrome. For diarrhea, it absorbs water and produces a formed stool. For constipation, chew tablet and follow with a full glass of water. *Pregnancy category:* C; PB: NA; t$^{1}/_{2}$: NA
methylcellulose (Cologel, Citrucel)	A: PO: 5-20 ml t.i.d. in 8-10 oz water C: 5-10 ml b.i.d. with 8 oz water	For constipation. Effects are similar to Metamucil. Mix in at least 8 oz of water and take immediately. *Pregnancy category:* UK; PB: NA; t$^{1}/_{2}$: NA
psyllium hydrophilic mucilloid (Metamucil)	See Prototype Drug Chart 45–5.	
Emollient: Stool Softeners		
docusate calcium (Surfak)	A: PO: 240 mg/d C: PO: 60-120 mg/d	Prevention of constipation. Softens the stool. Acts on the small and large intestines and has little absorption. When first used it may take 1 to 5 days for effectiveness. Available with calcium, potassium, or sodium. Drug should not be taken if CHF is present because of the sodium content. *Pregnancy category:* C; PB: NA; t$^{1}/_{2}$: NA
docusate potassium (Dialose)	A: PO: 100-300 mg/d	Same as docusate calcium.
docusate sodium (Colace)	A: PO: 50-300 mg/d C: >6 y: 40-120 mg/d	Same as docusate calcium.
docusate sodium with casanthranol (Peri-Colace)	A: PO: 1-2 cap/d C: PO: 1 cap/d	For preventing constipation. Combination drug: docusate sodium 100 mg with casanthranol 30 mg. *Pregnancy category:* C; PB: NA; t$^{1}/_{2}$: NA
Emollient: Lubricant		
mineral oil	A: PO: 15-45 ml/at bedtime C: 6-12 y: PO: 5-20 ml	Relief of constipation and fecal impaction. May be useful for those with cardiac disorder and following anorectal surgery. Avoid prolonged use because vitamins A, D, E, and K may be lost. *Pregnancy category:* UK; PB: NA; t$^{1}/_{2}$: NA
Evacuant/Bowel Preparation		
polyethylene glycol-electrolyte solution (Colyte, GoLYTELY)	Preparation for GI examination requires 4 h; fasting for 3-4 h A: PO: 240 ml q10-15 min for total of 4 L C: PO: 25-40 ml/kg/h for 4-10 h. Administer via NGT to those unable or unwilling to drink solution (prepared with tap water and refrigerated)	For bowel preparation before GI examination. *Pregnancy category:* C; PB: NA; t$^{1}/_{2}$: NA

A, Adult; *b.i.d.,* twice a day; *C*, child; *cap,* capsule; *CHF,* congestive heart failure; *d,* day; *h,* hour; *GI,* gastrointestinal; *max,* maximum; *min,* minute; *NA,* not applicable; *NGT,* nasogastric tube; *PB,* protein-binding; *PO,* by mouth; *q.i.d.,* four times a day; *t$^{1}/_{2}$,* half-life; *t.i.d.,* three times a day; *UK,* unknown; *y,* year; >, greater than.

Nursing Process

Laxative: Stimulant

ASSESSMENT

■ Obtain a history of constipation and possible causes such as insufficient water or fluid intake, diet deficient in bulk or fiber, or inactivity; a history of the frequency and consistency of stools; and the general health status.

■ Record baseline vital signs for identification of abnormalities and for future comparisons.

■ Evaluate renal function.

■ Assess electrolyte balance of clients who frequently use laxatives.

NURSING DIAGNOSES

■ Constipation
■ Nutrition, Imbalanced: Less than Body Requirements
■ Fluid Volume, Deficient, Risk for
■ Knowledge deficient related to overuse of laxatives
■ Health Maintenance, Ineffective

PLANNING

■ Client will have a normal bowel elimination pattern.
■ Client will exercise, eat foods high in fiber, and have adequate fluid intake to avoid constipation.

NURSING INTERVENTIONS

■ Monitor fluid intake and output. Note signs and symptoms of fluid and electrolyte imbalances that may result from watery stools. Habitual use of laxatives can cause fluid volume deficit and electrolyte losses. In addition, it can cause a loss of urge to defecate.

Client Teaching

General

• Encourage client to increase water intake, if not contraindicated, which will decrease hard, dry stools.

• Advise client to avoid overuse of laxatives, which can lead to fluid and electrolyte imbalances and drug dependence. Suggest exercise to help increase peristalsis.

• Instruct client not to chew the tablets but to swallow them whole.

• Direct client to store suppositories at <86° F (30° C).

• Tell client to take the drug only with water to increase absorption.

• Educate client not to take drug within 1 hour of any other drug.

• Remind client that drug is not for long-term use; tone of bowel may be lost.

• Warn client to time administration of drug so as not to interfere with activities or sleep.

Side Effects

• Guide client to discontinue use if rectal bleeding, nausea, vomiting, or cramping occurs.

Diet

• Inform client to increase foods rich in fiber such as bran, grains, and fruits.

Cultural Considerations ⊕

• Provide explanation and written information as needed to clients from various cultural groups related to the use and abuse of stimulant laxatives.

EVALUATION

■ Determine the effectiveness of nonpharmacologic methods for alleviating constipation.

■ Evaluate client's use of laxatives in managing constipation. Identify laxative abuse.

Nursing Process

Laxative: Bulk Forming

ASSESSMENT

■ Obtain a history of constipation and possible causes such as insufficient water or fluid intake, diet deficient in bulk or fiber, or inactivity; a history of the frequency and consistency of stools; and the general health status.

■ Record baseline vital signs for identification of abnormalities and for future comparisons.

■ Assess renal function, urine output, blood urea nitrogen (BUN), and serum creatinine.

NURSING DIAGNOSES

■ Constipation
■ Fluid Volume, Deficient, Risk for

PLANNING

■ Client will have a normal bowel elimination pattern.
■ Client will exercise, eat foods high in fiber, and have adequate fluid intake to avoid constipation.

NURSING INTERVENTIONS

■ Check fluid intake and output. Note signs and symptoms of fluid and electrolyte imbalances that may result from watery stools. Habitual use of laxatives can cause fluid volume deficit and electrolyte losses.

■ Monitor bowel sounds.

■ Identify the cause of constipation.

■ Avoid inhalation of psyllium dust.

Client Teaching

General
- Teach client to mix drug with water immediately before use.
- Instruct client *not* to swallow the drug in dry form.
- Direct client to avoid overuse of laxatives, which can lead to fluid and electrolyte imbalances and drug dependence. Suggest exercise to help increase peristalsis.
- Advise client to avoid inhaling psyllium dust; it may cause watery eyes, runny nose, and wheezing.

Side Effects
- Guide client to discontinue use if nausea, vomiting, cramping, or rectal bleeding occurs.

Diet
- Inform client to increase water intake, which will decrease hard, dry stools. Drink at least eight 8-oz glasses of fluids per day.
- Tell client to mix the drug in 8 to 10 oz of water, stir, and drink immediately. At least one glass of extra water should follow. Insufficient water can cause the drug to solidify and lead to fecal impaction.
- Encourage client to increase foods rich in fiber such as bran, grains, and fruits.

Cultural Considerations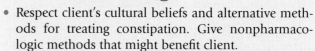
- Respect client's cultural beliefs and alternative methods for treating constipation. Give nonpharmacologic methods that might benefit client.
- Provide additional explanation and written information as needed to clients from various cultural groups related to the use and abuse of laxatives.

EVALUATION

- Determine the effectiveness of nonpharmacologic methods for alleviating constipation.
- Evaluate client's use of laxatives in managing constipation. Identify laxative abuse.

WEBSITES

For further information on *Drugs for Gastrointestinal Tract Disorders*, visit these Internet resources:

Promethazine:
www.wyeth-pharmaceutical.com/promethazine.htm

Ipecac:
www.maripoisoncenter.com/commonpoisons/ipecac.htm

Critical Thinking Case Study

C.S., age 34, has been vomiting for 48 hours. In the last 12 hours, C.S. has had diarrhea. Prochlorperazine (Compazine) 10 mg was administered intramuscularly.

1. What nonpharmacologic measures should the nurse suggest when vomiting occurs?

2. Why was C.S. given prochlorperazine intramuscularly and not orally or rectally? Prochlorperazine should be given deep intramuscularly. Why?

3. What electrolyte imbalances may occur as a result of vomiting and diarrhea? Explain how they can be replaced.

4. What are the side effects of prochlorperazine? Could these occur to C.S.? Explain.

5. Could a serotonin antagonist be given to C.S. instead of prochlorperazine? Explain.

C.S. was prescribed diphenoxylate with atropine (Lomotil) 2.5 mg t.i.d.

6. Is the Lomotil dosage for C.S. within the normal prescribed range? Explain.

7. What clinical conditions are contraindicated for the use of Lomotil?

8. What are some of the combination drugs that may be prescribed to control diarrhea? Give their advantages and disadvantages.

9. Explain the similarities of two over-the-counter antidiarrheals? Explain how frequently they should be administered.

10. Do you think C.S. should receive an adsorbent? Explain.

11. Explain the similarities and differences between ipecac and charcoal.

Study Questions

1. The client complains of motion sickness. What types of drugs might be suggested? What are the side effects?

2. Certain phenothiazines are prescribed for vomiting. What are the pharmacodynamics (actions)? Give examples of phenothiazine antiemetics.

3. What is ipecac syrup? How is it administered? For what conditions is ipecac contraindicated?

4. The client takes paregoric for diarrhea. How does this drug differ from opium tincture? What type of antidiarrheal is paregoric?

5. Diphenoxylate (Lomotil) is what type of drug? What are the side effects?

6. What is the difference between laxatives and cathartics? What is the action of contact (irritant) laxatives? What are the side effects?

7. The client takes a bulk-forming laxative. What instructions should be given?

46 Antiulcer Drugs

OBJECTIVES

- Identify the predisposing factors for peptic ulcers.
- Differentiate between peptic ulcer, gastric ulcer, duodenal ulcer, and gastroesophageal reflux disease.
- Describe the actions of seven groups of antiulcer drugs used in the treatment of peptic ulcer: tranquilizers, anticholinergics, antacids, histamine₂ blockers, proton pump inhibitors, pepsin inhibitor, and prostaglandin analogue antiulcer.
- Identify at least two drugs from each of the following drug groups: anticholinergics, antacids, and histamine₂ blockers.
- Differentiate between the side effects of anticholinergics and systemic and nonsystemic antacids.
- Describe the nursing processes, including client teaching, related to antiulcer drugs.

TERMS

antacids	gastric mucosal barrier	gastroesophageal reflux	hydrochloric acid (HCl)
duodenal ulcer	(GMB)	disease (GERD)	pepsin
esophageal ulcer	gastric ulcer	histamine₂ receptor	peptic ulcer
		antagonists	stress ulcer

Introduction

Peptic ulcer is a broad term for an ulcer occurring in the esophagus, stomach, or duodenum within the upper gastrointestinal (GI) tract. The ulcers are more specifically named according to the site of involvement: esophageal, gastric, and duodenal ulcers. Duodenal ulcers occur 10 times more frequently than gastric and esophageal ulcers. The release of **hydrochloric acid (HCl)** from the parietal cells of the stomach is influenced by histamine, gastrin, and acetylcholine. Peptic ulcers occur when there is a hypersecretion of hydrochloric acid and pepsin, which erode the GI mucosal lining.

The gastric secretions in the stomach strive to maintain a pH of 2 to 5. **Pepsin**, a digestive enzyme, is activated at a pH of 2, and the acid-pepsin complex of gastric secretions can cause mucosal damage. If the pH of gastric secretion increases to pH 5, the activity of pepsin declines. The **gastric mucosal barrier (GMB)** is a thick, viscous, mucous material that provides a barrier between the mucosal lining and the acidic gastric secretions. The GMB maintains the integrity of the gastric mucosal lining and is a defense against corrosive substances. The two sphincter muscles—the *cardiac*, located at the upper portion of the stomach, and the *pyloric*, located at the lower portion of the stomach—act as barriers to prevent reflux of acid into the esophagus and the duodenum. Figure 46–1 illustrates common sites of peptic ulcers.

An **esophageal ulcer** results from reflux of acidic gastric secretion into the esophagus as a result of a defective or incompetent cardiac sphincter. A **gastric ulcer** frequently occurs because of a breakdown of the GMB. A **duodenal ulcer** is caused by hypersecretion of acid from the stomach that passes to the duodenum because of (1) insufficient buffers to neutralize the gastric acid in the stomach, (2) a

defective or incompetent pyloric sphincter, or (3) hypermotility of the stomach. **Gastroesophageal reflux disease (GERD)** is inflammation or erosion of the esophageal mucosa caused by a reflux of gastric acid content from the stomach into the esophagus.

Predisposing Factors in Peptic Ulcer Disease

The nurse needs to assist the client in identifying possible causes of the ulcer and to teach ways to alleviate them. Predisposing factors include mechanical disturbances, genetic influences, bacterial organisms, environmental factors, and certain drugs. Healing of an ulcer takes 4 to 8 weeks. Complications can occur as the result of scar tissue. Table 46–1 lists the predisposing factors for peptic ulcers and their effects.

Table 46–1

Predisposing Factors in Peptic Ulcer Disease

Predisposing Factors	Effects
Mechanical disturbances	Hypersecretion of acid and pepsin. Inadequate GMB mucous secretion. Impaired GMB resistance. Hypermotility of the stomach. Incompetent (defective) cardiac or pyloric sphincter.
Genetic influences	Increased number of parietal cells in the stomach. Susceptibility of mucosal lining to acid penetration. Susceptibility to excess acetylcholine and histamine. Excess hydrochloric acid caused by external stimuli.
Environmental influences	Foods and liquids containing caffeine; fatty, fried, and highly spiced foods; alcohol. Nicotine products, including cigarettes. Stressful situations. Pregnancy, massive trauma, major surgery.
Helicobacter pylori	A gram-negative bacterium, *H. pylori* infects the gastric mucosa and can cause gastritis, gastric ulcer, and duodenal ulcer. If the *H. pylori* is not eradicated, peptic ulcer may return as frequently as every year. *H. pylori* can lead to atrophic gastritis in some clients. Serology and special breath tests can detect the presence of *H. pylori*.
Drugs	NSAIDs, including aspirin and aspirin compounds, ibuprofen (Motrin, Advil, Nuprin), and indomethacin (Indocin); corticosteroids (cortisone, prednisone); potassium salts; antineoplastic drugs.

GMB, Gastric mucosal barrier; *NSAIDs*, nonsteroidal antiinflammatory drugs.

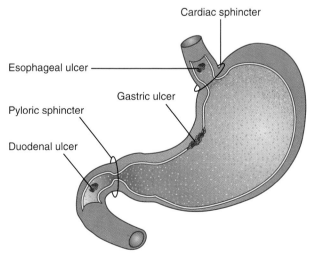

FIGURE 46–1 Common sites of peptic ulcers.

The classic symptom of peptic ulcers is gnawing, aching pain. With a gastric ulcer, pain occurs 30 minutes to 1.5 hours after eating, and with a duodenal ulcer, 2 to 3 hours after eating. Small, frequent meals of nonirritating foods decrease the pain. With treatment, pain usually subsides in 10 days; however, the healing process may take 1 to 2 months.

A **stress ulcer** usually follows a critical situation such as extensive trauma or major surgery (e.g., burns, cardiac surgery). Prophylactic use of antiulcer drugs decreases the incidence of stress ulcers.

Helicobacter pylori

Helicobacter pylori, a gram-negative bacillus, is linked with the development of peptic ulcer. *H. pylori* is known to cause gastritis, gastric ulcer, and duodenal ulcer. When a peptic ulcer recurs after antiulcer therapy, and the ulcer is not caused by nonsteroidal antiinflammatory drugs (NSAIDs) such as aspirin or ibuprofen, the client should be tested for the presence of the bacterium *H. pylori,* which may have infected the gastric mucosa. In the past, endoscopy and a biopsy of the gastric antrum were needed to check for *H. pylori.* Currently, a noninvasive breath test, the Meretek UBT, can detect *H. pylori.* This test consists of drinking a liquid containing ^{13}C urea and breathing into a container. If *H. pylori* is present, the bacterial urease hydrolyzes the urea, releasing $^{13}CO_2$, which is detected by a spectrometer. This test is 90% to 95% effective for detecting *H. pylori.* In addition, a serology test may be performed to check for antibodies of *H. pylori.*

There are various protocols for treating *H. pylori* infection. Antibacterial agents are the choice of treatment for *H. pylori.* The use of only one antibacterial agent is not effective for eradicating *H. pylori* because the bacterium can readily become resistant to that drug. Treatment to eradicate this bacterial infection includes using a dual, triple, or quadruple drug therapy program in a variety of drug combinations, such as amoxicillin (Amoxil), tetracycline (Achromycin V), clarithromycin (Biaxin), omeprazole (Prilosec), lansoprazole (Prevacid), metronidazole (Flagyl), bismuth subsalicylate (Pepto-Bismol), and ranitidine bismuth citrate (Tritec), on a 7- to 14-day treatment plan. The combination of drugs differs for each client according to the client's drug tolerance. A common treatment protocol is the triple therapy of metronidazole (or amoxicillin), omeprazole (or lansoprazole), and clarithromycin (MOC). The drug regimen eradicates more than 90% of peptic ulcer caused by *H. pylori.* (See Herbal Alert 46–1.)

One of the proton pump inhibitors (PPIs) (e.g., omeprazole, lansoprazole, etc.) is frequently used as one of the combination drugs because each suppresses the acid secretion by inhibiting the enzyme hydrogen or potassium ATPase, which makes gastric acid. These agents block the final steps of acid production. If triple therapy fails to eradicate *H. pylori,* then the quadruple therapy using two antibiotics, a PPI, and a bismuth or histamine$_2$ (H$_2$) blocker is recommended. After completion of the treatment regimen, 6 weeks of standard acid suppression, such as H$_2$ blocker therapy, is recommended. Table 46–2 lists various combinations of treatment regimens to eradicate *H. pylori,* and Table 46–3 lists data for the drugs used to treat *H. pylori.*

Gastroesophageal Reflux Disease

GERD, also called *reflux esophagitis,* is an inflammation of the esophageal mucosa caused by a reflux of gastric acid content into the esophagus. Its main cause is an incompetent lower esophageal sphincter. Smoking and obesity tend to accelerate the disease process. In the United States 40% to 44% of adults have heartburn, which in many cases is caused by GERD.

The medical treatment for GERD is similar to the treatment for peptic ulcers. This includes the use of the common antiulcer drugs to neutralize gastric contents and to reduce gastric acid secretion. Drugs used in treatment include H$_2$ blockers, such as ranitidine (Zantac), and PPIs, such as omeprazole (Prilosec), lansoprazole (Prevacid), rabeprazole (Aciphex), pantoprazole (Protonix), or esomeprazole (Nexium). A PPI relieves symptoms faster and maintains healing better than an H$_2$ blocker. Once the strictures are relieved by dilation, they are less likely to recur if the client was taking PPIs rather than an H$_2$ blocker.

GERD is a chronic disorder that requires continuous management. Effective management of GERD keeps the esophageal mucosa healed and the client free of symptoms.

Nonpharmacologic Measures for Managing Peptic Ulcer and Gastroesophageal Reflux Disease

With a GI disorder, nonpharmacologic measures, along with drug therapy, are an important part of the treatment. Once the GI problem is resolved, the client should continue to follow nonpharmacologic measures to avoid recurrence of the GI disorder.

Avoiding tobacco and alcohol can decrease gastric secretions. With GERD, nicotine relaxes the lower esophageal sphincter, thus permitting gastric acid reflux. Obesity enhances the problem of GERD; weight loss is helpful in decreasing symptoms. The client should avoid hot, spicy, and greasy foods, which could aggravate the gastric problem. NSAIDs, which include aspirin, should be taken with food or in a decreased dosage. Glucocorticoids can cause gastric ulceration therefore food should be taken with these drugs.

To relieve symptoms of GERD, the client should raise the head of the bed, not eat before bedtime, and wear loose-fitting clothing.

HERBAL ALERT 46-1

Tetracycline and Herbs

🌿 St. John's wort may increase the risk of photosensitivity when taken with tetracycline.

Table 46–2

Various Regimens Used to Eradicate Helicobacter pylori

Type of Therapy	Drugs	Treatment Duration	Eradication Rate
Dual therapy	Ranitidine bismuth citrate, 400 mg b.i.d.	2-4 wk	82%
	Clarithromycin, 500 mg t.i.d.		
	*Omeprazole, 40 mg/d	2-4 wk	64%–82%
	Clarithromycin, 500 mg t.i.d.		
	*Lansoprazole, 30 mg b.i.d.	14 d	72%
	Clarithromycin, 400 mg b.i.d.		
Triple therapy	Colloidal bismuth subcitrate, 120 mg q.i.d.	14 d	96%
	Metronidazole, 250 mg q.i.d.		
	Tetracycline, 250 mg q.i.d. OR tetracycline, 500 mg q.i.d.	7 d	83%
	Bismuth subsalicylate, 300 mg q.i.d.	14 d	84%
	Metronidazole, 500 mg t.i.d.		
	Amoxicillin, 500 mg t.i.d.		
	OR		
	Bismuth with clarithromycin, 500 mg t.i.d.	14 d	93%
	Tetracycline, 500 mg q.i.d.		
	Metronidazole, 500 mg b.i.d. OR amoxicillin, 1 g b.i.d.	7-14 d	>90%
	*Omeprazole, 20 mg b.i.d. OR lansoprazole, 30 mg b.i.d.		
	Clarithromycin, 500 mg b.i.d.		
	Combinations of:		
	Metronidazole, omeprazole, clarithromycin		
	Metronidazole, omeprazole, amoxicillin		
	*Lansoprazole, clarithromycin, metronidazole		
	*Lansoprazole, amoxicillin, clarithromycin		
	*Omeprazole, amoxicillin, clarithromycin		
Quadruple therapy	Colloidal bismuth subcitrate, 120 mg q.i.d.	7 d	98%
	Tetracycline, 500 mg q.i.d.		
	Metronidazole, 500 mg t.i.d.		
	*Omeprazole, 20 mg b.i.d.		
	Other combinations may be used		

b.i.d., Twice a day; *d,* day; *q.i.d.,* four times a day; *t.i.d.,* three times a day; *wk,* week; >, greater than.
*Other proton pump inhibitors may be substituted for omeprazole and lansoprazole.

Table 46–3

Pharmacologic Agents Used to Treat Helicobacter pylori

Generic (Brand)	Route and Dosage	Uses and Considerations
Antiinfective Agents		
metronidazole HCl (Flagyl, Protostat)	A: PO: 250-500 mg b.i.d., t.i.d., q.i.d.	To treat numerous organisms including *H. pylori.* Used in combination with other drugs to treat *H. pylori.*
amoxicillin (Amoxil)	A: PO: 500 mg t.i.d.	Used in triple or quadruple therapy for *H. pylori*
clarithromycin (Biaxin)	A: PO: 500 mg b.i.d.-t.i.d.	Used in dual and triple therapy for *H. pylori*
tetracycline	A: PO: 500 mg q.i.d.	Used in triple and quadruple therapy for *H. pylori*
Proton Pump Inhibitors (PPIs)		
omeprazole (Prilosec)	A: PO: 20 mg/d or 40 mg/d	Used in dual, triple, and quadruple therapy for *H. pylori*
lansoprazole (Prevacid)	A: PO: 30 mg b.i.d.	Used in dual and triple therapy for *H. pylori*
esomeprazole (Nexium)	A: PO: 20-40 mg/d	Used in therapy for *H. pylori*
pantoprazole (Protonix)	A: PO: 40-80 mg/d	Used in therapy for *H. pylori*
rabeprazole (Aciphex)	A: PO: 20 mg/d	Used in therapy for *H. pylori*
Antacids		
bismuth subsalicylate	A: PO: 300 mg q.i.d.	Used in combination with other drugs to treat *H. pylori*
colloidal bismuth subcitrate	A: PO: 120 mg q.i.d.	Used in combination with other drugs to treat *H. pylori*
ranitidine bismuth citrate (Tritec)	A: PO: 400 mg b.i.d.	Used in combination with other drugs to treat *H. pylori*

A, Adult; *b.i.d.,* twice a day; *d,* day; *PO,* by mouth; *q.i.d.,* four times a day; *t.i.d.,* three times a day.

Antiulcer Drugs

There are seven groups of antiulcer agents: (1) tranquilizers, which decrease vagal activity; (2) anticholinergics, which decrease acetylcholine by blocking the cholinergic receptors; (3) antacids, which neutralize gastric acid; (4) H_2 blockers, which block the H_2 receptor; (5) PPIs, which inhibit gastric acid secretion regardless of acetylcholine or histamine release; (6) the pepsin inhibitor sucralfate; and (7) the prostaglandin E_1 analogue misoprostol, which inhibits gastric acid secretion and protects the mucosa. Figure 46–2 il-

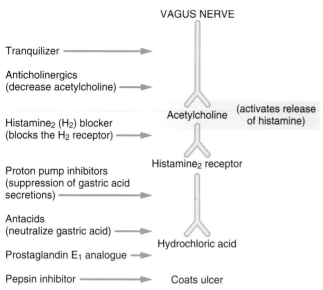

FIGURE 46–2 Actions of the seven antiulcer drug groups.

lustrates the action of the seven antiulcer drug groups, each of which is discussed separately.

Tranquilizers

Tranquilizers have minimal effect in preventing and treating ulcers; however, they reduce vagal stimulation and decrease anxiety. Librax, a combination of the anxiolytic chlordiazepoxide (Librium) and the anticholinergic clidinium bromide (Quarzan), may be used in the treatment of ulcers.

Anticholinergics

Anticholinergics (antimuscarinics, parasympatholytics) and antacids were the drugs of choice for peptic ulcers for many years. However, with the introduction of H_2 blockers in 1975, anticholinergic use has declined. These drugs relieve pain by decreasing GI motility and secretion; they act by inhibiting acetylcholine and blocking histamine and hydrochloric acid. Anticholinergics delay gastric emptying time, so they are used more frequently for duodenal ulcers than for gastric ulcers. An anticholinergic, propantheline bromine (Pro-Banthine), inhibits gastric secretions and is used to treat peptic ulcers.

Anticholinergics should be taken before meals to decrease the acid secretion that occurs with eating. Antacids can slow the absorption of anticholinergics and therefore should be taken 2 hours after anticholinergic administration.

Table 46–4 lists selected anticholinergic drugs used in the treatment of peptic ulcer. Anticholinergics should be used as adjunctive therapy and not as the only antiulcer drug. Anticholinergics are discussed in more detail in Chapter 18, Cholinergics and Anticholinergics.

Side Effects and Adverse Reactions

Anticholinergics have many side effects, including dry mouth, decreased secretions, headache, blurred vision, drowsiness, dizziness, lethargy, palpitations, bradycardia, tachycardia, urinary retention, and constipation. Because anticholinergics decrease GI motility, the gastric emptying time is delayed, which can stimulate gastric secretions and aggravate the ulceration.

Antacids

Antacids promote ulcer healing by neutralizing hydrochloric acid and reducing pepsin activity; they do not coat the ulcer. There are two types of antacids: those that have a *systemic* effect and those that have a *nonsystemic* effect.

Sodium bicarbonate, a systemically absorbed antacid, was one of the first antiulcer drugs. Because it has many side effects (sodium excess, causing hypernatremia and water retention; metabolic alkalosis caused by excess bicarbonate; and acid rebound [excess acid secretion]), sodium bicarbonate is seldom used to treat peptic ulcers. Examples of sodium bicarbonate compounds are Bromo-Seltzer and Alka-Seltzer.

Table 46–4

Antiulcer: Anticholinergics

Generic (Brand)	Route and Dosage	Uses and Considerations
belladonna tincture	A: PO: 0.6-1 ml t.i.d.-q.i.d. C: PO: 0.1 ml/kg/d in 3-4 divided doses *max*: 3.5 ml/d	For peptic ulcers; decreases gastric secretions. Contraindicated in clients with narrow-angle glaucoma, myasthenia gravis, paralytic ileus, and urinary retention. Dry mouth and constipation can occur. *Pregnancy category:* C; PB: UK; t $\frac{1}{2}$: 18-36 h
clidinium bromide and chlordiazepoxide HCl (Librax)	A: PO: 1-2 cap t.i.d.-q.i.d. a.c., at bedtime	Decreases anxiety and GI distress. Contains a benzodiazepine. *Pregnancy category:* C; PB: UK; t$\frac{1}{2}$: UK
glycopyrrolate (Robinul)	A: PO: 1-2 mg b.i.d.-t.i.d. IM/IV: 0.1-0.2 mg (100-200 mcg) t.i.d.-q.i.d.	For peptic ulcers and gastric disorder caused by hyperacidity. Used as one of the preanesthetic drugs. Same contraindications as belladonna. *Pregnancy category:* B; PB: UK; t$\frac{1}{2}$: UK
propantheline bromine (Pro-Banthine)	A: PO: 15 mg t.i.d. 30 min a.c. and 30 mg at bedtime; *max:* 120 mg/d Elderly: PO: 7.5 mg b.i.d.-t.i.d. a.c. *max:* 90 mg/d	For peptic ulcers; decreases gastric secretions, irritable bowel syndrome, pancreatitis, and urinary bladder spasm. Standard anticholinergic side effects. *Pregnancy category:* C; PB: UK; t$\frac{1}{2}$: 9 h
tridihexethyl chloride (Pathilon)	A: PO: 25-50 mg t.i.d.-q.i.d. a.c. and at bedtime	For peptic ulcers; decreases gastric secretions. *Pregnancy category:* C; PB: UK; t$\frac{1}{2}$: UK

A, Adult; *a.c.*, before meals; *b.i.d.*, twice a day; *C*, child; *cap*, capsule; *d*, day; *GI*, gastrointestinal; *h*, hour; *IM*, intramuscular; *IV*, intravenous; *max*, maximum; *PB*, protein-binding; *PO*, by mouth; *q.i.d.*, four times a day; *t$\frac{1}{2}$*, half-life; *t.i.d.*, three times a day; *UK*, unknown.

Calcium carbonate is most effective in neutralizing acid; however, one third to half of the drug can be systemically absorbed and can cause acid rebound. Hypercalcemia and "milk-alkali syndrome" can result from excessive use of calcium carbonate. Milk-alkali syndrome is intensified if milk products are ingested with calcium carbonate. It is identified by the presence of alkalosis, hypercalcemia, and in severe cases crystalluria and renal failure.

The nonsystemic antacids are composed of alkaline salts such as aluminum (aluminum hydroxide, aluminum carbonate) and magnesium (magnesium hydroxide, magnesium carbonate, magnesium trisilicate, magnesium phosphate). There is a small degree of systemic absorption with these drugs, mainly of aluminum. Magnesium hydroxide has greater neutralizing power than aluminum hydroxide. Magnesium compounds can cause diarrhea, and aluminum and calcium compounds can cause constipation with long-term use. A combination of magnesium and aluminum salts neutralizes gastric acid without causing severe diarrhea or constipation. Simethicone (an antigas agent) is found in many antacids, including Mylanta II, Maalox Plus, and Gelusil II (Figure 46–3).

Prototype Drug Chart 46–1 gives the drug data for aluminum hydroxide antacid.

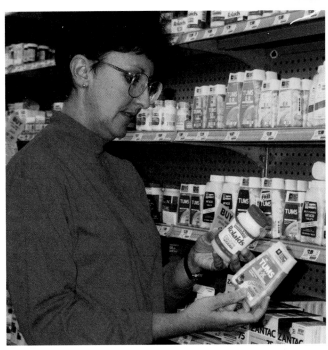

FIGURE 46–3 Numerous over-the-counter antacids are available. This client is deciding which of these antacids would best help relieve her upset stomach.

• PROTOTYPE DRUG CHART 46–1

ALUMINUM HYDROXIDE

Drug Class

Antiulcer: antacid
Trade Name: Amphojel, AlternaGEL, Alu-Tab
Pregnancy Category: C

Dosage

Antacid:
A: PO: 600 mg 1 h p.c. and at bedtime; chewed with water or milk
Susp: 5-10 ml 1 h p.c. and at bedtime
Hyperphosphatemia:
A: PO: 2 cap or 10-30 ml (regular carbonate suspension) t.i.d.-q.i.d. with meals

Contraindications

Hypersensitivity to aluminum products, hypophosphatemia
Caution: In older adults

Drug-Lab-Food Interactions

Drug: Decrease effects with tetracycline, phenothiazine, isoniazid, phenytoin, digitalis, quinidine, amphetamines; may *increase* effect of benzodiazepines
Lab: Increase urine pH

Pharmacokinetics

Absorption: PO: Small amount absorbed
Distribution: PB: UK
Metabolism: t½: UK
Excretion: In feces; small amount in urine

Pharmacodynamics

PO: Onset: 15-30 min
  Peak: 0.5 h
  Duration: 1-3 h

Therapeutic Effects/Uses

To treat hyperacidity, peptic ulcer, and reflux esophagitis; to reduce hyperphosphatemia
Mode of Action: Neutralizes gastric acidity

Side Effect

Constipation

Adverse Reactions

Hypophosphatemia; long-term use results in GI obstruction

A, Adult; *cap*, capsule; *GI*, gastrointestinal; *h*, hour; *min*, minute; *PB*, protein-binding; *p.c.*, after meals; *PO*, by mouth; *q.i.d.*, four times a day; *Susp*, suspension; *t½*, half-life; *t.i.d.*, three times a day; *UK*, unknown.

Pharmacokinetics

Aluminum hydroxide (Amphojel) was one of the first antacids used to neutralize hydrochloric acid. Aluminum products are frequently used to lower high serum phosphate (hyperphosphatemia). Because aluminum hydroxide alone can cause constipation and magnesium products alone can cause diarrhea, combination drugs, such as aluminum hydroxide and magnesium hydroxide (Maalox), have become popular because they decrease these side effects.

Only a small amount of aluminum hydroxide is absorbed from the GI tract. It is primarily bound to phosphate and excreted in the feces. The small portion that is absorbed is excreted in the urine.

Pharmacodynamics

Aluminum hydroxide neutralizes gastric acid, including hydrochloric acid, and increases the pH of gastric secretions (an elevated pH inactivates pepsin). The onset of action is fairly rapid, but the duration of action varies depending on whether the antacid is taken with or without food. If the antacid is taken after a meal, the duration of action may be up to 3 hours because food delays gastric emptying time. Frequent dosing may be necessary if the antacid is given during a fasting state or early in the course of treatment.

The ideal dosing interval for antacids is 1 and 3 hours after meals (maximum acid secretion occurs after eating) and at bedtime. Antacids taken on an empty stomach are effective for 30 to 60 minutes before passing into the duodenum. Chewable tablets should be followed by water. Liquid antacids should also be taken with water (2 to 4 oz) to ensure that the drug reaches the stomach; however, no more than 4 oz of water should be taken because water quickens gastric emptying time.

Antacids containing magnesium salts are contraindicated in clients with impaired renal function because of the risk of hypermagnesemia. Prolonged use of aluminum hydroxides can cause hypophosphatemia (low serum phosphate). If hyperphosphatemia occurs because of poor renal function, aluminum hydroxide can be given to decrease the phosphate level. In clients with renal insufficiency, aluminum salt ingestion can cause encephalopathy from accumulation of aluminum in the brain.

Table 46–5 lists the drug data for antacids.

Nursing Process

Antiulcer: Antacids

ASSESSMENT

■ Evaluate client's pain, including the type, duration, severity, and frequency.
■ Check client's renal function.
■ Assess for fluid and electrolyte imbalances, especially serum phosphate and calcium levels.
■ Obtain drug history; report probable drug-drug interactions.

NURSING DIAGNOSES

■ Pain
■ Knowledge deficit related to (mis)use of antacids

PLANNING

■ Client will be free of abdominal pain after 1 to 2 weeks of antiulcer drug management.

NURSING INTERVENTIONS

■ Avoid administering antacids with other oral drugs because antacids can delay their absorption. An antacid should definitely not be given with tetracycline, digoxin, or quinidine because it binds with and inactivates most of the drug. Antacids are given 1 to 2 hours after other medications.
■ Shake suspension well before administering; follow with water.
■ Monitor electrolytes and urinary pH, calcium, and phosphate levels.

Client Teaching
General
• Instruct client to report pain, coughing, or vomiting of blood.
• Encourage client to drink 2 oz of water after antacid to ensure that the drug reaches the stomach.
• Direct client to take the antacid 1 to 3 hours after meals and at bedtime. Do not take antacids at mealtime; they slow gastric emptying time, causing increased GI activity and gastric secretions.
• Advise client to notify the health care provider if constipation or diarrhea occurs; the antacid may have to be changed. Self-treatment should be avoided.
• Stress that antacids are not candy and that taking an unlimited amount is contraindicated.
• Warn client to avoid taking antacids with milk or foods high in vitamin D.
• Tell client to avoid taking antacids within 1 to 2 hours of other oral medications because there may be interference with absorption.
• Guide client to check antacid labels for sodium content if on a sodium-restricted diet.
• Alert client to consult with the health care provider before taking self-prescribed antacids for longer than 2 weeks.
• Inform client on the use of relaxation techniques.

Self-Administration
• Teach client how to take antacids correctly. Chewable tablets should be thoroughly chewed and followed with water. With liquid antacid, 2 to 4 oz of water should follow the antacid. Increased amount of water with antacids increases gastric emptying time.

Side Effects
• Direct client to avoid foods and liquids that can cause gastric irritation, such as caffeine-containing beverages, alcohol, and spices.
• Explain to client that stools may become speckled or white.

Cultural Considerations ⊕

- Respect client's cultural beliefs and alternative methods for treating GI discomfort. Discuss with client the safety of his or her methods and the use of drugs prescribed to heal and lessen the symptoms.
- Recognize that clients of various cultural backgrounds may need guidance in understanding the disease process of their GI disturbance. Use of a written plan of care with modification should be considered.

EVALUATION

■ Determine the effectiveness of the antiulcer treatment and the presence of side effects. Client should be free of pain, and healing should progress.

Histamine₂ Blockers

The histamine$_2$ (H$_2$) blockers (**histamine$_2$ receptor antagonists**) are popular drugs used in the treatment of gastric and duodenal ulcers. H$_2$ blockers prevent acid reflux in the

Table 46–5

Antiulcers: Antacids

Generic (Brand)	Route and Dosage	Uses and Considerations
aluminum carbonate (Basaljel)	A: PO: 10-30 ml or 2 tab/cap q2h Extra strength 5-15 ml	To alleviate gastric hyperacidity related to gastritis, gastric and duodenal ulcers, esophageal reflux, and hiatal hernia. Increases gastric pH and inhibits pepsin activity. Also used to decrease hyperphosphatemia for clients with renal dysfunction. Duration of action is 2 to 3 h when taken 1 h after meals. *Pregnancy category:* C; PB: UK; t½: UK
aluminum hydroxide (Amphojel, AlternaGEL)	See Prototype Drug Chart 46–1.	
calcium carbonate (Tums, Dicarbosil)	A: PO: 2 tab or 10 ml q2h; *max:* 12 doses/d	To alleviate heartburn, acid indigestion, esophagitis, and hiatal hernia caused by hyperacidity. Also treat hyperphosphatemia for clients with renal disorders. OTC drug. One third of the drug dose is absorbed from GI tract. Constipation can be a problem. *Pregnancy category:* C; PB: UK; t½: UK
dihydroxyaluminum sodium carbonate (Rolaids Antacid)	A: PO: Chew 1-2 tab PRN	Similar to calcium carbonate except it contains sodium instead of calcium. *Pregnancy category:* C; PB: UK; t½: UK
magaldrate (Riopan, Lowsium [plus simethicone])	A: PO: 5-15 ml, PRN; *max:* 100 ml/d; or 1-2 tab PRN; *max:* 20 tab/d	To alleviate heartburn, gastritis, esophagitis, and peptic ulcers caused by hyperacidity. Contains aluminum and magnesium hydroxide. Low sodium content. Simethicone decreases flatus. Drug is minimally absorbed. *Pregnancy category:* C; PB: UK; t½: UK
magnesium hydroxide and aluminum hydroxide (Maalox)	A: PO: 2-4 tab PRN; *max:* 16 tab/d or 10–30 ml, 1-3 h p.c. and at bedtime	Same as magaldrate. Caution for clients with renal disorder caused by the magnesium content. OTC drug. *Pregnancy category:* UK; PB: UK; t½: UK
magnesium hydroxide, aluminum hydroxide, and calcium carbonate (Camalox)	A: PO: 10-20 ml PRN; *max:* 80 ml/d; or 2-4 tab PRN; *max:* 16 tab	Same as magaldrate except it also contains calcium. *Pregnancy category:* UK; PB: UK; t½: UK
magnesium hydroxide and aluminum hydroxide with simethicone (Aludrox, Mylanta, Mylanta III, Maalox Plus, Gelusil-I, Gelusil-II, Gelusil-M, Di-Gel)	A: PO: 10-20 ml PRN; *max:* 120 ml/d; or 2-4 tab PRN; *max:* 24 tab	Same as magaldrate. It also contains simethicone, which decreases flatus. OTC drug. *Pregnancy category:* UK; PB: UK; t½: UK
magnesium trisilicate (Gaviscon)	A: PO: 1-2 tab PRN; *max:* 8 tab/d	To relieve gastric disorders caused by hyperacidity. OTC drug. Contains magnesium trisilicate and aluminum hydroxide. *Pregnancy category:* UK; PB: UK; t½: UK
sodium bicarbonate	A: PO: 0.5 tsp of powder in 8 oz water	Previously used for gastric hyperacidity. It is a short-acting, potent antacid that is systemically absorbed. Acid-base imbalance could occur. *Pregnancy category:* C; PB: UK; t½: UK

A, Adult; *cap,* capsule; *d,* day; *GI,* gastrointestinal; *h,* hour; *max,* maximum; *OTC,* over-the-counter; *PB,* protein-binding; *p.c.,* after meals; *PO,* by mouth; *PRN,* as needed; *t½,* half-life; *tab,* tablet; *tsp,* teaspoon; *UK,* unknown.

esophagus (reflux esophagitis). These drugs block the H_2 receptors of the parietal cells in the stomach, thus reducing gastric acid secretion and concentration. Antihistamines, used to treat allergic conditions, act against histamine$_1$ (H_1); they are not the same as H_2 blockers.

The first H_2 blocker was cimetidine (Tagamet), introduced in 1975. Cimetidine, which has a short half-life and a short duration of action, blocks about 70% of acid secretion for 4 hours. Good kidney function is necessary because approximately 50% to 80% of the drug is excreted unchanged in the urine. If renal insufficiency is present, cimetidine's dose and frequency may need to be reduced. Antacids can be given an hour before or after cimetidine as part of the antiulcer drug regimen; however, if they are given at the same time, the effectiveness of the H_2 blocker is decreased.

Three H_2 blockers, ranitidine (Zantac [1983]), famotidine (Pepcid [1986]), and nizatidine (Axid [1988]), are more potent than cimetidine. In addition to blocking gastric acid secretions, they promote healing of the ulcer by eliminating its cause. Their duration of action is longer, thus decreasing the frequency of dosing, and they have fewer side effects and fewer drug interactions than cimetidine. Prototype Drug Chart 46–2 gives the pharmacologic data for ranitidine (Zantac), the most frequently prescribed H_2 blocker.

PREVENTING MEDICATION ERRORS

Do not confuse...

- **ranitidine** (H_2 blocker) with **rimantadine** (an antiviral) or **amantadine** (an antiviral and antiparkinsonism agent). These drug names look alike but are from different classes and have different actions.

Pharmacokinetics

Ranitidine is 5 to 12 times more potent than cimetidine; however, it is less potent than famotidine. It is rapidly absorbed and reaches its peak concentration after a single dose in 1 to 3 hours. Ranitidine has a low protein-binding power and a short half-life. With liver disease, the half-life of ranitidine is prolonged. About 50% of the absorbed drug is excreted unchanged in the urine.

Ulcer healing occurs in 4 weeks for 70% of clients and in 8 weeks for 90% of clients taking ranitidine. Large doses of ranitidine are effective for controlling Zollinger-Ellison syndrome, whereas cimetidine is not effective in controlling the symptoms of this disorder.

Pharmacodynamics

Ranitidine inhibits histamine at the H_2 receptor site. The drug is effective in treating gastric and duodenal ulcers and can be used prophylactically. It is also useful in relieving symptoms of reflux esophagitis, preventing stress

---

PROTOTYPE DRUG CHART 46–2

RANITIDINE

Drug Class	**Dosage**
Antiulcer: histamine$_2$ blocker Trade Name: Zantac *Pregnancy Category:* B	A: PO: 150 mg q12h or 300 mg at bedtime; *maint:* 150 mg at bedtime IM: 50 mg q6-8h IV: 50 mg q6-8h diluted C: PO: 2-4 mg/kg/d divided q12h IV: 1-2 mg/kg/d divided q6-8h
Contraindications	**Drug-Lab-Food Interactions**
Hypersensitivity, severe renal or liver disease *Caution:* Pregnancy, lactation	*Drug:* Decrease absorption with antacids; *decrease* absorption of ketoconazole; *toxicity* with metoprolol *Lab:* Increase serum alkaline phosphatase
Pharmacokinetics	**Pharmacodynamics**

Absorption: PO: well absorbed, 50%
Distribution: PB: 15%
Metabolism: t½: 2-3 h
Excretion: In urine and feces
	PO: Onset: 15 min
	  Peak: 1-3 h
	  Duration: 8-12 h
	IM/IV: Onset: 10-15 min
	  Peak: 15 min
	  Duration: 8-12 h

Therapeutic Effects/Uses

To prevent and treat peptic ulcers, gastroesophageal reflux, and stress ulcers
Mode of Action: Inhibition of gastric acid secretion by inhibiting histamine at histamine$_2$ receptors in parietal cells

Side Effects	**Adverse Reactions**
Headache, confusion, nausea, vertigo, diarrhea or constipation, depression, rash, blurred vision, malaise	**Life-threatening:** Hepatotoxicity, cardiac dysrhythmias, blood dyscrasias

A, Adult; *C,* child; *d,* day; *h,* hour; *IM,* intramuscular; *IV,* intravenous; *maint,* maintenance; *min,* minute; *PB,* protein-binding; *PO,* by mouth; *t½,* half-life.

Table 46-6

Antiulcers: Histamine₂ Blockers

Generic (Brand)	Route and Dosage	Uses and Considerations
cimetidine (Tagamet)	A: PO: 300 mg q.i.d. with meals and at bedtime or 800 mg at bedtime; *maint:* 300 mg at bedtime IV: 300 mg q6-8h diluted in 50 ml (administered over 15-30 min) IV: continuous infusion: 37.5 mg/h over 24 h; *max:* 900 mg/d C: PO/IV: 10-40 mg/kg/d divided q6h	For peptic ulcers (gastric and duodenal). The first H₂ blocker marketed. Has many drug interaction and side effects. Duration of action is 4-6 h. *Pregnancy category:* B; PB: 20%; t½: 2 h
famotidine (Pepcid)	A: PO: 20 mg q12h or 40 mg at bedtime; *maint:* 20 mg at bedtime IV: 20 mg q12h diluted C: PO: 0.5-1 mg/kg/d divided q8-12h; *max:* 40 mg/d C: IV: 0.5 mg/kg/d divided q8-12h	For treatment of active duodenal ulcer. Inhibits gastric secretion. More potent than cimetidine. *Pregnancy category:* B; PB: 15%-20%; t½: 2.5-4 h
nizatidine (Axid)	A: PO: 150 mg q12h or 300 mg at bedtime; *maint:* 150 mg at bedtime	Same as famotidine. Also to treat gastroesophageal reflux. Give drug after meals or at bedtime. Do not give within 1 h of antacids. *Pregnancy category:* B; PB: 35%; t½: 1-2 h
ranitidine (Zantac)	See Prototype Drug Chart 46-2.	

A, Adult; *C,* child; *d,* day; *h,* hour; *IV,* intravenous; *maint,* maintenance; *max,* maximum; *PB,* protein-binding; *PO,* by mouth; *q.i.d.,* four times a day; *t½,* half-life.

---

ulcers that can occur following major surgery, and preventing aspiration pneumonitis that can result from aspiration of gastric acid secretions.

Ranitidine has a longer onset of action and duration of action (up to 12 hours) than cimetidine. Because cimetidine has a duration of action of only 4 to 5 hours, it is frequently given three to four times a day.

Famotidine (Pepcid) is 50% to 80% more potent than cimetidine and is five to eight times more potent than ranitidine. It is indicated for short-term use (4 to 8 weeks) for duodenal ulcer and for Zollinger-Ellison syndrome.

Nizatidine (Axid) is the latest H₂ blocker. It can relieve nocturnal gastric acid secretion for 12 hours. This drug is similar to famotidine and ranitidine, and none of these agents suppresses the metabolism of other drugs. To prevent recurrence of duodenal ulcers, administer nizatidine 150 mg per day at bedtime or famotidine 20 mg per day at bedtime. Both nizatidine and famotidine have similar protein-binding times and half-lives.

Table 46-6 lists the H₂ blockers and their dosages, uses, and considerations.

Side Effects and Adverse Reactions

Side effects and adverse reactions of H₂ blockers include headaches, dizziness, constipation, pruritus, skin rash, gynecomastia, decreased libido, and impotence. Ranitidine and famotidine have fewer side effects than cimetidine.

Drug and Laboratory Interactions

Cimetidine interacts with many drugs. By inhibiting hepatic drug metabolism, it enhances the effects of oral anticoagulants, theophylline, caffeine, phenytoin (Dilantin), diazepam (Valium), propranolol (Inderal), phenobarbital, and calcium channel blockers. Cimetidine can cause an increase in blood urea nitrogen (BUN), serum creatinine, and serum alkaline phosphatase. Neither cimetidine nor ranitidine should be taken with antacids because their H₂ blocking action could be decreased. Ranitidine can increase the effect of oral anticoagulants. Table 46-6 lists the drug data for the H₂ blockers.

Nursing Process

Antiulcer: Histamine₂ Blocker

ASSESSMENT

- Determine client's pain, including the type, duration, severity, frequency, and location.
- Evaluate GI complaints.
- Check mental status.
- Assess fluid and electrolyte imbalances, including intake and output.
- Monitor gastric pH (>5 is desired), blood urea nitrogen (BUN), and creatinine.
- Determine drug history; report probable drug-drug interactions.

NURSING DIAGNOSES

- Pain related to gastric dysfunction

PLANNING

- Client will no longer experience abdominal pain after 1 to 2 weeks of drug therapy.

NURSING INTERVENTIONS

- Do not confuse drug with alprazolam (Xanax).
- Administer drug just before meals to decrease food-induced acid secretion or at bedtime.
- Be alert that reduced doses of drug are needed by older adults, who have less gastric acid. Metabolic acidosis must be prevented.
- Administer drug IV in 20 to 100 ml of solution.

Client Teaching

General
- Instruct client to report pain, coughing, or vomiting of blood.
- Advise client to avoid smoking because it can hamper the effectiveness of the drug.
- Remind client that the drug must be taken exactly as prescribed to be effective.
- Direct client to separate ranitidine and antacid dosage by at least 1 hour, if possible.
- Warn client not to drive a motor vehicle or engage in dangerous activities until stabilized on the drug.
- Tell client that drug-induced impotence and gynecomastia are reversible.
- Educate client on the use of relaxation techniques to decrease anxiety.

Diet
- Teach client to eat foods rich in vitamin B_{12} to avoid deficiency as a result of drug therapy.

- Alert client to avoid foods and liquids that can cause gastric irritation, such as caffeine-containing beverages, alcohol, and spices.

Cultural Considerations
- Respect client's cultural beliefs and alternative methods for treating GI discomfort. Discuss with client the safety of his or her methods and the use of drugs prescribed to heal and lessen the symptoms.
- Recognize that clients of various cultural backgrounds may need guidance in understanding the disease process of their GI disturbance. Use of a written plan of care with modification should be considered.

EVALUATION

- Determine the effectiveness of the drug therapy and the presence of any side effects or adverse reactions. Client should be free of pain, and healing should progress.

PROTOTYPE DRUG CHART 46–3

LANSOPRAZOLE

Drug Class
Antiulcer: proton pump inhibitor
Trade Name: Prevacid
Pregnancy Category: C

Dosage
Erosive esophagitis:
A: PO: 30 mg daily for 8 wk then 15 mg daily
GERD
A: PO: 15 mg daily for up to wk
C: PO: 1-11 y: 1.5 mg/kg/d max: 30 mg/d
Helicobactor pylori:
A: PO: 30 mg b.i.d. for 2 wk in combination therapy
Duodenal ulcer:
A: PO: 15 mg daily for 4 wk

Contraindications
Hypersensitivity, pregnancy, lactation

Drug-Lab-Food Interactions
Drugs: May decrease theophylline levels, Sucralfate decreases lansaprazole bioavailability; may interfere with absorption of ampicillin, ketoconazole, digoxin
Food: Food decreases peak levels

Pharmacokinetics
Absorption: Rapidly absorbed in GI tract
Distribution: PB: 97%
Metabolism: t½: 1.5 h
Excretion: primarily in urine; also in bile and feces

Pharmacodynamics
PO: Onset: 2 h
Peak: 1.5-3 h
Duration: 24 h

Therapeutic Effects/Uses
To treat peptic and duodenal ulcers, GERD, erosive esophagitis, and H. pylori
Mode of Action: Suppression of gastric acid secretion by inhibiting the hydrogen/potassium ATPase enzyme in the gastric parietal cells

Side Effects
Headache, dizziness, fatigue, thirst, increased appetite, anorexia, nausea, diarrhea or constipation, and rash

Adverse Reactions
Elevated AST, ALT

A, Adult; ALT, alanine aminotransferase; AST, aspartate aminotransferase; ATP, adenosine triphospate; b.i.d., two times a day; C, child; d, day; GERD, gastroesophageal reflux disease; GI, gastrointestinal; h, hour; max, maximum; PB, protein-binding; PO, by mouth; t½, half-life; wk, week; y, year.

Proton Pump Inhibitors (Gastric Acid Secretion Inhibitors, Gastric Acid Pump Inhibitors)

The PPIs suppress gastric acid secretion by inhibiting the hydrogen/potassium adenosine triphosphatase (ATPase) enzyme system located in the gastric parietal cells. They tend to inhibit gastric acid secretion up to 90% greater than the H_2 blockers (histamine antagonists). These agents block the final step of acid production.

Omeprazole (Prilosec) was the first PPI marketed. Lansoprazole (Prevacid) became available in 1993. In the late 1990s, two new PPIs were approved: rabeprazole (Aciphex) and pantoprazole (Protonix). Esomeprazole (Nexium) received Food and Drug Administration (FDA) approval in 2001. These five agents are effective in suppressing gastric acid secretions and are used to treat peptic ulcers and GERD. With lansoprazole, ulcer relief usually occurs in 1 week. Rabeprazole is more effective in treating duodenal ulcers than gastric ulcers and is most effective for treating GERD and hypersecretory disease (Zollinger-Ellison syn-

drome). Pantoprazole, the fourth PPI developed, is prescribed to treat short-term erosive GERD. Intravenous pantoprazole is also reported as effective in treating Zollinger-Ellison syndrome. Esomeprazole, the newest PPI, has the highest success rate for healing erosive GERD, more so than omeprazole. Omeprazole promotes irreversible hydrogen or potassium ATPase inhibition until new enzyme is synthesized, which could take days, whereas rabeprazole causes reversible ATPase inhibition. All PPIs, in large doses, can be combined with antibiotics to treat *H. pylori*. See Prototype Drug Chart 46–3 for the pharmacologic data on lansoprazole.

Pharmacokinetics and Pharmacodynamics

The duration of action for omeprazole is 72 hours and 24 hours for lansoprazole. These drugs have a short-life and are highly protein bound (97%). PPIs should be taken before meals. Caution should be used in clients with hepatic impairment; liver enzymes should be monitored. Possible side effects include headache, dizziness, diarrhea, abdominal pain, and rash. Prolonged use of PPIs may increase the risk of cancer, although this has only been proven in mice, not humans.

Table 46–7 lists the PPIs and their dosages, uses, and considerations.

Table 46–7

Antiulcers: Pepsin Inhibitor, Proton Pump Inhibitors, and Prostaglandin Analogue

Generic (Brand)	Route and Dosage	Uses and Considerations
Pepsin Inhibitor		
sucralfate (Carafate)	See Prototype Drug Chart 46–3.	
Proton Pump Inhibitors (Gastric Acid Secretion Inhibitors)		
esomeprazole magnesium (Nexium)	A: PO: 20-40 mg/d	It is most effective for treating erosive GERD. Healing usually occurs in 4 to 8 wk. May be combined with amoxicillin or clarithromycin for treating *Helicobacter pylori*. *Pregnancy category:* UK; PB: 97%; $t^{1/2}$: 1-1.5 h.
lansoprazole (Prevacid)	*Duodenal ulcer:* A: PO: 15 mg/d a.c. for 4 wk *Erosive esophagitis:* A: PO: 30 mg/d a.c. for 8 wk	Short-term treatment for duodenal ulcer and erosive esophagitis. Used in drug combination for treatment of *H. pylori*. Also effective for treating Zollinger-Ellison syndrome. Swallow capsule whole (do not chew or crush). *Pregnancy category:* B; PB: 97%; $t^{1/2}$: 1.5 h
omeprazole (Prilosec)	*GERD and peptic ulcer:* A: PO: 20 mg/d for 4-8 wk *Hypersecretory:* A: PO: Initially: 60 mg/d; may increase to 120 mg t.i.d.	Treatment of GERD, including esophagitis, Zollinger-Ellison syndrome, and *H. pylori*. Poorly absorbed with only 35%-40% in circulation. Antacids can be taken with drug. *Pregnancy category:* C; PB: 95%; $t^{1/2}$: 0.5-1.5 h
pantoprazole (Protonix)	A: PO/IV: 40 mg/d	To treat gastric and duodenal ulcers and GERD. Action is the same as rabeprazole by suppressing gastric acid secretion. *Pregnancy category:* B; PB: UK; $t^{1/2}$: 1-2 h.
rabeprazole (Aciphex)	*Duodenal ulcer/GERD:* A: PO: 20 mg/d *Hypersecretory disease:* A: PO: 60 mg/d or 60 mg b.i.d.	To treat duodenal ulcer, GERD, and hypersecretory syndrome (Zollinger-Ellison syndrome). Decreases gastric acid production by inhibiting hydrogen/potassium ATPase enzyme at the gastric parietal cells. *Pregnancy category:* B: PB: UK: $t^{1/2}$: UK
Prostaglandin Analogue		
misoprostol (Cytotec)	A: PO: 100-200 mcg q.i.d. with food C: <18 y: PO: Safety and efficacy not established	Prevention of NSAID-induced gastric ulcer. May be taken during NSAID therapy, including with aspirin. Side effects include diarrhea, abdominal pain, flatulence, nausea and vomiting, constipation, and menstrual spotting. Has a short duration of action. *Pregnancy category:* X; PB: 85%; $t^{1/2}$: 1.5 h

A, Adult; *a.c.*, before meals; *ATP*, adenosine triphosphate; *b.i.d.*, two times a day; *C*, child; *d*, day; *GERD*, gastroesophageal reflux disease; *h*, hour; *IV*, intravenous; *NSAIDs*, nonsteroidal antiinflammatory drugs; *PB*, protein-binding; *PO*, by mouth; *q.i.d.*, four times a day; *t¹/₂*, half-life; *t.i.d.*, three times a day; *UK*, unknown; *wk*, week; *y*, year; *<*, less than.

Drug Interactions

Omeprazole can enhance the action of oral anticoagulants, certain benzodiazepines, and phenytoin because it interferes with the liver metabolism of these drugs. Lansoprazole may decrease the theophylline levels. With pantoprazole, no significant drug interactions are reported.

Pepsin Inhibitor (Mucosal Protective Drug)

Sucralfate (Carafate), a complex of sulfated sucrose and aluminum hydroxide, is classified as a pepsin inhibitor, or mucosal protective drug. It is nonabsorbable and combines with protein to form a viscous substance that covers the ulcer and protects it from acid and pepsin. This drug does not neutralize acid or decrease acid secretions.

The dosage of sucralfate is 1 g, usually four times a day before meals and at bedtime. If antacids are added to decrease pain, they should be given either 30 minutes before or after the administration of sucralfate. Because sucralfate is not systemically absorbed, side effects are few; however, it can cause constipation. If the drug is stored at room temperature in a tight container, it will remain stable for up to 2 years.

PREVENTING MEDICATION ERRORS

Do not confuse...

- **protonix** (a proton pump inhibitor) with **Lotronex** (serotonin 5–HT3 receptor antagonist). These drug names look alike but are from different classes and have different actions. Alosetron (Lotronex) is used to treat symptoms of severe irritable bowel syndrome that lasts longer than 6 months and are unresponsive to traditional therapy.

See Prototype Drug Chart 46–4 for the action and effects of sucralfate.

Pharmacokinetics

Less than 5% of sucralfate is absorbed by the GI tract. It has a half-life of 6 to 20 hours. Ninety percent of the drug is excreted in the feces.

Pharmacodynamics

Sucralfate promotes healing by adhering to the ulcer surface. The onset of action occurs within 30 minutes, and the duration of action is short. Sucralfate decreases the absorption of tetracycline, phenytoin, fat-soluble vitamins, and the antibacterial agents ciprofloxacin and norfloxacin. Antacids decrease the effects of sucralfate.

PROTOTYPE DRUG CHART 46–4

SUCRALFATE

Drug Class	**Dosage**
Antiulcer: pepsin inhibitor Trade Name: Carafate, ♣ Sulcrate *Pregnancy Category:* B	*Active disease:* A: PO: 1 g q.i.d. 1 h a.c. and at bedtime *Maintenance:* A: PO: 1 g b.i.d.
Contraindications	**Drug-Lab-Food Interactions**
Hypersensitivity *Caution:* Renal failure	*Drug: Decrease* effects with tetracycline, phenytoin, fat-soluble vitamins, digoxin; *altered absorption* with ciprofloxacin, norfloxacin, antacids
Pharmacokinetics	**Pharmacodynamics**
Absorption: PO: Minimal absorption (<5%) **Distribution:** PB: UK **Metabolism:** t½: 6-20 h **Excretion:** In urine	PO: Onset: 30 min Peak: UK Duration: 5 h

Therapeutic Effects/Uses

To prevent gastric mucosal injury from drug-induced ulcers (aspirin, NSAIDs); to manage ulcers
Mode of Action: In combination with gastric acid, forms a protective covering on the ulcer surface

Side Effects	**Adverse Reactions**
Dizziness, nausea, constipation, dry mouth, rash, pruritus, back pain, sleepiness	None significant

A, Adult; *a.c.,* before meals; *b.i.d.,* twice a day; *h,* hour; *min,* minute; *NSAIDs,* nonsteroidal antiinflammatory drugs; *PB,* protein-binding; *PO,* by mouth; *q.i.d.,* four times a day; *t½,* half-life; *UK,* unknown; ♣, Canadian drug name; <, less than.

Nursing Process

Antiulcer: Pepsin Inhibitor

ASSESSMENT

■ Evaluate client's pain, including the type, duration, severity, and frequency. Ulcer pain usually occurs after meals and during the night.
■ Determine client's renal function. Report urine output of <600 ml/d or <25 ml/h.
■ Assess for fluid and electrolyte imbalances.
■ Measure gastric pH (>5 is desired).

NURSING DIAGNOSES

■ Pain related to GI dysfunction

PLANNING

■ Client will be free of abdominal pain after 1 to 2 weeks of antiulcer drug management.

NURSING INTERVENTIONS

■ Administer drug on empty stomach.
■ Administer an antacid 30 minutes before or after sucralfate. Allow 1 to 2 hours to elapse between sucralfate and other prescribed drugs; sucralfate binds with certain drugs (e.g., tetracycline, phenytoin) thus reducing the effect of the other drugs.

Client Teaching
General
• Advise client to take drug exactly as ordered. Therapy usually requires 4 to 8 weeks for optimal ulcer healing. Advise client to continue to take drug even if feeling better.
• Increase fluids, dietary bulk, and exercise to relieve constipation.
• Instruct client on the use of relaxation techniques.
• Monitor for severe, persistent constipation.
• Stress need for follow-up medical care.
• Emphasize cessation of smoking as indicated.

Side Effects
• Direct client to report pain, coughing, or vomiting of blood.

Diet
• Teach client to avoid foods and liquids that can cause gastric irritation, such as caffeine-containing beverages, alcohol, and spices.

Cultural Considerations
• Greet the person by name with the appropriate title: Mr., Mrs., Miss, Ms., or Dr. Wait until client gives permission for you to use the first name.
• Males should not extend the hand in greeting to a female unless she extends her hand first.
• Orthodox males do not shake hands with females, and their failure to do so when one's hand is extended should not be interpreted as a sign of rudeness.

EVALUATION

■ Determine the effectiveness of the antiulcer treatment and the presence of any side effects. Client should be free of pain, and healing should progress.

Prostaglandin Analogue Antiulcer Drug

Misoprostol, a synthetic prostaglandin analogue, is a drug used to prevent and treat peptic ulcer. It appears to suppress gastric acid secretion and increase cytoprotective mucus in the GI tract. It causes a moderate decrease in pepsin secretion. Misoprostol is considered as effective as cimetidine. Clients who complain of gastric distress from NSAIDs, such as aspirin or indomethacin prescribed for long-term therapy, can benefit from misoprostol. When the client takes high doses of NSAIDs, misoprostol is frequently recommended for the duration of the NSAID therapy. Misoprostol is contraindicated during pregnancy and for women of childbearing age.

Table 46–7 lists the drug data for the pepsin inhibitors, PPIs, and prostaglandin analogue.

WEBSITES

For further information on *Antiulcer Drugs*, visit these Internet resources:

Ranitidine:
www.diseasesdatabase.com/sieve/item1.asp?glngUserChoice=29916

Esomeprazole:
www.nlm.nih.gov/medlineplus/druginfo/medmaster/a699054.html

Critical Thinking Case Study

J.H., age 48, complains of a gnawing, aching pain in the abdominal area that usually occurs several hours after eating. He said that Tums helps somewhat, but the pain has recently intensified. Diagnostic tests indicate that the client has a duodenal ulcer.

1. Differentiate between peptic ulcer, gastric ulcer, and duodenal ulcer. Explain.

2. What are the predisposing factors related to peptic ulcers? What additional information do you need from J.H.?

3. What nonpharmacologic measures can you suggest to alleviate symptoms related to peptic ulcer?

The health care provider prescribed Mylanta 2 tsp to be taken 2 hours after meals and ranitidine (Zantac) 150 mg b.i.d. The dose of Mylanta is to be taken either 1 hour before or 1 hour after the ranitidine.

4. J.H. asks the nurse the purposes for Mylanta and ranitidine. What would be the response?

5. The health care provider may suggest that the client take ranitidine with meals. Why? Why should Mylanta and ranitidine not be taken at the same time?

6. In what ways are ranitidine and cimetidine the same and how do they differ? Explain.

7. As part of client teaching, the nurse discusses side effects of ranitidine with J.H. What might be the most effective way to present this information? Develop a plan.

The client states that he drinks beer at lunch and has two gin and tonics in the midafternoon. He states that these drinks help him relax.

8. What nursing intervention should be taken in regard to his alcohol intake?

9. What foods should he avoid?

A week later the client states that he discontinued the prescribed medications because he "felt better." However, the pain recurred and he asked whether he should resume taking the medications.

10. What would be your response? What client teaching should be included?

Study Questions

1. What is the action of antacids used in the treatment and control of peptic ulcers?

2. Your client takes Maalox 15 ml four times a day. At what times should the drug be taken? What would the duration of action be if the drug were taken with and without food? How should it be taken?

3. What is a major side effect of antacids that contain aluminum salts and magnesium salts?

4. Your client takes ranitidine (Zantac). What type of drug is ranitidine?

5. What is sucralfate (Carafate)? What is its action in treating peptic ulcer?

6. What are the actions of omeprazole and misoprostol?

7. What are the similarities and differences between H_2 inhibitors and PPIs?

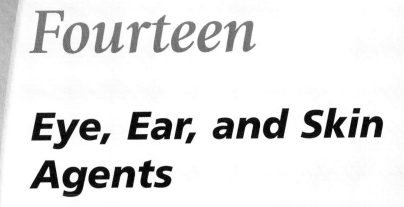

Fourteen

Eye, Ear, and Skin Agents

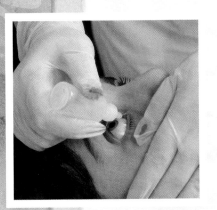

Many drugs used to treat eye and ear disorders are discussed in other chapters, such as the antibiotics covered in Chapters 28, Antibacterials: Penicillins and Cephalosporins, 29, Antibacterials: Macrolides, Tetracyclines, Aminoglycosides, and Fluoroquinolones, and 30, Antibacterials: Sulfonamides. Unit XI discusses in more detail the agents used to treat disorders of the eye and ear as well as the skin. Chapter 47, Drugs for Disorders of the Eye and Ear, presents medications used to treat eye disorders, particularly glaucoma and ocular infections. Drugs used to treat ear disorders are also covered. Chapter 48, Drugs for Dermatologic Disorders, presents the agents for dermatologic disorders.

Overview of the Eye

The eyeballs, protected within the orbits of the skull, are controlled by the third, fourth, and sixth cranial nerves and are connected to six extraocular muscles. The eye has three layers: (1) the cornea and sclera; (2) the choroid, iris, and ciliary body; and (3) the retina. Figure XIV–1 illustrates the basic structures of the eye.

The cornea, the anterior covering of the eye, is transparent, enabling light to enter the eye. It has no blood vessels and receives nutrition from the aqueous humor. An abraded cornea is susceptible to infection. Loss of corneal transparency is usually caused by increased intraocular pressure (IOP).

The sclera is the opaque, white fibrous envelope of the eye. Within the sclera are the posterior chamber and the anterior chamber. The posterior chamber has a blind spot, which is not sensitive to light, around the optic nerve. The lens, held in place by ligaments, separates these two chambers. The normally transparent lens focuses light on the retina by changing its shape through a process called *accommodation*.

The anterior chamber, filled with aqueous humor secreted by the ciliary body, lies in front of the lens. The fluid flows into the anterior chamber through a space between the lens and iris. The excess fluid drains into the canal of Schlemm. A rise in intraocular pressure, resulting in glaucoma, occurs with increased production or decreased drainage of aqueous humor.

The choroid, iris, and ciliary body (thickened part of vascular covering of the eye that provides attachment to ligaments and support to lens) constitute the second layer. The choroid absorbs light. The iris, which surrounds the pupil and gives the eye its color, controls the quantity of light reaching the lens through dilation and constriction.

The retina, the third layer, consists of nerves, rods, and cones that serve as visual sensory receptors. The retina is connected to the brain via the optic nerve.

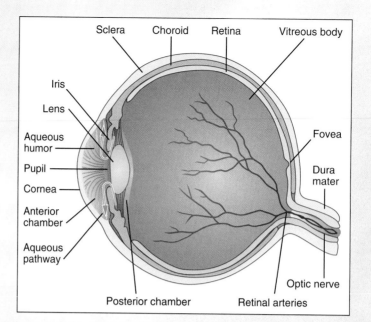

FIGURE XIV–1 Basic structures of the eye.

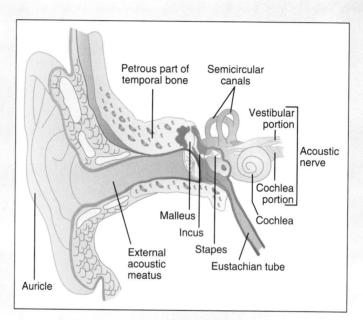

FIGURE XIV–2 Basic structures of the ear.

The eyebrows, eyelashes, eyelids, tears, and corneal and conjunctival reflexes all serve to protect the eye. Bilateral blinking occurs every few seconds during waking hours to keep the eye moist and free of foreign material.

Overview of the Ear

The ear is divided into the external, middle, and inner ear. Figure XIV–2 illustrates the ear's basic structures.

The *external ear* consists of the pinna and the external auditory canal. The external auditory canal transmits sound to the tympanic membrane (eardrum), a transparent partition between the external and middle ear. The eardrum in turn transmits sound to the bones of the middle ear; it also serves a protective function.

The *middle ear*, an air-filled cavity, contains three auditory ossicles (malleus, incus, and stapes) that transmit sound waves to the inner ear. The tip of the malleus is attached to the eardrum; its head is attached to the incus, which is attached to the stapes. The eustachian tube provides a direct connection to the nasopharynx and equalizes air pressure on both sides of the eardrum to prevent it from rupturing. Swallowing, yawning, and chewing gum help the eustachian tube relieve pressure changes on airplane flights.

The *inner ear*, a series of labyrinths (canals), consists of a bony section and a membranous section. The vestibule, cochlea, and semicircular canals make up the bony labyrinth. The vestibular area is responsible for maintaining equilibrium and balance. The cochlea is the principal hearing organ.

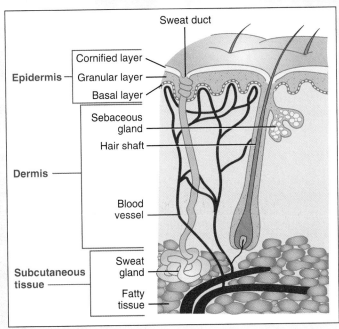

FIGURE XIV–3   Basic structures of the skin.

Professional evaluation of ear problems is essential because hearing loss can result from untreated disorders. Middle ear problems require prescription medications and are not treated with over-the-counter preparations.

Overview of the Skin

Skin, the largest organ of the body, consists of two major layers: the *epidermis* (the outer layer of the skin) and the *dermis* (the layer of skin beneath the epidermis). The functions of the skin include (1) protecting the body from the environment, (2) aiding in body temperature control, and (3) preventing body fluid loss.

The epidermis has four layers: (1) the basal layer (stratum germinativum), the deepest layer lying over the dermis; (2) the spinous layer (stratum spinosum); (3) the granular layer (stratum granulosum); and (4) the cornified layer (stratum corneum), the outer layer of the epidermis. As the epidermal cells migrate to the surface, they die and their cytoplasm converts to keratin (hard and rough texture), forming keratinocytes. Eventually the keratinocytes slough off as new layers of epidermal cells migrate upward.

The dermis has two layers: (1) the papillary layer, next to the epidermis, and (2) the reticular layer, which is the deeper layer of the dermis. The dermal layers consist of fibroblasts, collagen fibers, and elastic fibers. The collagen and elastic fibers give the skin its strength and elasticity. Within the dermal layer, there are sweat glands, hair follicles, sebaceous glands, blood vessels, and sensory nerve terminals. Figure XIV–3 shows the layers of the skin.

The subcutaneous tissue, primarily fatty tissue, lies under the dermis. Besides fatty cells, subcutaneous tissue contains blood and lymphatic vessels, nerve fibers, and elastic fibers. It supports and protects the dermis.

47 Drugs for Disorders of the Eye and the Ear

ELECTRONIC RESOURCES

Additional information can be found on the companion website at *http://evolve.elsevier.com/KeeHayes/pharmacology/* or on the companion CD-ROM, which includes:
- *NCLEX-style examination review questions*
- *Pharmacology animations*
- *Medication error and IV therapy checklists*
- *Medication calculation problems*
- *Electronic calculators*

OBJECTIVES

- Identify the medication groups commonly used for disorders of the eye and ear.
- List the mechanisms of action, route, side effects and adverse reactions, and contraindications for selected drugs in each group.
- Describe the content of teaching plans for the drug groups presented.
- Describe the nursing process, including client teaching, related to disorders of the eye and ear.

TERMS

carbonic anhydrase inhibitors

cerumen

ceruminolytic

conjunctivitis

cycloplegics

lacrimal duct

miosis

miotics

mydriatics

ophthalmic

optic

osmotics

otic

Introduction

This chapter describes the most commonly used drugs for eye and ear disorders. Many of these drugs have other uses and are discussed in greater detail in other chapters.

Drugs for Disorders of the Eye

The nurse must be alert to the fact that a variety of systemic diseases have ocular findings that are characteristic. Examples of these systemic disorders are acquired immunodeficiency syndrome (AIDS), coronary vascular disease, muscular and endocrine disorders, and hematologic and neurologic diseases.

Diagnostic Aids

Diagnostic aids are frequently used to locate lesions or foreign objects and to provide local anesthesia to the area. Drugs commonly used as diagnostic aids are presented in Table 47-1.

Topical Anesthetics

Topical anesthetics are used in selected aspects of a comprehensive eye examination and in the removal of foreign bodies from the eye. The two most common topical anesthetics are proparacaine HCl (Ophthaine, Ophthetic) and tetracaine HCl (Pontocaine).

Corneal anesthesia is achieved within 1 minute and generally lasts about 15 minutes. The blink reflex is temporarily lost; therefore the corneal epithelium is not kept moist. To protect the eye, a patch is usually worn over the eye until the effects of the drug are gone. These drugs are *not* to be self-administered by the client. Repeated doses are given only under strict medical supervision.

Antiinfectives and Antiinflammatories

Antiinfectives are frequently used for eye infections. Screen the client for previous allergic reactions. **Conjunctivitis** (inflammation of the delicate membrane covering the eyeball and lining the eyelid) and local skin and eye irritation are possible side effects of topical **ophthalmic** anti-infective drugs. Examples of frequently occurring ocular conditions treated with antiinfectives include the following:

- Conjunctivitis
- Blepharitis (infection of margins of eyelid)
- Chalazion (infection of meibomian glands of the eyelids that may produce cysts, causing blockage of the ducts)
- Endophthalmitis (inflammation of structures of the inner eye)
- Hordeolum (local infection of eyelash follicles and glands on lid margins)
- Keratitis (corneal inflammation)
- Uveitis (infection of vascular layer of eye [ciliary body, choroids, and iris])

Conjunctivitis is an eye infection that can be bacterial, viral, or allergic in origin. The common ophthalmic antihistamines used to treat allergic conjunctivitis include cromolyn sodium (Crolom), ketotifen fumarate (Zaditor), levocabastine (Livostin), lodoxamide tromethamine (Alomide), olopatadine (Patanol), and peritolast potassium (Alamast). Burning, headache, and stinging are the most frequent adverse effects.

See Chapters 28, Antibacterials and their Effects: Penicillins and Cephalosporins, 29, Antibacterials: Macrolides, Tetracyclines, Aminoglycosides, and Fluoroquinolones, and 30, Antibacterials: Sulfonamides, for more comprehensive information on anti-infectives. The drug data for **optic** (eye) anti-infectives are presented in Table 47-2. Optic antiinflammatories are presented in Table 47-3.

Lubricants

Both healthy and ill persons may need to use eye lubricants. Healthy clients who complain of "dryness of the eyes" use lubricants as artificial tears; lubricants are also used to moisten contact lenses or artificial eyes. Lubricants alleviate discomfort associated with dryness and maintain the integrity of the epithelial surface. They are also used during anesthesia and in acute or chronic central nervous system (CNS) disorders that result in unconsciousness or decreased blinking.

Table 47-1

Diagnostic Aids for Eye Disorders

Diagnostic Aid	Purpose
fluorescein sodium	Dye used to demonstrate defects in corneal epithelium. Corneal scratches turn bright green; foreign bodies are surrounded by green ring. Loss of conjunctiva shows orange-yellow. Dye appears in nasal secretions if lacrimal duct patent.
fluorescein sodium and benoxinate HCl (Fluress)	Dye and local anesthetic. Used for short corneal and conjunctival procedures, including removal of foreign bodies.
rose bengal	Preferred dye when superficial conjunctival tissue or corneal changes suspended.

Table 47–2

Ophthalmic: Antiinfectives

Generic (Brand)	Route and Dosage*	Uses and Considerations
Antibacterials		
chloramphenicol (AK-Chlor, Chloromycetin Ophthalmic)	A & C: Ophthalmic: Instill 1-2 gtt or 0.5-in oint q3-4h for 48 h; increase interval to b.i.d./t.i.d.	Effective against both gram-negative and gram-positive bacteria. For treatment of severe infections or when other antibacterials not effective. Continue treatment for at least 48 h after eye appears normal. *Pregnancy category:* C; PB: NA; $t\frac{1}{2}$: NA
ciprofloxacin (Cipro)	A & C >12 y: *Day 1:* 2 gtt q15min for 6 h then 2 gtt q30min for rest of day *Day 2:* 2 gtt qh *Days 3-14:* 2 gtt q4h	Effective against bacterial conjunctivitis. To treat corneal ulceration. Minimal absorption through cornea or conjunctiva. *Pregnancy category:* C; PB: NA; $t\frac{1}{2}$: NA
erythromycin (Ilotycin)	A & C >12 y: Oint: 0.5%: 0.5-1 cm daily/q.i.d.	Most commonly used antibacterial. For superficial ocular infections and prevention of ophthalmia neonatorum. *Pregnancy category:* B; PB: NA; $t\frac{1}{2}$: NA
gentamicin sulfate (Garamycin Ophthalmic)	A & C: Sol 0.3%: 1-2 gtt q4h; may increase to 2 gtt qh for severe infections Oint 0.3%: 0.5-in ribbon b.i.d./t.i.d.	For infections of the external eye: *Pregnancy category:* C; PB: NA; $t\frac{1}{2}$: NA
norfloxacin (Chibroxin)	A & C >1 y: Sol 3%: instill 1-2 gtt in affected eye(s) q.i.d. for 7 d	For treatment of conjunctivitis. *Pregnancy category:* C; PB: NA; $t\frac{1}{2}$: NA
silver nitrate 1% (Dey-Drop)	Neonate: Instill 2 gtt in each eye within 1 h of birth	For prevention and treatment of ophthalmia neonatorum. *Pregnancy category:* C; PB: NA; $t\frac{1}{2}$: NA
sulfacetamide (Bleph-10, Sulamyd)	A & C >12 y: Sol: 1 gtt q1-3h while awake; then q3-4h while sleeping	Effectiveness of sulfonamides decreased in the presence of PABA and purulent drainage, hence exudates should be removed before instilling drops. *Pregnancy category:* C; PB: NA; $t\frac{1}{2}$: NA
tobramycin (Nebcin, Tobrex)	A & C >12 y: Oint 0.3%: 0.5-in b.i.d./t.i.d. Sol 0.3%: 1-2 gtt q4h *For severe infections;* Oint: 0.5-in q3-4h Sol: 2 gtt q30-60 min until improvement, then decrease frequency	For external ocular infections. *Pregnancy category:* D; PB: NA; $t\frac{1}{2}$: NA
tetracycline HCl (Achromycin Ophthalmic)	A: Instill 1-2 gtt b.i.d./q.i.d. A: Instill 0.5-in q2-12h	Bacteriostatic action; alternative to silver nitrate for prevention of ophthalmia neonatorum. *Pregnancy category:* D; PB: NA; $t\frac{1}{2}$: NA
triple antibiotic ophthalmic ointment (Neomycin, Polymyxin B Sulfate, Bacitracin Ophthalmic)	A & C >12 y: 1 cm applied in conjunctival sac q3-4h	Combination dosage form effective against many gram-negative organisms. *Pregnancy category:* C; PB: NA; $t\frac{1}{2}$: NA
Antifungal		
natamycin (Natacyn Ophthalmic)	A & C: Sol 5%: 1 gt q2h for 3-4 d; then 1 gt q3h for 14-21 d	May cause transient stinging or temporary blurring of vision. *Pregnancy category:* C; PB: NA; $t\frac{1}{2}$: NA
Antiviral		
idoxuridine (IDU, Herplex Liquifilm)	A & C: Sol 1%: Initially: 1 gt q1h during the day and q2h at night; when definite improvement occurs, use 1 gt q2h during the day and q4h at night; continue 3-7 d after healing occurs Oint 0.5%: Place 0.5-in. q4h while awake	To treat cytomegalovirus or herpes simplex keratitis. Store in refrigerator; do not mix with boric acid. If no response in 1 wk, discontinue. *Pregnancy category:* C; PB: NA; $t\frac{1}{2}$: NA
trifluridine (Viroptic)	A: Sol 1%: Instill 1 gt into infected eye q2h while awake; *max:* 9 gtt/d until corneal ulcer reepithelialized; then 1 gt q4h for 7 d; *max:* 21 d of treatment	For treatment of herpetic ophthalmic infections and keratoconjunctivitis caused by HSV-1 and HSV-2. *Pregnancy category:* C; PB: NA; $t\frac{1}{2}$: NA
vidarabine monohydrate (Vira-A)	A & C: Oint 3%: 0.5-in. 5 × d at 3-h intervals	For treatment of keratoconjunctivitis and herpes simplex keratitis. *Pregnancy category:* C; PB: NA; $t\frac{1}{2}$: NA

*To minimize systemic absorption, gently apply pressure on inner canthus.

A, Adult; *b.i.d.,* twice a day; *C,* child; *d,* day; *HSV,* herpes simplex virus; *gt,* drop; *gtt,* drops; *h,* hour; *in,* inch; *max,* maximum; *NA,* not applicable; *oint,* ointment; *PABA,* paraaminobenzoic acid; *PB,* protein-binding; *q.i.d.,* four times a day; *sol,* solution; $t\frac{1}{2}$, half-life; *t.i.d.,* three times a day; *wk,* week; *y,* year; *>,* greater than.

Table 47-3

Ophthalmic: Antiinflammatories

Generic (Brand)	Route and Dosage*	Uses and Considerations
Nonsteroidals		
*diclofenac Na (Voltaren)	A: 1 gt to affected eye q.i.d. for 2 wk; start 24 h after cataract surgery	For postoperative inflammation and photophobia. *Pregnancy category:* B; PB: NA; t½: NA
*flurbiprofen Na (Ocufen)	A: Instill 1 gt q30min at 2 h before surgery; total dose is 4 gtt	To decrease corneal edema; miosis. *Pregnancy category:* C; PB: NA; t½: NA
*ketorolac tromethamine (Acular)	A: Sol 0.5%: Instill 1 gt q.i.d.	Efficacy has not been established beyond 1 wk of therapy. Used to relieve itching associated with seasonal allergic conjunctivitis. *Pregnancy category:* C; PB: NA; t½: NA
*suprofen (Profenal)	*Preoperative:* A: Instill 2 gtt in sac q4h while awake on day preceding surgery; instill 2 gtt in conjunctival sac at 3, 2, and 1 h before surgery	Used to prevent intraoperative miosis. *Pregnancy category:* C; PB: NA; t½: NA
Corticosteroids		
dexamethasone (AK-Dex Ophthalmic, Decadron, Maxidax)	A & C: Oint: Apply into conjunctival sac t.i.d./q.i.d.; gradually decrease to discontinue Susp: Instill 2 gtt qh while awake and q2h during night; taper to q3-4h; then t.i.d./q.i.d.	For uveitis, allergic conditions, and inflammation of conjunctiva, cornea, and lids. Should not be used for minor abrasions and wounds. *Pregnancy category:* C; PB: NA; t½: NA
medrysone (HMS Liquifilm)	A & C: Susp: Initially: Instill 1 gt in conjunctival sac q1-2h (1-2 d); then 1 gt b.i.d./q.i.d.	To treat allergic conditions, burns, inflammation of conjunctiva, cornea, and lids. *Pregnancy category:* C; PB: NA; t½: NA
prednisolone acetate (Econopred)	A: Initially instill 1-2 gtt in conjunctival sac qh while awake, q2h during night until desired effect; *maint:* 1 gt q4h Susp: 0.125% and 1%	To treat uveitis, allergic conditions, burns, and inflammation of conjunctiva, cornea, and lids. *Pregnancy category:* C; PB: NA; t½: NA
prednisolone Na phosphate (AK-Pred, Inflamase)	A & Elderly: Sol 0.125% and 1%: 1-2 gtt q1h during day; q2h during night; with response give 1 gt q4h, then 1 gt t.i.d./q.i.d. Oint: thin coat t.i.d./q.i.d.; with response Decrease to b.i.d., then daily	To prevent or decrease tissue response to inflammatory process.
Combination: tobramycin 0.3% and dexamethasone 0.1% (TobraDex)	A: 1-2 gtt q2-6h first 24-48h; then q4-6h or less until symptoms decrease; *max:* 20 ml for first treatment Oint: Apply to conjunctival sac up to t.i.d./q.i.d.; *max:* 8 g for initial treatment Drops and ointment not recommended for children.	Combines antiinflammatory power of dexamethasone with antibiotic. Increased tolerability and comfortable pH. For treatment of fungal, mycobacterial, or viral infection of eye.

*To minimize systemic absorption, gently apply pressure to inner canthus.
A, Adult; *b.i.d.*, twice a day; *C*, child; *d*, day; *gt*, drop; *gtt*, drops; *h*, hour; *maint*, maintenance; *max*, maximum; *min*, minute; *NA*, not applicable; *oint*, ointment; *PB*, protein-binding; *q.i.d.*, four times a day; *sol*, solution; *susp*, suspension; *t½*, half-life; *t.i.d.*, three times a day; *wk*, week.

Most lubricants are available over-the-counter (OTC) in both liquid and ointment form. Popular lubricants include Isopto Tears, Tearisol, Ultra Tears, Tears Naturale, Tears Plus, Lens Mate, and Lacri-Lube. Be alert to allergic reactions to preservatives in lubricants.

Antiglaucoma Agents

Pharmacotherapy is the primary approach used to treat glaucoma, which is an increased intraocular pressure (IOP) resulting from excessive production or diminished outflow of aqueous humor. Glaucoma is classified as either (1) *primary* (pathologic change within the eye) or (2) *secondary* (change associated with systemic disease and use of selected drugs). The angle of the anterior chamber also determines the type of glaucoma. The angle can be either *open angle* (diminished outflow of aqueous humor related to degenerative changes in the trabecular meshwork) or *closed angle* (triggered by emotions and drugs that dilate pupils).

Antiglaucoma drugs belong to the following categories: cholinergic and anticholinesterase miotics, beta-adrenergic blockers, carbonic anhydrase inhibitors, osmotics, and anticholinergics. See Herbal Alert 47–1.

HERBAL ALERT 47–1

Herbs and Antiglaucoma Agents

- Avoid the use of goldenseal in clients with glaucoma.
- Many herbs alter coagulation; therefore they generally are discontinued before ophthalmic or otic surgery.
- Consult health care provider prior to use of herbs.

Normal flow of aqueous humor

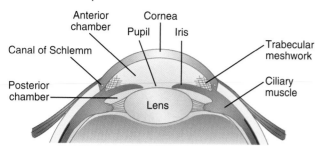

FIGURE 47–1 Increased intraocular pressure.

Impeded flow of aqueous humor,
resulting in intraocular pressure

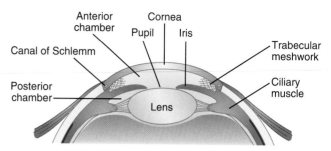

Obstructive flow to canal of Schlemm

Table 47–4

Miotics: Cholinergics and Beta-Adrenergic Blockers

Generic (Brand)	Route and Dosage	Uses and Considerations
Direct-Acting Cholinergics		
carbachol (Isopto-carbachol)	A: Ophthalmic: 1-2 gtt daily/q.i.d.	To reduce IOP, especially when pilocarpine is ineffective. *Pregnancy category:* C; PB: NA; t¹/₂: NA
pilocarpine HCl (Isopto Carpine)	See Prototype Drug Chart 47–1.	
pilocarpine nitrate (Ocusert Pilo-20, Pilo-40)	See Prototype Drug Chart 47–1.	
echothiophate iodide (Phospholine Iodide)	A: Sol 0.03%-0.25%: 1 gt daily/b.i.d.	Used to treat chronic open-angle glaucoma and glaucoma following cataract surgery. *Pregnancy category:* C; PB: NA; t¹/₂: NA
Indirect-Acting Cholinesterase Inhibitors		
Short Acting		
physostigmine salicylate (Isopto Eserine)	A & C: Oint 0.25%: 0.25-in up to daily/t.i.d. Sol 0.25-0.5%: 1-2 gtt daily/q.i.d.	For wide-angle glaucoma. *Pregnancy category:* C; PB: NA; t¹/₂: NA
Long Acting		
demecarium bromide (Humorsol)	A: Sol 0.125-0.25%: 1-2 gtt 2 × wk or 1-2 gtt b.i.d.	Used for open-angle glaucoma when shorter-acting agents have been unsuccessful. Also used for conditions affecting aqueous outflow and accommodative strabismus. *Pregnancy category:* C; PB: NA; t¹/₂: NA
Beta-Adrenergic Blockers		
betaxolol HCl (Betoptic)	A: Susp 0.25% or sol 0.5%: Usual dose 1 gt b.i.d.	Selective beta blocker. Used to decrease elevated IOP in chronic open-angle glaucoma and ocular hypertension. Contraindicated in clients with asthma caused by increased airway resistance from systemic absorption. Use caution in clients receiving oral beta-blockers. *Pregnancy category:* C; PB: NA; t¹/₂: NA
carteolol HCl (Ocupress)	A: Sol 1% sol: 1 gtt b.i.d.	Used for open-angle glaucoma. May potentiate effect of systemic beta-blockers.
levobetaxolol (Betaxon)	A: 1 gt 0.5% susp b.i.d.	Selective beta blocker
levobunolol HCl (Betagan Liquifilm, AKBeta)	A: Sol 0.25%-0.5%: 1-2 gtt daily/b.i.d.	Lowers IOP. *Pregnancy category* C; PB: NA; t¹/₂: NA
timolol maleate (Timoptic)	A: Sol 0.25%-0.5% initially: 1 gt b.i.d.; *maint:* 1 gt/d once response occurs with initial dosage	Reduces production of aqueous humor. Monitor vital signs during initial therapy. Concurrent use of similar drugs must be individualized. Blurred vision decreases with use. *Pregnancy category:* C; PB: NA; t¹/₂: NA

A, Adult; *b.i.d.,* twice a day; *C,* child; *d,* day; *gt,* drop; *gtt,* drops; *in,* inch; *IOP,* intraocular pressure; *maint,* maintenance; *NA,* not applicable; *oint,* ointment; *PB,* protein-binding; *q.i.d.,* four times a day; *sol,* solution; *susp,* suspension; *t¹/₂,* half-life; *t.i.d.,* three times a day; *wk,* week.

Cholinergic Agents (Miotics)

In open-angle glaucoma, **miotics** are used to lower the IOP, thereby increasing blood flow to the retina and decreasing retinal damage and loss of vision. Miotics cause a contraction of the ciliary muscle and widening of trabecu-

lar meshwork. The two types of miotics differ in their mechanism of action: (1) *direct-acting cholinergics* (similar to the neurotransmitter acetylcholine), which mediate transmission of nerve impulses at all parasympathetic (cholinergic) nerve sites; and (2) *indirect-acting anti-*

cholinesterase drugs, which inactivate cholinesterase, thereby inhibiting enzymatic destruction of acetylcholine and resulting in pupil constriction and ciliary muscle contraction. Figure 47–1 illustrates increased IOP resulting in glaucoma. Table 47–4 presents the drug data for commonly prescribed miotics.

Pharmacokinetics

Systemic absorption is possible but not common with the use of miotics. To reduce systemic absorption of eye drops, the client or nurse should gently apply pressure on the **lacrimal duct** (passage that carries tears into the nose). Pilocarpine, a direct-acting miotic, binds to the ocular tissues; its half-life is unknown. The metabolism and elimination of this drug are also currently unknown.

Pharmacodynamics

Pilocarpine produces **miosis** (contraction of the pupil) and decreases IOP. The onset of action, peak, and duration of action vary with the dose, desired effect, and form. When pilocarpine is administered to produce miosis, its onset of action is 10 to 30 minutes, its time of peak action is unknown, and its duration of action is 4 to 8 hours. When used to reduce IOP, ophthalmic pilocarpine has an unknown onset of action, a peak time of 75 minutes, and duration of action of 4 to 14 hours.

Ocusert is a wafer-thin disk impregnated with time-release pilocarpine. The disk is replaced every 7 days. Clients should check for the presence of the Ocusert disk in the conjunctival sac daily at bedtime and on awakening. With the ocular therapeutic system Ocusert, the onset of action is unknown, the peak is 1.5 to 2 hours, and the duration of action is 7 days.

The drug data for pilocarpine are shown in Prototype Drug Chart 47–1.

PROTOTYPE DRUG CHART 47–1

PILOCARPINE

Drug Class

Direct-acting miotic
Trade Name: Isopto Carpine, Pilopine HS, Ocusert Pilo-20 and -40
Pregnancy Category: C

Dosage

A & C: Sol: 1%-2%, 1-2 gtt, t.i.d./q.i.d.
Gel: Apply 0.5-in ribbon in lower eyelid at bedtime
Ocusert: Replace q7d

Contraindications

Retinal detachment, adhesions between iris and lens, acute ocular inflammation; must avoid systemic absorption of drug with coronary artery disease, obstruction of GI/GU tract, epilepsy, asthma

Drug-Lab-Food Interactions

Drug: Avoid use with carbachol and echothiophate; *decrease* antiglaucoma effects with belladonna alkaloids; *decrease* dilation with phenylephrine

Pharmacokinetics

Absorption: PO: Some systemic absorption
Distribution: PB: UK
Metabolism: t½: UK; binds to ocular tissue
Excretion: UK

Pharmacodynamics

Miosis:
Ophthalmic: Onset: 10-30 min
  Peak: 20 min
  Duration: 4-8 h
Reduce IOP:
Ophthalmic: Onset: 45-60 min
  Peak: 75 min
  Duration: 4-14 h
Ocusert: Onset: 1 h
  Peak: 1.5-2 h
  Duration: 7 d
Gel: Onset: 1 h
  Peak: 3-12 h
  Duration: 18-24 h

Therapeutic Effects/Uses

To induce miosis; to decrease IOP in glaucoma
Mode of Action: Stimulation of pupillary and ciliary sphincter muscles

Side Effects

Blurred vision, eye pain, headache, eye irritation, brow ache, stinging and burning, nausea, vomiting, diarrhea, increased salivation and perspiration, muscle tremors, contact allergy
Conjunctival irritation with Ocusert

Adverse Reactions

Dyspnea, hypertension, tachycardia, retinal detachment; *long term:* bronchospasm
Corneal abrasion and visual impairment potential with Ocusert

---

A, Adult; *C,* child; *d,* day; *GI,* gastrointestinal; *gtt,* drops; *GU,* genitourinary; *h,* hour; *in,* inch; *IOP,* intraocular pressure; *min,* minute; *PB,* protein-binding; *PO,* by mouth; *q.i.d.,* four times a day; *sol,* solution; *t½,* half-life; *t.i.d.,* three times a day; *UK,* unknown.

Side Effects and Adverse Reactions

Side effects from the use of miotics include headache, eye pain, decreased vision, brow pain, and, less frequently, hyperemia of the conjunctiva. Systemic absorption can cause nausea, vomiting, diarrhea, frequent urination, precipitation of asthmatic attacks, increased salivation, diaphoresis, muscle weakness, and respiratory difficulty. Manifestations of toxicity include vertigo, bradycardia, tremors, hypotension, syncope, cardiac dysrhythmias, and seizures. Atropine sulfate must be available in the case of systemic toxicity.

Drug Interactions

Ophthalmic epinephrine, timolol, levobunolol, betaxolol, and systemic carbonic anhydrase inhibitors have the added effect of lowering IOP. Cyclopentolate, ophthalmic belladonna alkaloids, and antidepressants antagonize the therapeutic effects of miotics.

Contraindications

Contraindications to pilocarpine include retinal detachment, adhesions between the iris and lens, and acute ocular infections. Caution is advised for clients with the following conditions: asthma, hypertension, corneal abrasion, hyperthyroidism, coronary vascular disease, urinary tract obstruction, gastrointestinal obstruction, ulcer disease, parkinsonism, and bradycardia.

Nursing Process
Miotics

ASSESSMENT

- Obtain medical, herbal, and drug history. Miotics are contraindicated in clients with narrow-angle glaucoma, acute inflammation of the eye, heart block, coronary artery disease, obstruction of the GI or urinary tract, and asthma.
- Check vital signs. Baseline vital signs can be compared with future findings.
- Assess client's level of anxiety. The possibility of diminished vision or blindness increases anxiety.
- Assess client's eye pigment; clients with dark, heavily pigmented irises may benefit from a pilocarpine concentration greater than 4%.

NURSING DIAGNOSES

- Disturbed sensory perception (visual)
- Risk for injury
- Anxiety related to possible diminished or loss of vision

PLANNING

- Client will take miotics as prescribed.
- Client's intraocular pressure (IOP) will decrease and be within the accepted range.

NURSING INTERVENTIONS

- Gently apply pressure to the inner canthus to prevent or minimize systemic absorption when administering eye drops.
- Monitor vital signs. Heart rate and blood pressure may decrease with large doses of cholinergics.
- Monitor for side effects such as headache, eye pain, and decreased vision.
- Monitor for postural hypotension. Instruct client to rise slowly from a recumbent position.
- Check breath sounds for rales and rhonchi; cholinergic drugs can cause bronchospasms and increase bronchial secretions.
- Maintain oral hygiene with excessive salivation.
- Keep atropine available as antidote for pilocarpine.

Client Teaching
General
- Instruct client or family on correct administration of eye drops and ointment; include return demonstration. See Figures 3–10 and 3–11.
- Advise client on need for regular and ongoing medical supervision.
- Inform client not to stop medication suddenly without prior approval of health care provider.
- Advise client to avoid driving or operating machinery while vision is impaired.
- Instruct client on use of relaxation techniques for decreasing anxiety, if appropriate.
- Instruct client with glaucoma to avoid atropine-like drugs and goldenseal, which increase IOP. Clients should check labels on OTC drugs or check with a pharmacist.
- Advise client that certain herbal products should be avoided before ophthalmic or otic surgery. See Herbal Alert 47–1.

Self-Administration
- Instruct client/family or both on the correct administration of eyedrops and ointment. Include return demonstration. Refer to Figures 3–10 and 3–11.
- Remove any exudates in eye before applying solution or ointment.
- Allow at least 5 minutes between instillation of another medication.

Ocular Therapeutic Systems (Ocusert)
- Store drug in refrigerator.
- Discard damaged or contaminated disks.
- Explain that the myopia is minimized by inserting the disk in the upper conjunctival sac at bedtime.
- For self-administration, advise clients to follow instructions related to insertion and removal.
- Instruct client to check for presence of disk in conjunctival sac at bedtime and when arising.
- Explain that temporary stinging is expected; notify health care provider if blurred vision or brow pain occurs.

Table 47-5

Prostaglandin Analogues Used to Treat Glaucoma

Generic (Brand)	Route and Dosage	Uses and Considerations
Latanoprost (Xalatan)	A: 1 gt 0.005% sol daily at bedtime	To lower IOP; generally well tolerated.
Bimatoprost (lumigan)	A: 1 gt 0.03% sol daily at bedtime	Increases outflow of aqueous humor through trabecular meshwork and uveoscleral routes. Onset is 4 h and peak action occurs in 4-12 h.
Travoprost (Travatan)	A: 1 gt 0.004% sol daily at bedtime	More effective in African American than non–African Americans. Increases uveoscleral outflow. Onset is 2 h with peak action occurring in 12 h.
Unoprostone (Rescula)	A: 1 gt 0.15% sol b.i.d.	Not recommended for children.

A, Adult; *b.i.d.,* twice a day; *gt,* drop; *h,* hour; *IOP,* intraocular pressure; *sol,* solution.

Cholinesterase Inhibitors

First dose should be administered by health care provider and followed by tonometry reading.

- Instruct client to tightly cap tube because ointment is inactivated by water.

Cultural Considerations

- Depending on client's culture, include the appropriate support person in health teaching and decisions. This need is heightened in conditions with possible loss or diminished vision.
- Use an interpreter as needed.

EVALUATION

- Evaluate the effectiveness of drug therapy and the presence of side effects. IOP will be within desired range or reduced.

Beta-Adrenergic Blockers

Beta-blockers are first-line drugs in the treatment of glaucoma. Six drugs—betaxolol, carteolol, levobetaxolol, levobunolol, metipranolol, and timolol—are approved for this indication by the Food and Drug Administration (FDA). Beta-adrenergic blockers decrease the production of aqueous humor. The exact mechanism of action is unknown for these agents. See Chapter 17, Adrenergics and Adrenergic Blockers, for a comprehensive discussion of adrenergic blockers. These agents are presented in Table 47-4.

Prostoglandin Analogues

Prostaglandin analogues are currently known to be as effective as beta-blockers in the treatment of glaucoma. Four FDA-approved analogues with fewer side effects than beta-blockers are presented in Table 47-5. When using additional topical ophthalmic agents, allow at least 5 minutes between instillations.

Side Effects and Adverse Reactions

Increased brown pigmentation is most noticeable in individuals with green-brown and yellow-brown irises. When the drug is stopped, the increased pigmentation remains. Systemic reactions are rare. Pigmentation of the eyelid and growth of eyelashes also may occur. Ocular hyperemia is the most common adverse effect; blurred vision, conjunctivitis, dry eye, tearing, and light intolerance were less commonly experienced.

Carbonic Anhydrase Inhibitors

Carbonic anhydrase inhibitors interfere with production of carbonic acid, which leads to decreased aqueous humor formation and decreased IOP. These drugs, initially developed as diuretics, are now also used for the long-term treatment of open-angle glaucoma. Their use is recommended only when pilocarpine, beta-blockers, epinephrine, and cholinesterase inhibitors have not been effective. Table 47-6 presents the drug data for commonly prescribed carbonic anhydrase inhibitors.

Side Effects and Adverse Reactions

Side effects include lethargy, anorexia, drowsiness, paresthesia, depression, polyuria, nausea, vomiting, hypokalemia, and renal calculi. Carbonic anhydrase inhibitors can also cause photosensitivity. Clients frequently discontinue these medications because of their side effects. These drugs are contraindicated during the first trimester of pregnancy. Do not use in persons allergic to sulfonamides.

Nursing Process

Carbonic Anhydrase Inhibitors

ASSESSMENT

- Obtain medical and drug history. Use is contraindicated during first trimester of pregnancy.
- Check vital signs. Baseline vital signs can be compared with future readings.
- Assess level of anxiety. Eye disorders carrying the possibility of blindness promote high anxiety state in clients.

NURSING DIAGNOSES

- Disturbed sensory perception (visual)
- Risk for injury
- Anxiety related to possible diminished or loss of vision

PLANNING

■ Client will take carbonic anhydrase inhibitors as prescribed.
■ Client's intraocular pressure (IOP) will decrease to within the desired range.

NURSING INTERVENTIONS

■ Monitor for side effects such as lethargy, anorexia, drowsiness, polyuria, nausea, and vomiting.
■ Monitor electrolytes because drug can cause hypokalemia.
■ Increase fluid intake, unless contraindicated. Record intake and output; weigh daily.
■ Maintain oral hygiene.

Client Teaching

General

● Encourage use of artificial tears for "dry eyes."
● Encourage client to maintain oral hygiene if mouth is dry; ice chips and sugarless gum are recommended.
● Instruct client not to abruptly discontinue medication. Clients frequently discontinue drug because of side effects.
● Inform client of need for regular and ongoing medical supervision.
● Advise client to avoid driving or operating hazardous machinery while vision is impaired.

Self-Administration

● Instruct client or family on the correct administration of eye drops and ointment. Include return demonstration. See Figures 3–10 and 3–11.
● Remove any exudate in eye before applying an antiinfective ointment or solution.
● Allow at least 5 minutes between instillation of another medication.

Side Effect

● Advise client to avoid prolonged exposure to sunlight because of the potential for photosensitivity.

Cultural Considerations ⊕

● Depending on client's culture, include the appropriate support person in health teaching and decisions. This need is heightened in conditions with possible loss or diminished vision.
● Use interpreter as needed.

EVALUATION

■ Determine effectiveness of drug therapy and presence of side effects. IOP will be within desired range.

Osmotics

Osmotics are generally used preoperatively and postoperatively to decrease vitreous humor volume, thereby reducing IOP. These drugs are primarily used in the emergency treatment of acute closed-angle glaucoma because of their

---

Table 47–6

Carbonic Anhydrase Inhibitors

Generic (Brand)	Route and Dosage	Uses and Considerations
acetazolamide (Diamox)	A: PO: 250-1000 mg/d given in divided doses for amounts >250 mg; doses >1000 mg show no increased benefit	To reduce aqueous humor formation thus lowering IOP. Monitor for dehydration and postural hypotension. Monitor electrolytes. Avoid hazardous activities if drowsy. Most frequently prescribed. *Pregnancy category:* C; PB: UK; $t^{1/2}$: 2-6 h
brinzolamide ophthalmic susp 1% (Azopt)	A: 1 gt t.i.d. C: not recommended	*Topical:* Treatment of elevated IOP in clients with ocular hypertension or open-angle glaucoma by suppressing production of aqueous humor. *Pregnancy category:* UK; PB: UK; $t^{1/2}$: UK
Cosopt (timolol/dorzolamide 0.5%/2%)	1 gt 0.25% in affected eye(s) b.i.d.	Decreases aqueous production. Contraindicated with sulfa allergy. Adverse effects include asthma, bronchospasm, bradycardia, and dyspnea.
dichlorphenamide (Daranide)	A: PO: Initially: 100-200 mg followed by 100 mg q12h until desired response is obtained	Same as brinzolamide. May cause confusion, especially in older adults. *Pregnancy category:* C; PB: UK; $t^{1/2}$: UK
dorzolamide (Trusopt)	A: Sol 2%: 1 gt t.i.d.	Do not use with oral carbonic anhydrase inhibitors. Side effects include burning, stinging, and bitter taste. *Pregnancy category:* UK; PB: UK; $t^{1/2}$: UK

A, Adult; *b.i.d.,* two times a day; *C,* child; *d,* day; *gt,* drop; *h,* hour; *IOP,* intraocular pressure; *PB,* protein-binding; *PO,* by mouth; $t^{1/2}$, half-life; *t.i.d.,* three times a day; *UK,* unknown; >, greater than.

Table 47-7

Osmotics

Generic (Brand)	Route and Dosage	Uses and Considerations
glycerin	A: PO: 1-1.5 g/kg given 1-1.5 h before surgery	Decreases volume of intraocular fluid thus lowering ocular tension. Carbohydrate; use with caution in clients with diabetes. *Pregnancy category:* C; PB: UK; t½: 30-45 min
isosorbide (Ismotic)	A: Sol 45%: 1.5-3 g/kg b.i.d./q.i.d.	Monitor I & O and electrolytes. *Pregnancy category:* C; PB: UK; t½: 5-9.5 h
mannitol (Osmitrol)	A: IV: Sol 15-20%, 1.5-2 g/kg over 0.5-1 h	Monitor I & O; weigh daily. Contraindicated in severe pulmonary congestion, anuria, and dehydration. Use with caution in clients with CHF. *Pregnancy category:* C; PB: UK; t½: 15-100 min

A, Adult; *b.i.d.*, twice a day; *C*, child; *CHF*, congestive heart failure; *h*, hour; *I & O*, intake and output; *IV*, intravenous; *min*, minute; *PB*, protein-binding; *PO*, by mouth; *q.i.d.*, four times a day; *sol*, solution; *t½*, half-life; *UK*, unknown.

ability to rapidly reduce IOP. Commonly prescribed osmotic drugs are presented in Table 47-7.

Side Effects and Adverse Reactions

Osmotic medications can cause headache, nausea, vomiting, and diarrhea. Disorientation resulting from electrolyte imbalances can result from use of mannitol and urea, especially in older adults.

Nursing Process

Osmotics

ASSESSMENT

■ Obtain medical and drug history.
■ Check vital signs. Baseline vital signs can be compared with future readings.
■ Assess level of anxiety. Eye disorders carrying the possibility of blindness promote high anxiety state in clients.

NURSING DIAGNOSES

■ Disturbed sensory perception (visual)
■ Risk for injury
■ Anxiety related to possible diminished or loss of vision

PLANNING

■ Client's intraocular pressure (IOP) will be lowered.

NURSING INTERVENTIONS

■ Monitor for side effects.
■ Monitor for potassium depletion and electrolyte imbalances.
■ Increase fluid intake, unless contraindicated.

■ Record input and output; weigh daily.
■ Monitor changes in level of orientation, especially in older adults.

Client Teaching

General

● Instruct client regarding side effects of drugs.
● Osmotics are usually administered intravenously in a health care setting.

Self-Administration

● Instruct client/family or both on the correct administration of eyedrops and ointment. Include return demonstration. Refer to Figures 3-10 and 3-11.
● Remove any exudates in eye before applying solution or ointment.
● Allow at least 5 minutes between instillation of another medication.

Cultural Considerations

● Depending on client's culture, include the appropriate support person in health teaching and decisions. This need is heightened in conditions with possible loss or diminished vision.
● Use an interpreter as needed.

EVALUATION

■ Determine the effectiveness of drug therapy and presence of side effects. IOP will be within desired range.

Anticholinergic Mydriatics and Cycloplegics

Mydriatics dilate the pupils; **cycloplegics** paralyze the muscles of accommodation. Both are used in diagnostic procedures and ophthalmic surgery. (See the Unit 5 opener for a review of the autonomic nervous system and a comprehensive discussion of anticholinergics.) Anticholinergics cause both dilation of the pupils and paralysis of the muscles of accommodation by relaxing the ciliary and dilator muscles of the iris by blocking acetylcholine. Commonly prescribed anticholinergic mydriatics and cycloplegics are presented in Table 47–8.

Side Effects and Adverse Reactions of Adrenergic Mydriatics

Side effects include headache, brow pain, allergic reaction, and worsening of narrow-angle glaucoma. Adrenergic mydriatics are contraindicated in clients with cardiac dysrhythmias and cerebral atherosclerosis and should be used with caution in older adults and clients with prostatic hypertrophy, diabetes mellitus, or parkinsonism. The health care provider should be notified of blurred vision

or loss of sight, difficult breathing, increased perspiration, or flush. The difference in the response of African American individuals to a mydriatic drug must be taken into consideration. Closely monitor African American clients for side effects. Filipino eye structure is such that it may be difficult for the health care provider to conduct selected assessments.

Side Effects and Adverse Reactions of Cycloplegics

Cycloplegics can cause tachycardia, photophobia, dryness of the mouth, edema, conjunctivitis, and dermatitis. Symptoms of atropine toxicity include dry mouth, blurred vision, photophobia, constipation, fever, tachycardia, confusion, hallucinations, delirium, and coma. Toxicity is treated with physostigmine. Cycloplegics are contraindicated in clients with glaucoma because they increase IOP.

Table 47–8

Mydriatics and Cycloplegics

Generic (Brand)	Route and Dosage*	Uses and Considerations
atropine sulfate (Atropisol, Isopto Atropine)	A: Sol 1%: 1-2 gtt up to q.i.d. C: Sol 0.5%: 1-2 gtt up to t.i.d. Oint 1%: Apply in lower eyelid sac up to t.i.d.	Most potent cycloplegic. For refraction, especially in children; for iritis and uveitis. *Not* for use with glaucoma or tachycardia. Wait 5 minutes before using other drugs. *Pregnancy category:* C; PB: NA; t½: NA
cyclopentolate HCl (AK-Pentolate, Cyclogyl, Pentolair)	A: Sol 0.5%-2%: 1-2 gtt; then 1 gt in 5 min C: 1-2 gtt × 1; may repeat × 1 in 5-10 min with 0.5% or 1% sol	Mydriasis and cycloplegia for eye examination. *Pregnancy category:* C; PB: NA; t½: NA
dipivefrin HCl (Propine)	A: Sol 0.1%: 1 gt q12h	Control of IOP in chronic open-angle glaucoma. *Pregnancy category:* B; PB: NA; t½: NA
epinephrine HCl (Epifrin, Glaucon)	A & C: Sol 0.1%-2%: 1-2 gtt d/b.i.d.	For open-angle glaucoma and during eye surgery. Discard brown or precipitate solution. *Pregnancy category:* C; PB: NA; t½: NA
epinephrine borate (Epinal)	*Surgery:* A: Sol 0.5-1%: Instill 1-2 gtt 3 × *Open-angle glaucoma:* A: Sol 0.5% or 1.0%: Instill 1 gt in eye b.i.d.	For treatment of open-angle glaucoma and during ocular surgery. Contraindicated in narrow-angle glaucoma. Monitor tonometer readings with long-term use. Increased pressor effects. *Pregnancy category:* C; PB: UK; t½: UK
homatropine hydrobromide (Isopto Homatropine)	A & C: Sol 2% and 5%: 1-2 gtt q3-4h Cy: Use only 2%	Similar to atropine but faster onset and shorter duration. Mydriasis and cycloplegia for eye examination. *Pregnancy category:* C; PB: NA; t½: NA
phenylephrine HCl (AK-Dilate)	*Mydriasis:* A & C: Sol 2.5% or 10%: Instill 1 gt in eye before examination *Mydriasis with vasoconstriction:* A & C >12 y: Instill 1 gt in eye; repeat × 1 in 1 h PRN Cy: 2.5% sol: Instill 1 gt in eye; repeat × 1 in 1 h PRN	For eye examination or surgery and treatment of wide-angle glaucoma and uveitis. *Pregnancy category:* C; PB: UK; t½: UK
scopolamine hydrobromide (Isopto Hyoscine)	A: Sol 0.25%: 1-2 gtt 1 h before examination; 1-2 gtt for treatment up to q.i.d.	Used for clients sensitive to atropine sulfate. More rapid onset and shorter duration than atropine. *Pregnancy category:* C; PB: NA; t½: NA
tropicamide (Mydriacyl Ophthalmic, Tropicacyl, Opticyl)	*Refraction:* A: 1%: 1-2 gtt; repeat in 5 min *Fundus examination:* 0.5%: 1-2 gtt 15-20 min before examination	Mydriasis and cycloplegia for eye examination. *Pregnancy category:* C; PB: NA; t½: NA

*To minimize systemic absorption, apply gentle pressure to lacrimal duct.

A, Adult; *b.i.d.,* twice a day; *C,* child; *Cy,* cycloplegic; *gt,* drop; *gtt,* drops; *h,* hour; *IOP,* intraocular pressure; *min,* minute; *oint,* ointment; *PB,* protein-binding; *PRN,* as needed; *q.i.d.,* four times a day; *sol,* solution; *t½,* half-life; *t.i.d.,* three times a day; *NA,* not applicable; *UK,* unknown; *y,* year; *>,* greater than.

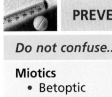

PREVENTING MEDICATION ERRORS

Do not confuse...	with
Miotics	
• Betoptic	• Betagan
• Timoptic	• Viroptic
• Ocupress	• Ocufen
Carbonic Anhydrase Inhibitors	
• Acetazolamide	• Acetohexamide
Ocular Lubricants	**Acular**
Antiinflammatories	
• Voltaren	• Verelan
• Maxidex	• Maxzide

Refer to Preventing Medication Errors box for examples of eye medications that are commonly confused with other agents.

Administration of Eyedrops and Ointments

The techniques for administering eyedrops and ointments are described in Chapter 3, Principles of Drug Administration, and Boxes 3–3 and 3–4 and illustrated in Figures 3–10 and 3–11. Individuals who wear contact lenses need to be knowledgeable about the products associated with some of the lenses (see Figure 47–2).

Clients with Eye Disorders: General Suggestions for Client Teaching

• Eye disorders carrying the possibility of blindness promote a high-anxiety state in clients. Provide time, instructions, and return demonstration in all teaching plans.

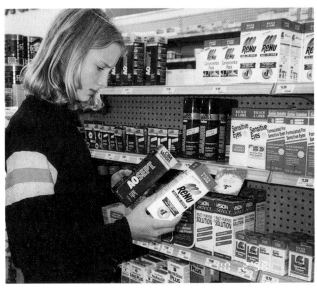

FIGURE 47–2 Clients who wear contact lenses should be knowledgeable about the products associated with some of the lenses.

• Use caution with confused or forgetful clients to prevent overdose.
• Instruct the client or family in the proper administration of eyedrops or ointment. Maintain sterile technique and prevent dropper contamination. Expect some blurriness from ointments. Apply at bedtime, if possible, to avoid safety problems from diminished vision.
• Instruct the client to report changes in vision, blurred vision, vision loss, breathing difficulties, or flush.
• Instruct the client to store the drug in a light-resistant container away from heat.
• Instruct the client not to stop medication suddenly without *prior* approval from the prescribing health care provider.
• Instruct the client to record medications administered. Prepare a chart so the client can record when eye medications are given.
• Instruct the client with glaucoma to avoid atropine-like drugs, which increase IOP. Some drugs for glaucoma are long acting and require only daily dosing if the client is forgetful or needs another person to administer the medicine.
• Clients should be alerted to check labels on OTC drugs with a pharmacist.
• Instruct the client to carry an identification card or wear a MedicAlert bracelet at all times if he or she is allergic to any medications.
• Encourage the client to keep health care appointments.
• Individuals who wear contact lenses need to be knowledgeable about the products associated with the care of the lenses.

Drugs for Disorders of the Ear

The medications most often used to treat **otic,** or ear, disorders are the same preparations (e.g., antiinfectives) used to treat similar problems in other areas of the body. Refer to appropriate chapters in the text for a comprehensive discussion of specific drug groups.

Antibacterials

Several antibacterials are commonly prescribed for external use for otic disorders. See the discussions of antibiotics in Chapters 28, Antibacterials: Penicillins and Cephalosporins, 29, Antibacterials: Macrolides, Tetracyclines, Aminoglycosides, and Fluoroquinolones, and 30, Antibacterials: Sulfonamides. Table 47–9 presents the drug data for selected antibacterial medications used to treat ear disorders.

Common conditions requiring antibacterial drugs are acute otitis media (AOM) and acute otitis externa (swimmer's ear). *Streptococcus pneumoniae* is the most common pathogen in children with AOM; no bacteria was found in 20% to 30% of children examined.

Side Effects and Adverse Reactions

Side effects include overgrowth of nonsusceptible organisms. Prior hypersensitivity is a contraindication.

Table 47–9

Otic: Antiinfectives

Generic (Brand)	Route and Dosage	Uses and Considerations
External		
acetic acid and aluminum acetate (Otic Domeboro)	A & C: Sol 2%: Insert saturated wick, keep moist × 24 h; instill 4-6 gtt q2-3h	Provides an acid medium; has antibacterial activity. Low cost. *Pregnancy category:* UK; PB: NA; t½: NA
boric acid (Ear-Dry), Carbamide peroxide (Debrox)	A & C >12 y: Instill 5-10 gtt b.i.d.; tilt head to unaffected side to keep gtt in ear or put cotton plug in outer ear	OTC preparations to dry the ear canal and to loosen and remove impacted wax (cerumen) from the ear canal. Debrox: instill for up to 4 days. If no improvement, call health care provider. *Pregnancy category:* C; PB: NA; t½: NA
chloramphenicol (Chloromycetin Otic)	A & C: Otic sol 0.5%: Instill 2-3 gtt into ear t.i.d.	Topically for infections of ear canal. *Pregnancy category:* C; PB: NA; t½: NA
polymyxin B	A & C: 3-4 gtt t.i.d./q.i.d. for 7-10 d	Usually given in combination with neomycin and hydrocortisone. For disorders of external ear. Discontinue after 10 days to prevent fungal overgrowth. *Pregnancy category:* B; PB: NA; t½: NA
tetracycline (Achromycin)	A & C: 1-2 gtt b.i.d./q.i.d.	Similar to polymyxin B. *Pregnancy category:* D; PB: NA; t½: NA
trolamine polypeptide oleate-condensate (Cerumenex)	A & C: Fill ear canal and insert cotton plug for 15-30 min; flush ear with lukewarm water; repeat × 1 if needed	To loosen and remove impacted wax (cerumen) from the ear canal. *Pregnancy category:* C; PB: NA; t½: NA
Internal		
amoxicillin (Amoxil, Augmentin)	A: PO: 250-500 mg q8h C: PO: 20-40 mg/kg/d in three divided doses	For treatment of otitis media. Mouth absorbs 80%; food does not prevent absorption. Long duration of action. *Pregnancy category:* B; PB: 20%; t½: 1-1.5 h
ampicillin trihydrate (Polycillin)	A: PO: 250-500 mg q6h IM/IV: 2-8 g/d in divided doses C: PO: 50-200 mg/kg/d in divided doses IM/IV: 50-200 mg/kg/d in divided doses	First broad-spectrum penicillin. GI tract absorbs 50%. Effective against gram-negative and gram-positive bacteria. Individuals allergic to penicillin may also be allergic to ampicillin. *Pregnancy category:* B; PB: 15%-28%; t½: 1-2 h
cefaclor (Ceclor)	A: PO: 250-500 mg q8h; *max,* 4 g/d C: PO: 20-40 mg/kg/d in three divided doses; *max:* 1 g/d	Second-generation cephalosporin. To treat ampicillin-resistant and gram-negative strains. Third-line drug for otitis media. Not for infants less than 1 month old. Monitor electrolytes in long-term therapy. *Pregnancy* category: B; PB: 25%; t½: 0.5-1 h

A, Adult; *b.i.d.,* twice a day; *C,* child; *d,* day; *GI,* gastrointestinal; *gtt,* drops; *h,* hour; *IM,* intramuscular; *IV,* intravenous; *max,* maximum; *min,* minute; *NA,* not applicable; *OTC,* over-the-counter; *PB,* protein-binding; *PO,* by mouth; *q.i.d.,* four times a day; *sol,* solution; *t½,* half-life; *t.i.d.,* three times a day; *UK,* unknown; *y,* year; >, greater than.

Nursing Process

Antiinfectives

ASSESSMENT

■ Obtain a medical and drug history including any allergies.
■ Check vital signs. Obtain baseline data that can be compared with future findings.

NURSING DIAGNOSES

■ Disturbed sensory perception (auditory)
■ Pain

PLANNING

■ Client will be free of ear infection after completion of drug regimen.

NURSING INTERVENTIONS

■ Complete culture and sensitivity before starting drug.
■ Monitor input and output.
■ Report hematuria or oliguria. High doses of antibacterials may be nephrotoxic.
■ Relief of associated pain, if present.
■ Monitor renal function, liver studies, and blood studies (white cell count, red cell count, hemoglobin and hematocrit, bleeding time), as appropriate.

Table 47–9

Otic: Antiinfectives—cont'd

Generic (Brand)	Route and Dosage	Uses and Considerations
Internal—cont'd		
erythromycin (E-Mycin)	A: PO: 250-500 mg q6h IV: 1-4 g/d in four divided doses C: PO: 30-50 mg/kg/d in four divided doses IV: 20-50 mg/kg/d in four divided doses	To treat gram-positive and gram-negative bacterial infections in clients allergic to penicillin. Enteric-coated tablet to prevent gastric acid from destroying drug. *Pregnancy category:* B; PB: 65%; t½: PO, 1-2 h; IV, 3-5 h
penicillin (Pentids, Pen-V)	*Penicillin G potassium (Pentids):* A: PO: 200,000-500,000 units q6h IM: 500,000-5 million units/d in divided doses IV: 4-20 million units/d in divided doses diluted in IV solution C: PO: 25,000-90,000 units/d in divided doses IV: 50,000-100,000 units/kg/d in divided doses *Penicillin V potassium (Pen-V):* A: PO: 125-500 mg q6h C: PO: 15-50 mg/kg/d in three to four divided doses	For otitis media and mastoiditis. Take before or after meals. Penicillin G: electrolytes should be monitored; injectable solution is clear. Penicillin V: not recommended in renal failure. *Pregnancy category:* B; PB: (G) 60%, (V) 80%; t½: (G) 0.5-1 h, (V) 0.5 h
sulfonamides (Azulfidine [sulfasalazine], Bactrim [trimethoprim and sulfamethoxazole])	Dose and route vary. See Chapter 29.	Most are highly protein-bound. Increase fluid intake to decrease crystalluria. Side effects include allergic response. Blood disorders may result from long-term use and high doses. Avoid in third trimester of pregnancy. *Pregnancy category:* B, D; PB: 50%-95%; t½: 4.5-12 h
clarithromycin (Biaxin)	A: PO: 250-500 mg q12h C: PO: 7.5 mg/kg q12h	For otitis media. Cautious use in renal impairment. Efficacy not established in children younger than 12 y. *Pregnancy category:* C; PB: UK; t½: 3-5 h
amoxicillin and potassium clavulanate (Augmentin)	A: PO: 250 mg q8h C: PO: 40 mg/kg/d divided q8h	For otitis media. Clavulanate inhibits beta lactamase degradation of amoxicillin. *Pregnancy category:* B; PB: UK; t½: 1-3 h
loracarbef (Lorabid)	A: PO: 200 mg q12h C: PO: 30 mg/kg/d q12h	For otitis media. Second-generation cephalosporin. Use caution in clients with renal impairment and seizures. *Pregnancy category:* B; PB: UK; t½: 45-60 min

■ Store medication in airtight container.
■ Report dizziness to health care provider.
■ Report fatigue, fever, or sore throat. Any of these symptoms could indicate superimposed infection.

Client Teaching

• Instruct client to complete entire course of medication (usually 10 to 14 days) and *not* to stop medication when he or she "feels better."
• Encourage client to eat yogurt or buttermilk to maintain intestinal flora.
• If client is prone to otitis after swimming or in warm weather, instruct him or her to keep ear canals dry; instillation of drops of alcohol into the ear canal may be helpful. Check with the health care provider.
• Instruct client to wear a MedicAlert bracelet at all times if allergic to medications.

Self-Administration

• Teach client or family about administration of eardrops. Include a return demonstration. Refer to Box 3–5 and Figure 3–12.

Cultural Considerations

• Depending on client's culture, include the appropriate support person in health teaching and decisions. This need is heightened in conditions with possible loss or diminished vision.
• Use interpreter as needed.

EVALUATION

■ Determine the effectiveness of drug therapy and the presence of side effects.

Antihistamine-Decongestants

Antihistamine-decongestants are thought to reduce nasal and middle ear congestion in acute otitis media. (See Chapter 38, Drugs for Common Upper Respiratory Disorders, for a comprehensive discussion of upper respiratory agents.) Reducing edema around the orifice of the eustachian tube promotes drainage from the middle ear. Numerous OTC antihistamine-decongestant medications are available, including Actifed, Allerest, Dimetapp, Drixoral, Novafed, Ornade, Phenergan, and Triaminic. Common side effects are drowsiness, blurred vision, and dry mucous membranes.

Combination Products

Combination products such as Cortisporin Otic are not held in high regard by most health care providers, who believe that multiple drugs are not necessary if one drug can successfully treat a disorder. These drugs combine local anesthetics or anti-inflammatory drugs with antiinfectives.

Ceruminolytics

Cerumen (earwax), produced by glands in the outer half of the ear canal, usually moves to the external os by itself and is washed away. However, **ceruminolytics** are sometimes needed to loosen and remove impacted cerumen from the ear canal. Irrigation with hydrogen peroxide solution (3% diluted to half-strength with water) can flush cerumen deposits out of the ear canal. For chronic impaction, one or two drops of olive oil or mineral oil soften the wax. Cerumenex (prescription) and Debrox (OTC) cost more and are no more effective than the hydrogen peroxide solution.

Administration of Ear Medications

Ear medications are generally contained in a liquid vehicle for ease of administration. Guidelines for the administration of eardrops are given in Box 3–5 and Figure 3–12.

Irrigation

Irrigations of the ear may also be ordered. Irrigation is best accomplished when there is direct visualization of the tympanic membrane (eardrum). It must be done *gently* to avoid damage to the eardrum. Frequently used irrigating solutions include Burow's solution, hydrogen peroxide 3% (with water), hypertonic sodium chloride solution 3%, and acetic acid (vinegar) solution. Contraindications include perforation of the eardrum and prior hypersensitivity.

Clients with Ear Disorders: General Suggestions for Client Teaching

- Instruct the client not to insert any foreign objects into the ear canal.
- Instruct the client to take the drug as prescribed.
- Instruct the client to keep the drug in a light-resistant container.
- Instruct the client about the expected drug effect, dosage, side effects, and when to notify the health care provider.
- Encourage the client to keep follow-up appointments.

WEBSITES

For further information on *Drugs for Disorders of the Eye and the Ear*, visit these Internet resources:

Eye disorders:
information/diagnosis/treatment/prevention
http://www.healthcyclopedia.com/eye-disorders.html

Eye care:
http://www.medicinenet.com/eye_care/article.htm

Ear Disorders Health Center:
http://my.webmd.com/medical_information/condition_centers/ear_disorders/default.htm

Critical Thinking Case Studies

M.H., age 70, has been on pilocarpine for several days (2% solution, four gtt q.i.d.). She says she must need new glasses because newsprint and the TV picture are a bit "fuzzy."

1. Is any action indicated? If so, what?

2. What additional advice would be appropriate if the client had coronary vascular disease and bradycardia?

3. Are there any expected effects on M.H.'s vital signs? If so, what?

4. What suggestions should M.H. be given to avoid systemic absorption of the medication?

M.Z. brings C.Z., age 7, to the HMO practice because he has been complaining of pain in his ear for 2 days. Following an assessment, the health care provider determines that C.Z. has an infection in the external right ear canal. Polymyxin B is prescribed to be administered three to four gtt t.i.d. for 14 days.

1. Is the drug regimen appropriate for C.Z.? What is the nurse's responsibility?

2. What is a consequence of long-term use of this drug?

3. What drug may be used in combination to decrease edema, itching, and redness?

Client teaching is an integral part of the therapeutic drug regimen. Explain the role of the nurse in relation to the following:

4. What position should C.Z. be in to receive the drugs?

5. What instructions should be given to M.Z. regarding the administration of eardrops, including the actual positioning of the ear before administering the drops? In what way should these instructions be modified if the child were 2 years old?

6. What advice should you give C.Z. about putting things in his ear?

Study Questions

1. Miotics are used to treat what disorders? What is the mechanism of action of miotics?

2. What information is required in a teaching plan for a client receiving pilocarpine?

3. What drug is the most potent cycloplegic? What are the nursing implications for the use of this medication?

4. The client, age 85, just began taking acetazolamide. What category of drug is this? What is the brand name? What are the nursing interventions associated with clients receiving this drug?

5. Mannitol is a commonly used osmotic. What are the contraindications for use of this drug?

6. Your client is being prepared for an eye examination. When taking the health history, the client says she is sensitive to atropine sulfate. What drug might be used instead for the examination?

7. What are the advantages and side effects of the prostaglandin analogues?

8. Describe appropriate general teaching strategies for clients with eye disorders.

9. What is a disadvantage to the use of combination products such as Cortisporin Otic?

10. What product is recommended to treat and prevent chronic impaction of cerumen?

11. What is included in the nursing assessment of the client before the start of an antibacterial drug for the treatment of an ear infection?

48 Drugs for Dermatologic Disorders

ELECTRONIC RESOURCES

Additional information can be found on the companion website at *http://evolve.elsevier.com/KeeHayes/pharmacology/* or on the companion CD-ROM, which includes:
* *NCLEX-style examination review questions*
* *Pharmacology animations*
* *Medication error and IV therapy checklists*
* *Medication calculation problems*
* *Electronic calculators*

OUTLINE

OBJECTIVES

* Differentiate acne vulgaris, psoriasis, drug-induced dermatitis, and contact dermatitis.
* Describe nonpharmacologic measures used to treat mild acne vulgaris.
* Describe three drugs that can cause drug-induced dermatitis and their characteristic symptoms.
* Compare the topical antibacterial agents used to prevent and treat burn tissue infection.
* Describe the nursing process, including client teaching, related to commonly used drugs for acne vulgaris, psoriasis, and burns.

TERMS

acne vulgaris
contact dermatitis
macules
papules
plaques
psoriasis
tinea capitis
tinea pedis
vesicles

Introduction

Numerous skin lesions and eruptions require mild to aggressive drug therapy. Some skin disorders include acne vulgaris, psoriasis, eczema dermatitis, contact dermatitis, drug-induced dermatitis, and burn infection. Skin eruptions may result from viral infections (e.g., herpes simplex, herpes zoster), fungal infections (e.g., **tinea pedis** [athlete's foot], **tinea capitis** [ringworm]), and bacterial infections. Please refer to Chapter 32 (Antiviral, Antimalarial, and Anthelmintic Drugs), Chapter 31 (Antitubercular Drugs, Antifungal Drugs, Peptides, and Metronidazole), and Chapters 28, 29, and 30 (Antibacterials and their Effects: Penicillins and Caphalosporins; Antibacterials: Macrolides, Tetracyclines, Aminoglycosides, and Fluoroquinolones; Antibacterials: Sulfonamides) for further information.

Most treatments for skin eruptions include topical creams, ointments, pastes, lotions, and solutions. Skin lesions may appear as **macules** (flat with varying colors), **papules** (raised, palpable, and less than 1 cm in diameter), **vesicles** (raised, filled with fluid, and less than 1 cm in diameter), or **plaques** (hard, rough, raised, and flat on top). Selected skin disorders and their drug therapy regimens are discussed separately.

Acne Vulgaris and Psoriasis

Acne Vulgaris

Acne is the most common skin disorder in the United States. **Acne vulgaris** is the formation of papules, nodules, and cysts on the face, neck, shoulders, and back resulting from keratin plugs at the base of the pilosebaceous oil glands near the hair follicles. Of persons with acne, 90% are adolescents. The increase in androgen production that occurs during adolescence increases the production of sebum, an oily skin lubricant. The sebum combines with keratin to form a plug, which results in acne.

Nonpharmacologic Approach

Nonpharmacologic measures should be tried before drug therapy is initiated. A prescribed or suggested cleansing agent is necessary for all types of acne. The skin should be gently cleansed several times a day. Vigorous scrubbing should be avoided. A well-balanced diet is indicated. Megadoses of vitamin A were once used to treat acne. Vitamin A is fat soluble and is retained in tissues, especially the liver, for long periods. Because excessive doses of vitamin A can be highly toxic, megadosing is no longer a valid therapy for treating acne. High doses of vitamin A may also cause teratogenic effects to a fetus. Decreasing emotional stress and increasing emotional support are suggested. If drug therapy is necessary, nonpharmacologic measures should be maintained.

Topical Antiacne Drugs

Mild acne may require gentle cleansing and the use of keratolytics (keratin dissolvers, such as benzoyl peroxide, resorcinol, salicylic acid). Benzoyl peroxide is applied as a cream, lotion, or gel once or twice a day. This agent loosens the outer, horny layer of the epidermis.

Tretinoin (Retin-A, Renova), a derivative of vitamin A, is a topical drug for mild to moderate acne that alters keratinization. There are additional antiacne agents, adapalene (Differin), azelaic acid (Azelex), and tazarotene (Tazorac) used to treat mild to moderate acne. Adapalene is similar in action to tretinoin. It has antiinflammatory and comedolytic (eliminates blackheads) properties and tends to be more effective than tretinoin in reducing the number of acne lesions. Adapalene should not be used before or after extended sun exposure or sunburn. It can increase the risk of sunburn and intensify an existing sunburn. Azelaic acid appears as effective as benzoyl peroxide and tretinoin. Adapalene and azelaic acid can cause burning, pruritus, and erythema after several applications; however, this is less common with azelaic acid. Adapalene and tazarotene bind to select retinoid receptors; thus fewer adverse effects are anticipated.

Moderate acne requires a stronger concentration of benzoyl peroxide (10%), and topical antibiotics (e.g., tetracycline, erythromycin, clindamycin, meclocycline) may be added to the treatment regimen. Erythromycin and clindamycin are the most frequently prescribed topical antibiotics and have the fewest side effects.

Systemic Antiacne Drugs

For severe acne, oral antibiotics (e.g., tetracycline [drug of choice] or erythromycin) and topical glucocorticoids may be prescribed. Tetracycline inhibits bacterial protein synthesis. It is used to treat acne with a lower maintenance dose over a period of months. Tetracycline should not be taken with antacids or milk products because they bind it into an insoluble compound, thus decreasing its absorption. A major side effect of tetracycline is photosensitivity. Exposure to the sun while taking tetracycline can result in severe sunburn. Pregnant women should not take tetracycline because of possible teratogenic effects on the fetus.

Isotretinoin (Accutane), a derivative of vitamin A, is used for severe cystic acne. It can be administered orally or topically. It decreases sebum formation and secretion, and it has antiinflammatory and antikeratinizing (keratolytic) effects. It can cause adverse reactions such as nosebleeds, pruritus, and inflammation of the eyes and lips. Isotretinoin must not be used during pregnancy because of teratogenic effects. Vitamin A and tetracycline may increase adverse effects. Do not confuse Accutane with Accupril. Baseline blood work is required before initiating Accutane. Monitoring of complete blood cell count (CBC), glucose and lipid levels, and urinanalysis on a regular basis is important. Isotretinoin must not be used during pregnancy; its pregnancy risk category is X. Based on this drug's teratogenicity, a system to manage Accutane-related teratogenicity (SMART) has been implemented, with the purpose that no woman be pregnant when treatment is initiated and no woman will become pregnant while taking this drug. This comprehensive program has rules for the health care provider, client, and pharmacist. The health care provider must read "Guide to Best Practices" and sign a letter of understanding. Once qualified, the health care provider must apply self-adhesive "Accutane Qualification Stickers" to each prescription (both new and refill). Women must receive warnings of tetragenicity both orally and in writing. Two negative pregnancy tests are required before starting the drug and one negative test before each monthly refill. Two effective methods of contraception are required 1 month before, throughout the duration of the drug, and 1 month after terminating drug. (Exceptions are abstinence or hysterectomy.) Viewing of the manufacturer's videotape on methods of contraception is required, along with signed informed consent. The pharmacist can fill only prescriptions carrying an "Accutane Qualification Sticker" when presented in person within 7 days. In addition, Accutane can elevate triglyceride levels. Table 48–1 lists the drugs commonly used to control acne vulgaris.

Table 48–1

Drugs for Acne Vulgaris and Psoriasis

Generic (Brand)	Route and Dosage	Uses and Considerations
Acne Vulgaris		
Systemic Preparations		
tetracycline (Sumycin)	A & C >12 y: PO: 250-500 mg b.i.d. *Mild acne:* 250 mg/d or q.o.d.	For moderate to severe acne. Inexpensive. Should not be taken during pregnancy. Should not be taken with milk products or antacids. *Pregnancy category:* D; PB: 65%; t½: 6-12 h
erythromycin (E-Mycin)	A: PO: 250-500 mg b.i.d.	For moderate to severe acne. A substitute for tetracycline. *Pregnancy category:* B; PB: 75%-90%; t½: 1.5-2 h
isotretinoin (Accutane)	A: PO: 0.5-1 mg/kg/d, in two divided doses, for 15 wk; *max:* 2 mg/kg/d in 2 divided doses	For severe acne. Decreases sebum secretion. Used when oral antibiotics have failed. Avoid use with tetracycline and vitamin A to reduce toxic effects. Monitor CBC, glucose, and lipid levels. *Pregnancy category:* X; PB: 99%; t½: 10-20 h
Topical Preparations		
Keratolytic Agents		
azelaic acid (Azelex)	A & C >12 y: Topical: cream 20%; apply b.i.d.	To treat mild to moderate acne. Inhibits hyperactivity of normal melanocytes. Mild pruritus, erythema, dryness, and peeling of skin might result. *Pregnancy* category: B; PB: UK; t½: 12 h
benzoyl-peroxide (Benzac, Persa-Gel)	A & C: 2.5%-10% one to four times/d (cream, gel, or lotion)	For mild to moderate acne. Promotes keratolysis (removal of horny layer of the epidermis). May cause skin irritation (burning, blistering, or swelling).
salicylic acid (Sebulex)	*Antiacne/antiseborrheic:* A & C: 2%-10% cream, gel, shampoo. Use as directed.	For mild to moderate acne; promotes desquamation.
resorcinol (Bicozene)	A & C: 1%-10% cream, ointment, lotion, shampoo	For mild to moderate acne.
resorcinol and sulfur	A & C: 2% resorcinol + 5% sulfur A & C: 2% resorcinol + 8% sulfur Use as directed.	For mild to moderate acne.
Antibiotics		
tetracycline	Ointment: 3% Sol: 2.2 mg/ml	For moderate acne. *Pregnancy category:* B
erythromycin	Ointment: 2% Gel: 1.5%-2%	For moderate acne.
clindamycin (Cleocin)	Gel: ⅕ Lotion: 1% Sol: 1%	For moderate acne.
meclocycline (Meclan)	Ointment, b.i.d.	For moderate acne.
tretinoin (Retin-A)	Cream: 0.05%-0.1% Gel: 0.025%-0.1% Liquid: 0.05% daily at bedtime	For mild to moderate acne. Vitamin A derivative. May be used with benzoyl peroxide or topical antibiotic. Should not be applied to open wounds. Area should be cleansed first. *Pregnancy category:* B
adapalene (Differin)	A & C >12 y: topical: 0.1% gel; apply daily at bedtime after washing	To treat mild to moderate acne. Do not use before or after extended sun exposure. It intensifies sunburn. Pruritus may occur. *Pregnancy* category: C; PB: UK; t½: UK

A, Adult; *b.i.d.*, twice a day; *b.i.w.*, twice a week; *C*, child; *d*, day; *DNA*, deoxyribonucleic acid; *FDA*, Food and Drug Administration; *h*, hour; *IV*, intravenous; *max*, maximum; *OC*, oral contraceptive; *PB*, protein-binding; *PO*, by mouth; *q.o.d.*, every other day; *sol*, solution; *subQ*, subcutaneous; *t½*, half-life; *tab*, tablet; *TNF*, tumor necrosis factor; *UK*, unknown; *wk*, week; *y*, year; *>*, greater than.

Table 48-1

Drugs for Acne Vulgaris and Psoriasis—cont'd

Generic (Brand)	Route and Dosage	Uses and Considerations
Oral Contraceptives		
Estrostep	A: PO: 1 tab daily × 21 d; no tab × 7d; Take as OC schedule	FDA approved for treatment of acne
Ortho Tri-Cyclen	A: PO: 1 tab daily × 21 d; then no tab × 7 d; take as OC schedule	FDA approved for treatment of acne
Psoriasis		
methoxsalen (Oxsoralen)	A: PO: 10-20 mg 2 h before exposure to therapeutic ultraviolet rays. Topical application before exposure to ultraviolet rays.	For severe psoriasis. Systemic antimetabolite drug. Avoid during pregnancy. Avoid sunlight during drug therapy; sunlight could cause burning and blistering. *Pregnancy category:* C; PB: 80%-90%; $t^{1/2}$: >2 h
etretinate (Tegison)	A: PO: 0.5-0.75 mg/kg/d, in divided doses, not to exceed 1.5 mg/kg/d	For recalcitrant psoriasis. Related to vitamin A. It may take up to 1-6 months for a response to treatment. *Pregnancy category:* X; PB: 99%; $t^{1/2}$: 4-8 d
Topical Preparations		
calcipotriene (Dovonex)	A: Topical: cream, ointment, and scalp; sol: 0.005%, daily or b.i.d.	To treat mild to moderate plaque psoriasis. Burning, stinging, and erythema may occur. Excess use may increase serum calcium level. *Pregnancy category:* C; PB: UK; $t^{1/2}$: UK
Coal tar (Estar, PsoriGel)	A: Topical: Shampoo, cream, gel, paste, soap, ointment, lotion, solution	For mild to moderate psoriasis. Suppresses DNA synthesis, decreasing mitotic activity. May stain clothing, skin, and hair.
anthralin (Anthra-Derm)	A: Topical: 0.1%-1.0% ointment and cream	For moderate psoriasis. It inhibits DNA synthesis thus suppressing proliferation of the epidermal cells. May stain clothing, skin, and hair.
tazarotene (Tazorac)	A: Topical: 0.05% and 0.1% gel. Apply in the PM to lesions.	Treatment for mild to moderate psoriasis; can also be used for acne. Reduces epidermal inflammation. Photosensitivity can occur.
alefacept (Amevive)	A: IV: 7.5 mg/wk Or 15 mg IM q wk	For treatment of severe chronic plaque psoriasis. Inhibits T-cell activation. *Pregnancy category:* B; PB: UK; $t^{1/2}$: 270 h
efalizumab (Raptiva)	A: subQ: 1 mg/kg q wk	For treatment of moderate to severe psoriasis. Inhibits T-cell migration & activation of CD 11a. *Pregnancy category:* PB: $t^{1/2}$
etanercept (Enbrel)	A: subQ: 25 mg b.i.w.	For moderate to severe psoriasis. *Pregnancy category:* B; PB: UK; $t^{1/2}$: 115 h
infliximab (Remicade)	A: IV: 3 mg/kg IV infusion (>120 min) days 0, 2, 6, then q 8 wk	In phase 3 psoriasis trials *Pregnancy category:* C; PB: UK; $t^{1/2}$: 9.5 d
adalimumab (Humira)	A: subQ: 40 mg q other wk	Human IgG1 monoclonal TNF-alpha antibody. In phase 3 psoriasis trials; approved for rheumatoid arthritis. *Pregnancy category:* B; PB: UK; $t^{1/2}$: 10-20 d
Keratolytic Drugs		
salicylic acid, sulfur, resorcinol		See acne vulgaris.

Psoriasis

Psoriasis is a chronic skin disorder that affects 1% to 2% of the U.S. population. It is more common in whites than African Americans. Onset of psoriasis usually appears before the age of 30 years, but it may occur as early as age 10. Psoriasis is characterized by erythematous papules and plaques covered with silvery scales (see Figure 48-1). It appears on the scalp, elbows, palms of the hands, knees, and soles of the feet. With psoriasis, epidermal cell growth, and epidermal turnover is accelerated to approximately five times the normal expected epidermal growth. Antipsoriatic drug therapy uses preparations such as coal tar products and anthralin to keep the psoriasis in check; however, there are usually periods of remission and exacerbation.

Topical and Systemic Preparations for Psoriasis

The psoriatic scales may be loosened with keratolytics (salicylic acid, sulfur). Topical glucocorticoids are sometimes used for mild psoriasis. Other topical preparations for psoriasis include anthralin (Anthra-Derm, Lasan) and coal tar (Estar, PsoriGel). Applications of 1% anthralin may cause erythema to occur. This agent can stain clothing, skin, and hair. Coal tar products are available in shampoos, lotions, and creams. They have an unpleasant odor and can cause burn-

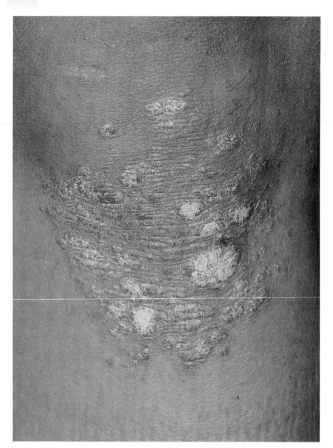

FIGURE 48–1 Psoriasis. Typical oval plaque with well-defined borders and silvery scale. (From Habif T: *Clinical dermatology*, St Louis, 2004, Mosby, p. 210.)

ing and stinging. Systemic toxicity does not occur with anthralin and coal tar. A topical product for mild to moderate psoriasis is calcipotriene (Dovonex), a synthetic vitamin D_3 derivative. It is useful for suppressing cell proliferation. This drug may cause local irritation, but the serious adverse effects are hypercalciuria and hypercalcemia (increased urine and serum calcium levels). A new topical antipsoriatic, tazarotene (Tazorac), is used to treat mild to moderate psoriasis. Photosensitivity is a side effect of tazarotene; therefore the client should use sunscreen to avoid severe sunburn.

The anticancer drug methotrexate is a systemic drug that slows high growth fraction. It is prescribed to decrease the acceleration of epidermal cell growth in severe psoriasis. Etretinate (Tegison) is used for severe pustular psoriasis, more so than the plaque-type psoriasis. It is used when other agents have failed to control psoriasis. Etretinate has an antiinflammatory effect and inhibits keratinization and proliferation of the epithelial cells. Ultraviolet A (UVA) may be used to suppress mitotic (cell division) activity. Photochemotherapy, a combination of ultraviolet radiation and the psoralen derivative methoxsalen (photosensitive drug), is used to decrease proliferation of epidermal cells. This type of therapy is called *psoralen and ultraviolet A (PUVA)*. PUVA permits lower doses of methoxsalen and ultraviolet A to be given.

High-cost biologic agents are helpful in the management of psoriasis in clients who are refractory to ultraviolet B (UVB) phototherapy and need improved control of disease. Four Food and Drug Administration (FDA)-approved agents include: alefacept (Amevive), efalizumab (Raptiva); etanercept (Enbrel), infliximab (Remicade). Another agent, adalimumab (Humira), is in phase 3 psoriasis trials and is approved for rheumatoid arthritis.

Alefacept (Amevive) is a recombinant protein that modifies the inflammatory process and inhibits the activation of memory effector T lymphocytes. No increased rate of opportunistic infections or malignancy has been observed. Weekly monitoring of T-cell counts is required; discontinue if the count is lower than 250 cells per liter.

Efalizumab (Raptiva) is a humanized therapeutic antibody to treat adults who have severe psoriasis with indication for systemic or phototherapy. Raptiva, a weekly subcutaneous injection, can be self-administered by the client or family. Maintained response is generally seen after 12 weeks of treatment. As an immunosuppressant agent, Raptiva may increase the risk of infection.

Etanercept (Enbrel) is a soluble recombinant human tumor necrosis factor (TNF)-alpha inhibitor. This agent worsens infections, especially tuberculosis (TB); thus PPD required prior to initiation of therapy. Etanercept may also worsen congestive heart failure (CHF).

Infliximab (Remicade) is a monoclonal antibody that neutralizes TNF-alpha purified protein derivative (PPD) before the start of therapy as a result of reactivation of TB. There are reports that this drug may initiate multiple sclerosis. Do not confuse with Reminyl.

Table 48–1 lists the drugs used to control psoriasis.

Side Effects and Adverse Reactions: Acne Vulgaris and Psoriasis

Acne Vulgaris

Benzoyl Peroxide

Dry and irritated skin with burning, scaling, and swelling.

Tretinoin

Skin irritation, such as burning, swelling, blistering, and peeling.

Adapalene

Burning, pruritus, erythema, dryness, and scaling, usually occurring during the second to fourth weeks of treatment, but subsiding later in treatment period. Severe sunburn can occur during extended exposure to the sun.

Tetracycline

Nausea, vomiting, diarrhea, rash, urticaria, and photosensitivity. **Adverse reactions:** oral candidiasis, superinfection, blood dyscrasias, hepatotoxicity, and nephrotoxicity.

Isotretinoin

Nosebleeds; dryness of the skin, nose, and mouth, especially in the corners of the mouth; inflamed eyes; pruritus; photosensitivity; anorexia, nausea, vomiting; and elevated liver enzymes. **Adverse reactions:** thrombocytopenia and hematuria. Monitoring of laboratory test results is required for duration of treatment.

Psoriasis

Anthralin

Erythema (redness) to normal skin, inflamed eyes, and staining effect.

Coal Tar

Skin irritation, such as burning; photosensitivity; and staining effect.

Etretinate

Anorexia, vomiting, dry skin and nasal mucosa, rash, pruritus, fatigue, bone or joint pain, peeling of skin, and photosensitivity. **Adverse reactions:** Alopecia, cardiac dysrhythmias, hepatitis, and hematuria.

Methoxsalen

Nausea, headache, vertigo, rash, pruritus, and burning and peeling of skin. **Adverse reactions:** Anemia, leukopenia, thrombocytopenia, ulcerative stomatitis, bleeding; alopecia, and cystitis.

Alefacept

Injection site reaction (erythema, itching, pain, swelling), dizziness, throat inflammation, nausea, muscle pain, and chills.

Efalizumab

Headache, chills, fever, nausea, myalgia, and potential of acute infection.

Etanercept

Injection site reaction (erythema, itching, pain, swelling).

Infliximab

Infusion reactions and infections, including reactivation of TB.

Nursing Process

Acne Vulgaris and Psoriasis

ASSESSMENT

- Obtain a history from client of the onset of skin lesions. Note whether there is a familial history of the skin disorder.
- Assess client's skin eruptions. Describe the lesions, location, and drainage, if present.
- Obtain a culture of a purulent draining skin lesion.
- Determine baseline vital signs. Report any elevation in temperature.
- Assess the psychologic effects of skin lesions and changes in body image.

NURSING DIAGNOSES

- Risk for impaired skin integrity
- Risk for infection
- Disturbed body image related to skin lesions
- Self-esteem

PLANNING

- Client's skin lesions will be decreased in size or will be absent after drug therapy and skin care.
- Client will report acceptance of body image.

NURSING INTERVENTIONS

- Establish rapport because client may be embarrassed.
- Apply topical medications to the skin lesions using aseptic technique.
- Monitor vital signs and report abnormal findings.
- Check the lesion sites during drug therapy for improvement or adverse reactions to the drug therapy, such as blistering, swelling, or scaling.

Client Teaching

General

- Instruct client not to use harsh cleansers on the skin. Tell client to clean the skin several times a day.
- Teach client how to apply topical ointments and creams using a clean technique.
- Inform client about the side effects and adverse reactions associated with the drugs taken.
- Tell client to report abnormal findings immediately. Inform client not to take milk or antacids with tetracycline.
- Instruct client to alert the health care provider if pregnant or if there is a possibility of pregnancy. Many agents used to treat acne can cause teratogenic effects on the fetus.
- Advise client to keep health care appointments and have laboratory tests performed as prescribed.

Self-Administration

- Instruct client and family about how to administer biologic agents given via the parenteral route (e.g., preparation and administration of Amevive: diluted solution to be stored in refrigerator and used within 4 hours; do not shake medication; rotate injection sites leaving at least 1 inch between sites).

EVALUATION

■ Evaluate the effectiveness of the drug therapy on the skin lesions. If improvement is not apparent, the drug therapy and skin care regimen may need to be changed.

Verruca Vulgaris (Warts)

The common wart is a hard, horny nodule that may appear anywhere on the body, particularly on the hands and feet. Warts are benign lesions. They may be removed by freezing, electrodesiccation, or surgical excision. Drugs used include salicylic acid, podophyllum resin, and cantharidin. Salicylic acid promotes desquamation. It can be absorbed through the skin, and salicylism (toxicity) might occur. Podophyllum resin is indicated mainly for venereal warts and is not as effective against the common wart. This drug also can be absorbed through the skin; toxic symptoms such as peripheral neuropathy, blood dyscrasias, and kidney impairment could result if a large area is treated. Podophyllum can cause teratogenic effects and should not be used during pregnancy. Imiquimod (Aldara) and podofilox (Condylox) may be prescribed as alternative agents for podophyllin. Both drugs may be used for topical treatment of external genital and perianal warts.

Cantharidin (Cantharone, Verr-Canth) is used to remove the common wart; however, it can be harmful to normal skin. For treating the common wart, cantharidin is applied to the wart and allowed to dry and then the wart is covered with a nonporous tape for 24 hours. The procedure can be repeated in 1 to 2 weeks.

Many OTC agents are used to remove warts. The efficiency of some of these is questionable; however, some that contain chemical compounds such as salicylic acid may be effective.

Drug-Induced Dermatitis

An adverse reaction to drug therapy may result in skin lesions that vary from a rash, urticaria, papules, and vesicles to life-threatening skin eruptions, such as erythema multiforme (red blisters over a large portion of the body) or Stevens-Johnson syndrome (large blisters in the oral and anogenital mucosa, pharynx, eyes, and viscera). A hyper-sensitive reaction to a drug is caused by the formation of sensitizing lymphocytes. If multiple drug therapy is used, the last drug given may be the cause of the hypersensitivity and skin eruptions. The usual skin reactions are a rash that may take several hours or a day to appear and urticarias (hives), which usually take a few minutes to appear. Certain drugs, such as penicillin, are known to cause hypersensitivity.

Other drug-induced dermatitides include discoid lupus erythematosus (DLE) and exfoliative dermatitis. Hydralazine hydrochloride (Apresoline), isoniazid (INH), phenothiazines, anticonvulsants, and antidysrhythmics, such as procainamide (Pronestyl), may cause lupuslike symptoms. If lupus symptoms occur, the drug should be discontinued. Certain antibacterials and anticonvulsants may cause exfoliative dermatitis, resulting in erythema of the skin, itching, scaling, and loss of body hair.

Contact Dermatitis

Contact dermatitis, also called *exogenous dermatitis,* is caused by chemical or plant irritation. A skin rash with itching, swelling, blistering, oozing, or scaling at the affected skin sites characterizes it. The chemical contact may include cosmetics, cleansing products (e.g., soaps, detergents), perfume, clothing, dyes, and topical drugs. Plant contacts include poison ivy, oak, or sumac.

Nonpharmacologic measures include avoiding direct contact with the causative irritant. Protective gloves or clothing may be necessary if the chemical is associated with work. Immediately cleanse the skin area that has been in contact with the irritant. Patch testing may be needed to determine the causal factor.

Treatment may consist of wet dressings containing Burow's solution (aluminum acetate); lotions, such as calamine, that contain zinc oxide; calcium hydroxide solution; and glycerin. Calamine lotion may contain the antihistamine diphenhydramine and is used primarily for plant irritations. If itching persists, antipruritics (topical or systemic diphenhydramine [Benadryl]) may be used. Topical antipruritics should not be applied to open wounds or near the eyes or genital area. Other agents used as antipruritics include the following:

- Systemic drugs, such as cyproheptadine hydrochloride (Periactin) and trimeprazine tartrate (Temaril)
- Antipruritic baths of oatmeal or Alpha-Keri
- Solutions of potassium permanganate, aluminum subacetate, or normal saline
- Glucocorticoid ointments, creams, or gels

Dexamethasone (Decadron) cream, hydrocortisone ointment or cream, methylprednisolone acetate (Medrol) ointment, triamcinolone acetonide (Aristocort), and flurandrenolide (Cordran) are examples of topical glucocorticoids that aid in alleviating dermatitis. Table 48–2 lists selected topical glucocorticoids according to their potency for relieving the itching and inflammation associated with dermatitis.

Table 48-2

Topical Glucocorticoids

Potency	Generic (Brand)	Drug Form
Extra-High	betamethasone dipropionate (diprolene) 0.05%	Cream, ointment, lotion
	clobetasol proprionate (Clobex, Temovate) 0.05%	Cream, ointment, lotion
	halobetasol proprionate (Ultravate) 0.05%	Cream, ointment
High	amcinonide 0.1% (Cyclocort)	Cream, ointment
	desoximetasone 0.25% (Topicort)	Cream, ointment
	desoximetasone 0.05%	Gel
	diflorasone diacetate 0.05% (Florone, Maxiflor)	Cream, ointment
	fluocinolone acetonide 0.025% (Synclor)	Cream, ointment
	halcinonide 0.1% (Halog)	Cream, ointment
	triamcinolone acetonide 0.5% (Aristocort A, Kenalog)	Cream, ointment
Moderate	betamethasone benzoate 0.025% (Uticort)	Lotion
	betamethasone valerate 0.1% (Valisone)	Cream, ointment, lotion
	clocortolone pivalate (Cloderm) 0.1%	Cream
	desoximetasone 0.05% (Topicort LP)	Cream, gel
	flurandrenolide 0.025% (Cordran, Cordran SP)	Cream, ointment, lotion
	halcinonide 0.025% (Halog)	Cream, ointment
	hydrocortisone valerate 0.2% (Westcort)	Cream, ointment
	mometasone furoate 0.1% (Elocon)	Cream, ointment, lotion
	triamcinolone acetonide 0.025%–0.1% (Aristocort A, Kenalog)	Cream, ointment, lotion
Low	dexamethasone 0.1% (Decadron)	Cream
	desonide 0.05% (Tridesilon)	Cream
	dexamethasone (Decaspray) 0.04%	Aerosol
	fluocinolone acetonide 0.01% (Flurosyn)	Cream, solution
	hydrocortisone 0.25%, 0.5%, 1.0%, 2.5% (Cortef, Hytone)	Cream, ointment
	methylprednisolone acetate 0.25%, 1.0% (Medrol)	Ointment

A portion of topical glucocorticoids can be systemically absorbed into the circulation; the amount and rate of absorption depend on the vehicle (cream, lotion), drug concentration, drug composition, and skin area to which the glucocorticoid is applied. Absorption is greater where the skin is more permeable—the face, scalp, eyelids, neck, axilla, and genital area. Side effects and adverse reactions may occur with prolonged use of the topical drug and if the drug is continuously covered with a dressing. Prolonged use of topical glucocorticoids can cause thinning of the skin with atrophy of the epidermis and dermis and purpura from small-vessel eruptions.

Hair Loss And Baldness

When the hair shaft is lost and the hair follicle cannot regenerate, male-pattern baldness, or *alopecia*, occurs. Permanent hair loss is associated with a familial history and occurs during the aging process, earlier in some individuals than others. Drugs also known to cause alopecia include the anticancer (antineoplastic) agents, gold salts, sulfonamides, anticonvulsants, aminoglycosides, and some of the nonsteroidal antiinflammatory drugs (NSAIDs), such as indomethacin. Severe febrile illnesses, pregnancy, myxedema (condition resulting from hypothyroidism), and cancer therapies are some of the health conditions contributing to temporary hair loss.

A 2% minoxidil (Rogaine) solution has been approved by the FDA for treating baldness for men and women. A 5% solution is approved for men only. Minoxidil causes vasodilation, thus increasing cutaneous blood flow. The increased blood flow tends to stimulate hair follicle growth. When the drug is discontinued, however, hair loss occurs within 3 to 4 months. Systemic absorption of minoxidil is minimal, so adverse reactions seldom occur. Occasionally, headaches and a slight decrease in systolic blood pressure occur.

Finasteride (Propecia) is an oral drug used for male baldness. It is available in 1-mg tablets. A 5-mg tablet is prescribed for benign prostatic hyperplasia (BPH). For growing hair, finasteride is effective in 50% of men. It has been reported that it is relatively ineffective in growing hair in older men, even with an increased dose.

Sunscreens

Ultraviolet radiation causes many problems, including premature aging of the skin, burns, and skin cancer. Sunscreens protect against sunburn photosensitivity to selected drugs but do not guard against melanoma and basal cell carcinoma. Sun protection factor (SPF) is a rating on sunscreen products of protection against UVB radiation. The highest rating approved by FDA is SPF 30+; SPF 15 is not one half the protection of SPF 30. A higher protection rating is not proportional to the number; for example, SPF 15 = 93% block of UVB and SPF 30 = 96.7% block.

Common sense is the best way to protect the skin. UVB radiation is most intense between 10:00 AM and 3:00 PM. Apply an appropriate sunscreen for the circumstances at least 30 minutes (sunscreens with PABA or padimate allow 2 hours) before going out in the sun. Each SPF is good for a certain time period, 2 hours, when applied properly and not exposed to moisture (through swimming or sweating). Wearing protective clothing, such as a wide-brimmed hat, sunglasses, and long-sleeve shirt is a good idea.

Burns and Burn Preparations

Burns from heat (thermal burns), electricity (electrical burns), and chemical agents (chemical burns) can cause skin lesions. Burns are classified according to degree and tissue depth of burns and are described in Table 48–3.

A moderately severe sunburn is an example of a *first-degree burn*. A severe sunburn can result in a *second-degree burn*. A burn needs immediate attention regardless of the degree and tissue depth of the burn.

For first-degree and minor burns, a cold wet compress should be applied to the burned area to constrict blood vessels and decrease swelling. This treatment also decreases the amount of pain. The quicker the burn area is cooled, the less tissue damage occurs. No greasy ointment, butter, or greasy dressing should be applied because they can inhibit heat loss from the burn and increase the damage to the tissues. A nonprescription antibiotic, such as bacitracin with polymyxin B (Polysporin), may be used for minor burns. Polymyxin B and neomycin, used separately, are not drugs of choice because they do not have a broad-spectrum effect. With chemical burns, the clothing should be removed immediately and the skin thoroughly flushed with water.

Persons with second- and third-degree burns that involve dermis and subcutaneous tissue should undergo treatment in a burn center or other hospital setting. Intravenous therapy is started immediately, and a nonnarcotic or narcotic analgesic is given for pain. Burn areas are cleansed with sterile saline solution and an antiseptic, such as povidone-iodine (Betadine). If a povidone-iodine solution is used, it should be determined that the client is not allergic to iodine or seafood. Broad-spectrum topical antibacterials, usually effective against many gram-positive and gram-negative as well as yeast infections, are applied to burn areas to prevent infection. Examples of these antibacterials include mafenide acetate (Sulfamylon), silver sulfadiazine (Silvadene), silver nitrate 0.5% solution, and nitrofurazone (Furacin). Prototype Drug Chart 48–1 lists the drug data for the antibacterial agent mafenide acetate (Sulfamylon).

Mafenide Acetate

Pharmacokinetics

Mafenide acetate is absorbed through the skin and is metabolized by the liver to a metabolite. The drug is excreted in the urine. The drug and its metabolite are strong carbonic anhydrase inhibitors, which may lead to acid-base imbalances (e.g., metabolic acidosis and respiratory alkalosis) and fluid loss from the mild diuretic effect. If respiration becomes rapid, labored, or shallow, the cream should be discontinued for a few days until the acid-base balance is restored.

Pharmacodynamics

Mafenide, a sulfonamide derivative, interferes with bacterial cell-wall synthesis and metabolism and is bacteriostatic. It is used as a topical water-soluble antibacterial agent to prevent or combat a burn infection. After the burn is cleansed and debrided, $1/16$ inch of mafenide cream is applied to the affected area one to two times daily and is covered lightly with a dressing. The client may complain of a burning sensation when the drug is applied.

Table 48–4 lists selected topical medications for burns and their strengths, uses, and considerations.

Silver Sulfadiazine

Silver sulfadiazine (Silvadene, SSD) is commonly used to prevent and treat sepsis in second- and third-degree burns. It acts on the cell membrane and cell wall to produce bactericidal effects. Unlike mafenide, it is *not* a carbonic anhydrase inhibitor. It is contraindicated at or near term pregnancy.

One percent or less of the silver is absorbed, and up to 10% of sulfadiazine is absorbed. Side effects and adverse reactions may include skin discoloration, burning sensation, rashes, erythema multiforme, skin necrosis, and possible leukopenia.

Table 48–3			
Degree and Tissue Depth of Burns			
Type	**Degree**	**Depth**	**Characteristics**
Superficial epidermal	First	Epidermis	Erythema (redness), painful
Partial thickness superficial	First-second	Epidermis, upper dermis	Blistering, very painful
Deep thickness	Second	Epidermis, lower dermis	Mottled, blistering, intense pain
Full thickness	Third	Epidermis, dermis, nerve ending involvement, subcutaneous tissue	Pearly white skin, charred, no pain

PROTOTYPE DRUG CHART 48-1

MAFENIDE ACETATE

Drug Class	**Dosage**
Topical antiinfective Trade Name: Sulfamylon *Pregnancy Category:* C	**A & C:** Topical: Apply ¹⁄₁₆-in layer evenly to affected area daily/b.i.d.; reapply as necessary
Contraindications	**Drug-Lab-Food Interactions**
Hypersensitivity, inhalation injury	None known
Pharmacokinetics	**Pharmacodynamics**
Absorption: Some absorbed **Distribution:** PB: UK **Metabolism:** t½: UK **Excretion:** In urine	**PO:** Onset: On contact Peak: 2-4 h Duration: As long as applied

Therapeutic Effects/Uses

To treat second- and third-degree burns; to prevent organism invasion of burned tissue areas; to treat burn infections
Mode of Action: Inhibits bacterial cell wall synthesis

Side Effect	**Adverse Reactions**
Rash, burning sensation, urticaria, pruritus, swelling	Metabolic acidosis, respiratory alkalosis, blistering, superinfection **Life-threatening:** Bone marrow suppression, fatal hemolytic anemia

A, Adult; *b.i.d.,* two times a day; *C,* child; *h,* hour; *in,* inch; *PB,* protein-binding; *PO,* by mouth; *t½,* half-life; *UK,* unknown.

Table 48-4

Topical Antiinfectives: Burns

Generic (Brand)	Route and Dosage	Uses and Considerations
nitrofurazone (Furacin)	0.2% cream, ointment, sol *Adjunctive therapy:* Apply directly or to dressing daily for second- to third-degree burns; q4-5d for second-degree burns with scant exudate	For second- and third-degree burns. Can cause photosensitivity; avoid sunlight. May cause contact dermatitis. *Pregnancy category:* C; PB: NA; t½: NA
mafenide acetate (Sulfamylon) silver nitrate	See Prototype Drug Chart 48-1. 0.5 sol; 10%, 25% sticks; apply only to affected area 2-3×/wk for 2-3 wk	For second- and third-degree burns. Dressings are soaked in 0.5% silver nitrate solution and then removed before they dry. Effective against some gram-negative organisms. May cause electrolyte imbalance (hypokalemia) if used extensively. *Pregnancy category:* C; PB: NA; t½: NA
silver sulfadiazine (Silvadene, SSD)	1% cream, apply daily-b.i.d. in ¹⁄₁₆-in layer	Prevent and treat infection of second- and third-degree burns. Ten percent of the drug is absorbed. Excessive use or extensive application area may cause sulfa crystals (crystalluria). *Pregnancy category:* C; PB: NA; t½: NA

b.i.d., Twice a day; *d,* day; *in,* inch; *NA,* not applicable; *PB,* protein-binding; *sol,* solution; *t½,* half-life; *wk,* week.

Nursing Process

Topical Antiinfectives: Burns

ASSESSMENT

■ Assess burned tissue for infection. Culture an oozing wound.
■ Check client's vital signs. Report abnormal findings, such as an elevated temperature.
■ Determine fluid status. Report signs and symptoms of hypovolemia or hypervolemia.

NURSING DIAGNOSES

■ Risk for infection related to loss of skin integrity
■ Pain related to thermal injury
■ Disturbed body image

PLANNING

■ Aseptic technique will be enforced when caring for burned tissue, and tissue will be free from infection.

NURSING INTERVENTIONS

■ Administer prescribed analgesia before application, if needed.
■ Cleanse burned tissue sites using aseptic technique.
■ Apply topical antibacterial drug and dressing with sterile technique.
■ Monitor client's fluid balance and renal function.
■ Monitor client for side effects and adverse reactions to topical drug.
■ Monitor client's vital signs and be alert for signs of infection. Use with caution in client with acute renal failure.
■ Closely monitor client's acid-base balance, especially in the presence of pulmonary or renal dysfunction.
■ Store drug in dry place at room temperature.

Client Teaching

General
• Instruct client and family about changes in respiratory status.

Self-Administration
• Explain to client and family the care given to the burned tissue areas, using aseptic technique.
• Instruct client and family how to apply topical agent and dressings to the burned areas.
• Instruct client and family on signs and symptoms of infection and to report them promptly to the health care provider.

Cultural Considerations
• In many cultures the extended family structure is important for health teaching and providing support.
• Do not assume that a positive response means a definite "yes" or understanding (it may be simply a show of politeness).

EVALUATION

■ Evaluate effectiveness of treatment interventions to burned tissue areas by determining whether healing is proceeding and sites are free from infection.

WEBSITES

For further information on *Drugs for Dermatologic Disorders,* visit these Internet resources:

Health Cyclopedia—Skin Disorders: *http://www.healthcyclopedia.com/skin-disorders.html*

The Merck Manual of Geriatrics—Chapter 123, Common Skin Disorders: *http://www.merck.com/mrkshared/mm_geriatrics/sec15/ch123.jsp*

Critical Thinking Case Study

M.G., age 15, complains about numerous black-heads and large raised pimples on her face. She seeks help from a health care provider.

1. To assist in identifying her skin problem, what should the health history and assessment include?

2. Which nonpharmacologic measures might you discuss with M.G. in caring for her facial skin condition?

   M.G.'s skin disorder does not improve. Her health care provider said she has acne vulgaris and has prescribed benzoyl peroxide and oral tetracycline.

3. M.G. asks the nurse how to use benzoyl peroxide. What should the explanation of the method and frequency for the use of benzoyl peroxide include?

4. What should be included in the client teaching related to the use of oral tetracycline?

5. What other agents for acne might M.G. use? Explain their uses and side effects.

6. M.G. asked if she would have to remain on benzoyl peroxide and oral tetracycline for the rest of her life. What is the answer or course of action? Explain.

Study Questions

1. What are the actions of keratolytics? Give examples of these agents and their actions.

2. What are the similarities and differences of the topical antiacne drugs tretinoin, adapalene, and azelaic acid?

3. What are the advantages and disadvantages for the use of the oral antiacne drugs isotretinoin and tetracycline?

4. What are at least three nursing implications for health teaching with clients taking Accutane?

5. T.H. has psoriasis. A coal-tar preparation has been suggested, and anthralin has been prescribed by the health care provider. T.H. asks how these agents will help him. What is the appropriate response?

6. What are the nursing implications of the new biologic agents for the management of psoriasis?

7. R.Q. has poison ivy. Poison ivy is classified as what type of skin disorder? What nondrug and drug regimens alleviate the poison ivy?

8. What drug is used to treat male-pattern baldness? How is it administered and how does it achieve hair follicle growth?

9. B.R. has second- and third-degree burns over 25% of his body. Mafenide acetate has been ordered. How is it administered? What care is taken before its administration? What acid-base imbalance can result from its use?

Fifteen

Endocrine Agents

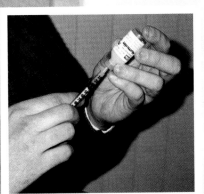

The endocrine system consists of ductless glands that secrete hormones into the bloodstream. *Hormones* are chemical substances synthesized from amino acids and cholesterol that act on body tissues and organs and affect cellular activity. Hormones can be divided into two categories: (1) proteins or small peptides and (2) steroids. Hormones from the adrenal glands and the gonads are steroid hormones; the others are protein hormones. The *endocrine glands* include the pituitary (hypophysis), thyroid, parathyroid, adrenal, gonads, and pancreas. Figure XV–1 illustrates the location and functions of these glands. This unit discusses the hormonal activity of the endocrine glands.

Pituitary Gland

The pituitary gland, or hypophysis, is located at the base of the brain and has two lobes, the anterior pituitary (adenohypophysis) and the posterior pituitary (neurohypophysis). The anterior pituitary gland is called the *master gland,* because it secretes hormones that stimulate the release of other hormones from target glands, including the thyroid, parathyroids, adrenals, and gonads. The posterior pituitary gland secretes two neurohormones—antidiuretic hormone (ADH), or vasopressin, and oxytocin. Figure XV–2 shows the anterior and posterior pituitary glands and the types of hormones secreted.

Anterior Pituitary Gland

The anterior pituitary hormones are (1) thyroid-stimulating hormone (TSH), (2) adreno-corticotropic hormone (ACTH), and (3) the gonadotropins (follicle-stimulating hormone [FSH] and luteinizing hormone [LH]). They control the synthesis and release of hormones from the thyroid, adrenals, and ovaries. Other hormones secreted from the anterior pituitary include growth hormone (GH), prolactin (PL), and melanocyte-stimulating hormone (MSH). The amount of each hormone secreted from the anterior pituitary is regulated by a negative feedback system. If excess hormone is secreted from the target gland, hormonal release from the anterior pituitary is suppressed. If there is a lack of hormone secretion from the target gland, there will be an increase in that particular anterior pituitary hormone.

Thyroid-Stimulating Hormone

The anterior pituitary gland secretes TSH in response to thyroid-releasing hormone (TRH) from the hypothalamus. TSH, or thyrotropic hormone, stimulates the release of thyroxine (T_4) and triiodothyronine (T_3) from the thyroid gland. Hypersecretion of TSH can cause hyperthyroidism and thyroid enlargement, and hyposecretion can cause hypothyroidism. Serum TSH levels should be checked to determine whether there is a TSH deficit or excess. TSH and T_4 levels are frequently measured to differentiate pituitary from thyroid dysfunction. A decreased T_4 level and a normal or elevated TSH level can indicate a thyroid disorder.

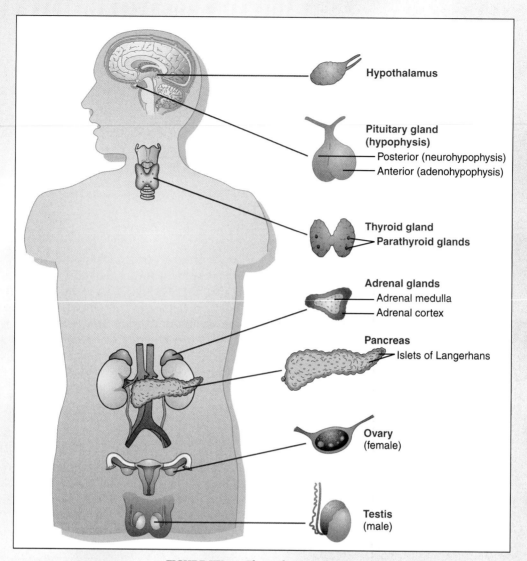

FIGURE XV–1   The endocrine glands.

FIGURE XV–2   The anterior and posterior pituitary glands. (*ACTH*, Adrenocorticotropic hormone; *ADH*, antidiuretic hormone; *FSH*, follicle-stimulating hormone; *GH*, growth hormone; *LH*, luteinizing hormone; *PL*, prolactin; *TSH*, thyroid-stimulating hormone.)

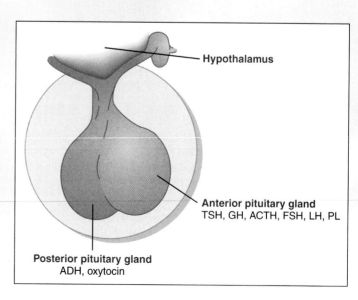

Adrenocorticotropic Hormone

Secretion of ACTH occurs in response to corticotropin-releasing factor (CRF) from the hypothalamus. ACTH from the anterior pituitary stimulates the release of glucocorticoids (cortisol), mineralocorticoids (aldosterone), and androgen from the adrenal cortex (adrenal glands). Elevated serum cortisol from the adrenal cortex inhibits ACTH and CRF release. When the cortisol level is low, ACTH secretion is stimulated, which in turn stimulates the adrenal cortex to release more cortisol. More ACTH is secreted in the morning than in the evening.

Gonadotropic Hormones

The gonadotropic hormones regulate hormone secretion from the ovaries and testes (the gonads). The anterior pituitary gland secretes the gonadotropic hormones FSH, LH, and prolactin. FSH promotes the maturation of follicles in the ovaries and initiates sperm production in the testes. LH combines with FSH in follicle maturation and estrogen production and promotes secretion of androgens from the testes. Prolactin stimulates milk formation in the glandular breast tissue after childbirth. Estrogen, progesterone, and testosterone are discussed in Chapters 54, Drugs Related to Women's Health and Disorders, and 55, Drugs Related to Reproductive Health: Male Reproductive Disorders, respectively.

Growth Hormone

GH, or somatotropic hormone (STH), acts on all body tissues, particularly the bones and skeletal muscles. The amount of GH secreted is regulated by growth hormone-releasing hormone (GH-RH) and growth hormone-inhibiting hormone (GH-IH, or somatostatin) from the hypothalamus. Sympathomimetics, serotonin, and glucocorticoids can inhibit the secretion of GH.

Posterior Pituitary Gland

The posterior pituitary gland (neurohypophysis) secretes ADH (vasopressin) and oxytocin. Interconnecting nerve fibers between the hypothalamus and the posterior pituitary gland allow ADH and oxytocin to be synthesized in the hypothalamus and stored in the posterior pituitary gland. ADH increases the reabsorption of water from the renal tubules thus returning it to the systemic circulation. Secretion of ADH is regulated by the serum osmolality (concentration of the vascular fluid). An increase in serum osmolality increases the release of ADH from the posterior pituitary; more water is then absorbed from the renal tubules to dilute the vascular fluid. Excess ADH can overload the vascular system. A decrease in serum osmolality decreases the release of ADH, promoting more water excretion from the renal tubules. Oxytocin stimulates contraction of the smooth muscles of the uterus; it is discussed in Chapter 52, Drugs Associated with the Female Reproductive Cycle II: Labor, Delivery, and the Preterm Neonate.

Thyroid Gland

Located anterior to the trachea, the thyroid gland has two lobes that are connected by a bridge of thyroid tissue. The thyroid gland secretes two hormones—thyroxine (T_4) and triiodothyronine (T_3 liothyronine). These hormones affect nearly every tissue and organ by controlling their metabolic rate and activity. Stimulation by the thyroid hormones results in an increase in cardiac output, oxygen consumption, carbohydrate use, protein synthesis, and breakdown of fat (lipolysis). Thyroid hormones also affect body heat regulation and the menstrual cycle. Thyroid hormone levels in the blood are regulated by negative feedback. The anterior pituitary gland secretes TSH, which stimulates the thyroid gland to produce T_4 and T_3. An increased amount of circulating thyroid hormones suppresses the release of TSH, and a decreased amount increases the release of TSH by the adenohypophysis.

Parathyroid Glands

There are four parathyroid glands (two pairs) that lie on the dorsal surface of the thyroid gland. The parathyroid gland secretes parathormone, or parathyroid hormone (PTH), which regulates calcium levels in the blood. A decrease in serum calcium stimulates the release of PTH. PTH increases calcium levels by (1) mobilizing calcium from the bone, (2) promoting calcium absorption from the intestine, and (3) promoting calcium reabsorption from the renal tubules. Calcitonin, a hormone produced primarily by the thyroid gland and to a lesser extent by the parathyroid and thymus glands, inhibits calcium reabsorption by bone and increases renal excretion of calcium. Calcitonin counteracts the action of PTH.

Adrenal Glands

The adrenal glands, located at the top of each kidney, consist of two separate sections—the adrenal medulla (the inner section) and the adrenal cortex (the section surrounding the adrenal medulla). The adrenal medulla releases the catecholamines epinephrine and norepinephrine and is linked with the sympathetic nervous system. The adrenal cortex produces two major types of hormones (corticosteroids)—glucocorticoids and mineralocorticoids. The principal glucocorticoid is cortisol, and the principal mineralocorticoid is aldosterone. In addition, the adrenal cortex produces small amounts of androgen, estrogen, and progestin. Glucocorticoids have a profound influence on electrolytes and the metabolism of carbohydrates, protein, and fat; glucocorticoids deficiencies can result in serious illness and even death.

Pancreas

The pancreas, located to the left of and behind the stomach, is both an exocrine and an endocrine gland. The exocrine section of the pancreas secretes digestive enzymes into the duodenum; these enzymes are discussed in Unit XIII, Gastrointestinal Agents. The endocrine section has cell clusters called *islets of Langerhans*. The alpha islet cells produce glucagon, which breaks glycogen down to glucose in the liver, and the beta cells secrete insulin, which regulates glucose metabolism. Insulin, an antidiabetic agent, is used to control diabetes mellitus. Antidiabetic agents are discussed in Chapter 50.

Drugs For Endocrine Disorders

Chapters 49, Endocrine Pharmacology: Pituitary, Thyroid, Parathyroids, and Adrenals, and 50, Antidiabetic Drugs, discuss the drugs used to diagnose and treat endocrine disorders. Chapter 49 discusses the agents for disorders involving the pituitary gland, thyroid gland, parathyroid gland, adrenal gland, and ADH. The parenteral and oral antidiabetic drugs (hypoglycemic drugs) are described in Chapter 50.

49 Endocrine Pharmacology: Pituitary, Thyroid, Parathyroids, and Adrenals

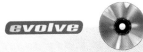

ELECTRONIC
RESOURCES

Additional information can be found on the companion website at *http://evolve.elsevier.com/KeeHayes/pharmacology/* or on the companion CD-ROM, which includes:
- *NCLEX-style examination review questions*
- *Pharmacology animations*
- *Medication error and IV therapy checklists*
- *Medication calculation problems*
- *Electronic calculators*

OBJECTIVES

- Define hormone, hypophysis, thyroxine, and glucocorticoids.
- Name the hormones secreted from the adenohypophysis and the neurohypophysis.
- Differentiate the actions, uses, and side effects of the pituitary hormones, thyroxine (T_4), triiodothyronine (T_3), parathyroid hormone (PTH), and glucocorticoids.
- Compare the nursing process, including client teaching, of drug therapy related to hormonal replacement or hormonal inhibition for the pituitary, thyroid, parathyroid, and adrenal glands.

TERMS

acromegaly
Addison's disease
adenohypophysis
adrenal glands
adrenocorticotropic hormone (ACTH)
antidiuretic hormone (ADH)

corticosteroids
cretinism
Cushing's syndrome
diabetes insipidus (DI)
endocrine
gigantism
glucocorticoids
Graves' disease

hyperthyroidism
hypophysis
hypothyroidism
mineralocorticoids
myxedema
neurohypophysis
parathyroid hormone (PTH)

thyroid-stimulating
  hormone (TSH)
thyrotoxicosis
thyroxine (T_4)
triiodothyronine (T_3)

Introduction

This chapter describes drugs used for hormonal replacement and for inhibition of hormonal secretion from the pituitary, thyroid, parathyroid, and adrenal glands. The gonadal, or sex, hormones are discussed in Chapters 54 (Drugs Related to Women's Health and Disorders) and 55 (Drugs Related to Reproductive Health: Male Reproductive Disorders). Before reading Chapters 49 (Endocrine Pharmacology: Pituitary, Thyroid, Parathyroids, and Adrenals) and 50 (Antidiabetic Drugs), the student or nurse should review the introduction to Unit XV (Endocrine Agents), which describes the locations of the endocrine glands and the hormones they secrete. Knowledge of the various **endocrine** hormones and their functions facilitates an understanding of the drugs that act on the endocrine glands.

Pituitary Gland

Anterior

The pituitary gland **(hypophysis)** has an anterior and a posterior lobe. The anterior pituitary gland, called the **adenohypophysis**, secretes the following various hormones that target glands and tissues:

- Growth hormone (GH), which stimulates growth in tissue and bone
- Thyroid-stimulating hormone (TSH), which acts on the thyroid gland
- Adrenocorticotropic hormone (ACTH), which stimulates the adrenal gland
- Gonadotropins (follicle-stimulating hormone [FSH] and luteinizing hormone [LH]), which affect the ovaries. (FSH and LH are discussed in Chapter 54, Drugs Related to Women's Health and Disorders).

The drugs with adenohypophyseal properties used to stimulate or inhibit glandular activity are discussed according to their drug use. The negative feedback system that controls the amount of hormonal secretion from the pituitary gland and the target gland is discussed in the introduction to Unit XV, Endocrine Agents.

Growth Hormone

Two hypothalamic hormones regulate GH: (1) growth hormone-releasing hormone (GH-RH) and (2) growth hormone-inhibiting hormone (GH-IH; somatostatin). GH does not have a specific target gland; it affects body tissues and bone. GH replacement stimulates linear growth when there is a GH deficiency. Enzymes in the gastrointestinal (GI) tract inactivate GH, thus requiring subcutaneous (subQ) or intramuscular (IM) administration of GH. GH drugs cannot be given orally because the drug is inactivated in the GI tract.

If a child's height is well below the standard for a specified age, GH deficiency may be diagnosed and dwarfism can result. Because GH replacement is very expensive (approximately $20,000 for 1 year), various tests are performed to determine whether this therapy is essential. Because GH acts on newly forming bone, it must be administered before the epiphyses are fused. Administration of GH over several years can increase height by a foot. Prolonged GH therapy can antagonize insulin secretion and eventually cause diabetes mellitus. Because of its effects on blood sugar and other side effects, athletes should be advised not to take GH to build muscle and physique.

Drug Therapy: Growth Hormone Deficiency

Somatrem (Protropin) and somatropin (Humatrope) are two growth hormones used to treat growth failure in children because of pituitary GH deficiency. Somatropin is a product that has the identical amino acid sequence as human growth hormone. Somatrem also has the identical sequence of pituitary GH plus an additional amino acid. Development of antibodies to somatrem has occurred in 30% to 40% of clients during the first 3 to 6 months of therapy, but in 95% of these clients, this has not decreased the effectiveness of the somatrem treatment. Somatropin is contraindicated in pediatric clients who have growth deficiency due to Prader-Willi syndrome and are severely obese or who have severe respiratory impairment because fatalities have been reported.

Drug Therapy: Growth Hormone Excess

Gigantism (during childhood) and **acromegaly** (after puberty) can occur with GH hypersecretion and are frequently caused by a pituitary tumor. If the tumor cannot be destroyed by radiation, the prolactin-release inhibitor bromocriptine can inhibit the release of GH from the pituitary.

Octreotide (Sandostatin) is a potent synthetic somatostatin used to suppress GH release. It can be used

Table 49–1

Anterior and Posterior Pituitary Hormones

Generic (Brand)	Route and Dosage	Uses and Considerations
Anterior		
Growth Hormone (GH)		
sermorelin acetate (Geref)	*Diagnostic:* A & C: IV: 0.3-1 mcg/kg	Diagnostic test to determine if the pituitary gland secretes growth hormone.
somatrem (Protropin)	*Growth hormone deficiency:* C: subQ/IM: 100 mcg/kg (0.1 mg/kg) 3 × wk or 0.2 units/kg 3 × wk; 48-h interval is recommended between doses	For growth hormone replacement for treating dwarfism. It affects growth of most body tissues and promotes bone growth at epiphyseal plates of long bones. *Pregnancy category:* C; PB: 20%-25%; $t\frac{1}{2}$: 20-30 min
somatropin (Humatrope, Nutropin, Genotropin)	C: subQ/IM: 60 mcg/kg (0.06 mg/kg) 3 × wk or 0.16 international units/kg 3 × wk; 48-h interval is recommended between doses	For treating growth hormone deficiency. Promotes bone growth at epiphyseal plates of long bones. *Pregnancy category:* D; PB: UK; $t\frac{1}{2}$: 15-60 min
Growth Hormone Suppressant Drugs		
bromocriptine mesylate (Parlodel)	A: PO: 1.25-2.5 mg daily × 3d; *range:* 10-30 mg/d; *max:* 100 mg/d	To treat acromegaly. Also used with pituitary radiation or surgery to decrease GH levels. This drug will decrease lactation and prolactinoma. *Pregnancy category:* C; PB: 93%; $t\frac{1}{2}$: 4.5 h (first phase), 45 h (last phase), average: 15 h
octreotide acetate (Sandostatin)	A: subQ: 50-100 mcg t.i.d.	For treatment of acromegaly and for clients with metastatic carcinoid tumors. *Pregnancy category:* B; PB: 65%; $t\frac{1}{2}$: 2.5 h
Thyroid-Stimulating Hormone (TSH)		
thyrotropin (Thytropar)	*Hypothyroidism and treatment of thyroid cancer:* A: subQ/IM: 10 international units/d for 1-3 d; cancer treatment: 3-8 d	For diagnosing cause of hypothyroidism (pituitary or thyroid). Radioiodine study follows last injection. *Pregnancy category:* C; PB: UK; $t\frac{1}{2}$: 35 min with normal thyroid
Adrenocorticotropic Hormone (ACTH)		
corticotropin (Acthar); corticotropin repository (Acthar gel)	See Prototype Drug Chart 49–1.	
cosyntropin (Cortrosyn)	A & C >2 y: IM/IV: 0.25 mg over 2 min C: <2 y: IM: 0.125 mg IV: 0.125 mg at 0.04 mg/h over 6 h	For diagnostic testing to differentiate between pituitary and adrenal cause of adrenal insufficiency. Obtain a plasma cortisol level before and 30 min after cosyntropin administration. *Pregnancy category:* C; PB: UK; $t\frac{1}{2}$: 15 min
Posterior		
Antidiuretic Hormone (ADH)		
desmopressin acetate (DDAVP)	*Diabetes insipidus (DI):* A: Intranasal: 0.1-0.4 ml/d in divided doses C: <12 y: Intranasal: 0.05–0.3 ml/d in divided doses	For treating DI, hemophilia A, von Willebrand's disease. Can have a long duration of action (5 to 21 h). *Pregnancy category:* B; PB: UK; $t\frac{1}{2}$: 1.25 h
desmopressin (Stimate)	A: subQ/IV: 2-4 mcg in 2 divided doses C: <12 y: Inf: 0.3 mcg/kg diluted in 10 ml of NSS over 15-30 min	Same as for desmopressin acetate.
lypressin (Diapid)	*Diabetes insipidus:* A & C: Intranasal: 1-2 sprays per nostril q.i.d.	Prevention or control of DI caused by insufficient ADH. To decrease polydipsia, polyuria, and dehydration. Duration of action is 3 to 8 hours. *Pregnancy category:* B; PB: UK; $t\frac{1}{2}$: 15 min
vasopressin (aqueous) (Pitressin)	*Diabetes insipidus:* A: subQ/IM: 5-10 units, b.i.d.-q.i.d. C: subQ/IM: 2.5-10 units, b.i.d.-q.i.d.	For treating DI. For relief of intestinal distention. Decreases GI bleeding from esophageal varices. Can also be given intranasally. Promotes reabsorption of water from the renal tubules. Duration of action is 2 to 8 h. *Pregnancy category:* X; PB: UK; $t\frac{1}{2}$: 15 min
vasopressin tannate/oil (Pitressin Tannate)	A: IM: 1.5-5.0 units, q2-3d C: IM: 1.25-2.5 units, q2-3d	Same as for vasopressin. Action is longer because of the oil.

A, Adult; *ADH*, antidiuretic hormone; *b.i.d.*, twice a day; *C*, child; *d*, day; *DI*, diabetes insipidus; *GI*, gastrointestinal; *h*, hour; *IM*, intramuscular; *inf*, infusion; *IV*, intravenous; *min*, minute; *NSS*, normal saline solution; *PB*, protein-binding; *PO*, by mouth; *q.i.d.*, four times a day; *subQ*, subcutaneous; *$t\frac{1}{2}$*, half-life; *t.i.d.*, three times a day; *UK*, unknown; *wk*, week; *y*, year; *>*, greater than; *<*, less than.

alone or with surgery or radiation. This drug is expensive. GI side effects are common. This drug can also be used for severe diarrhea resulting from carcinoid tumors.

Table 49–1 lists the drugs used to replace or inhibit GH.

Thyroid-Stimulating Hormone

The adenohypophysis secretes **thyroid-stimulating hormone (TSH)** in response to thyroid-releasing hormone (TRH) from the hypothalamus. TSH stimulates the thyroid gland to release thyroxine (T_4) and triiodothyronine (T_3, or liothyronine). Excess TSH secretion can cause hyperthyroidism, and a TSH deficit can cause hypothyroidism. Hypothyroidism may be caused by a thyroid gland disorder (primary cause) or a decrease in TSH secretion (secondary cause). Thyrotropin (Thytropar), a purified extract of TSH, is used as a diagnostic agent to differentiate between primary and secondary hypothyroidism (see Table 49–1).

Adrenocorticotropic Hormone

The hypothalamus releases corticotropin-releasing factor (CRF), which stimulates the pituitary corticotrophs to secrete **adrenocorticotropic hormone (ACTH).** ACTH secretion stimulates the release of glucocorticoids (cortisol), mineralocorticoids (aldosterone), and androgen from the adrenal cortex. Usually, ACTH and cortisol secretions follow a diurnal rhythm in which the ACTH and cortisol secretion is higher in the early morning and then decreases through the day. Stresses such as surgery, sepsis, and trauma override the diurnal rhythm, causing an increase in secretions of ACTH and cortisol.

The ACTH drug corticotropin (Acthar) is used to diagnose adrenal gland disorders, to treat adrenal gland insufficiency, and as an anti-inflammatory drug in the treatment of an allergic response. Administration of ACTH intravenously (IV) should increase the serum cortisol level in 30 to 60 minutes if the adrenal gland is functioning. If steroid deficiency is caused by pituitary insufficiency, ACTH should eventually stimulate cortisol production. ACTH decreases the symptoms of multiple sclerosis during its exacerbation phase. Prototype Drug Chart 49–1 lists the actions and effects of corticotropin (Acthar).

Pharmacokinetics

Corticotropin stimulates the adrenal gland to secrete corticosteroids. The aqueous and gel preparations are well absorbed into the circulation. Zinc is added to some formulations to slow the absorption rate. A portion of

---

PROTOTYPE DRUG CHART 49–1

CORTICOTROPIN, CORTICOTROPIN REPOSITORY, CORTICOTROPIN-ZINC HYDROXIDE

Drug Class

Pituitary adrenocorticotropic hormone
Trade Name:
corticotropin: Acthar, ACTH
corticotropin repository: Acthar Gel, Cortigel
corticotrophin-zinc hydroxide: Cortrophin zinc
Pregnancy Category: C

Dosage

Diagnostic testing:
A: IV: 10-25 units in 500 ml D_5W q8h
subQ/IM: 20 units, q.i.d.
Repository injection:
A: subQ/IM; 40-80 units, q24-72h
Acute multiple sclerosis:
A: subQ/IM: 80-120 units/d for 2-3 wk

Contraindications

Severe fungal infection, CHF, peptic ulcer
Caution: Hepatic disease, psychiatric disorders, myasthenia gravis

Drug-Lab-Food Interactions

Drug: *Increase* ulcer formation with aspirin; may *increase* effect of potassium-wasting diuretics; *decrease* effects of oral antidiabetics (hypoglycemics) or insulin

Pharmacokinetics

Absorption: IM: Well absorbed
Distribution: PB: UK
Metabolism: t½: 15-20 minutes
Excretion: In urine

Pharmacodynamics

IM: Onset: <6 h
    Peak: 6-18 h
    Duration: 12-24 h
IV: Onset: UK
    Peak: 1 h
    Duration: UK

Therapeutic Effects/Uses

To diagnose adrenocortical disorders; acts as an antiinflammatory agent; to treat acute MS
Mode of Action: Stimulation of the adrenal cortex to secrete cortisol

Side Effects

Nausea, vomiting, increased appetite, mood swing (euphoria to depression), petechiae, water and sodium retention, hypokalemia, hypocalcemia

Adverse Reactions

Edema, ecchymosis, osteoporosis, muscle atrophy, growth retardation, decreased wound healing, cataracts, glaucoma, menstrual irregularities
Life-threatening: Ulcer perforation, pancreatitis

A, Adult; *CHF*, congestive heart failure; *d*, day; *h*, hour; *IM*, intramuscular; *IV*, intravenous; *MS*, multiple sclerosis; *q.i.d.,* four times a day; *subQ*, subcutaneous; *PB*, protein-binding; *t½*, half-life; *UK*, unknown; *wk*, week; <, less than.

the drug is bound to protein; however, the percent is unknown. The half-life of the drug is 15 to 20 minutes. It is excreted in the urine.

Pharmacodynamics

Corticotropin suppresses the inflammatory and immune responses. It is also prescribed to treat adrenal insufficiency secondary to inadequate corticotropin secretion. The drug is administered intramuscularly (IM) and IV. Its onset of action, peak concentration time, and duration of action are prolonged when it is injected IM. The IV preparation is in an aqueous form; therefore its actions are faster than those of the gel and zinc- additive preparations.

Drug Interactions

Corticotropin has numerous drug interactions. Diuretics and anti-*Pseudomonas* penicillins such as piperacillin can decrease the serum potassium level (hypokalemia). If the client is taking a digitalis preparation and hypokalemia is present, digitalis toxicity can result. Phenytoin, rifampin, and barbiturates increase the metabolic rate, which can decrease the effect of the ACTH drug. Persons with diabetes may need increased insulin and oral antidiabetic (hypoglycemic) drugs because ACTH stimulates cortisol secretion, which increases the blood sugar level.

Posterior

The posterior pituitary gland, known as the **neurohypophysis**, secretes **antidiuretic hormone (ADH)** (vasopressin) and oxytocin. (Oxytocin is discussed in Chapter 52, Drugs Associated with the Female Reproductive Cycle II: Labor, Delivery, and the Preterm Neonate.)

ADH promotes water reabsorption from the renal tubules to maintain water balance in the body fluids. When there is a deficiency of ADH, large amounts of water are excreted by the kidneys. This condition, **diabetes insipidus (DI),** can lead to severe fluid volume deficit and electrolyte imbalances. Head injury and brain tumors resulting in trauma to the hypothalamus and pituitary gland can also cause DI. Fluid and electrolyte balance must be closely monitored in these clients, and ADH replacement may be needed. The ADH preparations vasopressin (Pitressin) and desmopressin acetate (DDAVP) can be administered intranasally or by injection.

Table 49–1 lists the drugs used for pituitary disorders and their dosages, uses, and considerations.

Nursing Process

Pituitary Hormones

ASSESSMENT

■ Obtain baseline vital signs for future comparison. Report abnormal results.
■ Determine client's urinary output and weight.
■ Assess client for an infectious process. Corticotropin can suppress signs and symptoms of infection.
■ Note client's physical growth. Compare child's growth with reported standards. Report findings.

NURSING DIAGNOSES

■ Ineffective health maintenance
■ Delayed growth and development

PLANNING

■ Client will be free of pituitary disorder with appropriate drug regimen.

NURSING INTERVENTIONS

Antidiuretic Hormone (ADH)

• Monitor vital signs. Increased heart rate and decreased systolic pressure can indicate fluid volume loss resulting from decreased ADH production. With less ADH secretion, more water is excreted, decreasing vascular fluid (hypovolemia).
• Record urinary output. Increased output can indicate fluid loss caused by a decrease in ADH.

Adrenocorticotropic Hormone (ACTH), Corticotropin

• Avoid administering corticotropin to clients with adrenocortical hyperfunction. Corticotropin stimulates the release of cortisol from the adrenal glands.
• Monitor the growth and development of a child receiving corticotropin.
• Observe client's weight. If a weight gain occurs, check for edema. A side effect of corticotropin (ACTH) is sodium and water retention.
• Watch carefully for adverse effects when corticotropin is discontinued. Dose should be tapered and not stopped abruptly because adrenal hypofunction may result.
• Check laboratory findings, especially electrolyte levels. Electrolyte replacement may be necessary.

Growth Hormone (GH)

• Monitor blood sugar and electrolyte levels in clients receiving GH. Hyperglycemia can occur with high doses.

Client Teaching

Adrenocorticotropic Hormone (ACTH)
• Advise client to adhere to the drug regimen. Discontinuation of certain drugs, such as corticotropin, can cause hypofunction of the gland being stimulated.
• Direct client to decrease salt intake to decrease or avoid edema. Potassium supplement may be needed.
• Instruct client to report side effects, such as muscle weakness, edema, petechiae, ecchymosis, decrease in growth, decreased wound healing, and menstrual irregularities.

Growth Hormone (GH)

- Advise athletes not to take GH because of its side effects. GH can be effective for children whose height is markedly below the expected norm for their age. Because GH acts on newly forming bone, it should be administered before the epiphyses are fused.
- Inform client with diabetes to closely monitor blood sugar levels. Insulin regulation may be necessary.
- Suggest that client or family monitor client's growth rate.

Cultural Considerations ⊕

- There is sometimes a lack of understanding in some cultural groups in regard to the purpose and use of GH. The health care provider needs to emphasize that these are not drugs for building muscles and that they can cause many serious side effects, such as diabetes mellitus, when abused.

EVALUATION

■ Evaluate the effectiveness of the drug therapy.

Thyroid Gland

Thyroxine (T_4) and triiodothyronine (T_3) are secreted by the thyroid gland. The functions of T_4 and T_3 are to regulate protein synthesis and enzyme activity and to stimulate mitochondrial oxidation. Approximately 20% of circulating T_3 is secreted from the thyroid gland, and 80% of T_3 comes from the degradation of about 40% of T_4, which occurs in the periphery. T_4 and T_3 are carried in the blood by thyroxine-binding globulin (TBG) and albumin, which protects the hormones from being degraded. T_3 is more potent than T_4, and only unbound free T_3 and T_4 are active and produce a hormonal response.

T_4 and T_3 secretion from the thyroid gland is regulated by the feedback mechanisms. The hypothalamus releases thyrotropin-releasing hormone (TRH), which stimulates the release of TSH from the pituitary gland. TSH stimulates the synthesis and release of T_4 and T_3 from the thyroid gland. Excess free T_4 and T_3 inhibit the hypothalamus-pituitary-thyroid (HPT) axis, which results in decreased TRH and TSH secretion. Likewise, too low an amount of T_4 and T_3 increases the function of the HPT axis.

For thyroid deficiency (hypothyroidism), synthetic T_4 and T_3 may be prescribed, either alone or in combination. When the thyroid gland secretes an overabundance of thyroid hormones (hyperthyroidism), antithyroid drugs are usually indicated.

Hypothyroidism

Hypothyroidism, a decrease in thyroid hormone secretion, can have either a primary cause (thyroid gland disorder) or a secondary cause (lack of TSH secretion). Primary hypothyroidism occurs more frequently. Decreased T_4 and elevated TSH levels indicate primary hypothyroidism, the causes of which are acute or chronic inflammation of the thyroid gland, radioiodine therapy, excess intake of antithyroid drugs, and surgery. **Myxedema** is severe hypothyroidism in the adult; symptoms include lethargy, apathy, memory impairment, emotional changes, slow speech, deep coarse voice, edema of the eyelids and face, thick dry skin, cold intolerance, slow pulse, constipation, weight gain, and abnormal menses. In children, hypothyroidism can have a congenital (**cretinism**) or prepubertal (juvenile hypothyroidism) onset. Drugs containing T_4 and T_3, alone or in combination, are used to treat hypothyroidism.

Drug Therapy: Hypothyroidism

Levothyroxine sodium (Levothroid, Synthroid) is the drug of choice for replacement therapy for the treatment of hypothyroidism. It increases the levels of T_3 and T_4. Levothyroxine is also used to treat simple goiter and chronic lymphocytic (Hashimoto's) thyroiditis.

Liothyronine (Cytomel) is a synthetic T_3 that has a short half-life and duration of action; it is not recommended for maintenance therapy. Liothyronine is better absorbed from the GI tract than levothyroxine, and because of its rapid onset of action and short half-life, it is frequently used as the initial therapy for treating myxedema.

Liotrix (Euthroid, Thyrolar) is a mixture of levothyroxine sodium and liothyronine sodium in a 4:1 ratio. There is no significant advantage to the use of liotrix for treating hypothyroidism over levothyroxine sodium used alone because levothyroxine converts T_4 to T_3 in the peripheral tissues.

The drug thyroid is seldom used. Some clients with hypothyroidism may benefit from this agent.

Prototype Drug Chart 49–2 presents the drug data for the synthetic thyroid drug levothyroxine.

Pharmacokinetics

Levothyroxine (T_4) is a synthetic thyroid hormone preparation. The GI mucosa absorbs 50% to 75% of levothyroxine. It is highly protein-bound, and when administered with other highly protein-bound drugs like oral anticoagulants, side effects can result. The half-life of levothyroxine is longer than that of liothyronine. Levothyroxine is excreted in the bile and feces.

Pharmacodynamics

Levothyroxine increases metabolic rate, cardiac output, protein synthesis, and glycogen use. The peak concentration time and duration of action are much longer with levothyroxine than with liothyronine. Liotrix is a combination of T_4 and T_3 with a greater concentration of T_4.

Drug Interactions

Many drug interactions are associated with T_4 and T_3 drugs. Thyroid preparations increase the effect of oral anticoagulants because of drug displacement from the protein-binding sites. When either of these drugs is taken with an adrenergic agent (e.g., decongestant or vasopressor), the cardiac and central nervous system (CNS) actions are increased. Levothyroxine and liothyronine can decrease the effectiveness of digitalis preparations. Estrogen can increase the effect of liothyronine. Insulin and oral antidiabetic drug dosages may need to be increased.

PROTOTYPE DRUG CHART 49-2

LEVOTHYROXINE SODIUM

Drug Class	**Dosage**
Thyroid hormone Trade Name: T$_4$, Synthroid, Levothroid; 🍁 Eltroxin *Pregnancy Category:* A	**A: PO:** Initially: 25-50 mcg/d (0.025-0.05 mg/d); *maint:* 50-200 mcg/d (0.05-0.2 mg/day) **IV:** 0.2-0.5 mg initial dose; 0.1-0.2 mg/d until stable and then PO **C: >3 y: PO:** 5-6 mcg/kg/d or 50-100 mcg/d (0.05-0.1 mg/d)

Contraindications	**Drug-Lab-Food Interactions**
Thyrotoxicosis, myocardial infarction (MI), severe renal disease *Caution:* Cardiovascular disease, hypertension, angina pectoris	*Drug:* *Increase* cardiac insufficiency with epinephrine; *increase* effects of anticoagulants, tricyclic antidepressants, vasopressors, decongestants; *decrease* effects of antidiabetics (oral and insulin), digitalis products; *decrease* absorption with cholestyramine, colestipol

Pharmacokinetics	**Pharmacodynamics**

Absorption: PO: 50%-75%
Distribution: PB: 99%
Metabolism: t½: 6-7 days
Excretion: In bile and feces
	PO: Onset: UK
	  Peak: 24 h-1 wk
	  Duration: 1-3 wk
	IV: Onset: 6-8 h
	  Peak: 24-48 h
	  Duration: UK

Therapeutic Effects/Uses

To treat hypothyroidism, myxedema, and cretinism
Mode of Action: Increase metabolic rate, oxygen consumption, and body growth

Side Effects	**Adverse Reactions**
Nausea, vomiting, diarrhea, cramps, tremors, nervousness, insomnia, headache, weight loss	Tachycardia, hypertension, palpitations **Life-threatening:** Thyroid crisis, angina pectoris, cardiac dysrhythmias, cardiovascular collapse

A, Adult; *C,* child; *d,* day; *h,* hour; *IV,* intravenous; *maint,* maintenance; *MI,* myocardial infarction; *PB,* protein-binding; *PO,* by mouth; *t½,* half-life; *UK,* unknown; *wk,* week; *y,* year; 🍁, Canadian drug name; >, greater than.

Table 49-2 lists the drug data for natural and synthetic thyroid preparations.

Hyperthyroidism

Hyperthyroidism is an increase in circulating T$_4$ and T$_3$ levels, which results from an overactive thyroid gland or excessive output of thyroid hormones from one or more thyroid nodules. Hyperthyroidism may be mild with few symptoms or severe, as in thyroid storm in which death may occur from vascular collapse. **Graves' disease,** or **thyrotoxicosis,** is the most common type of hyperthyroidism caused by the hyperfunction of the thyroid gland. It is characterized by a rapid pulse *(tachycardia),* palpitations, excessive perspiration, heat intolerance, nervousness, irritability, exophthalmos (bulging eyes), and weight loss.

Hyperthyroidism can be treated by surgical removal of a portion of the thyroid gland (subtotal thyroidectomy), radioactive iodine therapy, or antithyroid drugs, which inhibit either the synthesis or the release of thyroid hormone. Any of these treatments can cause hypothyroidism.

Propranolol (Inderal) can control the cardiac symptoms, such as palpitations and tachycardia, that result from hyperthyroidism. It does not lower T$_4$ and T$_3$.

Drug Therapy: Hyperthyroidism

The purpose of antithyroid drugs is to reduce the excessive secretion of thyroid hormones (T$_4$ and T$_3$) by inhibiting thyroid secretion. The use of surgery (subtotal thyroidectomy) and radioiodine therapy frequently leads to hypothyroidism. Thiourea derivatives (thioamides) are the drugs of choice used to decrease thyroid hormone production. This drug group interferes with synthesis of thyroid hormone. Thiourea derivatives do not destroy thyroid tissue but rather block the thyroid hormone action.

Propylthiouracil (PTU) and methimazole (Tapazole) are effective thioamide antithyroid drugs. They are useful for treating thyrotoxic crisis and in preparation for subtotal thyroidectomy. Methimazole does not inhibit peripheral conversion of T$_4$ to T$_3$ as does PTU; however, it is 10 times more potent and it has a longer half-life than PTU.

Table 49-2

Thyroid Hormone: Replacements and Antithyroid Drugs

Generic (Brand)	Route and Dosage	Uses and Considerations
Thyroid Replacements: Hypothyroidism		
levothyroxine sodium (Synthroid)	See Prototype Drug Chart 49–2.	
liothyronine sodium (Cytomel)	A: PO: Initially: 5-25 mcg/d; *maint:* 25-75 mcg/d C: PO: Initially: 5 mcg/d, >3 y: 25-75 mcg/d	For hypothyroidism. Synthetic T_3 drug. Faster acting than other thyroid drugs. Effects seen in 24 to 72 h. Cardiac side effects. *Pregnancy category:* A; PB: 99%; $t^1/_2$: 1-1.5 h
liotrix (Euthroid, Thyrolar)	A: PO: Initially: 15-30 mcg/d, increased q2-3wk; *maint:* 60-120 mcg/d C: PO: Initially: same as adult	For hypothyroidism. Synthetic T_4 and T_3 drug; 4:1 ratio. Onset of action is immediate. Duration of action is 72 h. Common side effects include irritability, nervousness, insomnia, tachycardia, weight loss. *Pregnancy category:* A; PB: 99%; $t^1/_2$: <7 d
thyroid (Armour Thyroid, Thyrar)	A: PO: Initially: 15-60 mg/d, increased monthly as needed; *maint:* 60-180 mg/d C: PO: 15 mg/d, increased q2wk as needed	For hypothyroidism to reduce goiter size. Natural form obtained from animals. T_4 and T_3: 4:1 ratio. Onset of action is slow; long duration of action (weeks). Common side effects include irritability, nervousness, insomnia, tachycardia, and weight loss. *Pregnancy category:* A; PB: 99%; $t^1/_2$: <7 d (T_3: 1-2 h; T_4: 6-7 h)
Antithyroid Drugs: Hyperthyroidism		
Thioamides		
methimazole (Tapazole)	A: PO: Initially: 15-60 mg/d in 3 divided doses; *maint:* 5-15 mg q8h C: PO: Initially: 0.4 mg/kg/d in divided doses; *maint:* 0.2 mg/kg/d in 3 divided doses	For treating hyperthyroidism. Inhibits thyroid hormone synthesis. Onset of action: 1 wk for effect. Rash, urticaria, headache, and GI upset may occur. *Pregnancy category:* D; PB: 0%; $t^1/_2$: 5-13 h
propylthiouracil (PTU)	A: PO: Initially: 300-450 mg/d in divided doses; *maint:* 150-300 mg/d C: 6-10 y: PO: 50-150 mg/d in divided doses C: >10 y: PO: Same as adult or 150 mg/m²/d	For hyperthyroidism to treat Graves' disease. Inhibits conversion of T_4 and T_3. May be used before surgery or radioactive iodine treatment and palliative control of toxic goiter. *Pregnancy category:* D; PB: 75%-80%; $t^1/_2$: 1-2 h
Iodine		
Strong iodine solution (Lugol's solution, potassium iodide solution)	A & C: PO: 0.1-0.3 ml (3-5 gtt) t.i.d. *Thyroid crisis:* A & C: PO: 1 ml in water p.c. t.i.d.	For hyperthyroidism. To reduce size and vascularity of thyroid gland. Dilute drug and administer after meals; sip through straw to avoid discoloration of teeth. Maximum effect after 10 to 15 days. *Pregnancy category:* D; PB: UK; $t^1/_2$: UK

A, Adult; *C*, child; *d*, day; *GI*, gastrointestinal; *gtt*, drops; *h*, hour; *maint*, maintenance; *PB*, protein-binding; *p.c.*, after meals; *PO*, by mouth; $t^1/_2$, half-life; T_4, thyroxine; T_3, triiodothyronine; *t.i.d.*, three times a day; *UK*, unknown; *wk*, week; *y*, year; >, greater than; <, less than.

Prolonged use of thioamides may cause a goiter because of the increased TSH secretion and inhibited T_4 and T_3 synthesis. Minimal doses of thioamides should be given when indicated to avoid goiter formation.

Strong iodide preparations such as Lugol's solution have been used to suppress thyroid function for clients who have undergone subtotal thyroidectomy as a result of Graves' disease. Sodium iodide administered IV is useful for the management of thyrotoxic crisis. Table 49–2 gives the drug data for the antithyroid drugs used to treat hyperthyroidism.

Drug Interactions

Thyroid drugs interact with many other drugs. When used with oral anticoagulants (e.g., warfarin [Coumadin]), they can cause an increase in the anticoagulating effect. In addition, thyroid drugs decrease the effect of insulin and oral antidiabetics; digoxin and lithium increase the action of thyroid drugs; and phenytoin (Dilantin) increases serum T_3 level.

Nursing Process

Thyroid Hormone: Replacement and Antithyroid Drugs

ASSESSMENT

■ Determine baseline vital signs to compare with future data. Report abnormal results.

■ Check serum T_3, T_4, and thyroid-stimulating hormone (TSH) levels. Report abnormal results.

Thyroid Replacement

- Obtain a history of drugs client currently takes. Be aware that thyroid drugs enhance the action of oral anticoagulants, sympathomimetics, and antidepressants and decrease the action of insulin, oral hypoglycemics, and digitalis preparation. Phenytoin and aspirin can enhance the action of thyroid hormone.

Antithyroid Drugs

- Assess for signs and symptoms of a thyroid crisis (thyroid storm), which includes tachycardia, cardiac dysrhythmias, fever, heart failure, flushed skin, apathy, confusion, behavioral changes, and later hypotension and vascular collapse. Thyroid crisis can result from a thyroidectomy (excess thyroid hormones released), abrupt withdrawal of antithyroid drug, excess ingestion of thyroid hormone, or failure to give antithyroid medication before thyroid surgery.

NURSING DIAGNOSES

- ■ Ineffective health maintenance
- ■ Ineffective tissue perfusion
- ■ Activity intolerance

PLANNING

- ■ Client's signs and symptoms of hypothyroidism will be alleviated within 2 to 4 weeks with prescribed thyroid drug replacement, and the client will not experience side effects.
- ■ Client's signs and symptoms of hyperthyroidism will be alleviated in 1 to 3 weeks with the prescribed antithyroid drug.

NURSING INTERVENTIONS

- ■ Record vital signs. With hypothyroidism, the temperature, heart rate, and blood pressure are usually decreased. With hyperthyroidism, tachycardia and palpitations usually occur.
- ■ Monitor client's weight. Weight gain commonly occurs in clients with hypothyroidism.

Client Teaching

Thyroid Drug Replacement for Hypothyroidism
- Encourage client to take the drug at the same time each day, preferably before breakfast. Food will hamper absorption rate.
- Teach client to check warnings on OTC drug labels. Avoid OTC drugs that caution against use by persons with heart or thyroid disease.
- Direct client to report symptoms of hyperthyroidism (tachycardia, chest pain, palpitations, excess sweating) caused by drug accumulation or overdosing.

- Suggest that client carry a MedicAlert card, tag, or bracelet with the health condition and thyroid drug used.

Diet: Hypothyroidism
- Caution client to avoid foods that can inhibit thyroid secretion, such as strawberries, peaches, pears, cabbage, turnips, spinach, kale, Brussels sprouts, cauliflower, radishes, and peas.

Antithyroid Drugs for Hyperthyroidism
- Instruct client to take the drug with meals to decrease gastrointestinal symptoms.
- Advise client about the effects of iodine and its presence in iodized salt, shellfish, and OTC cough medicines.
- Emphasize the importance of drug compliance; abruptly stopping the antithyroid drug could bring on a thyroid crisis.
- Teach client the signs and symptoms of hypothyroidism: lethargy, puffy eyelids and face, thick tongue, slow speech with hoarseness, lack of perspiration, and slow pulse. Hypothyroidism can result from treatment of hyperthyroidism.
- Advise client to avoid antithyroid drugs if pregnant or breastfeeding. Antithyroid drugs taken during pregnancy can cause hypothyroidism in the fetus or infant.

Self-Administration

- Demonstrate to client how to take a pulse rate. Instruct client to monitor the pulse rate and report increases or marked decreases in pulse rate.

Side Effects

- Teach client the side effects of antithyroid drugs, such as skin rash, hives, nausea, alopecia, loss of hair pigment, petechiae or ecchymoses, and weakness.
- Advise client to contact the health care provider if a sore throat and fever occur while taking antithyroid drugs. A serious adverse reaction of antithyroid drugs is agranulocytosis (loss of white blood cells). A complete blood count should be monitored for leukopenia.

Cultural Considerations ⊕

- Recognize that various cultural groups may need guidance in understanding the disease process of hypothyroidism or hyperthyroidism. Support client and family member who may be dismayed about the symptoms of either of these health problems and who lack knowledge of the prescribed drug therapy for management of the thyroid condition. Additional time in explanations and a written plan of care may be necessary for non–English-speaking persons.

EVALUATION

Thyroid Replacement

- Evaluate the effectiveness of the thyroid drug and drug compliance.

- Continue monitoring for side effects from drug accumulation or overdosing.

Antithyroid Drugs

- Evaluate the effectiveness of the antithyroid drug in decreasing signs and symptoms of hyperthyroidism. If signs and symptoms persist after 2 to 3 weeks of therapy, other methods for correcting hyperthyroidism may be necessary.

Parathyroid Glands

The parathyroid glands secrete **parathyroid hormone (PTH)**, which regulates calcium levels in the blood. A decrease in serum calcium stimulates the release of PTH. Calcitonin decreases serum calcium levels by promoting renal excretion of calcium. The functions of PTH and calcitonin are discussed in the introduction to Unit XV, Endocrine Agents.

PTH agents treat hypoparathyroidism and synthetic calcitonin treats hyperparathyroidism. Hypocalcemia (serum calcium deficit) can be caused by PTH deficiency, vitamin D deficiency, renal impairment, or diuretic therapy. PTH replacement helps correct the calcium deficit. PTH promotes calcium absorption from the GI tract, promotes reabsorption of calcium from the renal tubules, and activates vitamin D.

Calcitriol

Calcitriol is a vitamin D analogue that promotes calcium absorption from the GI tract and secretion of calcium from bone to the bloodstream. Prototype Drug Chart 49–3 describes the drug data related to calcitriol.

Pharmacokinetics

Calcitriol is readily absorbed from the GI tract. Its half-life is moderate (3 to 8 hours). Most of the drug is excreted in the feces.

Pharmacodynamics

Calcitriol is given for the management of hypocalcemia. It increases serum calcium levels by promoting calcium absorption from the intestines and from the renal tubules. Calcitriol has a long onset of action, peak action, and duration of action.

Hyperparathyroidism can be caused by malignancies of the parathyroid glands or ectopic PTH hormone secretion from lung cancer, hyperthyroidism, or prolonged immobility during which calcium is lost from bone. Table 49–3 lists the drugs used to treat hypoparathyroidism and hyperparathyroidism.

Nursing Process

Parathyroid Hormone Insufficiencies

ASSESSMENT

■ Note serum calcium level. Report abnormal results.

PROTOTYPE DRUG CHART 49–3

CALCITRIOL

Drug Class	**Dosage**
Vitamin D analogue Trade Name: Rocaltrol *Pregnancy Category:* C	A: PO: 0.25 mcg/d

Contraindications	**Drug-Lab-Food Interactions**
Hypersensitivity, hypercalcemia, hyperphosphatemia, hypervitaminosis D, malabsorption syndrome *Caution:* Cardiovascular disease, renal calculi	*Drug:* Increase cardiac dysrhythmias with digoxin, verapamil; *decrease* calcitriol absorption with cholestyramine *Lab:* Increase serum calcium with thiazide diuretics, calcium supplements

Pharmacokinetics	**Pharmacodynamics**
Absorption: PO: Well absorbed Distribution: PB: UK; crosses the placenta Metabolism: t½: 3-8 h Excretion: Mostly in feces	PO: Onset: 2-6 h Peak: 10-12 h Duration: 3-5 d

Therapeutic Effects/Uses

To treat hypoparathyroidism and manage hypocalcemia in chronic renal failure
Mode of Action: Enhancement of calcium deposits in bones

Side Effects	**Adverse Reactions**
Anorexia, nausea, vomiting, diarrhea, cramps, drowsiness, headache, dizziness, lethargy, photophobia	Hypercalciuria, hyperphosphatemia, hematuria

A, Adult; *d,* day; *h,* hour; *PB,* protein-binding; *PO,* by mouth; *t½,* half-life; *UK,* unknown.

■ Assess for symptoms of tetany in hypocalcemia: twitching of the mouth, tingling and numbness of the fingers, carpopedal spasm, spasmodic contractions, and laryngeal spasm.

NURSING DIAGNOSES

■ Risk for impaired tissue integrity
■ Ineffective health maintenance

PLANNING

■ Client's serum calcium level will be within the normal range.

NURSING INTERVENTIONS

■ Monitor the serum calcium level. Normal reference value is 8.5 to 10.5 mg/dl, or 4.5 to 5.5 mEq/L. A serum calcium level <8.5 mg/dl, or <4.5 mEq/L, indicates hypocalcemia, and a serum calcium level >10.5 mg/dl, or >5.5 mEq/L, indicates hypercalcemia. Serum ionized calcium levels are usually used because much of the calcium is protein-bound and is nonionized and nonactive.

Client Teaching

Hypoparathyroidism

• Direct client to report symptoms of tetany (see Assessment).

Hyperparathyroidism

• Advise client to report signs and symptoms of hypercalcemia: bone pain, anorexia, nausea, vomiting, thirst, constipation, lethargy, bradycardia, and polyuria.
• Instruct women to inform their health care provider about pregnancy status before taking calcitonin preparation.
• Encourage client to check over-the-counter drugs for possible calcium content, especially if client has an elevated serum calcium level. Some vitamins and antacids contain calcium. Tell client to contact the health care provider before taking drugs with calcium.

Cultural Considerations ⊕

• Obtain an interpreter when necessary; do not rely on family members, who may not fully disclose because of honor and shame.

EVALUATION

■ Monitor the effectiveness of drug therapy.
■ Continue monitoring for signs and symptoms of hypocalcemia (tetany) when commercially prepared calcitonin has been given.

Adrenal Glands

The paired **adrenal glands** consist of the adrenal medulla and the adrenal cortex. The adrenal cortex produces two types of hormones, or corticosteroids: glucocorticoids

---

Table 49–3

Drug Therapies for Parathyroid Disorders

Generic (Brand)	Route and Dosage	Uses and Considerations
Treatment for Hypoparathyroidism and Hypocalcemia: Vitamin D Analogues		
calcifediol (Calderol)	A: PO: Initially: 300-350 mcg/wk PO: 50-100 mcg/d or 100-200 mcg every other day	For bone disease and hypocalcemia associated with chronic renal disease and dialysis. *Pregnancy category:* C; PB: UK; t$^{1}/_{2}$: 12-22 d
calcitriol (Rocaltrol)	See Prototype Drug Chart 49–3.	
dihydrotachysterol (Hytakerol)	A: PO: 0.75-2.5 mg/d for 4 d, then 0.2-1 mg/d C: PO: 1-5 mg/d for 4 d, then 0.5-1.5 mg/d	For treatment of hypoparathyroidism associated with hypocalcemia and for pseudohypoparathyroidism. Serum calcium levels should be monitored weekly during early therapy. Clients should avoid taking thiazide diuretics to prevent causing possible hypercalcemia. *Pregnancy category:* A; PB: UK; t$^{1}/_{2}$: UK
ergocalciferol (Drisdol)	A & C: PO/IM: 50,000-200,000 international units/day or 1.25-5.0 mg/d	For hypoparathyroidism and rickets. A larger dose may be required in vitamin D-resistant rickets. It enhances calcium and phosphorus absorption. It has a long duration of action. *Pregnancy category:* C; PB: UK; t$^{1}/_{2}$: 12-24 h
Treatment for Hyperparathyroidism and Hypercalcemia		
calcitonin (human) (Cibacalcin); calcitonin (salmon) (Calcimar)	*Human:* A: subQ: Initially: 0.5 mg/d; *maint:* 0.25 mg/d-0.5 mg b.i.d. *Salmon:* A: subQ/IM: Initially: 4 international units/kg/d; *maint:* 4-8 international units/kg q12h	For treating Paget's disease of the bone (osteitis deformans), hyperparathyroidism, and hypercalcemia. Calcitonin salmon is more potent than calcitonin human. Calcitonin decreases serum calcium by binding at receptor sites on osteoclast. *Pregnancy category:* C; PB: UK; t$^{1}/_{2}$: 1-1.5 h
etidronate (Didronel)	A: PO: 5-10 mg/kg/d; *max:* 20 mg/kg/d	For Paget's disease; for hypercalcemia caused by antineoplastic therapy. *Pregnancy category:* B; PB: UK; t$^{1}/_{2}$: 6 h

A, Adult; *b.i.d.*, two times a day; *C*, child; *d*, day; *h*, hour; *IM*, intramuscular; *maint*, maintenance; *max*, maximum; *PB*, protein-binding; *PO*, by mouth; *subQ*, subcutaneous; *t$^{1}/_{2}$*, half-life; *UK*, unknown; *wk*, week.

(cortisol) and mineralocorticoids (aldosterone). Cortisol secreted by the adrenal glands is in response to the hypothalamus-pituitary-adrenal (HPA) axis as a result of the feedback mechanism. A decrease in the serum cortisol levels increases CRF and ACTH secretions, which stimulate the adrenal glands to secrete and release cortisol. An increased serum cortisol level exerts the negative feedback mechanism, which inhibits the HPA axis resulting in less cortisol being released. Additional physiologic functions related to the hormones secreted from the adrenal medulla and adrenal cortex are described in the introduction to Unit XV, Endocrine Agents.

The **corticosteroids** promote sodium retention and potassium excretion. A sodium ion is reabsorbed from the renal tubules in exchange for a potassium ion; the potassium ion is then excreted. Because of their influence on electrolytes and carbohydrate, protein, and fat metabolism, a deficiency of corticosteroids can result in serious illness or death. A decrease in corticosteroid secretion is called *adrenal hyposecretion* (adrenal insufficiency, or **Addison's disease**) and an increase in corticosteroid secretion is called *adrenal hypersecretion* (**Cushing's syndrome**).

Glucocorticoids

Glucocorticoids are influenced by ACTH, which is released from the anterior pituitary gland. They affect carbohydrate, protein, and fat metabolism as well as muscle and blood cell activity. Because of their many mineralocorticoid effects, glucocorticoids can cause sodium absorption from the kidney, resulting in water retention, potassium loss, and increased blood pressure. Cortisol, the main glucocorticoid, has antiinflammatory, antiallergic, and antistress effects. Indications for glucocorticoid therapy include trauma, surgery, infections, emotional upsets, and anxiety. Table 49–4 lists the physiologic aspects of adrenal hyposecretion (Addison's disease) and hypersecretion (Cushing's syndrome).

Most of the wide variety of glucocorticoid drugs, frequently called *cortisone* drugs, are synthetically produced. These drugs have several routes of administration: oral, parenteral (IM or IV), topical (creams, ointments, lotions), and aerosol (inhaler) (see Chapter 38, Drugs for Common Upper Respiratory Disorders). The IM route, although seldom used, should be administered deep in the muscle. The subQ route is not recommended. The topical glucocorticoids are listed in Chapter 48, Drugs for Dermatologic Disorders.

Glucocorticoids are used to treat many diseases and health problems including inflammatory, allergic, and debilitating conditions. Among the inflammatory conditions that may require glucocorticoids are autoimmune disorders (e.g., multiple sclerosis, rheumatoid arthritis, myasthenia gravis); ulcerative colitis; glomerulonephritis; shock; ocular and vascular inflammations; head trauma with cerebral edema; polyarteritis nodosa; and hepatitis. Allergic conditions include asthma, drug reactions, contact dermatitis, and anaphylaxis. Debilitating conditions are mainly caused by malignancies. Organ transplant recipients may require glucocorticoids to prevent organ rejection.

There are many glucocorticoids—some more potent than others. Dexamethasone (Decadron) has been used for severe inflammatory response as a result of head trauma or allergic reactions. An inexpensive glucocorticoid frequently prescribed is prednisone. Prototype Drug Chart 49–4 describes the pharmacologic data for prednisone.

Pharmacokinetics

Prednisone is readily absorbed from the GI tract. It has a short half-life of 3 to 4 hours, and it has a moderately high protein-binding power. Prednisone is excreted primarily in the urine.

Table 49–4

Physiologic Data: Adrenal Hyposecretion and Hypersecretion

Body System	Systemic Effects	
	Adrenal Hyposecretion	**Adrenal Hypersecretion**
Metabolism:		
Glucose	Hypoglycemia	Hyperglycemia
Protein	Muscle weakness	Muscle wasting; thinning of the skin; poor wound healing; osteoporosis; fat accumulation in face, neck, and trunk (protruding abdomen, buffalo hump); hyperlipidemia; high cholesterol
Fat		
Central nervous system	Apathy, depression, fatigue	Increased neural activity; mood elevation; irritability; seizures
Gastrointestinal	Nausea, vomiting, abdominal pain	Peptic ulcers
Cardiovascular	Tachycardia, hypotension, cardiovascular collapse	Hypertension; edema; heart failure
Eyes	None	Cataract formation
Fluids and electrolytes	Hypovolemia; hyponatremia; hyperkalemia	Hypervolemia; hypernatremia; hypokalemia
Blood cells	Anemia	Increased red blood cell count and neutrophils; impaired clotting

PROTOTYPE DRUG CHART 49–4

PREDNISONE

Drug Class

Adrenal hormone: glucocorticoid
Trade Name: Deltasone, Meticorten, Orasone, Panasol-S, ✦ Apo-Prednisone, Winpred
Pregnancy Category: C

Dosage

A: PO: 5-60 mg/d in divided doses
C: PO: 0.1-0.15 mg/kg/d in 2-4 divided doses or 4-5 mg/m²/d in 2 doses

Contraindications

Hypersensitivity, psychosis, fungal infection
Caution: Diabetes mellitus

Drug-Lab-Food Interactions

Drug: *Increase* effect with barbiturates, phenytoin, rifampin, ephedrine, theophylline; *decrease* effects of aspirin, anticonvulsants, isoniazid (INH), antidiabetics, vaccines

Pharmacokinetics

Absorption: PO: Well absorbed
Distribution: PB: 65%-91%; crosses the placenta
Metabolism: t½: 3-4 h
Excretion: In urine

Pharmacodynamics

PO: Onset: UK
  Peak: 1-2 h
  Duration: 24-36 d

Therapeutic Effects/Uses

To decrease inflammatory occurrence; as an immunosuppressant; to treat dermatologic disorders
Mode of Action: Suppression of inflammation and adrenal function

Side Effects

Nausea, diarrhea, abdominal distention, increased appetite, sweating, headache, depression, flush, mood changes

Adverse Reactions

Petechiae, ecchymosis, hypertension, tachycardia, osteoporosis, muscle wasting
Life-threatening: GI hemorrhage, pancreatitis, circulatory collapse, thrombophlebitis, embolism

A, Adult; *C,* child; *d,* day; *GI,* gastrointestinal; *h,* hour; *PB,* protein-binding; *PO,* by mouth; *t½,* half-life; *UK,* unknown; ✦, Canadian drug names.

Pharmacodynamics

The major actions of prednisone are to suppress an acute inflammatory process and for immunosuppression. It prevents cell-mediated immune reactions. Do not confuse prednisone with prednisolone. Peak action occurs in 1 to 2 hours, and its duration of action is long (1 to 1.5 days).

Commonly used glucocorticoid drugs are listed in Table 49–5. Most of the glucocorticoids are pregnancy category C drugs. Agents used for adrenocortical insufficiency contain both glucocorticoids and mineralocorticoids, whereas drugs for antiinflammatory or immunosuppressive use contain mostly glucocorticoids.

Side Effects and Adverse Reactions

The side effects and adverse reactions of glucocorticoids that result from high doses or prolonged use include increased blood sugar, abnormal fat deposits in the face and trunk (moon face and buffalo hump), decreased extremity size, muscle wasting, edema, sodium and water retention, hypertension, euphoria or psychosis, thinned skin with purpura, increased intraocular pressure (glaucoma), peptic ulcers, and growth retardation. Long-term use of glucocorticoid drugs can cause adrenal atrophy (loss of adrenal gland function). When drug therapy is discontinued, the dose should be tapered to allow the adrenal cortex to produce cortisol and other corticosteroids. Abrupt withdrawal of the drug can result in severe adrenocortical insufficiency.

Drug Interactions

Glucocorticoids increase the potency of drugs taken concurrently, including aspirin and nonsteroidal anti-inflammatory drugs (NSAIDs), thus increasing the risk of GI bleeding and ulceration. Use of potassium-wasting diuretics (e.g., HydroDiuril, Lasix) with glucocorticoids increases potassium loss, resulting in hypokalemia. Glucocorticoids can decrease the effect of oral anticoagulants (e.g., warfarin [Coumadin]).

Barbiturates, phenytoin, and rifampin decrease the effect of prednisone. Prolonged use of prednisone can cause severe muscle weakness.

Dexamethasone, a potent glucocorticoid, interacts with many drugs. Phenytoin, theophylline, rifampin, barbiturates, and antacids decrease the action of dexamethasone, whereas NSAIDs, including aspirin, and estrogen increase its action. Dexamethasone decreases the effects of oral anticoagulants and oral antidiabetics. When the drug is given with diuretics or anti-*Pseudomonas* penicillin preparations, the serum potassium level may decrease markedly. Gluco-

Table 49–5

Adrenal Hormones: Glucocorticoids, Mineralocorticoid, and Glucocorticoid Inhibitors

Generic (Brand)	Route and Dosage	Uses and Considerations
Glucocorticoids		
Short Acting		
cortisone acetate (Cortone Acetate, Cortistan)	A: PO/IM: 20-300 mg/d; decrease dose periodically	For adrenocortical insufficiency. Contains glucocorticoid and mineralocorticoid. Decreases inflammatory process. Oral dose is rapidly absorbed from the GI tract. Administer deep intramuscularly. With oral dose, give with food. *Pregnancy category:* C; PB: UK; t½: 0.5-12 h
hydrocortisone (Cortef, Hydrocortone)	A: PO: 20-240 mg/d in 3-4 divided doses IV: 15-240 mg (phosphate) q12h Rectal supp: 10-25 mg	For adrenocortical insufficiency and inflammation. Hydrocortisone sodium phosphate is parenteral form. Acetate form of drug may be injected into joints. Available in cream, ointment, lotion, and spray. *Pregnancy category:* C; PB: 79%; t½: 2-12 h
Intermediate Acting		
methylprednisolone (Medrol, Solu-Medrol [sodium succinate] Depo-Medrol [acetate])	A: PO: 4-48 mg/d in one or more divided doses IM/IV: Succinate: 10-40 mg q4h-q6h IM: Acetate: 40-80 mg/wk	For treating inflammatory conditions such as arthritis, bronchial asthma, allergic reactions, and cerebral edema. *Pregnancy category:* C; PB: UK; t½: 3.5 h
prednisolone (Delta-Cortef, Hydeltrasol [phosphate])	A: PO: 2.5-15 mg b.i.d.-q.i.d. IV: Phosphate: 2-30 mg q12h C: PO: 0.14-2 mg/kg/d in a single or divided doses	For antiinflammatory or immunosuppressive effect. For parenteral use. It can be injected into joints and soft tissue. Potent steroid. *Pregnancy category:* C; PB: 80%-90%; t½: 3.5 h (tissue: 18-36 h)
prednisone	See Prototype Drug Chart 49–4.	
triamcinolone (Aristocort, Kenacort, Azmacort, Kenalog)	A: PO: 4-48 mg/d in 2-4 divided doses Inhal: 2 puffs t.i.d.-q.i.d. Topical preparations: cream, ointment	For antiinflammatory or immunosuppressive effect. *Pregnancy category:* C; PB: UK; t½: 2-5 h
Long Acting		
beclomethasone dipropionate (Vanceril, Beclovent)	A: Inhal: 2 puffs b.i.d.-q.i.d.	Inhalation for treating bronchial asthma and bronchial inflammation. Also to treat seasonal rhinitis. *Like all glucocorticoid inhalants, it is for prophylactic use and not for acute asthmatic attack. Pregnancy category:* C; PB: 87%; t½: 5-15 h
betamethasone (Celestone, Celestone Phosphate)	A: PO: 0.6-7.2 mg/d in single or divided doses IM/IV: 1-9 mg/d; *max:* IM: 12 mg/d	Potent antiinflammatory steroid drug. It may be injected in joints. Effective for treating bronchial asthma, arthritis, severe allergic reactions, and cerebral edema. Should be taken with food. *Pregnancy category:* C; PB: 64%-90%; t½: 3-5 h
dexamethasone (Decadron)	*Inflammation:* A: PO: 0.25-4 mg b.i.d.-q.i.d. IM: 4-16 mg q1-3wk C: PO: 0.2 mg/kg/d in divided doses *Shock:* A: IV: 1-6 mg/kg as a single dose (IV push in IV fluids)	Potent antiinflammatory drug. For acute allergic disorders, asthmatic attack, cerebral edema, and unresponsive shock. For diagnosis of Cushing's syndrome and depression. Can be administered by IV push or in IV fluids. With oral dose, give with food. *Pregnancy category:* C; PB: 80%-90%; t½: 3-4 h

A, Adult; *ACTH,* adrenocorticotropic hormone; *b.i.d.,* twice a day; *C,* child; *d,* day; *GI,* gastrointestinal; *h,* hour; *IM,* intramuscular; *inhal,* inhalation; *IV,* intravenous; *PB,* protein-binding; *PO,* by mouth; *q.i.d.,* four times a day; *t½,* half-life; *t.i.d.,* three times a day; *UK,* unknown; *wk,* week.

corticoids can increase blood sugar levels; thus insulin or oral antidiabetic drug dosage may need to be increased.

Glucocorticoid Inhibitors

The antifungal drug ketoconazole (Nizoral) and the antineoplastic hormone antagonists mitotane (Lysodren) and aminoglutethimide (Cytadren) inhibit glucocorticoid synthesis. Ketoconazole is effective in treating clients with Cushing's syndrome and is useful as an adjunct to surgery or radiation. High doses should be avoided because this drug can induce fatal ventricular dysrhythmias. Amino-

glutethimide is frequently prescribed for temporary treatment of selected clients with Cushing's syndrome, especially clients with adrenal adenoma or carcinoma, ectopic ACTH-producing tumors, or adrenal hyperplasia.

Mineralocorticoids

Mineralocorticoids, the second type of corticosteroid, secrete aldosterone. Aldosterone is controlled by the renin-angiotensin system, not by ACTH. These hormones maintain fluid balance by promoting the reabsorption of sodium from the renal tubules. Sodium attracts water, re-

Table 49-5

Adrenal Hormones: Glucocorticoids, Mineralocorticoid, and Glucocorticoid Inhibitors—cont'd

Generic (Brand)	Route and Dosage	Uses and Considerations
Glucocorticoids—cont'd		
Long Acting		
paramethasone acetate (Haldrone)	A: PO: 0.5-6 mg t.i.d-q.i.d. C: PO: 58-200 mcg/kg/d in 3-4 divided doses	For treating inflammatory conditions and allergic reactions. Similar to prednisone. Give with food. Do not abruptly stop dosing with long-term therapy. *Pregnancy category*: C; PB: 95%; $t\frac{1}{2}$: 3-45 h
Mineralocorticoid		
fludrocortisone acetate (Florinef Acetate)	A & C: PO: 0.1-0.2 mg/d	For treating adrenocortical insufficiency as in Addison's disease. Also for salt-losing adrenogenital syndrome. Used only for its mineralocorticoid effects. *Pregnancy category*: C; PB: 92%; $t\frac{1}{2}$: 3.5 h
Glucocorticoid Inhibitors		
aminoglutethimide (Cytadren)	*Cushing's syndrome:* A: PO: 250 mg q6h; *max:* 2 g/d	This agent is a hormonal antagonist. May be used to treat Cushing's syndrome associated with adrenal adenoma or carcinoma and ACTH-secreting tumors. It blocks the first step in steroid synthesis. *Pregnancy category*: D; PB: UK; $t\frac{1}{2}$: 13 h
ketoconazole (Nizoral)	A: PO: 200-400 mg/d	Usually used in conjunction with surgery or radiation to inhibit glucocorticoid synthesis. Needs a higher dose to suppress steroid synthesis than for a fungal infection. *Pregnancy category*: C; PB: UK; $t\frac{1}{2}$: 8 h
Mitotane and Diagnosis for Adrenal Gland Dysfunction		
mitotane (Lysodren)	A: PO: 2-6 g/d, q6-8h. Dose may be increased; *max:* 16 g/d	An antineoplastic agent that suppresses the action of the adrenal gland. Used to treat Cushing's syndrome. *Pregnancy category*: C; PB: UK; $t\frac{1}{2}$: 18-160 d
Diagnosis for Adrenal Gland Dysfunction		
metyrapone (Metopirone)	A: PO: 30 mg/kg at midnight or 750 mg q4h × 6 doses, 4 days before ACTH administration C: PO: 15 mg/kg q4h × 6 doses	For diagnosing secondary adrenal insufficiency. It blocks cortisol synthesis in adrenals. **Caution:** may cause acute adrenal insufficiency. *Pregnancy category*: UK; PB: UK; $t\frac{1}{2}$: 1-2.5 h
corticotropin (Acthar)	Diagnostic test for adrenal and pituitary function	See Prototype Drug Chart 49-1.
cosyntropin (Cortrosyn)	Diagnostic test for adrenal and pituitary function	See Table 49-1.

sulting in water retention. When *hypovolemia* (decrease in circulating fluid) occurs, more aldosterone is secreted to increase sodium and water retention and to restore fluid balance. With sodium reabsorption, potassium is lost and hypokalemia (potassium deficit) can occur. Some glucocorticoid drugs also contain mineralocorticoids; these include cortisone and hydrocortisone. A severe decrease in the mineralocorticoid aldosterone leads to hypotension and vascular collapse, as seen in Addison's disease. Mineralocorticoid deficiency usually occurs with glucocorticoid deficiency, frequently called *corticosteroid deficiency*.

Fludrocortisone (Florinef) is an oral mineralocorticoid that can be given with a glucocorticoid. It can cause a negative nitrogen balance; therefore a high-protein diet is usually indicated. Because potassium excretion occurs with the use of mineralocorticoids and glucocorticoids, the serum potassium level should be monitored.

Nursing Process

Adrenal Hormone: Glucocorticoids

ASSESSMENT

■ Note baseline vital signs for future comparison.

■ Assess laboratory test results, especially serum electrolytes and blood sugar. Serum potassium level usually decreases and blood sugar level increases when a glucocorticoid such as prednisone is taken over an extensive period.

■ Obtain client's weight and urine output to use for future comparison.

■ Assess client's medical and herbal history. Report if client has glaucoma, cataracts, peptic ulcer, psychiatric problems, or diabetes mellitus. Glucocorticoids can intensify these health problems.

NURSING DIAGNOSES

- Deficient knowledge
- Fluid volume excess
- Risk for impaired tissue integrity

PLANNING

- Client's inflammatory process will abate. Side effects of glucocorticoid will be minimal.

NURSING INTERVENTIONS

- Determine vital signs. Glucocorticoids such as prednisone can increase blood pressure and sodium and water retention.
- Administer glucocorticoids only as ordered. Routes of administration include oral, intramuscular (not in the deltoid muscle), intravenous, aerosol, and topical. Topical glucocorticoid drugs should be applied in thin layers. Rashes, infection, and purpura should be noted and reported.
- Record weight. Report weight gain of 5 lbs in several days; this would most likely be caused by water retention.
- Monitor laboratory values, especially serum electrolytes and blood sugar. Serum potassium level could decrease to <3.5 mEq/L, and blood sugar level would probably increase.
- Watch carefully for signs and symptoms of hypokalemia, such as nausea, vomiting, muscular weakness, abdominal distention, paralytic ileus, and irregular heart rate.
- Assess for side effects from glucocorticoid drugs when therapy has lasted more than 10 days and the drug is taken in high dosages. The cortisone preparation should not be abruptly stopped because adrenal crisis can result.
- Monitor older adults for signs and symptoms of increased osteoporosis. Glucocorticoids promote calcium loss from the bone.
- Report changes in muscle strength. High doses of glucocorticoids promote loss of muscle tone.

Client Teaching

General
- Advise client to take the drug as prescribed. Caution client *not* to abruptly stop the drug. When the drug is discontinued, the dose is tapered over 1 to 2 weeks.
- For short-term use (<10 days) of glucocorticoids such as prednisone or other cortisone preparations, the drug dose still needs to be tapered. Prepare a schedule for client to decrease the dose over 4 to 5 days. For example, take one tab q.i.d.; the next day, take one tab t.i.d.; the next day, take one tab b.i.d.; and then take one tab daily.

- Direct client not to take cortisone preparations (oral or topical) during pregnancy unless necessary and prescribed by the health care provider. These drugs may be harmful to the fetus.
- Inform client that certain herbal laxatives and diuretics may interact with a glucocorticoid drug and may increase the severity of hypokalemia. See Herbal Alert 49–1.
- Instruct client to avoid persons with respiratory infections because these drugs suppress the immune system. This is especially important if client is receiving a high dose of glucocorticoids.
- Teach client receiving glucocorticoids to inform other health care providers of all drugs taken, especially before surgery.
- Encourage client to have a MedicAlert card, tag, or bracelet stating the glucocorticoid drug taken.

Self-Administration
- Instruct client how to use an aerosol nebulizer. Warn client against overuse of the aerosol to avoid possible rebound effect.

Side Effects
- Teach client to report signs and symptoms of drug overdose or Cushing's syndrome, including a moon face, puffy eyelids, edema in the feet, increased bruising, dizziness, bleeding, and menstrual irregularity.

Diet
- Instruct client to take cortisone preparations at mealtime or with food. Glucocorticoid drugs can irritate the gastric mucosa and cause a peptic ulcer.
- Advise client to eat foods rich in potassium, such as fresh and dried fruits, vegetables, meats, and nuts. Prednisone promotes potassium loss and thus hypokalemia.

Cultural Considerations ⊕

- Recognize that various cultural groups need guidance in understanding the disease process of Cushing's disease. Explain to the family that their family member is not "dumb or disinterested" but has an adrenal problem. Explain that the symptoms do not "go away" and may be progressive if prescribed therapy is not followed.

EVALUATION

- Evaluate the effectiveness of glucocorticoid drug therapy. If the inflammation has not improved, a change in drug therapy may be necessary.
- Continue monitoring for side effects, especially when client is receiving high doses of glucocorticoids.

HERBAL ALERT 49-1

Herbs and Corticosteroids

☙ Herbal laxatives *(cascara, senna)* and herbal diuretics *(celery seed, juniper)* can decrease the serum potassium levels. When these herbs are taken with corticosteroids, hypokalemia can become more severe.

☙ *Ginseng* taken with corticosteroids may cause central nervous system stimulation and insomnia.

☙ *Echinacea* may counteract the effects of corticosteroids.

☙ *Licorice* potentiates the effect of corticosteroids that may cause a substantial decrease in the serum potassium level.

WEBSITES

For further information on *Endocrine Pharmacology,* visit these Internet resources:

Somatropin:
www.fda.gov/medwatch/SAFETY/2003/genotropin_pi.pdf

Vasopressin:
www.med/umich.edu/ccmu/vasopressin.htm

Levothyroxine:
www.nlm.nih.gov/medlineplus/druginfo/medmaster/a682461.html

Critical Thinking Case Study

M.P., age 68, had a severe allergic reaction to shellfish. She was taken to the emergency room. A single dose of dexamethasone 100 mg IV (direct IV over 30 seconds) was ordered. M.P. weighs 65 kg.

1. Why is M.P. receiving dexamethasone IV? Is the dosage of dexamethasone within safe therapeutic range? Explain.

2. Describe the various ways for administering dexamethasone IV. By what other routes can dexamethasone be administered?

3. What additional health information and assessment may aid the health care provider in treating M.P.'s serious health problem?

   Twenty-one tablets of prednisone, 5 mg each, were prescribed to be taken over 5 days, with tapering daily doses. The first day would be 10 mg q.i.d.; the second day, 10 mg t.i.d.; the third day, 10 mg b.i.d.; the fourth day, 10 mg once daily; and the fifth day, 5 mg once daily.

4. Why was prednisone ordered and not oral dexamethasone? Explain.

5. What is the purpose for tapering prednisone doses? Explain.

6. Is the drug dose within safe therapeutic range? Explain.

7. Should M.P. have side effects such as peripheral edema caused by water and sodium retention as a result of tapered prednisone doses? Explain.

8. What is the difference between prednisone and prednisolone?

9. What are the adverse reactions from prolonged use of prednisone?

10. What are the nursing interventions and client teaching for M.P. and clients who take prednisone?

Study Questions

1. What hormones are secreted by the anterior pituitary gland (adenohypophysis) and what are their functions?

2. What is the action of ACTH? What are the nursing interventions and client teaching for clients receiving ACTH?

3. The client has diabetes insipidus. Is this the same as diabetes mellitus? Explain. What are the symptoms of diabetes insipidus? What drug is used to control this health problem?

4. What are the two hormones secreted by the thyroid gland? Differentiate between levothyroxine (Synthroid) and liothyronine (Cytomel). What are their actions?

5. For what disorders are the antithyroid drugs used? What severe side effects can result from their use?

6. What electrolyte is directly influenced by parathyroid hormone?

7. What are the physiologic effects of hypersecretion and hyposecretion of parathyroid hormone?

8. What are the subgroups of corticosteroids? What are four signs and symptoms of prolonged use of corticosteroids (cortisone)? What are the nursing implications of discontinuing a cortisone preparation? What instructions should the client receive?

9. A deficiency of the hormone cortisol leads to what health problem? What are the symptoms of this disease? What type of drug is used to control this disease?

50 Antidiabetic Drugs

OUTLINE

OBJECTIVES

- Compare type 1 and type 2 diabetes mellitus.
- Identify the symptoms of diabetes mellitus.
- Explain a hypoglycemic reaction and describe the symptoms.
- Differentiate among rapid-acting, intermediate-acting, and long-acting insulins and combination mix.
- Determine the peak concentration time for four types of insulin action and when a hypoglycemic reaction is most likely to occur.
- Identify the action of oral antidiabetic drugs and their side effects.
- Describe the nursing process, including client teaching, for insulin and oral antidiabetic agents.
- Differentiate between the action of insulin, oral antidiabetic agents, and glucagon.

TERMS

diabetes mellitus
hypoglycemic reaction
insulin
insulin-dependent diabetes mellitus (IDDM)
insulin shock
ketoacidosis
lipodystrophy
non-insulin-dependent diabetes mellitus (NIDDM)
oral antidiabetic drugs
oral hypoglycemic drugs
polydipsia
polyphagia
polyuria
type 1 diabetes mellitus
type 2 diabetes mellitus

Introduction

About 18.5 million persons in the United States have diabetes mellitus, of which approximately 6 million adults are unaware that they have this disease. Complications from uncontrolled diabetes are the third leading cause of death. In the sixteenth century, diabetes was traced to Egyptian writings about "honeyed urine." Insulin, the protein hormone used to control diabetes, was not available for client use until 1921. In the 45 to 65 age group, Native Americans, Hispanics, and African Americans have a two to three times higher incidence of developing diabetes mellitus than whites.

Antidiabetic drugs are used primarily to control diabetes mellitus, a chronic disease that affects carbohydrate metabolism. There are two groups of antidiabetic agents: (1) insulin and (2) oral hypoglycemic (antidiabetic) drugs. **Insulin,** a protein secreted from the beta cells of the pancreas, is necessary for carbohydrate metabolism and plays an important role in protein and fat metabolism. The beta cells make up 75% of the pancreas, and the alpha cells that secrete glucagon, a hyperglycemic substance, occupy approximately 20% of the pancreas. **Oral hypoglycemic drugs,** also known as **oral antidiabetic drugs,** which is the term frequently used to avoid the confusion of the term *hypoglycemic reaction,* are synthetic preparations that stimulate insulin release or otherwise alter the metabolic response to hyperglycemia.

Diabetes Mellitus

Diabetes mellitus, a chronic disease resulting from deficient glucose metabolism, is caused by insufficient insulin secretion from the beta cells.* This results in high blood sugar *(hyperglycemia).* Diabetes mellitus is characterized by the three *p's:* **polyuria** (increased urine output), **polydipsia** (increased thirst), and **polyphagia** (increased hunger).

The four types of diabetes are presented in Table 50–1. Viral infections, environmental conditions, and genetic factors contribute to the onset of **type 1 diabetes mellitus.**

---

*Diabetes *mellitus* is a disorder of the pancreas; diabetes *insipidus* is a disorder of the posterior pituitary gland.

Type 2 diabetes mellitus is the most common type of diabetes. Some sources suggest that heredity and obesity are the major factors that cause type 2 diabetes. With type 2 diabetes, there is some beta-cell function with varying amounts of insulin secretion. Hyperglycemia may be controlled for some type 2 diabetes with oral antidiabetic *(hypoglycemic)* drugs and a diet prescribed by the American Diabetic Association; however, about one third of clients with type 2 diabetes need insulin. Clients with type 2 diabetes who use one or two oral antidiabetic drugs may become insulin-dependent years later.

Certain drugs increase blood sugar and can cause hyperglycemia in prediabetic persons. These include glucocorticoids (cortisone, prednisone), thiazide diuretics (hydrochlorothiazide [HydroDiuril]), and epinephrine. Usually the blood sugar level returns to normal after the drug is discontinued.

During the second and third trimesters of pregnancy, the levels of the hormones progesterone, cortisol, and human placental lactogen (hPL) increase. These increased hormone levels can inhibit insulin usage. This is a contributing factor for the occurrence of gestational diabetes mellitus (GDM) during pregnancy. Glucose is then mobilized from the tissue and lipid storage sites. After pregnancy, the blood glucose level may decrease; however, some clients may develop diabetes, whereas others may develop type 2 diabetes in later years.

Insulin

Insulin is released from the beta cells of the islets of Langerhans in response to an increase in blood glucose. Oral glucose load is more effective in raising the serum insulin level than an intravenous (IV) glucose load. Insulin promotes the uptake of glucose, amino acids, and fatty acids and converts them to substances that are stored in body cells. Glucose is converted to glycogen for future glucose needs in the liver and muscle, thereby lowering the blood glucose level. The normal range for blood glucose is 60 to 100 mg/dl and 70 to 110 mg/dl for serum glucose. When the blood glucose level is greater than 180 mg/dl, *glycosuria* (sugar in the urine) can occur. Increased blood sugar acts as an osmotic diuretic, causing polyuria. When blood sugar remains elevated (>200 mg/dl), diabetes mellitus occurs.

Table 50–1

Types and Occurrences of Diabetes Mellitus

Types of Diabetes Mellitus	Additional Names	Percentage of Occurrences
Type 1	Insulin-dependent diabetes mellitus (IDDM); also called *juvenile-onset diabetes*	10%-12%
Type 2	Non-insulin-dependent diabetes mellitus (NIDDM); also called *maturity-onset* or *adult-onset diabetes*	85%-90%
Secondary diabetes (medications, hormonal changes)		2%-3%
Gestational diabetes mellitus (GDM)		<1% (2% to 5% of all pregnancies)

<, Less than.

Beta Cell Secretion of Insulin

The beta cells in the pancreas secrete approximately 0.2 to 0.5 units/kg/daily. A client weighing 70 kg (154 pounds) secretes 14 to 35 units of insulin a day. More insulin secretion may occur if the person consumes a greater caloric intake. A client with diabetes mellitus may require 0.2 to 1.0 units/kg/daily. The higher range may be because of obesity, stress, or tissue insulin resistance.

Commercially Prepared Insulin

Parenteral (injectable) insulin is obtained from pork and beef pancreas when the animals are slaughtered. Pork insulin is closely related to human insulin, having only one different amino acid; beef insulin has four different amino acids. Human insulin (Humulin) was introduced in 1983 and is produced by two separate methods: (1) changing the different amino acid of pork insulin or (2) using deoxyribonucleic acid (DNA) technology. Pork insulin is a weaker allergen than beef insulin, and the use of human insulin has a low incidence of allergic effects and insulin resistance. Insulin is made more pure than previously, especially the Humulin produced by DNA technology, which results in fewer side effects. Human insulins administered subcutaneously (subQ) are absorbed faster and have a shorter duration than animal insulins. Newly diagnosed clients with insulin-dependent diabetes are usually prescribed human insulin. In addition, clients in whom hyperglycemia develops during pregnancy or who already have diabetes and become pregnant are usually prescribed human insulin. If a client has been taking animal (pork or beef) insulin without experiencing any untoward effects, it is not necessary to change to human insulin.

The concentration of insulin is 100 units/ml or 500 units/ml (U100/ml, U500/ml), and the insulin is packaged in a 10-ml vial (see the figures on insulin in Chapter 4D, Calculations for Injectable Dosages). Insulin 500 units is seldom used except in emergencies and for clients with serious insulin resistance (>200 units/daily). Insulin 40 units is no longer used in the United States, although it is still used in other countries. Insulin syringes are marked in units of 100 units per 1 ml for insulin U100. Insulin syringes must be used for accurate dosing. To prevent dosage errors, the nurse must be certain that there is a match of the insulin concentration with the calibration of units on the insulin syringe. Before use, the client or nurse must roll, not shake, cloudy insulin bottles to ensure that the insulin and its ingredients are well mixed. Shaking a bottle of insulin can cause bubbles and an inaccurate dose. Insulin requirements vary; usually less insulin is needed with increased exercise, and more insulin is needed with infections and high fever.

Administration of Insulin

Insulin is a protein and *cannot* be administered orally because gastrointestinal (GI) secretions destroy the insulin structure. It is administered subQ, at a 45- to 90-degree angle. The 90-degree angle is made by raising the skin and fatty tissue; the insulin is injected into the pocket between the fat and the muscle. In a thin person with little fatty tissue, the 45- to 60-degree angle is used. Regular insulin is the *only* type that can be administered IV.

The site and depth of insulin injection affect absorption. Insulin absorption is greater when given in the deltoid and abdominal areas than when given in the thigh and buttock areas. Insulin administered subQ has a slower absorption rate than if it is administered IM. Heat and massage could increase subQ absorption. Cooling the subQ area can decrease absorption.

Insulin is usually given in the morning before breakfast. It can be given several times a day. Insulin injection sites should be rotated to prevent **lipodystrophy** (tissue atrophy or hypertrophy), which can interfere with insulin absorption. *Lipoatrophy* (tissue atrophy) is a depression under the skin surface that primarily occurs in females and children. A frequent cause of an atrophied area is caused by the use of animal insulins (beef and pork). *Lipohypertrophy* (tissue hypertrophy) is a raised lump or knot on the skin surface that is more common in males. It is frequently caused by repeated injections into the same subQ site. The client needs to develop a "site rotation pattern" to avoid lipodystrophy and to promote insulin absorption. There are various insulin rotation programs, such as an 8-day rotation schedule (insulin is given at a different site each day). The American Diabetic Association suggests that insulin be injected daily at a chosen site for 1 week. Injections should be 1.5 inches apart (a knuckle length) at a site area each day. If a client requires two insulin injections a day (morning and evening), one site should be chosen on the right side (morning) and one site on the left side (evening). Figure 50–1 illustrates

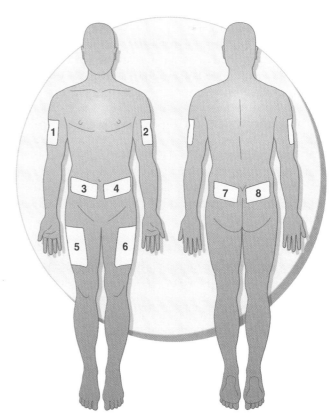

FIGURE 50–1 Sites for insulin injection.

sites for insulin injections. A record of injection area sites and dates administered should be kept.

Illness and stress increase the need for insulin. Insulin doses should *not* be withheld during illness, including infections and stress. Hyperglycemia and ketoacidosis may result from withholding insulin.

Types of Insulin

There are several standard types of insulin: rapid acting, short acting, intermediate acting, long acting, and combinations. Rapid and short-acting insulins are in clear solution without any added substance to prolong the insulin action. Intermediate-acting insulins are cloudy and may contain protamine, a protein that prolongs the action of insulin or zinc, which also slows the onset of action and prolongs the duration of activity.

Rapid-acting insulins include lispro and regular insulins. Lispro insulin (Humalog) is a rapid-acting insulin approved for use in 1996. The action of lispro begins in 5 to 15 minutes, and the duration of action is 2 to 4 hours. Lispro insulin acts faster than regular insulin; thus it MUST NOT be administered more than 5 minutes before mealtime, whereas regular insulin is given 30 minutes before meals. Lispro insulin is formed by reversing two amino acids in human regular insulin (Humulin). Regular (unmodified, crystalline) insulin is the only type of insulin that can be administered IV and subQ. Clients who are insulin dependent and who take a rapid-acting insulin usually require an intermediate-acting insulin.

Short-acting insulin has an onset of action in 30 minutes to 1 hour. The peak action occurs in 2 to 4 hours, and the duration of action is 6 to 8 hours.

Intermediate-acting insulins include neutral-protamine-Hagedorn (NPH), Lente, Humulin N, and Humulin L. NPH and Humulin N contain protamine, a protein that prolongs the action of the insulin. Lente and Humulin L contain zinc, which also prolongs the insulin action time. The onset of intermediate-acting insulin is 1 to 2 hours; peak action occurs in 6 to 12 hours; and the duration of action is 18 to 24 hours.

A long-acting insulin is Humulin U Ultralente. This insulin is absorbed slower than other insulins because of its large crystals, which dissolve slowly and prolong the duration time. Use of protamine-zinc-insulin (PZI) has been discontinued. Long-acting insulin acts in 4 to 8 hours, peaks in 14 to 20 hours, and lasts for 24 to 36 hours.

A newer long-acting insulin is Lantus, an insulin glargine that is an analogue of human insulin. Lantus is the first long-acting recombinant DNA (rDNA) human insulin approved by the Food and Drug Administration (FDA) for clients with types 1 and 2 diabetes. It has a 24-hour duration of action; thus it is administered once a day, usually at bedtime. Some clients complain of more pain at the injection site with the administration of Lantus than with NPH insulin. Lantus is available in a 3-ml cartridge, "OptiPen," or insulin pen. Incidence of nocturnal hypoglycemia is not as common as with other insulins because of its continuous sustained release.

Combination insulins are commercially premixed. These include Humulin 70/30, Novolin 70/30, Humulin 50/50, and Humalog 75/25. These combinations are widely used. The Humulin 70/30 vials or prefilled disposable pens contain 70% of human insulin isophane (intermediate-acting insulin, NPH) and 30% regular (fast-acting) insulin. The exterior of the insulin pens resembles fountain pens. The Humulin 50/50 vial or pen contains 50% of isophane (NPH) insulin and 50% regular insulin. The Humalog 75/25 mix is available as a prefilled disposable pen only and contains 75% lispro protamine insulin and 25% lispro "rapid" insulin. Humalog 75/25 helps prevent hypoglycemia, which could occur with the 70/30 or 50/50 combination insulins and helps control hyperglycemia more effectively. The 75/25 pen contains 300 units of insulin and does not require refrigeration after first use. It can be stored at room temperature for up to 10 days. With these combinations of insulin, the client does not have to mix regular and NPH insulins as long as one of these combinations are effective. However, some clients need less than 25% or 30% regular insulin and more intermediate-acting insulin; such a client needs to mix the two insulins in the prescribed proportions.

Regular insulin can be mixed with protamine or zinc insulin in the same syringe. Mixing insulin can alter the absorption rate. When regular insulin is mixed with Lente insulin, a portion of the effect of regular insulin is lost. Less regular insulin is in effect decreased when mixed with NPH than when mixed with Lente. However, Lente insulin causes less allergic response than NPH.

Insulin Resistance

Antibodies develop over time in persons taking animal insulin. This can slow the onset of insulin action and extend its duration of action. Antibody development can cause insulin resistance and insulin allergy. Obesity can also be a causative factor of insulin resistance. Skin tests with different insulin preparations may be performed to determine whether there is an allergic effect. Human and regular insulins produce fewer allergens.

Storage of Insulin

Unopened insulin vials are refrigerated until needed. Once an insulin vial has been opened, it may be kept (1) at room temperature for 1 month or (2) in the refrigerator for 3 months. Insulin is less irritating to the tissues when injected at room temperature. Insulin vials should not be put in the freezer. In addition, insulin vials should not be placed in direct sunlight or in a high-temperature area. Prefilled syringes should be stored in the refrigerator and should be used within 1 to 2 weeks. Opened insulin vials lose their strength after approximately 3 months.

Prototype Drug Chart 50–1 compares regular insulin with NPH insulin.

PROTOTYPE DRUG CHART 50–1

INSULINS

Drug Class

Antidiabetic: insulins
Humalog (Lispro)—rapid acting
Regular Humulin R—short acting
Humulin N—intermediate acting
Glargine (Lantus)—long acting
Pregnancy Category: B

Dosage

Varies according to client's blood sugar

Contraindications

Hypersensitivity to beef, pork, zinc, protamine insulins
Caution: Hypersensitivity

Drug-Lab-Food Interactions

Drug: Increased hypoglycemic effect with aspirin, oral anticoagulant, alcohol, oral hypoglycemics, beta-blockers, tricyclic antidepressants, MAOIs, tetracycline; *decreased* hypoglycemic effect with thiazides, glucocorticoids, oral contraceptives, thyroid drugs, smoking

Pharmacokinetics

Absorption: Lispro and Humulin R rapidly absorbed from subQ injection site.
Humulin N is absorbed at a slower rate.
Glargine is absorbed at a slow evenly distributed rate.
Distribution: PB: UK
Metabolism: t½: varies with type of insulin
Excretion: Mostly in urine

Pharmacodynamics

Humalog (Lispro):
subQ: Onset: 5-15 min
  Peak: 30-60 min
  Duration: 3-4 h
Regular Humulin R:
subQ: Onset: 30-60 min
  Peak: 2-3 h
  Duration: 4-8 h
Humulin N:
subQ: Onset: 1-2 h
  Peak: 4-12 h
  Duration: 18-24 h
Glargine (Lantus):
subQ: Onset: 1 h
  Peak: None
  Duration: 24 h

Therapeutic Effects/Uses

To control diabetes mellitus; to lower blood sugar
Mode of Action: Insulin promotes use of glucose by body cells

Side Effects

Confusion, agitation, tremors, headache, flushing, hunger, weakness, lethargy, fatigue, urticaria; redness, irritation or swelling at insulin injection site

Adverse Effects

Tachycardia, palpitations, hypoglycemic reaction, rebound hyperglycemia (somogyi effect), lipodystrophy
Life-threatening: Shock; anaphylaxis

h, Hour; *MAOI,* monoamine oxidase inhibitor; *min,* minute; *PB,* protein-binding; *subQ,* subcutaneous; *t½,* half-life; *UK,* unknown.

Pharmacokinetics

All insulins can be administered subQ, but only regular insulin can be given IV. The half-life varies. Insulin is metabolized by the liver and muscle and excreted in the urine.

Pharmacodynamics

Insulin lowers blood sugar by promoting use of glucose by the body cells. It also stores glucose as glycogen in muscles. The onset of action of regular insulin given subQ is 30 minutes to 1 hour and 10 to 30 minutes given IV. The onset of action of intermediate-acting insulin is 1 to 2 hours. The peak action of insulins is important because of the possibility of hypoglycemic reaction (insulin shock) occurring during that time. The peak time for regular insulin is 2 to 4 hours and 6 to 12 hours for intermediate-acting insulin. The nurse needs to assess for signs and symptoms of hypoglycemic reaction, such as nervousness, tremors, confusion, sweating, and increased pulse rate. Orange juice, sugar-sweetened beverages, or hard candy should be kept available and given if a reaction occurs.

Regular insulin can be given several times a day, especially during the regulation of insulin dosage. Intermediate- and long-acting insulins are usually administered once a day. Regular insulin (3 to 15 units) can be mixed with an intermediate-acting insulin (Humulin N), especially if rapid onset of action is needed. Ultralente insulin is seldom ordered because its peak action time occurs during the night or early morning. When switching from pork to human insulin, the client may require an adjustment of insulin dose because human insulin has a shorter duration of action.

Sliding-Scale Insulin Coverage

Insulin may be administered in adjusted doses that depend on individual blood glucose test results. When the diabetic client has extreme variances in insulin requirements (e.g., stress from hospitalization, surgery, illness, infection), adjusted dosing or sliding scale insulin coverage provides a more constant blood glucose level. Blood glucose testing is performed several times a day at specified intervals (usually before meals). A preset scale usually involves directions for the administration of rapid- or short-acting insulin.

Drug Interactions

Drugs such as thiazide diuretics, glucocorticoids (cortisone preparations), thyroid agents, and estrogen increase the blood sugar; therefore insulin dosage may need adjustment. Drugs that decrease insulin needs are tricyclic antidepressants, monoamine oxidase (MAO) inhibitors, aspirin products, and oral anticoagulants.

Table 50–2 lists the drug data for the rapid-acting, intermediate-acting, and long-acting insulins.

Side Effects and Adverse Reactions: Hypoglycemic Reactions and Ketoacidosis

When more insulin is administered than is needed for glucose metabolism, a **hypoglycemic reaction,** or **insulin shock,** occurs. The person may exhibit nervousness, trembling, and lack of coordination, with cold and clammy skin, and may complain of a headache. Some clients become

Table 50–2

Antidiabetics: Insulins

Generic (Brand)	Route and Dosage	Pregnancy Category	Half-Life	Protein-Binding	Action Onset	Action Peak	Action Duration
Rapid Acting							
lispro (Humalog)	A: subQ: 5-10 units, dose individualized	B	<13 h	UK	5 min	0.5-1 h	2-4 h
Short Acting							
regular	A & C: subQ/IV: 100 units/ml; dose is individualized according to blood sugar	B	10 min-1 h	UK	0.5-1 h	2-4 h	6-8 h
Humulin R	Same as regular insulin						
Intermediate Acting							
NPH insulin	See Prototype Drug Chart 50-1	B	13 h	UK	1-2 h	6-12 h	18-24 h
Humulin N insulin	Same as NPH insulin.	B	13 h	UK	1-2 h	8-12 h	18-24 h
Lente insulin	A & C: subQ: 100 units/ml; dose is individualized according to blood sugar	B	13 h	UK	1-2 h	8-12 h	18-28 h
Humulin L insulin	Same as Lente.	B	13 h	UK	1-2 h	8-12 h	18-28 h
Long Acting							
Ultralente insulin	Same as Lente.	B	13 h	UK	5-8 h	14-20 h	30-36 h
Lantus (Insulin Glargine)	Dose individualized	C	UK	UK	UK	UK	24 h
Combinations*							
Humulin 70/30 (isophane NPH 70%, regular 30%)	Dose individualized	B	13 h	UK	0.5 h	4-8 h	22-24 h
Humulin 50/50 (isophane NPH 50%, regular 50%)	Dose individualized	B	13 h	UK	0.5 h	4-8 h	24 h
Humalog 75/25 (lispro protamine 75%, lispro 25%)	Dose individualized	B	<13 h	UK	15 min	0.5-6 h	20-24 h

A, Adult; C, child; h, hour; IV, intravenous; min, minute; NPH, neutral-protamine-Hagedorn; subQ, subcutaneous; UK, unknown; <, less than.
*Protamine and zinc suspensions are added to regular insulin.

combative and incoherent. Giving sugar orally or IV increases the use of insulin, and the symptoms disappear immediately.

In response to an excessive dose of insulin, diabetic clients may develop the somogyi effect. This hypoglycemic condition usually occurs in the predawn hours of 2:00 to 4:00 AM. When the somogyi effect occurs, a rapid decrease in blood glucose during the night hours stimulates a release of hormones (e.g., cortisol, glucagon, epinephrine) to increase blood glucose by lipolysis, gluconeogenesis, and glycogenolysis. Management of the somogyi effect involves monitoring blood glucose between 2:00 AM and 4:00 AM and reducing the bedtime insulin dosage.

Hyperglycemia on awakening is known as the *dawn phenomenon*. The client usually awakens with a headache and reports night sweats and nightmares. Management of the dawn phenomenon involves increasing the bedtime dose of insulin.

With an inadequate amount of insulin, the sugar cannot be metabolized and fat catabolism occurs. The use of fatty acids (ketones) for energy causes **ketoacidosis** (diabetic acidosis or diabetic coma). Table 50–3 gives the signs and symptoms of hypoglycemic reaction and ketoacidosis.

Insulin Pen Injectors

An insulin pen resembles a fountain pen. The pen contains a disposable needle and a disposable insulin-filled cartridge. The insulin pens come in two types: prefilled and reusable. These insulin-filled pens are considered to deliver an insulin dose more accurate than the traditional 100 unit syringe and vial. In Europe more clients with diabetes mellitus use the insulin pens than do clients in the United States.

To operate the insulin pen, the insulin dose is obtained by turning the dial to the number of insulin units needed. The capacity of these prefilled and reusable insulin pens is 150 to 300 units, or 1.5 to 3 ml. Some insulin pens can measure the insulin dose to as low as 0.5 to 2 units. Eli Lilly manufactures two types of prefilled insulin pens: the Humulin (NPH) 70/30 and the Humalog 75/25. The Novo Nordisk produces the Novolin prefilled pen, NPH 70/30. The new insulin-made product, Lantus (a long-term acting insulin), can be administered by the pen injector. Both the Humalog and Lantus are more expensive.

The use of insulin pens increases the client's compliance with the insulin regimen. The convenience of the pen is most appealing. The client may choose to use the insulin pen for its portability (e.g., at work or while traveling). The traditional method for administering insulin may be used at other times. The cost of insulin in vials is somewhat less than the prefilled insulin pens. Most clients state that less injection pain is associated with the insulin pens than with the traditional insulin syringe.

Figure 50–2 demonstrates the technique for administering insulin using a prefilled insulin pen.

Insulin Pumps

There are two types of insulin pumps: implantable and portable. The implantable insulin pump is surgically implanted in the abdomen. It delivers basal insulin infusion

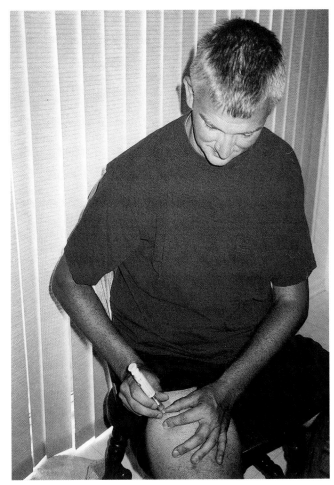
FIGURE 50–2   The client administers Humulin 70/30 using a prefilled insulin pen.

Table 50–3	
Hypoglycemic Reaction and Diabetic Ketoacidosis	
Reaction	**Signs and Symptoms**
Hypoglycemic reaction (insulin shock)	Headache, light-headedness; Nervousness, apprehension; Tremor; Excess perspiration; cold, clammy skin; Tachycardia; Slurred speech; Memory lapse, confusion, seizures; Blood sugar level <60 mg/dl
Diabetic ketoacidosis (hyperglycemic reaction)	Extreme thirst; Polyuria; Fruity breath odor; Kussmaul breathing (deep, rapid, labored, distressing, dyspnea); Rapid, thready pulse; Dry mucous membranes, poor skin turgor; Blood sugar level >250 mg/dl

>, Greater than; <, less than.

and bolus doses with meals, administered either intraperitoneally or IV. With the use of implantable insulin pumps, fewer hypoglycemic reactions occur and the blood glucose levels are controlled. Long-term effectiveness of the pump is under study.

The portable or external insulin pumps, also called *continuous subQ insulin infusion* (CSII), have been available since 1983. The external insulin pump keeps the blood glucose levels as close to normal as possible. The insulin pump is a battery-operated device that uses regular insulin, which is stored in a reservoir syringe placed inside the device. The syringe is the size of a "pager" and weighs about 3.5 ounces. It delivers both basal insulin infusion (continuous release of a small amount of insulin) and bolus doses with meals. Infusions are programmed by the client. About three basal rates are programmed a day; however the client can adjust the rate according to changes in activity. The insulin can be delivered by bolus (the client pushes a button to deliver a bolus dose at meals).

Insulin is delivered from the device through a plastic tube with a metal or plastic needle placed subQ by the client. The needle can be inserted into the abdomen, upper thigh, or upper arm. Only regular insulin is used. Modified insulins (NPH and Lente) are not used because of unpredictable control of blood sugars. The pump delivers exactly as much regular insulin as the client programs.

The ongoing insulin delivery therapy helps to decrease the risk of severe hypoglycemic reaction and maintains glucose (glycemic) control. Glucose levels should be monitored at least daily with or without an insulin pump.

Most insulin pumps have a memory of the last 24 boluses (time and day). An alarm is sounded when insulin is not delivered. The pump can be disconnected from the insertion site for bathing, swimming, and the like; however, it is recommended that it not be discontinued for longer than 1 to 2 hours. Portable insulin pumps are expensive ($3000 to $5000).

Success of insulin pump therapy depends on the client and his or her knowledge and compliance related to insulin use and the diabetic state. The person with type 1 diabetes mellitus may benefit most from the use of insulin pump therapy. This insulin delivery method is considered more effective and lessens the long-term diabetic complications than the use of multiple injections of regular and modified types of insulins. Figure 50–3 shows an example of an insulin pump.

Intranasal Insulin

Administration of insulin intranasally is in the experimental stage. This route of insulin administration causes a rapid onset and has a short duration of action. This method is used primarily to provide mealtime insulin supplements and is not used to meet basal insulin needs. Intermediate-acting insulin would still be needed. Only about 10% of the insulin is absorbed through the

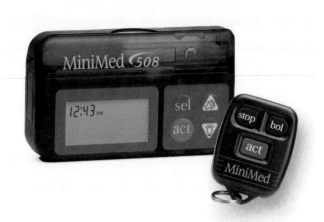

FIGURE 50–3   Insulin pump. (Courtesy MiniMed Inc., Sylmar, California.)

nasal membrane; thus the intranasal insulin dose is 10 times greater than a subQ dose. In addition, the nasal mucous membranes can become irritated. Intranasal insulin is expensive.

Insulin Jet Injectors

Insulin jet injectors shoot insulin, without a needle, directly through the skin into the fatty tissue. Because the insulin is delivered under high pressure, stinging, pain, burning, and bruising may occur. This method of insulin insertion is not indicated for children or older adults. This type of device is also expensive, costing approximately 2 to 10 times as much as the subQ dose.

Nursing Process

Antidiabetics: Insulin

ASSESSMENT

■ Identify the drugs that client currently takes. Certain drugs such as alcohol, aspirin, oral anticoagulants, oral antidiabetics, beta-blockers, tricyclic antidepressants, monoamine oxidase inhibitors (MAOIs), and tetracycline increase the hypoglycemic effect when taken with insulin. Note that thiazides, glucocorticoids, oral contraceptives, thyroid drugs, and smoking can increase blood sugar.

■ Assess the type of insulin and dosage. Note whether it is given once or multiple times a day.

■ Note vital signs and blood sugar levels. Report abnormal findings.

■ Determine client's knowledge of diabetes mellitus and the use of insulins.

■ Check for signs and symptoms of a hypoglycemic reaction (insulin shock) and hyperglycemia or ketoacidosis.

NURSING DIAGNOSES

■ Risk for impaired tissue integrity
■ Imbalanced nutrition: more or less than body requirements
■ Risk for injury

PLANNING

■ Client's blood sugar will be within the normal values (70 to 110 mg/dl).

NURSING INTERVENTIONS

■ Monitor vital signs. Tachycardia can occur during an insulin reaction.
■ Determine blood glucose levels and report changes. The reference value is 60 to 100 mg/dl for blood glucose and 70 to 110 mg/dl for serum glucose.
■ Prepare a teaching plan based on the client's knowledge of the health problem, diet, and drug therapy.

Client Teaching

General

• Instruct client to report immediately symptoms of a hypoglycemic (insulin) reaction, such as headache, nervousness, sweating, tremors, and rapid pulse, and symptoms of a hyperglycemic reaction (diabetic acidosis), such as thirst, increased urine output, and sweet fruity breath odor.
• Advise client that hypoglycemic reactions are more likely to occur during the peak action time. Most diabetics know whether they are having a hypoglycemic reaction; however, some have a higher tolerance to low blood sugar and can have a severe hypoglycemic reaction without realizing it.
• Explain that orange juice, sugar-containing drinks, and hard candy may be used when a hypoglycemic reaction begins.
• Teach family members to administer glucagon by injection if client has a hypoglycemic reaction and cannot drink sugar-containing fluid.
• Inform client that certain herbs may interact with insulin and oral antidiabetic drugs. A hypoglycemic or hyperglycemic effect might occur. See Herbal Alert 50–1.
• Instruct client about the necessity for compliance to prescribed insulin and diet.
• Advise client to obtain a MedicAlert card, tag, or bracelet indicating the health problem and insulin dosage.

Self-Administration

• Direct client how to check the blood sugar with a glucometer, such as the Sure Touch, One Step, or Accu-Chek. Figure 50–4 illustrates the use of a glucometer.

• Instruct client in the care of the insulin bottle and syringes. Inform client taking NPH or Lente insulin with regular insulin that the regular insulin should be drawn up before the NPH or Lente insulin.

Diet

• Advise client taking insulin to eat the prescribed diet on a consistent schedule. The diet information may be obtained from the American Diabetic Association or a nutritionist.

Cultural Considerations ⊕

• Provide additional explanation as needed to clients from various cultural groups related to insulin action and administration, insulin reactions, and possible complications.
• Follow-up by a community health nurse is needed to determine client's compliance with insulin use, diet, and exercise regimens.
• Explain the composition of insulin because client may prefer to avoid pork insulins for religious reasons.

EVALUATION

■ Evaluate the effectiveness of the insulin therapy by noting whether blood sugar level is within the accepted range.
■ Determine client's knowledge of the signs and symptoms of hypoglycemic or hyperglycemic reaction.

Oral Antidiabetic Drugs (Oral Hypoglycemic Drugs)

First- and Second-Generation Sulfonylureas

Oral antidiabetic drugs, also called *oral hypoglycemics,* were discovered in the 1950s. Persons with type 2 diabetes use these drugs; persons with type 1 diabetes should *not* use them. Clients with type 2 diabetes have some degree of insulin secretion by the pancreas. The sulfonylureas, a group of antidiabetics chemically related to sulfonamides but

---

HERBAL ALERT 50–1

Antidiabetic Agents

🌿 *Chromium* may decrease insulin requirements.
🌿 *Black cohosh* may potentiate the hypoglycemic effects of insulin and oral antidiabetic drugs.
🌿 *Garlic, bitter melon, aloe,* and *gymnema* can increase insulin levels and therefore may cause hypoglycemia when used with insulin or oral antidiabetic drugs. They can have a direct hypoglycemic effect.
🌿 *Ginseng* can lower the blood glucose levels and, when taken with insulin or an oral antidiabetic (hypoglycemic) drug, hypoglycemic effects or reaction may occur.
🌿 *Bilberry* may increase hypoglycemia when it is taken with insulin or oral antidiabetics.
🌿 *Cocoa, rosemary,* and *stinging nettle* decrease therapeutic effect of insulin and oral antidiabetic drugs thus they can have a hyperglycemic effect.

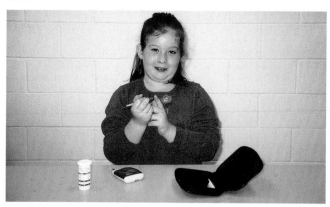

FIGURE 50–4 A 10-year-old child uses a glucometer to check her blood sugar level.

lacking antibacterial activity, stimulate the beta cells to secrete more insulin. This increases the insulin cell receptors thus increasing the ability of the cells to bind insulin for glucose metabolism. Acetohexamide (Dymelor) is a first-generation sulfonylurea. Do not confuse acetohexamide with acetazolamide, an anticonvulsant.

The sulfonylureas are classified as first- and second-generation. The first-generation sulfonylureas are divided into short-acting, intermediate-acting, and long-acting antidiabetics.

The second-generation sulfonylureas were first used in Europe; in 1984 they were approved by the FDA for use in the United States. The newer sulfonylureas increase the tissue response to insulin and decrease glucose production by the liver. They have a greater hypoglycemic po-

Table 50–4

Oral Antidiabetics

Generic (Brand)	Route and Dosage	Uses and Considerations
First-Generation: Short Acting		
tolbutamide (Orinase)	A: PO: 500-3000 mg/d in 2-3 divided doses	For managing type 2 diabetes. Drug is chemically related to sulfonamides with no antiinfective effect. Hypoglycemic reaction may occur if overdosed. *Pregnancy category:* C; PB: >90%; t½: 4-7 h
First-Generation: Intermediate Acting		
acetohexamide (Dymelor)	A: PO: 250 mg/d before breakfast; *max:* 1.5 g/d	For managing mild to moderately severe type 2 diabetes mellitus. *Pregnancy category:* C; PB: UK; t½: 5-6 h
tolazamide (Tolinase)	A: PO: 100-250 mg/d in 1-2 divided doses; *max:* 1 g/d	Same as acetohexamide (see Prototype Drug Chart 50–2). Diet and exercise should be a part of diabetic therapy. Duration of action is 10 to 20 hours. *Pregnancy category:* C; PB: 90%; t½: 7 h
First-Generation: Long Acting		
chlorpropamide (Diabinese)	A: PO: Initially: 100-250 mg/d; *maint:* 100-500 mg/d in 1-2 divided doses; *max:* 750 mg/d	For managing type 2 diabetes. May be given to selected type 1 clients for reducing insulin doses. Diet and exercise should be a part of diabetic therapy. Duration of action is 24 h. May cause water and sodium retention. *Pregnancy category:* C; PB: 95%; t½: 36 h
Second Generation		
glipizide (Glucotrol)	See Prototype Drug Chart 50–2.	
glyburide nonmicronized (DiaBeta, Micronase)	A: PO: Initially: 1.25-5 mg/d; *maint:* 1.25-20 mg q.i.d./b.i.d.; *max:* 20 mg/d	Same as chlorpropamide. Potent drug. Duration of action is 10 to 24 h. *Pregnancy category:* B; PB: 90%-95%; t½: 10 h
glyburide micronized (Glynase)	A: PO: 1.5-3 mg/d in AM; *maint:* 3-4.5 mg/d; *max:* 12 mg/d in 1 or 2 divided doses	For type 2 diabetes. Same as glyburide nonmicronized.
glimepiride (Amaryl)	A: PO: Initially: 1-2 mg a.c.; *maint:* 1-4 mg/d a.c.; *max:* 8 mg/d a.c.	To treat clients with type 2 diabetes. May be used in combination with insulin. Can lower the 2-hour postprandial glucose levels significantly. GI disturbances may occur. *Pregnancy category:* C; PB: 99.5%; t½: 5-9 h
Nonsulfonylurease		
Biguanides		
metformin (Glucophage)	See Prototype Drug Chart 50–3.	
Alpha-Glucosidase		
Inhibitors		
acarbose (Precose)	A: PO: Initially 25 mg 1-3 × daily with meals; *max:* 150 mg/d <60 kg, 300 mg/d if >60 kg	For managing hyperglycemia in type 2 diabetes mellitus. Used as monotherapy or in combination with a sulfonylurea. *Pregnancy category:* B; PB: UK; t½: 2 h

A, Adult; *a.c.,* before meals; *b.i.d.,* twice a day; *d,* day; *GI,* gastrointestinal; *h,* hour; *maint,* maintenance; *max,* maximum; *PB,* protein-binding; *PO,* by mouth; *q.i.d.,* four times a day; *t½,* half-life; *t.i.d.,* three times a day; *UK,* unknown; >, greater than; <, less than.

tency than the first-generation sulfonylureas. Effective doses for the second-generation drugs are less than the dosages of the first generation. They have a longer duration and cause fewer side effects. The second-generation drugs have less displacement potential from protein-binding sites by other highly protein-bound drugs, such as salicylates and warfarin (Coumadin), than those of the first-generation drugs. The second-generation sulfonylureas should not be used when liver or kidney dysfunction is present. A hypoglycemic reaction is more likely to occur in older adults.

Second-generation sulfonylureas include glimepiride (Amaryl) and glipizide (Glucotrol), which directly stimulate the beta cells to secrete insulin, thus decreasing the blood glucose level. Glimepiride improves the postprandial glucose levels. It may be used in combination with insulin in persons with type 2 diabetes. Side effects include GI disturbances such as nausea, vomiting, diarrhea, and abdominal pain. Do not confuse Amaryl with Altace or Amerge, an antimigraine medication.

Table 50–4 lists the drug data for the sulfonylureas. Prototype Drug Chart 50–2 lists the actions and effects of the second-generation, sulfonylurea glipizide. Do not confuse glipizide with glyburide.

Pharmacokinetics

Acetohexamide (Dymelor) is well absorbed from the GI tract and is highly protein bound. Acetohexamide is metabolized by the liver, with 50% converted to a metabolite. There are two half-lives: the half-life of the drug metabolite is three times as long as that of the pure drug. The kidneys excrete acetohexamide unchanged in the urine.

Pharmacodynamics

Glipizide XL is the most common sulfonylurea drug prescribed for type 2 diabetes mellitus. It lowers the blood sugar by stimulating the beta cells in the pancreas to secrete insulin.

Table 50–4

Oral Antidiabetics—cont'd

Generic (Brand)	Route and Dosage	Uses and Considerations
Alpha-Glucosidase—cont'd		
Inhibitors—cont'd		
miglitol (Glyset)	A: PO: 25-100 mg t.i.d. with meals	For managing type 2 diabetes. May be taken with a sulfonylurea or as monotherapy with diet and exercise. GI disturbances may occur. *Pregnancy category:* B; PB: <4%; t$\frac{1}{2}$: 2 h
Thiazolidinediones (Insulin-Enhancing Agents)		
pioglitazone HCl (Actos)	A: PO: 15-45 mg/d	Management of type 2 diabetes. It improves glycemic control and decreases insulin resistance. It inhibits gluconeogenesis and increases sensitivity to insulin in muscle and fatty tissues. For monotherapy; can be combined with sulfonylurea or insulin. Liver enzymes should be monitored. *Pregnancy category:* C; PB: 99%; t$\frac{1}{2}$: 3-7 h
rosiglitazone maleate (Avandia)	A: PO: 4-8 mg/d; or 2-4 mg b.i.d.	Management for type 2 diabetes. Improves blood glucose control and increases insulin sensitivity. Can increase resumption of ovulation in premenopausal women. For monotherapy use; maybe combined with metformin. Diet, exercise, and monitoring liver enzymes are suggested. Replaced troglitazone (Rezulin), which was removed from the market because it caused severe liver problems. *Pregnancy category:* C; PB: 99.8%; t$\frac{1}{2}$: 3-4 h
Meglitinides		
repaglinide (Prandin)	A: PO: 0.5-4 mg a.c. b.i.d., t.i.d., q.i.d.; *max:* 16 mg/d	To manage type 2 diabetes. May be taken alone or in combination with metformin. Similar in action to sulfonylureas but not in structure. Increases beta-cell secretion of insulin. *Pregnancy category:* C; PB: 98%; t$\frac{1}{2}$: 1 h
nateglinide (Starlix)	A: PO: 60-120 mg a.c. t.i.d.; *max:* 540 mg/d	To treat type 2 diabetes. It increases the release of insulin from the beta cells. This drug may be used alone or in combination with metformin. *Pregnancy category:* UK; PB: 98%; t$\frac{1}{2}$: 1.5 h
Fixed Combination of Oral Antidiabetic Drug		
glyburide/metformin (Glucovance)	A: PO: Initially: 1.25/250 mg (glyburide/ metformin) daily or b.i.d. with meals. Increase dose at 2-wk intervals; *maint:* 2.5/ 500 mg or 5/500 mg/d or b.i.d. with meals; *max:* 20/2000 mg/d	For managing type 2 diabetes. May be used when glucose is not controlled with either drug alone. Contraindicated for clients with renal insufficiency because of the risk of developing lactic acidosis. *Pregnancy category:* B-D; PB: UK; t$\frac{1}{2}$: UK

PROTOTYPE DRUG CHART 50–2

GLIPIZIDE

Drug Class	**Dosage**
Glipizide: sulfonylurea, first-generation Trade Name: Glucotrol, Glucotrol XL *Pregnancy Category:* C	A: PO: Initially 2.5-5 mg before meals daily; mainte- nance: 10-15 mg daily before meals; (dose should be divided if >15 mg); *max:* 40 mg/d A: PO: SR: 5-10 mg/d
Contraindications	**Drug-Lab-Food Interactions**
Diabetic ketoacidosis *Caution:* Hepatic or renal dysfunction, elderly, debilitated or malnourished, adrenal or pituitary insufficiency	***Drug:*** Alcohol may produce a disulfiram-like reaction (flushing, headache, sweating, nausea, violent vomit- ing, weakness); Hypoglycemia may be potentiated by oral anticoagulants, MAO inhibitors, salicylates, probenecid, sulfonamides, cimetidine, clofibrate, phenylbutazone ***Lab:*** Altered liver function tests ***Food:*** None known
Pharmacokinetics	**Pharmacodynamics**
Absorption: Rapidly absorbed from GI **Distribution:** PB: 90-95% **Metabolism:** t½: 3-5 h **Excretion:** Primarily in urine	**PO:** Onset: 15-30 min Peak: 1-2 h Duration: 24 h

Therapeutic Effects/Uses

To control hyperglycemia in type 2 diabetes mellitus
Mode of Action: Directly stimulates beta cells in pancreas to secrete insulin, indirectly alters sensitivity of peripheral
insulin receptors allowing increased insulin binding

Side Effects	**Adverse Effects**
Drowsiness, headache, confusion, visual disturbances, anxiety, hunger, anorexia, nausea, constipation, diarrhea	Hypoglycemia, tachycardia **Life-threatening:** Seizures, coma, respiratory depression

A, Adult; *d,* day; *GI,* gastrointestinal; *h,* hour; *MAO,* monoamine oxidase; *max,* maximum; *min,* minute; *PB,* protein-binding; *PO,* by
mouth; *SR,* sustained release; *t½,* half-life; >, greater than.

The onset of action of acetohexamide usually occurs within 1 hour, and the peak action time is between 2 and 6 hours. Acetohexamide is normally given once a day in the morning because of its long duration of action.

Side Effects, Adverse Reactions, and Contraindications

The side effects of most oral antidiabetic drugs are similar to those of insulin. Taking antidiabetic drugs without adequate food can lead to an insulin reaction with signs and symptoms such as nervousness, tremors, and confusion. Adverse reactions are those of hematologic disorders: aplastic anemia, leukopenia, and thrombocytopenia. Sulfonylureas are contraindicated in type 1 diabetes (no functioning beta cells), pregnancy, and breastfeeding and during stress, surgery, or severe infection.

The major side effect of acetohexamide is hypoglycemic reaction. Acarbose does not cause hypoglycemia unless it is taken with a sulfonylurea drug. It can cause an increase of flatulence (gas).

Drug Interactions

Aspirin, anticoagulants, anticonvulsants, sulfonamides, and some NSAIDs can increase the action of sulfonylureas, especially first generation, by binding to the plasma protein and displacing sulfonylureas. Because this causes increased free sulfonylurea, an insulin reaction can result. Sulfonylureas also enhance the action of thiazide diuretics, phenothiazines, and barbiturates. Sulfonylureas decrease the action of thyroid replacement drugs. Clients should be alerted not to drink alcohol while taking sulfonylureas because alcohol increases the half-life and a hypoglycemic reaction can result.

Many drug interactions are associated with acetohexamide. Glucocorticoids (cortisone), thiazide diuretics, calcium channel blockers, thyroid drugs, estrogen, and phenytoin (Dilantin) can decrease the effectiveness of acetohexamide. A hypoglycemic reaction can occur when acetohexamide is taken with sulfonamides, aspirin, NSAIDs, monoamine oxidase inhibitors (MAOIs), cimetidine (Tagamet), alcohol, or insulin.

Nonsulfonylureas

Expanding knowledge of glucose metabolism has revealed new mechanisms for the management of type 2 diabetes. The drugs metformin and acarbose use different methods to control serum glucose levels following a meal. Unlike the sulfonylureas, which enhance insulin release and receptor interaction, these drugs affect the hepatic and GI production of glucose.

Biguanides: Metformin (Glucophage)

Metformin is a biguanide compound that acts by decreasing hepatic production of glucose from stored glycogen. This diminishes the increase in serum glucose following a meal and blunts the degree of postprandial hyperglycemia. Metformin also decreases the absorption of glucose from the small intestine. There is also evidence that it increases insulin receptor sensitivity as well as peripheral glucose uptake at the cellular level. Unlike sulfonylureas, metformin does not produce hypoglycemia or hyperglycemia. It can cause GI disturbances.

Metformin is 50% to 60% bioavailable and is absorbed primarily from the small intestine. It does not undergo hepatic metabolism and is eliminated unchanged in the urine. It is not recommended for clients with renal impairment. Monotherapy with metformin is effective; however, when combined with a sulfonylurea, the drug is useful in cases resistant to oral antidiabetics (oral hypoglycemics). Withhold metformin therapy for 48 hours before and after the client undergoes IV contrast dye because lactic acidosis or acute renal failure may develop. Do not confuse glucophage with glutofac.

Alpha-Glucosidase Inhibitors: Acarbose (Precose) and Miglitol (Glyset)

Acarbose acts by inhibiting the digestive enzyme in the small intestine responsible for the release of glucose from the complex carbohydrates (CHO) in the diet. By inhibiting alpha glucosidase, the CHO cannot be absorbed and therefore pass into the large intestine. Acarbose has no demonstrated systemic effects and is not absorbed into the body in significant amounts. It does not cause a hypoglycemic reaction. Acarbose is intended for use in clients who do not achieve results with diet alone. Miglitol (Glyset), like acarbose, inhibits alpha glucosides. Miglitol is absorbed from the GI tract. This drug will not cause hypoglycemia; however, if it is taken with a sulfonylurea or insulin, hypoglycemia could occur.

Thiazolidinediones

Troglitazone (Rezulin) was the first drug in this group approved by the FDA in 1997. Because of the severe liver problems and deaths associated with this drug, it was removed from the market in early 2000. Pioglitazone (Actos) and rosiglitazone (Avandia) recently received FDA approval and are considered safer thiazolidinedione drugs. Do not confuse Avandia with Prandin. See Prototype Drug Chart 50–3. These two drugs can be prescribed for monotherapy or combined with other oral antidiabetic drugs. Pioglitazone can be taken in combination with sulfonylurea or insulin, and rosiglitazone may be combined with metformin. These drugs do not induce hypoglycemic reactions if taken alone. They decrease insulin resistance and improve blood glucose control.

Meglitinides

Repaglinide (Prandin) and nateglinide (Starlix) are classified as meglitinide oral antidiabetic agents that stimulate the beta cells to release insulin. The action of repaglinide and nateglinide is similar to that of sulfonylureas. They can be used alone or in combination with metformin for clients with type 2 diabetes mellitus. They are short-acting antidiabetic drugs. These drugs should not be prescribed for clients with liver dysfunction because of a possible decreased liver metabolism rate. More of the drug could remain in the body, which may cause a hypoglycemic reaction.

Guidelines for Oral Antidiabetic (Hypoglycemic) for Type 2 Diabetes

The following are criteria for the use of oral antidiabetic drugs:

- Onset of diabetes mellitus at age 40 years or older
- Diagnosis of diabetes for less than 5 years
- Normal weight or overweight
- Fasting blood glucose equal to or less than 200 mg/dl
- Less than 40 units of insulin required per day
- Normal renal and hepatic function

Nursing Process

Oral Antidiabetics

ASSESSMENT

- Identify the drugs client currently takes. Aspirin, alcohol, sulfonamides, oral contraceptives, and monoamine oxidase inhibitors (MAOIs) increase the hypoglycemic effect; a decrease in oral antidiabetic drug may be needed. Glucocorticoids (cortisone), thiazide diuretics, and estrogen increase blood sugar.
- Note vital signs and blood sugar levels. Report abnormal findings.
- Determine client's knowledge of diabetes mellitus and the use of oral antidiabetics.

NURSING DIAGNOSES

- Risk for impaired tissue integrity
- Imbalanced nutrition: more or less than body requirements
- Deficient knowledge

PLANNING

- Client's blood sugar will be within normal serum levels (70 to 110 mg/dl).
- Client will adhere to prescribed diet, blood testing, and drug.

NURSING INTERVENTIONS

■ Determine vital signs. Oral antidiabetics increase cardiac function and oxygen consumption, which can lead to cardiac dysrhythmias.

■ Administer oral antidiabetics with food to minimize gastric upset.

■ Monitor blood glucose levels and report changes. The reference value is 60 to 100 mg/dl for blood glucose and 70 to 110 mg/dl for serum glucose.

■ Prepare a teaching plan based on client's knowledge of health problems, diet, and drug therapy.

Client Teaching

General

• Advise client that hypoglycemic (insulin) reaction can occur when taking an oral hypoglycemic drug, especially the sulfonylureas. This drug stimulates the release of insulin from the beta cells of the pancreas.

Oral antidiabetics are *not* insulin. Normally, clients with diabetes mellitus type 1 do not have functioning beta cells and should *not* take oral antidiabetics, only insulin. Sulfonylureas are prescribed for clients with diabetes mellitus type 2.

• Teach client to recognize symptoms of hypoglycemic reaction (headache, nervousness, sweating, tremors, rapid pulse) and symptoms of hyperglycemic reaction (thirst, increased urine output, sweet fruity breath odor).

• Explain that insulin might be needed instead of an oral antidiabetic drug during stress, surgery, or serious infection. Blood sugar levels are usually elevated during stressful times.

• Instruct client about the necessity for compliance to diet and drug.

• Advise client to obtain a MedicAlert card, tag, or bracelet indicating the health problem and insulin dosage.

PROTOTYPE DRUG CHART 50–3

METFORMIN

Drug Class

Metformin: Biguanide
Trade Name: Glucophage, Glucophage XL
Pregnancy Category: B

Dosage

A: PO: Initial: 500 mg/d-t.i.d. with meals; increase dose gradually; *max:* 2500 mg/d
A: PO: SR: 500 mg/day with evening meal; *max:* 2000 mg/d

Contraindications

Hypersensitivity, concurrent infection, hepatic or renal dysfunction, cardiopulmonary insufficiency, alcoholism
Caution: Pregnancy, lactation

Drug-Lab-Food Interactions

Drug: Hypoglycemia may be potentiated by captopril, nifedipine, procainamide, quinidine, digoxin, furosemide, triamterene, cimetidine, ranitidine, azole antifungals, trimethoprim, vancomycin, quinine; Iodinated contrast dyes may lead to lactic acidosis or acute kidney failure
Lab: Altered liver function tests
Food: None known

Pharmacokinetics

Absorption: 50-60% absorbed
Distribution: PB: 0%
Metabolism: $t\frac{1}{2}$: 6.2-17.6 h
Excretion: Primarily in urine

Pharmacodynamics

PO: Onset: UK
  Peak: 1-3 h
  Duration: UK

Therapeutic Effects/Uses

To control hyperglycemia in type 2 diabetes mellitus
Mode of Action: Increases binding of insulin to receptors, improves tissue sensitivity to insulin, increases glucose transport into skeletal muscles and fatty tissues, suppresses gluconeogenesis

Side Effects

Dizziness, fatigue, headache, agitation, bitter or metallic taste, anorexia, nausea, vomiting, diarrhea

Adverse Effects

Lactic acidosis; malabsorption of amino acids, vitamin B_{12}, and folic acid
Life-threatening: None known

A, Adult; *d*, day; *h*, hour; *max*, maximum; *PB*, protein-binding; *PO*, by mouth; *SR*, sustained release; *t½*, half-life; *t.i.d.*, three times a day; *UK*, unknown.

Self-Administration
- Direct client how to check the blood sugar level with a glucometer. Client should record and report abnormal results.

Side Effects
- Advise client to report side effects, such as vomiting, diarrhea, and rash.

Diet
- Instruct client not to ingest alcohol with antidiabetic drugs to avoid a hypoglycemic reaction. Food taken with oral antidiabetics will decrease gastric irritation.
- Advise client taking oral antidiabetics to eat the prescribed diet on schedule. Delaying or missing a meal can cause hypoglycemia.
- Explain the use of orange juice, sugar-containing drinks, or hard candy when a hypoglycemic reaction begins. Report to the health care provider of the health problem.
- Direct client to take oral antidiabetics with food to decrease gastric irritation.

Cultural Considerations

- Respect client's cultural beliefs and alternative method for treating "sugar in the urine" and elevated blood sugar levels. Discuss with client (the use of an interpreter may be necessary) the safety of the methods and the use of oral antidiabetic drugs to correct the problem. If client takes an oral antidiabetic drug to decrease the blood glucose level, emphasize the importance of checking the blood sugar levels daily or as indicated. Hypoglycemic reaction can result from increased doses of oral antidiabetic agents and insufficient dietary intake.

EVALUATION

- Evaluate the effectiveness of drug therapy by noting whether blood sugar levels are within the accepted range.

Hyperglycemic Drugs

Glucagon

Glucagon is a hyperglycemic hormone secreted by the alpha cells of the islets of Langerhans in the pancreas. Glucagon increases blood sugar by stimulating glycogenolysis (glycogen breakdown) in the liver. It protects the body cells, especially those in the brain and retina, by providing the nutrients and energy needed to maintain body function.

Glucagon is available for parenteral use (subQ, IM, and IV). It is used to treat insulin-induced hypoglycemia when other methods of providing glucose are not available. For example, the client may be semiconscious or unconscious and unable to ingest sugar-containing products. Clients with diabetes who are prone to severe hypoglycemic reactions (insulin shock) should keep glucagon in the home,

and family members should be taught how to administer subQ or IM injections during an emergency hypoglycemic reaction. The blood glucose level begins to increase within 5 to 20 minutes after administration. Recently, IV glucagon has been used in the acute treatment of beta-blocker overdose and profound shock.

Diazoxide

Oral diazoxide (Proglycem), which is chemically related to thiazide diuretics, increases blood sugar by inhibiting insulin release from the beta cells and stimulating release of epinephrine (Adrenalin) from the adrenal medulla. This drug is not indicated for hypoglycemic reactions; rather, it is used to treat chronic hypoglycemia caused by hyperinsulinism because of islet cell cancer or hyperplasia. The parenteral form of diazoxide (Hyperstat) is prescribed for malignant hypertension. Hypotension usually does not occur with oral diazoxide.

Diazoxide has a long half-life and is highly protein bound. Its onset of action is 1 hour, and the duration of action is 8 hours. Most of the drug is excreted unchanged in the urine.

Other Agents

Exenatide (Byetta) is an antidiabetic agent from Amylin Pharmaceuticals and Eli Lilly and Company that was approved by the FDA in April 2005. This agent has been placed in a new classification of drugs known as *incretin mimetic* that improves beta-cell responsiveness, which improves glucose control in people with type 2 diabetes mellitus. The actions of exenatide are to enhance insulin secretion, increase beta-cell responsiveness, suppress glucoagon secretion, slow gastric emptying, and reduce food intake. Exenatide is not a substitute for insulin and should not be administered to patients with type 1 diabetes mellitus, diabetic ketoacidosis, severe renal dysfunction, or severe GI disease. Common adverse effects that occur with exenatide include headache, dizziness, jitteriness, nausea, vomiting, and diarrhea. Exenatide is administered by injectable prefilled pens in twice-a-day dosing and has significantly improved A1C levels and weight loss in many individuals.

Pramlintide acetate (Symlin) is another antidiabetic agent from Amylin Pharmaceuticals and approved by the FDA in March 2005 for adults with type 1 and type 2 diabetes mellitus. The primary purpose of pramlintide is to improve postprandial glucose control in diabetic patients who are using insulin but are unable to achieve and maintain glucose control. The actions of pramlintide are to suppress glucagon secretion, slow gastric emptying, and modulate appetite by inducing satiety. Suppression of glucagon secretion reduces postprandial hepatic glucose for approximately 3 hours. By slowing gastric emptying, the absorption rate of glucose is reduced. Satiety promotes reduced food intake. Common adverse effects include dizziness, anorexia, nausea, vomiting, and fatigue. Pramlintide is administered by injection subcutaneously before meals in the abdomen or thigh; it is never given in the arm.

Critical Thinking Case Study

T.C., age 32, was diagnosed with diabetes mellitus after the birth of her first child; her blood sugar level was 180 mg/dl. Her serum glucose level has been maintained within the normal range with aceto-hexamide (Dymelor) 250 mg/daily.

1. Why was T.C., at her age, taking an oral antidiabetic drug instead of insulin?

2. Acetohexamide is indicated for what type of diabetes mellitus? When should acetohexamide not be taken?

3. Should acetohexamide be taken with sulfon-amides, aspirin, NSAIDs, cimetidine, alcohol, or insulin? Why or why not?

4. Why should T.C. monitor her blood sugar using a home glucometer?

Two years later, T.C. became pregnant again. Aceto-hexamide was discontinued, and Humulin N insulin 25 units was prescribed. Since the birth of her second child, she has remained on Humulin N 25 U daily.

5. Give a possible reason why the health care provider changed the antidiabetic drug to insulin when T.C. became pregnant.

6. Humulin N is similar to what other type of insulin? How do these two types differ?

7. Give the onset, peak, and duration of action for Humulin N insulin. When is an insulin reaction most likely to occur with Humulin N?

8. What are the pros and cons for T.C. to receive Humulin 70/30 insulin?

9. What are the signs and symptoms of a hypo-glycemic reaction?

10. What should be included in client teaching?

T.C. asks the nurse if she can take acetohexamide again instead of insulin because she is eating the "right foods."

11. What should the response be?

Study Questions

1. V.A., age 13, was recently diagnosed with diabetes mellitus. She receives 35 units of NPH insulin a day. She asks why she has to take insulin when other diabetics she knows do not. What should the response be?

2. Prepare a teaching plan for V.A. that includes the type of insulin, injection sites, how to check her blood sugar, and the signs and symptoms of a hy-poglycemic reaction.

3. What are the pros and cons for the use of prefilled insulin pens?

4. S.Y. takes the sulfonylurea tolbutamide (Orinase). What generation and type of sulfonylurea is tolbutamide?

5. Develop a nursing plan for S.Y. focusing on tol-butamide. What are the side effects of this drug? How often is it usually taken? To what types of drug interactions should she be alerted?

6. How do acarbose and rosiglitazone differ from acetohexamide?

Sixteen

Reproductive and Gender-Related Agents

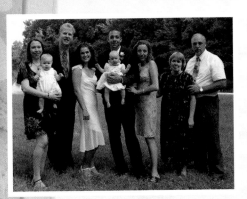

This unit comprises five chapters that focus on reproductive and gender-related drugs. Chapters 51, 52, 53, and 54 address agents specifically associated with female health and disorders. Drugs used throughout the female reproductive cycle, including pregnancy and preterm labor, are comprehensively discussed in Chapter 51, Drugs Associated with the Female Reproductive Cycle I: Pregnancy and Preterm Labor. Chapter 52, Drugs Associated with the Female Reproductive Cycle II: Labor, Delivery, and the Preterm Neonate, covers labor and delivery. Chapter 53, Drugs Associated with the Postpartum and Newborn, focuses on the pharmacology of the postpartum and neonatal period. Chapter 54, Drugs Related to Women's Health and Disorders, details the variety of oral contraceptive products and the drugs used to treat uterine dysfunction, including premenstrual syndrome, endometriosis, and menopausal discomforts. Chapter 55, Drugs Related to Reproductive Health: Male Reproductive Disorders, describes androgens and anabolic steroids, antiandrogens, and other drugs related to male reproductive health and disorders. Chapter 56, Drugs Related to Reproductive Health: Infertility and Sexually Transmitted Diseases, concludes this unit with a discussion of drugs used for infertility and sexually transmitted diseases.

Female Reproductive Processes

The uterus is a pear-shaped, hollow, very muscular organ located in the pelvic cavity between the rectum and the bladder; it is connected to the vagina by the cervix (Figure XVI–1). Three distinct layers compose the uterine wall: the outer layer (perimetrium); the muscular middle layer (myometrium); and the inner mucosal layer (endometrium).

The myometrium is a network of involuntary (smooth) muscles divided into three layers, with the muscles of each layer configured in different patterns. For example, the outer muscles are arranged longitudinally to assist with cervical effacement (thinning and shortening) and to expel the fetus at the time of delivery. Muscles in the middle layer are arranged in a figure-8 design. These muscles are extremely important in the control of bleeding (hemostasis). Blood vessels are threaded throughout these muscles, and when a contraction occurs, the vessels are compressed, creating a hemostatic effect. Circular muscle fibers are found in the area of the internal os and help control its sphincter. These circular muscles keep the fetus contained in the uterus for the normal gestational period. It is these muscles that stretch (dilate) the cervix to a diameter of 10 cm during labor. When all three muscle layers work together during labor, contractions cause cervical dilation and descent and delivery of the infant.

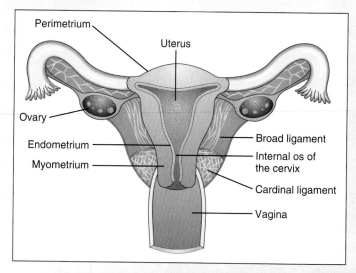

FIGURE XVI–1 Anatomy of the female reproductive system.

The Menstrual Cycle

The reproductive cycle is hormonally controlled by interactions between the endocrine and reproductive systems. The hypothalamus secretes gonadotropin-releasing hormone (Gn-RH), which stimulates the anterior pituitary to synthesize and release follicle-stimulating hormone (FSH) and luteinizing hormone (LH). These gonadotropins stimulate the ovaries to produce estrogen and progesterone, respectively.

In most women the menstrual cycle lasts 28 days (range of 22 to 34 days). The ovarian hormones estrogen and progesterone regulate the cycle, which has three ovarian phases: follicular, ovulatory, and luteal. Endometrial phases occur simultaneously with these ovarian phases.

The *follicular phase* occurs during days 1 to 14 of the cycle. Days 1 to 6 of this period constitute the menstrual phase and days 7 to 14, the proliferative phase. During the total 14-day period, FSH increases and follicles begin to mature within the ovary. One graafian follicle from the group matures and swells by days 10 to 13, ruptures on day 14, and releases the ovum to the fallopian tube. The *ovulatory phase* occurs on day 14 when the ovum is released. The *luteal phase* occurs from days 15 to 28 and includes the secretory phase of the endometrial cycle. During this period, estrogen and progesterone are produced by the ovarian corpus luteum (the ruptured graafian follicle), reaching peak levels 8 days into the phase. Changes occur in the endometrium for optimal implantation of a fertilized ovum. FSH and LH levels decrease, mediated by dopamine, norepinephrine, and serotonin. Estrogen and progesterone are withdrawn immediately before menstruation, and the endometrial prostaglandin level increases. The cycle begins anew with the follicular phase. In cycles that are nonovulatory, hormonal secretion of estrogen, FSH, and LH is erratic; there is also an alteration in the usual amount of progesterone. These physiologic alterations become the basis for planning and implementing pharmacologic interventions.

Male Reproductive Processes

There are three male reproductive processes: *spermatogenesis,* or sperm production; regulation of male sexual functioning; and sexual intercourse.

Male Reproductive Anatomy and Physiology

The anatomy of the male sexual organs is depicted in Figure XVI–2. The external reproductive organs include the penis, the scrotum, and the testes. The penis consists of three cylindrical bodies of erectile tissue: two corpora cavernosa and the corpus spongiosum. With sexual excitement, the vascular spaces fill with blood to produce an erection (Figure XVI–3).

The scrotum has two compartments, each of which holds a testis, epididymis, and spermatic cord. The spermatic cord supports the testis and includes the vas deferens, blood vessels, nerves, and muscle fibers.

Each testis contains seminiferous tubules in which spermatogenesis occurs. The sperm then move into the epididymis. This leads into the vas deferens, the source of about 20% of ejaculate, or semen. On either side of the prostate gland, a seminal vesicle empties seminal fluid into the ampulla. Seminal fluid contains fructose to provide energy for the sperm, prostaglandins, fibrinogen, and a sperm-activating factor.

The contents of the ampulla and the seminal vesicles empty into an ejaculatory duct that leads through the body of the prostate to empty into the urethra. Prostatic fluid, which constitutes about 20% of semen, empties from the prostate gland into the ejaculatory duct. The urethra carries semen to its distal end. The urethral glands along the length of the urethra and the bulbourethral glands near the prostatic end of the urethra supply the urethra with mucus. The bulbourethral glands secrete alkaline preejaculatory fluid to protect sperm from the acidity of the urethra.

Hormonal Regulation of Male Reproductive Functioning and Spermatogenesis

Gn-RH from the hypothalamus stimulates the anterior pituitary gland to secrete two major gonadotropins, LH and FSH, in both men and women. LH stimulates the interstitial Leydig cells of the testes to mature and produce testosterone. There is a direct relationship between the amount of circulating LH and the amount of testosterone produced. Testosterone is also produced to a lesser extent in the adrenal cortex and in the ovaries of women.

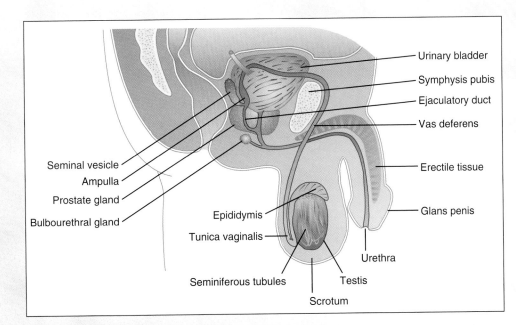

FIGURE XVI–2 Anatomy of the male reproductive system.

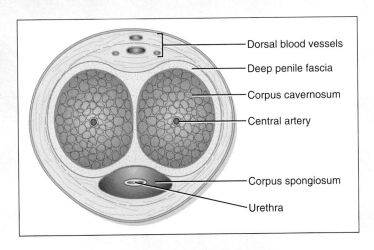

FIGURE XVI–3 Erectile tissue of the penis.

In men, FSH stimulates the Sertoli cells to begin conversion of spermatids into mature sperm. In addition, the Sertoli cells are stimulated to secrete estrogens, which may promote spermatogenesis. For spermatogenesis to be complete, testosterone must be secreted simultaneously by the Leydig cells and diffused into the seminiferous tubules.

Testosterone is the precursor of two classes of sex steroids: 5-alpha-reduced androgens and estrogens. The net effect of endogenous androgens is the sum of the effects of the 5-alpha-reduced metabolite *dihydrotestosterone* and its estrogen derivative, *estradiol*. Most testosterone is loosely bound by plasma protein and circulates for 15 to 30 minutes before it is fixed to target tissues or metabolized. Most testosterone fixed to target cells is then converted to its active form, dihydrotestosterone.

The rate of testosterone production is controlled by a negative feedback loop. With increased testosterone, the hypothalamus decreases production of Gn-RH (Figure XVI–4). In addition, with sperm production, the Sertoli cells release a hormone called *inhibin*, which suppresses FSH production by the anterior pituitary thus maintaining

a constant rate of spermatogenesis. It is not known how, before puberty, the brain stimulates the hypothalamus to begin Gn-RH secretion, but if the brain is not intact, this may not occur.

Sexual Function

The human sexual response cycle consists of five phases: desire, excitement, plateau, orgasm, and resolution. Sexual desire is the stimulus that causes an individual to initiate or be receptive to sexual activity. During the excitement phase, the man experiences penile erection. Men are incapable of engaging in sexual intercourse without this arousal. The plateau phase is characterized by genital enlargement, mucous secretion, generalized muscle tension, hyperventilation, tachycardia, and increased blood pressure. During the orgasmic phase, the vas deferens, seminal vesicles, ejaculatory duct, and penile urethra contract three or four times over a few seconds causing the man to ejaculate. During resolution, there is a refractory period in which pelvic vasocongestion declines and generalized muscle relaxation takes place.

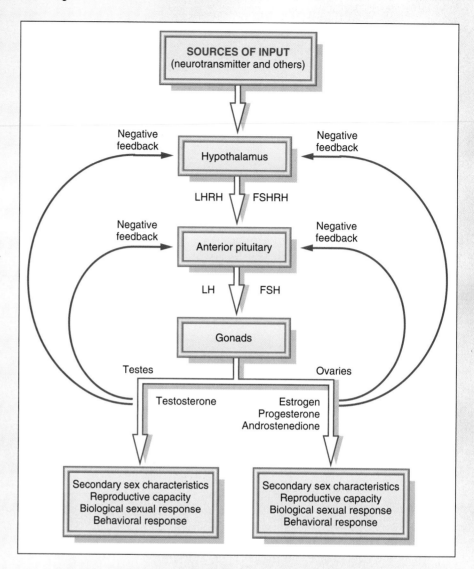

FIGURE XVI–4 Hypothalamic-pituitary-gonadal feedback loops. (From Fogel CI, Lauver D: *Sexual health promotion,* Philadelphia, 1990, Saunders, p. 339.)

Process Of Fertilization

Fertilization, or *conception,* occurs when a sperm penetrates an ovum, usually in the distal third of the fallopian tube.

In a single ejaculation, between 200 and 400 million spermatozoa are deposited in the vagina. Sperm move up the female reproductive tract using the flagellar motion of their tails. It takes an average of 4 to 6 hours for the sperm to reach the distal fallopian tube. Semen contains prostaglandins that may enhance uterine motility to facilitate sperm migration. The ciliary action of the fallopian tubes enhances migration of the ovum to the uterus and of sperm toward the ovary.

Uterine enzymes capacitate the sperm by altering their glycoprotein coat. In an acrosomal reaction, the sperm release the enzyme hyaluronidase, which breaks through the outer layer of the ovum. The moment one sperm penetrates the ovum, a chemical reaction occurs that blocks other sperm from entering. Cellular division begins immediately in what is now called the *zygote,* or fertilized egg.

After 3 days, the zygote enters the uterus. It has now differentiated into an inner solid mass of cells, the *blastocyst,* and an outer layer, the *trophoblast.* Progesterone secreted by the corpus luteum of the ovary maintains a favorable uterine environment to nourish the blastocyst until *implantation* in the uterine lining occurs. The blastocyst develops into the embryo and the amniotic membrane, whereas the trophoblast develops into the chorionic membrane and the fetal side of the placenta. The maternal portion of the placenta develops under the site of the blastocyst's implantation. The *placenta* is the structure through which oxygen, nutrients, and metabolic wastes pass between the maternal and fetal circulations for the duration of pregnancy. The placenta begins to function by the fourth week of pregnancy. Within the first 8 weeks of pregnancy, organ systems are differentiated, and it is during this period that the fetus is most threatened by teratogens. Growth of the fetus throughout pregnancy depends on adequate oxygenation and nutrition, the metabolic environment, freedom from infection, and integrity of the mother's reproductive tract.

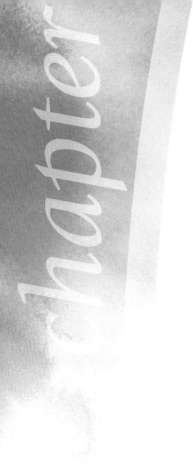

51

Drugs Associated with the Female Reproductive Cycle I: Pregnancy and Preterm Labor

ROBIN WEBB CORBETT AND LAURA K. WILLIFORD OWENS

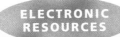

Additional information can be found on the companion website at *http://evolve.elsevier.com/KeeHayes/pharmacology/* or on the companion CD-ROM, which includes:
- *NCLEX-style examination review questions*
- *Pharmacology animations*
- *Medication error and IV therapy checklists*
- *Medication calculation problems*
- *Electronic calculators*

OUTLINE

OBJECTIVES

- Explain potential health-promoting and detrimental effects of substances ingested by the woman during the prenatal period.
- Describe the drugs that alter uterine muscle contractility.
- Describe drug therapy used during preterm labor to decrease the incidence or severity of neonatal respiratory dysfunction.
- Describe systemic and regional medications for pain control during labor.
- Describe the drugs used in pregnancy-induced hypertension.
- Describe the nursing process, including client teaching, associated with the drugs used during pregnancy and preterm labor.

TERMS

eclampsia
HELLP syndrome
L/S (lecithin/sphingo-
    myelin) ratio

neural tube defects
preeclampsia
pregnancy-induced
    hypertension (PIH)

preterm labor (PTL)
progesterone

teratogens
tocolytic therapy

Introduction

This chapter focuses on the pharmacologic aspects of pregnancy in cycle I and labor and delivery in cycle II. Topics include prenatal health promotion and drugs used for uterine dysfunction during labor and delivery, pain control during labor, and pregnancy-induced hypertension (PIH).

Physiology of Pregnancy

Because pregnancy is a change in the normal physiology of the body, the normal and expected pharmacokinetics and pharmacodynamics of medications also change. Some of the changes in drug action during pregnancy include (1) the effect of circulating steroid hormones on the liver's metabolism of drugs, (2) increased glomelular filtration rate and increased renal perfusion resulting in more rapid renal excretion of drugs, (3) expanded maternal circulating blood volume resulting in dilution of drugs, and (4) alteration in the clearance of drugs in later pregnancy resulting in a decrease in serum and tissue concentrations of drugs. Because of the alteration in the normal physiology of the body, medications should not be ordered in lower doses with longer intervals between doses because of the possibility of subtherapeutic serum and tissue concentrations.

In addition to the aforementioned effects on medication during pregnancy, other factors, such as late pregnancy and labor, can alter the half-lives of some medications. Antibiotics and barbiturates are examples of medications that have shorter half-lives during pregnancy. In contrast to later pregnancy, labor can actually increase the half-life of some medications, such as analgesics, hypnotics, and antibiotics. Labor affects half-life because it is believed that drug clearance decreases as a result of transient reduced blood flow associated with uterine contractions when the mother is in a supine position. In certain disease states during pregnancy, concern arises as to the effects of these conditions on medication. For example, disorders such as diabetes and PIH may result in decreased renal perfusion and subsequent drug accumulation.

The placenta plays an important role in drug use and metabolism; it was thought for some time that the placenta played a barrier role, but it is now known that the placenta plays a major role in the metabolism and the use of medication during pregnancy. It allows some substances to transfer quickly or slowly between mother and fetus, depending on variables such as (1) maternal and fetal blood flow, (2) the molecular weight of the substance (low-molecular-weight substances cross more readily than do higher-molecular-weight substances, and most medications fall into the low-molecular-weight class, which means they would readily cross the placenta), (3) the degree of ionization of the drug molecule (the more ionized the molecule, the less readily it crosses the placenta), (4) the degree of protein binding (highly bound drugs do not cross readily), (5) the metabolic activity of the placenta (the metabolic activity can biotransoform molecules into active metabolites that can affect the fetus).

Guidelines for medication administration during pregnancy must include determination that the benefits of prescribing a drug outweigh potential short- or long-term risks to the maternal-fetal system. Careful selection and monitoring for the minimum effective dose for the shortest interval in the therapeutic range are required. Consideration must be given to alterations related to the physiologic changes of pregnancy.

Liver metabolism of medications is much slower in the fetus as a result of the immaturity of the liver. Therefore drug metabolism is slower in the fetus, which can cause more evident or longer drug effects than on the mother. The degree of fetal exposure to a drug and its breakdown products are more important to fetal outcome than the rate at which the drug is transported to the fetus.

The mechanisms by which drugs cross the placenta are analogous to the way in which drugs infiltrate breast tissue. Lactation results in increased blood flow to the breasts, and drugs accumulate in adipose breast tissue through simple diffusion. Long-term effects on infants from drugs in breast milk are unknown, but medications that do accumulate in breast milk are known, and the breastfeeding mother should be alerted to the potential accumulation.

Despite prenatal education, public service announcements, and information conveyed through the media, use of legal and illicit drugs by pregnant women continues. In addition, health care providers may prescribe drugs for maternal disorders that indirectly affect the fetus. It is estimated that half of the medications taken by pregnant women are over-the-counter (OTC) drugs. The drugs most commonly ingested during pregnancy (other than illicit drugs) are iron and vitamins, antiemetics, antacids, nasal decongestants, mild analgesics, and antibiotics. Pregnant women who use OTC medications should be discouraged from using such medications and consult their health care provider.

Drugs determined conclusively to be safe for the embryo are limited in number. Clinical trials can be recourses for reliable drug information; however it is unethical to test for the safety and efficacy of medications in pregnant women. For this reason the number of medications determined conclusively to be safe for the embryo is limited. Animal studies are required during drug testing, but the information obtained from such studies is difficult to extrapolate to humans. Additionally, case reports are used for such information, but the information contained can in these reports be of limited value because of the isolated occurrence. There are many known **teratogens** (substances that cause developmental abnormalities). Timing, dose, and duration of exposure are of crucial importance

in determining the teratogenicity of a given drug. In humans, the teratogenic period begins after the first 2 weeks. During the first 2 weeks, the embryo is not susceptible to teratogenesis. At this time of development, exposure to teratogens may result in either death of the embryo or minor cellular damage without congenital birth defects. From 2 gestational weeks through the next 10 weeks is the period of organogenesis (development of major structures and organs). Examples of adverse effects of selected illicit substances commonly used during pregnancy are presented in Table 51–1.

Table 51–1

General Adverse Effects of Selected Substances Commonly Abused During Pregnancy

Substance	Maternal Effects	Fetal Effects*
Alcohol (high risk: 6 oz or more/d)	1 oz (2 drinks) absolute alcohol 2 ×/wk: increased risk of spontaneous abortion (2-4 times)	Fetal alcohol syndrome (FAS): mild to moderate mental retardation, altered facial features, growth retardation, low birth weight, small head circumference, hypotonia, and poor motor coordination. Full FAS seen only in some children; others display only fetal alcohol effect (FAE).
Caffeine	2 cups increase epinephrine concentrations after 30 min and decrease intervillous blood flow with potential for spontaneous abortion (dosage and gestational period related)	Excess consumption (>6-8 cups/d) likely toxic to embryo. No evidence of teratogenicity.
Cocaine	48-h clearance via urine. Increased incidence of spontaneous abortion in first trimester. Continued use or sporadic use related to premature delivery and abruptio placentae secondary to placental vasoconstriction and hyperextension.	4-5 d clearance time via urine of newborn because of liver immaturity and lack of cholinesterase. Intrauterine growth retardation, decreased head circumference, intrauterine cerebral infarction. No true withdrawal syndrome but increased irritability, hyperreflexia, and tremulousness. Deficient organization and interactive abilities. By month 4, still exhibits hypertonicity, tremulousness, and impaired motor development. By month 6, effects may appear to be self-limited, but long-term research needed.
Heroin	First trimester spontaneous abortion, premature delivery, inadequate maternal calorie and protein intake.	Neonatal meconium aspiration syndrome; decreased weight and length through postnatal month 9 (weight and length catch up by month 12); smaller head circumference (with no catch up); impaired interactive abilities (hard to console and engage); inconsistent behavioral responses; increased tremulousness and irritability.
Marijuana	Heavy use (5 or more marijuana cigarettes per week): shortened gestation (<37 wk), may hasten delivery through uterine stimulation.	No higher incidence of serious birth defects caused solely by marijuana. Higher incidence of meconium passage during labor.
Tobacco/nicotine	Degenerative placental lesions with areas of poor oxygen exchange; higher incidence of abruptio placentae; placenta previa, vaginal bleeding during pregnancy; possible PROM; possible amnionitis; less likely to choose to breastfeed.	Short stature, smaller head and arm circumferences; no increase in mortality rate or congenital anomalies (some evidence of increased oral clefts); increased respiratory infections beyond the perinatal period; possible shorter attention span beyond perinatal period.
Methadone	If taken before pregnancy, will need to slow detoxification during pregnancy and decrease dose 5 mg every 2 wk. Do not detoxify before week 14 of gestation because of increased risk of spontaneous abortion.	Smaller weight and length through postnatal month 9 (catch up on weight and length by month 12); smaller head circumference (no catch up); withdrawal-induced fetal distress if mother detoxifies after week 32 of gestation.

*Narcotic-exposed infants show a downward trend in development score by age 2, suggesting that lack of environmental stimulation may be the major variable based on the Bayley Scales of Development.
CNS, Central nervous system; *d,* day; *h,* hour; *min,* minute; *PROM,* premature rupture of fetal membranes; *wk,* week; <, less than; >, greater than.

Continued

Table 51–1

General Adverse Effects of Selected Substances Commonly Abused During Pregnancy—cont'd

Substance	Maternal Effects	Fetal Effects*
Barbiturates	CNS depression; lethargy; sleepiness; subtle mood alterations and impaired judgment/fine motor skills for 24 h. No known inhibitory effect on uterine tone or contractility. Selective anticonvulsant activity without anesthesia effects may warrant use in pregnancy for seizure disorders. Active labor with imminent delivery is a contraindication because no antagonist drug is available.	Rapidly cross placenta and cause CNS depression with excessive use/high doses leading to respiratory depression, hyperactivity, and decreased sucking reflex.
Tranquilizers	Dose-dependent; toxic reactions include ataxia, syncope, vertigo, and drowsiness; control of acute eclamptic seizures during labor.	Benzodiazepine (diazepam [Valium]) use in first trimester not associated with oral clefts or other anomalies. Chronic third trimester or labor exposure in high doses associated with hypotonia, hypothermia, hyperbilirubinemia, and poor sucking reflex. Effects may be enhanced if systemic analgesics also given to mother. Fetal effects are prolonged.

Therapeutic Drug and Herbal Use in Pregnancy

The most common indications for use of drugs and herbs during pregnancy are nutritional supplementation with iron, vitamins, and minerals and treatment of nausea and vomiting, gastric acidity, and mild discomforts. See Herbal Alert 51–1.

Iron

During pregnancy approximately twice the normal amount of iron is needed to meet fetal and maternal daily requirements, 27 mg daily during pregnancy compared with 18 mg daily for nonpregnant women 19 to 30 years of age. Supplementation with iron is not generally necessary until the second trimester, when the fetus begins to store iron; the goal is to prevent *maternal* deficiency, not to supply the fetus. The fetus is adequately supplied through the placenta, although the mother is deficient. The time of greatest iron demand is during the third trimester, 22.4 mg daily compared with 6.4 mg daily and

HERBAL ALERT 51–1

Pregnancy

Just as prescription and over-the-counter (OTC) medications are not generally recommended during pregnancy, herbal preparations are also to be avoided. The following herbs in particular should be avoided:

- *Sage:* stimulates uterus
- *Kava kava:* decreases platelets
- *Garlic* and *gingko biloba:* increase bleeding when used with anticoagulants
- *Ginseng:* may decrease action of anticoagulants

Use of these herbal products may be especially deleterious during pregnancy.

18.8 mg daily for the first and second trimesters respectively (National Academy of Sciences, 2000, p. 347).

Although a normal diet generally provides the 18-mg recommended daily allowance (RDA) of iron for nonpregnant clients, nonanemic pregnant women usually are instructed to supplement using a dosage that provides 60 mg of elemental iron; anemic clients should receive 120 mg of elemental iron. The elemental iron content of the most common iron salts includes ferrous sulfate 20% (300 mg of ferrous sulfate is equivalent to 60 mg elemental iron), ferrous sulfate (exsiccated) 30%, ferrous gluconate 12%, and ferrous fumarate 33%. The net iron cost of pregnancy is estimated as approximately 8000 mg. This iron cost is calculated as 250 mg (basal losses) + 320 mg (deposition in fetal and placental tissue) + 500 mg (increased hemoglobin mass) − 350 mg (iron loss in blood associated with delivery (National Academy of Sciences, 2000, p. 345-346). Clients are advised to continue supplements during the 6 weeks postpartum.

Pregnant women generally have a decreased hematocrit early in the third trimester; those with levels less than 30% will have their supplemental iron dosages increased and complete blood counts with platelet and ferritin measured. In those found to have true iron-deficiency anemia, response to iron supplementation is usually noted in 5 to 7 days with a modest reticulocytosis and a rise in the hemoglobin in 3 weeks. No teratogenic effects have been reported with physiologic doses. Numerous OTC and prescription iron products are available in varying dosages, which differ in the amount of elemental iron contained in the form of iron salt. Examples are listed in Table 51–2.

Adverse Reactions

Common side effects of iron supplements include nausea, constipation, black or red tarry stools, epigastric pain, vomiting, and diarrhea.

Table 51–2

Iron Products

Generic (Brand)	Route and Dosage	Uses and Considerations
Ferrous sulfate (Fer-In-Sol, Feosol, Fero-Gradumet, Mol-Iron, Fer-Iron)	A: PO: 300-600 mg/d in divided doses 325 mg/d sufficient to meet needs of noniron deficient pregnant client; with iron deficiency, should receive 325 mg 2-3 ×/d	Hematinic; for iron deficiency anemia; prophylaxis for iron deficiency in pregnancy. Replaces iron stores needed for RBC development. Absorption PO is 5%-30% in intestines; therefore GI side effects. Toxic reactions include pallor, hematemesis, shock, cardiovascular collapse, and metabolic acidosis. Contraindicated in hypersensitivity and peptic ulcer. Decreased absorption of tetracycline, penicillamine, and antacids; increased absorption with ascorbic acid; decreased absorption with eggs, milk, coffee, and tea. Can reduce availability of zinc from the diet. *Nursing implications:* Taking iron at bedtime helps to avoid GI upset. Absorption of iron is promoted when taken with orange juice or other vitamin C source. Use straw (elixir); swallow tablet/capsule whole; take with water on empty stomach. Sit upright 30 min after dose to decrease reflux. Increase fluids, activity, and dietary bulk. Keep away from children. Peak reticulocytosis: 5-10 d; hemoglobin values increase: 2-4 wk *Pregnancy category:* A; PB: UK; $t^{1/2}$: UK; onset: 4 d; duration: 3-4 mo
Ferrous gluconate (Fergon)	A: PO: 200-600 mg t.i.d.	Same as above.
Ferrous fumarate (Fumasorb, Femiron, Feostat, Fumerin)	A: PO: 200 mg t.i.d. or q.i.d.	Same as above.

A, Adult; *d,* day; *GI,* gastrointestinal; *min,* minute; *mo,* month; *PB,* protein-binding; *PO,* by mouth; *q.i.d.,* four times a day; *RBC,* red blood cell; *$t^{1/2}$,* half-life; *t.i.d.,* three times a day; *UK,* unknown; *wk,* week.

Nursing Implications

Liquid forms can cause temporary discoloration of the teeth and therefore should be diluted and administered through a plastic straw. Additionally, iron supplementation may inhibit the absorption of several medications, and appropriate separation of the doses should be followed. For example, iron supplementation should be administered 2 hours before or 4 hours after antacids. Additional examples of such medications that may require separation in dose include levodopa, levothyroxine, methyldopa, penicillamine, quinolones, and tetracyclines. For the same reasons, do not administer with milk.

Folic Acid

The ingestion of folic acid as a part of preconception planning improves the outcomes of pregnancy. During pregnancy, folic acid (vitamin B_6, folacin) is needed in increased amounts. Folic acid deficiency early in pregnancy can result in spontaneous abortion or birth defects (e.g., **neural tube defects**), premature birth, low birth weight, and premature separation of the placenta (*abruptio placentae*). In the United States, approximately 4000 pregnancies are affected by neural-tube defects. Controlled clinical trials have demonstrated that folic acid supplementation can reduce this incidence by as much as 50%.

The RDA for folic acid in the nonpregnant client is 180 mcg; it is recommended, however, that all women of childbearing age ingest 400 mcg of folic acid daily to reduce the risk in potential offspring. In contrast, during pregnancy the RDA for pregnancy is 600 mcg. The reason behind this recommendation is because of the high incidence of unplanned and unrecognized pregnancies. The neural tube closes within the first 4 weeks of pregnancy; therefore it is important that women consume the recommended amounts of folic acid per day. For women who have had a pregnancy that was affected by a neural tube defect, higher doses of folic acid are recommended; the recommended dose for women in this category is 4 mg starting 1 to 3 months before conception. In contrast, during pregnancy the RDA for pregnancy is 600 mcg.

The recommended amount should be ingested from folate-enriched foods and supplementation because the amount of naturally occurring folic acid ingested in foods will vary from day to day, and the folic acid from these sources is not well absorbed. Examples of folate-enriched foods include bread, rolls, flour, cornmeal, rice, pasta, and cereals.

Adverse Reactions

Side effects are not common but include allergic bronchospasm, rash, pruritus, erythema, and general malaise. Clients should be aware that folic acid supplementation may cause their urine to turn more intensely yellow.

Multiple Vitamins

Prenatal vitamin preparations are routinely recommended for pregnant women. These preparations generally supply vitamins A, D, E, C, B complex (B_1, B_2, B_3, B_5, B_6), B_{12}, iron, calcium, and other minerals. The role of prenatal vitamins in preventing congenital defects (e.g., cleft lip or palate, limb defects) remains undetermined.

Poor food habits cannot be rectified through supplements alone; vitamins are used most effectively by the body when taken with meals. Calories and protein are not supplied by supplements.

Megadoses of vitamins and minerals during pregnancy will not improve health and may cause harm to the fetus, the pregnant client, or both. Large doses of vitamin A can be teratogenic, and excessive ingestion of vitamins D, E, and K may also be toxic.

Practitioners should consider cultural food practices and beliefs in regard to the use of prenatal vitamins. For example, in Mexico, some people view vitamins as a *hot* food that should not be ingested during pregnancy. Cultural sensitivity is important in assessment and teaching regarding herbs, foods, and nonprescription and prescription drugs.

Drugs for Minor Discomforts of Pregnancy

The average prenatal client uses three drugs during pregnancy, two of which are vitamin and mineral supplements. Drug ingestion is most likely during the first and the third trimesters, when the minor discomforts of pregnancy tend to be most bothersome. Many of the complaints associated with pregnancy will be related to the gastrointestinal (GI) tract (nausea and vomiting, heartburn, constipation). The etiology of nausea and vomiting is unclear. Physiologically, nausea is purported to be related to increased human chorionic gonadotropin (hCG) levels of pregnancy. The increased progesterone of pregnancy, which relaxes smooth muscle, contributes to the discomforts of heartburn and constipation. The physiologic reason is that the elevated female sex hormones during pregnancy change the motility of the GI tract. Additionally, the enlarging uterus displaces the bowel.

Nausea and Vomiting

Nausea and vomiting (morning sickness) during early pregnancy are major complaints for most (about 88%) pregnant women, but *hyperemesis gravidaum* (severe nausea and vomiting requiring hospitalization for hydration and nutrition) occurs in a much lower incidence (1% to 3%). Nausea and vomiting are common possibly because of increased levels of hCG, changes in the metabolism of carbohydrates, and emotional changes. Nonpharmacologic measures to decrease nausea and vomiting include (1) eating crackers, dry toast, or bread, dry cereal, or other complex carbohydrates before rising; (2) avoiding fatty or highly seasoned foods; (3) eating small, frequent meals; (4) drinking fluids between rather than with meals; (5) drinking apple juice or flat carbonated beverages between meals; (6) eating a high-protein bedtime snack; (7) stopping or cutting down on smoking; and (8) taking an iron supplement at bedtime. These measures work well for most women, but if vomiting is severe, fluid replacement and pharmacologic measures may be necessary.

The Food and Drug Administration (FDA) has *not* approved any drug for morning sickness, nor is there consensus among health care providers who do prescribe drug therapy as to the best agents. Antiemetic drug studies often find that affected women rate even placebo agents as helpful. Examples of commonly used antiemetics include phenothiazines (promethazine), antihistamines (doxylamine), anticholinergics (scopolamine), prokinetic agents (metoclopramide), and ginger. Table 51–3 presents examples of the most commonly used drugs for management of nausea and vomiting during pregnancy.

Many women may choose to use ginger to help treat nausea and vomiting associated with pregnancy. However, there is insufficient evidence to determine the safety and efficacy of the use of ginger during pregnancy. Recent studies suggest that ginger can be safely used, but as with all medications and herbal supplements, encourage the pregnant client to discuss the use of ginger with her health care provider.

Women who experience nausea and vomiting may experience gastric distress if they are also taking supplemental iron; temporary suspension of iron therapy may help. It is suggested that prenatal vitamins be taken at the time of day the client is least likely to experience emesis because there is a high incidence of nausea and vomiting associated with prenatal vitamins. In addition, taking iron with meals or at bedtime has been shown to decrease gastric distress. For clients with continued iron-induced gastric distress, many health care providers recommend taking two Flinstones vitamins with iron. Salting food to taste may help to replace vomited chloride; foods rich in potassium and magnesium may also help replace lost nutrients.

Clients whose symptoms persist and who experience weight loss and dehydration may require intravenous (IV) rehydration, including replacement of electrolytes and vitamins. Antiemetic therapy (probably with phenothiazines) may be used.

Heartburn

Heartburn (*pyrosis*) is a burning sensation in the epigastric and sternal regions that occurs with reflux of acidic stomach contents. The incidence of heartburn during pregnancy is common, up to 80%. Pregnant clients experience decreased motility in the GI tract as a result of the normal increase in the hormone **progesterone.** Progesterone also relaxes the cardiac sphincter (the sphincter leading into the stomach from the esophagus also called the *lower esophageal sphincter*), making reflux activity (*reverse peristalsis*) more likely. Digestion and gastric emptying are slower than in the nonpregnant state. Heartburn is common when a pregnant client sits or lies down soon after eating a normal meal, only to have her gravid uterus exert upward force on her stomach, causing increased reflux activity and the perception of hyperacidity. Heartburn is a disorder of the second and third trimesters of pregnancy.

Nonpharmacologic measures are preferred in the management of heartburn. These include (1) limiting the size of meals; (2) avoiding highly seasoned, fried, or greasy

Table 51-3

Drugs for Management of Nausea and Vomiting During Pregnancy (Recommendation Not Implied)

Generic (Brand)	Route and Dosage	Uses and Considerations
Antihistamines		
meclizine (Antivert, Bonine, Vergon)	PO: 20-50 mg/d	No evidence of teratogenesis. In use since 1956. Considered mild; available as OTC drug. Site of action is labyrinth and CNS. Blocks CTZ, which acts on vomiting center. Metabolized in liver and excreted unchanged in feces and as metabolites in urine. Increased effect of alcohol, tranquilizers, and narcotics. *Side effects:* Dizziness, drowsiness, dry mouth and nose, blurred vision, diplopia, urinary retention, urticaria, rash, and headache. Cardiovascular effects can include hypotension, palpitations, and tachycardia. *Contraindications:* Hypersensitivity to drug or any component. *Warnings/precautions:* Use with closed-angle glaucoma. *Pregnancy category:* B; $t^1/_2$: 6 h; onset: 1-2 h; duration: 8-24 h.
Phenothiazine		
promethazine (Phenergan)	PO, IV, IM, PR: 12.5-25 mg q4-6h prn	*Mechanism of action:* Blocks postsynaptic mesolimbic dopaminergic receptors in the brain; exhibits a strong alpha-adrenergic blocking effect and depresses the release of hypothalamic and hypophyseal hormones; competes with histamine for the H_1 receptor. *Adverse reactions:* Dizziness, drowsiness, excitation, fatigue, insomnia, photosensitivity reactions, nausea, vomiting, and constipation. *Contraindications:* Hypersensitivity to drug or any component of the formulation; CNS depression or coma. *Warnings/precautions:* Use caution in cardiovascular disease, not for subQ or intra-arterial administration; injection may contain sulfites which may cause allergic reactions in some clients. *Pregnancy category:* C, $t^1/_2$: 9-16 h; onset IM 20 min, IV 3-5 min, duration 2-6 h
Anticholinergic		
scopolamine (Scopace)	IM, IV, subQ 0.3-0.65 mg q4-6h	*Mechanism of action:* Antagonizes histamine and serotonin *Adverse reactions:* Confusion, drowsiness, headache, fatigue, dry skin, constipation, vomiting, bloated feeling. Cardiovascular side effects include orthostatic hypotension, ventricular fibrillation, tachycardia, palpitations. *Contraindications:* Hypersensitivity to the active ingredient or any component of the formulation. Narrow-angle glaucoma, acute hemorrhage, GI or GU obstruction, tachycardia secondary to cardiac insufficiency, and myasthenia gravis. *Warnings/precautions:* Use with caution in hepatic or renal impairment. *Pregnancy category:* C; onset IM 0.5-1 h, duration 4-6 h.
Prokinetic Agents		
metoclopramide (Reglan)	PO: 10-15 mg QID 30 min a.c.	*Mechanism of action:* Blocks dopamine receptors in chemoreceptor trigger zone of the CNS, causes enhanced motility and accelerated gastric emptying without stimulating secretions. *Adverse reactions:* Restlessness, drowsiness, diarrhea, weakness, insomnia. *Contraindications:* Hypersensitivity to metoclopramide or any component of the formulation. GI obstruction, perforation or hemorrhage; pheochromocytoma; history of seizure disorder. *Pregnancy category:* B; $t^1/_2$ 4-7 h; onset 0.5-1 h, duration 1-2 h
Other		
trimethobenzamide (Tigan, T-Gen)	200 mg rectally, q6-8h	Obscure action; may be mediated through CTZ. Does not inhibit direct impulse to vomiting center. Chemically classified as an ethanolamine derivative. Precautions include use in client with cardiac dysrhythmias, narrow-angle glaucoma, asthma, and pyloroduodenal obstruction. Rectal doses of the drug are more unpredictable. *Side effects:* Drowsiness, headache, blurred vision, diarrhea, depression, hypotension, muscle cramps, allergic reactions, and extrapyramidal symptoms; blood dyscrasias *Contraindications:* Benzocaine, hypersensitivity to drug. Use suppository form in neonates or preterm infants. *Warning/precaution:* Avoid use in acute emesis to avoid masking of symptoms. *Drug interactions:* Phenothiazines/barbiturates, belladonna *Pregnancy category:* C; $t^1/_2$: UK; onset: PO/PR: 10-40 min; IM: 15-35 min; duration: 3-4 h

a.c., Before meals; *CNS,* central nervous system; *CTZ,* chemoreceptor trigger zone; *d,* day; *GI,* gastrointestinal; *GU,* genitourinary; *H_1,* histamine 1; *h,* hour; *IM,* intramuscular; *IV,* intravenous; *min,* minute; *OTC,* over-the-counter; *PO,* by mouth; *PR,* by rectum; *PRN,* as needed; *subQ,* subcutaneous; *$t^1/_2$,* half-life; *UK,* unknown.

foods; (3) avoiding gas-forming foods (e.g., cabbage, beans, onions); (4) eating slowly and chewing thoroughly; (5) avoiding citrus juices; (6) drinking adequate fluids but not with meals; and (7) avoiding reclining immediately after eating.

Antacids should be considered first line of therapy if the client does not respond to nonpharmacologic therapy. The antacids of choice for the pregnant client include nonsystemic low-sodium products (those considered dietetically sodium free) containing aluminum and magnesium (in the form of hydroxide) in combination. These two ingredients can also be found in the combined form of magaldrate (also called *hydroxymagnesium aluminate*). Discourage the long-term use or large doses of magnesium antacids because fetal renal, respiratory, cardiovascular, and muscle problems may result. Some products also include simethicone (Mylicon), an antiflatulent used to decrease the surface tension of GI gas bubbles, burst the bubbles, and promote rapid gas expulsion. Additionally, sucralfate is likely safe during pregnancy because the drug is not systemically absorbed. Calcium carbonate antacid preparations may be avoided in pregnancy because of the rebound effect following acid neutralization by the antacid. Tums are frequently taken by pregnant women for heartburn. Because Tums are calcium based, excessive use may further contribute to the constipation of pregnancy.

Most clients do not realize that remedies commonly used by nonpregnant women (e.g., baking soda [sodium bicarbonate], antacids such as Alka-Seltzer, Bromo-Seltzer, Rolaids) can be harmful during pregnancy. Selection of the wrong antacid can result in diarrhea, constipation, or electrolyte imbalance. The combination of nonpharmacologic measures plus minimal use of safe antacids should effectively meet the pregnant client's needs.

Liquid antacids are the preparations most commonly used in pregnancy because of their uniform dissolution, their rapid action, and their greater activity. Tablets are also acceptable, particularly for convenience, provided these are thoroughly chewed and the client maintains an adequate fluid intake.

Histamine$_2$ receptor antagonists (H$_2$RAs) can be used during pregnancy, but only if the client has failed initial treatment with antacids, and their use is recommended by a health care provider. The teratogenicity of these medications is unknown; however, cimetidine, ranitidine, famotidine, and nizatidine have received the FDA's pregnancy category B rating. H$_2$RAs work by competitively and reversibly binding to the histamine receptors of the parietal cells, causing a reduction in gastric acid secretion. The onset of action is generally in 1 hour and can persist for 6 to 12 hours.

There is even less experience with the use of proton pump inhibitors. These medications work by suppressing gastric acid secretion by inhibiting the proton pump on the surface of the parietal cells. With the recent release of Prilosec OTC (omeprazole), pregnant clients may be inquisitive about its use for heartburn during pregnancy. Encourage clients to discuss the options with their provider. Currently the use of omeprazole is limited to cases in which the benefits of therapy far outweigh the risks.

Table 51–4 presents medications for heartburn commonly used during pregnancy.

Constipation

Constipation is a frequent occurrence during pregnancy. Its cause may be related to hormonal changes, specifically progesterone, which decreases GI motility. Like heartburn, nonpharmacologic treatments for constipation should be tried first. These include (1) increasing fluid intake, (2) increasing dietary fiber intake, and (3) physical exercise.

If the aforementioned methods do not work, treatment is indicated, and the safest agent is considered the bulk-forming preparations containing fiber (for example, Metamucil). This is because these agents are not systemically absorbed. Also, docusate sodium, a stool softener, would be appropriate as first-line treatment during pregnancy. Agents that should be reserved for occasional use include milk of magnesia, magnesium citrate, lactulose, sorbitol, bisacodyl, and senna.

Castor oil should be avoided during pregnancy because it can cause uterine contractions. Mineral oil should also be avoided because it can reduce the absorption of fat-soluble vitamins such as vitamin K; low levels of vitamin K in the neonate can result in hemorrhage.

Pain

Headaches (up through week 26 resulting from hormonally induced body changes, sinus congestion, or eye strain), backaches, joint pains, round ligament pain resulting in mild abdominal aches and pains, and minor injuries are common in pregnancy. Nonpharmacologic pain relief measures should be tried initially. These include rest, nonstimulatory environment, relaxation exercises, alteration in routine, mental imagery, ice packs, warm moist heat, postural changes, correct body mechanics, and changes in the height and style of footwear.

Acetaminophen. Acetaminophen (Tylenol, Datril), a para-aminophenol analgesic, is a pregnancy category B drug. It is the most commonly ingested nonprescription drug during pregnancy. Acetaminophen is commonly used during all trimesters of pregnancy in therapeutic doses on a short-term basis, generally for its analgesic and antipyretic effects. The drug is a weak prostaglandin inhibitor and does not have significant anti-inflammatory effects. Chapter 21, Drugs for Pain Management: Nonnarcotic and Narcotic Analgesics, presents a drug chart for in-depth review of pharmacokinetics.

Pharmacokinetics.

The rate of absorption is dependent on the rate of gastric emptying. Acetaminophen is 20% to 50% protein bound and crosses the placenta during pregnancy; it also is found in low concentrations in breast milk. Acetaminophen is partially hepatically metabolized into inactive metabolites; however, a highly active metabolite (N-acetyl-p-benzoquinone) is produced only in large doses and can have potential liver and kidney toxicity. The half-life is 2 to 3 hours. To date there is no concrete evidence of fetal anomalies associated with the use of the drug, and no adverse effects have been noted in breastfed infants of mothers who used the drug while pregnant or breastfeeding.

Table 51–4

Over-the-Counter Antacids Commonly Used in Pregnancy

Generic (Brand)	Route and Dosage	Uses and Considerations
aluminum hydroxide (Amphojel)	A: PO: As directed*	Contains aluminum hydroxide gel (320 mg) per 300 mg tablet or per 5 ml; ANC 8; contains saccharin and sorbitol. OTC preparation. *Use:* For heartburn secondary to reflux. *Action:* Neutralization of gastric acidity. *Side effects:* Constipation. *Adverse reactions:* Dehydration, hypophosphatemia (long-term use), GI obstruction. *Drug interactions:* Decreased effects with tetracycline, phenothiazine, benzodiazepines, isoniazid, digoxin; follow dose with water. *Pregnancy category:* C; PB: UK; $t^{1}/_{2}$: UK; onset: 15-30 min; peak: 0.5 h; duration: 1-3 h
magnesium hydroxide and aluminum hydroxide with Simethicone (Maalox Plus, Extra Strength Maalox Plus Suspension, Mylanta Liquid, Mylanta II)	As directed*	*Maalox Plus Tablets:* Each tablet contains magnesium hydroxide (200 mg), aluminum hydroxide (200 mg), and Simethicone (25 mg); ANC 11, 4; chewable; contains saccharin and sorbitol; OTC *Extra Strength Maalox Plus Suspension:* Each 5 ml contains magnesium hydroxide (450 mg), aluminum hydroxide (500 mg), and Simethicone (40 mg); ANC 28; contains saccharin and sorbitol; OTC. *Mylanta Liquid:* Each 5 ml contains magnesium hydroxide (200 mg), aluminum hydroxide (200 mg), and Simethicone (25 mg); ANC 12.7; contains sorbitol; OTC. *Mylanta II:* Each 5 ml contains magnesium hydroxide (400 mg), aluminum hydroxide (400 mg), and Simethicone (40 mg); ANC 23; OTC. *Use:* Same as above with addition of antiflatulence action. *Drug interactions:* Same as above, with addition of allopurinol, quinolones, ketoconazole. *Pregnancy category:* C; PB: UK; $t^{1}/_{2}$: UK.
magaldrate with Simethicone (Riopan Plus Tablets, Riopan Plus Suspension)	As directed*	*Riopan Plus Tablets:* Each contains Magaldrate (480 mg) and Simethicone (20 mg); ANC 13.5; chewable; contains sorbitol. *Riopan Plus Suspension:* Each 5 ml contains magaldrate (540 mg) and Simethicone (20 mg); ANC 15; contains saccharin. *Use:* Same as above. *Action:* Same as above. *Side effects:* Same as above. *Adverse reactions:* Same as above. *Drug interactions:* Decreased absorption of phenothiazines, isoniazid, fluoroquinolones, tetracyclines *Pregnancy category:* C; $t^{1}/_{2}$: UK; PB: UK; onset: immediate; peak: UK; duration: prolonged.

*Dosage recommendations for antacid preparations should be clarified by the health care provider; however, as a general rule, no more than 12 tablets or 12 tsp should be taken in a 24-hour period depending on the strength of the product. Major side effects are a change in bowel habits (diarrhea or constipation), nausea, vomiting, alkalosis, and hypermagnesemia. Antacids figure in numerous drug interactions owing to their action on gastric pH (increased) and their propensity to bind with other drugs to form poorly absorbed complexes. Antacids should not be given within 2 hours of iron, digitalis products, or tetracycline. Likewise, when a client takes a phenothiazine as an antiemetic, 2 hours should elapse between administration of these drugs.

A, Adult; ANC, acid-neutralizing capacity (per tablet or 5 ml); GI, gastrointestinal; h, hour; min, minute; OTC, over-the-counter; PB, protein-binding; PO, by mouth; $t^{1}/_{2}$, half-life; tsp, teaspoon; UK, unknown.

Pharmacodynamics

Use of acetaminophen during pregnancy should not exceed 12 tablets per 24 hours of a 325-mg formulation (regular strength) or 8 tablets per 24 hours of a 500-mg (extra strength) formulation (because of the potential for kidney and liver toxicity). The drug should be taken at 4- to 6-hour intervals. Onset of effects following oral ingestion is within 10 to 30 minutes; peak action occurs at 1 to 2 hours; duration lasts from 3 to 5 hours.

Adverse Reactions

Most clients *without* preexisting renal or hepatic disease tolerate acetaminophen well. Clients with hypersensitivity to the compound should not use it. Acetaminophen should be used cautiously in clients at risk for infection because of the possibility of masking signs and symptoms. The most frequent side effects are skin eruptions, urticaria, unusual bruising, erythema, hypoglycemia, jaundice, hemolytic anemia, neutropenia, leukopenia, pancytopenia, and thrombocytopenia.

Aspirin. Aspirin (ASA, Bayer, Ecotrin, Halfprin), a salicylate, is classified as a mild analgesic. Aspirin is a pregnancy category C drug (which changes to category D if full-dose aspirin is used in the third trimester). Aspirin is discussed in Chapter 21, Drugs for Pain Management: Nonnarcotic and Narcotic Analgesics.

Aspirin is a prostaglandin synthetase inhibitor that has antipyretic, analgesic, and anti-inflammatory properties. Teratogenic effects have not been shown conclusively, and the risk of anomalies is perceived to be small.

Aspirin can inhibit the initiation of labor and actually prolong labor through its effects on uterine contractility; therefore its use is not recommended during pregnancy. In addition, aspirin use late in pregnancy is associated with greater maternal blood loss at delivery. There may be increased risk of anemia in pregnancy and of antepartum hemorrhage as well. Hemostasis is affected in the newborn whose mother ingested aspirin during the last 2 months of pregnancy (even without use during the actual week of delivery). The platelets are unable to aggregate to form clots, and it appears that this is not a reversible effect after delivery; the infant has to wait for its own bone marrow to produce new platelets.

Nursing Process
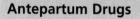

Antepartum Drugs

ASSESSMENT

■ Gather comprehensive medical, drug (illict, nonpharmcologic and pharmacologic), and herbal history.
■ Obtain baseline vital signs.
■ Identify clients at risk for substance abuse and collaborate with other professionals to plan strategies to minimize risks.
■ Assess drug history to determine whether antacid use will interfere with absorption.
■ Review history of aspirin use when admitting a client in labor. If aspirin has been used, alert the staff and monitor for increased bleeding.
■ Ascertain any medical history of alcoholism, liver disease, viral infection, and renal deficiencies. Acetaminophen should be used cautiously in these clients.

NURSING DIAGNOSES

■ Deficient knowledge related to health maintenance needs during pregnancy
■ Deficient knowledge related to potential fetal outcomes from exposure to teratogens.

PLANNING

■ Client will use and avoid various drugs during pregnancy as advised.
■ Client will discuss drugs (illict, nonpharmcologic and pharmacologic), and herbal use with health care provider or pharmacist prior to use.

NURSING INTERVENTIONS

General

■ Be cognizant that drug use may be part of multiple substance abuse and may also involve maternal-neonatal infections.
■ Stress the importance of prenatal care, and discuss fears client may have about health care professionals and concerns about legal action in the event of substance abuse.

Specific

■ Instruct on nonpharmacologic and pharmacologic measures to relieve common pregnancy discomforts.
■ Refer to tobacco, alcohol, or drug treatment program if appropriate.
■ Instruct on nutritional and therapeutic supplements needed during pregnancy.
■ Monitor hemoglobin/hematocrit of prenatal clients per agency protocol.

Iron

■ Question client about nausea, constipation, and bowel habit changes if taking iron preparations.
■ Give diluted liquid iron preparation through a plastic straw to prevent discoloration of teeth.
■ Store iron in a light-resistant container.
■ Be cognizant that client may have false-positive result of occult blood in stool if taking iron.

Client Teaching

General
• Advise pregnant woman that tobacco, alcohol, and heavy caffeine use may have adverse effects on the fetus.
• Instruct client that before taking drugs (illicit, OTC, prescribed) to discuss with health care provider secondary to teratogenic potential.
• Advise client planning to breastfeed to discuss drugs (illicit, OTC, prescribed) with health care provider.

Aspirin/Acetaminophen
• Advise client not to take aspirin during pregnancy, particularly during the third trimester.

Antepartum Drugs
• Instruct client not to take nonsteroidal antiinflammatory drugs (NSAIDs) with acetaminophen.

Caffeine/Alcohol/Nicotine
• Advise client to limit coffee and caffeine ingestion from none to 1 to 2 cups per day and to limit other sources of caffeine (tea, cola, soft drinks, chocolate, certain drugs).

- If caffeine is allowed by the health care provider, teach client to space limited caffeine intake evenly throughout the day because caffeine passes readily to the fetus, who cannot metabolize it. Caffeine can decrease intervillous placental blood flow.
- Advise client to use decaffeinated products or dilute caffeinated products.
- Suggest that client use herbal products carefully because of occasionally harmful ingredients. (See Herbal Alert 51–1.)
- If client plans to breastfeed, tell her that 1% of the caffeine she consumes will appear in her breast milk within 15 minutes. Therefore, although a cup of coffee is not a problem, it is not wise to drink several cups of coffee in succession; excess caffeine will accumulate in the infant's tissues. The infant lacks enzymes to adequately clear the caffeine for 7 to 9 months after birth.
- Instruct client not to drink alcohol if she is pregnant because no safe level of alcohol has been determined and even minimal exposure has resulted in fetal alcohol effect and moderate/excess exposure has resulted in fetal alcohol syndrome.
- Advise client that smoking can cause the loss of nutrients such as vitamins A and C, folic acid, cobalamin, and calcium. Tobacco use may contribute to a shortened gestation and low-birth-weight infants.

Antacids
- Advise that antacids should not be taken within 1 hour of taking an enteric-coated tablet because the acid-resistant coating may dissolve in the increased alkaline condition of the stomach, and the medication will not be released in the intestine as intended. Stomach upset may result.
- Advise client to store antacid liquid suspension at room temperature, not to let it freeze, and to shake the bottle well before pouring.

Iron
- Instruct client about dietary sources of iron, which include organ meats (liver), red meat, nuts and seeds, wheat germ, spinach, broccoli, prunes, and iron-fortified cereals.
- Explain to client that if supplemental iron is taken between meals, increased absorption (and also increased side effects) may result. Taking iron 1 hour before meals is suggested. Give with juice or water but not with milk or antacids.

Self-Administration for Iron and Antacids
- Advise client to swallow the iron tablets whole, not to crush them. Liquid iron preparations should be taken with a plastic straw to avoid staining the teeth.

- Caution client not to take antacids with iron because antacids impair absorption and are generally discouraged during pregnancy. Iron and antacids should be taken 2 hours apart if both are prescribed.

Side Effects for Iron and Antacids
- Advise client to keep *iron* tablets away from children. Iron tablets look like candy, and death has been reported in small children who have ingested 2 g or less of ferrous sulfate.
- Advise client that there may be a change in bowel habits when taking *antacids*. Aluminum products can cause constipation, whereas magnesium products can cause diarrhea. Many antacids contain both ingredients.

EVALUATION

- Evaluate the effectiveness of the prescribed drug therapy. Report side effects.
- Evaluate client's understanding of possible effects on the fetus with maternal use of drugs (pharmacologic, OTC, and illicit) and the use of tobacco and alcohol.

Drugs that Decrease Uterine Muscle Contractility

Preterm Labor

Preterm labor (PTL) is labor that occurs between 20 and 37 weeks of pregnancy involving a fetus with an estimated weight between 500 and 2499 g. Regular contractions occur at less than 10-minute intervals over 30 to 60 minutes and are strong enough to result in 2-cm cervical dilation and 80% effacement. PTL occurs in approximately 8% to 10% of all pregnancies. Preterm infants who survive very early delivery have significant physiologic challenges to overcome. PTL that progresses to preterm delivery accounts for most perinatal morbidity and mortality (excluding fetuses with anomalies) in the United States.

Although PTL has no single known cause, certain risk factors have been identified: maternal age younger than 18 or older than 40 years, low socioeconomic status, previous history of preterm delivery (17% to 37% chance of recurrence), intrauterine infections (i.e., bacterial vaginosis), polyhydramnios, multiple gestation, uterine anomalies, antepartum hemorrhage, smoking, drug use, urinary tract infections, and incompetent cervix. Attempts to arrest PTL are *contraindicated* in (1) pregnancy of less than 20 weeks' gestation (confirmed by ultrasound), (2) bulging or premature rupture of membranes (PROM), (3) confirmed fetal death or anomalies incompatible with life, (4) maternal hemorrhage and evidence of severe fetal compromise, and (5) chorioamnionitis.

Nonpharmacologic treatment measures for PTL include bed rest, hydration (ingestion of six to eight glasses of fluids daily or more, IV fluid bolus), pelvic rest (no sexual intercourse or douching), and screening for intrauterine and urinary tract infections. Client assessment will include uterine activity (frequency, duration, and intensity), vaginal bleeding or discharge, and fetal monitoring.

Tocolytic Therapy

When clients in true PTL (with cervical change) have no contraindications, they become candidates for **tocolytic therapy** (drug therapy to decrease uterine muscle contractions) using beta-adrenergic receptor agonists (e.g., terbutaline [Brethine]) or the calcium antagonist magnesium sulfate. The goal in tocolytic therapy is to interrupt or inhibit uterine contractions to create additional time for in utero fetal maturation, to delay delivery so antenatal corticosteroids can be delivered to facilitate fetal lung maturation, or to allow safe transport of the mother to an appropriate facility.

Table 51–5 lists the most commonly used drugs to decrease preterm uterine contractions.

Beta-Sympathomimetic Drugs

Beta-sympathomimetic drugs act by stimulating beta$_2$-receptors on smooth muscle. The frequency and intensity of uterine contractions decrease as the muscle relaxes. Terbutaline (Brethine) is commonly used. It is approved for medicinal use but not specifically as a tocolytic. Terbutaline can effectively decrease uterine contractions; however, the literature indicates that knowledge about the long-term effects of this drug is still lacking.

Pharmacokinetics

Clients with mild contractions may be given subcutaneous terbutaline (Brethine) initially, followed by a series of subcutaneous (subQ) injections of terbutaline. Clients are monitored to determine whether and when contractions diminish or cease. It is minimally protein bound (25%) and metabolized via the liver to inactive metabolites. Terbutaline's half-life is 11 to 16 hours. Oral therapy or subcutaneous pump therapy with terbutaline may be prescribed for longer-term maintenance.

Pharmacodynamics

Oral terbutaline has an onset of action of 30 to 45 minutes, a peak plasma/serum concentration of 1 to 2 hours, and a duration of action of 4 to 8 hours. IV and subcutaneous terbutaline have an onset of action

Table 51–5

Drugs Used to Decrease Uterine Contractility

Generic (Brand)	Route and Dosage	Uses and Considerations
Beta-Adrenergic Agent terbutaline (Brethine)	Follow agency protocols for specific directives plus individual health care provider's order; may be given subQ; usually therapy is 0.25 mg subQ to 0.5 mg subQ every 3 to 4 h.	Sympathomimetic beta$_2$-adrenergic agonist. Partially metabolized in the liver; excreted by the kidneys. 40%-50% rate of tocolytic breakthrough and recurrence of preterm labor 3 wk after start of PO therapy may require repeat therapy (may be due to desensitization of beta receptors over time). Current research focused on use of low-dose continuous subQ pumps that are portable and can deliver intermittent bolus doses based on data reflecting peak need periods. Pumps are cost-effective with high client satisfaction. Increases in maternal pulse and FHR. Rapidly crosses placenta; breastfeeding not contraindicated because of short half-life. *Drug interactions:* Additive effect with CNS depressants (narcotics, sedative-hypnotics) and neuromuscular blocking agents. *Pregnancy category:* B; t$_{1/2}$: 11-16 h; onset: 15 min IV/subQ and 30-45 min PO; duration: 4-8 h PO and 1.5-4 h subQ; peak serum levels: 0.5-1 h IV/subQ and 1-2 h PO.
Calcium Antagonist magnesium sulfate	Follow agency protocols for specific directives plus individual physician orders for concentration and ml/h IV: usual LD: 4-6 g in 100 ml over 15-20 min; *maint:* 40 g in 1 L of IVF at 2-4 g/h. Dose based on serum magnesium levels, deep tendon reflex assessment, and uterine response	Calcium antagonist and CNS depressant. Relaxes uterine smooth muscle through calcium displacement. Must be given by infusion pump for accurate dosage. Freely crosses placenta. Few contraindications allow for use in clients who exhibit life-threatening complications. Maternal magnesium levels monitored through serum analyses, DTR, respiratory rate, and urinary output. Elevated levels may be evident in newborn for 7 d; observe newborn for 24-48 h for signs of toxicity if mother treated close to delivery; breastfeeding not contraindicated. *Antidote:* calcium gluconate 1 g given IV over 3 min. *Pregnancy category:* B; onset: immediate by IV; duration: 30 min.

CNS, Central nervous system; *d,* day; *DTR,* deep tendon reflex; *FHR,* fetal heart rate; *h,* hour; *IV,* intravenous; *IVF,* intravenous fluid; *LD,* loading dose; *maint,* maintenance; *min,* minute; *PO,* by mouth; *subQ,* subcutaneous; *t$_{1/2}$,* half-life; *wk,* week.

within 15 minutes, a peak serum concentration level in 30 to 60 minutes, and a duration of action of 1.5 to 4 hours subQ.

Adverse Reactions

Maternal side effects include tremors, malaise, weakness, dyspnea, tachycardia (maternal and fetal), increased systolic pressure and decreased diastolic pressure, chest pain, nausea, vomiting, diarrhea, constipation, erythema, sweating, hyperglycemia, and hypokalemia. Many of these effects are associated with terbutaline's cross-reactivity with beta$_1$-adrenergic receptors. More serious adverse reactions include pulmonary edema, dysrhythmias, ketoacidosis, and anaphylactic shock.

Fetal side effects include tachycardia and potential hypoglycemia resulting from fetal hyperinsulinemia caused by maternal hyperglycemia.

Drug Interactions

The increased effects of general anesthetics can produce additive hypotension. Pulmonary edema can occur with concurrent use of corticosteroids. Cardiovascular effects may be additive with other sympathomimetic drugs, such as epinephrine, albuterol, and isoproterenol. Beta-adrenergic blocking agents, such as propranolol HCl, nadolol, pindolol, timolol maleate, and metoprolol tartrate, antagonize beta-sympathomimetics.

Magnesium Sulfate

Magnesium sulfate, a calcium antagonist and central nervous system depressant, relaxes the smooth muscle of the uterus through calcium displacement. Administered IV, the drug has a direct depressant effect on uterine muscle contractility. The drug increases uterine perfusion, which has a therapeutic effect on the fetus. This drug, which is also less expensive, may be safer to use than the beta-sympathomimetics because it has fewer adverse effects; it can also be used when beta-sympathomimetics are contraindicated (e.g., in women with diabetes and cardiovascular disease). The drug is excreted by the kidneys and crosses the placenta. The maintenance dose must be titrated to keep uterine contractions under control, and magnesium levels are drawn based on the clinical response of the client. Magnesium sulfate therapy is contraindicated in clients who have myasthenia gravis; impaired kidney function and recent myocardial infarction are relative contraindications. Clients with renal impairment may require adjusted dosages. Do not confuse magnesium sulfate with manganese sulfate.

Adverse Reactions

Dosage-related side effects in the maternal client include flush, feelings of increased warmth, perspiration, dizziness, nausea, headache, lethargy, slurred speech, sluggishness, nasal congestion, heavy eyelids, blurred vision, decreased GI action, increased pulse rate, and hypotension. Increased severity is evidenced by depressed reflexes, confusion, and magnesium toxicity (respiratory depression and arrest, circulatory collapse, cardiac arrest). Side effects in the fetus are decreased fetal heart rate variability and, in the neonate, slight hypotonia with diminished reflexes and lethargy for 24 to 48 hours.

If maternal neurologic, respiratory, or cardiac depression is evidenced, the antidote is calcium gluconate (10 mg IV push over 3 minutes).

Nursing Process

Beta$_2$-Adrenergic Agonists: Brethine (Terbutaline)

ASSESSMENT

■ Identify risks for preterm labor (PTL) early in pregnancy.
■ When a client has preterm uterine contractions, obtain a history, complete physical assessment, vital signs, fetal heart rate (FHR), and urine specimen for screening for intrauterine infection and urinary tract infection.

NURSING DIAGNOSES

■ Risk for activity intolerance
■ Ineffective health maintenance
■ Deficient knowledge related to etiology and nonpharmacologic and pharmacologic interventions for PTL
■ Fear related to potential for early labor and birth

PLANNING

■ Client's preterm uterine contractions will cease by resting in left side-lying position, increasing fluid intake, assuming pelvic rest, and following tocolytic therapy as directed.
■ Client has no progressive cervical change.

NURSING INTERVENTIONS

■ Monitor and assess uterine activity and FHR.
■ Maintain client in left lateral position as much as possible to facilitate uteroplacental perfusion.
■ Monitor vital signs per unit protocol, specifically maternal pulse. Report maternal heart rate greater than 110 beats/min.
■ Report auscultated cardiac dysrhythmias. An electrocardiogram (ECG) may be ordered.
■ Auscultate breath sounds every 4 hours. Notify health care provider if respirations are more than 30 per minute or if there is a change in quality (wheezes, rales, coughing).
■ Monitor daily weight to assess fluid overload; strict input and output (I & O) measurement.
■ Report baseline FHR that is more than 180 beats/min or any significant increase in uterine contractions from pretreatment baseline.
■ Report persistence of uterine contractions despite tocolytic therapy.

■ Report leaking of amniotic fluid, any vaginal bleeding or discharge, or complaints of rectal pressure.

■ Be alert to presence of hypoglycemia and hypoglycemia in the newborn delivered within 5 hours of discontinued beta-sympathomimetic drugs.

■ Assist clients on bed rest and home tocolytic therapy to plan for assistance with self-care and family responsibilities.

Client Teaching

General

* Inform client of the signs and symptoms of PTL (menstrual-type cramps, sensation of pelvic pressure, low backache, increased vaginal discharge, and any abdominal discomfort).
* Instruct client that if she experiences PTL contractions, initially she should void, recline on her left side to increase uterine blood flow, and drink extra fluids. Emphasize that she should notify her health care provider if the uterine contractions do not cease or if they increase in frequency.
* Explain side effects of beta-sympathomimetic drugs. Report heart palpitations or dizziness to health care provider.
* Instruct client to take drugs regularly and as prescribed.
* Advise client to contact the health care provider before taking any other drugs while on tocolytic drug therapy.

Cultural Considerations ⊕

* Provide an interpreter with the same ethnic background and gender if possible, especially with sensitive topics and stress situations.

EVALUATION

■ Evaluate the effectiveness of the tocolytic drug by noting six or fewer uterine contractions in 1 hour or per provider order.

■ Evaluate client's understanding of nonpharmacologic measures for decreasing preterm contractions, such as bed rest, increasing oral fluid intake, pelvic rest, and lying on her left side.

■ Continue monitoring client's vital signs, FHR, and uterine activity. Report any change immediately.

Tocolytic Therapy: Magnesium Sulfate

* Monitor vital signs, FHR, and uterine activity as ordered. Report respirations fewer than 12 per minute, which may indicate magnesium sulfate toxicity.
* Monitor I & O. Report urinary output less than 30 ml/h.
* Assess breath and bowel sounds as ordered or at least every 4 hours.

* Assess deep tendon reflexes (DTR) and clonus before initiation of therapy and as ordered. Notify health care provider of changes in DTR (areflexia or hyporeflexia) and clonus.
* Weigh daily.
* Monitor serum magnesium levels as ordered (therapeutic level is 4 to 7 mg/dl).
* Have calcium gluconate (1 g given IV over 3 minutes) available as an antidote.
* Observe newborn for 24 to 48 hours for magnesium effects if drug was given to mother before the delivery.

Corticosteroid Therapy in Preterm Labor

The desired outcome from tocolytic therapy is prevention or cessation of PTL. Clients (24 to 34 weeks' gestation) at risk for preterm delivery should receive antenatal corticosteroid therapy with betamethasone (Celestone) or dexamethasone. Administration of corticosteroids accelerates lung maturation with resultant surfactant development in the fetus in utero, thereby decreasing the incidence and severity of respiratory distress syndrome (RDS) with increased survival of preterm infants. Antenatal therapy decreases infant mortality, RDS and intraventricular bleeds in neonates born between 24 to 34 gestational weeks (Chan & Johnson, 2004, p. 145). The effects and benefits of corticosteroid administration are believed to begin 24 hours after administration and last for up to 1 week.

Surfactant is made up of two major phospholipids: sphingomyelin and lecithin. Sphingomyelin develops in greater quantity initially (from about the 24th week) than lecithin. However, by the 33rd to 35th weeks of gestation, lecithin production peaks, making the ratio of the two substances about 2 : 1 in favor of lecithin. This is called the **L/S (lecithin/sphingomyelin) ratio**, measured in the amniotic fluid. The L/S ratio is a predictor of fetal lung maturity and risk for neonatal RDS.

Clients with PIH, PROM, placental insufficiency, some types of diabetes, or narcotic abuse may have amniotic fluid with higher than expected L/S ratios for the gestational date because of a stress-induced increase in endogenous corticosteroid production.

Betamethasone (Celestone)

When PTL occurs before the 33rd week of gestation, corticosteroid therapy with betamethasone may be prescribed, 12 mg intramuscularly (IM) every 24 hours for two doses.

Adverse Reactions

Side effects of betamethasone are rare but include seizures, headache, vertigo, edema, hypertension, increased sweating, petechiae, ecchymoses, and facial erythema.

Table 51-6

Prenatal Therapy for Surfactant Development

Generic (Brand)	Route and Dosage	Uses and Considerations
Betamethasone (Celestone) Dexamethasone (Decadron)	IM: 12 mg IM q24h × 2 doses IM: 6 mg q12h × 4 doses	Corticosteroid. Given to prevent RDS in preterm infants by injecting mother before delivery to stimulate surfactant production in the fetal lung. Not effective in treating preterm infant after delivery. Most effective if given at least 24 h (preferably 48-72 h) but less than 7 d before delivery in week 33 or before. Contraindicated in severe PIH and in systemic fungal infection. Simultaneous use with terbutaline may enhance risk of pulmonary edema. Drug can mask signs of chorioamnionitis; therefore drug not usually given with ruptured membranes. Metabolized in the liver and excreted by the kidneys; crosses the placenta; enters breast milk. Therapy less effective with multifetal birth and with male infants. No data available related to breastfeeding. *Pregnancy category:* C; PB: 64%; t½: 6.5 h; onset: 1-3 h; peak: 10-36 min IV; duration: 7-14 d

d, Day; *h,* hour; *IM,* intramuscular; *IV,* intravenous; *min,* minute; *PB,* protein-binding; *PIH,* pregnancy-induced hypertension; *RDS,* respiratory distress syndrome; *t½,* half-life.

Dexamethasone

In clinical controlled trials, there is insufficient evidence to recommend betamethasone over dexamethasone because the two have not been compared. Dexamethasone has a rapid onset of action and a shorter duration of action; therefore, it must be prescribed in a shorter frequency compared with betamethasone. The recommended anetepartum regimen for dexamethasone is 6 mg IM every 12 hours for four doses. *Do not confuse dexamethasone with desoximetasone.*

Adverse Reactions

The potential adverse reactions associated with dexamethasone therapy include insomnia, nervousness, increased appetite, headache, hypersensitivity reactions, and arthralgias. Table 51-6 provides the information for the reviewed corticosteroids.

Nursing Process

Betamethasone (Celestone)

ASSESSMENT

- ■ Assess for history of hypersensitivity.
- ■ Assess vital signs; report abnormal findings.
- ■ Assess fetal heart rate (FHR).

NURSING DIAGNOSES

- ■ Fear related to potential for preterm labor and birth with uncertain fetal outcome secondary to fetal immaturity
- ■ Risk for infection

PLANNING

- ■ Client will not deliver within 24 hours of receiving betamethasone (Celestone).

NURSING INTERVENTIONS

- ■ Shake the suspension well. Avoid exposing to excessive heat or light.
- ■ Inject into large muscle, but not the deltoid, to avoid local atrophy.
- ■ Monitor maternal vital signs.
- ■ Maintain accurate intake and output.
- ■ Check blood glucose if used for client with diabetes.

Cultural Considerations ⊕

- • Provide an interpreter with the same ethnic background and gender if possible, especially when dealing with sensitive topics and stress situations.

EVALUATION

- ■ Continue monitoring client's vital signs. Report changes.
- ■ Continue monitoring FHR. Report changes.
- ■ Monitor neonate for hypoglycemia and presence of neonatal sepsis.

Drugs for Pregnancy-Induced Hypertension

Pregnancy-induced hypertension (PIH), the most common serious complication of pregnancy, can have devastating maternal and fetal effects. However, with proper management, the prognosis for both mother and infant is good. Hypertensive disorders are reported in 6% to 30% of all pregnant clients, with 3% to 8% of all pregnancies reflecting incidence of PIH. The condition is most often observed after 20 weeks' gestation intrapartum and during the first 72 hours postpartum. The cause of PIH remains unknown, although numerous hypotheses exist. The pathophysiology of preeclampsia-eclampsia is believed to be related to decreased levels of vasodilating prostaglandins with resulting vasospasm.

Predisposing Factors in Pregnancy-Induced Hypertension

- African American
- Primigravida (first pregnancy)
- History of preclampsia
- Younger than 20 or older than 35 years of age (especially as primigravida)
- Multifetal gestation
- Family history of pregnancy-induced hypertension
- Lower socioeconomic class
- Gestational trophoblastic disease
- Pregestational diabetes mellitus
- Preexisting hypertensive, vascular, or renal disease
- Underweight or overweight

The major predisposing risk factors for the development of PIH are listed in Box 51–1.

The two categories of PIH—preeclampsia and eclampsia—are based on clinical manifestations. **Preeclampsia** is the presence of hypertension (systolic blood pressure >140 mm Hg or diastolic blood pressure >90 mm Hg) and proteinuria (i.e., >300 mg in 24-hour urine collection) in a normotensive prepregnant client after the 20th week of gestation. Preeclampsia is subdivided into *mild* preeclampsia and *severe* preeclampsia (see Table 51–7 for comparison).

About 5% of preeclamptic clients, notably those without adequate prenatal care, progress to **eclampsia,** in which seizure activity occurs and the perinatal mortality rate is about 20%. Early diagnosis of PIH with appropriate treatment keeps most preeclamptic clients from progressing to this stage. About 25% of eclampsia occurs postpartum.

A severe sequela of PIH is known as **HELLP syndrome** (defined by *H*emolysis, *E*levated *L*iver enzymes, and *L*ow *P*latelet count), which occurs in about 2% to 12% of clients with PIH. Clients who manifest severe preeclampsia are most likely to also have HELLP syndrome.

Two primary treatment goals in PIH, in addition to delivery of an uncompromised fetus and psychological support for the client and her family, are reduction of vasospasm and prevention of seizures.

Delivery of the infant and placenta (products of conception) is the only known cure for PIH. Vaginal delivery is preferred so that anesthesia or surgical risks will not be added. Labor induction via cervical ripening may be initiated to facilitate labor. For a vaginal delivery, an epidural or combined epidural and spinal anesthesia is frequently performed for pain management while promoting uteroplacental circulation. Maternal hypotension is a significant concern for hypertensive clients who have epidurals. In contrast, parturients with worsening PIH or fetal distress may be delivered via cesarean section. Clients with HELLP syndrome may have their labor induced for a vaginal delivery at 32 or more weeks' gestation. For clients with HELLP syndrome who are at less than 32 weeks' gestation, a cesarean delivery may be considered.

If a client's disease progresses to the point of eclampsia (maternal seizure), delivery is generally postponed for 1 to 3 hours if fetal status allows. The labor induction or cesarean delivery is an additional stressor for the client who exhibits acidosis and hypoxia resulting from seizure. Ideally, once vital signs are stabilized with improved urinary output and decreased acidosis/hypoxia, delivery is pursued.

Potential nonmedication treatments for preeclampsia include activity reduction, lying on the left side, increased

Table 51–7

Comparison of Mild and Severe Preeclampsia and Eclampsia

Mild Preeclampsia	Severe Preeclampsia	Eclampsia
Blood pressure increase to >140 and/or >90 diastolic but <160 systolic	Blood pressure increase of >160/110 on two occasions at least 6 h apart (client on bed rest)	Signs and symptoms of mild or severe PIH and 1 seizure
Proteinuria >500 mg in 24 h or +1 ± 2; edema not generalized; noted in hands, feet	Proteinuria .5 g in 24 h or 13 or 14; edema generalized; found in face (periorbital, coarse features), hands, lower extremities (ankles), abdomen, and dependent areas	
Weight gain >1 lb/wk before 32 wk or >2.5 lb/wk after 34 wk	Weight gain up to 10 lb in 1 wk	
Deep tendon reflexes in arms and legs only slightly increased (0: no response; 1+: sluggish/low; 2+: normal active; 3+: brisk)	Deep tendon reflexes in arms and legs hyperactive (4+: hyperactive/transient clonus; 5+: brisk; clonus sustained)	
Adequate urinary output (1 ml/kg/h)	Oliguria present (<400 ml per 24 h)	
No major cerebral or visual symptoms	Cerebral or visual symptoms, particularly blurred vision, spots, flashing lights, and/or persistent and severe headache in frontal area	
May have mild frontal headache		
No epigastric pain	Epigastric pain may be present; pulmonary edema, cyanosis	

h, Hour; *PIH,* pregnancy-induced hypertension; *wk,* week; >, greater than; <, less than.

dietary protein (supplemental 90 g/day), psychosocial therapy, and biofeedback. The aforementioned recommendations have been studied and have been shown not to have clinically beneficial effects. Therefore, drug therapy is commonly used for treatment.

Methyldopa (Aldomet), hydralazine (Apresoline), and Labetalol (Trandate) are considered first-line therapy for preeclampsia because they have been most widely used in pregnant women and their established safety and efficacy for mother and fetus. Additional alternatives include beta-blockers, prazosine, nifedipine, and clonidine. Beta-blockers are generally considered safe, but there is potential impairment of fetal growth if used early in pregnancy. Nifedipine, a calcium channel blocker, has been used with no major problems. Diuretics should be avoided because of the potential alteration in plasma volume; additionally, angoitensin-converting enzyme inhibitors should be avoided in the second and third trimesters because of the potential for fetal renal toxicity.

Table 51–8 presents the drug data for the two most commonly used drugs for treating PIH: magnesium sulfate and hydralazine.

Adverse Reactions of Methyldopa (Aldomet)

Observe the client for peripheral edema, anxiety, nightmares, drowsiness, headache, dry mouth, drug fever, and mental depression. These are the most common potential adverse reactions.

Adverse Reactions of Hydralazine (Apresoline)

Observe the client for headache, nausea, vomiting, nasal congestion, dizziness, tachycardia, palpitations, and angina pectoris. Avoid a sudden decrease in maternal blood pressure, which may cause fetal hypoxia. Hydralazine has no known direct adverse effects on the fetus.

Adverse Reactions of Magnesium Sulfate

Early signs of increased magnesium levels include lethargy, flush, feelings of increased warmth, perspiration, thirst, sedation, heavy eyelids, slurred speech, hypotension, depressed deep tendon reflexes (DTR), and decreased muscle tone. Adverse reactions generally occur with serum magnesium sulfate levels greater than 10 mg/dl. Therapeutic levels are 4 to 8 mg/dl. Loss of DTR is often the first sign of magnesium toxicity and may be seen at 9 to 12 mg/dl. Respiratory depression may manifest at levels greater than 15 mg/dl

PREVENTING MEDICATION ERRORS

Do not confuse...

- **Terbutaline (Brethine)** with **methylergonovine (Methergine).** These drugs have the same packaging but opposite actions! Both are amber ampules with colored neckbands wrapped in foil and amber plastic packaging. Do not store together.

and cardiac arrest at levels greater than 30 mg/dl. Heart block has been reported occasionally with levels lower than 10 mg/dl.

Decreased variability is commonly seen on the fetal heart rate tracing. If the client received magnesium sulfate close to the time of delivery, the neonate may exhibit low Apgar scores, hypotonia, lethargy, weakness, and potential respiratory distress. The fetal level of magnesium generally reaches more than 90% of maternal levels within 3 hours of administration. There is no evidence linking congenital defects and maternal hypocalcemia or hypermagnesemia. The greater risk to the fetus is from maternal PIH with resulting decreased placental blood flow and intrauterine growth retardation.

Nursing Process

Pregnancy-Induced Hypertension

ASSESSMENT

- Review baseline vital signs from early pregnancy and BP readings during prenatal visits.
- Identify client history that may predispose client to pregnancy-induced hypertension (PIH).

NURSING DIAGNOSES

- Deficient fluid volume related to shift of intravascular fluid to extravascular space as outcome of vasospasm with subsequent elevated arterial hypertension
- Deficient knowledge related to PIH, diagnosis, treatment modalities, common outcomes for mother and infant
- Risk for inadequate placental perfusion and risk to fetal well-being secondary to vasospasm
- Risk for maternal injury related to seizure activity
- Risk for maternal injury related to magnesium toxicity
- Anxiety related to possible preterm hospitalization and delivery with possible adverse fetal or maternal outcomes

PLANNING

- Client's blood pressure will be maintained within acceptable ranges.
- Client will verbalize understanding of PIH, etiology, signs and symptoms and nonpharmacologic and pharmacologic treatment measures.
- Client will comply with planned PIH treatment regimen.
- Fetus will tolerate impaired uteroplacental perfusion and subsequent delivery without injury.
- Therapeutic magnesium levels will be maintained.
- Plan for magnesium sulfate infusion for at least 24 hours postpartum.

Continued on p. 813

Table 51–8

Drugs Used in Severe Preeclampsia

Generic (Brand)	Route and Dosage	Uses and Considerations
magnesium sulfate	LD: 6 g in 20 min IV; piggyback via infusion pump; *maint:* 2/h IV via infusion pump	Prevention and treatment of seizures related to PIH. Acts as CNS depressant. Decreases acetylcholine from motor nerves, which blocks neuromuscular transmission and decreases incidence of seizures. A secondary effect is the reduction in the blood pressure as magnesium sulfate relaxes smooth muscle.
		Secondarily affects peripheral vascular system with increased uterine blood flow caused by vasodilation and some transient BP decrease during first hour; also inhibits uterine contractions. Depresses DTRs and respiration; maintenance dose depends on reflexes, respiratory rate, urinary output, and magnesium level. Production of abnormally high magnesium level is main risk.
		Therapeutic levels range from 4-8 mg/dl; levels of 4-7.5 mg/dl are effective in preventing seizures. Client is at risk if respiratory rate <12, urinary output <30 ml/h, DTR is absent or hyporeflexic. DTR disappears with serum magnesium levels of 9-12 mg/dl. Maternal respiratory depression may occur with levels greater than 15 mg/dl and cardiac arrest with levels >30 mg/dl. Notify health care provider of any of the above.
		Can be given IV or IM (infrequent). Should not be given parenterally to clients with heart block, myocardial damage, or renal impairment.
		Absorbed magnesium is excreted by kidneys; excreted in breast milk, but not a contraindication to breastfeeding.
		Contraindications: myasthenia gravis. Relative contraindications—myocardial damage or heart block.
		Antidote: calcium gluconate 1 g slow IV push over 3 min.
		Pregnancy category: B; PB: UK; t$\frac{1}{2}$: UK; onset: IV immediate, IM 1 h; duration: IV 30 min, IM 3-4 h; infusion usually stopped 24 h postpartum.
hydralazine hydrochloride (Apresoline)	IV: 100 mg in 1000 ml normal saline by infusion pump titrated at 6-12 mg/h to maintain elected BP IV Push: 5 mg IV, repeat 5-10 mg IV every 20 min to maximum cumulative dose of 20 mg or until BP is controlled IM & PO routes not usually used	Antihypertensive agent. Acts by causing arteriolar vasodilation. Usually lowers diastolic BP more than systolic BP. Objective of treatment is to maintain diastolic BP between 90 and 110 mmHg. Usually not given to pregnant PIH client with diastolic BP >105 mmHg because of risk of reduced intervillous blood flow. Clients with impaired renal function may require lower doses. *Parenteral: onset:* 5-20 min; peak: 10-80 min; duration: 2-6 h; well tolerated; maternal tachycardia and increased cardiac output and oxygen consumption may occur. *Oral: onset:* 20-30 min; peak: 1-2 h; duration: 2-4 h.
methyldopa (Apo-Methyldopa/Aldomet)	IV: 250-1000 mg every 6-8 h, *max:* 1 g every 6 h PO: 25 mg b.i.d., *max:* 4 g/d	*Mechanism of action:* Stimulates the central alpha-adrenergic receptors that results in a decreased sympathetic outflow to the heart, kidneys, and peripheral vasculature. *Contraindications:* Hypersensitivity to methyldopa (Apo-Methyldopa/Aldomet) or any component of the formulation. Active hepatic disease, liver disorders previously associated with the use of methyldopa, concurrent use with MAO inhibitors. *Warnings/precautions:* Sedation is usually transient during initial treatment and dosage increases.
Labetalol (Trandate)	IV: 20 mg IV, followed by 40 mg, then 80 mg, then 80 mg every 10 min until blood pressure is controlled or maximum cumulative dose of 220 mg is given	*Pregnancy category:* B; t$\frac{1}{2}$: 75-80 min, onset 3-6 h; duration 12-24 h.

b.i.d., Two times a day; *BP,* blood pressure; *CNS,* central nervous system; *d,* day; *DTR,* deep tendon reflex; *h,* hour; *IM,* intramuscular; *IV,* intravenous; *LD,* loading dose; *maint,* maintenance; *MAO,* monoamine oxidase; *min,* minute; *PB,* protein-binding; *PIH,* pregnancy-induced hypertension; *PO,* by mouth; *t$\frac{1}{2}$,* half-life; *UK,* unknown; *>,* greater than; *<,* less than.

Client Teaching

General

*   Teach client about PIH and implications for mother, fetus, and newborn.
*   Provide client with information about nonpharmacologic and pharmacologic treatment measures for PIH.

Safety

*   Instruct client to lie in the left lateral recumbent position and the rationale.
*   Teach client signs and symptoms of progressive PIH and when to seek medical assistance and rationale.
*   Explain to client that fetal well-being will be assessed through biophysical profile (BPP), nonstress (NST), or contraction stress test at frequent intervals depending on the health care provider and PIH severity (i.e., NST or BPP 1-2 ×/week.
*   Educate family regarding possibility of seizures and appropriate actions to take if seizures occur.

Diet

*   Provide nutritional counseling in regard to need for additional protein intake (90 g) because of urinary protein losses, normal sodium diet, and importance of adequate fluid intake.
*   Explain to client the rationale for daily weights.

Magnesium Sulfate

*   Explain to client why she will have a Foley catheter, infusion pump, continuous fetal monitoring, and assessment of deep tendon reflex (DTR) and clonus and that therapy will extend into the postpartum period × 24 to 48 hours, dependent on the agency and health care provider.
*   Explain to client about visitor restrictions and that she will be in a low-stimulation environment.
*   Tell client that she will likely experience flush, warm sensation, and possibly nausea and vomiting during the initial loading dose.
*   Tell client that evidence of magnesium levels that are within therapeutic range include decreased appetite, some speech slurring, double vision, and weakness.

Hydralazine

*   Explain to client that nurses will be monitoring pulse and BP almost constantly until it becomes stable after administration and then every 15 minutes. Explain that an electronic BP monitor may be used to obtain constant readings.
*   Explain to client the need for careful measuring of I & O.
*   Tell client she may experience headache as a side effect of the drug.

NURSING INTERVENTIONS

Magnesium Sulfate

*   Continuous electronic fetal monitoring.
*   Monitor for maternal toxicity. Lethargy and weakness result from the blocking of the neuromuscular transmission. Diaphoresis, flush, feeling of warmth, and nasal congestion are the results of the vasodilation from relaxation of smooth muscle.
*   Have airway suction, resuscitation equipment and emergency drugs available.
*   Have antidote available. Calcium gluconate (1 g) IV is given over 3 minutes.
*   Maintain client in left lateral recumbent position in low-stimulation environment. Provide close observation.
*   For IM administration, use Z-track technique and rotate sites (drug is painful and irritating). Infrequent administration.
*   Monitor BP, pulse, and respiratory rate per agency protocol, DTR, clonus, and hourly I & O with urimeter for output.
*   Monitor temperature, breath sounds, and bowel sounds every 4 hours.
*   Check urine for protein every hour.
*   Assess for epigastric pain (heralds impending seizure), headache, visual symptoms (blurred vision and scotoma), sensory changes, edema, level of consciousness, and seizure activity on ongoing basis.
*   Monitor serum magnesium levels according to agency protocol for range between 4 and 7 mg/dl.
*   Notify physician if following are observed:
    Respirations less than 12/min
    Absence of DTR
    Urinary output less than 30 ml/h
    Systolic BP greater than or equal to 160 mm Hg, unless ordered otherwise
    Magnesium level greater than 7 mEq/L
    Absent bowel sounds or altered breath sounds
    Epigastric pain, headache, visual symptoms (blurred) vision and scotoma), sensory changes, change in affect or level of consciousness, seizure activity
*   Monitor laboratory reports: evidence of low platelet count, and, if present, observe for excessive bleeding.
*   Monitor fetal status. FHR baseline should remain 110 to 160.
*   Monitor laboratory results: 24 hours urinary protein results if ordered (>300 mg/24 h is abnormal).
*   Monitor client for magnesium toxicity.
*   Monitor newborn for effects of placental exposure to excess magnesium sulfate. Although infrequent, newborn side effects include lethargy, neurologic or respiratory depression, and muscle hypotonia.

Hydralazine

- Take pulse and BP every 5 minutes when drug is administered or monitor with an electronic BP device until stabilized and then every 15 minutes.
- Maintain diastolic BP between 90 and 110 mm Hg or as ordered.
- Observe for change in level of consciousness and headache.
- Monitor I & O to avoid hypotensive episodes or overload.
- Monitor fetal heart rate (FHR).

Cultural Considerations ⊛

- Provide an interpreter with the same ethnic background and gender if possible, especially with sensitive topics and stress situations.

Client Teaching

General
- Instruct client to avoid exposure to infection.
- Remind client with diabetes to check her glucose level as ordered.

Side Effects
- Instruct client to report immediately any breathing difficulty, weakness, or dizziness.
- Instruct client to report changes in stool, easy bruising, bleeding, blurred vision, unusual weight gain, and emotional changes.

EVALUATION

- ▣ Evaluate the effectiveness of therapy to reduce BP (hydralazine).
- ▣ Continue monitoring vital signs. Report changes.
- ▣ Document the effect of teaching and learning opportunities on client's knowledge deficit about PIH treatment modalities and outcomes.
- ▣ Note fetal well-being secondary to treatment with drugs as evidenced by fetal monitoring and fetal movement assessment.
- ▣ Monitor changes that occur in magnesium level per laboratory results compared with physiologic measures.
- ▣ Continue monitoring FHR. Report changes.

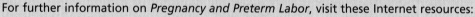

WEBSITES

For further information on *Pregnancy and Preterm Labor*, visit these Internet resources:

American College of Obstetricians and Gynecologists:
http://www.acog.org

American Pregnancy Association:
http://www.americanpregnancy.org/duringpregnancy/fetallifesupportsystem.html

Centers for Disease Control and Prevention (CDC):
http://www.cdc.gov/nccdphp

Center for CAM Research in Women's Health,
Columbia University:
http://cpmcnet.columbia.edu/dept/rosenthal/

Center for the Evaluation of Risks to Human Reproduction:
http://cerhr.niehs.nih.gov/genpub/topics/ccae_index.html

Clinical Trials in Pregnancy:
http://clinicaltrials.gov/ct/gui/action

Clinical Trials-Pregnancy Complications—NIH:
http://clinicaltrials.gov/ct/gui/action

Drugs:
www.drugs.com

ePregnancy:
http://www.epregnancy.com

Healthy Pregnancy:
http://www.4woman.gov/Pregnancy/

Mayo E Clinic:
http://www.mayoclinic.com

National Center for Complementary
and Alternative Medicine:
http://altmed.od.nih.gov

National Institutes of Health—National Institute
of Child Health & Human Development:
http://www.nichd.nih.gov/womenshealth

National Library of Medicine & NIH—Medline Plus:
http://www.nlm.nih.gov/medlineplus/prenatalcare.html

Organization of Teratology Information Services:
http://www.otispregnancy.org/

Pregnancy and drugs:
http://www.fda.gov

Pregnancy organization:
http://www.pregnancy.org

Pregnancy Today:
http://pregnancytoday.com

The National Academies Press:
http://www.nationalacademies.org/health

Critical Thinking Case Study

T.A. (gravida 3, para 0) has a history of spontaneous abortion at 10 weeks' gestation and a preterm delivery and demise of a neonate at 21 weeks' gestation. At her 28-week prenatal visit, she reports increased clear vaginal discharge and feelings of pelvic pressure. Examination of her cervix reveals 2-cm dilation and a presenting fetal part low in the pelvis. T.A. is admitted to the hospital and uterine activity is documented. Terbutaline therapy is ordered for treatment of preterm labor. The nurse prepares for terbutaline administration by the subQ route.

1. How will terbutaline therapy be initiated? What intervals and dosages should be anticipated?

2. What maternal and fetal side effects should the nurse expect to observe?

3. What should T.A. be told about the drug effects she will experience?

4. How should the nurse respond to T.A.'s questions about the risks of preterm delivery?

After 24 hours of terbutaline subQ therapy, uterine contractions have been reduced to two to three per hour. T.A. is to be discharged home after oral terbutaline therapy is initiated. The nurse is preparing T.A.'s discharge teaching.

5. What dose and administration schedule would the nurse expect to be ordered?

6. What should T.A. be advised to do if she forgets or misses an oral dose of terbutaline?

7. What instructions should be given to T.A. about her activity and diet?

8. T.A. asks whether the side effects of terbutaline will continue. What is an appropriate nursing response?

9. What signs and symptoms should T.A. be advised to report?

Study Questions

1. What is the main reason drug use is discouraged during pregnancy?

2. What are six suggestions to decrease nausea and vomiting during early pregnancy?

3. What are three suggestions to alleviate headache during early pregnancy?

4. What are known risk factors for preterm labor?

5. What are the nursing responsibilities associated with the administration of drugs used for tocolysis?

6. What are two drugs commonly used to treat pregnancy-induced hypertension? What is the mode of action of each drug?

7. What are four signs of worsening pregnancy-induced hypertension?

8. What observations are indications to discontinue administration of magnesium sulfate?

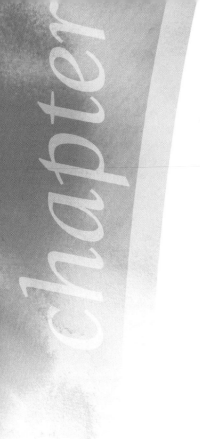

52 Drugs Associated with the Female Reproductive Cycle II: Labor, Delivery, and the Preterm Neonate

ROBIN WEBB CORBETT AND LAURA K. WILLIFORD OWENS

ELECTRONIC RESOURCES

Additional information can be found on the companion website at *http://evolve.elsevier.com/KeeHayes/pharmacology/* or on the companion CD-ROM, which includes:
* *NCLEX-style examination review questions*
* *Pharmacology animations*
* *Medication error and IV therapy checklists*
* *Medication calculation problems*
* *Electronic calculators*

OUTLINE

OBJECTIVES

- Discuss systemic and regional medications for pain control during labor, their action, side effects, and nursing implications.
- Describe the nursing process, including client teaching, associated with the drugs used during labor and delivery.
- Discuss drugs used to enhance uterine contractility during labor and following placental expulsion, their action, side effects, and nursing implications.
- Describe the nursing process associated with the administration of surfactant therapy for preterm neonates.

TERMS

Bishop's score	ergotism	labor induction	surfactant
cervical ripening	labor augmentation	respiratory distress syn-	uterine contractility
ergot alkaloids		drome (RDS)	uterine inertia

Drugs for Pain Control During Labor

Labor and delivery are divided into four stages. The first three stages are specific to labor and delivery. During the *first stage,* the dilating stage, cervical effacement and dilation occur; the cervix becomes fully dilated at 10 cm. The first stage consists of three phases categorized by cervical dilatation. These three phases are the latent phase (0 to 4 cm), active phase (4 to 7 cm), and the transition phase (8 to 10 cm). The *second stage,* the pelvic stage, begins with the complete dilatation and ends with delivery of the newborn (Figure 52–1). During the *third stage,* the placenta separates from the uterine wall and is delivered. The *fourth stage* of labor, or the first 1 to 4 hours postpartum, is a period of physiologic stabilization for the mother and initiation of familial attachment.

During the first stage of labor, uterine contractions produce progressive cervical effacement and dilatation. As

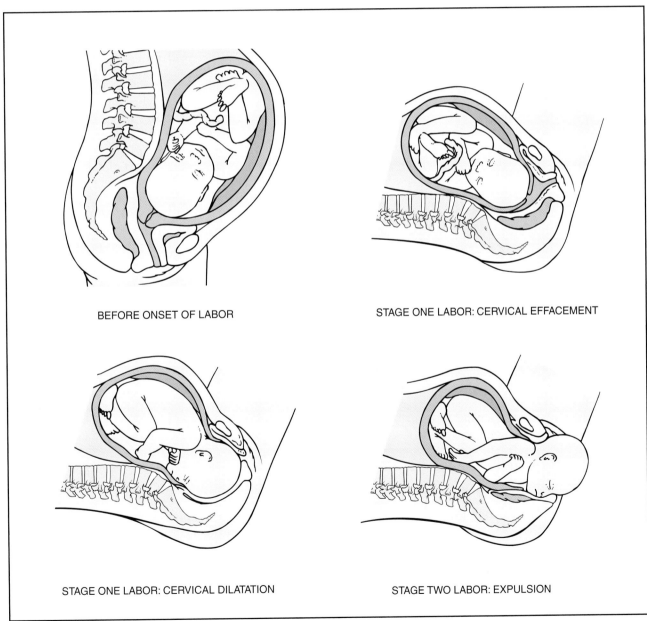

BEFORE ONSET OF LABOR

STAGE ONE LABOR: CERVICAL EFFACEMENT

STAGE ONE LABOR: CERVICAL DILATATION

STAGE TWO LABOR: EXPULSION

FIGURE 52–1 First and second stages of labor. (From Nichols F, Zwelling E: *Maternal-newborn nursing: theory and practice,* Philadelphia, 1997, Saunders.)

the first stage of labor progresses, uterine contractions become stronger, longer, and more frequent, and discomfort increases. Pain and discomfort in labor are caused by uterine contraction, cervical dilatation and effacement, hypoxia of the contracting myometrium, and perineal pressure from the presenting part. Pain perception is influenced by physiologic, psychologic, social, and cultural factors. In particular, the woman's past experience with pain, anticipation of pain, fear and anxiety, knowledge deficit of the labor and delivery process, and involvement of support persons.

Before administering pharmacologic treatment, nonpharmacologic measures should be initiated. Nonpharmacologic measures for pain relief during labor include (1) ambulating, (2) positioning supportive of the gravid uterus and promoting uterine perfusion, (3) using touch and massage, (4) using hygiene and comfort measures, (5) involving support persons, (6) using breathing and relaxation techniques, (7) transcutaneous electrical nerve stimulation, (8) hypnosis, (9) acupuncture, and (10) using hydrotherapy (warm water tubs and showers).

Other nonpharmacologic measures include alternative and complementary medicine. Of particular concern is the use of herbal supplements by the pregnant client later in pregnancy to stimulate labor. For example, some women ingest pregnancy toner tea, which includes the components raspberry, nettles, dandelion, alfafa, and peppermint leaf. Other herbal supplements used include blue cohosh, castor oil, red raspberry leaf, and evening primrose oil. Pregnant women may self-administer, or the practice may be part of their traditional beliefs and framework of health. Concerns with herbal supplements are related to the often numerous physiologic active components of the herbs, adulterants, inconsistent dosing, and lack of proven efficacy. Herbs taken in later pregnancy may contribute to preterm labor or increased bleeding at delivery. Nurses must be culturally sensitive to the use of herbal supplements and health practices during pregnancy and specifically in the later gestational weeks.

When pharmacologic intervention is needed for pain relief, drugs are used as an adjunct to nonpharmacologic measures. Drugs should be selected to not only decrease the client's pain but also minimize side effects for the fetus or newborn and mother. Pain relief in labor can be obtained with systemic analgesics and regional anesthesia. Analgesics alter the client's perception and sensation of pain without producing unconsciousness.

Analgesia/Sedation

Systemic medications used during labor include sedative-tranquilizers, narcotics agonists, and mixed narcotic agonist-antagonists and may be administered orally (sedative-hypnotic drugs), intravenously (IV) or intramuscularly (IM) (Table 52-1). Because of the variable response and blood levels with intramuscular administration, these drugs are more commonly administered intravenously. These medications should be administered at the onset of the uterine contrac-tion. Parenteral administration at the onset of the contraction decreases neonatal drug exposure as blood flow is decreased to the uterus and fetus.

The sedative-tranquilizer drugs are most commonly given for false labor, latent labor, or with ruptured membranes without true labor. In addition, these drugs may be administered to minimize maternal anxiety and fear. These drugs promote rest and relaxation and decrease fear and anxiety, but they do not provide pain relief. The sedative drugs most commonly used are barbiturates or hypnotics—generally secobarbital sodium (Seconal) and pentobarbital sodium (Nembutal). Other drugs, such as phenothiazine derivatives and hydrozyzine, can be given alone during early labor or in combination with narcotic agonists when the client is in active labor. In addition to decreasing anxiety and apprehension, these drugs potentiate the analgesic action of the opioids and minimize emesis. These drugs include promethazine (Phenergan), a phenothiazine, and hydroxyzine hydrochloride (Vistaril, Atarax), a sedative-hypnotic. Do not confuse promethazine hydroxyzine with promazine hydralazine.

The second group of drugs given for active labor are narcotic agonists. These drugs may be administered parenterally or via regional blocks. When administered with neuraxial anesthesia, a lower dose of anesthetic is required for effective pain relief, thereby minimizing side effects. These drugs interfere with pain impulses at the subcortical level of the brain. To effect pain relief, opioids interact with mu and kappa receptors. For example morphine sulfate activates both mu and kappa receptors.

Meperidine (Demerol) is the most commonly prescribed synthetic opioid for pain control during labor. A second narcotic agonist used for pain relief during labor is fentanyl (Sublimaze). Fentanyl is a short-acting synthetic opioid that is best administered IV because of its short duration of action. Morphine sulfate may also be used for pain control in active labor, but it is less frequently used. High doses of opioids are required for effective labor analgesia when administered parenterally.

The third group of systemic medications used for pain relief in labor is the opioids with mixed narcotic agonist-antagonist effects. These drugs exert their effects at more than one site—often an agonist at one site and an antagonist at another. The two most commonly used narcotic-agonist–antagonist drugs are butorphanol tartrate (Stadol) and nalbuphine (Nubain). A primary advantage of these drugs is their *dose ceiling effect*. This means additional doses do not increase the degree of respiratory depression, so there is less respiratory depression with these drugs than with opioids. The respiratory depression ceiling effect is believed to result from activation of kappa agonists and weak U antagonists.

Adverse Reactions

Adverse effects of sedative-hypnotic drugs (secobarbital, pentobarbital) include paradoxically increased pain and excitability, lethargy, subdued mood, decreased sensory

Table 52–1

Common Systemic Medications Used for Pain Relief in Labor

Generic (Brand)	Route and Dosage	Uses and Considerations
Sedative-Hypnotics		
secobarbital (Seconal)	IM: 50-100 mg PO: 100-200 mg	Used to decrease anxiety during latent phase of labor. Onset: 10-30 min; peak: 20-30 min; duration: 4-8 h. No effects on uterine tone or contractility; rapidly crosses placenta; can cause decreased variability in FHR because of decreased CNS control over heart rate. No antagonist for barbiturates, so secobarbital administered only if delivery not expected for 24-48 h. May have prolonged depressant effects on neonate. Excreted into breast milk. Compatible with breast-feeding. May increase CNS depression with alcohol, narcotics, antihistamines, tranquilizers, and MAOIs. *Pregnancy category:* D; PB: UK; $t\frac{1}{2}$: 15-30 h
pentobarbital (Nembutal) phenothiazine derivative	PO: 20-30 mg IM/IV: 12.5-50 mg q3-4h or IM: 25-50 mg with 25-75 mg meperidine or IV: 15-25 mg with 25-75 mg meperidine; repeat if needed; *max:* 100 mg in 24 h	Short-acting barbiturate. *Pregnancy category:* D. See Prototype Drug Chart 17–1. A phenothiazine antihistamine; used as adjunct to narcotic analgesics during first stage of labor; antiemetic properties. Onset: PO: 20 min; IM: 3-5 min; IV: 1-2 min. Do not give subcutaneously. Used alone to promote rest and sleep; potentiates action of narcotic agonists reducing narcotic doses. May cause decreased variability in FHR; contraindicated during lactation. At term, rapidly crosses placenta; fetal and maternal blood concentrations in equilibrium in 15 min, with infant levels persisting for 4 h. Transient hypotonia, lethargy, and electroencephalographic changes for 3 d in newborn. May cause maternal tachycardia; may impair newborn platelet aggregation. If given with meperidine, give slowly at beginning of contraction over several minutes to decrease amount of drug perfused immediately to the fetus via placenta. *Adverse reactions:* dizziness, dry mouth, excessive sedation, weakness, blurred vision, and restlessness. *Pregnancy category:* C; PB: UK; $t\frac{1}{2}$: UK
promethazine HCl (Phenergan)	IM: 25-50 mg q4-6 h; repeat if needed	Antianxiety agent; antihistamine; antiemetic; sedative-hypotonic. Used alone early in labor or later to potentiate action of narcotic agonists. Onset: 15-30 min; peak: <2 h; duration: 4-6 h. Use Z-track injection for IM to reduce pain. Intraarterial, subQ, or IV administration *not* recommended (thrombus and digital gangrene can occur). Extravasation can result in sterile abscesses and marked tissue induration. Use with caution in clients with chronic obstructive pulmonary disease and asthma. Can cause decreased variability in FHR. No data available about breastfeeding. No effect on labor or neonatal Apgar scores. *Adverse reactions:* hypotension, drowsiness, dizziness, ataxia; may cause CNS depression with alcohol, analgesics, barbiturates, narcotics; may decrease effects of epinephrine. *Pregnancy category:* C; PB: UK; $t\frac{1}{2}$: 3 h
hydroxyzine pamoate (Vistaril)	IV: 25-50 mg IV q 3-4 h	Opioid agonist; 100 times more potent than morphine sulfate. Analgesic activity of 100 mcg is equivalent to 10 mg morphine or 75 mg meperidine. Binds with opiate receptors in the CNS, altering perception of and emotional response to pain through an unknown mechanism. Onset: 1-2 min; peak: 3-5 min; duration: 30-60 min. Only staff trained in administration of IV anesthetics and management of their potential adverse effects should administer IV fentanyl. Often used IV with droperidol to produce neuroleptanalgesia. Have resuscitation equipment and opiate antagonist (naloxone) readily available. *Adverse reactions:* sedation, somnolence, clouded sensorium, euphoria, dizziness, headache, confusion, asthenia, nervousness, hallucinations, anxiety, depression, seizures; hypotension, hypertension, arrhythmias, chest pain; nausea, vomiting, constipation, ileus, abdominal pain, dry mouth, anorexia, diarrhea, dyspepsia, urine retention; respiratory depression, hypoventilation, dyspnea, apnea. *Pregnancy category:* C; PB: UK; $t\frac{1}{2}$: 3.6 h
Narcotic Agonists		
fentanyl citrate (Sublimaze)	IM/IV: 25-50 mcg or IM 50-100 mcg	subQ onset: 5-30 min; peak: 50-90 min; duration: 4-5 h. IM onset: 5-30 min; peak: 30-60 min; duration: 3-7 h. Administer drug slowly and rotate injection sites to avoid irritation of local tissue. Crosses placenta and found in breast milk. Watch for respiratory depression in neonates of mothers who receive this drug in labor. May see withdrawal symptoms in neonate if mother was regular opioid user during pregnancy. Be alert to risk of overdose in clients with circulatory impairment. Use with extreme caution in clients with asthma, respiratory depression, anoxia, seizures, shock, and acute alcoholism. *Pregnancy category:* C; PB: UK; $t\frac{1}{2}$: 2.5-3 h

CNS, Central nervous system; *d,* day; *FHR,* fetal heart rate; *h,* hour; *IM,* intramuscular; *IV,* intravenous; *MAOI,* monoamine oxidase inhibitor; *max,* maximum; *min,* minute; *PB,* protein-binding; *PO,* by mouth; *PRN,* as needed; *subQ,* subcutaneous; $t\frac{1}{2}$, half-life; *UK,* unknown; <, less than.

Continued

Table 52–1

Common Systemic Medications Used for Pain Relief in Labor—cont'd

Generic (Brand)	Route and Dosage	Uses and Considerations
Narcotic Agonists—cont'd		
morphine sulfate	IM/IV: 5-10 mg or IV 2-5 mg	Potent nonnarcotic analgesic (2-mg dose approximately equivalent to 10-15 mg morphine); has mixed narcotic agonist-antagonist mechanism of action with central analgesic actions; binds to CNS opiate receptors and inhibits ascending pain pathways. Used for relief of moderate to severe pain, for preoperative medication, and as supplement to anesthesia. Onset: IM 10-30 min, IV 1-2 min; peak: IM 0.5-1 h, IV 4-5 min; duration: IM 3-4 h, IV 2-4 h. Do not give subQ. Have naloxone available as antidote. Additive effects with CNS depressants. May see withdrawal symptoms in narcotic-dependent clients; may cause drowsiness and respiratory depression, sedation, euphoria, hallucinations, headache, palpitations. Do not give if respirations <12/min. Use with caution in clients delivering preterm infant because fetus may exhibit decreased beat-to-beat variability on FHR monitor. Newborn may have moderate CNS depression, hypotonia at birth, and mild behavioral depression. *Pregnancy category:* B (D, if prolonged use or high at-term dose); PB: 20%-35%; t½: 2.5-4 h
Mixed Narcotic Agonist-Antagonists		
butorphanol tartrate (Stadol)	IV: 0.5-1 mg IV q 1.5-2h	
nalbuphine (Nubain)	IV: 10 mg	Limited respiratory depression. Less analgesic effect than morphine. About 10%-15% of laboring women experience hallucinations with nalbuphine. Toxicity can be reversed with naloxone. *Pregnancy category:* B; PB: UK; t½: 5 h

perception, and hypotension. Fetal and neonatal side effects include a decreased fetal heart rate (FHR) variability and neonatal respiratory depression, sleepiness, hypotonia, and delayed breastfeeding with a poor sucking response for up to 4 days.

The side effects of phenothiazine derivatives and antiemetic/antihistamine (promethazine, hydroxyzine) include confusion, disorientation, excess sedation, dizziness, hypotension, tachycardia, blurred vision, headache, restlessness, weakness, and urinary retention with *promethazine;* drowsiness, dry mouth, dizziness, headache, blurred vision, dysuria, urinary retention, and constipation with *hydroxyzine.* Decreased FHR variability occurs, and the neonate can experience moderate central nervous system (CNS) depression, hypotonia, lethargy, poor feeding, and hypothermia.

The adverse effects of opioids depends on the responses activated by the mu and kappa receptors. Activation of mu receptors result in analgesia, decreased gastrointestinal (GI) motility, euphoria, respiratory depression, sedation and physiologic dependence. In contrast, activation of kappa receptors results in analgesia, decreased gastrointestinal motility, miosis, and sedation. When parenterally administered, the side effects of opioids include nausea, vomiting, sedation, orthostatic hypotension, pruritis, and maternal and neonatal respiratory depression. The associated nausea and vomiting result from stimulation of the chemoreceptor trigger zone

in the medulla. Motor block is another concern. Mothers may not walk after delivery until they are able to maintain a straight leg raise against downward pressure as applied by the practitioner. Fetal and neonatal effects include a diminished FHR variability and depression of neonatal respirations and Apgar scores. Depression of neonatal neurobehavior is evidenced by lowered Apgar scores. For example, with meperidine, neonatal respiration occurs within 2 to 3 hours after administration. Neonatal respiratory depression may require reversal by administration of naloxone (Narcan). Through inhibition of both mu and kappa receptors, naloxone (Narcan) may reverse the effects of opioids. Note with maternal administration of naloxone (Narcan) there will be a subsequent increase in pain. See Chapter 18, Cholinergics and Anticholinergics, for a discussion of neonatal naloxone dosing and administration.

Narcotic agonist drugs (morphine, fentanyl) can cause orthostatic hypotension, nausea, vomiting, headache, sedation, hypotension, and confusion. Decreased FHR variability and neonatal CNS depression can occur with meperidine. Do not confuse fentanyl with alfentanil.

Mixed narcotic agonist-antagonist drugs (Stadol, Nubain) can cause nausea, clamminess, sweating, sedation, respiratory depression, vertigo, lethargy, headache, and flush. Side effects in the fetus and neonate include decreased FHR variability, moderate CNS depression, hypotonia at birth, and mild behavioral depression.

Nursing Process

Pain Control Drugs

ASSESSMENT

■ Assess client's level of pain using agency pain scale.

■ Assess client's cultural framework to determine the use of complementary and alternative medicine in later pregnancy and specifically beliefs regarding laboring.

■ Assess the laboring client's behavior for relaxation and progress of labor in relation to expected norms.

■ Assess client's verbal and nonverbal behavior for data supportive or nonsupportive of coping with labor.

■ Obtain baseline vital signs, BP, breath sounds, quality of uterine contractions, degree of effacement and dilation, and fetal heart rate (FHR) before administering the analgesic to determine effectiveness of pain management.

■ Question client regarding use of complementary and alternative medicine to include herbal supplements during pregnancy.

■ Screen for drug history to ascertain potential for drug-drug interactions.

■ Assess cultural expectations related to pain experiences.

NURSING DIAGNOSES

■ Acute pain related to progressive labor

■ Fear of pain related to labor

■ Anxiety related to uncertainty about labor experience and personal coping ability

PLANNING

■ Client will verbalize a level of pain she is comfortable with during the labor and delivery process.

■ Client will demonstrate minimal to no side effects of pain control drugs during labor.

■ Client will verbalize a decrease in pain on a scale of 1 to 10 or per agency pain scale.

NURSING INTERVENTIONS

■ Incorporate client's cultural beliefs and framework of health in plan of care as possible.

■ Offer appropriate analgesia for stage and phase of labor and the anticipated method of delivery. Encourage client and her support persons to participate in the decision-making about analgesia.

■ Document administration of the drug per agency protocol.

■ Provide appropriate safety measures after administration of drugs.

■ Check compatibility chart for any mixing of drugs.

■ Verify that correct antidote drugs are available.

■ Within agency protocols, safe obstetric practice, and client preferences, administer drugs before maximum intensity of pain and anxiety.

■ Assess client's level of pain using agency appropriate pain scale within 30 to 60 minutes after analgesic administration.

Sedative-Hypnotics: Barbiturates

• Do not give if active labor is imminent.

• Monitor FHR; expect decreased variability.

Phenothiazine Derivative

Promethazine (Phenergan)

• If administered by IV route, give at onset of the uterine contraction. Administer at a rate not to exceed 25 mg/min.

• Monitor amount of promethazine client receives in 24 hours; monitor maternal heart rate following administration.

Hydroxyzine (Vistaril)

• Administer IM (Z-track technique) only. Do not give subQ or IV.

Narcotic Agonists and Mixed Narcotic Agonist-Antagonists

• Assess client parity, obstetrical delivery history and anticipated time until delivery.

• Do not administer when delivery is likely within 1 to 3 hours, as there is a greater chance of a depressed fetus or neonate (i.e., birth should occur within 1 hour or after 3 to 4 hours after administration).

• Monitor urine output.

• Monitor FHR assessing for fetal well-being before and during drug administration.

Fentanyl (Sublimaze)

• Generally not given before active labor. Have Naloxone (Narcan) available as antidote if needed.

• If drug is administered IV, administer slowly at beginning of a contraction over several minutes to decrease the amount of drug perfused to the fetus via the placenta.

• Assess respirations. Must be >12 before administration.

• Provide restful environment as adjunctive therapy.

• Keep bed rails up when client is nonambulatory and have client solicit assistance with ambulation.

• Monitor FHR assessing for fetal well-being before and during drug administration.

• Have neonatal naloxone (Narcan) available.

Butorphanol Tartrate (Stadol)

• Monitor for signs of narcotic withdrawal in narcotic-dependent clients.

• Monitor for respiratory depression.

- Assess respirations. Must be >12 before administration.
- IM: inject deep into muscle. If given IV, give slowly at onset contraction. Do not administer subQ.
- Provide restful environment as adjunctive therapy.
- Monitor FHR tracing assessing for fetal well-being before and during drug administration.
- Keep bed rails up when client is nonambulatory, and have client solicit assistance with ambulation.
- Have naloxone (Narcan) available.

Client Teaching
General
- Instruct client concerning the following: (1) drugs ordered, (2) route of administration and reason, (3) expected effects of drug on labor, and (4) potential drug effects on client and fetus or newborn.
- Tell client that most drugs used for pain relief in labor and delivery are not given by mouth because the gastrointestinal tract functions more slowly during labor. Thus drug absorption is decreased, making the oral route ineffective.

Safety
- Instruct client about safety precautions that will be used while receiving the drug, including the following: (1) positioning in bed, (2) side rails, (3) assistance with ambulation.

Cultural Considerations
- Acknowledge and incorporate client's cultural belief framework in nursing care.
- Assess client's use of complementary and alternative medicine, to include herbal supplements during pregnancy and labor.
- Recognize cultural influence on client's perception of and expression of discomfort and pain.
- Provide an interpreter as appropriate.

EVALUATION

- Evaluate effectiveness of the drug in lessening or alleviating the pain.
- Evaluate fear and anxiety in regard to pain and ability to cope with the labor experience.
- Monitor maternal respirations, heart rate, BP, uterine contractions, dilatation and effacement, and FHR for alterations from baseline. Report deviations beyond those expected with a normally progressing labor.
- Document findings using agency protocols and obstetric nursing standards of care.

Anesthesia

Anesthesia in labor and delivery represents the loss of painful sensations with or without the loss of consciousness. There are two types of pain experienced in childbirth. *Visceral pain* from the cervix and uterus is carried by sympathetic fibers and enters the neuraxis at the thoracic 10, 11, 12, and lumbar 1 spinal levels. Early labor pain is transmitted to T11 to T12 with later progression to T10 and L1. *Somatic pain* caused by pressure of the presenting part and stretching of the perineum and vagina. This pain is the pain of the transition phase and the second stage of labor and is transmitted to the sacral 2, 3, and 4 areas by the pudendal nerve.

Regional Anesthesia

Regional anesthesia achieves pain relief during labor and delivery without loss of consciousness. Injected local anesthetic agents temporarily block conduction of painful impulses along sensory nerve pathways to the brain (Table 52-2). Regional anesthesia allows the client to experience labor and birth with relief from discomfort in the blocked area. There are primarily two types of anesthesia: (1) local anesthetic agents for local infiltration (i.e., episiotomy) and (2) regional blocks (i.e., epidural).

Table 52–2

Anesthetic Agents Used in Obstetrics

Anesthetic Agent	Usual Concentration	Usual Dose (mg)	Onset	Average Duration (minutes)	Clinical Use
Chloroprocaine	1-2	400-600	Rapid	15-30	Local or pudenal
	2-3	300-750		30-60	Epidural
Tetracaine	0.2	4	Slow	70-150	Low spinal block
	0.5	7-10	Fast	75-150	Spinal for cesarean
Lidocaine	1	200-300	Rapid	30-60	Local or pudenal block
	2	300-450		60-90	Epidural for cesarean
	5	50-75		45-60	Spinal for cesarean, PP tubal ligation, and vaginal delivery
Bupivacaine	0.5	75-100	Slow-Moderate	90-150	Epidural for cesarean
	0.25	20-25	Moderate	60-90	Epidural for labor
	0.75	7.5-11		60-120	Spinal for cesarean
Ropivacaine	0.5	75-100	Slow-Moderate	90-150	Epidural for cesarean
	0.25	20-25	Slow-Moderate	60-90	Epidural for labor

PP, Postpartum.

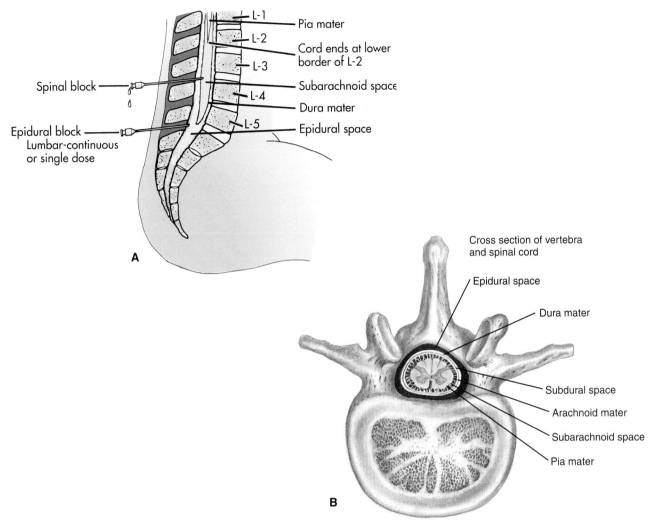

FIGURE 52–2   A, Membranes and spaces of spinal cord and levels of sacral, lumbar, and thoracic nerves. **B,** Cross-section of vertebra and spinal cord. (From Lowdermilk D, Perry S: *Maternity and women's health care*, St Louis, 2004, Mosby.)

The most common peridural anesthesias include spinal, epidural, and combined spinal-epidural and pudenal (Figure 52–2). Other less commonly administered regional blocks include caudal and paracervical blocks.

Women receiving parenteral analgesic for labor and delivery may require more focused anesthesia for episiotomies and for repair of perineal lacerations. Local anesthestic agents may be administered alone, and the anesthetic agent primarily administered is lidocaine. Burning at the site of injection is the most common side effect.

Spinal anesthesia, also known as a saddle block, is injected in the subarachnoid space at the T10 to S5 dermatone (Figure 52–3). This anesthesia may be a single dose or administered as a combined spinal epidural. Spinal anesthesia is administered immediately before delivery or late in the second stage when the fetal head is on the perineal floor. Drugs frequently administered either alone or in combination with the local anesthetic for a vaginal delivery include lidocaine (20 to 40 mg), bupivacaine (1.25 to 2.5 mg) with sufentanil (10 mcg), or fentanyl (25 mcg). Dosages vary de-

pending on administration of the anesthetic agent plain or with epinephrine. Spinal anesthesia has a rapid onset, requires less local anesthetic, and may be used with high risk obstetric and obese clients. Postdural puncture headache is a primary concern, occurring 6 to 48 hours after dural puncture and may occur with spinal and with accidental dura puncture with epidural anesthesia. Treatment for postdural headaches includes analgesics, increased fluids, and bed rest. With resistant headaches, 500 mg of caffeine in 500 ml normal saline may be given over 2 hours and blood patching. Autologous blood patching (10 to 20 ml) is the most effective means to treat post dural headache.

Lumbar epidurals may be administered as a single injection; intermittent injections; continuous, patient-controlled epidural anesthesia (PCEA); and as a combined spinal-epidural (see Figure 52–3). Epidurals may be administered as a single anesthetic agent or with opioids or epinephrine. Single-dose epidural anesthesia is infrequently used as analgesia and is limited to the single dosing action. Intermittent epidural bolus dosing was used for pain relief. Doses of the

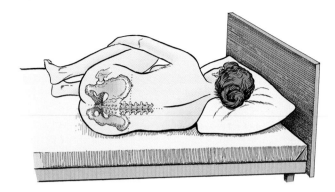

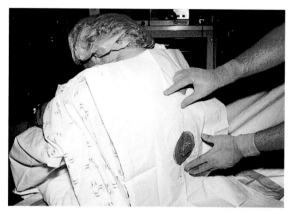

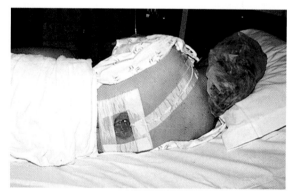

FIGURE 52–3   Positions for epidural blocks. (Photos courtesy of Michael S. Clement, MD, Mesa, Arizona. From Lowdermilk D, Perry S: *Maternity and women's health care,* St Louis, 2004, Mosby.)

local anesthetic were injected intermittently via an epidural catheter. Limitations of this method include the need for frequent injections and decreased pain control because of the dosing schedule. Most frequently, clients receive a continuous epidural infusion, which provides more consistent drug levels and more effective pain relief. Rescue doses are given as necessary to achieve pain relief.

Opioids are administered with the local anesthetic to control more effectively the somatic pain of transition and second-stage labor pain. The opioids most frequently used in combination with the local anesthetic (e.g., 0.125% bupivacaine or 0.2% ropivacaine) are fentanyl or sufentanil. Fentanyl or sufentanil are lipophilic opioids, which are commonly used with continuous or PCEA epidural. These opioids have a rapid analgesia and fewer side effects than hydrophilic opioids. In contrast, morphine sulfate and hydromorphone are hydrophilic opioids. They have a slower onset of action, variable duration and increased side effects, specifically respiratory depression (see Table 52–3).

Another additive to the local anesthetic is epinephrine. Epinephrine increases the duration and decreases the uptake and clearance of the local anesthetic from the central spinal fluid (CSF) while enhancing the intensity of the neural blockade. Single and intermittent injections have wide variations in drug levels and less-controlled pain. A continuous lumbar epidural allows a more evenly spaced drug level; less anesthestic is required and it provides more effective pain control. PCEA is administered by continuous infusion and allows the client control of the anesthesia with a basal infusion rate of 6 ml/h, a 5-ml bolus dose, with a 10-minute lockout. Frequently, single, intermittent, and PCEA will require rescue doses to improve analgesia.

Lastly, the combined spinal-epidural (CSE) analgesia allows the rapid analgesia and the specificity of catheter placement associated with spinal anesthesia and the continuous infusion via catheter of epidurals providing pain relief for later labor.

Controversy exists regarding the effect of regional analgesia, specifically epidurals on the progress of labor. Some

Table 52–3

Parenteral Opioids for Labor and Delivery

Opioid	Dosage	Analgesic Effect Begins	Peak Analgesic Effect	Duration of Action
meperidine (Demerol)	IM 50-100 mg	IM 10-45 min	IM 40-50 min	IM & IV 3-4 h
	IV 25-50 mg	IV 5 min	IV 5-10 min	IM 1-2 h
fentanyl (Sublimaze)	IM 50-100 mcg	IM 7-8 min	IM 30 min	IV 30-60 min
	IV 25-50 mcg	IV Almost immediately	IV 3-5 min	IM & IV 4-6 h
morphine sulfate	IM 5-10 mg	IM 15-60 min	1-2 hours–IM	IM & IV 3-6 h
	IV 2-5 mg	IV 5-10 min	20 min–IV	IM & IV 3-4 h
nalbuphine (Nubain)	IM 10-20 mg	IM <15 min	IM 60 min	
	IV 10 mg	IV 12-30 min	IV 30 min	
butorphanol (Stadol)	IM 1-4 mg	IM 5-10 min	IM 30-60 min	
	IV 2 mg	IV <10 min	IV 30-60 min	

h, Hour; *IM,* intramuscular; *IV,* intravenous; *min,* minute.

studies indicate no significant effect on labor, whereas other research has demonstrated a decreased maternal urge to push and increased length of labor. Single-dose epidural anesthesia is infrequently used as analgesia and is limited to the single dosing action. Later, intermittent epidural bolus dosing was used for pain relief. Doses of the local anesthetic were injected intermittently via an epidural catheter. Limitations of this method included the need for frequent injections and decreased pain control as a result of the dosing schedule. Most frequently, clients receive a continuous epidural infusion, which provides more consistent drug levels and more effective pain relief. Rescue doses are given as necessary to achieve pain relief.

Anesthesia for cesearean deliveries may be general, spinal, or epidural. General anesthesia is generally for emergency deliveries when spinal or epidural anesthesias are contraindicated. It allows for rapid anesthesia induction and control of the airway. Before the administration of general anesthesia, Bicitra 30 ml is orally administered to decrease gastric acidity. Other medications that may be used in place of Bicitra are cimetidine 300 mg, ranitidine 50 mg, or metoclopraminde 10 mg.

More commonly, epidural or spinal anesthesia is administered for cesaren births. Spinal anesthesia is the more common choice for cesareans because of rapid onset, increased reliability, and improvement in spinal needle design (smaller gauge and shape [strotte needle]) with subsequent reduction in postdural headaches. For epidural inductions, the test dose is given, followed by administration of the local anesthetics: lidocaine 1.5% to 2%, bupivacaine 0.5%, or chloroprocaine 3%. Epinephrine may be added, as have the opioids of fentanyl 50 to 100 mcg, sufentanil 10 to 20 mcg, or duramorph 3 to 5 mg, which is administered after clamping of the cord. Epidural provides pain relief for 18 to 24 hours. With spinal anesthesia, the local anesthetics most commonly administered are lidocaine 5% (60 to 75 mg), bupivacaine 0.75% (8 to 15 mg), or tetracaine 1% (7 to 10 mg). Epinephrine 0.2 mg and the opioids fentanyl 10-25 mg or sufentanil 10 mcg or duramorph 0.10 to 0.25 mg may also be administered. With the additives, spinal anesthesia also provides 18 to 24 hours of pain relief.

Contraindications to peridural anesthesia are clients with skin infection at the injection site, coagulopathies, active neurologic disease, severe aortic or mitral stenois, prior sensitivity to anesthetic agent, and hypovolemia. Of particular importance is client understanding of the procedure and consent.

Adverse effects from local anesthetic agents depend on their chemical properties but primarily affect the CNS and cardiovascular systems. CNS generally precede cardiovascular effects, with the exception of bupivacaine, in which adverse effects occur at the same drug level. Maternal systemic hypotension is the most frequent complication of regional anesthesia. Adverse CNS effects include dizziness, confusion, headache, slurred speech, metallic taste, nausea, vomiting, seizures, and coma. Cardiovascular symptoms include hypertension and tachycardia initially and followed by hypotension, cardiac arrhythmias and cardiac arrest. Fetal distress is secondary to maternal hypotension and the subsequent reduced uretroplacental perfusion.

Adverse effects from regional anesthetics vary depending on the agent and mode of delivery. With spinal and epidural anesthesia, a primary concern is maternal hypotension. Hypotension is defined as a decrease in systolic blood pressure greater than 20% to 30% of the baseline blood pressure or below 100 mmHg. To decrease maternal hypotension before epidural placement, an IV fluid bolus of 500 to 1000 ml of crystalloids is given. Women with hypotension are turned on their left side to facilitate placental perfusion and rapidly bolused with a crystalloid IV solution. If the maternal hypotension is resistant to fluid bolusing, then ephedrine 5 to 15 mg is administered IV. Maternal block is a primary consideration and is decreased with administration of lower concentrations of the regional local anesthetics.

Nursing Process

Regional Anesthetics

ASSESSMENT

- Check history for drug sensitivity to local anesthetic agents.
- Assess client's "labor plan" with expectations for coping with labor and beliefs about use of analgesia and anesthesia.
- Assess knowledge about regional anesthesia.
- Assess cervical dilation and effacement and labor progress.
- Monitor fetal status.
- Review history for presence of any contraindications to regional anesthesia; notify anesthesia provider.

NURSING DIAGNOSES

- Acute pain related to progressive labor with diminished coping ability
- Deficient knowledge related to inexperience with regional anesthesia/analgesia
- Risk for impaired gas exchange to fetus with maternal hypotension secondary to epidural block
- Impaired physical mobility secondary to regional anesthesia
- Risk for urinary retention secondary to regional anesthesia

PLANNING

- Client will verbalize desired amount of pain relief during labor.
- Client will remain normotensive and maintain a normal pulse rate; fetal heart rate (FHR) will remain within normal parameters.

■ Client will not experience bladder distention.
■ Client will be able to discuss use of regional anesthesia for labor and delivery pain control.

NURSING INTERVENTIONS

General

- Assess hydration status before regional anesthesia is given because of the hypotensive effects. Provide bolus IV fluids as ordered, usually 500-1000 ml prior to regional anesthesia administration.
- Position and support client on her left side or as instructed by the anesthesia provider.
- Monitor the progress of labor for any decrease in frequency or intensity of uterine contractions. Monitor maternal vital signs and FHR.
- Have emergency drugs and ephedrine, antihistamines, oxygen, and resuscitation equipment available.
- Be aware of how to place client in Trendelenburg's position if necessary.
- Monitor for postdura headache; notify anesthesia provider.

Spinal

- Assess uterine contractions, as the anesthetic agent must be given immediately after a contraction.
- Monitor BP for hypotensive effects per agency protocol after administration. Have oxygen with positive pressure ventilation equipment readily available.
- Assess level of analgesia following administration and sensory and motor status following delivery.
- Document procedure per agency protocol.

Epidural

- Ensure that client has 500 to 1000 ml IV bolus of an isotonic solution before the procedure to increase circulatory volume and prevent maternal hypotension.
- Monitor FHR and progress of labor and keep in mind that anesthetic can inhibit fetal descent.
- Monitor blood pressure (BP) for hypotensive effects per agency protocol after administration.
- Assess level of analgesia following administration.
- If maternal hypotension occurs, maintain client on left side and increase rate of IV fluids. Notify health care provider.
- Assess for bladder distention. If voiding cues (e.g., placement in semi-Fowler's position, privacy, running water over the perineum, running water over the hand) are unsuccessful then catheterize.
- Before allowing client to ambulate after delivery, assess sensory and motor status.
- Conduct ongoing pain assessment. If nature of pain changes, contact the anesthesia provider to evaluate anesthesia needs.
- Document procedure per agency protocol.

Caudal

- Place client in position requested by anesthesia provider for administration.

Paracervical Block

- Maintain continuous FHR monitoring for fetal bradycardia after administration.
- Monitor maternal BP.

Client Teaching

- Discuss technique, potential benefits, and side effects of client's particular method of anesthesia.

Side Effects
- Instruct client that regional anesthetics may slow labor and that some clients may need a drug to enhance uterine contractions.
- Assess client for a postdura headache after spinal anesthesia or accidental dura puncture with an epidural. Instruct client that bed rest, oral analgesics, caffeine, or a autologous blood patch may be used for headache pain relief.

Skill
- Instruct client how to curl into position for *epidural* administration. Instruct client that forceps or vacuum extraction may be needed for delivery (because of the reduction of the "urge to push" sensation).
- Instruct client how to assume the left lateral or other position as requested by anesthesia provider for *caudal* anesthesia.

Safety
- Instruct client receiving epidural anesthesia that she will have an IV and close monitoring of FHR and uterine contractions secondary to anesthesia.

EVALUATION

■ Evaluate BP compared with preprocedure baseline; also evaluate FHR for alterations in variability and for decelerations.
■ Evaluate the effectiveness of the anesthetic in relief of discomfort; also evaluate for uniformity of anesthesia; lateralization or if "patchy" notify anesthesia provider.
■ Assess for bladder distention. If voiding cues (e.g., placement in semi-Fowler's position, privacy, running water over the perineum, running water over the hand) are unsuccessful, then catheterize.
■ Before allowing client to ambulate after delivery, assess sensory and motor status.
■ Evaluate the fundus for firmness.

Spinal Block (Subarachnoid Block). *Adverse reactions:* **Client:** Hypotension; paresthesia or nerve injury, high/spinal block (respiratory muscles are impaired by block), (post dural headache, neuritis, block failure. Note: Headache is less common because of the small size (25 gauge) of needle used; client may have nausea, vomiting, backache, urinary retention, apnea with total spinal, or infection. **Fetus or neonate:** None, unless secondary to maternal hypotension and then FHR late decelerations.

Normal dose: **For vaginal delivery:** Bupivacaine 1.25-2.5 mg (with sufentanil 10 mcg or fentanyl 25 mcg) or 5% lidocaine 20-40 mg injected intrathecally; **for cesarean delivery:** Lidocaine 5% (60-75 mg), Bupivacaine 0.75% (8-15 mg), tetracaine 1% (7-10 mg) with epinephrine 0.2 mg and/or fentanyl 10-25 mcg or sufentanil 10 mcg or duramorph 0.10-0.25 mg.

Nursing implications: Client needs to be well hydrated, bolus with 500-1000 ml crystalloid solution. Cervix should be fully dilated before administration. Anesthetic is given immediately after a contraction to avoid impairing respiratory efforts. Client generally is sitting or in curled side-lying position for administration. Monitor blood pressure every 1 to 2 minutes for the first 10 minutes. After administration monitor BP every 5 to 10 minutes. Assess level of analgesia. Treat maternal hypotension with uterine displacement by placing a wedge under hip.

Contraindications: Infection at site, increased intracranial pressure, allergy to local anesthetics, coagulopathies, severe hypovolemia, severe aortic or mitral stenosis, or lack of client consent.

Indication: Need for high degree of pain relief for delivery. Used primarily for cesarean delivery, forceps delivery, or in the postpartum period for repair of traumatic lacerations of the perineal or removal of the retained placenta, and infrequently used for labor.

When given: Immediately before delivery; late in second stage when fetal head is on the perineum (for vaginal delivery).

Area blocked: Umbilicus to toes with vaginal delivery. Immediately below xyphoid process to toes with cesearean delivery.

Injection site: Place client in sitting or side-lying position; inject anesthetic into subarachnoid space at L4–L5.

Lumbar Epidural

Lumbar Epidural Block (Single Dose). *Adverse reactions:* Hypotension; paresthesia or nerve injury, neuritis, post dural headache with accidental puncture of dura, epidural hematoma, and high/total block (respiratory muscles are impaired by block). Note: Headache is less common because of the small size (25 gauge) of needle used; client may have nausea, vomiting, backache, urinary retention, infection, catheter complications, intravascular injection, direct spinal cord injury and bloody tap. **Fetus or neonate:** Few, unless secondary to maternal hypotension and then FHR late decelerations.

Normal dose: **For vaginal delivery:** bupivacaine 0.125-0.25%, lidocaine 1%, or chloroprocaine 2% (8-15 ml), or sufentanil 10-15 mcg or 100-200 fentanly in 10 ml of slaine, or Bupivacaine 0.0625% + fentanyl 50 mcg or sufentanil 10 mcg; **for cesarean delivery:** lidocaine 1.5-2% or bupivacaine 0.5% or chloroprocain 3% with epineph-

rine or sodium bicarbonate 1 ml/10 ml local anesthetic and/or fentanyl 50-100 mcg or sufentanil 10-20 mcg or duramorph 3-5 mg given after the umbilical cord is clamped.

Nursing implications: Note: Before epidural, client is well hydrated with 500-1000 ml of dextrose free intravenous fluids. Test dose (3 ml of lidocaine 1.5% epinephrine) is used to confirm correct placement of catheter; if local anesthetic is injected into vein, client may experience dizziness, ringing in ears, numb mouth, metallic taste, or toxic response. Loss or reduction of bearing-down reflex means low forceps or vacuum extraction may be needed for delivery. May slow progress of labor. Maternal lateral positioning is done to prevent aortocaval compression. Maternal diastolic blood pressure should be less than 110 mmHg before initiating the epidural. When maternal hypotension occurs, place the client on her left side, infuse IV fluids rapidly, and administer ephedrine 5-15 mg IV. Monitor BP every 1 to 2 minutes for the first 10 minutes and then every 10-30 minutes until the block wears off. Assess level of analgesia. After delivery assess motor strength prior to ambulation after administration. If unilateral analgesia occurs, client is turned to opposite side and more anesthetic is injected.

Contraindications: Infection at site, increased intracranial pressure, allergy to local anesthetics, coagulopathies, severe hypovolemia, severe aortic or mitral stenosis, or lack of client consent.

Indication: Pain relief in first and second stages of labor.

When given: Active labor. 5-6 cm dilated in a primipara, 3-4 cm in a multipara.

Area blocked: T12–S5 (entire pelvis) in area of dorsal root ganglion with varying degrees of motor and sensory loss depending on dosage and agent injected.

Injection site: Epidural space (potential space between the dura mater and vertebral canal from cranium to sacrum) between L2–L3 or L3–L5 or L4–L5; *not* in the dura. Never injected above L1 where the spinal cord ends. Nerves run off and down the spinal canal where they free-float and are easily moved aside by the epidural needle. The goal is to bathe the nerves with the dispersed local anesthetic.

Continuous Lumbar Epidural Block Using Indwelling Catheter in Epidural Space. *Adverse reactions:* Hypotension; paresthesia or nerve injury, post dural headache with accidental puncture of dura. Note: Headache is less common because of the small size (25 gauge) of needle used; client may have nausea, vomiting, backache, urinary retention, infection, catheter complications, intravascular injection, direct spinal cord injury and bloody tap. **Fetus or neonate:** Few, unless secondary to maternal hypotension and then FHR late decelerations.

Normal dose: Continuous infusions options (rate is 8-15 ml/hr). Bupivacaine 0.04-0.125% + fentanyl 1-2 mcg/ml or sufentanil 0.1-0.3 mcg/ml or Bupivacaine 0.125% without opiate

Nursing implications: Before epidural, client is well hydrated with 500-1000 ml of dextrose-free IV fluids. Test dose (3 ml of lidocaine 1.5% epinephrine) is used to confirm correct placement of catheter; if local anesthetic is injected into vein, client may experience dizziness, ringing in ears, numb mouth, metallic taste, or toxic response. Loss or reduction of bearing-down reflex means low forceps or vacuum extraction may be needed for delivery. May slow progress of labor. Maternal lateral positioning is done to prevent aortocaval compression. Maternal diastolic blood pressure should be less than 110 mmHg before initiating the epidural. When maternal hypotension occurs, place the client on her left side, infuse IV fluids rapidly, and administer ephedrine 5-15 mg IV. Monitor BP every 1-2 minutes for the first 10 minutes and then every 10-30 minutes until the block wears off. Assess level of analgesia. After delivery assess motor strength prior to ambulation after administration. Breakthrough pain is treated by increased infusion rate of rescue dose of anesthetic.

Indication: Pain relief during first and second stages. Useful for prolonged labor.

When given: Progressive, active labor. Active labor. 5-6 cm dilated in a primipara, 3-4 cm in a multipara. This is the most widely used anesthesia method for labor pain management.

Area blocked: Same as for lumbar epidural block.

Injection site: Same as for lumbar epidural block.

Advantages: Provides continuous anesthesia from stage 1 through delivery and perineal repair. Client can feel movement and pressure but no pain. Can be used for vaginal delivery or cesarean birth. Sensory level can be altered and density of the block can be manipulated. Can be used to deliver epidural morphine PF (Duramorph) or fentanyl (Sublimaze) into epidural space for regional analgesia (highly effective). Clients may experience pruritus, which may be effectively relieved with diphenhydramine (Benadryl) or naloxone (Narcan) infusions.

Considerations: Loss or reduction of bearing-down reflex means that forceps or a vacuum extraction may be needed for delivery. Requires an increased amount of local anesthestic agent. Bupivacaine is used in low concentration (as low as $1/_{16}$%) and may be combined with fentanyl (Sublimaze).

Complications: Same as for lumbar epidural block.

Side effects: Pruritus (in 2 to 3 hours when drug reaches upper thoracic segments), urinary retention, and nausea and vomiting related to ineffective hydration to prevent hypotension during labor.

PCEA (Patient Controlled Epidural Administration). *Adverse reactions:* Hypotension; paresthesia or nerve injury, post dural headache with accidental puncture of dura. Note: Headache is less common because of the small size (25 gauge) of needle used; client may have nausea, vomiting, backache, urinary retention, infection, catheter complications, intravascular injection, direct spinal cord injury and bloody tap. **Fetus or neonate:** Few, unless secondary to maternal hypotension and then FHR late decelerations.

Nursing implications: Before epidural, client is well hydrated with 500-1000 ml of dextrose-free IV fluids. Test

dose (3 ml of lidocaine 1.5% epinephrine) is used to confirm correct placement of catheter; if local anesthetic is injected into vein, client may experience dizziness, ringing in ears, numb mouth, metallic taste, or toxic response. Loss or reduction of bearing-down reflex means low forceps or vacuum extraction may be needed for delivery. May slow progress of labor. Maternal lateral positioning is done to prevent aortocaval compression. Maternal diastolic blood pressure should be less than 110 mmHg before initiating the epidural. When maternal hypotension occurs, place the client on her left side, infuse IV fluids rapidly, and administer ephedrine 5-15 mg IV. Monitor BP every 1 to 2 minutes for the first 10 minutes and then every 10-30 minutes until the block wears off. Assess level of analgesia. After delivery assess motor strength prior to ambulation after administration. Breakthrough pain is treated by increased infusion rate of rescue dose of anesthetic.

Indication: Pain relief during first and second stages. Useful for prolonged labor.

When given: Progressive, active labor. Active labor. 5-6 cm dilated in a primipara, 3-4 cm in a multipara.

Area blocked: Same as for lumbar epidural block.

Injection site: Same as for lumbar epidural block.

Advantages: Provides continuous anesthesia from stage 1 through delivery and perineal repair. Client can feel movement and pressure but no pain. Client in control of treatment and dose self titrated specific to client's pain. Sensory level can be altered and density of the block can be manipulated. Can be used to deliver epidural morphine PF (Duramorph) or fentanyl (Sublimaze) into epidural space for regional analgesia (highly effective). Clients may experience pruritus, which may be effectively relieved with diphenhydramine (Benadryl) or naloxone (Narcan) infusions.

Considerations: Loss or reduction of bearing-down reflex means that forceps or a vacuum extraction may be needed for delivery. Requires an increased amount of local anesthestic agent. Bupivacaine is used in low concentration (as low as $1/_{16}$%) and may be combined with fentanyl (Sublimaze).

Complications: Same as for lumbar epidural block.

Side effects: Pruritus (in 2 to 3 hours when drug reaches upper thoracic segments), urinary retention, and nausea and vomiting related to ineffective hydration to prevent hypotension during labor.

Combined Spinal-Epidural. *Adverse reactions:* Hypotension; paresthesia or nerve injury, post dural headache. Note: Headache is less common because of the small size (25 gauge) of needle used; client may have nausea, vomiting, backache, urinary retention, infection, catheter complications, intravascular injection, direct spinal cord injury and bloody tap. Proper catheter placement not assured and problem if epidural catheter needed for emergency analgesic administration. **Fetus or neonate:** Few, unless secondary to maternal hypotension and then FHR late decelerations.

Normal dose: **Spinal:** 25 mcg fentanyl or 10 mcg Sufentanil in 1 ml PF saline; epidural is inititated with Bupivacaine 0.04%-0.125% + fentanyl 1-2 mcg/ml or sufentanil 0.1-0.3 mcg/ml or Bupivacaine 0.125% without opiate.

Nursing implications: Before epidural, client is well hydrated with 500-1000 ml of dextrose-free IV fluids. Test dose (3 ml of lidocaine 1.5% epinephrine) is used to confirm correct placement of catheter; if local anesthetic is injected into vein, client may experience dizziness, ringing in ears, numb mouth, metallic taste, or toxic response. Loss or reduction of bearing-down reflex means low forceps or vacuum extraction may be needed for delivery. May slow progress of labor. Maternal lateral positioning is done to prevent aortocaval compression. Maternal diastolic blood pressure should be less than 110 mmHg before initiating the epidural. When maternal hypotension occurs, place the client on her left side, infuse IV fluids rapidly, and administer ephedrine 5-15 mg IV. Monitor BP every 1 to 2 minutes for the first 10 minutes and then every 10-30 minutes until the block wears off. Assess level of analgesia. After delivery assess motor strength prior to ambulation after administration. Breakthrough pain is treated by increased infusion rate of rescue dose of anesthetic.

Indication: Pain relief during first and second stages. Spinal can help with early labor pain and epidural for pain management during active labor.

When given: Progressive, active labor.

Area blocked: Same as for spinal and lumbar epidural block.

Injection site: Same as for spinal and lumbar epidural block.

Advantages: Provides continuous anesthesia from stage 1 through delivery and perineal repair. Client can feel movement and pressure but no pain. Sensory level can be altered and density of the block can be manipulated. Can be used to deliver epidural morphine PF (Duramorph) or fentanyl (Sublimaze) into epidural space for regional analgesia (highly effective). Clients may experience pruritus, which may be effectively relieved with diphenhydramine (Benadryl) or naloxone (Narcan) infusions. Adminstration of a combination of local anesthetic and opioid more effectively blocks the somatic pain of transition and second-stage labor.

Considerations: Loss or reduction of bearing-down reflex means that forceps or a vacuum extraction may be needed for delivery. Requires an increased amount of local anesthetic agent. Bupivacaine is used in low concentration (as low as $\frac{1}{16}$%) and may be combined with fentanyl (Sublimaze).

Complications: Same as for lumbar epidural block.

Side effects: Pruritus (in 2 to 3 hours when drug reaches upper thoracic segments), urinary retention, and nausea and vomiting related to ineffective hydration to prevent hypotension during labor.

Caudal (A Type of Epidural Anesthesia)

Indication: Pain in first and second stages of labor.

When given: Active labor.

Area blocked: Perineum; masks uterine contractions.

Injection site: Epidural space through sacral hiatus (S4).

Advantages: Useful for women with metabolic, lung, and heart disease. Very rapid perineal anesthesia and muscle relaxation. Can be used continuously.

Considerations: Increased need to use forceps or vacuum extraction because there is a loss of urge to push. Risk of systemic toxic reactions; level of anesthesia is more difficult to obtain.

Paracervical Block

Indication: Pain during first stage. Due to high incidence of fetal bradycardia, paracervical block is infrequently administered.

When given: Active phase of first stage; may be repeated periodically until 8-cm dilated.

Area blocked: Uterus, cervix, and vagina; masks uterine contractions.

Injection site: Submucosa of the fornix of the vagina lateral to the cervix.

Advantages: Rapid onset. Lasts 60 to 90 minutes. Relieves pain of cervical dilation and contractions. Does not block lower vagina or perineum.

Considerations: Rapid absorption (because injected into a very vascular area). Does not provide anesthesia for delivery or episiotomy repair. Has variable effects on labor progress.

Side effects: **Client:** Hematomas in tissue around injection site. **Fetus:** Mild to severe bradycardia or prolonged FHR deceleration common with decreased variability.

Pudendal Block

Indication: For low forceps deliveries, episiotomy, and laceration repair.

When given: Immediately before birth.

Area blocked: Perineum; pudendal nerves.

Injection site: Transvaginally behind each sacrospinous ligament to block pudenal nerves.

Considerations: None. Not useful for pain management in first stage of labor.

Side effects: None.

Local Infiltration

Indication: For episiotomy and perineal laceration repair.

When given: Just before delivery or repair.

Area blocked: Local area adjacent to injection.

Injection site: Perineal subcutaneous tissue.

Advantage: No effect on FHR or client's vital signs.

Considerations: May not obtain complete relief of pain and may need additional injections; requires large amount of local anesthetic agent.

Side effects: **Client:** Mild discomfort and/or burning during injection. **Fetus or neonate:** None.

Contraindications

The following are relative contraindications to regional anesthesia:

- Morbid obesity
- Severe pregnancy-induced hypertension (PIH) (caused by increased risk of profound hypotension, associated with underlying disease state) and a risk of bleeding secondary to decreased platelets

- Coagulation disorders (client should have a normal partial thomboplastin time and platelet count)
- Generalized sepsis or local infection at needle insertion site

Drugs that Enhance Uterine Muscle Contractility

Uterotropic drugs enhance **uterine contractility** by stimulating the smooth muscle of the uterus. Oxytocin, the ergot alkaloids, and some prostaglandins constitute the uterotropics.

Oxytocin is synthesized in the hypothalamus and is transported to nerve endings in the posterior pituitary. The hormone is released by the nerve endings under appropriate stimulation; capillaries absorb the substance and carry it into the general circulation, where it facilitates uterine smooth muscle contraction.

In the presence of adequate estrogen levels (those normally achieved by the third trimester), IV oxytocin stimulates uterine contraction. Oxytocin, prepared in synthetic form and marketed as Pitocin, is approved by the Food and Drug Administration (FDA) for labor induction and labor augmentation. Do not confuse oxytocin (Pitocin) with Pitressin. Box 52–1 presents common medical reasons for induction.

Before **labor induction** begins, risks and benefits and the status of the mother and fetus must be assessed. The gestational age of the fetus must be considered together with the position of the fetus (head down and deep in the pelvis) and the size of the fetus in relation to the client's pelvis. The client's **cervical ripening** is also assessed; the cervix is ripe, and thus ready for induction, when it is soft and progressing in effacement and partial dilation. An objective scoring system called the **Bishop score** is used to assess readiness for induction. Elements assessed in the modified Bishop Scoring System are dilatiation, effacement, station, cervical consistency, and cervical position. Modified Bishop scores of 9 or greater are associated with a successful labor induction.

Some clients are not suitable candidates for labor induction because the risks of the procedure outweigh the potential benefits. Box 52–2 presents some major contraindications to labor induction.

Two approaches of labor induction are used to ripen, efface, and begin cervical dilation in pregnant women at term (or near term) with a medical or obstetric indication for labor induction. *Mechanical methods* and *prostaglandins* may be used to induce labor.

One mechanical method involves insertion of a Foley catheter through an undilated cervix and internal os with subsequent inflation of the bulb. The Foley catheter bulb provides a mechanical stimulation similar to "stripping of the membranes." When the Foley "falls out," the client is started on IV oxytocin. Secondly, an extra-amniotic saline infusion with a balloon catheter may be used to induce labor. A third mechanical method is membrane "stripping." With membrane stripping, there is release of prostagladin F_2 from the decidua or prostanglandin E_2 from the cervix. Spontaneous labor has been within 72 hours with membrane stripping with no increase in infection. Finally an amniotomy, artificial rupture of membranes is commonly used and is performed in women with a partially dilated and effaced cervix. When done at 5 cm, dilated spontaneous labor is shortened by 1 to 4 hours without an increase in maternal or fetal complications. Chorioamnionitis and cord compression have been reported.

The second approach uses administration of dinoprostone, the naturally occurring form of prostaglandin $E_2(PGE_2)$. It is thought that intracervically or intravaginally administered PGE_2 acts to create cervical effacement and softening by a combination of contraction-inducing and cervical-ripening properties, possibly secondary to an increased submucosal water content and collagen degradation resulting from collagenase secretion in response to PGE_2. One approach uses prefilled syringes of commercially prepared dinoprostone cervical gel 0.5 mg. (Prepidil gel); the gel is introduced just inside the cervical os. A second approach is the placement in the posterior vaginal fornix of a vaginal insert

---

BOX 52–1

Indications for Labor Induction

- Pregnancy-induced hypertension
- Chronic hypertension
- Membrane rupture >24 hours
- Chorioamnionitis
- Postdates (>42 weeks' gestation)
- Intrauterine growth retardation (IUGR)
- Positive contraction stress test (CST)
- Maternal diabetes mellitus (classes B–F)
- Maternal renal disease
- Isoimmunization
- Intrauterine fetal death

BOX 52–2

Contraindications to Labor Induction

- Disproportion between fetal head and pelvis (cephalopelvic disproportion)
- Nonfavorable fetal presentation (transverse or breech)
- Documented fetal intolerance of uterine contractions
- Prematurity
- Placenta previa or suspected abruptio placentae
- Severe pregnancy-induced hypertension
- Multiparity (6 or more)
- Multifetal gestation
- History of uterine trauma
- Previous major surgery in the area of the cervix or uterus
- Prior classical uterine incision
- Active genital herpes infection
- Umbilical cord prolapse
- Excessive amniotic fluid causing overdistended uterus

Table 52–4

Dinoprostone for Cervical Ripening

Generic (Brand)	Route and Dosage	Uses and Considerations
dinoprostone cervical gel, 0.5 mg (Prepidil gel)	Intracervical: Prepidil contains 0.5 mg of dinoprostone in 2.5 ml of gel for intracervical use. Repeat in 6-12 h if negative cervical or uterine response. The maximum 24 h dose is 1.5 mg, supplied in 3 doses. Before beginning oxytocin after the Prepidil administration there should be a 6- to 12-h delay.	A naturally occurring form of prostaglandin E_2 (PGE_2). Used to ripen unfavorable cervix at or near term in pregnant women needing labor induction. Metabolized in lung, liver, and kidney; eliminated by kidney. Must be administered in a hospital. Clients may have a reactive nonstress test before first dose. Monitor uterine activity and FHR; suggest a 20-min FHR strip before doses. Gel must be at room temperature before administration and is administered by sterile technique. Gel must *not* be placed above level of cervical os. Client is to remain recumbent 15-30 min following administration of gel and 2 h after insert administration. Drug may augment other oxytocic agents; therefore no concomitant use; sequential use 6-12 h after gel is recommended. Insert may be inserted with minimal amount of water solute lubricant. Wear gloves when administering gel or insert. Must be used with caution in clients with renal or hepatic dysfunction. Contraindicated in clients with sensitivity to drug hypersensitivity, cephalopelvic (CPD), ruptured membranes, and unexplained vaginal bleeding. Use gel and insert with caution in clients with asthma, seizures, glaucoma, increased intraocular pressure, cardiovascular, renal or hepatic disease. Not recommended for clients in whom oxytocic drugs are contraindicated or with prolonged uterine contractions; not recommended in clients with placenta previa or active genital herpes (vaginal delivery not indicated). *Adverse reactions:* uterine hyperstimulation, nausea, vomiting, diarrhea, back pain, warm feeling in vagina, and dinoprostone-induced fever, fetal distress. Treat dinoprostone-induced fever, which occurs in about 50% of clients with tepid baths and increased fluids. Fever is not to be treated with aspirin. *Pregnancy category:* C; PB: UK; $t^{1/2}$: UK; onset: 10-60 min; peak: UK; duration: 12 h
dinoprostone (Cervidil vaginal inserts)	Vaginal: Cervidil contains 10 mg of dinoprostone in a timed release insert, releasing 0.3 mg/h. Insert is left in place for 12 h. Oxytocin may be started 30-60 min after removal of the insert. In contrast to the gel, the insert may be removed with FHR decelerations or uterine hyperstimulation. Ripening unfavorable cervix: Intravaginal: 10 mg over 12 h; remove 12 h after insertion or at onset of active labor.	Have oxygen or beta-adrenergic drugs to treat uterine hyperstimulation. Use suppository at room temperature. Provider should wear gloves to decrease risk of absorption as inserted high into the vagina. Assess vaginal dilatation and effacement at the time of suppository insertion. After administration, client remains in lying position for 10 min. Have medication available for frequent gastrointestinal side effects of abdominal cramping, diarrhea, nausea, and vomiting. Provide emotional support.

FHR, Fetal heart rate; *h,* hour; *min,* minute; *PB,* protein-binding; $t^{1/2}$, half-life; *UK,* unknown.

(Cervidil) containing 10 mg of controlled-release dinoprostone at 0.3 mg/h. Do not confuse dinoprostone (prepidil Gel) with bepridil.

Table 52–4 presents the dosage, uses, and considerations for administration of dinoprostone for cervical ripening.

Oxytocin

In addition to labor induction, IV oxytocin can also be used for **labor augmentation.** It facilitates smooth-muscle contraction in the uterus of a client already in labor but experiencing inadequate uterine contractility. The client with **uterine inertia** may be more responsive to oxytocin than the client who has not begun labor; therefore a lower starting dose will be needed.

In both labor induction and labor augmentation, oxytocin is infused at a prescribed individualized dosage rate, and this rate is increased, decreased, or maintained at fixed intervals based on uterine and fetal response. The objective is to establish an adequate contraction pattern that promotes labor progress, generally represented by contractions every 2 to 3 minutes that last for 50 to 60 seconds with moderate intensity. It is important that the client receiving oxytocin not experience uterine hyperstimulation, which causes markedly increased pain and nonreassuring FHR patterns secondary to impaired placental perfusion. Continuous nursing observation during labor induction or augmentation is critical. The need for an accurate infusion rate requires the use of an infusion pump with oxytocin as an IV piggyback line. Once cervical dilation has reached 5 to 6 cm and an adequate contraction pattern is evident, the rate of oxytocin infusion can often be slowed or stopped.

Following delivery, oxytocin, 10 to 20 mg is usually added to an existing IV solution to help the uterus stay contracted and thus close the uterine sinuses at the placental site. The drug can also be given IM after delivery of the placenta.

Prototype Drug Chart 52–1 shows the actions and effects of oxytocin.

Oxytocin (Pitocin, Syntocinon) is well absorbed from the nasal mucosa when administered intranasally for milk letdown. The protein-binding percent is low, and the half-life is 1 to 9 minutes. It is rapidly metabolized and excreted by the liver.

The onset of action of oxytocin administered IM is in 3 to 5 minutes, the peak concentration time is unknown, and the duration of action is 2 to 3 hours. The onset of action of oxytocin administered by IV is immediate, the peak concentration time is unknown, and the duration of action is 1 hour. The onset of action of intranasally administered oxytocin is a few minutes, the peak concentration time is unknown, and the duration of action is 20 minutes.

The medication is diluted and administered IV piggyback for induction or augmentation of labor. Pitocin is diluted in a variety of ways and administered via infusion pump in ml/min dosing with the volume determined by the dilution. IV administration of undiluted oxytocin is not recommended because of the risk of a sudden, acute hypotensive response.

Concurrent use of vasopressors can result in severe hypertension. Hypotension can occur with concurrent use of cyclopropane anesthesia and with undiluted IV push administration.

Nursing Process

Enhancement of Uterine Contractility: Oxytocins

ASSESSMENT

For induction or augmentation of labor:
■ Confirm term gestation before inducing or augmenting labor.
■ Collect accurate baseline data before beginning infusion, including maternal pulse and blood pressure (BP), uterine history, uterine activity, and fetal heart rate (FHR) pattern.
■ Interview client and review history to ascertain that there are no contraindications.

NURSING DIAGNOSES

■ Deficient knowledge related to drugs used to promote uterine contractility

PLANNING

■ Oxytocin will enhance uterine contractions without adverse maternal or fetal effects.
■ Client's vital signs will be within acceptable ranges throughout labor, delivery, and postpartum period.
■ FHR will demonstrate normal rate, pattern, and variability throughout labor and delivery.

NURSING INTERVENTIONS

■ Have tocolytic agents and oxygen readily available.
■ Monitor intake and output.
■ Monitor maternal pulse and BP, uterine activity, and FHR during oxytocin infusion.
■ Maintain client in sitting or lateral recumbent position to promote placental infusion.
■ Monitor for signs of uterine rupture, which include FHR decelerations, sudden increased pain, loss of uterine contractions, hemorrhage, and rapidly developing hypovolemic shock.

Client Teaching

• Instruct client the drug is given IV and the dosage is adjusted in response to uterine contraction pattern.
• For milk letdown, teach client timing and method of nasal administration.

EVALUATION

■ Evaluate for effective labor progress.
■ Monitor maternal vital signs and FHR. Report changes in vital signs and FHR, specifically late decelerations and any vaginal bleeding.

Ergot Alkaloids

The **ergot alkaloids** act by direct smooth-muscle-cell receptor stimulation. These drugs are not used during labor because they can cause sustained uterine contractions (tetanic contractions), which would result in fetal hypoxia and possibly in rupture of the uterus. The uterus becomes more sensitive to these drugs too. After delivery, however, these sustained contractions are effective in the prevention or control of postpartum hemorrhage and the promotion of uterine involution.

The two most commonly used ergot derivatives are ergonovine maleate (Ergotrate) and methylergonovine maleate (Methergine). These preparations can be given IV, IM, or by mouth. If methylergonovine maleate (Methergine) is given IV, administer 0.2 mg over 1 minute. IV administration is not recommended and is given only in emergency situations. Transient significant elevations in BP can occur, particularly after IV infusion of either drug, and clients with pregnancy-induced hypertension, or peripheral vascular dis-

PROTOTYPE DRUG CHART 52–1

OXYTOCIN

Drug Class

Oxytocic drug
Trade Name: Pitocin, Syntocinon
Pregnancy Category: X

Dosage

For induction or augmentation of labor:
A: IV: 10 units (1 amp) diluted in 1000 ml lactated Ringer's to 10 mU/ml; connect to primary IV line close to the needle site as a piggyback line. (Resulting concentration is 10 mU oxytocin per 1 ml of IV fluid.) The low-dose oxytocin regimen is to start the oxytocin at 0.5-1 or 1-2 mU/min with an incremental dose of 1-2 mU per min and a maximum dose of 20 mU/min. The high-dose oxytocin regimen is to begin oytocin at 6 mU/min IV with an increase in dose by 6 mU/min every 15 min. The maximum dose is 40 mU/min.
Postdelivery:
A: IV: 10-20 units added to 1000 ml electrolyte or dextrose solution; infuse at rate to prevent uterine atony
IM: 10 units after delivery of the placenta
Nasal spray: One spray into one or both nostrils 2-3 min before nursing or pumping; not for use during pregnancy

Contraindications

Proven cephalopelvic disproportion, fetal intolerance of labor, hypersensitivity, anticipated nonvaginal delivery, pregnancy (intranasal spray)

Drug-Lab-Food Interactions

Drug: Hypertension with vasopressors, cyclopropane anesthetics

Pharmacokinetics

Absorption: PO: Not well absorbed, intranasal and IM very rapidly
Distribution: PB: Low; widely distributed in extracellular fluid; minute amounts in fetal circulation
Metabolism: $t\frac{1}{2}$: 1-9 min; rapidly metabolized by liver
Excretion: In urine

Pharmacodynamics

IM: Onset: 3-5 min
 Peak: 40 min
 Duration: 2-3 h
IV (infusion): Onset: Within 1 min
 Peak: UK
 Duration: 1 h
Intranasal: Onset: Few minutes
 Peak: UK
 Duration: UK

Therapeutic Effects/Uses

To induce or augment labor contractions; to treat uterine atony; milk letdown (intranasal spray)
Mechanism of Action: Promotes uterine contractions by increasing intracellular concentrations of calcium in uterine myometrial tissue, thereby increasing the activity of the calcium-dependent phosphorylating enzyme myosin light-chain kinase. The nasal spray works by forcing milk into larger ducts and sinuses. This occurs because oxytocin promotes milk ejection by causing contraction of the smooth-muscle fibers surrounding the breast alveoli and lactiferous ducts.

Side Effects

Maternal effects with undiluted IV use only: hypotension, dysrhythmias, tachysystole, and uterine hyperstimulations. Tachysystole is 6 or more uterine contractions in a 20-min window. Hyperstimulation is defined as uterine contractions lasting at least 2 min or 5 or greater contractions in a 10-min window.

Adverse Reactions

Seizures, water intoxication if given in electrolyte-free solution or at a rate greater than 20 mU/min. Water intoxication is manifested by nausea, vomiting, hypotension, tachycardia, and cardiac arrhythmias.
Life-threatening: *Client:* Intracranial hemorrhage, cardiac dysrhythmias, asphyxia. *Fetus:* jaundice, hypoxia

---

A, Adult; *amp,* ampule; *h,* hour; *IM,* intramuscular; *IV,* intravenous; *min,* minute; *PB,* protein-binding; *PO,* by mouth; *t½,* half-life; *UK,* unknown.

Table 52–5

Uterotonic Drugs Commonly Used to Enhance Uterine Contractility

Generic (Brand)	Route and Dosage	Uses and Considerations
oxytocin (Pitocin, Syntocinon)	See Prototype Drug Chart 52–1.	
ergonovine maleate (Ergotrate)	PO: 0.2-0.4 mg (1-2 tablets) q6-12h over 48 h IM: 0.2 mg q2-4 h; *max:* 5 doses IV: 0.2 mg over 1 min while BP is monitored (IV route for acute emergencies only [e.g., bleeding])	Oxytocic; ergot alkaloid. Used to stimulate directly vascular smooth muscle to vasoconstrict peripheral and cerebral vessels; used to prevent and treat postpartum or post-abortion hemorrhage caused by uterine atony or subinvolution. IV onset: immediate; duration: 45 min. IM onset: 2–5 min; duration: 3 h. PO onset: 6-15 min; duration: 3 h. Use IV only for true emergencies. Metabolized in liver; excreted in urine. Do not use in clients with coronary artery disease, hypertension, PIH; contraindicated before delivery of placenta. Use with caution in clients with sepsis or hepatic or renal impairment. *Adverse reactions:* diaphoresis, palpitations, transient chest pain, thrombophlebitis, seizures, cerebrovascular accidents, dizziness, headache, nausea, vomiting, tinnitus, dyspnea. *Pregnancy category:* X; PB: UK; $t^{1}/_{2}$: 2 h
methylergonovine maleate (Methergine)	PO: 0.2-0.4 mg, q6-12 h; *max:* 1 wk IM: 0.2 mg after delivery of anterior shoulder (if full obstetric supervision), after delivery of placenta, or postpartum; repeat q2-4 h; oral doses may follow parenteral IV: Same as for IM; but slowly over 1 min with careful monitoring of BP (IV route for acute emergencies only [e.g., bleeding])	Prevention and treatment of postpartum hemorrhage; subinvolution and postabortion hemorrhage. Exhibits similar smooth-muscle action to ergotamine but affects primarily smooth muscle, producing *sustained* contractions and thus shortening third stage of labor. IV onset: immediate; duration: 45 min. IM onset: 2-5 min; duration: 3 h. PO onset: 5-25 min; duration: 3 h. Metabolized in liver; eliminated in urine. Not routinely administered IV because of possible sudden hypertensive and cerebrovascular accidents; limit use with clients with hypertension (especially IV). Contraindicated with maternal sepsis, labor induction, threatened spontaneous abortion; do not use with vasodepressors, other ergot alkaloids, or vasoconstrictors. Appears in breast milk, but interference with breastfeeding is less than with ergonovine. *Adverse reactions:* transient hypertension, diaphoresis, palpitations, dizziness, headache, nausea, vomiting, tinnitus, transient chest pain, dyspnea. *Pregnancy risk factor:* C; PB: UK; $t^{1}/_{2}$: biphasic: *initial:* 1-5 min; *terminal:* 30 min-2 h

BP, Blood pressure; *h,* hour; *IM,* intramuscular; *IV,* intravenous; *max,* maximum; *min,* minute; *PB,* protein-binding; *PO,* by mouth; $t^{1}/_{2}$, half-life; *UK,* unknown; *wk,* week.

eases should not receive ergot derivatives. Table 52–5 presents the most commonly used uterotonic drugs.

Side Effects and Adverse Reactions

Side effects of ergot alkaloids include uterine cramping, nausea and vomiting, dizziness, hypertension with IV administration, sweating, tinnitus, chest pain, dyspnea, itch-

PREVENTING MEDICATION ERRORS

Do not confuse...

- **Methylergonovine (Methergine)** with **terbutaline sulfate (Brethine).** These drugs have opposite actions! Be alert to packaging, which is very similar. Both are amber ampules with colored neckbands wrapped in foil and amber plastic packaging. Do not store these drugs together.

ing, and sudden severe headache. Signs of ergot toxicity **(ergotism)** include pain in arms, legs, and lower back; numbness; cold hands and feet; muscular weakness; diarrhea; hallucinations; seizures; and blood hypercoagulability.

Nursing Process

Other Oxytocics: Ergonovine and Methylergonovine

ASSESSMENT

Ergonovine (Ergotrate) and Methylergonovine (Methergine)

■ Assess lochia and uterine tone before giving ergonovine or methylergonovine.
■ Assess effectiveness of uterine massage and oxytocin administration on local flow and uterine tone.

■ Recognize that these two drugs have a vasoconstrictive effect, which may cause hypertension. Ergonovine is more vasoconstrictive than methylergonovine.

■ Obtain baseline BP before administration.

NURSING INTERVENTIONS

Ergonovine (Ergotrate) and Methylergonovine (Methergine)

• Monitor client's BP per agency protocol.
• Protect drugs from exposure to light.
• Monitor for side effects or symptoms of ergot toxicity (ergotism). Notify physician if systolic BP increases by 25 mmHg or diastolic BP by 20 mmHg over baseline.

Client Teaching

Ergonovine and Methylergonovine

• Instruct client that she will feel more intense uterine cramps after receiving the drug but may receive analgesics for pain.

Safety

• Instruct client to avoid smoking. Nicotine increases the vasoconstrictive properties of these drugs.

Side Effects

• If client is breastfeeding, explain that the drug lowers serum prolactin levels with the potential to inhibit postpartum lactation; note that ergonovine has an increased potential to inhibit lactation than methylergonovine.

Cultural Considerations

• Recognize cultural influence on client's expression or lack of expression of discomfort and/or pain.
• Provide an interpreter, as appropriate.

EVALUATION

■ Evaluate the effectiveness of the drug via assessment of lochia and uterine tone. Count and weigh perineal pads as appropriate.

■ Continue monitoring maternal vital signs, specifically pulse and BP. Report changes in maternal vital signs, continued excessive vaginal bleeding, or uterine atony.

Surfactant Therapy in Preterm Birth

Synthetic Surfactant

One approach to respiratory difficulties in the preterm infant is **surfactant** replacement therapy. This is used to prevent the development of **respiratory distress syndrome (RDS)**. Surfactant replacement therapy is also used to decrease the severity of RDS following diagnosis. Supplementing the amount of endogenous surfactant available to maintain distention of the alveolar sacs is the focus of this therapy.

Currently the FDA has approved the use of beractant (Survanta), calfactant (Infasurf), and poractant alfa (Curosurf). Beractant (Survanta) lowers alveolar surface tension during respiration and stabilizes alveoli. Beractant (Survanta) intratracheal suspension, a natural bovine-lung extract, contains phospholipids, neutral lipids, fatty acids, and surfactant-associated proteins to which solfosceril palmitate (DPPC), palmitic acid, and tripalmitin are added. Beractant (Survanta) does not require reconstitution. Calfactant (Infasurf) is a calf-lung surfactant that can be used preventilatory for prevention of RDS or postventilatory for treatment. Poractant alfa (Curosurf) is porcine-lung surfactant and is indicated for rescue treatment. All three of these products define *prophylactic* and *rescue* use differently (Table 52–6) and have different dosing and administration requirements for each use.

All products require a patent endotracheal (ET) tube for administration and specified alterations in positioning the infant throughout the procedure to ensure even drug dispersion. These precise position changes allow gravity to assist in the distribution of the product in the lungs, particularly at the alveolar surface.

Rales and moist breath sounds may be a transient finding following administration of these products, particularly with beractant (Survanta). Additionally, transient oxygen desaturation has occurred with poractant alfa (Curosurf), and airway obstruction has occurred in 39% of infants in clinical studies with calfactant (Infasurf). Unless obvious signs of airway obstruction are noted, suctioning should not be performed for 2 hours after administration.

Surfactant replacement therapy has been found effective in reducing the severity of RDS; rapid improvements in lung compliance and oxygenation may require immediate decreases in ventilator settings to prevent lung overdistention and pulmonary air leak.

Adverse Reactions

Side effects during administration have included incidents of reflux of product up the ET tube with decreases in oxygenation. Dosing is slowed or halted if the infant (1) becomes dusky colored, (2) becomes agitated, (3) experiences transient bradycardia, (4) has oxygen saturation increases of more than 95%, (5) experiences improved chest expansion, or (6) has arterial or tracutaneous CO_2 levels less than 30 mm Hg. Pulmonary hemorrhage has been seen in infants treated with Exosurf. Suctioning before dosing decreases the chance for ET tube blockage during dosing. No long-term complications or sequelae of synthetic surfactant therapy have been reported.

Nursing Process

Beractant (Survanta), Calfactant (Infasurf), and Poractant Alfa (Curosurf)

ASSESSMENT

■ Assess for informed consent. Separate consents are needed for multifetal birth.

Table 52–6

Postnatal Surfactant Therapy for Prevention and Treatment of Respiratory Distress Syndrome

Generic (Brand)	Route and Dosage	Uses and Considerations
Beractant (Survanta) Intratracheal suspension	4 ml/kg per dose ET (divided into 4 quarter doses and give each quarter dose with infant in different position) in one of two modes: *Prophylaxis:* 1 dose within 15 min of birth if possible; repeat in 6 h if respiratory distress continues; maximum 4 doses in 24 h (6 h apart). *Rescue:* 4 ml/kg intratracheally (also divided into 4 quarter doses and give each quarter dose with different infant positioning). Give dose as soon as RDS is diagnosed, preferably within 8 h of birth. Repeat in 6 h, giving a maximum of 4 doses in 24 h.	Beractant (Survanta) contains phospholipids, neutral lipids, fatty acids, and surfactant-associated proteins to which colfosceril palmitate (DPPC), palmitic acid, and tripalmitin are added. Each 1 ml contains 2.5 mg phospholipids. Must be given by health care personnel experienced with ventilators as *prevention* or *rescue* in treatment of RDS. Administered through a 5 French end-hole catheter as a dosing catheter inserted into ET tube. Following administration of each quarter dose, catheter removed from ET tube and infant ventilated for 30 sec until stable. *Prophylaxis* defined as use in infants less than 1250 g at high risk for RDS or larger infants with evidence of pulmonary immaturity. *Rescue* defined as treatment of infants with moderate to severe RDS. Biophysical effects occur at the alveolar surface; lowers surface tension on alveolar surfaces during respiration and stabilizes alveoli against collapse at resting pressures. Infants should be frequently monitored with arterial or transcutaneous measurement of systemic oxygen or carbon dioxide. Does not require reconstitution. Drug should appear off-white to light brown. Swirl vial gently; DO NOT SHAKE. Foam at surface normal. Store at 36-46° F (2-8° C); warm 20 min at room temperature or in hand for at least 8 min. Do not artificially warm. For prevention dose, begin preparation before infant's birth. Do not warm or return drug to refrigerator more than once. Protect from light. No known contraindications. *Adverse reactions:* transient bradycardia, oxygen desaturation (associated with dosing procedure); ET tube reflux; ET blockage, pallor, vasoconstriction, hypotension, hypocarbia, hypercarbia, and apnea. All reactions resolve with symptomatic treatment.
Calfactant (Infasurf)	3 ml/kg of birth weight as soon as possible after birth. Give as 2 doses of 1.5 ml/kg each every 12 h for total of 3 doses.	Must be given by health care personnel experienced with ventilators and RDS. Stabilization of the premature infant with hypoxemia should occur before administration of calfactant therapy. Give preferably within 30 min after birth. Give through an ET tube. Draw dose with 20-G needle; avoid foaming. Does not require reconstitution. Do not dilute or shake. Gently agitate for dispersion of drug. Drug does not have to be warmed before administration. Refrigerate at 36-46° F (2-8° C) and protect from light. No known contraindications. Adverse reactions: bradycardia, airway obstruction, apnea, hypoventilation, cyanosis, ET tube reflux, ET blockage.
Poractant alfa (Curosurf)	2.5 ml/kg of birth weight. Up to 2 additional doses of 1.25 ml/kg birth weight can be every 12 h; maximum dose 5 ml/kg.	Administered via 5 French catheter inserted into ET tube. Administer $\frac{1}{2}$ dose into each main bronchus with the infant positioned with either right or left side dependent. Must be given by health care personnel experienced with ventilators and RDS. Do not suction airways for 1 h after surfactant instillation unless airway obstruction occurs. Multiple-dose regimen has evidenced efficacy. Ventilator inspiratory pressures should be reduced immediately if chest expansion improves substantially after dosing. Contraindications are previous hypersensitivity to any component of poractant alfa formulations. Adverse reactions: increased incidence of patent ductus arteriosus, hypotension, transient oxygen desaturation, apnea, and flushing.

ET, Endotracheal; *h,* hour; *min,* minute; *RDS,* respiratory distress syndrome; *sec,* second; $t^{1}/_{2}$, half-life; *UK,* unknown.

■ Assess infant's vital signs.

NURSING DIAGNOSES

■ Impaired gas exchange related to inadequate lung surfactant

PLANNING

■ Infant's oxygen requirement and respiratory effort will decrease.
■ Infant's need for mechanical ventilation will be quickly reduced.
■ Infant will experience no respiratory distress within 1 hour of surfactant administration.

NURSING INTERVENTIONS

Beractant (Survanta) Intracheal Suspension

• Prepare drug in adequate time for drug to warm to room temperature for 20 minutes or in hand for at least 8 minutes. Do not artificially warm drug.
• Do not shake drug.
• Provide only off-white to light brown product for use in procedure.
• Assist with the positioning of the infant after each quarter dose as detailed in protocol.

Calfactant (Infasurf)

• Avoid excessive foaming.
• Draw up dose using 20-g or larger needle.
• Administer through side port of endotracheal (ET) tube.
• Administer medication with infant on one-for-one dose, and turn to opposite side for subsequent dose.
• Administer while ventilation is continued over 20 to 30 breaths for each dose, with small bursts during inspiratory cycles.

Beractant (Survanta) Intracheal Suspension and Calfactant (Infasurf)

• Monitor infant carefully for chest expansion, color, arterial blood gases, oxygen saturation, heart rate, facial expression, ET tube patency, BP, and electrocardiogram.
• Monitor ventilator pressure readings and breath sounds.
• Expect the infant's lungs to sound wet after administration; do not suction through the endotracheal tube for 2 hours.

Poractant Alfa (Curosurf)

• Draw up doses using 20-g or larger needle.
• Suction before dosing.
• Mucous plugging of the ET tube can occur during or after dosing.
• Do not suction airways for 1 hour after surfactant instillation unless signs of airway obstruction are present.

• Monitor ventilator inspiratory pressures, which should be reduced immediately if chest expansion improves after dosing administration.

Client Teaching

General
• Explain to parents what respiratory distress syndrome is and how surfactant helps the infant.
• Explain to parents the purpose of multiple monitoring devices to reduce unrealistic fears about the neonate's condition.
• Ensure informed consent for usage.

Side Effects
• Encourage parents to verbalize understanding about risks associated with use of the drug.

EVALUATION

■ Evaluate preadministration breath sounds and ventilator pressure readings to compare with postadministration findings.

WEBSITES

For further information on *Labor, Delivery, and the Preterm Neonate*, visit these Internet resources:

American College of Obstetricians and Gynecologists: *http://www.acog.org*

American Society of Anesthesiologists: *http://www.asahg.org/index.htm*

Centers for Disease Control and Prevention (CDC): *http://www.cdc.gov/nccdphp*

Center for Complementary Alternative Medicine Research in Women's Health, Columbia University: *http://cpmcnet.columbia.edu/dept/rosenthal/*

Childbirth organizations: *www.childbirth.org*

Clinical Trials in Pregnancy: *http://clinicaltrials.gov/ct/gui/action*

Clinical Trials-Pregnancy Complications—NIH: *http://clinicaltrials.gov/ct/gui/action*

Drugs: *www.drugs.com*

Mayo E Clinic: *http://www.mayoclinic.com*

National Center for Complementary and Alternative Medicine: *http://atmed.od.nih.gov*

National Library of Medicine & NIH—Medline Plus: *http://www.nlm.nih.gov/medlineplus/prenatalcare.htm*

The National Academies Press: *http://www.nationalacademies.org/health*

Critical Thinking Case Study

T.A. (gravida 3, para 0) is at 42 weeks' gestation. At her prenatal visit, her health care provider notes signs and symptoms of pregnancy-induced hypertension and advises T.A. of the plan to induce labor after administration of prostaglandin gel. T.A. asks the nurse, "Can you help me understand all this?"

1. What objective tool (scoring system) can be used to predict the extent to which T.A.'s cervix is "ripe" and therefore favorable for successful induction?

T.A.'s health care provider orders Prepidil gel for use in the cervix.

2. What will be accomplished with the use of the gel?

3. Who will administer the gel?

4. How often can the gel be administered?

5. How long after the last dose of gel can the IV oxytocic medication be started to induce labor?

6. Why is there a waiting period before starting the oxytocin?

7. Further questioning reveals that T.A. has been ingesting a pregnancy tonic that includes herbal supplements since she was 36 weeks' gestation. List three concerns specific to pregnancy.

It is now 16 hours since T.A. first had the gel inserted. When responding to T.A.'s call light, the nurse finds her in the bathroom upset that she feels nauseous, occasionally vomiting a little stomach fluid, and complaining that her stool is "really watery." "Is something wrong?" T.A. asks.

8. Analysis of the data about T.A.'s symptoms support what conclusion?

9. What nursing actions might be taken to support T.A.?

10. When T.A. returns to bed and the external fetal monitor is reapplied, what data should the nurse collect, record, and report to the obstetric provider?

It is now 24 hours since T.A. had her first gel instillation; it has been 6 hours since her last insertion. A vaginal examination reveals that T.A.'s cervix is soft, 50% effaced, 3 cm dilated, and the presenting part is at −2 station. Contractions are 5 minutes apart and mild. The health care provider elects to begin an oxytocin infusion.

11. T.A. asks how a medicine "running into my arm is able to make my uterus contract." How would one explain the mode of action of oxytocin to T.A.?

12. Why is the oxytocin infusion run through a secondary line, which is attached as a "piggyback" to the primary line? At which port along the primary line is the piggyback inserted and why?

13. Why is oxytocin administered via an infusion pump? What is the measurement for dosing?

14. What actions in regard to the IV equipment setup should be taken as safety measures before starting the oxytocin?

15. What drugs should be nearby in the event of an emergency with the oxytocin?

16. What information should be recorded during the infusion?

17. While setting up the oxytocin infusion, a nurse in training asks what criteria to use to know when to slow the rate or stop the infusion. You correctly respond that contractions would be _____ minutes apart with _____ intensity and the cervix would be dilated at least _____ cm.

18. If uterine hyperstimulation occurs, explain how to handle the situation. Address the following:
Position T.A. _____
    Rationale _____
IV Fluids
    Rationale _____
Oxygen
    Rationale _____

19. T.A. asks what side effects can occur if she receives a continuous lumbar epidural. What is the appropriate response?

Study Questions

1. What are the potential complications of epidural analgesia or anesthesia?

2. What client teaching should precede administration of regional anesthesia during labor?

3. What is an indication to administer oxytocin or ergotamine following placental expulsion?

4. What route of administration is appropriate for giving ergonovine maleate (Ergotrate) to a woman with pregnancy-induced hypertension?

5. Why would beractant (Survanta) be administered to a neonate born at 31 weeks' gestation?

6. What are the potential complications of herbal supplement use during pregnancy and later gestation?

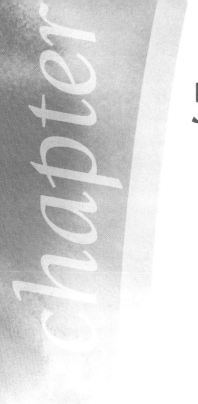

53 Drugs Associated with the Postpartum and the Newborn

ROBIN WEBB CORBETT AND LAURA K. WILLIFORD OWENS

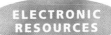

ELECTRONIC RESOURCES

evolve

Additional information can be found on the companion website at *http://evolve.elsevier.com/KeeHayes/pharmacology/* or on the companion CD-ROM, which includes:

• *NCLEX-style examination review questions*
• *Pharmacology animations*
• *Medication error and IV therapy checklists*
• *Medication calculation problems*
• *Electronic calculators*

OBJECTIVES

• Discuss the purpose, action, side effects, and nursing implications of the drugs commonly administered during the postpartum period, their action, side effects, and nursing implications.

• Discuss the purpose, action, side effects, and nursing implications of the drugs administered to the newborn.

• Describe the nursing process, including client teaching, related to drugs used during the postpartum period and drugs administered to the newborn immediately after delivery.

TERMS

antiflatulents	flatus	ophthalmia neonatorum	Rh_0 (D) immune globulin
congenital rubella syn-	folliculitis	perineal	(RhoGAM)
drome	lactation	puerperium	urticaria
contact dermatitis	necrosis	Rh sensitization	
episiotomy	occlusive		

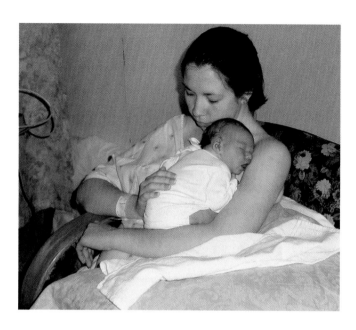

Introduction

This chapter focuses on the pharmacologic considerations for mothers and infants after delivery. Nonpharmacologic measures and pharmacologic agents related to the relief of common discomforts during the postpartum period are described. In addition, drugs commonly administered to newborns immediately after delivery are included.

It is important to note that for some cultures, pregnancy is perceived as a cold state, so warm foods and activities are encouraged to balance the body; it is believed, failure to do so may contribute to later poor health. For example, women of Mexican American ethnicity need to avoid chilling and exposure to drafts. Therefore perineal cold compresses may not be accepted by these women. Japanese women may prefer to take their postpartal medications with warm water rather than cold water. Cultural values also influence infant care. It is important that nurses are culturally sensitive to the pregnant client's cultural belief framework and try to include this framework in establishing rapport with the client and provision of care.

Drugs Used During the Postpartum Period

During the **puerperium** (the period from delivery until 6 weeks postpartum), the maternal body physically recovers from antepartal and intrapartal stressors and returns to its prepregnant state.

Pharmacologic and nonpharmacologic measures commonly used during the postpartum period have five primary purposes: (1) to prevent uterine atony and postpartum hemorrhage (see Chapter 51, Drugs Associated with the Female Reproductive Cycle I: Pregnancy and Preterm Labor); (2) to relieve pain from uterine contractions, perineal wounds, and hemorrhoids; (3) to enhance or suppress lactation; (4) to promote bowel function; and (5) to enhance immunity (Box 53–1).

BOX 53–1

Routine Postpartum–Vaginal Delivery and Cesarean Birth Medication Orders

Standing Orders

Oxytocin (Pitocin) 20 units in 1 L D5LR or 10 units IM
$FeSO_4$ 325 mg PO b.i.d.-t.i.d.
Prenatal vitamin 1 tab PO daily
Motrin 800 mg t.i.d.

PRN Orders

Docusate sodium (Colace) 100 mg PO b.i.d. PRN constipation OR
Dulcolax suppository PR PRN for constipation
Rubella vaccine if nonimmunized
Cesarean Delivery

Routine Postpartum–Cesearean Birth Medication Orders

Standing Orders

Cefazolin (Ancef) 1 g IVP × 1
Oxytocin (Pitocin) 20 units in 1 L D5LR or 10 units IM
POD 1
$FeSO_4$ 325 mg PO b.i.d.-t.i.d.
Prenatal vitamin 1 tab PO daily
Motrin 800 mg t.i.d.

PRN Orders

POD 1
Acetaminophen/codeine (Tylenol #3) 1-2 tab PO q 4-6 h PRN for pain OR
Oxycodone/acetaminophen (Percocet) 1 tab PO q 6 h PRN for pain
POD 2
Bisacodyl (Dulcolax) suppository PR PRN for constipation OR
Magnesium hydroxide (Milk of Magnesia) 30 ml PO t.i.d. PRN
Simethicone (Mylicon) 80 mg PO q.i.d. PRN for flatus
Rubella vaccine (Meruzax 2) subQ if nonimmunized

From Chan PD, Johnson SM: *Gynecology and obstetrics*, Laguna Hills, Calif, 2004, Current Clinical Strategies Publishing.
b.i.d., Twice a day; *h*, hour; *IM*, intramuscular; *IVP*, intravenous pyelogram; *PO*, by mouth; *PRN*, as needed; *q.i.d.*, four times a day; *subQ*, subcutaneous; *tab*, tablet; *t.i.d.*, three times a day.

HERBAL ALERT 53-1

Use of Herbs During Lactation

Herbal supplements are not generally recommended during lactation. The herbal supplements listed below are contraindicated for breastfeeding women:

Aloe
Buckthron bark
Cascara sagrada bark
Coltsfoot leaf
Senna leaf, peppermint oil, and caraway oil
Kava Kava
Petasites root
Indian snakeroot
Rhubarb root
Senna leaf
Uva ursi

BOX 53-2

Commonly Used Postpartum Systemic Analgesics

Acetaminophen (Tylenol)
Acetaminophen/codeine (Tylenol #3)
Acetaminophen/propoxyphene (Darvocet N50/Darvocet N-100)
Ibuprofen (Motrin)
Codeine sulfate
Ketorolac tromethamine (Toradol)
Meperidine (Demerol)
Morphine sulfate
Nalbuphine (Nubain)
Oxycodone acetaminophen (Percocet)

Whenever possible, nonpharmacologic measures are preferred to the use of drugs or are used in conjunction with drugs. See Herbal Alert 53–1 regarding the use of herbs during the postpartum period.

Postpartum nursing care ideally occurs as a partnership between the nurse and the new family. To enhance health and wellness, the nurse collaborates with the mother and family to strengthen the new mother's self-confidence and ability to handle her own health challenges. The nurse's role in this system is threefold:

1. To assess and provide postpartual physical changes and pain management with the client to determine both healing progress within a standard and effectiveness of medications
2. To teach the client and administer postpartal medications
3. To teach the client and administer narcotic analgesics (as prescribed) when pain control by nonnarcotic products is ineffective;

Pain Relief for Uterine Contractions

"Afterbirth pains" may occur during the first few days postpartum when uterine tissue experiences ischemia during contractions, particularly in multiparous women and when breastfeeding. Nonsteroidal agents may be used to control postpartal discomfort and pain with narcotic agents reserved for more severe pain such as that experienced by the client after cesarean delivery, tubal ligation, or extensive perineal laceration. Box 53–2 presents a list of systemic analgesics commonly used during the postpartum period.

Because some systemic analgesics (e.g., codeine, meperidine, oxycodone) can cause decreased alertness, it is important for the nurse to observe the client as she cares for her newborn to ensure safety. Clients who receive opioids, such as morphine sulfate or codeine sulfate, should be assessed for bowel function and respirations. With continued opioid use, client assessment of bowel history is necessary because these drugs can exacerbate the constipation from pregnancy. Intrapartally, women are NPO (nothing by mouth) or ingest limited liquids and are nonambulatory, all factors which contribute to decreased bowel activity. In addition, respiratory assessment is important in clients receiving opioids as respiratory depression may occur.

Frequently, nonsteroidal agents, such as (Ibuprofen) Motrin, and ketorolac tromethamine (Toradol) are used to control postpartum discomfort and pain. Nonsteroidal antiinflammatory drugs (NSAIDs) inhibit the enzyme cyclo-oxygenase (COX), of which there are two isoenzymes, COX-1 or COX-2; both decrease prostaglandin synthesis. These drugs are effective in relieving mild to moderate pain, including postpartum uterine contractions, episiotomy, hemorrhoids, and perineal wounds. NSAIDs commonly cause gastrointestinal (GI) irritation, and it is recommended that clients take with a full glass or water or with meals to minimize GI distress. With administration of NSAIDs, a lower narcotic dosage may control pain as a result of the additive analgesic effect. The use of NSAIDS requires an ongoing assessment for GI bleeding. These drugs inhibit platelet synthesis and may prolong bleeding time. Client teaching with this category of drugs is important because some NSAIDS may be purchased over the counter (OTC). Client teaching includes avoidance of these drugs while pregnant; symptoms of GI bleeding (dark, tarry stools, blood in urine, and coffee-ground emesis); and avoidance of the concurrent use of alcohol, aspirin, and corticosteroids, which may increase the risk of GI toxicity.

Pain Relief for Perineal Wounds and Hemorrhoids

Pregnancy and the delivery process increase the pressure on **perineal** soft tissue. The tissue may become ecchymotic or edematous. Increased edema, ecchymosis, and pain may occur if an **episiotomy** (incision made to enlarge the vaginal opening to facilitate newborn delivery) or perineal laceration is present. In addition, hemorrhoids that developed during pregnancy may be exacerbated secondary to the pushing during labor. Comfort measures (ice packs immediately after birth, tightening of the buttocks before sitting, use of peribottles and cool and warm sitz baths) and selected topical agents (witch hazel and Nupercainal ointment) may relieve pain and minimize discomfort (Table 53–1). Note that rectal suppositories should not be used by women with fourth-degree perineal lacerations.

Table 53-1

Drugs Used to Relieve Pain from Perineal Wounds and Hemorrhoids

Generic (Brand)	Route and Dosage	Uses and Considerations
Perineal Wounds (Episiotomy or Laceration)		
benzocaine (Americaine, Dermoplast OTC)	Spray liberally t.i.d. or q.i.d. 6-12 in from perineum following perineal cleansing. Supplied as aerosol; benzocaine 20%	Local anesthetic inhibits impulses from sensory nerves as a result of a decrease in the permeability of cell membrane to sodium ions. Apply 6-12 in from affected area. Peak: 1 min; duration: 30-60 min. Hydrolyzed in the plasma and liver (to lesser extent) by cholinesterase; eliminated as metabolites in urine. Well absorbed from mucous membranes and traumatized skin. Contraindicated in secondary bacterial infection of tissue and known hypersensitivity.
witch hazel pads (Tucks [50% witch hazel with glycerine, water, and methylparaben])	Apply premoistened pads t.i.d. or q.i.d. to wound site	Precipitates protein, causing tissue to contract. May be chilled/refrigerated in original container for additional comfort. If liquid, pour over ice and dip absorbent pads into solution; change when diluted. Medical intervention should be sought if rectal bleeding is present. *Side effect:* local irritation (discontinue use).
Hemorrhoids		
hydrocortisone acetate 10 mg (Anusol HC, Anusol Ointment [Promoxine HCl 1%, mineral oil 46.7%, zinc oxide 12.5%])	1 suppository b.i.d. for 3-6 d	Relieves pain and itching from irritated anorectal tissue. Contains hydrocortisone acetate. Acts as an antiinflammatory agent. Available without hydrocortisone. Wear gloves. Onset: UK; peak: UK; duration: UK. Contraindicated with hypersensitivity. If second infection in tissue, discontinue. If anorectal symptoms do not improve in 7 d or if bleeding, protrusion, or seepage occurs, inform health care provider. Not to be used if fourth-degree perineal laceration. Not known if excreted in breast milk; use cautiously. *Pregnancy category:* C
hydrocortisone acetate 1% and promazine HCl 1% topical aerosol (Proctofoam-HC)	1 applicator transferred to a 2 × 2 in pad and placed against rectum inside peripad b.i.d. or t.i.d. and after bowel movements	Topical corticosteroid aerosol foam with same action and considerations as above. Also available in nonsteroidal preparation. Shake foam aerosol before use. Onset: UK; peak: UK; duration: UK. Extent of percutaneous absorption of topical cortico-steroids is determined by vehicle integrity of epidermal barrier and use of occlusive dressings (not known if any quantity detectable in breast milk). *Side effects:* burning, itching, irritation; dryness, infrequent folliculitis reactions.
dibucaine ointment, USP 1% (Nupercaine)	Apply as above t.i.d. or q.i.d., using no more than 1 tube in 24 h	Local anesthetic ointment containing dibucaine 1%. Action same as benzocaine. Onset: within 15 min; peak: UK; duration: 2-4 h. Do not use if rectal bleeding is present. Do not use near eyes or over denuded surfaces or blistered areas. Do not use if known hypersensitivity to amide-type anesthetics. *Side effects:* burning, tenderness, irritation, inflammation, contact dermatitis, urticaria, cutaneous lesions, edema. *Pregnancy category:* C

b.i.d., Two times a day; *d*, day; *h*, hour; *in*, inch; *min*, minute; *q.i.d.*, four times a day; *t.i.d.*, three times a day; *UK*, unknown.

Side Effects and Adverse Reactions

The most commonly reported side effects of topical or local agents (e.g., witch hazel) include burning, stinging, tenderness, edema, rash, tissue irritation, sloughing, and tissue **necrosis** (death of tissue caused by disease or injury). The most commonly reported side effects of hydrocortisone local or topical drugs include burning, pruritus, irritation, dryness, **folliculitis** (inflammation of hair follicle), allergic **contact dermatitis**, and secondary infection. These side effects are more likely to occur when **occlusive** (i.e., obstructive) dressings are used.

Nursing Process

Pain Relief for Perineal Wounds and Hemorrhoids

ASSESSMENT

- Assess client's cultural framework for health.
- Assess client's pain using agency pain scale.
- Assess the perineal area for wounds and hemorrhoids (size, color, location, pain scale, REEDA (*r*edness, *e*cchymosis, *e*dema, *d*ischarge, *a*pproximation).

■ Check the expiration dates on topical spray cans, bottles, and ointment tubes.

■ Assess for presence of infection in perineal site; avoid use of benzocaine on infected perineal tissue.

NURSING DIAGNOSES

■ Impaired comfort: pain related to episiotomy, perineal laceration, or hemorrhoids

■ Deficient knowledge related to etiology of pain and discomfort and treatment measures, nonpharmacologic and pharmacologic

PLANNING

■ Client's perineal discomfort will be alleviated by use of topical sprays, compresses, sitz baths and ointment.

NURSING INTERVENTIONS

■ Incorporate client's cultural framework of help in nursing plan of care.

■ Do not use benzocaine spray when perineal infection is present.

■ Shake benzocaine spray can. Administer 6 to 12 inches from perineum with client lying on her side with top leg up and forward to provide maximum exposure. This can also be done with one foot on the toilet seat after voiding.

■ Use witch hazel compresses (Tucks or witch hazel solution) with an ice pack and a peri-pad to apply cold to the affected area in addition to the active agent.

■ Store Anusol HC suppositories below 86° F (30° C) but protect from freezing. Use gloves for administration. If client is breastfeeding, assess to determine whether client is ready to switch to nonhydrocortisone preparation (goal is to discontinue use of suppositories as quickly as possible).

■ Check lot numbers and expiration date.

■ Use of Proctofoam-HC needs to be explained carefully to client because directions instruct the client to place the agent inside the anus, which is not generally done with obstetric clients because they may have perineal wounds that extend into the anus.

■ Do not use rectal suppositories in client with fourth-degree perineal laceration.

Client Teaching: Perineal Wounds: Topical Spray Containing Benzocaine

General
• Describe the process of perineal wound healing.
• Explain expected action and side effects.

• Instruct client that the drug is not for prolonged use (no more than 7 days) or for application to a large area.

• Instruct client with bleeding hemorrhoids to use the drug carefully and to keep her health care provider informed if condition exacerbates or does not improve within 7 days.

Self-Administration
• Apply three to four times daily or as directed.
• Apply without touching sensitive area.
• Hold can 6 to 12 inches from affected area. Administer the spray by either lying on the side in bed while spraying the treatment from behind or by standing with one foot on a chair or toilet seat.

Safety
• Assess use of complementary and alternative medicine to include herbal supplements.
• Avoid contact of the medication with eyes.
• Instruct client not to use a perineal heat lamp following application because this could cause tissue burns.
• If condition exacerabates or symptoms recur within a few days, notify the health care provider and discontinue use until directed.
• Keep medication out of the reach of children in postpartum unit and later at home. If ingested, contact poison control center immediately.
• Store below 120° F (49° C).
• Dispose of empty can without puncturing or incinerating.

Client Teaching: Witch Hazel Compresses

General
• Explain expected action and side effects of product. These may provide relief of itching, burning, and irritation in episiotomy site or from hemorrhoids with cooling, soothing sensation.
• Notify health care provider if condition exacerabates or does not improve within 7 days.

Self-Administration
• Pour liquid witch hazel over chipped ice; place soft, clean, absorbent squares in solution; squeeze square to eliminate excess moisture; fold and place moist square against episiotomy site or hemorrhoids.
• If using commercial medicated pads, entire container may be placed in the refrigerator.
• Avoid touching the surface of the pad placed next to the perineal wound.
• Instruct client when to change the compress and show how to place ice bag and peri-pad over the compress.

Safety
• Do not insert medicated pads into the rectum.

- Keep product away from children.
- Do not use if rectal bleeding is present.

Side Effects
- Discontinue use if local irritation occurs.

Client Teaching: Hemorrhoids: Anusol Ointment and Anusol Suppositories (HC and Plain)

General
- Explain expected effects of product use. These include relief of burning, itching, and discomfort from irritated anorectal tissues while soothing, lubricating, and coating mucous membranes.
- Explain that topical analgesia lasts for several hours after use.
- Tell client to store below 86° F (30° C) so suppositories do not melt but do not freeze.

Self-Administration
- Apply *ointment* externally in postpartum period.
- Place *suppository* in lower portion of anal canal. *Caution:* products usually are not inserted rectally if fourth-degree lacerations are present.
- Apply small quantity *ointment* onto 2 × 2 inch gauze square; place inside peripad against swollen anorectal tissue approximately 5 times per day.
- If *suppository* is ordered, tell client to keep refrigerated but not frozen. Remove wrapper before inserting in rectum (hold suppository upright and peel evenly down sides). Do not hold suppository for prolonged period because it will melt. If suppository softens before use, hold in foil wrapper under cold water for 2 to 3 minutes.

Safety
- Ascertain client hypersensitivity to any of the components of the ointment (e.g., promazine HCl 1%, mineral oil 46.7%, zinc oxide 12.5%).
- Avoid contact of the medication with eyes.

Side Effects
- Ointment may occasionally cause burning sensation in some clients, especially if anal tissue is *not* intact.
- If erythema, irritation, edema, or pain develops or increases, discontinue use and consult health care provider.
- Notify health care provider if bleeding occurs.

Client Teaching Promazine and Hydrocortisone (Proctofoam-HC) and Promazine Hydrochloride (ProctoFoam [OTC])

General
- Explain expected action and side effects of product.
- Explain that promazine HCl is not chemically related to "caine" type local anesthetics and there is decreased chance of cross-sensitivity reactions in clients allergic to other local anesthetics.

Self-Administration
- Tell client that product is for anal or perianal use only and is not to be inserted into rectum.
- Shake can vigorously before use.
- Fully extend applicator plunger; hold can upright to fill applicator.
- Express contents of applicator onto a 2 × 2-inch gauze pad and place inside peripad against rectum.
- Use two to three times daily and after bowel movements.
- Take the applicator apart after each use and wash with warm water.

Safety
- Keep aerosol container away from children in postpartum unit and later at home.
- Store below 120° F (49° C).
- Dispose of aerosol container without puncturing or incinerating.
- Avoid contact of the medication with eyes.

Side Effects
- Tell client it is unknown whether topical administration of corticosteroids could result in sufficient systemic absorption to produce detectable quantities in breast milk.
- Burning, itching, irritation, dryness, and folliculitis occasionally occur, especially if occlusive dressings are used.

Client Teaching: Dibucaine Ointment 1% (Nupercainal Ointment)

General
- The ointment is poorly absorbed through intact skin but is well absorbed through mucous membranes and excoriated skin.
- Effects should be perceived within 15 minutes and last for 2 to 4 hours.

Self-Administration
- Express ointment from the applicator on a tissue or 2 × 2-inch pad and place against the anus. Do not insert the applicator into the rectum.

Safety
- Do not use product near the eyes, over denuded surface or blistered areas, or if there is rectal bleeding.
- Do not use more than one tube (30-g size) in 24 hours.
- Keep medication out of the reach of children.

Side Effects
- Ask client if there is any known hypersensitivity to amide-type anesthetics; if so, product is contraindicated.
- Local effects may include burning, tenderness, irritation, inflammation, and contact dermatitis; inform health care provider if these occur.

- Other side effects may include edema, cutaneous lesions, and urticaria.

Cultural Considerations ⊕

- Provide an interpreter with the same ethnic background and gender if possible, especially with sensitive topics.

EVALUATION

▦ Reevaluate pain using a agency pain scale following use of nonphramacologic and pharmacologic measures.

▦ Identify need for additional client teaching.

▦ Reassess perineal and anal tissues for integrity, healing, and any side effects.

Lactation Suppression

In the past, **lactation** was commonly controlled through drug therapy with one of three agents: chlorotrianisene (Tace), Deladumone OB (combination of estrogen plus androgen in the form of estradiol valerate and testosterone enanthate), or bromocriptine mesylate (Parlodel). Estrogenic substances are much less popular than in the past because of the increased incidence of thrombophlebitis associated with the high dosage needed to suppress lactation as well as concerns about potential carcinogenic effects. Although these drugs are not used now, your clients and their families may ask about these medications, which were given in the past for lactation suppression. Presently, nonpharmacologic measures (wearing a supportive bra 24 h/day for 10 to 14 days, breast binding, and axillary ice packs) are recommended for lactation suppression (Table 53–2).

Table 53–2

Nonpharmacologic Measures for Common Postpartum Needs

Indication	Measure
Uterine contractions	Client positioned on abdomen with pillow under abdomen × 20-30 min for 3-4 d
	Distraction, breathing techniques, therapeutic touch, relaxation, guided imagery, ambulation
	No heat to abdomen because of risk of uterine relaxation and increased bleeding
Perineal wound resulting from episiotomy or laceration	Ice packs/glove (covered in thin, absorbent material to protect tissue) for 6-8 h after delivery
	Client positioned on side as much as possible with pillow between legs
	Early and frequent ambulation
	Perineal exercises
	Cool sitz bath 2-3 h after delivery
	Warm sitz bath 12-24 h after delivery 3-4 × per d
	Area cleansed front to back using perispray squeeze bottle, cleansing shower, or Surgi-Gator
	Client tightens buttocks or squeezes buttocks together before sitting and sits tall and flat, not rolled back onto coccyx
	No tampons, douche, or feminine hygiene sprays
	No intercourse until after lochia has ceased or as advised by health care provider
Hemorrhoids	As above but particularly:
	Ice
	Sims' position to help increase venous return
	Warm, moist heat; sitz bath
	Witch hazel pads (e.g., Tucks)
Lactation suppression	Tight bra or binder worn continuously for 10-14 d
	Normal fluid intake
	No manipulation or stimulation of breasts
Engorgement	As above, plus ice to axillary area of breasts if client is bottle feeding the newborn, or apply warm compresses if client is breastfeeding
	Express a small amount of colostrum or milk (if breastfeeding) by hand expression before putting infant to breast to facilitate latching on
Sore or cracked nipples	Absorbent breast pads worn to keep moisture away from nipples
	No soap on nipples
	Air-dry nipples after nursing
	Express a small amount of breast milk on nipples to be used as a protective lubricant
	Apply hypoallergenic purified lanolin (Lansinoh, PureLan) or similar cream or ointment to the nipples, which may be used as a protective lubricant and promote healing
	No nipple shields because they can promote chafing
	Do not limit infant's "nursing" time at breast; otherwise nonemptying of milk ducts and increased pressure may occur
	Proper positioning for feeding; nursing begun on the less sore nipple
	Suction broken with little finger after feeding to prevent pulling on nipple

d, Day; *h*, hour; *min*, minute.

Promotion of Bowel Function

Constipation is common during the postpartum period because of the residual effects of progesterone on smooth muscle coupled with decreased peristalsis, decreased liquid intake during labor, decreased activity, and relaxation of the abdominal muscles. Clients who deliver by cesarean section are at increased risk of constipation and **flatus.** Nonpharmacologic measures (e.g., high-fiber foods, early ambulation, drinking at least 64 oz of fluids a day, and promptly responding to the defecation urge) are generally instituted after delivery.

Pharmacologic measures include the use of stool softeners, laxative stimulants, and, for the postcesarean client, **antiflatulents** (Table 53–3). (See Chapter 45, Drugs for Gastrointestinal Disorders, for additional information).

Side Effects and Adverse Reactions

The following side effects have been reported:

- **Docusate sodium (Colace):** Bitter taste, throat irritation, rash
- **Casanthranol and docusate sodium (Peri-Colace):** Nausea, abdominal cramping, diarrhea, and rash

Table 53–3

Drugs Used to Promote Postpartum Bowel Function

Generic (Brand)	Route and Dosage	Uses and Considerations
docusate sodium (Colace) 100-mg capsule docusate calcium (Surfak) 240-mg capsule	100 mg PO b.i.d. 50-400 mg PO daily in 1-4 divided doses	Reduces surface tension of the oil-water interface of the stool, resulting in enhanced incorporation of water and fat, allowing for stool softening. Onset: 12-72 h. Docusate salts are interchangeable (amount of Na, Ca, or K per dosage is clinically insignificant). Do not use concomitantly with mineral oil. Contraindicated if intestinal obstruction, acute abdominal pain, nausea, or vomiting is present. Do not use >1 wk. Prolonged, frequent, or excessive use may cause bowel dependence or electrolyte imbalance. Compatible with breastfeeding. *Side effects:* rash. *Pregnancy category:* C; PB: NA; t½: NA
casanthranol with docusate sodium (Peri-Colace); docusate sodium, 100 mg; casanthranol, 30 mg	1-2 capsules PO usually at bedtime	Mild stimulant laxative. Should be taken with full glass of water. Onset: 8-12 h but may require up to 24 h. Do not use if abdominal pain, nausea, or vomiting present. Compatible with breastfeeding. *Adverse reactions:* rash, abdominal cramping, diarrhea, nausea. *Pregnancy category:* C; PB: NA; t½: NA
docusate potassium (Dialose)	1 capsule PO daily or b.i.d.	Stool softener. Sodium free. Onset: 12-72 h. *Pregnancy category:* C. See docusate sodium for additional information.
casanthranol with docusate potassium (Dialose Plus)	1 capsule PO b.i.d.	Mild stimulant laxative. Sodium. Onset: 8-12 h, but may require up to 24 h. *Pregnancy category:* C. See casanthranol with docusate sodium for additional information.
bisacodyl USP (Dulcolax) (suppository 10 mg or tablet 5 mg)	2-3 tablets PO or 1 suppository	Stimulant laxative. Irritates smooth muscle of the intestine, possibly the colon and intramural plexus; alters water and electrolyte secretion, increasing intestinal fluid and producing laxative effect. Onset PO: 6-10 h; rectally: 15 min-1 h. Absorption: 5% absorbed systemically following oral or rectal form. Metabolized in the liver to conjugated metabolites; eliminated in breast milk, bile, and urine. Do not crush tablets (enteric coated). Do not administer within 1 h of milk or antacid because enteric coating may dissolve, resulting in abdominal cramping and vomiting. *Side effects:* abdominal cramps, nausea, vomiting, rectal burning, electrolyte and fluid acidosis or alkalosis, hypocalcemia. *Pregnancy category:* C
magnesium hydroxide (Milk of Magnesia)	30 ml PO PRN t.i.d. or q.i.d.	Laxative. Acts by increasing and retaining water in intestinal lumen, causing distention that stimulates peristalsis and bowel elimination. Onset: 4-8 h. Excreted by kidneys (absorbed portion); unabsorbed portion excreted in feces. Poses risk to client with renal failure because 15%-30% of magnesium is systemically absorbed. Use with caution in clients with impaired renal function because hypermagnesemia and toxicity may occur as a result of decreased renal clearance of absorbed magnesium. Contraindicated in clients with colostomy, ileostomy, abdominal pain, nausea, vomiting, fecal impaction, and renal failure. Drug interactions may occur with tetracyclines, digoxin, indomethacin, or iron salts, isoniazid. Milk of Magnesia concentrate is 3× as potent as regular-strength product. *Side effects:* abdominal cramps, nausea. *Adverse reactions:* hypotension, hypermagnesemia, muscle weakness, and respiratory depression. *Pregnancy category:* B

b.i.d., Twice a day; *d,* day; *h,* hour; *min,* minute; *NA,* not applicable; *PB,* protein-binding; *p.c.,* after meals; *PO,* by mouth; *q.i.d.,* four times a day; *t½,* half-life; *t.i.d.,* three times a day; *UK,* unknown; >, greater than.

Table 53-3

Drugs Used to Promote Postpartum Bowel Function—cont'd

Generic (Brand)	Route and Dosage	Uses and Considerations
magnesium hydroxide with mineral oil (Haley's M-O)	30-60 ml PO	Mild saline laxative. Acts by drawing water into gut, increasing intraluminal pressure and intestinal motility. Onset: 0.5-6 h. *Pregnancy category:* B. Equivalent to magnesium hydroxide.
mineral oil	15-45 ml PO daily or in divided doses	Lubricant laxative eases passages of stool by decreasing water absorption and lubricating the intestine. Onset: 6-8 h; peak: UK; duration: UK. May impair absorption of fat-soluble vitamins (A, D, E, K), oral contraceptives, coumarin, and sulfonamides. Generally recommend avoidance of bedtime doses because of risk of aspiration (lipid pneumonitis). Do not give with food or meals because of risk of aspiration and decreased fat-soluble vitamin absorption. Contraindicated in clients with ileostomy, colostomy, appendicitis, ulcerative colitis, and diverticulitis. Best administered on an empty stomach. *Side effects:* nausea, vomiting, diarrhea, and abdominal cramps. *Pregnancy category:* C; PB: NA; $t^{1/2}$: NA
senna (Senokot)	10-15 ml syrup at bedtime.; 2-4 tablets PO b.i.d.	Stimulant laxative. Acts by local irritant effect on colon to promote peristalsis and bowel evacuation. Also increases moisture content of stool by accumulating fluids in intestine. Onset: 6-24 h. Metabolized in liver; eliminated in feces (viable) and urine. Drug interactions may occur with monoamine oxidase (MAO) inhibitors, disulfiram, metronidazole, and procarbazine. May discolor urine or feces. Liquid syrups contain 7% alcohol. May create laxative dependence and loss of bowel function with prolonged use. Contraindicated in clients with fluid and electrolyte disturbances, abdominal pain, and nausea and vomiting. Excreted in breast milk. *Pregnancy category:* C; $t^{1/2}$: NA
simethicone (Mylicon) (chewable tablets 40 mg, 80 mg)	1 tablet q.i.d. p.c. and at bedtime up to 6× per d as needed	Antiflatulent. Acts by dispersing and preventing formation of mucus-surrounded gas pockets in GI tract; changes surface tension of gas bubbles and allows them to coalesce, making them easier to eliminate as belching and rectal flatus. Must be chewed thoroughly before swallowing; suggest client drink a full glass of water after tablets are chewed. Onset: UK. Excreted unchanged in the feces. May interfere with results of guaiac tests of gastric aspirates. Double doses should not be taken to make up for missed doses. Store below 104° F (40° C) in well-closed container. No known side effects. *Pregnancy category:* C; $t^{1/2}$: UK

- **Bisacodyl suppositories Dulcolax):** Proctitis and inflammation
- **Magnesium hydroxide (Milk of Magnesia):** Abdominal cramps and nausea
- **Senna (Senokot):** Nausea, vomiting, diarrhea, abdominal cramps; can also cause diarrhea in breastfed infants
- **Mineral oil:** Nausea, vomiting, diarrhea, abdominal cramps; if aspirated, lipid pneumonitis may occur

Nursing Process

Laxatives

ASSESSMENT

■ Note time of delivery, predelivery food and fluid intake, ambulation and activity, and predelivery bowel habits.
■ Obtain history of bowel problems.

■ Assess client's bowel sounds × 4 (particularly postcesarean delivery) and abdominal distention.
■ Assess the perineal area for wounds, hemorrhoids, and episiotomy (REEDA).

NURSING DIAGNOSES

■ Risk for constipation related to perineal discomfort, decreased peristalsis, and use of opioids
■ Fear of impaired discomfort with first postdelivery bowel movement (especially if episiotomy, hemorrhoids, or perineal wounds are present)

PLANNING

■ Client will have a bowel movement by 2 to 4 days postpartum.
■ Client will resume normal prepregnancy bowel elimination pattern within 4 to 6 weeks.

NURSING INTERVENTIONS

Docusate Sodium (Colace) and Casanthranol with Docusate Sodium (Peri-Colace); Casanthranol with Docusate Potassium (Dialose Plus)

• Store at room temperature.
• If a liquid preparation is ordered, give with milk or fruit juice to mask bitter taste.
• Take with a full glass of water.
• Assess client for any history of laxative dependence.
• Drug interaction may occur with mineral oil, phenolphthalein, or aspirin.

Bisacodyl USP (Dulcolax)

• Store tablets and suppositories below 77° F (25° C) and avoid excess humidity.
• Do not crush tablets.
• Do not administer within 1 to 2 hours of milk or antacid because enteric coating may dissolve, resulting in abdominal cramping and vomiting.
• Take with a full glass of water.

Mineral Oil

• Do not give with or immediately after meals.
• Give with fruit juice or carbonated drinks to disguise taste.

Magnesium Hydroxide (Milk of Magnesia)

• Shake container well.
• Do not give 1 to 2 hours before or after oral drugs because of effects on absorption.
• Take with a full glass of water.
• Note that milk of magnesia concentrate is three times as potent as regular-strength product.
• Give laxative 1 hour before or 1 hour after any oral antibiotic.

Senna (Senokot)

• Protect from light and heat.

Simethicone (Mylicon)

• Administer after meals and at bedtime.
• If chewable tablets ordered instruct client to chew tablets thoroughly before swallowing.

Client Teaching: General

• Instruct client that stool softeners are given to provide for a bowel movement without straining.
• Instruct clients that continued laxative use may result in laxative dependence.
• Instruct client that measures to prevent and treat constipation include drinking 6-8 glasses of fluid/day, ingesting foods high in fiber (bran, fruits, vegetables), and increasing daily ambulation and activity.
• Instruct clients to avoid/minimize ingestion of gas forming foods (cabbage, onions) and to increase ambulation/activity.

• Instruct clients regarding temperature and storage requirements for particular drugs.

Client Teaching: Docusate Sodium (Colace) and Casanthranol with Docusate Sodium (Peri-Colace) and Casanthranol with Docusate Potassium (Dialose Plus)

• Drink at least six 8-oz glasses of liquid daily. Drink one glass of fluid with each dose.
• Take liquid forms with milk or fruit juice to mask bitter taste.
• Explain that many laxatives contain sodium. Tell client to check with health care provider or pharmacist before using laxative if on a low-sodium diet.
• Do not take drug if already taking mineral oil or having acute abdominal pain, nausea, vomiting, or signs of intestinal obstruction.
• Do not use products for longer than 1 week. Advise that prolonged, frequent, or excessive use may result in dependence on drug or electrolyte imbalance.
• Report to health care provider if skin rash occurs or if stomach or intestinal cramping occurs and does not diminish.

Client Teaching: Senna (Senokot)

• Instruct client that drug may discolor urine or feces to yellow-green.
• Instruct client to discontinue the drug if abdominal pain, nausea, or vomiting occurs.
• Instruct client that syrup form is 7% alcohol.

Client Teaching: Mineral Oil

• Instruct client not to take other laxatives (e.g., docusate products) if she is already taking mineral oil.
• Instruct client to take mineral oil on an empty stomach; do not take with food or meals because of risk of aspiration and decreased fat-soluble vitamin absorption.
• Avoid bedtime doses because of risk of aspiration.
• Instruct client to report nausea, vomiting, diarrhea, or abdominal cramping.

Client Teaching: Magnesium Hydroxide (Milk of Magnesia)

• Laxative action generally occurs in 4 to 8 hours.
• Take with a full glass of water.
• Note whether dose is regular strength or concentrated form of drug, because concentrate is three times as potent as regular strength.
• Drug may interact with tetracyclines, digoxin, indomethacin, iron salts, isoniazid; notify health care provider if any of these drugs are used.
• Instruct client to report any muscular weakness, diarrhea, or abdominal cramps.

Client Teaching: Simethicone (Mylicon)

• Drug will help relieve flatus and associated pain.

- Take after meals. If chewable tablets are ordered, instruct client to chew tablets thoroughly, drink a full glass of water.
- If a dose is missed, take it as soon as possible; however, if the time is close to the next scheduled dose, skip the missed dose and take the scheduled dose. Do not take double doses.

Cultural Considerations (·:·)

- Provide an interpreter with the same ethnic background and gender if possible, especially with sensitive topics.

EVALUATION

■ Evaluate for return of prepregnancy regular bowel function.

Immunizations

Rh$_0$ (D) Immune Globulin

An Rh-negative client who lacks the Rh factor in her own blood may carry a fetus who is either Rh negative or Rh positive. During pregnancy, minimal amounts of fetal blood may cross the placenta. Also, an abortion (spontaneous, therapeutic or induced), amniocentesis, ectopic pregnancy, previa, and abruption result in some mixing of maternal and fetal blood. Subsequently, anti-D antibodies develop in a Rh-negative mother with a Rh-positive fetus; with the development of these antibodies, the mother becomes sensitized (Figure 53–1). If the mother and fetus are both Rh negative, there is no difficulty. However, if the fetus is Rh positive, the Rh-negative mother is at risk for **Rh sensitization** (i.e., the development of protective antibodies against Rh-positive blood). The immunoglobulin IgM is formed and cannot cross the placenta. Later IgD antibodies develop, which may cross the placenta with isoimmunization to the D antigen and subsequent hemolysis of fetal red blood cells. Prenatal D isoimmunization occurs in approximately 1% to 2% of Rh-negative women. In later exposure, as with subsequent pregnancies, there is a more rapid IgG (secondary) immune response and an increased potential for fetal hemolysis in an Rh-positive fetus. The protective antibodies, once formed, remain throughout life and may result in hemolytic difficulties for fetuses in subsequent pregnancies. Maternal blood is assessed for the D antibody at the ini-

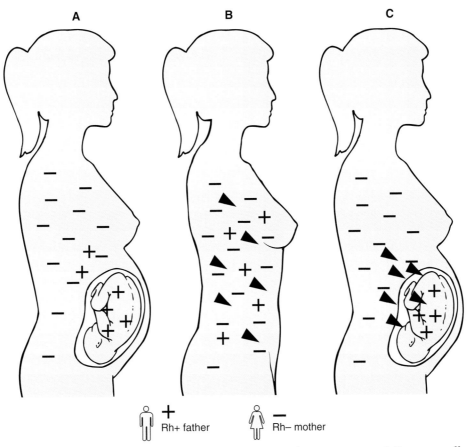

FIGURE 53–1 Understanding Rh isoimmunization. **A,** During pregnancy or delivery, a small amount of fetal blood may enter the mother's circulation. **B,** When the mother is Rh negative and is pregnant with an Rh-positive fetus, the mother's immune system responds by producing anti-Rh$_0$ (D) antibodies. **C,** In subsequent pregnancies, these antibodies cross the placenta and enter the fetal circulation; when the fetus is Rh positive, the anti-Rh$_0$ (D) antibodies will attack the fetal red blood cells and cause hemolysis. (From Nichols F, Zwelling E: *Maternal-newborn nursing: theory and practice,* Philadelphia, 1997, Saunders.)

Table 53–4

Rh_0 (D) Immune Globulin (RhoGAM)

Route and Dosage	Uses and Considerations
IM in deltoid	A sterile concentrated solution of gamma globulin prepared from human serum containing antibodies to the Rh factor (D antigen), also expressed as anti-Rh_0 (D). Administered to nonsensitized Rh-negative clients. Action is to suppress active antibody response and formation of anti-Rh_0 (D) in Rh-negative clients exposed to fetal Rh-positive blood. Promotes destruction of Rh-positive fetal cells in maternal serum before mother can make antibodies that would cause hemolysis of fetal RBCs in Rh-positive fetuses and newborns in subsequent pregnancies. Use with caution in clients with thrombocytopenia, bleeding disorders, and IgA deficiency. Contraindicated in clients with known hypersensitivity to immune globulins or thimerosal, transfusion of Rh_0 (D)-positive blood in previous 3 mo or previous sensitization to Rh_0 (D). 1 vial (300 mcg) prevents maternal sensitization if fetal RBC volume that entered maternal circulation is <15 ml. If the estimated fetal blood and maternal mixing is ≥30 ml, then an additional 300 mcg is administered. When 15 ml maternal fetal blood mixing has occurred, a fetal RBC should be performed to determine the appropriate dose. Appears in breast milk (not absorbed by infant). *Adverse reactions:* lethargy, splenomegaly, elevated bilirubin, myalgia, temperature elevation; most commonly (rare) fever and pain at injection site. *Pregnancy category:* C; $t^{1/2}$: 23-26 d
300 mcg (1 vial) (standard dose)	Given at 28 wk gestation as prophylaxis and again after normal delivery (within 72 h) with negative direct and indirect Coombs' test. Also 300 mcg (standard dose) given after amniocentesis. Larger than standard dose may be given if the Kleihauer Betke analysis show large fetal-maternal blood transfusion has occurred.
50 mcg (1 vial) (microdose)	Given after abortion, ectopic pregnancy before 13 gestational wk. Because it is a blood product, some clients may refuse because of their religious beliefs

d, Day; *IgA,* immunoglobulin A; *IM,* intramuscular; *mo,* month; *RBC,* red blood cell; $t^{1/2}$, half-life; *wk,* week; >, greater than; <, less than.

tial prenatal laboratory evaluation and at 28 to 29 gestational weeks. D immunoglobulin (RhoGAM, Rho(D) immunoglobulin) is routinely administered to women with maternal/fetal blood mixing, such as following an abortion, ectopic pregnancy, or amniocentesis. Dosage depends on gestation: 50 mcg (a microdose) of D immunoglobin is administrated before 13 gestational weeks and 300 mcg is given thereafter. Postpartally, the D immunoglobulin should be administered within 72 hours. For women with abruption, previa, cesarean births, or manual placental removal, a Kleihauer-Betke analysis should be done because greater than 30 ml of fetal maternal bleeding may have occurred, necessitating an increased dose of D immunoglobulin. In this case, 300 mcg of D immunoglobulin is given for each 30 ml of "estimated fetal whole blood" in the maternal circulation. Therefore, one full dose (300 mcg) provides enough antibody to prevent Rh sensitization if the volume of red blood cells entering the circulation is 15 ml or less. When 15 ml or more is suspected, a fetal red cell count should be performed to determine the appropriate dose.

The Rh sensitization process can be prevented through the administration of **Rh_0 (D) immune globulin (RhoGAM)** to nonsensitized Rh-negative clients after each actual or potential exposure to Rh-positive blood (Table 53–4).

Adverse Reactions

Adverse reactions include hypotension, chills, dizziness, fever, headache, pruritus, rash, abdominal pain, diarrhea, and injection site reactions (discomfort, mild pain, redness, and swelling).

Nursing Process

Rh_0 (D) Immune Globulin

ASSESSMENT

■ Determine blood type and Rh status of all prenatal clients.

■ Assess client for her understanding of her Rh status and her partner's Rh status.

■ Ask client whether she has had previous pregnancies and their outcome; ask whether she has ever received Rh_0 (D) immune globulin.

■ Follow agency protocols for Rh blood testing for client and infant at time of delivery.

■ Assess client's religious beliefs because some clients may refuse Rh(D) immune globulin based on their religious beliefs considering it to be a blood product.

■ Postpartum, assess data about newborn's Rh type (if infant is Rh negative, no need for drug; if infant is Rh positive [mother negative], and mother is *not* sensitized [indirect Coombs' test negative] and the infant is direct Coombs' test negative, the mother is a candidate to receive the injection [to *prevent* antibody production or "sensitization"]).

■ Obtain client's written consent before administration. A refusal form is required in some agencies if the drug is declined.

■ Assess for history of allergy to immune globulin products.

NURSING DIAGNOSES

■ Deficient knowledge related to Rh incompatibility and sensitization
■ Deficient knowledge related to Rh_0 (D) immunoglobulin (RhoGAM) purpose, action, and side effects

PLANNING

■ Client will receive Rh_0 (D) immune globulin (RhoGAM) as indicated within 72 hours after delivery or abortion.
■ Client will be able to discuss Rh sensitization and actions indicated during subsequent pregnancies.

NURSING INTERVENTIONS

■ Document Rh workup and eligibility of client to receive drug in client record using agency protocol. Convey information in verbal report.
■ Check lot numbers on vial and laboratory slip for agreement before administration; check expiration date. Check identification band and laboratory slip for matching number. Return required slips to laboratory or blood bank.
■ Administer Rho(D) immune globulin, dose (microdose/standard dose) according to gestational weeks and exposure and route according to provider orders and agency.
■ Administer intramuscularly, usually administered in deltoid within 72 hours following delivery. If after 72 hours, administer as soon as possible up to 28 days.
■ Rho(D) immune globulin (IV) administration is possible though infrequent. Check provider orders and dose. If IV administration then reconstitute with normal saline.
■ Store at 36° F to 46° F (2° C to 8° C).
■ Have epinephrine available to treat anaphylaxis.

Client Teaching

General
• Explain the action, purpose, and side effects of the drug.
• Instruct client to avoid live virus vaccines for 3 months following administration.
• Provide written documentation of date of administration for client's personal health record.

Cultural Considerations ⊕
• Provide an interpreter with the same ethnic background and gender if possible, especially with sensitive topics.

EVALUATION

■ Evaluate client's understanding of the need for Rh_0 (D) immune globulin.

Rubella Vaccine

Maternal rubella is a potentially devastating infection for the fetus, depending on gestational age. If a nonimmunized woman (**rubella titer <1:10**) contracts the virus during the first trimester, a high rate of abortion and neurologic and developmental sequelae associated with **congenital rubella syndrome** may result. Cataracts, glaucoma, deafness, heart defects, and mental retardation are seen with this syndrome. When infection occurs after the first trimester, there is less risk of fetal damage because of the developmental stage of the fetus. There is no treatment for maternal or congenital rubella infection. The goals are immunization and prevention of rubella in women of childbearing age (Table 53–5).

Adverse Reactions

Side effects are generally mild and temporary. Burning or stinging at the injection site is caused by the acidic pH of the vaccine. Regional lymphadenopathy, **urticaria** (i.e., skin rash caused by an allergic reaction), rash, malaise, sore throat, fever, headache, polyneuritis, arthralgia, and moderate fever are occasionally seen.

Table 53–5

Rubella Virus Vaccine, Live, MSD (Meruvax II) (Ra27/3 Strain)

Route and Dosage	Uses and Considerations
Given subQ: 0.5 ml into outer upper arm	Live virus vaccine for immunization against German measles. Dose is same for all persons, using either single dose or multidose vials. Do not give immune serum globulin (ISG) concurrent with vaccine. Contraindicated in pregnant women and clients with anaphylactoid reactions to neomycin, febrile respiratory illness or other febrile infection, active untreated tuberculosis, or immune deficiency conditions. Vaccinated persons can shed but not transmit the virus. Defer vaccination for 3 mo after blood or plasma transfusions and also after human serum immune globulin. Postpartum clients who received blood products may be vaccinated if repeat titer is drawn 6-8 wk later to ensure that seroconversion occurred. Excreted in breast milk; use caution. Important for client to use contraceptive method for three months following administration as rubella is tetratogenic. Rubella titer may be assessed approximately 3 mo after administration. *Side effects:* burning, stinging at injection site; malaise; fever; headache; slight rash 2-4 wk after injection; joint pain 1-3 d within 1-10 wk of injection. *Pregnancy category:* C

d, Day; *mo*, month; *subQ*, subcutaneous; *wk*, week.

Nursing Process

Rubella Vaccine

ASSESSMENT

■ Review history and laboratory results to determine need for rubella vaccine.

■ A rubella titer of less than 1:8/1:10 (agency lab), negative, or nonimmunized indicates need for rubella vaccine administration.

■ Rubella vaccine is contraindicated if the client verbalizes or if chart review indicates any of the following:
  * Pregnant
  * Receipt of whole blood transfusions, plasma transfusion, or human immune serum globulin within the past 3 months
  * History of anaphylactic or anaphylactoid reactions to neomycin (dose contains 25 g of heomycin)
  * Received other virus vaccines within 1 month (Do not give less than 1 month before or after other virus vaccines.)
  * Immunosuppressed, radiation therapy, untreated, active tuberculosis (TB), AIDS or symptomatic HIV
  * Blood dyscrasias, leukemia, lymphomas of any type, or other malignant neoplasms affecting bone marrow or lymphatic system
  * Any febrile or respiratory illness or other acute illness

■ Determine whether client is also a candidate to receive Rh_0 (D) immune globulin (RhoGAM). Administration of both drugs may result in suppression of rubella antibodies with need to recheck rubella titer in approximately 3 months.

NURSING DIAGNOSES

■ Deficient knowledge related to risk of rubella infection and benefit of prevention

■ Risk of injury related to rubella infection in subsequent pregnancy secondary to lack of immunity

PLANNING

■ Client will receive rubella vaccine to protect against rubella (German measles).

■ Client will plan to prevent pregnancy for 3 months following subQ injection.

NURSING INTERVENTIONS

■ Protect vaccine from light and store at 35.6° F to 46.4° F (2° C to 8° C) before reconstitution.

■ Reconstitute with dilutent provided and administer within 8 hours.

■ Administer 0.5 ml vaccine subQ in upper outer arm. Do not administer IV.

■ If tuberculin skin test is to be done, administer it before or simultaneously with rubella vaccine (may have temporary depression in tuberculin skin sensitivity).

Skill: Reconstitution

* Single-dose vial: withdraw entire amount of diluent into syringe.
* Inject total volume into vial of lyophilized vaccine and agitate to mix thoroughly.
* Withdraw entire contents into syringe and inject total volume of restored vaccine.
* Have epinephrine readily available in case of anaphylactic reaction.
* Clearly convey in writing and verbal report that vaccination has occurred.
* Record date of administration, lot number, manufacturer, name, and title to comply with agency policy.

Client Teaching

General
* Discuss the importance of immunity to rubella with client and help her understand the need to obtain titers to determine immune status.
* Discuss the importance for use of effective contraception for 3 months after vaccine injection. Identify method of choice and document instruction.
* Reassure client that there is no risk to her from being near small children who received the injection even if she is pregnant and not immune.
* Instruct parents regarding the drug action, purpose, and side effects.

Safety
* Recommend that client have titer rechecked in 3 months if she also received RhoGAM.

Side Effects
* The most common side effect is burning or stinging at injection site; some also experience malaise, fever, headache, and slight rash about 2 to 4 weeks after injection. About 1 to 10 weeks after injection, some may experience joint pain that lasts 1 to 3 days.

Cultural Considerations
* Provide an interpreter as appropriate.

EVALUATION

■ Evaluate the need for rubella vaccine and administration to women with titer less than 1:8/1:10 (agency lab), nonimmunized, or negative titer.

Table 53–6

Drugs Administered to the Newborn Immediately After Delivery

Generic (Brand)	Route and Dosage	Uses and Considerations
erythromycin ophthalmic ointment (Ilotycin Ophthalmic)	$\frac{1}{2}$-in ribbon of ointment placed in lower conjunctival sac of each eye, beginning with the inner canthus within 1 h of delivery	Prevention of gonococcal conjunctivitis and chlamydial conjunctivitis (**ophthalmia neonatorum**), which can cause blindness. Source of infection is birth canal. Contains antibiotic (erythromycin) in sterile base of mineral oil and white petrolatum. Has bactericidal or bacteriostatic action based on concentration per gram and the target organisms present. Mandatory administration in the U.S. *Side effects:* Chemical conjunctivitis (swelling, inflammation 24-48 h)
phytonadione (Vitamin K₁, Mephyton, Aqua-MEPHYTON)	0.5-1 mg IM in vastus lateralis (preferably) or rectus femoris within 1 h after birth (Check care provider or agency standing orders for dosage)	Prevention of hemorrhagic disease of the newborn. Anticoagulant antagonist. An aqueous colloidal solution of vitamin K₁. Newborn does not receive adequate vitamin K transplacentally and is unable to synthesize vitamin initially because of limited intestinal flora; therefore production of clotting factors in liver is hindered and low prothrombin levels are evidenced. Phytonadione facilitates production of clotting factors equal to natural vitamin K. Newborns of mothers who received oral anticoagulants, anticonvulsants, antituberculosis drugs or recent antibiotics during pregnancy may need higher dosage 6-8 h after the first injection. *Side effects:* Pain and edema at injection site; possible allergic reactions include urticaria and rash; those who receive larger doses may exhibit hyperbilirubinemia and jaundice.

h, Hour; *IM,* intramuscular; *in,* inch.

Drugs Administered to the Newborn Immediately After Delivery

Drugs administered to the newborn in the immediate postbirth period are (1) erythromycin ophthalmic ointment to provide prophylaxis against eye infections (required by U.S. public health law and all states) and (2) vitamin K to prevent hemorrhagic disease of the newborn (Table 53-6). Anti-infective agents may be applied to the cord stump, as alcohol or Triple Dye, during the first few hours after birth; however, current literature supports "dry cord care" with no agents applied.

Side Effects and Adverse Reactions

Erythromycin Ophthalmic Ointment. Side effects include chemical conjunctivitis in about 20% of newborns, which manifests as edema and inflammation lasting about 24 to 48 hours. This may interfere slightly with eye-to-eye contact between parents and the newborn.

Phytonadione Vitamin K1, (Aqua-Mephyton). Side effects include pain and edema at the injection site. Some allergic reactions, manifested by urticaria and rash, have been reported. Newborns who receive larger doses may exhibit hyperbilirubinemia and jaundice resulting from competition for binding sites. Do not confuse mephyton with mephytoin.

Nursing Process

Drugs Administered to the Newborn After Delivery

ASSESSMENT

Erythromycin Ophthalmic Ointment (Ilotycin Ophthalmic)

• Assess newborn for signs of hypersensitivity.

Phytonadione (Vitamin K₁, Mephyton, Aqua-MEPHYTON)

• Assess newborn for bleeding from umbilical cord, circumcision site, nose, and gastrointestinal tract, and for generalized ecchymoses.

NURSING DIAGNOSIS

■ Risk of injury related to infectious process (congenital) or transient low prothrombin levels in the newborn

PLANNING

■ Newborn will experience minimal or no side effects from drugs routinely administered after delivery.

NURSING INTERVENTIONS

Erythromycin Ophthalmic Ointment

- See Chapter 3, Principles of Drug Administration, for the procedure for administration of eye ointment.
- Promote bonding by facilitating eye contact between parents and the infant during this period but delay instillation no longer than 1 hour after delivery.
- Wear gloves for administration of eye ointment.
- Do not place tube of ointment under radiant warmer with infant before administration.
- Following administration, close eyes to more evenly distribute ointment. After 1 minute, may remove excess ointment. Do not irrigate eyes following instillation.

Phytonadione (Vitamin K₁, Mephyton, Aqua-MEPHYTON)

- Protect drug from light because of photosensitivity of the preparation.
- Cleanse anterolateral site before injecting drug, if alcohol is used allow to dry prior to drug administration.
- Observe injection site for edema and inflammation. (See Figure 53–2 and Chapter 3, Principles of Drug Administration, for site.)
- Administer phytonadione prior to circumcision.

Client Teaching: Erythromycin Ophthalmic Ointment (Ilotycin Ophthalmic)

- Instruct parents regarding the drug action, purpose, and side effects.

- Instructing parents about drug administration is mandatory in United States.
- Tell parents that any edema around eyes usually disappears within 24 to 48 hours.
- Explain that administration of eye prophylaxis is federally and state mandated and that there is no risk to vision from the ointment.

Client Teaching: Phytonadione (Vitamin K1, Mephyton, Aqua-MEPHYTON)

- Instruct parents regarding the drug action, purpose and side effects.

EVALUATION

- Evaluate for newborn bleeding, specifically days 2 and 3 after administration of phytonadione (Vitamin K, Mephyton, Aqua-MEPHYTON).
- Evaluate for drug hypersensitivity or side effects.
- Evaluate parents' understanding about medications administered to their newborns.

Immunization During the Newborn Period Before Discharge

The American Academy of Pediatrics and the Centers for Disease Control and Prevention (CDC) have recommended that immunization against hepatitis B virus (HBV) begin in the newborn period. The HBV infection may result in serious long-term liver disease, cancer, and death in adulthood. The goal of immunization is to reduce the number of chronic carriers of the virus in the population, thus preventing HBV infection.

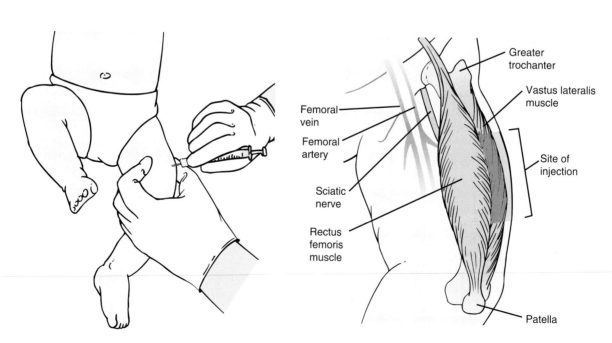

FIGURE 53–2 Site for giving an intramuscular injection to a newborn shortly after birth. (From Nichols F, Zwelling E: *Maternal-newborn nursing: theory and practice*, Philadelphia, 1997, Saunders.)

Table 53–7

Hepatitis B Immunization in the Newborn Period

Generic (Brand)	Route and Dosage	Uses and Considerations
Hepatitis B vaccine (Engerix-B, Recombivax HB)	For newborns of HBsAg-negative, HBsAg-positive mothers and unknown hepatitis B status: Engerix-B 0.5 ml (10 mcg) IM within 12 h after birth (first dose); repeated at 1 mo and 6 mo. Recombivax HB-0.5 ml (5 mcg) IM within 12 h after birth (first dose), repeated at 1 mo and 6 mo. For newborns of HBsAg-*negative* mothers: 0.5 ml (10 mcg) IM before discharge but no later than 2 mo of age; followed by repeat doses at 1-2 mo and 6-18 mo. (If unlikely to return for routine immunizations, may give repeat doses at 4 mo and 6-18 mo.)	Hepatitis B vaccine is a recombinant vaccine that provides passive immunization against all subtypes of HBV. Given to all infants regardless of HBsAg status of mother. Unvaccinated infants *younger than* 12 mo old with a mother or primary care giver with acute hepatitis B should be given HBIG because of risk of becoming an HBV carrier following infection (also start HBV vaccine series). Must be injected IM into rectum femoris preferably, or rectus femoris; never inject IV. Following three doses, >90% of infants and children will seroconvert 95-99%. Protection in those who seroconvert will last 3-7 y with a single booster. Contraindicated if hypersensitivity to any component of vaccine or yeast. *Neonatal side effects:* soreness at injection site with edema, warmth, erythema, and induration. *Pregnancy category:* C Newborns of HBsAg-positive mothers should also receive HBIG. HBIG 0.5 ml IM within 12 h of birth. It is given concurrently with first dose of hepatitis B vaccine for infants of HBsAg positive mothers in separate sites (thighs). Newborns of mothers with HBsAg-unknown status whose maternal results are positive within 7 d of birth should receive HBIG (0.5 ml) IM in the opposite thigh.

h, Hour; *HBIG,* hepatitis B immune globulin; *HBsAg,* hepatitis B surface antigen; *HBV,* hepatitis B virus; *IM,* intramuscular; *IV,* intravenous; *mo,* month; *y,* year; >, greater than.

In pregnancy, HBV transmission occurs vertically, primarily at the time of delivery. The recombinant hepatitis B (Engerix-B, Recombivax HB) provides passive immunization for the newborn (Table 53–7). The current recommendation is that newborns receive recombinant hepatitis B (Engerix-B, Recombivax HB) and, if appropriate, hepatitis B immunoglobulin (HBIG) injections intramuscularly (IM) in the anterolateral thigh following a protocol based on the mother's HBsAg-positive or -negative status. These injections require signed maternal consent prior to administration. Do not confuse Hepatitis B vaccine (Engerix-B, Recombivax) with Hepatitis B immunoglobulin (HBIG).

Infants born to HBsAg-negative mothers will receive only the recombinant hepatitis B (Engerix-B, Recombivax HB). In contrast, infants born to HBsAg-positive mothers will receive concurrent injections of both HBIG and hepatitis B vaccine (Engerix-B, Recombivax HB) in separate sites because it is believed that infection can be prevented in 90% of newborns.

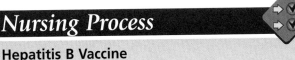

Nursing Process

Hepatitis B Vaccine

ASSESSMENT

■ Review prenatal record laboratory data for maternal HBsAg status.

■ Validate whether infant is to receive hepatitis B vaccine singly or in concert with hepatitis B immune globulin (HBIG).
■ Assess parental knowledge of immunizations, purpose and childhood immunization schedule.
■ Assess for hypersensitivity to yeast (recombinant HB).
■ Assess for written maternal consent for newborn vaccine before administration.

NURSING DIAGNOSES

■ Risk for injury related to hepatitis B infection
■ Deficient knowledge related to hepatitis B, maternal prophylaxis, and pediatric immunization schedule

PLANNING

■ The newborn will receive correct dosage of hepatitis B vaccine before discharge, including HBIG, if indicated.
■ The newborn's caregiver will go to primary health care provider and verbalizes plans to continue childhood immunizations as recommended by the current immunization schedule.

NURSING INTERVENTIONS

Skill

• Shake vial well before withdrawal of medication.
• Discard if other than slightly opaque white suspension.

- Cleanse anterolateral site before injecting drug, if alcohol is used, allow to dry prior to drug administration.
- Inject complete contents of vial; do not dilute.
- Have epinephrine available for allergic reaction.
- If mother refuses heptatitis B vaccine (Engerix-B, Recombivax HB) or HBIG, note in maternal and newborn chart. Assess agency protocol as some agencies document medication refusal.
- Monitor newborn's temperature post injection per agency protocol.

Safety

- Give IM in vastus lateralis (preferably) or rectus femoris.
- Document site in chart.
- Record lot number, expiration date, name, and title in chart.
- Store product at 35.6° F to 46.4° F (2° C to 8° C).
- Do not freeze (because freezing destroys potency).
- Do not confuse hepatitis B vaccine (Engerix-B, Recombivax) because these drugs have different dosages.
- Do not confuse hepatitis B vaccine (Engerix-B, Recombivax) and HBIG.

Client Teaching

General

- Inform mother of implications of her hepatitis B surface antigen (HBsAg)-positive or HBsAg-negative status for her newborn and recommend interventions.
- Have mother read literature and sign consent for vaccine administration. Place original/copy in newborn's chart as per agency protocol.
- Instruct parents regarding childhood immunizations as recommended by the current immunization schedule.
- Inform mother when repeat doses need to be given.

EVALUATION

- Evaluate mother's understanding of the need for hepatitis B vaccine for her newborn.

WEBSITES

For further information on *Postpartum and the Newborn,* visit these Internet resources:

American College of Obstetricians and Gynecologists: *http://www.acog.org*

Centers for Disease Control and Prevention (CDC): *http://www.cdc.gov/nccdphp*

CDC—Birth Defects: *http://www.cdc.gov/ncbddd/bd/abc.htm*

Center for Complementary Alternative Medicine Research in Women's Health, Columbia University: *http://cpmcnet.columbia.edu/dept/rosenthal/*

Drugs: *www.drugs.com*

March of Dimes Birth Defects Foundation: *www.marchofdimes.com*

Mayo E Clinic: *http://www.mayoclinic.com*

National Center for Complementary and Alternative Medicine: *http://atmed.od.nih.gov*

National Institutes of Health—National Institute of Child Health & Human Development: *http://www.nichd.nih.gov/womenshealth*

National Library of Medicine & NIH—Medline Plus: *http://www.nlm.nih.gov/medlineplus/prenatalcare.htm*

The National Academies Press: *http://www.nationalacademies.org/health*

Critical Thinking Case Study

T.A., age 17 (gravida 4, para 1), is the same client treated in Chapters 51, Drugs Associated with the Female Reproductive Cycle I: Pregnancy and Preterm Labor, and 52, Drugs Associated with the Female Reproductive Cycle II: Labor, Delivery, and the Preterm Neonate. T.A. came to the hospital for labor induction/augmentation at 42 weeks' gestation because of her prolonged pregnancy and signs and symptoms of pregnancy-induced hypertension. T.A.'s mother arrived at the hospital when T.A. was 8 cm dilated, in time for the latter stages of T.A.'s labor. Her mother remained as T.A.'s support person throughout the delivery, which occurred at 6:00 AM by vacuum extraction. T.A. had a continuous epidural for her labor and delivery. An episiotomy was done at the time of delivery, and a fourth-degree laceration occurred. A cluster of hemorrhoids was evident. Baby J.A., weighing 8 lbs 7 oz, had Apgar scores of 7 and 9. The infant is alert and active. T.A. lives with her mother and has been going to high school while working part time in an automotive parts store. T.A. wants to keep her infant and to breastfeed "for at least 3 months." She plans to finish school and return to work in 6 weeks.

Immediately after the delivery, you conduct an assessment of T.A., analyze the data, and determine and prioritize her nursing care needs. The same is done for the newborn.

1. Based on the data supplied about her delivery, what is the priority nursing diagnosis for T.A.?

2. What is an outcome-based goal for the diagnosis given?

3. How should the nurse intervene in regard to the episiotomy during the early postpartum period, integrating both pharmacologic and nonpharmacologic measures? Orders include benzocaine spray, witch hazel pads, Proctofoam-HC, and ibuprofen tablets (200 mg) at the bedside.

4. T.A verbalizes that her grandmother wants her to eat warm soup that she will bring to the hospital. She also told T.A not to take a shower for 4 weeks. What further assessment is necessary?

Baby J.A.'s newborn medications must be administered within the first hour following delivery. Bonding for T.A. and J.A. should also be promoted at this time.

5. Within the standard, how should bonding be promoted, including eye contact between mother and infant, while eye prophylaxis is also administered?

6. What steps should be followed to instill the ointment into the infant's eyes, including safety aspects for the nurse administering the ointment?

7. What should T.A. be taught about the side effects of eye prophylaxis?

8. How should the reason for the vitamin K_1 injection for the infant be explained to T.A. in terms she can understand?

9. What steps should be followed to prepare and give the vitamin K_1 injection, including safety aspects for the nurse administering the injection?

T.A. is Rh negative. The blood type of the infant's father is unknown. A cord blood was drawn on the infant at the time of delivery. Based on T.A.'s historical data, answer the following:

10. What is a concern in terms of defining T.A. as a likely or unlikely Rh_0 (D) immune globulin candidate? What information about the mother and infant is needed to aid in the decision?

Assuming T.A. is a Rh_0 (D) immune globulin candidate, answer the following:

11. What is a nursing diagnosis for T.A.?

12. What is an outcome-based goal for the diagnosis given?

13. What is the timeframe in which Rh_0 (D) immune globulin should be administered? Explain the rationale for this timeframe.

14. What are appropriate verbal and written documentation in regard to Rh_0 (D) immune globulin administration, both before and after administration?

15. T.A.'s chart reveals that her rubella titer is 1:6. What orders should be expected in regard to rubella vaccine?

16. Neomycin is listed as a known allergy in T.A.'s medication administration record. Considering T.A.'s titer, the standing health care provider's order, and knowledge about this vaccine, how should this situation be handled?

17. In a situation in which a mother is both a rubella and Rh_0 (D) immune globulin candidate, with both products being administered, what is the focus of client teaching for T.A. in regard to the rubella titer?

Because of her episiotomy, T.A. is concerned about her first postdelivery bowel movement. It is explained to her that the docusate with casanthranol product in her self-administered medication packet will help.

18. T.A. says that she does not want to take the docusate because she plans to breastfeed. What is the appropriate nursing diagnosis based on T.A.'s communication?

19. How should T.A.'s concerns be addressed based on knowledge of the product and breastfeeding?

Continued

Critical Thinking Case Study—cont'd

T.A. asks what can be done about her hemorrhoids. The mode of action of the ordered pharmacologic products is explained to her. She then states, "So I just have to insert this syringe-type applicator into my rectum once I fill it from the big can?"

20. Analyze T.A.'s statement. What is correct and incorrect concerning the knowledge?

21. What nursing diagnosis is appropriate for T.A. based on the information supplied?

22. What client teaching is needed for T.A.?

Baby J.A. is ordered to receive hepatitis B vaccine before discharge. T.A. is HBsAg negative.

23. Which newborns are eligible to receive hepatitis B vaccine?

24. How many doses constitute the total series, and what is the duration for these?

25. Why is this vaccine given to newborns? Why is this important in today's society?

26. T.A. asks how long the infant's immunity should last. How should she be answered?

27. Where would one expect to find the vaccine stored?

28. What is the written documentation required with administration of this vaccine?

Study Questions

1. A client was supposed to chew her simethicone tablets at 8:00 AM, but she forgot. It is now 11:15 AM. She asks if she should chew them now or wait and take extra tablets at the scheduled noon dose. What is the appropriate response? Explain the rationale.

2. Describe what a newly admitted postpartum (vaginal delivery) client should be told about the process of self-administered drugs and the specific products included. Why would this material be selected?

3. What client data are required before postpartum administration of ergot derivatives (e.g., methyl-ergonovine [Methergine])? (See Chapter 51, Drugs Associated with the Female Reproductive Cycle I: Pregnancy and Preterm Labor.)

4. What should the nurse assess before advising a postpartum client to initiate use of laxative products?

5. S.H., age 24, delivered her infant 24 hours ago. She has a history of drug and alcohol abuse. Her health care provider ordered senna syrup for her as a stimulant laxative. What action should be taken? Why?

6. Why are bedtime doses of mineral oil not generally recommended?

7. A postpartum client complains of "pain in my bottom where the doctor cut me." Her chart states that she has a fourth-degree laceration. What pharmacologic products are available to help this client, in addition to nonpharmacologic comfort measures? How will these help the client?

8. M.Y., a postpartum client, has an order for promazine and hydrocortisone. She has the product at her bedside but has not used it. When questioned, M.Y. said, "Oh, I forgot to tell you—I'm allergic to things like lidocaine, benzocaine." What is the appropriate response to M.Y.?

9. What are three factors to evaluate concerning drugs and products used to relieve pain from perineal wounds and hemorrhoids?

10. A client says she sees no reason to use her dibucaine ointment because it "feels like nothing on my hand—not cooling or soothing—so it probably won't help my bottom." How should one correctly respond with factual information?

11. What is the purpose for newborn injection of vitamin K_1 following delivery?

12. What agent is used for newborn eye prophylaxis? In what time frame should it be given? How is it administered?

13. What injection site should be used to administer hepatitis B vaccine to a newborn?

14. E.S., age 18, is of Japanese ethnicity. What would your cultural assessment include?

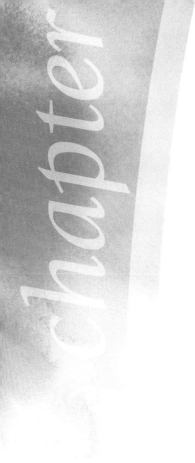

54 Drugs Related to Women's Health and Disorders

SANDRA ELLIOTT

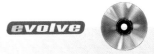

ELECTRONIC RESOURCES

Additional information can be found on the companion website at *http://evolve.elsevier.com/KeeHayes/pharmacology/* or on the companion CD-ROM, which includes:

- *NCLEX-style examination review questions*
- *Pharmacology animations*
- *Medication error and IV therapy checklists*
- *Medication calculation problems*
- *Electronic calculators*

OBJECTIVES

- Describe the types, expected actions, and side effects of oral contraceptive products.
- Recognize new hormonal/pharmacologic products related to conception control.
- Explain the expected effects of medications used to treat dysfunctional uterine bleeding, premenstrual syndrome, endometriosis, menopausal symptoms, and osteoporosis.
- Describe the nursing process, including client teaching, associated with drugs used for women's health and disorders.

TERMS

dysfunctional uterine
   bleeding
dyspareunia
endometriosis
estrogen replacement
   therapy (ERT)

follicular phase
hormone replacement
   therapy (HRT)
luteal phase

menopause
oral contraceptives
osteoporosis

premenstrual syndrome
   (PMS)
progestin

Introduction

Oral contraceptive products and medications used for uterine dysfunction and menopause are described in this chapter. Nursing interventions and client teaching are emphasized.

Oral Contraceptive Products

Among the various methods of contraception available, the **oral contraceptives** that use hormone therapy enjoy wide popularity because of their ease of use and high degree of effectiveness with relative safety for most women. The effectiveness of oral contraceptives can be compromised by concurrent use of some medications (i.e., antibiotics) or herbal products (see Herbal Alert 54–1). When these steroidal agents were first approved for use by the Food and Drug Administration (FDA) in 1960, little was known about the best combinations of drugs to use or their optimum doses. Adverse side effects, particularly circulatory disorders, were frequent. Subsequent research has resulted in lower-dose drugs. Research continues to focus on actual and potential short- and long-term benefits and risks associated with use of low-dose oral contraceptives and new administration forms (e.g., long-acting progestin-releasing subcutaneous implants), particularly in the areas of circulatory risks and carcinogenesis. Immunologic methods of contraception are another area of current research.

There are two main types of oral contraceptives: the estrogen-progestin combination products, often called *"the pill,"* and the progestin-only products, sometimes called *the minipill*. The combination products have the lowest pregnancy rate.

Estrogen-Progestin Combination Products

Combined estrogen-progestin oral contraceptive products prevent pregnancy by suppressing pituitary release of follicle-stimulating hormone (FSH) and luteinizing hormone (LH),

which are needed to mature a graafian follicle in the ovary, thereby inhibiting ovulation. These agents also create changes in the endometrium that make it less favorable for implantation of a fertilized ovum. In addition, the quantity and viscosity of the cervical mucus is changed by progestins, making it hostile to sperm. Alterations in motility within the fallopian tube may also impede the movement of the ova.

The most commonly prescribed oral contraceptive products are the estrogen-progestin combinations. These formulations are differentiated based on the strength of the individual components and whether estrogen or progesterone effects predominate. The amount of estrogen varies among the available products. Low-dose combination products have 35 mcg or less of ethinyl estradiol or 50 mcg or less of mestranol. The synthetic progesterone **progestin** incorporated in the combination products reduces the effects of estrogen. The goal of therapy is to identify the product that offers the best contraceptive protection throughout the menstrual cycle that also has the fewest unwanted side effects as a result of either the estrogen or the progestin component.

There are three types of combination products: monophasic, biphasic, and triphasic. The *monophasics*, the most common, provide a fixed ratio of estrogen to progestin throughout the menstrual cycle. In *biphasics*, the amount of estrogen is fixed throughout the cycle, but the amount of progesterone varies (reduced in the first half and increased in the second half) to provide for proliferation of the endometrium and secretory development similar to the physiologic process. Ortho-Novum 10/11–21 is an example of a biphasic. The *triphasics*, the newest combination products, deliver low doses of both hormones with minimal side effects, including breakthrough bleeding. With triphasics, the amount of either estrogen or progesterone varies throughout the cycle in different ratios during three phases.

Ortho Tri-Cyclen is an example of a triphasic pill that varies the dosage of progestin. Estrostep is an example of a triphasic pill that varies the dosage of estrogen. Both have FDA indications for the treatment of acne.

Seasonale is the first and only FDA-approved extended-cycle birth control pill. The 91-day regimen (84 active pills/ 7 placebo pills) of Seasonale reduces a woman's periods from 13 to just 4 per year. Women who may benefit from an extended cycle regimen include women with menstrual disorders such as endometriosis, dysmenorrhea, and ovarian cysts.

HERBAL ALERT 54–1

St. John's Wort

❧ St. John's Wort *(Hypericum perforatum)* may reduce the effectiveness of contraceptive steroids. This may also result in breakthrough bleeding.

Progestin-Only Products

The progestin-only oral contraceptive, called "the mini-pill," acts primarily by altering the cervical mucus and secondarily by altering the endometrium to inhibit implantation. Ovulation is also inhibited in some clients through blockage of LH release. These products were designed to further decrease circulatory side effects. There is, however, a lower pregnancy prevention rate, which increases further if a client misses a pill, because these drugs do not suppress activity of the hypothalamus and pituitary to the same degree as the combination products. If the minipill is taken more than 3 hours late, a back-up contraceptive method should be used for 48 hours. There are no placebo pills in a pack of progestin only pills. All 28 pills contain active hormones. An increase in the amount of breakthrough bleeding is also noted. Examples of progestin-only products include Ovrette, Micronor, and Nor-QD. Table 54–1 presents selected examples of the various oral contraceptive formulations.

Pharmacokinetics

Combination Products. Ethinyl estradiol is rapidly absorbed orally. It undergoes significant first-pass metabolism and elimination via the liver. Mestranol is converted in the liver to ethinyl estradiol, which is 97% to 98% bound to plasma proteins. The half-life varies from 6 to 20 hours. Excretion is via bile and urine in a conjugated form. There is some enterohepatic recirculation.

Progestin-Only Products. Progestins are also well absorbed orally. Peak plasma levels occur from 0.5 to 4 hours after ingestion, depending on the particular compound. Norethynodrel and ethynodiol diacetate are converted to norethindrone. Levonorgestrel is bioavailable and does not undergo first-pass liver metabolism; norethindrone undergoes first-pass metabolism and is 65% available. The progestins are bound to plasma proteins and to sex hormone-binding globulin. The half-life of norethindrone varies from 5 to 14 hours; the half-life of levonorgestrel is 11 to 45 hours.

Table 54–1

Oral Contraceptives

Product	Amount of Estrogen (mcg)	Amount of Progestin (mg)
Combination Products: Listed by Decreasing Estrogen Content		
Monophasic Products		
Norinyl 1 + 50 (21 days)	50 mestranol	1 norethindrone
Genora 1/50	50 mestranol	1 norethindrone
Ovcon 50	50 ethinyl estradiol	1 norethindrone
Norlestrin 1/50	50 ethinyl estradiol	1 norethindrone acetate
Demulen 1/50	50 ethinyl estradiol	1 ethynodiol diacetate
Norlestrin 21 2.5/50	50 ethinyl estradiol	2.5 norethindrone acetate
Ovral	50 ethinyl estradiol	0.5 norgestrel
Genora 1/35	35 ethinyl estradiol	1 norethindrone
Norcept-E 1/35	35 ethinyl estradiol	1 norethindrone
Ortho-Novum 1/35	35 ethinyl estradiol	1 norethindrone
N.E.E. 1/35	35 ethinyl estradiol	1 norethindrone
Norethin 1/35 E	35 ethinyl estradiol	1 norethindrone
Norinyl 1 + 35	35 ethinyl estradiol	1 norethindrone
Modicon	35 ethinyl estradiol	0.5 norethindrone
Brevicon	35 ethinyl estradiol	0.5 norethindrone
Nelova	35 ethinyl estradiol	0.5 norethindrone
Ovcon 35	35 ethinyl estradiol	0.4 norethindrone
Demulen 1/35	35 ethinyl estradiol	1 ethynodiol diacetate
Desogen	30 ethinyl estradiol	0.15 desogestrel
Loestin Fe 21 1.5/30	30 ethinyl estradiol	1.5 norethindrone acetate
Lo/Ovral	30 ethinyl estradiol	0.3 norgestrel
Levlen	30 ethinyl estradiol	0.15 levonorgestrel
Nordette	30 ethinyl estradiol	0.15 levonorgestrel
Levlite	20 ethinyl estradiol	0.10 levonorgestrel
Loestrin 21 1/20	20 ethinyl estradiol	1 norethindrone acetate
Biphasic Products		
Jenest 28	*Phase I (7 days):* 35 ethinyl estradiol	0.5 norethindrone
	Phase II (14 days): 35 ethinyl estradiol	1 norethindrone
N.E.E. 10/11	*Phase I (10 days):* 35 ethinyl estradiol	0.5 norethindrone
	Phase II (11 days): 35 ethinyl estradiol	1 norethindrone
Ortho-Novum 10/11	Same formulation as above but different colors for tablets	

Continued

Table 54–1

Oral Contraceptives—cont'd

Product	Amount of Estrogen (mcg)	Amount of Progestin (mg)
Combination Products: Listed by Decreasing Estrogen Content—cont'd		
Triphasic Products		
Tri-Norinyl	*Phase I (7 days):*	
	35 ethinyl estradiol	0.5 norethindrone
	Phase II (9 days):	
	35 ethinyl estradiol	1 norethindrone
	Phase III (5 days):	
	35 ethinyl estradiol	0.5 norethindrone
Ortho Tri-Cyclen	*Phase I (7 days):*	
	35 ethinyl estradiol	0.18 norgestimate
	Phase II (7 days):	
	35 ethinyl estradiol	0.215 norgestimate
	Phase III (7 days):	
	35 ethinyl estradiol	0.25 norgestimate
Ortho-Novum 7/7/7	*Phase I (7 days):*	
	35 ethinyl estradiol	0.5 norethindrone
	Phase II (7 days):	
	35 ethinyl estradiol	0.075 norethindrone
	Phase III (7 days):	
	35 ethinyl estradiol	1 norethindrone
Tri-Levlen	*Phase I (6 days):*	
	30 ethinyl estradiol	0.05 levonorgestrel
	Phase II (5 days):	
	40 ethinyl estradiol	0.075 levonorgestrel
	Phase III (10 days):	
	30 ethinyl estradiol	0.125 levonorgestrel
Triphasil	Same as above	
Progestin-Only Products: Listed by Decreasing Progestin Content		
Micronor		0.35 norethindrone
Nor-QD		0.35 norethindrone
Ovrette		0.075 norgestrel

Dosage Schedule

Combination Products

Most monophasic products are available in 21- and 28-tablet packages. The 28-tablet packages include seven non-hormone-containing tablets (some contain iron) so that the client continues to take one tablet each day rather than having to remember starting and stopping times. Clients are instructed to take one tablet every day at approximately the same time each day. Many products require the client to start the tablets on the Sunday following the first day of menstruation. If menstruation actually starts on Sunday, the client starts her tablets that day. Other products instruct the client to start her tablets on day 5 of the menstrual cycle (day 1 is the day she begins menstruation). If the client is on a 21-day regimen, she restarts her next cycle following a 7-day break whether her bleeding has stopped or not. If a Sunday start is used, a backup method (such as condoms or a diaphragm) needs to be used for a minimum of 7 days. Other products instruct the client to start her tablets on day 1 of the menstrual cycle (which is the day she begins menstruation). A backup method is not needed with this method.

The biphasic and triphasic products are taken in phases and are color-coded to assist the client. They, too, are available in 21- and 28-day regimens and are started within the guidelines previously presented. For example, the biphasic Ortho-Novum 10/11 requires 10 white tablets for 10 days, followed by 11 peach tablets for 11 days. With a 21-day regimen, the client stops for 7 days; with a 28-day regimen, the client takes seven green inert tablets during this period before beginning the next cycle. The triphasic Ortho-Novum 7/7/7 works similarly. White tablets are taken for 7 days, light peach for 7 days, darker peach for 7 days, followed by 7 days off or 7 green inert tablets. Exceptions to these guidelines include the triphasics Triphasil 21 and Tri-Levulen 21, which are started on the first day of the menstrual cycle with the designated color code followed for 6 days, 5 days, and 10 days, respectively. These, too, are available in 21- and 28-day packaging.

A new product, drospirenone/ethinyl estradiol (Yasmin 28), is the first oral contraceptive with progestin to reduce water retention. Dosage is drospirenone/ethinyl estradiol 3 mg/0.03 mg daily for 21 days; then one inert tablet daily (white tablet) for 7 days. It is contraindicated in women with renal, hepatic or adrenal insufficiency. Monitor potassium level during first cycle if risk of hyperkalemia (taking drugs that increase potassium, such as angiotensin-converting enzyme [ACE] inhibitors, angiotension receptor blockers, nonsteroidal antiinflammatory drugs [NSAIDs], potassium sparing diuretics). Potential adverse effects include headache, menstrual disorder, and breast pain.

Progestin-Only Products

The progestin-only products are taken one tablet at the same time daily without interruption. The tablets should begin being taken on the first day of menstruation.

Missed Doses

Clients occasionally miss a tablet. If only one tablet is missed, it is unlikely that ovulation will occur. However, the risk increases with each additional missed dose.

Table 54–2 presents guidelines for missed doses of oral contraceptives.

Contraindications

Not every client is a candidate for use of oral contraceptives. Box 54–1 lists contraindications to their use.

Drug Interactions

The effectiveness of some drugs is impaired by oral contraceptives; other drugs impair the effectiveness of oral contraceptives. Box 54–2 lists examples of drugs for which the nurse should maintain a high index of suspicion for interactive effects with oral contraceptives. Clients receiving low-dose formulations of oral contra-

---

Table 54–2

Guidelines for Missed Doses of Oral Contraceptives

Missed Dose	Recommendations
Combination Products	
One tablet	Take tablet as soon as realized OR take two tablets the next day OR take one tablet and discard missed tablet and continue schedule but use secondary form of contraception until menses begin.
Two tablets	Take two tablets as soon as realized with next tablet at the usual time OR take two tablets daily for the next 2 days and resume regular schedule plus use a secondary form of contraception for the rest of the cycle.
Three tablets	Start a new package of tablets 7 days after the last tablet was taken. Use another form of contraception until tablets have been taken for 7 consecutive days.
Progestin-Only Products	
One tablet	Take tablet as soon as realized; follow with next tablet at regular time PLUS
Two tablets	If taken more than 3 h late, use back-up method for 48 h.
Three tablets	If taken more than 3 h late, use back-up method for 48 h.

h, hour.

BOX 54–1

Contraindications for Oral Contraceptives

Absolute Contraindications

Pregnancy (known or suspected)
Breastfeeding <6 weeks postpartum
Hypertension 160/100 or with vascular disease
Heavy smokers (>15 cig/day) over the age of 35 y
Migraine with aura
Diabetic nephropathy/retinopathy/neuropathy, or diabetes of >20 y duration
Vascular disease
Past or current history of deep venous thrombosis (DVT)/pulmonary embolism (PE)
Past or current history of stroke
Major surgery with prolonged immobilization or any surgery on the legs
Current history is ischemic heart disease, valvular heart disease
Multiple risk factors for cardiovascular disease (e.g., older age, smoking, diabetes, hypertension)
Active viral hepatitis
Cirrhosis

Benign or malignant liver tumors
Breast cancer of <5 y duration
Known or suspected endometrial cancer

Cautious Use

Undiagnosed genital bleeding
Postpartum <21 d
Over the age of 35 and smokes <15 cig/d
Under the age of 35 and smokes >15 cig/d
Gallbladder disease
Past history of breast cancer >5 y ago
Use of drugs that affect liver enzymes (e.g., anticonvulsants, rifampicin, griseofulvin)
Mild hypertension without other risk factors for cardiovascular disease
Hyperlipidemia
Non-insulin-dependent diabetes
Known hyperlipidemias

cig, Cigarettes; *d,* day; *y,* year; >, greater than; <, less than.

BOX 54–2

Drug Interactions with Oral Contraceptives

Enzyme-Inducing Drugs (Use Higher Dose Pill or Alternative Form of Contraception)
   Rifampin
   Rifabutin
   Griseofulvin
   Dilantin
   Phenobarbital
   Topirimate
   Tegretol
Non-Enzyme-Inducing Drugs (Use Back-up Method for Duration of Treatment Plus 7 Days)
   Ampicillin
   Doxycycline
   Tetracycline

ceptives need to be particularly cautious about potential interactions.

Side Effects and Adverse Reactions

The risk of death from the use of oral contraceptives is less than the risk from pregnancy, especially if the client does not exhibit contraindications listed in Box 54–1. Most side effects are related to differences in the estrogen-progestin ratio of the products and the client's response.

Side effects primarily caused by an excess of estrogen include nausea, vomiting, dizziness, fluid retention, edema, bloating, breast enlargement, breast tenderness, chloasma (slightly more in dark-skinned clients exposed to sunlight on higher dose tablets), leg cramps, decreased tearing, corneal curvature alteration, visual changes, vascular headache, and hypertension (in about 1% to 5% of previously normotensive clients within the first few months).

Side effects primarily caused by estrogen deficiency include vaginal bleeding (breakthrough bleeding, especially in the first few cycles after starting therapy) that lasts several days (usually during days 1 to 14), oligomenorrhea (especially after long-term use), nervousness, and **dyspareunia** (painful sexual intercourse) secondary to atrophic vaginitis.

Side effects primarily caused by an excess of progestin include increased appetite, weight gain, oily skin and scalp, acne, depression, vaginitis from yeast *(Candida)*, excess hair growth, decreased breast size, and amenorrhea after cessation of use (1% to 2% of clients).

Side effects primarily caused by progestin deficiency include dysmenorrhea, bleeding late in the cycle (days 15 to 21), heavy menstrual flow with clots, or amenorrhea. There may also be changes in laboratory values, including thyroid and liver function, blood glucose, and triglycerides.

The combined oral contraceptive pill may increase the vascularity of the cervical epithelium, extend the area of cervical ectopy, and alter certain immune parameters. Advise pill users to use male or female latex or polyurethane condoms unless they are confident that both partners are free of human immunodeficiency virus (HIV) and other sexually transmitted infections.

Adverse reactions of a more severe nature include increased risk of superficial and deep venous thrombosis, pulmonary embolism, cerebrovascular accident (thrombotic stroke), myocardial infarction, and acceleration of preexisting but nondiagnosed breast tumors.

Nursing Process

Oral Contraceptives

ASSESSMENT

■ Obtain a record of client's drug and herbal use.
■ Obtain baseline BP and weight. Report abnormal findings. Determine pregnancy status.
■ Assess for history of smoking, hypertension, and all contraindications listed in Box 54–1.
■ Recognize the need for periodic reassessment of baseline data and side effects. Most clients should be seen in 1 to 3 months after beginning regimen.

NURSING DIAGNOSES

■ Deficient knowledge related to fertility pattern
■ Deficient knowledge related to oral contraceptive method(s)
■ Noncompliance with oral contraceptive method selected

PLANNING

■ Client will take oral contraceptives as prescribed and will report side effects that occur.

NURSING INTERVENTIONS

■ Separate personal views from those of client regarding contraception and use of specific products.
■ Recognize that many clients on oral contraceptives abandon the method within a year; therefore plan to provide client with alternatives.
■ Nonnursing mothers can begin combination oral contraceptives 3 to 4 weeks postpartum, regardless of whether menstruation has spontaneously occurred.

Client Teaching

General

• Remind client that these drugs should be used only under a health care provider's direction.
• Inform client that concurrent use of some drugs and herbal products decreases the effectiveness of oral contraceptives. Client should use a second form of contraception during these times. See Herbal Alert 54–1.
• Review with client the following aspects of oral contraceptives:

Advantages

- Easy to use and has low failure rate
- Minimal risks for women who do not smoke
- Contraception is not linked to the sexual act
- Decreased pregnancy fears may increase sexual responsiveness
- Suppressed pain at ovulation
- Decreased dysmenorrhea
- Regular, predictable menses
- Lighter, shorter menstrual flow
- Decreased iron-deficiency anemia resulting from decreased menstrual flow
- 80% to 90% reduced risk of functional ovarian cysts
- May provide protection against benign breast lesions and uterine and ovarian cancers
- Reduced risk of pelvic inflammatory disease
- Lower risk of ectopic pregnancy
- Decreased menstrual migraine-type headache
- No evidence that breast cancer is caused or increased by use of oral contraceptives
- Decreased chance of endometrial cancer (possibly because of progestin) in younger women not past menopause; protection may last up to 10 years after pills have been stopped if a client has used them long-term
- Thromboembolism risk does not appear related to duration of oral contraceptive use but rather to the dose of estrogen (lower-dose products less risky).

Disadvantages

- If nonmonogamous, increased risk of acquiring sexually transmitted diseases (STDs), because no barrier is involved
- Bothersome side effects
- Requires medical follow-up after first 3 to 6 months, which may, in addition to cost of pills, be perceived as expensive in terms of time and money
- Requires daily administration
- Expense

Safety

- Counsel client not to smoke tobacco because of the increased cardiovascular risks.
- Advise client to use barrier method of contraception during the first month of oral contraceptive use and for 3 months after discontinuing use and before trying to conceive.
- Provide instructions about dealing with "missed pills" (see Table 54-2).
- Tell client to report any effects from the pill to a health professional so that the therapy can be adjusted to suit her own particular needs. Encourage her not to give up and discontinue use of the pills.
- Tell client to report breakthrough bleeding or spotting, because she may need a change in dose of oral contraceptive.
- Tell client to always report that she takes oral contraceptives when seeing a health care provider because of possible synergistic or antagonistic responses to other therapies.
- Nursing mothers should delay use of oral contraceptives until after breastfeeding is completed; another method should be selected.

Side Effects

- Acquaint client with the rare but possible side effects that are considered serious, including thrombophlebitis, pulmonary embolus, myocardial infarction, cerebral vascular accident, and retinal vein thrombosis.
- As an outcome of discussion about serious side effects, teach client the acronym ACHES for dangerous side effects that must be reported to a health care provider:

A = *A*bdominal pain (severe)

C = *C*hest pain or shortness of breath

H = *H*eadaches that are severe; dizziness, weakness, numbness, speech difficulties

E = *E*ye disorders including blurring or loss of vision

S = *S*evere leg pain or swelling in the calf or thigh

More Common Side Effects

- Inform client that her menstrual flow may be less in amount and duration because of thinning of the endometrial lining.
- Determine whether client wears contact lenses and discuss how to handle dry eyes caused by decreased tearing and alterations in the shape of the cornea.
- Tell client who experiences postpill amenorrhea that 95% of women have regular periods within 12 to 18 months. In addition, tell her that those who participate in endurance fitness activities may have increased postpill amenorrhea.
- Inform client of a possible decrease in libido caused by alteration in vaginal secretions and decreased levels of testosterone.

Skill

- Teach client to do a monthly breast self-examination.

Diet

- Counsel client to moderate caffeine intake because elimination of caffeine may be decreased because of oral contraceptives.
- Tell client to take her pill with a snack at night or after meals to help eliminate nausea and also to take the pill at the same time each day.

Cultural Considerations ⊕

- Be aware of different cultures' contraception practices.
- Consider the role of each partner in the specific culture regarding decision making of contraception method.

EVALUATION

■ Evaluate client's compliance with the oral contraceptive regimen.

Alternative Methods of Contraception

Alternative methods of contraception are suited to clients who select not to take a pill on a daily basis or who are unable to comply with the daily dosing.

Norplant

Other forms of hormonal therapy that have long-lasting but reversible contraceptive effects include Norplant (approved in December 1990), which uses low-dose levonorgestrel in six matchstick-shaped Silastic implants placed under the skin of the upper arm. Norplant is considered effective for 5 years and has the advantage of not requiring conscious daily awareness of contraception. Side effects that include reports of visibility of implant rods and of rods traveling up the arm, scars on the arm, breakthrough and uncontrolled bleeding, hirsutism, hair loss, weight gain, increased ovarian cysts, and difficulty with removal that requires a minor surgical procedure. The Norplant is no longer available because of manufacturing problems.

Implanon

The newest implant, Implanon, was scheduled to become available in 2005. It is a single implant containing the progestin etonogestrel. It is effective for 3 years. Amenorrhea may occur in about 20% of clients. The single implant is easier and faster to insert and remove. Its advantages include decreased menstrual and ovulatory cramping or pain. The Implanon has less bleeding than with the Norplant.

Depo-Provera

Long-acting injectable progestin, known as *medroxyprogesterone acetate (Depo-Provera)*, is gaining favor because it requires only one injection every 3 months. The injection acts by suppressing ovulation and changing the pH of the vaginal mucosa to an environment less hospitable to sperm. The injection (150 mg, given deep intramuscularly [IM] in the gluteus) is relatively inexpensive. The site of the injection is documented so that injection sites are rotated. The client is given a personalized calendar for subsequent doses. Like oral contraceptives, there is no protection against sexually transmitted diseases (STDs). The method is safe for postpartum clients to receive before discharge following delivery; clients may also breastfeed while using this contraceptive. The most common side effects reported include initially irregular menstruation and spotting (menstruation may cease in about 1 year). Women who smoke may complain of headaches (usually relieved by acetaminophen). In addition, other side effects include weight gain, bloating, decreased libido, hair loss, and depression. In rare instances, serious side effects may occur, including chest pain, hemoptysis, abdominal pain, shortness of breath, and numbness in the extremities. The drug is contraindicated in cases of undiagnosed vaginal bleeding or known or suspected pregnancy. When injections are discontinued, some clients may experience delayed resumption of fertility for a year or more.

Depo-subQ provera 104 is now also available. The medroxyprogesterone acetate injectable suspension is now in a subQ form administered at 104 mg/0.65 mL to women every 3 months (12 to 14 weeks). Depo-subQ provera 104 is indicated for the prevention of pregnancy in women of childbearing potential. Women who use either depo-subQ provera 104 or IM depo-provera long-term should be counseled about the loss of bone mineral density (BMD). The new black box warning further notes that bone loss is greater with increased duration of use and may not be completely reversible and that depo-provera should be used as a long-term birth control method (e.g., longer than 2 years) only if other birth control methods are "inadequate." If abnormal bleeding associated with depo-subQ provera 104 is severe, appropriate investigation and treatment should be instituted.

Lunelle

Lunelle (a combination of medroxyprogesterone acetate and estradiol cypionate) is a contraceptive that inhibits secretion of gonadotropin, thereby preventing follicular maturation and ovulation. Inject IM medroxyprogesterone acetate 25 mg and estradiol cypionate 5 mg per 0.5 ml suspension every 28 to 30 days, not to exceed 33 days. Shake the solution vigorously before administering to distribute the two medications evenly. Administer the first dose during the first 5 days of a normal menstrual period to ensure nonpregnant status. If the time between injections is more than 33 days, the medication is not administered until pregnancy is ruled out. It is not administered earlier than 4 weeks after delivery if the mother is not breastfeeding or 6 weeks after delivery if the mother is breastfeeding. It is not recommended for clients who smoke. Clients should be aware that this contraceptive does not protect against STDs or HIV infection. Lunelle was taken off the market in 2001 because of manufacturing problems.

NuvaRing

NuvaRing, a newer form of birth control, was recently approved by the FDA. A 2-inch diameter ring is inserted in the vagina to release estrogen and progestin in quantities comparable with oral contraceptives. Effectiveness is reported at 98%, reflecting a rate similar to other leading contraceptives. The client inserts the ring during the first 5 days of the menstrual cycle. The client then removes the ring after 3 weeks, remains "ring-free" for 1 week, and then inserts a new ring. Backup contraception is recommended during the first 7 days after the first ring is placed. During this time, the hormones reach an appropriate protective level. Then contraception is expected to be continuous, provided the ring is correctly inserted. If the ring slips out and remains out for more than 3 hours, additional contraception is required until the ring has been in place for 7 days. Possible side effects include vaginal discharge, irritation, or infection. There is some risk of blood clots or heart attack, which is increased in clients who smoke (similar to that associated with other hormonal contraceptives). NuvaRing does not protect against STDs or HIV infection. Its price is reported to be comparable with name-brand oral contraceptives.

Today Sponge

The Today Sponge is a polyurethane sponge impregnated with nonoxynol 9. This contraceptive product was discontinued in 1995 because of manufacturing problems, but is now available again over the counter in stores.

Intrauterine Devices

Other alternatives to oral contraceptives are intrauterine devices (IUDs). Currently two IUDs are on the market. The ParaGard T380A releases copper, which interferes with sperm motility and fertilization as a result of inflammation of the endometrium. The ParaGard may increase the average monthly blood loss during menses by about 35%; NSAIDs may diminish this effect. It may also increase dysmenorrhea. ParaGard can remain in place for up to 10 years.

The Mirena levonorgestrel-releasing intrauterine system (LNG-IUS) causes cervical mucus to become thicker, so sperm cannot enter the upper reproductive tract or reach the ovum. Changes in uterotubal fluid also impair sperm migration. Alteration of endometrium prevents implantation of the fertilized ovum. The Mirena has some anovulatory effect. Menorrhagia improves by 90%. There is an improvement in dysmenorrhea. There is a 20% chance of amenorrhea by 1 year and 60% by 5 years. The Mirena is as effective as female sterilization, it may decrease a woman's risk of pelvic inflammatory disease (PID) by 60%, and it has a decreased risk of ectopic pregnancy. The Mirena is effective for 5 years. IUDs are safe for use in women who are at low risk for acquiring STDs.

Nonoxynol-9-based spermicide products are no longer advised for STI protection. The spermicide can cause vulvovaginal abrasions and altered vaginal flora, which could increase the susceptibility to HIV.

The Patch

Ortho Evra is the first weekly form of birth control. The patch consists of a norelgestromin/ethinyl estradiol transdermal system. It is a thin plastic patch placed on the skin of the buttocks, stomach, upper outer arm, or upper torso once a week for 3 weeks in a row. A new patch is used each week for 3 weeks. The fourth week is patch free to allow for menses. The patch releases combined estrogen and progesterone that protect against pregnancy for 1 month.

The patch prevents ovulation, thickens cervical mucus to prevent fertilization, and prevents a fertilized egg from implanting in the uterus. It is up to 99.7% effective, but it is not effective against STDs. Advantages include having no pill to take daily; the ability to become pregnant returns quickly when use is stopped; there is less menstrual flow and cramping, acne, iron deficiency anemia, excess body hair, premenstrual symptoms, and vaginal dryness; it reduces the risk of ovarian and endometrial cancers, pelvic inflammatory disease, breast cysts, ovarian cysts,

and osteoporosis; and there are fewer occurrences of ectopic pregnancy.

Disadvantages of the patch include skin reaction at the site of application, menstrual cramps, a change in vision or the inability to wear contact lenses, and it may not be as effective for women who weigh more than 198 pounds. Serious side effects are similar to the pill, including blood clots, heart attack, and stroke; women who are over 35 and smoke are at a greater risk. Other side effects include temporary irregular bleeding, weight gain or loss, breast tenderness, nausea.

Medical Abortion

Medical abortion is a way to end a pregnancy that is less than 63 days from the first day of the last period (LMP). Methotrexate stops the pregnancy in the uterus. It may also be used to treat ectopic pregnancy. Mifepristone (RU486) blocks the hormone progesterone. Without progesterone, the lining of the uterus breaks down, ending the pregnancy. Misoprostol is then given to cause the uterus to contract and empty.

Emergency Contraception

Emergency contraception (EC) has been available for more than 25 years. EC, also called *postcoital contraception*, can prevent pregnancy after unprotected intercourse. It may be prescribed in two ways: using hormonal contraceptive pills or inserting a copper-releasing IUD (ParaGard).

The ECPs contain hormones that reduce the risk of pregnancy when started within 120 hours (5 days) of unprotected intercourse. The treatment is more effective the sooner it begins. The only documented contraindication to oral EC is an established pregnancy because ECPs are ineffective in these cases.

The Yuzpe regimen, named after Canadian professor A. Albert Yuzpe, consists of 0.1 mg dl-norgestrel (or its equivalent), followed by a second dose 12 hours later. The Yuzpe regimen prevents about 60% to 75% of expected pregnancies. About 50% of users experience nausea and 20% report vomiting, which can reduce client adherence.

The Preven Emergency Contraceptive Kit, produced by Gynétics, Inc., contains Yuzpe regimen ECPs (two pills per dose, taken 12 hours apart), a pregnancy test, and instructions for use. It is approved by the FDA and was the first product specifically labeled and marketed for emergency contraception. It is no longer available.

The EC pills delay or prevent ovulation; interfere with tubal transport of the embryo, egg, or sperm; and change the hormones necessary for the preparation of the uterine lining. They decrease the risk of pregnancy by 75% for each act of unprotected sexual intercourse; birth control pills have a much higher rate of effectiveness—almost 100%. The major side effect is nausea; an over-the-counter (OTC) antinausea medicine (e.g., diphenhydramine, 25 to 50 mg) may be helpful if taken 1 hour before the EC. Irregular menstrual bleeding is another side effect. If a woman does

Table 54–3

Emergency Contraception: The Yuzpe Regimen

Pill Brand	Manufacturer	Pills per Dose (Every 12 h for 2 Doses)
Alesse	Wyeth-Ayerst	5 pink pills
Aviane	Duramed	5 orange pills
Cryselle	Barr	4 white pills
Enpress	Barr	4 orange pills
Lessina	Barr	5 pink pills
Levlen	Berlex	4 light orange pills
Levlite	Berlex	5 pink pills
Levora	Watson	4 white pills
Lo/Ovral	Wyeth-Ayerst	4 white pills
Low-Ogestrel	Watson	4 white pills
Nordette	Wyeth-Ayerst	4 light orange pills
Ogestrel	Watson	2 white pills
Ovral	Wyeth-Ayerst	2 white pills
Portia	Barr	4 pink pills
Seasonale	Barr	4 pink pills
Tri-Levlen	Berlex	4 yellow pills
Triphasil	Wyeth-Ayerst	4 yellow pills
Trivora	Watson	4 pink pills
Progestin-Only Pills		
Ovrette	Wyeth-Ayerst	20 yellow pills *or* 40 yellow pills in one dose
Plan B	Barr	1 white pill *or* 2 white pills in one dose

h, Hour.

not begin menstruation within a few days of the expected time, she should take a pregnancy test. Clients who are unable to take estrogen should not take the usual EC pill dosage. See Table 54–3 for combined oral contraceptives used for EC.

If pregnancy is already established or if implantation occurred since the unprotected sexual intercourse, the pregnancy is not disrupted. EC pills do not result in an abortion, and there are no reports of harm to the fetus. EC can be used when needed. EC is not as effective as taking oral contraceptives or using condoms as directed (i.e., consistently and correctly).

On July 28, 1999, the FDA approved the first progestin-only ECP available in the U.S. Produced by Barr Pharmaceuticals, known as Plan B, it consists of two pills, taken 12 hours apart, and it contains only the hormone levonorgestrel, a progestin. Plan B contains no estrogen. Progestin-only ECPs cause less nausea and may reduce a risk of pregnancy by 89%. If taken within 24 hours of unprotected intercourse, they were found to reduce the risk of pregnancy by 95%. The two 0.75-mg doses of levonorgestrel may be combined into a single more-convenient 1.5-mg dose with no effect on efficacy or side effects.

A copper IUD may be inserted within 5 days of unprotected intercourse and removed after the woman's next menstrual period, or it may remain in place as a method of birth control for up to 10 years.

The hotline for EC information is (888) NOT-2-LATE, and the website is *http://ec.princeton.edu.*

Drugs Used to Treat Hormone Dysfunction

Uterine dysfunction is common in premenstrual syndrome, endometriosis, and menopause. This section describes these entities and presents current pharmacologic approaches to management. The menstrual cycle is described in this unit's introduction.

Premenstrual Syndrome

Premenstrual syndrome (PMS), first formally described and named in 1931, comprises a collection of varied physical, emotional, and behavioral symptoms. Box 54–3 lists commonly reported physical and psychobehavioral symptoms of PMS. More than 150 symptoms have been reported in the literature.

PMS can result in decreased work effectiveness and impaired interpersonal relationships. PMS affects 40% of all adult women (four to five million in the United States) to some degree, with about 5% exhibiting debilitating symptoms. There is a family history associated with the syndrome, but it is not hereditary. The syndrome is seen most commonly in women in their thirties and early forties, but it also affects adolescents. PMS occurs in a repetitive regular pattern during the **luteal phase** (days 15 to 28) of the menstrual cycle; it decreases during the **follicular phase** (days 1 to 14).

BOX 54–3

Symptoms of Premenstrual Syndrome

- Bloating in lower abdomen
- Weight gain
- Headache (migraine)
- Increased appetite
- Cravings for foods high in sugar or salt
- Breast soreness
- Fatigue
- Sleep disorders
- Backaches
- Acne
- Joint pain
- Constipation
- Feelings of being out of control
- Emotional lability
- Tension
- Anxiety
- Difficulty with concentration
- Irritability
- Agitation
- Depression
- Suicidal thoughts
- Rage

Nursing Process

Premenstrual Syndrome

ASSESSMENT

■ Obtain history of premenstrual syndrome (PMS) symptoms such as bloating, weight gain, headache, and increased appetite. See Box 54-3.

NURSING DIAGNOSES

■ Deficient knowledge related to the menstrual cycle and etiology of related alterations in mood and comfort
■ Ineffective coping
■ Interrupted family processes

PLANNING

■ Client will verbalize relief from PMS from nonpharmacologic and pharmacologic measures.

NURSING INTERVENTIONS

■ Provide quality client and family education in a supportive manner that encourages family communication.

Client Teaching

General

* Express that symptoms are real and that "crazy feelings" do not mean client is crazy.
* Explain menstrual cycle and current knowledge about PMS verbally, in writing, and graphically.
* Share current research findings regarding PMS and known treatment modalities with client, her family, and community groups.
* Encourage client to include aerobic exercise in her regular activity pattern three to five times each week.
* Describe and discuss stress-reduction activities.
* Encourage family communication regarding PMS symptoms experienced by client so that the family understands client's behavior.
* Suggest sources for, and potential value of, support groups.

Self-Administration

* Have client keep a log of symptoms experienced during her menstrual cycle to better link events with symptoms.
* If alprazolam (Xanax) is ordered, discuss issues of dependency and withdrawal.
* If danazol (Danocrine) is ordered, see the guidelines for use of this drug in the Nursing Process box on endometriosis and Table 54-4.

Diet

* Encourage client to take nontoxic doses of vitamin and mineral supplements with meals.

* Encourage a low-fat, low-salt, high-carbohydrate diet. Suggest four to six small meals and portable snacks (bagels, rice cakes).
* Decrease caffeine intake and increase water consumption.
* Limit alcoholic beverages; these may precipitate headaches.

EVALUATION

■ Evaluate the effectiveness of the nonpharmacologic and pharmacologic measures for relief of PMS.

There is no universal agreement about the definition, etiology, symptoms, or treatment of PMS. The most widely held theory is that PMS is linked to estrogen and progesterone levels and the relationship of these hormones to other brain chemicals. The symptoms are observed during the luteal phase when levels are high and decrease when drugs that inhibit gonadotropin-releasing hormone (Gn-RH) and ovulation are used. Other hypotheses center on the release of endogenous opiates (beta-endorphins), disruptions in central nervous system neurotransmitters (resulting in mood swings), and the role of prolactin secretion.

Diagnosis of PMS is made when the client's symptoms are documented as consistently occurring at about the same time and in the same way during a defined number of menstrual periods. Other endocrine abnormalities need to be ruled out. One difficulty with diagnosis is that PMS is not consistent, because every cycle is not the same; therefore measurement is problematic, particularly because every symptom that occurs associated with a menstrual cycle is not PMS.

Treatment of PMS includes nonpharmacologic and pharmacologic measures. There is not one curative therapy or a way to know what therapy may be best for a particular client other than trial and error.

Nonpharmacologic treatment includes expression of empathy, support from family and others, correction of knowledge deficits about PMS and the menstrual cycle, exercise, and dietary changes (e.g., limiting salty foods, alcohol, caffeine, chocolate, concentrated sweets; eating four to six small high-carbohydrate, low-fat meals, which help stabilize blood sugar levels and enhance mood). Stress reduction is helpful, as is aerobic exercise, which is believed to have a regulatory effect on estrogen and progesterone secondary to hypothalamic stimulation. These measures may help the client feel proactive regarding her situation, give her a sense of overall well being, and improve her general health. In addition, endorphin levels are heightened, which is found to be helpful.

Pharmacologic treatment remains largely empirical because research has not consistently been done under double-blind, placebo-controlled conditions. Some clients experience improvement with selected symptoms through use of vitamin B_6 (popular with self-help groups but not

Table 54-4

Drug Therapy for Endometriosis

Generic (Brand)	Route and Dosage	Uses and Considerations
danazol (Danocrine)	PO: 400 mg b.i.d. for 4-6 mo; can extend to 9 mo; can restart if symptoms return	Pituitary gonadotropin inhibitory agent. No estrogenic or progestational action. Suppresses and atrophies intra- and extrauterine tissue. Menses cease during therapy and no ovulation occurs; pain is relieved. Ovulation/menses usually recur within 90 d after treatment. Therapy started during menstruation or after pregnancy. If therapy is for fibrocystic breast disease, breast carcinoma must also be ruled out before treatment. Commonly used for women with infertility associated with endometriosis. Used for PMS on investigational basis. *Contraindications:* pregnancy; breastfeeding; abnormal genital bleeding; impaired heart, liver, or kidney function; severe hypertension. Can alter some laboratory values (e.g., decreased HDL, increased LDL). Can increase insulin requirements and, if given with warfarin, cause a prolonged PT. *Adverse effects:* thrombocytopenia, hypertension, depression, headache, *hot flashes, weight gain,* androgenic effects, hemorrhagic cystitis, hematuria, hepatotoxicity, cholestatic hepatitis, acne, rashes, oily skin, hirsutism, bloating, *muscle cramps,* voice deepening (irreversible), hearing loss, mood swings, anxiety, fatigue, nausea, vomiting, diarrhea, constipation. Also produces atherogenic lipid profile. Many clients cannot tolerate side effects and discontinue drug. Alternate doses may be used for clients with hereditary angioedema and fibrocystic breast disease. *Pharmacokinetics:* Therapeutic effects occur within 3 wk of daily therapy. Absorbed well orally; peak action: 2-4 h. Biotransformed by the liver; excreted in the urine. *Pregnancy category:* X; $t^{1}/_{2}$: 4.5 h
Gonadotropin-Releasing Hormone (Gn-RH) Agonists		
leuprolide acetate for depot suspension (Lupron Depot 3.75)	IM: 3.75 mg q mo for up to 6 mo	As an agonist, initially stimulates FSH and LH, but over time, creates prolonged suppression, which causes decreased ovarian secretion of estrogen/progesterone, resulting in a hypoestrogenic state. Lack of hormonal stimulation causes regression of displaced endometrial tissue. Contains no androgen. Found as effective as danazol in reducing extent of endometriosis. Initial dose best given during day 1-3 of menstrual cycle to avoid affecting a pregnancy. Barrier contraceptives should be used during treatment because pregnancy is possible. Minimal changes produced in lipid profile. Normal function returns in 4 to 12 wk after treatment discontinued. Retreatment not recommended because safety data beyond 6 mo are not available. *Contraindications:* actual or potential pregnancy, undiagnosed vaginal bleeding, and breastfeeding because it is unknown if excreted in breast milk. *Side effects:* hot flashes, headaches, decreased libido, dry vagina, night sweats, mood changes, mild bone loss (usually regained within 6 mo of finishing treatment). FDA classification 3B.* *Pharmacokinetics:* Therapeutic levels detected for at least 4 wk after injection; 85%-100% released within 4 wk with no accumulation. *Pregnancy category:* X; PB: 46%; $t^{1}/_{2}$: 3-4.2 h
nafarelin acetate (Synarel Nasal Solution)	400 mcg daily, administered as one spray (200 mcg) into one nostril in morning and one spray (200 mcg) into other nostril in the evening for up to 6 mo	Contains no androgen. Controlled studies comparing nafarelin (400 µg) and danazol (600 or 800 mcg/d) found higher hypoestrogenic (therapeutic state) but less androgenic side effects. Found comparable in reducing extent of endometriosis and in effect on associated client symptoms. Maintains LDL/HDL ratio. Return of normal function in 4-12 wk after treatment discontinued. *Contraindications:* clients sensitive to Gn-RH, Gn-RH analogs, or inert substances included in product; actual or potential pregnancy; undiagnosed vaginal bleeding; breastfeeding. Clients with rhinitis should have a topical decongestant prescribed by health care provider and use at least 30 min after nafarelin. *Side effects:* effects seen in a natural menopause caused by a hypoestrogenic state, notably hot flashes, vaginal dryness, decreased libido, headaches, and emotional lability. FDA classification 1B.† *Pharmacokinetics:* peak action: 10-40 min. Drug elimination after intranasal administration has not been studied. PB: 80%; $t^{1}/_{2}$: approximately 30 h (range 0.8-10 h)

*A new formulation of a compound already on the market that offers a modest therapeutic gain over currently available agents.
†A new chemical entity that offers a modest therapeutic gain over currently available agents.
b.i.d., Twice a day; *d,* day; *FDA,* Food and Drug Administration; *FSH,* follicle-stimulating hormone; *Gn-RH,* gonadotropin-releasing hormone; *h,* hour; *HDL,* high-density lipoproteins; *IM,* intramuscular; *LDL,* low-density lipoproteins; *LH,* luteinizing hormone; *min,* minute; *mo,* month; *PB,* protein-binding; *PMS,* premenstrual syndrome; *PO,* by mouth; *PT,* prothrombin time; *t¹/₂,* half-life; *wk,* week.

found superior to placebo) or vaginal or rectal progesterone suppositories (200 to 400 mg twice daily), which are commonly used but not documented as effective and have some long-term effects. In addition, individuals who exhibit depressive symptoms tend to get worse with progesterone use because of its depressant effects. Other pharmacologic trials include diuretics (not recommended) and prostaglandin inhibitors; bromocriptine (Parlodel) (2.5 mg twice daily started on day 10 of cycle and taken until menstruation begins) for breast soreness; and alprazolam (Xanax) (0.25 mg three times daily from day 20 of cycle to day 2 of menses, followed by one tablet per day) for treatment of anxiety, irritability, and depression. Oral contraceptives have been used experimentally as a form of anovulatory therapy but are not approved for this purpose. Reducing dietary caffeine decreases breast tenderness more than by pharmacologic intervention.

A theory under study is that stronger antiprostaglandins (e.g., NSAIDs) will prove useful when taken in conjunction with vitamin therapy that contains magnesium, calcium, pyridoxine, vitamin E, and zinc. This drug regimen should begin when PMS symptoms start and continue through the beginning of the menstrual period.

Serafem (fluoxetine hydrochloride) is an FDA-approved prescription treatment that relieves the mood and physical symptoms of premenstrual dysphoric disorder (PMDD), a severe form of PMS. It is a selective seratonin reuptake inhibitor (SSRI). Symptom relief includes a decrease in irritability, mood swings, fatigue, tension, and breast tenderness. SSRIs block the uptake of seratonin into human platelets and regulate seratonin use by the brain.

Two other forms of experimental (not approved by the FDA) hormonal anovulatory treatment are danazol (Danocrine) and Gn-RH agonists. These formulations, which are also approved for treatment of endometriosis, are presented in Table 54–4.

Endometriosis

Endometriosis is the abnormal location of endometrial tissue outside of the uterus, in the pelvic cavity; it has no single, clearly identifiable cause. Possible etiologies are retrograde menstruation (backward movement of endometrial cells through the fallopian tubes out into the abdomen) or spread through the lymphatic or vascular systems. Regardless of cause, the displaced endometrial tissue is found affixed to the ovaries, the posterior surface of the uterus, the uterosacral ligaments, the broad ligaments, or the bowel. The displaced tissue responds to hormonal control, particularly estrogen from the ovaries, in the same way as the tissue inside the uterus. Thus, when menstruation occurs, this extrauterine tissue also bleeds. As the number of menstrual cycles increases, inflammation, scar tissue formation, and adhesions result.

Clients with endometriosis may be symptomatic (about 75%) or asymptomatic (those diagnosed during infertility work-ups). The diagnosis is based on symptoms and laparoscopic evidence of endometrial tissue. Symptoms include severe low-back and pelvic pain that increases with menstruation. Painful, sometimes bloody, bowel movements during menstruation have been reported, as has painful sexual intercourse (dyspareunia). Irregular bleeding (spotting) before and after menses is common. Long term, there is an association with primary or secondary infertility; about 25% to 40% of infertile women exhibit the condition. Endometriosis may obstruct or affect the motility of the fallopian tubes. There is also a risk that nearby organs (e.g., urinary and gastrointestinal tracts) may become obstructed by invasion of endometrial tissue.

Endometriosis is found most often in women who have delayed childbearing until their thirties, although it may occur during adolescence. There is an increased prevalence rate of 7% for siblings and daughters of affected women. Approximately five million women in the United States have endometriosis. Affected women may exhibit increased ectopic pregnancy rates and difficult pregnancies and labors.

Some success for the treatment of endometriosis has been seen with the use of a laser during laparoscopy to remove or destroy endometrial growths.

Three drugs are approved for use in endometriosis: danazol (Danocrine) and two Gn-RH agonists, leuprolide acetate (Lupron Depot) and nafarelin acetate (Synarel). Danazol has been the drug of choice, but use of the Gn-RH agonists is increasing. These drugs are presented in Table 54–4.

In long-term and highly painful endometriosis that has not been controlled with drug therapy or laparoscopy, hysterectomy (including ovary removal) may be elected.

Nursing Process

Endometriosis

ASSESSMENT

- Obtain a complete client history, including menstrual history.
- Identify client's fertility plans.
- Review chart for baseline liver function studies and pregnancy test.

Leuprolide Acetate

- Review client's history for risk factors associated with major bone loss; the drug may pose an additional risk.

NURSING DIAGNOSES

- Pain (acute and chronic) related to hormonally controlled displaced endometrial tissue
- Activity intolerance secondary to painful menstrual cycles
- Deficient knowledge related to menstrual cycle, displaced endometrial tissue, etiology of pain, and treatment options

PLANNING

■ Client will be free of pain/discomfort resulting from endometriosis with the use of danazol, leuprolide acetate, or nafarelin acetate.

NURSING INTERVENTIONS

Danazol

- Observe client for signs of anxiety about potential loss of fertility and time involved in treatment.
- Recall that the drug must be started during client's menstrual period.

Leuprolide Acetate

- Store product and diluent at room temperature.
- Must be reconstituted and used immediately (no preservatives). Reconstituted product must be shaken to create a milky suspension.

Client Teaching: Danazol

General
- Discuss the purpose, action, and side effects of the drug with client. Explain that the medication is expensive. Explain length of treatment.
- Plan with client for the use of a back-up nonhormonal form of birth control.
- Tell client that menses will usually return in 2 to 3 months after treatment.
- Tell client to have one menstrual cycle after treatment is completed before trying to conceive.

Side Effects
- Suggest for client to wear minipads for spotting during the first month of therapy and to report any bleeding to her health care provider.
- Discuss removal of unwanted hair and skin care for acne prevention. If acne occurs, consult a dermatologist.
- Suggest for client to wash her face and hair more often because of oily scalp and skin and to use oil-free makeup and shampoo.
- If muscle cramps occur, advise client to do warm-up exercises before active workout and to gradually increase exertion.

Diet
- Ask client to keep a food history. Suggest increased exercise to help offset weight gain that is experienced by 75% (average, 4 kg); suggest caloric control plan based on history.
- Increase water consumption.

Skill
- Review breast self-examination with client.

Client Teaching: Leuprolide Acetate

General
- Explain to client that the drug causes a temporary state of menopause.

- Explain that the treatment process requires one injection each month.
- Explain that the drug is palliative and temporarily effective in reducing symptoms. It does not create a change in basic physiology, metabolism, or hormone production. When treatment is complete, whatever is normal for client will return over time.
- Advise client that initially there may be an increase in clinical signs and symptoms of endometriosis, but these will disappear.
- Explain that 6 months is the accepted duration of therapy for gonadotropin-releasing hormone (Gn-RH) agonists. Safety data are available only for 6-month use. Retreatment is not recommended.

Self-Administration
- Remind client that she must use a nonhormonal contraceptive method during treatment.

Side Effects
- If client is concerned about potential bone loss, state that one 6-month course of treatment has been found to cause only a small loss. However, clients who are at higher risk for bone loss caused by chronic alcoholism, tobacco use, strong family history of osteoporosis, or chronic use of anticonvulsants or corticosteroids should carefully discuss the decision for or against therapy with this drug. Suggest client add weight-bearing exercise and walking or low-impact aerobics to offset bone loss.
- Stress that client must be consistent in receiving her doses of the drug; otherwise breakthrough bleeding or ovulation can occur.
- Tell client to inform the health care provider if menstruation persists while being treated.
- Discuss mood changes secondary to hormonal changes with drug and possible emotional lability; suggest support network and resource groups.
- If vaginal dryness occurs, suggest client use water-based lubricants and try alternate sexual positions for intercourse.
- If night sweats occur, suggest cotton bedclothes and change of clothes; resist chills by gradually exposing body from under bed covers to room air. Contact health care provider if sleep disturbances persist.

Diet
- Suggest increased calcium-based food products.

Client Teaching: Nafarelin Acetate

General
- Explain that precise guidelines must be followed by client if the treatment is to be effective.
- Ask client if she is allergic to any component of the drug including nafarelin base, benzalkonium chloride, acetic acid, sodium hydroxide, hydrochloride, or sorbitol.

- Tell client that the action of the drug, guidelines for birth control use, hypoestrogenic effects, and return of normal function are the same as for leuprolide acetate.
- Advise client that the medication is expensive, is provided as a 30-day supply, and needs to be continued for 6 months of therapy without interruption.

Self-Administration

- Stress that client must use the drug twice a day (every 12 hours) for the full duration of treatment.
- Tell client to start the drug between days 2 and 4 of the menstrual period.
- Client must be told of the need to prime the spray pump only before the first use. The sprayer is designed to deliver the exact dose each time. A fine spray will occur after 7 to 10 pushes on the pump. If a thin stream occurs, she should call her pharmacist immediately.
- Tell client to store the bottle upright, below 86° F (30° C), and out of light. Because she must use it every 12 hours, it is suggested she put it near her toothbrush or other regularly used product (morning and night).
- Tell client to record each dose on the supplied chart and to refill prescription so as not to miss any doses.
- Tell client it is permissible to use a nasal decongestant spray (with health care provider's knowledge) while on nafarelin. Use the nafarelin spray first and allow 30 minutes to elapse before using the decongestant spray.
- Instruct client to blow her nose to clear both nostrils before using the drug. She should bend forward and place the spray tip in one nostril aimed at the back and outer side of her nose. She should close the other nostril with her finger and then spray one time while sniffing gently, then tilt her head back to spread the drug over the back of the nose. She must be told *not* to spray in the second nostril unless told to do so by her doctor. Alternate nostrils are used for each dose.

Side Effects

- Advise client that she may note irregular vaginal spotting or bleeding, which should decrease and stop unless doses are missed.
- See Leuprolide—similar effects and potential remedial actions.

Diet

- Suggest increased calcium-based food products.

EVALUATION

■ Evaluate the effectiveness of the drug regimen. If pain or discomfort persists, notify the health care provider. Drug dose adjustment may be necessary.

Menopause

The transitional process experienced by women as they move from the reproductive into the nonreproductive stage of life is called the *female climacteric*, a natural event.

Women perceive the "change of life" experience in an individualized way on a continuum from no difficulty to severe difficulty. This phase of life occurs for most women somewhere between their late thirties to late fifties. The climacteric has three stages—premenopause, menopause, and postmenopause—during which certain physiologic events occur.

The premenopausal period may last for more than 5 years before true menopause occurs. During this period, menstrual variations become evident. For example, menstrual periods may occur as usual, be lighter in flow, or last a shorter time. They may begin, stop, and then start again or be of longer duration with a heavier flow that may contain blood clots. Sudden episodes of vasodilation (hot flashes) also begin to occur in some women. Others experience vaginal dryness. These unpredictable changes may last for several years and are probably caused by alterations in the hypothalamic-pituitary-ovarian feedback system.

Menopause is defined as the permanent end of menstruation caused by decreased ovarian function. This natural event is documented as having occurred once a woman has had no menstrual periods for 1 year. The triggering event for the onset of natural menopause is not known. The average age at menopause is about 50 years (range 45 to 55 years). Women who experience menopause before age 40 are said to have had *premature menopause*. Menopause can also occur abruptly as a secondary effect of surgical removal of the ovaries (oophorectomy), radiologic procedures in which ovarian function is destroyed, severe infection, ovarian tumors, or as a temporarily induced state for treatment of conditions such as endometriosis.

Postmenopause is the stage when the body adapts to a new hormonal environment. Although the production of estrogen and progesterone from the ovaries decreases during the late premenopausal and early postmenopausal periods, the ovary is able to secrete androgens (testosterone) in varying amounts as a result of the influence of increased LH levels. During postmenopause, androstenedione (the main androgen secreted by the ovaries and adrenal cortex, which is present in reduced amounts postmenopause) is converted into estrone, a naturally occurring estrogen formed in extraglandular tissue of the brain, liver, kidney, and adipose tissue. This represents the main source of available estrogen once the ovaries lose the ability to produce estradiol. Table 54–5 presents common physical effects associated with the climacteric.

Hormone and Estrogen Replacement Therapy

Hormone replacement therapy (HRT) is the most prevalent treatment for the relief of vasomotor symptoms and vaginal dryness. Oral estrogen, most commonly in the form of conjugated estrogens, is taken by the client together with the synthetic hormone progestin in one of several treatment regimens. The progestin is added to minimize the risk of endometrial hyperplasia and endometrial cancer from the use of estrogen alone. The progestin, however, has potential negative effects, including potential

Table 54–5

Common Physical Effects Associated with the Female Climacteric

Hypoestrogenic State	Effects
Irregular menstruation	Variable frequency, duration, flow
Vasodilation	Hot flashes with transient sensations of intense heat in upper chest, neck, and head; visible flushing; sweating; chills; tachycardia; sleep disruption
Vaginal alterations	Dryness; decreased lubrication during sexual stimulation; thinning. Decreased acidity and increased irritation response to stressors such as intercourse can cause increased vaginitis (itching, burning, discharge). Increased incidence of prolapse/cystocele
Decreased bone mass (osteoporosis)	Backache, reduced height, and sudden fracture particularly in thin, fair, small-boned women and those with a family history, no pregnancies, sedentary lifestyle, inadequate diet, smoking, alcohol use, or use of drugs that increase calcium loss (anticonvulsants, corticosteroids). Most rapid decrease in mass (particularly in hips, spine, and torso) occurs in first 3-5 y postmenopause and slows after age 65 years

Additional Effects Caused by Menopause Combined with Natural Aging

Urethral disorders	Loss of urethral tone, painful urination, frequency, and stress incontinence
Decreased breast size	
Decreased skin elasticity	Facial, neck, and hand wrinkling; variations in quantity and distribution of body hair
Lower HDL levels	Increased risk (3×) for cardiovascular disease as LDL levels increase
Abdominal fat development	Greater degree of central android abdominal fat accumulates because of altered peripheral resistance to insulin and increase in type II diabetes as aging progresses (lower incidence in estrogen users)
Hyperinsulinemia	Signs and symptoms of low blood sugar
Short-term memory loss	

HDL, High-density lipoproteins; LDL, low-density lipoproteins; y, year.

PMS-type symptoms, breast pathology, and alterations in lipid metabolism. Thus progestin partially blunts the beneficial effects of estrogen. The client has much to consider when deciding on a course of action.*

The Women's Health Initiative (WHI) was a randomized, controlled primary prevention trial that recruited 16,608 women between 1993 and 1998. The WHI focused on risk and benefit strategies that could reduce the incidence of heart disease, breast and colorectal cancer, and fractures in postmenopausal women. Results of the first arm of the WHI were released in May 2002. The results concluded that HRT should *not* be prescribed for long-term prevention of chronic diseases. HRT is associated with increased risk of breast cancer, thromboembolism, coronary heart disease, and stroke. HRT should *only* be used for the treatment of menopausal symptoms, at the lowest dose possible, for the shortest duration possible, usually less than 5 years.

Hormone therapy is no longer recommended *solely* for the purpose of preventing osteoporosis, although the study demonstrated a reduction in hip and vertebral fractures by one third using HRT. Other medications can help prevent osteoporosis and fractures, and these agents appear to carry lower risks for conditions such as breast cancer or heart disease. Other drug therapies include bisphosphonates, which can reduce the breakdown of bone. Another class of drug, selective estrogen receptor modulators, or SERMs, are a new class of synthetic estrogens that act like estrogens in certain parts of the body (such as the

bones) while leaving other parts unaffected. Evista is an example of a SERM used to treat osteoporosis.

For all women, lifestyle recommendations for healthy bones include a diet high in calcium (postmenopausal women should be taking 1200 to 1500 mg of calcium per day), a multivitamin containing vitamin D, and regular weight-bearing exercise such as walking.

In the United States the typical approach to HRT is to take oral estrogen in the lowest dose to control symptoms for days 1 to 25 of the month, with the addition of progesterone (Provera) 10 mg from days 16 to 25 or estrogen and progesterone to be taken together every day without any days off.

Currently, there is no absolutely correct HRT management regimen. Health care providers may prescribe either cyclic or continuous estrogen with progestin or a combined continuous approach. Other regimens are also used.

Dosage forms for the various types of HRT include oral, transdermal, vaginal cream or suppositories, injections, pellets, or vaginal rings. The natural or biologic estrogens are composed of estrones (including conjugated equine estrogens, esterified estrogens, and piperazine estrone sulfate) and estradiols (including micronized estradiol and estradiol valerate or 17 β-estradiol). These are preferred for use in postmenopausal clients rather than the synthetic estrogens (ethinyl estradiol, mestranol) used for oral contraception. Synthetic estrogens are believed to be more taxing to the renal and hepatic systems than are biologic estrogens. Conjugated estrogens, mixtures of natural estrogens isolated from the urine of pregnant mares, are the most commonly used preparations for **estrogen replacement therapy (ERT)**.

---

*Consult health care provider on latest research.

PROTOTYPE DRUG CHART 54–1

CONJUGATED ESTROGENS

Drug Class

Estrogen replacements
Trade Name: Premarin, PMB, Milprem-400
Pregnancy Category: X

Dosage

A: PO: 0.3–1.25 mg/d cyclically (with or without progestins); most often, 0.625 mg/d

Contraindications

Breast or reproductive cancer, undiagnosed genital bleeding, pregnancy, lactation, thromboembolitic disorders, smoking
Caution: Cardiovascular disease, severe renal or hepatic disease, smoking, diabetes mellitus

Drug-Lab-Food Interactions

Drug: *Increase* effects with corticosteroids; *decrease* effects of anticoagulants, oral hypoglycemics; *decrease* effects with rifampin, anticonvulsants, barbiturates; *toxicity* with tricyclic antidepressants

Pharmacokinetics

Absorption: PO: Well absorbed
Distribution: PB: Widely distributed; crosses placenta and enters breast milk
Metabolism: t½: UK
Excretion: In urine and bile

Pharmacodynamics

PO/IV: Onset: Rapid
  Peak: UK
  Duration: UK
IM: Onset: Delayed
  Peak: UK
  Duration: UK

Therapeutic Effects/Uses

To relieve vasodilation, hot flashes, and vaginal dryness
Mode of Action: Development and maintenance of female genital system, breast, and secondary sex characteristics; increased synthesis of protein

Side Effects

Nausea, vomiting, fluid retention, breast tenderness, leg cramps and breakthrough bleeding, chloasma

Adverse Reactions

Jaundice, thromboembolic disorders, depression, hypercalcemia, gallbladder disease
Life-threatening: Thromboembolism, cerebrovascular accident, pulmonary embolism, myocardial infarction, endometrial cancer

A, Adult; *d,* day; *IM,* intramuscular; *IV,* intravenous; *PB,* protein-binding; *PO,* by mouth; *t½,* half-life; *UK,* unknown.

Premarin, the most frequently used conjugated estrogen product, is presented in Prototype Drug Chart 54–1.

Dosage Forms

The oral route is most commonly used; it is well tolerated by most clients and relatively easy to use but does require daily dosing. Some clients experience gastrointestinal (GI) upsets, particularly nausea and vomiting. A client with GI disorders such as colitis, irritable bowel syndrome, peptic ulcer, or malabsorption may receive inconsistent doses with oral administration, necessitating the use of another dosage form. Oral estrogens have a particularly beneficial effect on lipids by increasing high-density lipoproteins. Although the oral route does result in complete absorption from the GI tract, there is greater impact upon liver proteins.

Medroxyprogesterone acetate (Provera), the progestin most often administered in combination with the estrogen, is taken orally. Examples of progestin products are given in Table 54–6.

The transdermal skin patch (the Estraderm Transdermal System) is a convenient method because it does not require daily dosing. The patch is applied to intact skin in the prescribed dosage. Generally the lower abdomen is used, but other sites (except for the breasts) may be used. The patch is applied twice a week for 3 weeks, with rotation of sites, followed by 1 week without use of the patch to allow for normal withdrawal bleeding. The transdermal patch allows for absorption of the estrogen (17 β-estradiol) directly into the bloodstream through a membrane that limits the absorption rate. The advantage is that the GI tract and liver are bypassed initially, which results in less nausea and vomiting and less impact on liver proteins.

Climara Pro is a thin translucent patch containing 0.015 mg/day of levonorgestrel and 0.045 mg/day of estradiol. It is the first once-a-week combined hormone therapy approved to treat menopausal symptoms such as hot flashes. The transdermal patch allows for continuous delivery of hormones at much lower doses than in oral HRT.

Table 54–6

Estrogens and Progestins

Generic (Brand)	Route and Dosage	Pregnancy Category
Conjugated Estrogens		
Premarin	See Prototype Drug Chart 54–1.	
Steroidal Estrogens		
estradiol (Estrace, Estraderm)	*Menopausal/hypogonadism:* PO: 1-2 mg/d for 21 d, then 7-10 d off cycle; may repeat cycle. *Patch:* 10-20 cm² system 2×/wk, in above cycle. *Breast cancer:* 10 mg t.i.d. *Prostate cancer:* 1-2 mg t.i.d. *Atrophic vaginitis:* Cream: 2-4 g/d for 1-2 wk; *maint:* 1 g 2×/wk	X
estradiol cypionate (Depo-Estradiol Cypionate)	*Menopausal symptoms:* IM: 1-4 mg q3-4 wk. *Hypogonadism:* IM: 1.5-2 mg q mo	X
esterified estrogens (Estratab, Menest)	*Menopausal symptoms:* PO: 0.3-1.25 mg/d for 3 wk, then 7-10 d off cycle. *Breast cancer:* PO: 10 mg t.i.d. *Prostate cancer:* 1.25-2.5 mg t.i.d.	X
estrone (Theelin)	*Hypogonadism:* 0.1-2 mg/wk. *Prostate cancer:* 2-4 mg 3×/wk	X
estropipate SO₄ (Ogen)	*Hypogonadism:* 1.25-7.5 mg/d for 3 wk, then 7-10 d off cycle	X
Nonsteroidal Estrogens		
chlorotrianisene (Tace)	*Menopausal/hypogonadism:* 12-25 mg/d for 21 d, then 10 d off cycle; repeat cycle. *Prostate cancer:* 12-25 mg/d	X
dienestrol (DV)	*Atrophic vaginitis:* Cream: Apply daily/ b.i.d. for 1-2 wk; *maint:* 1-3×/wk	X
diethylstilbestrol	*Breast cancer:* 15 mg/d. *Prostate cancer:* 1-3 mg t.i.d.	X
Progestins	*Menopausal/hypogonadism:* 100 mcg daily for 7 d, then 7 d off cycle; *maint:* q wk	X
progesterone	*DUB:* IM: 5-10 mg/d for 7 d. *Amenorrhea:* IM: 5-10 mg/d for 6-8 d	X
medroxyprogesterone acetate (Amen, Curretab, Provera, Cycrin, Depo-Provera)	*DUB/amenorrhea:* 5-10 mg/d for 5-10 d. *Endometriosis:* IM: 150 mg q3mo	X
megestrol acetate (Megace)	*Breast cancer:* PO: 40 mg q.i.d. *Endometrial cancer:* 40-320 mg/d in divided doses	X
norethindrone (Norlutin)	*DUB/amenorrhea:* 5-20 mg/d on days 5-25 of menstrual cycle	X

b.i.d., Twice a day; *d,* day; *DUB,* dysfunctional uterine bleeding; *IM,* intramuscular; *maint,* maintenance; *mo,* month; *PO,* by mouth; *q.i.d.,* four times a day; *t.i.d.,* three times a day; *wk,* week.

Vaginal cream preparations are used in the treatment of vaginal atrophy, which causes painful intercourse and urinary difficulties. These preparations contain conjugated estrogens and are rapidly absorbed into the bloodstream via the mucous membranes that lines the vagina. Vaginal creams may be used in conjunction with another method, such as tablets or the transdermal patch.

Estring is an elastomer ring containing 2 mg of 17 beta-estradiol, the major naturally occurring estrogen produced in the ovaries of fertile women. The Estring ring is inserted into the upper portion of the vagina, where it releases 50% to 60% of the estradiol, providing a consistent low dose of estrogen for 3 months. Estring is used to treat local symptoms of urogenital atrophy, which affects 20% to 40% of postmenopausal women

Femring is the first and only vaginal ERT to treat moderate to severe hot flashes, night sweats, and vaginal dryness in menopause. Femring contains estradiol acetate, an estrogen, contained in a soft, flexible silicone ring. It is inserted into the upper vagina for 3 months. It may be left in place during intercourse and treatment for vaginal infections.

EstroGel 0.06% is a synthetic, plant-based transdermal estradiol gel applied once daily for the treatment of moderate to severe vasomotor symptoms. A thin film is applied to one arm from the shoulder to wrist. The gel dries in 2 to 5 minutes. EstroGel is packaged in a non-aerosol, metered dose pump that is designed to deliver 1.25 g of gel per compression. A progestin should be used with an intact uterus.

Estrasorb is the first prescription topical emulsion for estrogen therapy. Estrasorb delivers consistent levels of estradiol into the bloodstream in a lotion-like emulsion, applied daily to the skin on the legs for the relief of moderate to severe vasomotor symptoms. Estrasorb should be applied in a comfortable sitting position to clean, dry skin on both legs each morning. A progestin should be used with an intact uterus.

Contraindications

Contraindications to ERT include pregnancy, history of endometrial or breast cancer within the last 5 years, history of thromboembolic disorders, acute liver disease or chronic impaired liver function, gallbladder or pancreatic disease, poorly controlled hypertension, undiagnosed genital bleeding, and endometriosis. Lifestyle factors, such as smoking, known to enhance the risk of thromboembolism should be considered in the treatment decision. The client with a history of fibroid tumors is not started on ERT for a full year after the last menstruation because estrogen would likely result in tumor growth. The hypoestrogenic state associated with natural menopause usually causes existing fibroids to shrink. The presence of fibrocystic breast disease, diabetes, or obesity may require extra caution.

Contraindications to HRT in conjunction with estrogen are the same as those for ERT. It is important to rule out the presence of known or suspected breast cancer before progestins are used.

Pharmacokinetics

The natural estrogens are completely and rapidly absorbed from the GI tract and rapidly metabolized by the liver, necessitating daily doses when oral products that are nonesterified (a process that delays metabolism and lengthens action) are used. About 80% of estradiol is bound to sex hormone-binding globulin, with 2% unbound and the rest bound to albumin. Estradiol is converted to estrone in the enterohepatic circulation and is conjugated and excreted via the urine. Progestin (Provera) is rapidly absorbed and metabolized primarily in the liver with excretion via the kidney; distribution of the agent is not well described.

Osteoporosis

Over half of U.S. women over the age of 50 have **osteoporosis** or osteopenia, placing them at risk for a bone fracture. The most serious fracture site is the hip. Hip fracture is the second most common reason for older women being placed in nursing homes, exceeded only by Alzheimer's disease.

Nursing Interventions

Prevention of osteoporosis includes 1200 mg of calcium daily if not taking estrogen; those taking hormones need only 1000 mg. Vitamin D supplementation (400 international units/day) is needed for women who do not receive daily doses of sunlight. Smoking cessation should be encouraged because smoking interferes with vitamin D absorption. Daily weight-bearing exercise strengthens the bones, increases muscle strength, and enhances balance. To prevent falls, loose rugs should be removed, adequate lighting provided, and handrails installed where appropriate. Caution should be used in clients who are prescribed medications that cause hypotension or dizziness.

Medications

Estrogen is no longer recommended for the sole treatment and prevention of osteoporosis because other medications are available that have a lower risk of cardiac disease, breast cancer, and blood clots.

Menostar (estradiol transdermal system) is 14 mcg of estrogen in a transdermal, once-a-week patch for prevention of postmenopausal osteoporosis. This estrogen patch is the lowest transdermal dose available. It is available for women who are unable to tolerate alternative therapies. For women with an intact uterus, a progestin is only recommended every 6 to 12 months.

Alendronate (Fosamax) is a bisphosphonate used to treat osteopenia and osteoporosis. It is available in a daily or weekly dose. It must be taken with 8 oz of water, 30 minutes before ingesting any food, liquids, or medication, and the client must remain upright for 30 minutes. Once-a-week dosing has made this a first-line therapy. Common side effects include abdominal pain and acid reflux.

Ibandronate sodium (Boniva) is a new, once-a-month bisphosphonate indicated for the treatment and prevention of osteoporosis in postmenopausal women. It has the same directions for use and side effects as the other biphosphonates.

Risedronate (Actonel) is also available in a daily or weekly dose. It has similar directions for use and side effects as the biphosphonates.

Raloxifene (Evista) is a selective estrogen receptor modulator (SERM) that increases bone mineral density, decrease bone turnover and reduces vertebral fractures. A secondary analysis of women with breast cancer in osteoporotic women treated with raloxifene showed a decrease in the risk of breast cancer. Side effects include hot flashes and increased risk of DVT.

Calcitonin and parathyroid hormone are used only for the treatment, not prevention, of osteoporosis.

Nursing Process

Estrogen Replacements

ASSESSMENT

- Assess the following baseline data:
  - Height and weight
  - Usual physical activity
  - Diet
  - Family history and personal risk factors regarding osteoporosis and cardiovascular disease
  - Client's menstrual history
  - Nature of the family members' climacteric experience
  - Current experience with the climacteric and the drugs client uses
- Assess client's perception of menopause.
- Assess client's attitude toward resumption of menstrual periods.

NURSING DIAGNOSES

- Sexual dysfunction
- Disturbed body image
- Health-seeking behaviors

PLANNING

- Client will verbalize menopausal symptoms and the nonpharmacologic and pharmacologic measures that may aid in alleviating symptoms.

NURSING INTERVENTIONS

- Educate women about the nature of the climacteric, its potential effects, and nonpharmacologic as well as pharmacologic treatment. Place current educational materials in health and community sites.
- Indicate on the laboratory slip or specimen that client takes hormone replacement therapy (HRT).
- Administer IM at bedtime to decrease adverse effects.

Client Teaching

General

- Review the risk-to-benefit ratio for use of estrogen replacement therapy (ERT).
- Review the contraindications to HRT.
- Advise client to have a breast examination, pelvic examination, Pap test, and endometrial biopsy before starting HRT.
- Tell client that warm weather and stress exacerbate vasodilation/hot flashes.
- Advise client to use a fan, drink cool liquids, wear layered cotton clothes, decrease intake of caffeine and spicy foods, and talk with her health care provider about the use of vitamin E to cope more comfortably with vasodilation. Individuals with diabetes, hypertension, or rheumatic heart disease should use vitamin E in low doses with the health care provider's approval.
- Encourage client on HRT to have medical follow-up every 6 to 12 months, including a blood pressure check and breast and pelvic examinations.
- Suggest that client carry sanitary pads or tampons for breakthrough bleeding or irregular menstruation.
- Stress the need to use nonhormonal birth control because irregular menstruation may create anxiety about pregnancy. Tell client to plan to use birth control for 2 years. If she has progesterone-induced bleeding, the only way to determine whether she is truly menopausal is by hormone assay.
- Suggest to client that she use a water-soluble vaginal lubricant to reduce painful intercourse (dyspareunia) and prevent trauma.
- Advise client to decrease use of antihistamines and decongestants if she experiences vaginal dryness.
- Advise client to wear cotton underwear and pantyhose with a cotton liner and to avoid douches and feminine hygiene products.
- Suggest that client take Premarin with progestin after meals to avoid nausea and vomiting.
- Tell client to report any heavy bleeding (flooding) and to have her hematocrit and hemoglobin evaluated.
- Tell client to report bleeding that occurs between menstruation or return of bleeding after cessation of menstruation.
- Advise client starting on HRT that the withdrawal bleeding that occurs from days 25 to 30 is normal and not the same as cyclic menstrual periods. Tell her that this bleeding will usually last only 2 to 3 days and that she will not experience the same degree of premenstrual symptoms she may have had with regular menstruation.
- Advise client to report if bleeding occurs other than on days 25 to 30 once she has started on HRT.
- Tell client that the withdrawal bleeding does not signify that she can become pregnant.
- Advise client that after HRT is discontinued, there may be a recurrence of menopausal signs and symptoms such as hot flashes.

Self-Administration

- Teach client to perform regular breast self-examination.
- If client uses vaginal cream, review the application procedure and suggest that she wear minipads.
- If client uses the transdermal patch, tell her to open the package and apply it immediately, holding it in place for about 10 seconds; to check the edges to ensure adequate contact; to use the abdomen (except waistline) for the patch; to rotate the sites with at least 1 week before reuse of a site; to not use the breast as a site; to not put the patch on an irritated or oily area; to reapply the patch if it loosens or apply a new one; and to follow the same cycle schedule.

Diet

- Discuss the use of yogurt containing *Acidophilus* or *Lactobacillus* as a way of maintaining normal bacterial flora in the vagina.
- Tell client that she may experience an occasional hot flash on days 25 to 30 when she goes through withdrawal bleeding. Instruct client to stop treatment and contact a health care provider if she has headache, visual disturbances, signs of thrombophlebitis, heaviness in legs, chest pain, or breast lumps.
- Tell client that if she wants to stop HRT, she should do so with the guidance of her health care provider.
- Suggest that client at risk for osteoporosis (1) exercise consistently (e.g., walking or bicycling), (2) eat a well-balanced diet (low in red meat and sugar) with 1200 mg calcium/d if premenopausal or 1200 to 1500 mg/d if menopausal, and (3) avoid smoking and alcohol.

EVALUATION

- Evaluate the effectiveness of the nonpharmacologic or pharmacologic measures for premenopausal symptoms.
- Determine whether side effects occur. Plan with the client alternative measures to control menopausal symptoms.

WEBSITES

For further information on *Women's Health and Disorders*, visit these Internet resources:

American College of Obstetricians and Gynecologists: *www.acog.org*

Femring: *www.femring.com*

Ortho Evra: *www.orthoevra.com*

Planned Parenthood: *www.plannedparenthood.org*

Seasonale: *www.seasonale.com*

The Contraception Report: *www.contraceptiononline.org/contrareport*

The Women's Health Initiative Study: *www.whi.org*

Critical Thinking Case Study

T.A. (gravida 3, para 1), the client discussed in Chapters 51 through 53, is ready to leave the hospital following her delivery of baby J.A. Pregnancy-induced hypertension had developed during the pregnancy, but she had no prior history of hypertension. She plans to breastfeed for 3 months. She desires contraception and asks questions about hormonally controlled birth control methods.

1. T.A. asks whether she can take combination birth control pills while breastfeeding. What is a nursing diagnosis for T.A. based on her communication?

2. The nurse tells her that she may breastfeed and start using combination pills in about 6 weeks once the milk flow is established. This information is:
   a. Correct: Why?
   b. Incorrect: Why?

3. T.A. asks if there are any advantages to the use of oral contraceptives over a diaphragm. What are four advantages and four disadvantages that a nurse could include in her discussion?

4. T.A. tells you that she smokes ¾ of a pack of cigarettes per day. How does this information impact the decision for or against oral contraceptive use?

5. T.A. starts to use combination birth control pills and calls the clinic upset that she has forgotten to take one pill. What would the clinic nurse correctly tell T.A. to do? How might the nurse in the postpartum unit have better prepared T.A. for this situation?

6. Because milk flow needs to be established before starting on combination birth control pills, what should be recommended to T.A. about contraception upon leaving the hospital? Consider that T.A. had a fourth-degree episiotomy and hemorrhoids.

7. T.A. states that when she has "bad allergies" she sometimes takes OTC antihistamines. How should T.A. be advised?

8. How should T.A. be advised to take her birth control pills?

9. Injectable progestin (Depo-Provera) is recommended as an alternative method for contraception. What advantage might this product have for T.A. over the oral products?

10. What should T.A. be advised about regarding the use of Depo-Provera while breastfeeding?

11. What implication does T.A.'s smoking have in regard to known side effects with Depo-Provera?

12. Why should the site in which a Depo-Provera injection is given be documented?

13. How should the way Depo-Provera works be explained to T.A.?

14. T.A. asks how long it will take to regain her fertility once she stops using the Depo-Provera injection. What is the correct response to her question?

Study Questions

1. What key factors should the nurse cover in a teaching plan for oral contraceptive use? What is the degree of effectiveness of oral contraceptives? What are the advantages and disadvantages of this method?

2. What are some common symptoms associated with PMS? What are effective treatment modalities for the symptoms?

3. What are the expected effects of drug therapy for endometriosis using danazol and gonadotropin-releasing hormone agonists?

4. A client asks about hormone replacement therapy. What information should be shared with her in regard to (a) indications for hormone therapy, (b) routes of administration, (c) types of therapy, (d) expected duration of therapy, (e) contraindications, and (f) side effects?

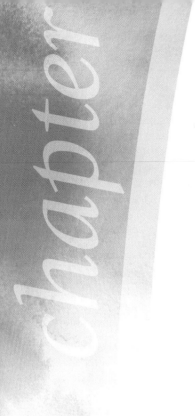

55 Drugs Related to Reproductive Health: Male Reproductive Disorders

KATHLEEN J. JONES

ELECTRONIC RESOURCES

evolve

Additional information can be found on the companion website at *http://evolve.elsevier.com/KeeHayes/pharmacology/* or on the companion CD-ROM, which includes:

- *NCLEX-style examination review questions*
- *Pharmacology animations*
- *Medication error and IV therapy checklists*
- *Medication calculation problems*
- *Electronic calculators*

OUTLINE

OBJECTIVES

- Describe the feedback loop comprising hypothalamic, anterior pituitary, and gonadal hormones.
- Describe the role of testosterone in development of primary and secondary male sex characteristics and in spermatogenesis.
- Differentiate common conditions for which androgen therapy and antiandrogen therapy are indicated.
- Identify clients for whom androgen therapy is particularly risky.
- Assess clients for therapeutic and adverse effects of androgen therapy.
- Compare and contrast commonly prescribed medications that can impair male sexual function.
- Explain the nursing process, including client teaching, related to drugs used to treat male reproductive disorders.

TERMS

Addison's disease	delayed puberty	hypogonadism	spermatogenesis
anabolic steroids	ejaculatory dysfunction	hypothyroidism	testosterone
androgens	erectile dysfunction	inhibited sexual desire	virilization
antiandrogens	gynecomastia	oligospermia	
cryptorchidism	hirsutism	priapism	

Introduction

This chapter discusses drug regimens for various alterations in male reproductive health other than the sexually transmitted diseases (STDs), which, because of their association with infertility, particularly among women, are addressed in Chapter 56, Drugs Related to Reproductive Health: Infertility and Sexually Transmitted Diseases.

Reproductive health requires the production of adequate quantities of various hypothalamic, pituitary, and gonadal hormones as well as the appropriate hormone receptors. It requires normal development and patency of the reproductive tract. In addition, reproductive health implies that men and women of developmentally appropriate life stages are fertile (i.e., able to produce gametes [sperm or eggs]). Finally, reproductive health entails the ability to engage in sexual intercourse with ejaculation by the male.

Alterations in reproductive health reflect a wide range of developmental, endocrine, infectious, inflammatory, hypertrophic, malignant, and psychoemotional processes. To gain a better understanding of ways in which reproductive health is affected, reproductive processes are reviewed.

The male reproductive processes, including anatomy and physiology, sperm production, regulation of male sexual functioning, and sexual intercourse, are discussed in the introduction to Unit XVI, Reproductive and Gender-Related Agents.

The drug family most clearly associated with male reproductive processes is the androgens. Because anabolic steroids and antiandrogens impact male reproduction, they are also discussed.

Substances Related to Male Reproductive Disorders

Androgens

Androgens, or male sex hormones, affect sexual processes, accessory sexual organs, cellular metabolism, and bone and muscle growth. The actions and effects of natural androgens are listed in Prototype Drug Chart 55–1. **Testosterone,** the main androgen, is synthesized primarily in the testes and, to a lesser extent, in the adrenal cortex. In women, the ovaries synthesize small amounts of testosterone. In men, normal plasma concentrations of testosterone are 250 to 1000 mg/dl, with circadian fluctuations.

Pharmacokinetics

In men, about 98% of circulating testosterone is bound to protein. It is the unbound fraction that is biologically active. Estrogen elevates the production of sex hormone-binding globulin; therefore more circulating testosterone is bound in women.

The half-life of endogenous free testosterone in the blood is 10 to 20 minutes. Exogenous testosterone is absorbed orally, but because as much as 50% is metabolized on its first pass through the hepatic circulation, high doses are needed to achieve effective plasma levels. Synthetic androgens have longer half-lives. Testosterone can be combined with esters to form esterified testosterone, in an oil base, to achieve a duration of action of up to 4 weeks.

Testosterone is excreted mainly in the urine as the metabolites androsterone and etiocholanolone. About 6% of the hormone is excreted unaltered in the feces. Synthetic androgens may be excreted as unaltered hormone or as metabolites. In some tissues, the action of testosterone depends on its reduction to 5-alpha-dihydrotestosterone, whereas in other tissues testosterone itself is the active hormone. In the central nervous system, the metabolite estradiol affects hormonal action.

Pharmacodynamics

Testosterone is responsible for the development of male characteristics. These include the fetal development and the maturation of the male reproductive system and the development of secondary sex characteristics such as pubic hair growth, beard and body hair growth, baldness, deepening of the male voice, thickening of the skin, sebaceous gland activity, increased musculature, bone development, and red blood cell formation.

The mechanism for these effects may be increased protein formation in the target cells. Dehydrotestosterone with its receptor acts at binding sites on the chromosomes. Increased ribonucleic acid (RNA) polymerase activity and increased synthesis of specific RNA and proteins result, accounting for the anabolic effects of testosterone.

The testes produce testosterone in utero. After birth until just before puberty, production is negligible. During puberty, testosterone production increases rapidly and continues until later adulthood. As men age, the number of Leydig cells decreases, sperm production declines, and luteinizing hormone (LH) and follicle-stimulating hormone (FSH) levels rise. Levels of unbound testosterone are reduced in older men to one third to one fifth the peak value. "Andropause" is beginning to receive attention as a health issue affecting older men, particularly those older than 70 years. If men experience osteoporosis and anemia, and if their testosterone levels are less than or equal to 300 ng/dl, testosterone replacement therapy should be considered.

Indications for Androgen Therapy

Various androgens and their uses are identified in Table 55–1.

Hypogonadism. The clearest indication for androgen therapy is insufficient testosterone production by the testes, or **hypogonadism.** Hypogonadism can be primary, reflecting testicular abnormality, or secondary, reflecting hypothalamic or pituitary failure. Severely affected boys do not experience puberty. Mild hypogonadism may result. Lack of libido, impotence, decreased bone density, or the onset of vasomotor flushing also can occur. The timing and extent of treatment depend on the clinical manifestations.

Artificial induction of puberty is undertaken after boys reach 15 to 17 years of age. Hypothalamic and pituitary function is assessed. A 4- to 6-month trial of androgen therapy is implemented, followed by a like period of rest

PROTOTYPE DRUG CHART 55–1

TESTOSTERONE

Drug Class

Androgens
Trade Name: Andro-Cyp 100, depAndro 100,
    Depotest-100, Duratest-100, Depo-Testosterone,
    Testred Cypionate 200, Virilon, depAndrogyn, Everone
Pregnancy Category: X
CSS III

Dosage

Androgen replacement:
PO: 10-40 mg/d
Buccal: 5-20 mg/d
subQ: 150-450 mg q3-6 mo
IM: 10-30 mg 2-3 times/wk
Metastatic carcinoma of the breast:
PO: 200 mg/d
Buccal: 200 mg/d
IM: 100 mg 3 times/wk

Contraindications

Pregnancy, nephrosis, hypercalcemia, pituitary insuffi-
    ciency, hepatic dysfunction, benign prostatic hyper-
    trophy, prostatic cancer, history of myocardial infarc-
    tion, prepubertal status, non–estrogen-dependent
    breast cancer
Caution: Hypertension, hypercholesterolemia, coronary
    artery disease, gynecomastia, renal disease, seizure
    disorders; prepubescent clients, older adults

Drug-Lab-Food Interactions

Drug: Increases effects of anticoagulants; *decreases* ef-
    fect with barbiturates, phenytoin, phenylbutazone;
    antagonizes calcitonin, parathyroid; corticosteroids
    exacerbate edema
Lab: Decreases blood glucose in diabetics; *increases*
    serum cholesterol, thyroid, liver function, hematocrit

Pharmacokinetics

Absorption: IM: Well absorbed
Distribution: PB: 98%
Metabolism: t½: 10-100 min
Excretion: In urine and bile

Pharmacodynamics

IM: Onset: UK
    Peak: UK
    Duration: cypionate enanthate: 2-4 wk
    Base, propionate: 1-3 d

Therapeutic Effects/Uses

To achieve normal androgen levels; to slow progress of estrogen-dependent breast cancers
Mode of Action: Development and maintenance of male sex organs and secondary sex characteristics

Side Effects

Abdominal pain, nausea, diarrhea, constipation, hives,
    irritation at injection site, increased salivation, mouth
    soreness, increased or decreased libido, insomnia,
    aggressive behavior, weakness, dizziness, pruritus

Adverse Reactions

Acne, masculinization, irregular menses, urinary ur-
    gency, gynecomastia, priapism, red skin, jaundice,
    sodium and water retention, allergic reaction, depres-
    sion, habituation
Life-threatening: Hepatic necrosis, hepatitis, hepatic
    tumors, respiratory distress

CSS, Controlled Substances Schedule; *d,* day; *IM,* intramuscular; *min,* minute; *mo,* month; *PB,* protein-binding; *PO,* by mouth; *subQ,*
subcutaneous; *t½,* half-life; *UK,* unknown; *wk,* week.

---

for reevaluation. If prolonged therapy is required, testosterone cypionate or testosterone enanthate is given, starting with 100 mg given intramuscularly (IM) every 2 weeks
for 6 to 12 months, with a gradual increase to 200 mg
every 2 weeks. It takes 3 or 4 years for sexual development
to occur. Plasma testosterone levels should be monitored
and dosages adjusted as needed to maintain normal levels.

Another form of treatment is transdermal testosterone
skin patches that are applied daily either scrotally or non-
scrotally. The patches eliminate the need for injections and
provide circadian fluctuations in dosage.

Constitutional Growth Delay. A height of two or more
standard deviations below the mean for age and sex occurs
in 2.5% of normal children. This tends to be of greater

concern for boys. Delay in bone growth seems to be of little consequence by the time boys reach the age of 20 years;
however, in some families, delayed growth causes significant emotional distress despite reassurance from health
professionals. The etiology may be a deficiency of growth
hormone, which can be associated with androgen deficiency, or it may be solely androgen deficiency. Treatment
is not initiated before the age of 14 years. Therapy for 3 to
6 months or less before epiphyseal closure may result in
linear growth without adverse permanent effects on hypothalamic, pituitary, or gonadal maturation. It is not known
whether treatment has an effect on final adult height.

The selection of an androgen or anabolic steroid depends on the balance of growth and sexual maturation
that is desired, as well as the preferred route of adminis-

Table 55–1

Androgens

Generic (Brand)	Route and Dosage	Uses and Considerations
Natural Androgens		
testosterone (Histerone, Tesamone, Testopel pellets, testosterone aqueous, testosterone powder)	IM: 10-25 mg 2-3 × wk subQ: 150-450 mg q3-6mo	Androgen replacement, delayed puberty, senile or postmenopausal osteoporosis. Started at full dose and adjusted according to tolerance and therapeutic response.
	IM: 100 mg 3 × wk	Carcinoma of the breast. Therapy may be lifelong. *Pregnancy category:* X; PB: 98%; t^1/$_2$: 10-100 min
testosterone cypionate (Andro-Cyp, Andronate, depAndro, Depotest, Depo-Testosterone, Duratest, Testred cypionate, Virilon IM)	IM: 50-400 mg q2-6wk	Androgen replacement, delayed puberty. Therapy generally lasts 3-4 y. *Pregnancy category:* X; PB: 98%; t^1/$_2$: 10-100 min
testosterone enanthate (Andro, Andropository, Delatest, Delatestryl, Durathate, Everone, Testrin)	IM: 50-400 mg q2-6wk	Androgen replacement, delayed puberty. *Pregnancy category:* X; PB: 98%; t^1/$_2$: 10-100 min
testosterone propionate (Testex, testosterone propionate powder)	IM: 50 mg 3 × wk	Androgen replacement. *Pregnancy category:* X; PB: 98%; t^1/$_2$: 10-100 min
transdermal testosterone (patch)	2.5 mg/24 h 5 mg/24 h	Apply to nonscrotal skin; avoid bony areas (Androderm)
testoderm testodermiss androderm	Apply to scrotal skin Apply to nonscrotal skin	Uses and considerations: Same
Synthetic Androgens		
danazol (Danocrine)	PO: 100-800 mg/d divided in 2 doses initially	Endometriosis, fibrocystic breast disease, angioedema. Initial doses are gradually reduced on an individual basis. Endometriosis therapy lasts 6-9 mo; fibrocystic breast disease therapy lasts 4-6 mo. *Pregnancy category:* X; PB: UK; t^1/$_2$: 4.5 h
fluoxymesterone (Halotestin)	PO: 10-30 mg/d divided in 1-4 doses	Androgen deficiency, carcinoma of the breast. *Pregnancy category:* X; PB: 98%; t^1/$_2$: 20-100 min
methyltestosterone (Android, Oreton Methyl, Testred, Virilon)	PO: 10-50 mg/d in divided doses initially, reduced for maintenance Buccal: 5-25 mg/d in divided doses	Androgen deficiency
	PO: 50-200 mg/d Buccal: 2-25 mg/d in divided doses	Carcinoma of the breast. *Pregnancy category:* X; PB: UK; t^1/$_2$: UK
Anabolic Steroids		
nandrolone decanoate (Androlone-D, Deca-Durabolin, Hybolin Decanoate, Neo Durabolic)	IM: 50-200 mg q1-4wk C: IM: 25-50 mg q3-4wk	Anemia of renal disease. *Pregnancy category:* X; PB: UK; t^1/$_2$: UK
nandrolone phenpropionate (Durabolin, Hybolin improved, Nandrobolic LA)	IM: 50-100 mg/wk	Carcinoma of the breast. *Pregnancy category:* X; PB: UK; t^1/$_2$: 1-9 h
oxandrolone (Oxandrin)	PO: 5-20 mg/d, divided C: PO: 0.1 mg/kg/d	Delayed growth/puberty, osteoporotic pain, short stature, Turner's syndrome, alcoholic hepatitis. *Pregnancy category:* X; PB: UK; t^1/$_2$: 1-9 h
oxymetholone (Anadrol-50)	PO: 1-5 mg/kg/d	Anemias of deficient RBC production. *Pregnancy category:* X; PB: UK; t^1/$_2$: 9 h
stanozolol (Winstrol)	PO: 2-6 mg/d	t^1/$_2$: UK

C, Child; *d,* day; *h,* hour; *IM,* intramuscular; *min,* minute; *mo,* month; *PB,* protein-binding; *PO,* by mouth; *RBC,* red blood cell; *subQ,* subcutaneous; *t^1/$_2$,* half-life; *UK,* unknown; *wk,* week; *y,* year.

tration. Oxandrolone, an orally active testosterone analog, is effective for treating boys. Oxandrolone stimulates the onset of puberty. It is classified as an anabolic steroid and is regulated as such. The daily dosage is less than or equal to 0.1 mg/kg.

Studies have shown that men treated with human growth hormone (hGH) for nongrowth hormone-dependent short stature, showed reduced testicular volume and hyper gonadotropic hypogonadism. They also have impaired spermatogenesis and altered testicular texture by ultrasound. Although no clinical or laboratory findings showed testicular dysfunction, an unfavorable gonadal outcome could occur in boys given growth hormone who did not have growth hormone deficiency.

Other Uses. Other uses of androgens include treatment of refractory anemias in men and women, the hereditary autosomal clotting disorder angioneurotic edema, tissue wasting associated with severe or chronic illness, advanced carcinoma of the breast in women, and endometriosis. The effectiveness of androgens for treatment of **cryptorchidism** (undescended testis) and impotence has not been established. Androgens may be used in combination with estrogens for management of severe menopausal symptoms in women (see Chapter 54, Drugs Related to Women's Health and Disorders).

Side Effects

Side effects of androgen therapy include abdominal pain, nausea, insomnia, diarrhea or constipation, hives or redness at the injection site, increased salivation, mouth soreness, and increased or decreased sexual desire. If side effects persist, worsen, or disturb the individual, the health care provider should be notified.

Adverse Reactions

Virilizing effects (the development of secondary male sex characteristics) are inappropriate when the client is not a hypogonadal man. Women who use androgen therapy risk such manifestations, including acne and skin oiliness, the growth of facial hair, and vocal huskiness. Menstrual irregularities or amenorrhea, suppressed ovulation or lactation, baldness or increased hair growth (**hirsutism**), and hypertrophy of the clitoris may develop in women undergoing androgen therapy. Although most adverse effects slowly reverse themselves after short-term therapy is completed, vocal changes may be permanent. With long-term therapy, as in the treatment of breast cancer, adverse effects may be irreversible.

Children may experience profound **virilization** or feminization, as well as impaired bone growth. During pregnancy, androgens can cross the placenta and cause masculinization of the fetus.

Hypogonadal men may experience frequent or continuous erection (**priapism**), **gynecomastia** (breast swelling or soreness), and urinary urgency. Continued use of androgens by normal men can halt **spermatogenesis** (formation of spermatozoa). The sperm count may be low (**oligospermia**) for 3 or more months after therapy is stopped. For this reason, androgens for contraceptive use by men are currently in development.

Less frequent adverse effects include dizziness, weakness, changes in skin color, frequent headaches, confusion, respiratory distress, depression, pruritus, allergic skin rash, edema of the lower extremities, jaundice, bleeding, paresthesias, chills, polycythemia, muscle cramps, and sodium

and water retention. Hepatic carcinoma can occur in clients who have received 17-alpha-alkyl substituted androgens over prolonged periods (i.e., 1 to 7 years).

Serum cholesterol may become elevated during androgen therapy. Other alterations in laboratory tests include altered thyroid and liver function tests, elevated urine 17-ketosteroids, and increased hematocrit.

Rare complications of long-term therapy include hepatic necrosis, hepatic peliosis, hepatic tumors, and leukopenia.

Contraindications

Androgen therapy is contraindicated during pregnancy and in individuals with nephrosis or the nephrotic phase of nephritis, hypercalcemia, pituitary insufficiency, hepatic dysfunction, benign prostatic hypertrophy, or prostate cancer. Men with breast cancer are not treated with androgens, nor are women whose breast cancer is not estrogen dependent. A history of myocardial infarction is a contraindication.

Caution must be exercised when using androgen therapy in individuals with hypertension, hypercholesterolemia, coronary artery disease, gynecomastia, renal disease, or seizure disorder. It is used with caution in infants and prepubertal children because of the potential for growth disturbances and in older men because of their increased risk for benign prostatic hypertrophy and prostate cancer.

Drug Interactions

Androgens potentiate the effects of oral anticoagulants, necessitating a decrease in anticoagulant dosage. Androgens antagonize calcitonin and parathyroid hormones. Because androgens can decrease blood glucose in clients with diabetes, dosages of insulin or other antidiabetic agents may need to be reduced. Concurrent use of corticosteroids exacerbates the edema that can occur with androgen therapy. Barbiturates, phenytoin, and phenylbutazone decrease the effects of androgens.

Nursing Process

Androgens

ASSESSMENT

■ Assess the reason for androgen therapy and the client's perception of it. If delayed puberty is the indication, the nurse will assess client's and family's attitudes about the condition.

■ Monitor client's weight, blood pressure, liver and thyroid function, hemoglobin and hematocrit, creatinine, clotting factors, glucose tolerance, serum lipids and electrolytes, and blood count before and throughout treatment. The presence of liver or endocrine dysfunction should be noted.

■ Determine the pregnancy status of women of child-bearing age. Concomitant anticoagulant therapy should be noted. When a prepubertal child is treated, radiographs are obtained before, every 6 months during, and after treatment to monitor growth.

■ Appraise client's affect during therapy, particularly aggressiveness in clients taking large doses. Self-concept is an important consideration in client on androgen therapy, particularly in children with delayed puberty and in women.

NURSING DIAGNOSES

■ Disturbed body image
■ Delayed growth and development
■ Situational chronic low self-esteem
■ Sexual dysfunction
■ Ineffective sexuality patterns
■ Deficient knowledge regarding treatment protocol

PLANNING

■ Clients will adhere to the prescribed regimen for taking the medication and for monitoring.
■ Client will appropriately use the medication, avoid preventable adverse effects, and maintain a positive self-concept during long-term treatment.

NURSING INTERVENTIONS

Client Teaching

General

• Instruct client and family on proper administration of the medications, their reasons for use, and potential undesired effects. Inform them of which effects warrant prompt medical attention (e.g., urinary problems, priapism, respiratory distress).

• Teach client that an intermittent approach to treatment allows for monitoring of endocrine status between courses of androgen therapy. Explain the need to return to the health care facility for monitoring, and determine client's ability to do so. Make social service referrals if necessary.

• Instruct families pursuing treatment for a client with delayed puberty about the range of normal development.

• Urge individuals being treated for tissue wasting to reduce environmental stressors and promote rest and relaxation, because stress hormones are catabolic. Muscle strength will be monitored during treatment.

Self-Administration

• Oral androgens should be taken with food to decrease gastric distress.

Side Effects

• Women and prepubertal clients need instruction on good skin hygiene to decrease the severity of acne.

• Men undergoing androgen therapy are instructed to report priapism (painful, continuous erection) promptly. The drug dosage will be reduced to avoid subsequent erectile dysfunction. In addition, they are taught to report decreased urinary stream promptly because androgens can stimulate prostatic hypertrophy.

Diet

• The nutritional intake of individuals with anemia, osteoporosis, or tissue wasting is assessed and revised as needed to ensure adequate intake of calories, protein, vitamins, iron, and other minerals.

• Sodium may need to be restricted if edema develops. Client will be instructed to record body weight several times per week.

• Individuals with elevated serum calcium need 3 to 4 L of fluid per day to prevent kidney stones. Individuals on bed rest need range-of-motion exercises, whereas ambulatory clients need to engage in active weight bearing. Indicators of hypercalcemia are shown in Box 55–1. Hypercalcemia needs prompt medical attention because it can lead to cardiac arrest.

Cultural Considerations ⊕

• Asses how the person's cultural group regards the expression of sexuality.

• Ascertain any culturally defined expectations about male-female or male-male relationships, including the health care relationship.

• Determine whether the person has any restrictions related to sexuality, exposure of body parts, or discussion of sexual functioning.

• If an interpreter is needed, meet these guidelines if possible:

Use a trained medical interpreter from your agency if possible. A medical interpreter can help with advice about the cultural appropriateness of client's health care plan

Use a family member only if absolutely necessary. Be aware that there may be limitations if the family member does not understand medical terms or is a different age or gender from the client. Family members may not be aware of medical procedures or medical ethics.

Use simple language; try to use as few medical terms as possible.

Speak in one or two sentences to allow easier translation.

EVALUATION

■ Client's ability to adhere to the treatment regimen and response to prescribed drugs will be monitored.

■ Client will be asked about therapeutic and adverse drug effects on follow-up visits. Monitoring of weight, blood pressure, and laboratory tests will continue throughout therapy, with alterations in the plan of care as needed.

■ Children and women who experience virilizing effects or acne will be periodically assessed for the ability to cope with these changes and maintain a positive self-concept.

■ Sexual function is assessed when appropriate.

■ Client's ability to adhere to the treatment plan and to discuss the treatment and its effects knowledgeably suggests that teaching has been effective and that client accepts the treatment.

Anabolic Steroids

Anabolic steroids are synthetic derivatives of testosterone developed to maximize the anabolic effects of androgens and to minimize their androgenic effects. Testosterone precursors available as nutritional supplements include androstenediol, androstenedione, and dehydroepiandrosterone (DHEA). Older teens are the heaviest users, but more than a half a million junior high school students use them. Marketed as "sport supplements" or "teen formulas," they can be purchased without a prescription in grocery stores, health food markets, and sports stores and on the Internet. Side effects include water retention, which overloads the kidneys, and cardiac damage. The adverse effects may not be recognized until years later.

Two other steroids that have gained popularity, especially with athletes, are human chorionic gonadotropin (hCG, Pregnyl, Novarel, Ovidrel) a hormone used to treat infertility, which also stimulates testosterone production, and tetrahydrogestrinone (THG), a potent androgen developed to escape urine detection. THG has not been approved by the Food and Drug Administration (FDA) and is not legally marketed. All major athletic organizations prohibit the use of anabolic steroids.

Antiandrogens

Antiandrogens, or androgen antagonists, block the synthesis or action of androgens (Table 55–2). These drugs may be useful in the management of benign prostatic hypertro-

BOX 55–1

Signs of Hypercalcemia

- Nausea and vomiting
- Lethargy
- Decreased muscle tone
- Polyuria
- Increased urine and serum calcium

Table 55–2

Antiandrogens

Mechanism	Drugs
Elevation of Gn-RH level	goserelin (Zoladex) nafarelin (Synarel) leuprolide acetate (Lupron, Lupron Depot)
Inhibition of testosterone synthesis	ketoconazole (Nizoral)
Blocks conversion of testosterone to dihydrotestosterone	finasteride (Proscar)
Receptor inhibitors	cyproterone, cyproterone acetate (orphan drug status in the United States) flutamide (Eulexin) spironolactone (generic, Aldactone)

Gn-RH, Gonadotropin-releasing hormone.

phy and carcinoma of the prostate. They have been used to treat male-pattern baldness, acne, hirsutism, virilization syndrome in women, and precocious puberty in boys, although their effectiveness is not well established. The effectiveness of these drugs to inhibit the sex drive of men who are sex offenders is controversial and not well documented.

Gonadotropin-releasing hormone (Gn-RH), or an analogue such as leuprolide, is the most effective inhibitor of testosterone synthesis. When such agents are given over time, LH and testosterone levels fall. Ketoconazole, an antimycotic, is used for treatment of prostatic carcinoma because of its inhibition of adrenal and gonadal steroid synthesis.

Two types of drugs have been developed to block testosterone action: androgen-receptor antagonists and agents that block conversion of testosterone to its active form, dihydrotestosterone. Cyproterone acetate, an orally active progesterone, is a potent androgen antagonist. It also suppresses LH and FSH secretion and has progestational qualities. Cyproterone acetate competes with dihydrotestosterone for binding to the androgen receptor. Cyproterone acetate can stunt growth in young people. Acne and baldness have been reported.

Flutamide (Eulexin) is a nonsteroidal drug that competes with androgens at androgen receptor sites. Men receiving flutamide show elevations in plasma LH and testosterone levels. Flutamide is used with Gn-RH blockade or estrogen to treat prostate cancer. Spironolactone also competes with dihydrotestosterone at the receptor site. It is used in doses of 50 to 100 mg/daily to treat hirsutism in women.

Finasteride, a steroid, inhibits conversion of testosterone to dihydrotestosterone. This orally active agent decreases the concentration of dihydrotestosterone in plasma and in the prostate without elevated plasma concentrations of LH or testosterone. Finasteride is used to treat benign prostatic hypertrophy. Other uses are under investigation. The recommended dose (for benign prostatic hypertrophy [BPH]) of 5 mg/daily needs to be reevaluated at 6 months and periodically thereafter. Women of childbearing potential should not be exposed to broken or crushed tablets. Adverse reactions include impotence, decreased libido, and decreased ejaculate.

Drugs Used in Other Male Reproductive Disorders

Developmental Disorders

Undescended testes are associated with subsequent infertility and testicular cancer. The primary treatment is orchidopexy (surgical placement of the testicle into the scrotum), which is usually performed by the time the child is 18 months old.

Delayed Puberty

In up to 5% of cases of **delayed puberty** (no signs of puberty by age 14 in a boy), there is insufficient secretion of Gn-RH, LH, or FSH. Once the cause is determined, Gn-RH, LH, or FSH replacement therapy is instituted.

Pituitary, Thyroid, and Adrenal Disorders

Inadequate pituitary function can result in hypogonadism. In a prepubertal boy, it results in lack of secondary sex characteristics and infertility; adult men may experience testicular atrophy and decreases in libido, potency, beard growth, and muscle tone. Menotropins (Pergonal), one ampule of which contains 75 international units each of LH and FSH, can stimulate testosterone production when injected intramuscularly (IM) three times a week over a period of years. Menotropins is indicated when both LH and FSH levels are low. It is given concomitantly with hCG 2000 international units IM twice a week for at least 3 months. Adverse effects include nausea, vomiting, diarrhea, gynecomastia, and fever. The drug is reconstituted with 1 to 2 ml sterile saline and must be used immediately.

Hypothyroidism, a deficiency in thyroid hormone, can be the result of insufficient thyroid hormone production or resistance to its effects at the target organs. The problem could be congenital. It can cause inhibited sexual desire and erectile dysfunction. In **Addison's disease,** there is a deficit of both cortisol and the mineralocorticoid aldosterone. Men with Addison's disease may experience inhibited sexual desire, erectile dysfunction, or diminished fertility. Both these conditions are highly responsive to replacement therapy with the appropriate hormones (see Chapter 49, Endocrine Pharmacology: Pituitary, Thyroid, Parathyroids, and Adrenals).

The successful treatment of cancer with chemotherapy in boys and in young adults can be associated with impaired gonadal function as a result of damage to the Leydig cells, which can cause impaired spermatogenesis or sterility. Abnormalities of endocrine function and growth are common problems following bone marrow and peripheral stem cell transplantation in children. About 25%

of children who receive total body irradiation experience hypothyroidism. Gonadal dysfunction is prevalent and most males experience oligoazospermia. At this time, the only clinical option for preserving male fertility is cryopreserving sperm, that is, sperm-banking, before the initiation of cancer therapy.

For young men with sickle cell disease, priapism is a complication that, left untreated, can result in irreversible fibrosis and impotency. The most common age for the first episode of priapism is 12, and most episodes are nocturnal. If an episode of priapism persists longer than 2 hours, the client should go to the emergency room for intravenous (IV) fluids and narcotics. After 4 hours, intracavernosal aspiration and instillation of an alpha-agonist should be performed.

Sexual Dysfunction

Sexual dysfunction is the inability to experience sexual desire, erection, ejaculation, and detumescence—the phases of the sexual response cycle. **Inhibited sexual desire** can result from androgen deficiency, an affective disorder, or discord in the sexual relationship. **Erectile dysfunction** may be caused by psychoemotional problems, diabetes, hypertension, lower urinary tract symptoms, and history of pelvic surgery, vascular insufficiency, neurologic disorders, androgen deficiency or resistance, or diseases of the penis. **Ejaculatory dysfunction** can be psychogenic or a result of drug therapy, androgen deficiency, or sympathetic degeneration. Failure of detumescence (reduction of penile swelling) is most commonly caused by penile disease or systemic disease. Male sexual dysfunction may result from the use of various drugs, as listed in Table 55-3.

Levodopa (L-Dopa), used to treat Parkinson's syndrome, has shown effectiveness in stimulating libido and treating erectile dysfunctions in non-Parkinson's clients. Individuals who experience premature ejaculation related to excessive anxiety about sexual intercourse may be helped by treatment with one of the monoamine oxidase (MAO) inhibitors in conjunction with psychotherapy (see Chapter 21, Drugs for Pain Management: Nonnarcotic and Narcotic Analgesics). Erectile dysfunction caused by vascular insufficiency is occasionally treated on a short-term basis by local vasoactive drugs, including papaverine, phentolamine, prostaglandin E, nitroglycerin, or yohimbine, a systemic vasoactive drug.

A recently developed class of drugs, the phosphodiesterase (PDE) inhibitors is now available. PDEs facilitate erections by enhancing blood flow to the penis. The first drug of this group available is sildenafil citrate (Viagra). The PDE inhibitors potentiate the hypotensive effects of nitrates and are contraindicated for use by any client using organic nitrates in any form. Organic nitrates include nitroglycerin, isosorbide mononitrate, isosorbide nitrate, pentaerythritol tetranitrate, erythrityl tertanitrate, isosorbide disitrate/phenobarbital, and illicit substances (amyl nitrate/nitrite, butyl nitrate). PDE inhibitors are contraindicated in clients with significant cardiovascular dis-

Table 55–3

Drugs Causing Sexual Dysfunction in Males

Drug Category	Drugs or Drug Families
Anticholinergics	atropine
	scopolamine
	benztropine
	trihexyphenidyl
Antidepressants	tricyclic antidepressants
	monoamine oxidase inhibitors
	serotonin reuptake inhibiting antidepressants (SSRIs)
Antihistamines	cimetidine
	diphenhydramine
	hydroxyzine
Antihypertensives	central sympathetic ganglion blockers
	postganglionic blockers
	alpha- and beta-receptor blockers
	diuretics
Antipsychotics	phenothiazines
	thioxanthenes
	butyrophenone
	lithium
Sedatives and social drugs	alcohol
	barbiturates
	diazepam
	chlordiazepoxide
	Cannabis
	cocaine
	opiates
	methadone
Others	aminocaproic acid
	baclofen
	steroids
	ethionamide
	perhexiline
	digoxin
	chemotherapeutic agents

ease (sildenafil citrate) or who have anatomic deformities or conditions predisposing them to priapism.

Newer phospodiesterase inhibitors are vardenafil (Levitra) and tadalafil (Cialis). Studies have shown that the newer agents are safe for clients with congestive heart failure or a history of myocardial infarctions. Thus more men have the option of using a PDE inhibitor for the treatment of erectile dysfunction. Like sildanafil, they are contraindicated if the client is taking nitrate-containing medications. Common side effect of the drugs are headache (most common), dyspepsia, nasal congestion, and nasopharyngitis. Other rare side effects can also occur, and the client should be taught about them; these effects include blurred vision; photosensitivity; changes in color perception (especially blue and green); and urinary tract symptoms such as frequency, painful urination, and cloudy or bloody urine). Clients are instructed to notify their health care provider of any side effects they experience.

The PDE inhibitors are taken before sexual activity. The differences are in the amount of time needed for the medication to start being effective and in the duration of the medication. Sildenafil has an onset of 30 to 60 minutes and a duration of 4 hours. Vardenafil's onset is 25 to 30 minutes and also has duration of 4 to 5 hours. Tadalafil has a quicker onset of 16 to 60 minutes but has a duration of up to 36 hours.

For men who do not respond to oral medications or in whom those medications are contraindicated, drugs for both intracavernous and nonintracavernous administration are available. Sublingual apomorphine (Uprima) and phentolamine (Vasomax) are examples of these medications. Some young hypogonadal men are able to resolve erectile dysfunction with testosterone replacement therapy by IM injection (testosterone cypionate, testosterone enanthate) or transdermal patches (Testoderm, Androderm, Testoderm TTS). Since the 1980s, intracavernous injection using prostaglandin E (alprostadil), papaverine with phentolamine, or a combination of all three has been a successful treatment. Intraurethral prostaglandin E (Muse) has also been effective in some men. Given the success and high efficacy of the PDE inhibitors, the use of cavernous and intraurethral medications has decreased. Vasoactive drug injections may be associated with hypotension, dizziness, pain, and priapism. Papaverine can cause hepatotoxicity.

Certain drugs are often abused by individuals seeking a heightened sexual experience. Amyl nitrate is commonly believed to be an aphrodisiac. Sudden death, myocardial infarction, and methemoglobinemia have been reported with its use. Cantharides (Spanish fly) causes bladder and urethral irritation, accounting for its use as a sexual stimulant. Permanent penile damage has been reported with its use.

Natural Products. To self-treat sexual problems or to enhance their sexual performance, clients use a wide variety of herbs and plant-derived compounds (phytochemicals). Despite new scientific-based therapies, men are attracted to phytochemicals because they are easy to obtain and may be cheaper than prescription medications, therapies, procedures, or surgeries not covered by insurance. The client may perceive natural products as providing health benefits beyond sexual performance because they can be purchased at "nutrition centers" or "health food stores."

Some common herbs used for sexual health and performance are yohimbine, ginseng, damiana, ginkgo biloba, saw palmetto, muira pauma, and tribulus terrestris. With the exception of yohimbine, which has been scientifically studied, the other compounds do not have benefits proven by research. Rather, their benefits appear to reflect popular or cultural beliefs. Reports in health magazines, booklets, and television/radio advertising are anecdotal and based on a small number of users or health care professionals.

Yohimbine, which is obtained from the bark of the African yohimbe tree, is an alpha-adrenergic antagonist that affects both the central and peripheral nervous system. Studies have shown that men experience a positive effect or improvement in erection. The side effects are headache, hypertension, sweating, anxiety, and sleeplessness. Men who have cardiovascular neurologic and psychologic problems should not take yohimbine.

Saw palmetto, a small palmlike plant found in southeast United States, has been used to treat BPH. Studies show that it is helpful in reducing the symptoms of BPH (difficult or frequent urination) and can help shrink enlarged prostate glands. Although effective in the treatment of prostate enlargement, it has not shown to exert a positive effect on sexual response in men, except if erections are inhibited by an enlarged prostate gland. In fact, saw palmetto may reduce androgen action and could cause an antisexual effect.

Ginkgo biloba leaves have been shown to treat peripheral vascular disease and enhance cerebral blood flow. Recent research suggests that ginkgo biloba may reduce antidepressant (SSRI)-induced sexual dysfunction. It is not known how it achieves these effects, and further research is needed to substantiate its use.

Ginseng has been shown to improve sexual functioning in animals, but research in humans is contradictory. Like ginkgo biloba, further human research is warranted.

Nonsexually Transmitted Infections

Urinary tract infections are addressed in Chapter 33, Drugs for Urinary Tract Disorders. If left untreated, acute or chronic prostatitis, orchitis, or epididymitis can develop.

Benign Prostate Hyperplasia

As a male ages, the glandular units in the prostate gland begin to undergo tissue hyperplasia (abnormal increase in the number of cells), resulting in prostatic hypertrophy (enlargement of the gland). The exact cause of BPH is unknown, but its development is almost universal in older men. The enlargement of the prostate gland causes pressure on the man's bladder, and he experiences lower urinary tract symptoms, such as a sensation of bladder fullness, frequency, nocturia, and hesitation, when trying to begin urinating, dribbling of urine, and erectile dysfunction. Because these are the same symptoms that prostate cancer may cause, the client will have a prostate-specific antigen (PSA) blood test and may undergo a prostate biopsy to make sure no cancer is present. Traditionally, the only effective treatment was surgical, but now drug therapy has become the initial treatment of BPH.

Finastride (Proscar) may be prescribed to shrink the prostate gland and relieve the client's symptoms. Finastride lowers the client's level of dehydrotestosterone (DHT) a major cause of prostate growth. Decreasing DHT levels may shrink the size of the prostate gland. The client is taught that it may take as long as 6 months before the client experiences relief of his symptoms.

The prostate gland has alpha-adrenergic receptors in the prostatic smooth muscle. When alpha-blocking agents are given, the prostate gland constricts, thereby decreasing the size of the gland, reducing urethral and bladder pressure, and improving urine flow.

The client with an enlarged prostate is to avoid medications that can cause urinary retention, such as anticholinergics, antihistamines, and decongestants.

Various medications used in the treatment of BPH are identified in Table 55–4.

Malignant Tumors

Prostatic cancer accounts for about 10% of all cancer deaths among American men. Most prostatic cancers are adenocarcinomas. Metastasis to lymph nodes, bone, lungs, liver, and adrenal glands is common. Prostatic cancer is often asymptomatic, but urinary obstruction is commonly

Table 55–4

Medications Used for the Treatment of Benign Prostatic Hyperplasia

Generic (Brand)	Route and Dosage	Side Effects
5 Alpha-Reductase Inhibitors		
Finasteride (Proscar)	A: PO: 5 mg daily	Decreased libido, erectile dysfunction
Duastride (Avodart, Duagen)	A: PO: 0.5 mg daily	
Alpha-Adrenergic Blocking Agents		
Tamsulosin (Flomax)	A: PO: 0.4 mg daily 30 min after a meal	Hypotension, dizziness, fatigue
Doxazosin (Cardura)	A: PO: Start 1 mg by mouth at bedtime; titrate up to 8 mg/d at bedtime	
Terazosin (Hytrin)	A: PO: Start 1 mg by mouth at bedtime; titrate up to 10 mg/d with a maximum dose of 20 mg/d	
Alfuzosin (Uroxatral)	A: PO: 10 mg daily after a meal	Postural hypotension, dizziness, fatigue
Safety in Administration		
Because the alpha-adrenergic blocking agents are also used to control blood pressure, be sure to monitor the client's medications before adding another antihypertensive medication to prevent the client from experiencing a hypotensive episode.		

d, Day; *min*, minute.

the first sign. Treatment may include a combination of surgical resection, cryotherapy, antiandrogen administration, radiation therapy, chemotherapy, and pain relief.

Testicular tumors peak in early adulthood. They include malignant germinal cell tumors and benign Leydig or Sertoli cell tumors. Treatment depends on the type and stage of tumor. Surgical excision, radiation therapy, and chemotherapy are used alone or in combination.

Of breast cancer cases, 1% occur in men—most commonly after the age of 60 years. Treatment, which is similar for men and women, entails surgery, radiation therapy, chemotherapy, and endocrine therapy. Carcinoma of the penis represents less than 1% of all malignancies among men. In situ, treatment entails local excision, radiation therapy, and local application of 5-fluorouracil cream or solution. Invasive carcinoma is treated by surgical resection of the penis and involved nodes. Radiation and chemotherapy follow as needed. Antineoplastic therapies are discussed in Unit IX, Immunologic Agents.

WEBSITES

For further information on *Drugs Related to Reproductive Health: Male Reproductive Disorders,* visit these Internet resources:

American Academy of Pediatrics: *www.aap.org*

American Cancer Society: *www.cancer.org*

American Urological Association: *www.auanet.org*

Ethnic Medicine Information: *www.ethnomed.org*

Medscape: *www.medscape.com*

National Institutes of Health: *www.health.nih.gov*

Nursing Center: *www.nursingcenter.com*

Office of Minority Health Resource Center: *www.omhrc.gov*

Sexuality Information and Education Council of the United States: *www.siecus.org*

Transcultural Nursing Society: *www.tcns.org*

Critical Thinking Case Studies

M.T., age 16, is a high school junior who is 5'3" and weighs 126 lb. He has increased feelings of discomfort about not fitting in with other students in his school because he has not yet begun sexual maturation. He is a good student and an accomplished violinist in the school orchestra. His only brother is younger than he is. His father states that he also was a "late bloomer," but he and his wife are concerned about their son's increasing social withdrawal and seem determined to seek medical intervention for him. The nurse in the clinic assesses the needs and status of M.T. and his family.

1. What is the client's primary complaint? What concerns his family?

2. What information must be included in the history and physical examination?

3. What teaching should the nurse do before the parents decide whether to start their son on androgen therapy?

The decision is made to prescribe methyltestosterone 5 mg/d by buccal tablet (held inside the cheek until it dissolves). M.T. will be on this regimen for 4 months, during which time he is to come to the clinic at monthly intervals.

4. M.T. asks why he will be treated for 4 months. What will the nurse reply?

5. About what adverse effects do M.T. and his parents need to be taught?

6. What physical and psychosocial parameters will be monitored at his monthly visits?

7. What special hygiene needs does M.T. have while on this regimen?

8. When should he have radiographs taken? Why?

9. During a clinical visit, M.T. mentions that he has heard that the use of anabolic steroids might improve his chances of making the wrestling team. What should he be told about the safety and efficacy of anabolic steroid use?

Mr. J. is a 70-year-old Hispanic man who came into the urgent care clinic complaining of being unable to empty his bladder. He has noticed over the past few months that he has had to get up two or three times during the night to urinate; sometimes he dribbles urine after he finishes urinating. He also mentions that his "plumbing isn't what it used to be" but does not seem to want to discuss it. He asks whether a male doctor is on duty today.

1. When interviewing this client, what should be the focus of the assessment?

2. How would you explain his symptoms to him?

3. What are some of the age and cultural related issues affecting this client's ability to communicate?

4. What laboratory tests would be appropriate for this client?

5. What are some of the drug options available to Mr. J.?

Study Questions

1. What are the relationships among gonadotropin-releasing hormone, follicle-stimulating hormone, luteinizing hormone, and the gonadal hormones?

2. What are some desired effects of androgen therapy?

3. Why would healthy adolescents abuse androgens?

4. What is the role of androgen therapy in the treatment of breast cancer?

5. What physical parameters are measured during androgen therapy?

6. In what clients must extra care be taken when androgen therapy is used?

7. What is an indication for antiandrogen therapy?

8. What are two reasons for treatment of cryptorchidism early in life?

9. What are the stages of the sexual response cycle? Which stages are most important for fertility in men and women?

10. What are 10 commonly used medications that can impair male sexual function?

11. What two precautions should men be taught when they are prescribed sildenafil citrate (Viagra)?

12. What are some of the symptoms of an enlarged prostate?

13. What are some of the medications that can be used to shrink the prostate?

14. What herbal medications might a man use in an attempt to enhance his sexual performance?

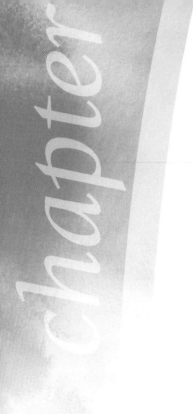

56 Drugs Related to Reproductive Health: Infertility and Sexually Transmitted Diseases

SANDRA ELLIOTT

ELECTRONIC RESOURCES

Additional information can be found on the companion website at *http://evolve.elsevier.com/KeeHayes/pharmacology/* or on the companion CD-ROM, which includes:

- *NCLEX-style examination review questions*
- *Pharmacology animations*
- *Medication error and IV therapy checklists*
- *Medication calculation problems*
- *Electronic calculators*

OUTLINE

OBJECTIVES

- Describe male, female, and couple causes of infertility.
- Instruct couples on the relationships among ovulatory stimulation therapy, fertility awareness, and timing of coitus.
- Describe the way in which ovulatory stimulants promote fertility.
- Identify clients at risk for acquiring sexually transmitted diseases (STDs).
- Describe the relationship among STDs and infertility.
- Instruct clients in regimens for common STDs.
- Plan management for STDs for which cures do not exist.
- Counsel health care workers about management of worksite exposure to blood-borne STDs.
- Describe the nursing process, including client teaching, related to drugs used for infertility and STDs.

TERMS

endometritis
epididymitis
infertility
orchitis

ovulation
pelvic inflammatory
    disease (PID)
perinatal infection

pregnancy wastage
primary infertility
prostatitis
secondary infertility

sexually transmitted
    diseases (STDs)
vertical transmission

Introduction

This chapter discusses drug regimens for two broad categories of reproductive health alterations that are often interrelated: infertility and sexually transmitted diseases (STDs). Alterations in fertility reflect a wide range of developmental, endocrine, infectious, inflammatory, hypertrophic, and psychoemotional processes. Drug therapies used in the management of female and, briefly, male infertility are addressed, with emphasis on ovulation stimulants.

The broad category of diseases that are sexually transmitted constitutes a threat to reproductive tract integrity and functioning, as well as to neonatal health. Some STDs, such as the human immunodeficiency virus (HIV), are life-threatening in and of themselves. Drug therapies for these conditions are briefly reviewed.

Drugs Related to Infertility Treatment

Infertility is defined as the inability to conceive a child after 12 months of unprotected sexual intercourse. Women older than 35 years of age may be considered infertile after a shorter trial. Infertility is considered **primary infertility** if a couple has never conceived and **secondary infertility** if

they have conceived. **Pregnancy wastage** exists if the woman has conceived but never produced a live birth.

Most pharmacologic approaches today are **ovulation** inducing agents; that is, they stimulate the maturation and release of eggs.

Assessing Infertility

Causes of infertility (Table 56–1) are numerous. In about 15% of cases, no specific cause can be found. Up to 40% of cases are the result of STDs, which may result in neonatal death or altered reproductive tract integrity. Treatment of infertility depends on assessment of the cause.

General health is assessed; nutritional, reproductive, social drugs, and sexual histories are taken; and physical examinations with routine laboratory tests are conducted on both partners. Common tests to determine the specific causes of infertility are listed in Table 56–2.

Induction of Ovulation

Clomiphene citrate (Serophene, Clomid), an estrogen antagonist, blocks the negative hypothalamic-pituitary-gonadal feedback loop. The feedback mechanism is altered as clomiphene binds to estrogen receptors, resulting in increased gonadotropin-releasing hormone

Table 56-1

Causes of Infertility

Female Factors	
Genetic	Chromosomal abnormalities, enzyme defects
Tubal or peritoneal	Infection, occlusion, fimbrial damage, pelvic adhesions, endometriosis
Ovarian	Anovulation, oligo-ovulation, inadequate luteal phase, polycystic ovarian syndrome (PCOS)
Cervical	Cervicitis, poor-quality cervical mucus, diethylstilbestrol exposure
Uterine	Uterine fibromas, congenital malformations, adhesions, endometrial abnormalities
Endocrine	Panhypopituitarism, hypothyroidism, adrenal insufficiency, congenital adrenal hyperplasia, Cushing's disease, cirrhosis, hyperprolactinemia, hormone receptor defects
Other	Age, drugs, malnutrition, excess alcohol intake, tobacco use
Male Factors	
Genetic	Chromosomal genetic abnormalities
Seminal	Failure of semen to liquefy, inadequate volume, low sperm count, decreased or erratic sperm motility, sperm dysmorphology, varicocele
Transport	Hypospadias, micropenis, retrograde ejaculation, epididymitis, impotence, ductal occlusion, ductal adhesions
Testicular	Oligospermia/azoospermia, cryptorchism, testicular agenesis, history of high fever, postpubertal orchitis, testicular injury/surgery, varicocele
Endocrine	Panhypopituitarism, hypothyroidism, adrenal insufficiency, congenital adrenal hyperplasia, Cushing's disease, cirrhosis, hormone receptor abnormalities
Other	Age, drugs, excess alcohol intake, tobacco use, pollution, malnutrition, scrotal heat exposure, autoimmunity to sperm, infectious processes, allergies
Couple Factors	Sexual technique, frequency or timing of intercourse, immune response to sperm

Table 56–2

Common Tests for Infertility

Test	Purpose
Physical examination	Assess secondary sex characteristics, reproductive tract function, and patency by gross examination
Hematology, liver and renal function	Rule out disease processes
Hysterosalpingogram, tubal insufflation	Evaluate fallopian tube patency
Cervical mucus test	Assess viscosity of mucus and its effect on sperm motility
Plasma progesterone	Assess function of corpus luteum
Endometrial biopsy	Assess ovulatory status or adequacy of corpus luteum
Semen analysis	Check number, structure, movement of sperm
Basal body temperature	Determine whether ovulation occurs; document temperatures daily in chart
Sperm penetration assay	Determine ability of sperm to penetrate and fertilize ovum
Laparoscopy	Visualize female pelvic organs
Hysteroscopy	Visualize uterus
Echohysteroscopy	Assess structure of woman's internal reproductive organs
Hormone assays	Gn-RH, FSH, LH, progesterone, estrogen, prolactin, testosterone, thyroid hormone levels
Immunologic testing	Assess cervical immunity against sperm, seminal fluid immunity against sperm, serum antisperm antibodies in either partner
Imaging	Pituitary integrity

FSH, Follicle-stimulating hormone; *Gn-RH*, gonadotropin-releasing hormone; *LH*, luteinizing hormone.

(Gn-RH) release and then increased luteinizing hormone (LH) and follicle-stimulating hormone (FSH) output. It is the most commonly used ovulation stimulant (Prototype Drug Chart 56–1). Some women may need concurrent treatment of hyperinsulinemia. Women with high circulatory androgens may be concurrently treated with dexamethasone.

Recombinant FSH and LH as well as human chorionic gonadotropin (hCG) are now available to normalize hormone levels with minimal adverse effects (Table 56–3). These drugs normalize FSH and LH levels to stimulate follicle maturation, ovulation, and development of the corpus luteum. The replacement of FSH or LH is enhanced in a few women by the use of leuprolide acetate before the administration of hCG and, in other women, by the use of a Gn-RH agonist such as progesterone after ovulation. In a small percentage of amenorrheic women, an elevated level of prolactin is the causative factor. A portion of these women can be treated with the ergot derivative bromocriptine (taken 2.5 mg twice daily). Bromocriptine binds to dopamine receptors in the pituitary and inhibits prolactin secretion; treatment continues until pregnancy is confirmed. Clomiphene can be introduced if needed after 2 months.

Pharmacokinetics

Data on the pharmacokinetics of clomiphene citrate are limited, but clomiphene is readily absorbed from the gastrointestinal (GI) tract. It is partially metabolized in the liver and excreted in the feces via biliary elimination. Clomiphene has a half-life of about 5 days.

Pharmacodynamics

The mechanism of action of clomiphene is unknown, but it is hypothesized that it competes with estrogen at receptor sites. The perception of decreased circulating estrogen by the hypothalamus and pituitary triggers the negative feedback response that increases the secretion of FSH and

LH. The results are ovarian stimulation, maturation of the ovarian follicle, and development of the corpus luteum.

Side Effects

Side effects of clomiphene citrate include breast discomfort, fatigue, dizziness, depression, nausea, vomiting, increased appetite, weight gain, dermatitis, urticaria, anxiety, restlessness, weakness, heavier menses, vasomotor flushing, abdominal bloating or pain, and gas (see Prototype Drug Chart 56–1). Antiestrogenic effects include interference with endometrial maturation and cervical mucus production. Paradoxically, this may interfere with fertilization or implantation.

Adverse Reactions

Adverse reactions include photophobia, mastalgia, diplopia, and decreased visual acuity. Ovarian hyperstimulation may result in ovarian enlargement, midcycle ovarian pain, and cysts. Reversible hair loss has been noted. Multiple gestation occurs in up to 12% of women who become pregnant. The effect of clomiphene citrate on fetal development is unclear. Neural tube defects have been reported but have not been confirmed by controlled studies. Adverse reactions of other ovulatory stimulants are listed in Table 56–4.

Contraindications

Contraindications for treatment with clomiphene citrate include undiagnosed vaginal bleeding, pregnancy, uterine fibroids, mental depression, history of hepatic dysfunction or thromboembolic disease, and primary pituitary or ovarian failure. If the woman has ovarian cysts, clomiphene citrate may cause them to enlarge. Contraindications to the use of other ovulatory stimulants are listed in Table 56–4.

PROTOTYPE DRUG CHART 56–1

CLOMIPHENE CITRATE

Drug Class	**Dosage**
Ovulation stimulant Trade Name: Clomid, Milophene, Serophene *Pregnancy Category:* X	**A: PO:** 50-100 mg/d for days 5-9 of cycle If ovulation does not occur with 50 mg/d, increase next course to 100 mg/d.
Contraindications	**Drug-Lab-Food Interactions**
Pregnancy, undiagnosed vaginal bleeding, depression, fibroids, hepatic dysfunction, thrombophlebitis, primary pituitary or ovarian failure	***Drug:*** None are significant; danazol may inhibit re- sponse; *decrease* effects of ethinyl estradiol **Lab:** *Increase* in serum thyroxine
Pharmacokinetics	**Pharmacodynamics**
Absorption: Readily absorbed from GI tract **Distribution:** PB: UK **Metabolism:** t½: 5-8 d **Excretion:** In feces	**PO:** Onset: 5-14 d Peak: UK Duration: UK

Therapeutic Effects/Uses

To stimulate ovarian follicle growth
Mode of Action: Stimulates release of follicle-stimulating hormone (FSH) and luteinizing hormone (LH)

Side Effects	**Adverse Reactions**
Breast discomfort, fatigue, dizziness, depression, anxiety, nausea, vomiting, constipation, increased appetite, headache, flatulence, multiple gestation, hot flashes, fluid retention	Visual disturbances, abdominal pain, weight gain, hair loss, ovarian hyperstimulation, anxiety, ovarian cysts, ectopic pregnancy

A, Adult; *d,* day; *GI,* gastrointestinal; *PB,* protein-binding; *PO,* by mouth; *t½,* half-life; *UK,* unknown.

Table 56–3

Ovulatory Stimulants

Generic (Brand)	Route and Dosage	Use and Considerations
bromocriptine mesylate (Parlodel)	Up to 7.5 mg/d in divided doses	Normalizes prolactin levels. Possibly teratogenic. *Pregnancy category:* C; PB: 92%; t½: 50 h
clomiphene citrate (Clomid, Serophene)	See Prototype Drug Chart 56–1.	
Gn-RH	1-10 mcg/60-120 min via pump	Induces ovulation in women with hypothalamic amenorrhea. Ovarian hyperstimulation is a risk. Pregnancy loss is common. *Pregnancy category:* X; PB: UK; t½: 11-23 h
recombinant FSH (Puregon, Gonal-F, Follistim), recombinant LH (LHadi), recombinant hCG (Ovidrel)	IM: 1-2 ampules/d × 5-12 d until follicle maturation; next day, hCG (5000-10,000 interna- tional units IM) administered	Ovarian hyperstimulation remains a risk, though min- imal, with recombinant products. Multiple gesta- tion is a risk, which is reduced by careful monitor- ing. PB: UK; t½: 23-77 h IM, 13-35 h subQ

d, Day; *FSH,* follicle-stimulating hormone; *Gn-RH,* gonadotropin-releasing hormone; *h,* hour; *hCG,* human chorionic gonadotropin; *IM,* intramuscular; *LH,* luteinizing hormone; *min,* minute; *subQ,* subcutaneous; *t½,* half-life; *UK,* unknown.

Drug Interactions

There are no known significant drug interactions with
clomiphene citrate. Danazol may inhibit client response to
clomiphene citrate, and clomiphene citrate may suppress
response to ethinyl estradiol. There are no known drug interactions with human menopausal gonadotropin (hMG)
or hCG.

Other Drug Treatments

Other pharmacologic approaches for the treatment of
women with infertility include the use of pulsatile exogenous Gn-RH. In addition, hypothyroidism or hyperthyroidism and adrenal dysfunction must be treated. Endometriosis can be treated with a course of danazol to
suppress gonadotropin output. Women with inadequate

Table 56–4

Side Effects, Adverse Reactions, and Contraindications for Selected Infertility Drugs

Side Effects	Adverse Reactions	Contraindications
Human Chorionic Gonadotropin		
Headache, irritability, restlessness, fatigue, depression, fluid retention, pain at injection site	Ovarian hyperstimulation syndrome, rupture of ovarian cysts, multiple births, arterial thromboembolism	Androgen-dependent neoplasms. Caution in clients with asthma, cardiac or renal disease, epilepsy, migraine
Bromocriptine Mesylate		
Nausea, vomiting, headache, dizziness, drowsiness, fatigue, light-headedness, nasal congestion, diarrhea, insomnia, depression	Confusion, visual disturbances, vertigo, shortness of breath, abdominal discomfort, involuntary movements, hypotension, anxiety, dysphagia, paresthesia, blepharospasm, mottling, urinary frequency, epileptiform seizures, ergotism. Transient elevations in BUN, SGOT, SGPT, creatine phosphokinase, alkaline phosphatase, serum uric acid	Ischemic heart disease, peripheral vascular disease, pregnancy, lactation, ergot nervousness, sensitivity. Caution in hypotension, epilepsy, psychoses, cardiac arrhythmia, impaired hepatic or renal function

BUN, Blood urea nitrogen; *SGOT,* serum glutamic-oxaloacetic transaminase; *SGPT,* serum glutamate pyruvate transaminase.

HERBAL ALERT 56–1

Herbs and Male Infertility

🔹 *Saw palmetto* may cause metabolic changes in the sperm.
🔹 *St. John's wort* may cause effects on sperm cells, decreased sperm motility, and decreased viability.

luteal-phase progesterone output are treated with progesterone 25 mg twice daily intravaginally or 12.5 mg intramuscularly (IM).

Drug Therapy for Male Infertility

For most infertile men, no specific causal factor can be identified. These clients are identified as having idiopathic oligospermia and asthenospermia. There is no documented cost-effective treatment for this large group of men. Most drug regimens used have shown little promise in controlled studies, with the exception of using testosterone (or other hormonal) therapy to attain physiologic levels. Assisted reproductive techniques currently appear to hold more promise than drug therapy. In addition, some herbal products contribute to male infertility problems (Herbal Alert 56–1).

Nursing Process

Infertility

■ Infertility management is a highly specialized field. Nurses are most likely to encounter clients when they are in the process of trying to identify the possible causes of their infertility. Nurses need to be sensitive to the guilt, decreased self-esteem, and embarrassment that infertility may cause. Treatment of infertility requires that the health care team direct a couple's sexual life. Evaluation and

intervention are often uncomfortable and expensive, and there is no guarantee that a viable pregnancy will result. The process drains the couple emotionally and economically.

ASSESSMENT

■ A general health history, including documenting drug and herbal product use, and physical examination are required. Clients' reproductive and sexual histories are assessed, with attention to the timing and technique of coitus.
■ The couple undergoes an exhaustive battery of diagnostic tests to evaluate the cause of infertility. Once this is determined, conditions that contraindicate the treatment of choice are ruled out.
■ It is particularly important that the couple's interpretation of their infertility be explored, along with its impact on their relationship. The nurse should help the couple discuss their feelings in a safe, supportive environment.

NURSING DIAGNOSES

■ Ineffective sexuality patterns
■ Disturbed body image
■ Situational low self-esteem
■ Deficient knowledge related to treatment regimen

PLANNING

■ Short-term goals include clients' adherence to the medical regimen with minimal adverse effects.
■ The long-term goal is the achievement of pregnancy or the consideration of alternatives to pregnancy with the partners' self-esteem and relationship intact.

NURSING INTERVENTIONS

General

- Interventions are aimed at helping clients understand the interrelationships among and timing of menses, ovulation, and coitus as they relate to conception. In addition, they need to know sexual techniques that enhance fertilization, such as the placement of a pillow under the woman's hips during coitus and the placement of the woman in a supine position with the hips elevated for about 30 minutes after her partner ejaculates. In addition, clients and their partners need to understand the treatment regimen.

Specific

- Female client is taught to report adverse effects such as abdominal pain or visual disturbances to her infertility specialist at once and to be cautious with tasks that require alertness. If she misses a dose of her medication, she should call her infertility specialist.
- Clients need to understand that treatment increases the chance of multiple births.

Client Teaching

- Couples need to be taught how to evaluate and record on a chart the basal body temperature and changes in the cervical mucus. The first day of menses is day 1 of the cycle. Ovulation is predicted by a 0.5° F drop in basal body temperature followed by a 1° F rise. In addition, over-the-counter diagnostic kits for assessing ovulatory status can be used to time coitus. The couple is advised to engage in coitus no more frequently than every other day from 4 days before to 3 days after ovulation to maximize the man's sperm count (Figure 56–1).
- The man is advised to wear boxer shorts during infertility treatment because briefs hold the scrotum close to the body and the heat reduces the sperm count. For the same reason, if he is seated all day in his work, he is counseled to take breaks every hour or so to walk about. Some women have conceived by taking guaifenesin (Robitussin) because it thins the cervical mucus.
- The man is advised to avoid the use of certain herbs that impact sperm production. See Herbal Alert 56–1.
- The woman is advised to take her medication at the same time each day to maintain steady blood levels.

Cultural Considerations ⊕

- Because of their modesty, many Chinese and Filipino women will only be examined by a female health care provider. Individuals frequently combine traditional Chinese medicine with western medicine.
- Amish view pregnancy (and the anticipated baby) as a gift from God and want to have many gifts. They may be reluctant to seek help for infertility, especially to go to a health care provider "outside the community." They often use herbal remedies and folk practices.
- Use an interpreter as appropriate; one of the same gender and culture is preferred for sensitive topics.
- In male-dominated cultures, the male may be unwilling to undergo an infertility evaluation because it is seen only as a female problem.

EVALUATION

- ■ Successful outcomes of fertility treatment include avoidance of ovarian hyperstimulation as well as other untoward effects. The achievement of pregnancy that results in the birth of a live infant fulfills the objectives of treatment. If pregnancy is not achieved, intervention is aimed at helping the couple consider alternatives to childbearing without adverse impact on their self-esteem or harm to their relationship.

Drugs Used in the Treatment of Sexually Transmitted Diseases

Sexually transmitted diseases (STDs) are infections that are transmitted during sexual contact. Some pathogens are spread primarily through sexual contact. Others, such as *Shigella*, hepatitis A, or *Candida*, are transmitted primarily by other ways but can also be spread sexually. Pathogens implicated in STDs are listed in Table 56–5. Depending on the causative organism, STDs may be localized in lesions of the skin or mucosa. They may spread upward through the reproductive tract, resulting in **pelvic inflammatory disease (PID)** or **endometritis** (intrauterine infection) in women or in **prostatitis** (infection of the prostate), **epididymitis** (infection of the epididymis), or **orchitis** (infection of the testicles) in men. Finally, blood and secretions may spread STDs. If not treated, STDs can result in (1) damage to the male and female reproductive tracts, thus impairing fertility; (2) life-threatening illness and death; and (3) neonatal illness and death. The past 30 years have seen a dramatic increase in this problem. The emergence of STDs that are incurable or lethal in adults, such as genital herpes and HIV infection, has led to growing awareness of the seriousness of STDs, even in affluent, industrialized countries. Several infections, including those caused by HIV, human papillomavirus (HPV), human T-lymphotrophic virus, and Epstein-Barr virus, are associated with malignancies. *Chlamydia trachomatis* has been linked to heart disease and cervical cancer.

Transmission and Risk

Sexual transmission of pathogens can occur through breaks in the vaginal or cervical mucosa or the skin covering the shaft or glans of the penis. Each act of coitus results in tiny, friction-induced fissures on these surfaces. This problem is exacerbated by inadequate vaginal lubrication, which may occur postmenopausally, postpartally, just following menses, or when the woman is not sufficiently aroused before penetration.

1. Purchase a special thermometer calibrated in tenths of degrees between 96° and 100° F.
2. Place the thermometer under the tongue for at least a full 3 minutes (preferably 5 minutes) after waking in the morning and before *any* activity (e.g., lifting your head off the pillow, shaking thermometer down, intercourse, or urinating) **or before you eat or drink anything.**
3. If you forget to take your temperature and have already gotten up, *do not take it.* Write *missed* on that day.
4. Take your temperature in the same manner about the same time each day.
5. Carefully record the reading on the graph by placing a dot at the proper location. Start this chart on the first day of your period.
6. Insert the month and day in the space provided.
7. The first day of menstrual flow is considered to be the start of a cycle (day 1). Each day of flow should be indicated with an M on the graph, starting at extreme left under number 1 day of cycle.
8. Record any obvious reason for temperature variation such as a cold, flu, or infection on the graph above the reading for that day.
9. If you are placed on medication, please indicate it in the space labeled medications on the days you take it.
10. If you feel you have menstrually related symptoms, such as breast tenderness or cramping, note these also.
11. If intercourse has taken place during the previous 24 hours, mark it with an (X).

Calendar for Thermal Method of Fertility Awareness

Day of Cycle: 1 2 3 4 5 6 7 8 9 10 11 12 13 14 15 16 17 18 19 20 21 22 23 24 25 26 27 28 29 30 31

Temperature
   99.0
   98.8
   98.6
   98.4
   98.2
   98.0
   97.8
   97.6
   97.4
   97.2
   97.0

Menses (M):
Intercourse (X):

Mucus
   Color
   Consistency
   Amount

Other factors
   Medications
   Breast tenderness
   Cramps

FIGURE 56-1 Instructions for keeping a sympothermal record. (Adapted from Fogel CI, Lauver D: *Sexual health promotion*, Philadelphia, 1990, Saunders.)

Table 56-5

Pathogens Causing Sexually Transmitted Diseases

Pathogen	Mode of Transmission		
	Predominantly Sexual	**Can Be Sexual**	**Sexual Contact with Oral-Fecal Exposure**
Bacteria	*Calymmatobacterium granulomatis*	*Escherichia coli*	*Shigella*
	Chlamydia trachomatis	*Gardnerella vaginalis*	*Campylobacter*
	Haemophilus ducreyi	Other vaginal bacteria	
	Neisseria gonorrhoeae	Group B streptococcus	
	Treponema pallidum	*Mycoplasma hominis*	
	Ureaplasma urealyticum		
Viruses	Cytomegalovirus	Human T-lymphotrophic virus-1	Hepatitis A
	HIV-1, HIV-2	Hepatitis C, D	
	Hepatitis B	Herpes simplex virus type 1	
	Herpes simplex virus type 2	Epstein-Barr virus	
	Human papillomavirus		
	Molluscum contagiosum virus		
Protozoa, fungi, ectoparasites	*Trichomonas vaginalis*	*Candida albicans*	*Giardia lamblia*
	Phthirus pubis		*Entamoeba histolytica*
	Sarcoptes scabiei		

HIV, Human immunodeficiency virus.

Semen, sperm cells themselves, vaginal secretions, blood, and other body fluids can carry pathogens. Skin and mucosal lesions cannot only be penetrated by microorganisms but also shed them. Sexual contact can involve skin to skin, mouth to mouth, oral-genital, oral-anal, or hand-anal transmission of pathogens through breaks in the skin or mucosal surfaces or from inoculation by infectious body fluids. Anal penetration is particularly risky because of the likelihood of tissue trauma that results in the partner's exposure to enteric microorganisms.

One practice that places individuals at high risk for the transmission of STDs, particularly HIV, is engaging in sexual activity with multiple partners. Investigators at the National Institutes of Health suggest that the risk of acquiring STDs is markedly increased among individuals who have more than one sexual partner per year versus those who have fewer partners. Other high-risk practices are anal or vaginal intercourse without a condom, hand-anal contact, blood contact during sexual activity during menses, the use of an enema before anal intercourse, and urination on broken skin or inside the body. Risk-reducing behaviors are listed in Box 56–1.

STDs are often manifested as multiple infections. Individuals undergoing treatment for one STD should be assessed for others, including HIV. This is especially true if genital or perianal ulcerations are present.

Vertical transmission, or **perinatal infection,** occurs when a fetus or neonate is infected by the mother. Microbes can travel up the reproductive tract from the vagina or cervix and enter the intrauterine environment. Organisms

---

BOX 56–1

Risk-Reducing Behaviors for Avoidance of STDs

- Sexual abstinence or sexual contact with one faithful partner
- Washing and urinating before and after intercourse
- Consistently using a condom
- Avoiding sex with someone who has genital or anal lesions
- Reducing use of alcohol or drugs, both of which impair judgment about sexual risk and immune response
- Avoiding sexual contact with HIV-infected persons, users of intravenous drugs, immigrants from high-prevalence regions, or sexual partners of all such individuals
- Never sharing hypodermic needles or razors

---

that are of little consequence to healthy adults can be devastating to a fetus. Transmission can occur through contact with the mother's blood at birth or through breast milk, as in the case of HIV and hepatitis B virus. Many STDs, such as syphilis, are transmitted transplacentally. Others, such as infection with herpes simplex virus type 2 (HSV-2), require actual contact by the infant with microorganisms in the birth canal. Because of the risk of blindness caused by *Chlamydia trachomatis* and *Neisseria gonorrhoeae*, erythromycin is routinely used to treat the eyes of neonates.

Common STD syndromes and their causative pathogens are listed in Table 56–6. Current guidelines from the Centers for Disease Control and Prevention (CDC) for the primary treatment of various STDs are listed in Table 56–7. All sexual

---

Table 56–6

Common Sexually Transmitted Disease Syndromes and Their Causative Pathogens

Syndrome	Pathogens
Acute arthritis	*Neisseria gonorrhoeae, Chlamydia trachomatis,* hepatitis B virus (HBV), human immunodeficiency virus (HIV)
Acquired immunodeficiency virus	HIV-1, HIV-2, and opportunistic pathogens
Cervicitis	*C. trachomatis, N. gonorrhoeae,* herpes simplex virus (HSV), *Candida albicans*
Cystitis, urethritis (female)	Gram-negative bacilli, gram-positive cocci, *C. trachomatis, N. gonorrhoeae*
Epididymitis	*C. trachomatis, N. gonorrhoeae*
Genital, anal warts	Human papillomavirus (HPV)
Lymphadenopathy	Cytomegalovirus (CMV), HIV, Epstein-Barr virus (EBV)
Neoplasias	HPV
Squamous cell cancers of cervix, anus, vulva, penis; Kaposi's sarcoma; lymphoid neoplasia, hepatocellular carcinoma	HIV, EBV HIV, human T-lymphotrophic virus (HTLV-1)
Pelvic inflammatory disease	*Trichomonas vaginalis, N. gonorrhoeae, C. trachomatis, Bacteroides* spp, peptostreptococci, *Escherichia coli,* streptococci groups B and D, bacterial vaginitis-associated pathogens
Proctitis, proctocolitis or enterocolitis, enteritis	*N. gonorrhoeae,* HSV, *C. trachomatis, Treponema pallidum, Giardia lamblia, Campylobacter* spp, *Shigella* spp, *Entamoeba histolytica, Mycobacterium avium-intracellulare, Salmonella* spp, *Cryptosporidium, Isospora* (ingestion of intestinal flora)
Pubic lice	*Phthirus pubis*
Scabies	*Sarcoptes scabiei*
Ulcerative lesions of the genitalia	HSV-1, HSV-2, *T. pallidum, C. trachomatis, Calymmatobacterium granulomatis,* HPV, *Haemophilus ducreyi,* molluscum contagiosum virus
Urethritis, male	*N. gonorrhoeae, C. trachomatis, T. vaginalis,* HSV, *Ureaplasma urealyticum, Mycoplasma hominis, Bacteroides urealyticum*
Vulvovaginitis	Bacterial vaginosis: *Gardnerella vaginitis (Haemophilus vaginalis), M. hominis, U. urealyticum, Mobiluncus curtisii, Mobiluncus mulieris, Bacteroides* spp, peptostreptococci, *T. vaginalis, C. albicans, Torulopsis glabrata*

Table 56–7

Current Guidelines for Primary Therapies for Common Sexually Transmitted Diseases

Disease	Primary Therapy	Notes
Acute urethral syndrome	doxycycline 100 mg PO b.i.d. × 7 d *or* sulfamethoxazole 1.6 g plus trimethoprim 320 mg PO single dose	
Bacterial vaginosis	metronidazole 500 mg PO b.i.d. × 7 d *or* 2 g PO single dose *or* vaginal gel b.i.d. × 5 d	Avoid alcohol during therapy; contraindicated in pregnancy.
Candidiasis	fluconazole 150 mg PO × 1 dose *or* miconazole nitrate 200 mg vaginal suppository qhs × 3 d *or* miconazole nitrate 2% vaginal cream, 5 g, qhs × 3 d *or* clotrimazole 200 mg, vaginal suppository, daily × 3 d	Recurrent candidiasis may be indicative of other disease, such as diabetes or HIV infection.
Chancroid	azithromycin 1 g PO × 1 dose *or* ceftriaxone 250 mg IM × 1 *or* erythromycin base 500 mg PO q.i.d. × 7 d	Use compresses to remove necrotic material; clean ulcerative lesions t.i.d.
Chlamydia	A: doxycycline 100 mg PO b.i.d. × 7-10 d *or* azithromycin 1 g PO × 1	
	C: <45 kg: erythromycin 50 mg/kg/d PO divided in 4 doses × 10-14 d	
	C: >45 kg: erythromycin base 500 mg PO q.i.d. × 7 d *or* erythromycin succinate 800 mg PO b.i.d. × 7 d	
	Infants: erythromycin 50 mg/kg/d PO divided into 4 doses × 10-14 d	A second course of therapy may be required.
Epididymitis	ceftriaxone 250 mg IM × 1 *and* doxycycline 100 mg PO b.i.d. × 10 d *or* ofloxacin 300 mg b.i.d. × 10 d	Treat for gonorrhea, then follow with treatment for nongonococcal urethritis.
Genital warts	Cryotherapy *or* cryoprobe *or* podofilox 0.5% solution b.i.d. × 3 d, then 4 days off; repeat cycle × 4 *or* podophyllin 10%-25% in compound tincture of benzoin × 1/wk × 6 wk	Nothing eradicates HPV; podophyllin contraindicated during pregnancy.
	Imiquimod 5% cream, applied once daily at bedtime, 3/wk for up to 16 wk. Treatment should be washed with soap and water 6-10 h after the application.	Safety during pregnancy has not been established
Gonorrhea	ceftriaxone 125 mg IM × 1 *or* ciprofloxacin 500 mg PO × 1 *or* ofloxacin 400 mg PO × 1 *or* levofloxacin 250 mg PO × 1	*Plus* Azithromycin 1 g PO × 1 *or* Doxycycline 100 mg PO b.i.d. × 7 *if chlamydia is not ruled out*
	C: <45 kg: ceftriaxone 125 mg IM × 1 *or* ceftriaxone 50 mg/kg IM/IV (*max:* 1 g) daily × 7 d	Ciprofloxacin or ofloxacin should not be used in men who have sex with men, or if they, or their partners have traveled to Asia, the Pacific Islands, and the Pacific coastal states of the U.S.
		Pregnant women: see complete CDC guidelines Treat for *Chlamydia* as well.
	Ophthalmia neonatorum: ceftriaxone 25-50 mg/kg IM/IV × 1 (*max:* 125 mg)	Neonate may also have scalp abscess at site of fetal monitors, rhinitis, anorectal infection.
	Ophthalmia neonatorum prophylaxis: silver nitrate (1%) aqueous × 1 *or* erythromycin (0.5%) ophthalmic ointment × 1 *or* tetracycline ophthalmic ointment (1%) × 1	
Granuloma inguinale	doxycycline 100 mg PO b.i.d. × 7-28 d *or* erythromycin 500 mg q.i.d. PO × 14 d	
Hepatitis A	No specific therapy exists	Vaccine available. Should be offered to high-risk individuals (men who have sex with men, or injection drug users).
Hepatitis B	HAV and HBV are the only two STDs for which a vaccine exists	The CDC recommends vaccination of all infants and adolescents. ACIP recommends vaccination of all persons with recent STD and those with more than one partner in the last 6 mo. A combined hepatitis A and B vaccine has been developed for adults.
Hepatitis C	Alpha interferon and oral agent ribavirin may be used to treat HCV chronic liver disease	No vaccine available.

A, Adult; *ACIP*, Advisory Committee on Immunization Practices; *b.i.d.*, twice a day; *C*, child; *CDC*, Centers for Disease Control and Prevention; *d*, day; *GI*, gastrointestinal; *h*, hour; *HAV*, hepatitis A virus; *HBV*, hepatitis B virus; *HCV*, hepatitis C virus; *HIV*, human immunodeficiency virus; *HPV*, human papillomavirus; *IM*, intramuscular; *IUD*, intrauterine device; *IV*, intravenous; *max*, maximum; *min*, minute; *mo*, month; *PO*, by mouth; *qhs*, every hour of sleep; *q.i.d.*, four times a day; *STD*, sexually transmitted disease; *t.i.d.*, three times a day; *wk*, week; *y*, year; >, greater than; <, less than. The most recent guidelines and alternative treatments are available from *www.cdc. gov/STD/treatment/*.

Table 56–7

Current Guidelines for Primary Therapies for Common Sexually Transmitted Diseases—cont'd

Disease	Primary Therapy	Notes
Genital herpes simplex	*First episode:* acyclovir 400 mg PO t.i.d. × 7-10 d *or* famciclovir 250 mg PO t.i.d. x 7-10 d *or* valacyclovir 1 g PO b.i.d. × 7-10 d *Recurrent episode:* acyclovir 400 mg PO t.i.d. × 5 d *or* famciclovir 125 mg PO b.i.d. × 5 d *or* valacyclovir 500 mg PO b.i.d. × 3-5 d *Suppressive therapy:* acyclovir 400 mg PO b.i.d. QD *or* famciclovir 250 mg b.i.d. QD *or* valacyclovir 500 mg PO QD *Severe:* acyclovir 5-10 mg/kg IV q8h × 5-7 d *Immunocompromised:* acyclovir 400 mg PO × 3-5/d until resolution *Neonatal:* acyclovir 30 mg/kg/d	Types 1 and 2 cannot be distinguished clinically. No cure is known. Systemic disease is life-threatening to neonates, and neurologic damage may result. Viral shedding is most prevalent when symptomatic; sexual relations should be avoided at that time.
Lymphogranuloma venereum	doxycycline 100 mg PO b.i.d. × 21 d *or* erythromycin 0.5 gm PO q.i.d. × 21 d	
Molluscum contagiosum	Cryoanesthesia and curettage *or* caustic chemicals (podophyllin, trichloroacetic acid, silver nitrate) and cryotherapy	If all lesions not eradicated, may recur.
Mucopurulent cervicitis	doxycycline 100 mg PO b.i.d. × 7-10 d	
Nongonococcal urethritis	doxycycline 100 mg PO b.i.d. × 7 d *or* erythromycin 500 mg PO q.i.d. × 7 d *or* azithromycin 1 g PO × 1 dose	
Pelvic inflammatory disease (PID)	*Inpatient:* doxycycline 100 mg IV b.i.d. *and* cefoxitin 2 g IV q.i.d. *or* cefotetan 2 g IV q.i.d. *48 h after clinical improvement:* doxycycline 100 mg PO b.i.d. for total of at least 14 d therapy *Ambulatory care:* ofloxacin 400 mg b.i.d. *plus* metronidazole 500 mg b.i.d. × 14 d *or* ceftriaxone 250 mg IM × 1 *plus* doxycycline 100 mg PO b.i.d. × 14 d *or* trovafloxacin 200 mg PO × 14 d	Often polymicrobial. This regimen may not treat anaerobes, pelvic mass, or IUD-associated PID.
Proctitis	ceftriaxone 125 mg IM × 1 *and* doxycycline 100 mg PO b.i.d. × 7 d	
Pubic lice	permethrin 1% cream rinse, apply for 10 min	Use lindane only if other therapy fails. Decontaminate clothes and bedding. Second treatment 7-10 d after first to kill newly hatched lice. If pubic lice, treat partner also.
Scabies	permethrin cream 5% applied to all affected areas from neck down for 8-14 min *or* lindane 1% applied to all affected areas from neck down for 8 h	
Sexual assault	ceftriaxone 125 mg IM × 1 *and* metronidazole 2 g PO × 1 *and* doxycycline 100 mg PO b.i.d. × 7 d	Tetanus-booster and gamma globulin as well as baseline HIV testing and follow-up are recommended.
Syphilis	*Primary, secondary, or <1 y duration:* benzathine penicillin G, 2.4 million units IM *Unknown duration or >1 y:* benzathine penicillin G, 7.2 million units divided in 2.4 million IM weekly × 3 *Allergic to penicillin:* doxycycline 100 mg PO b.i.d. × 14-28 d *C:* benzathine penicillin G 50,000 units/kg IM × 1, up to 2.4 million units; repeat × 3 if unknown or >1 y duration	Pregnant women who are allergic to penicillin should be desensitized.
Trichomoniasis	metronidazole 2 g PO × 1 *or* metronidazole 500 mg PO b.i.d. × 7 d	Pregnant women can be treated after the first trimester.

Continued

Table 56–7

Current Guidelines for Primary Therapies for Common Sexually Transmitted Diseases—cont'd

Disease	Primary Therapy	Notes
Trichomoniasis—cont'd	Tindamax (tinidazole tablets); second-generation nitroimidazole for the treatment of trichomoniasis, giardiasis, amebiasis, and amebic liver abscess; synthetic antiprotozoal agent with a longer half-life than metronidazole and has a lower incidence of GI side effects; should be taken with food, and clients should abstain from drinking alcohol for 72 h following therapy; because trichomoniasis is a sexually transmitted disease with potentially serious sequelae, partners of infected clients should be treated simultaneously to prevent reinfection.	Tindamax is contraindicated during the first trimester of pregnancy.

contacts of an infected individual should be informed of their exposure so they can be treated. Partners should refrain from sexual activity until each is clear of infection on follow-up evaluation or, at the very least, condoms should be used.

HIV Disease

Chapter 34, HIV and AIDS-Related Agents, is devoted to the presentation of drugs used to treat HIV and acquired immunodeficiency syndrome (AIDS). These conditions involve the immune system and can be transmitted by means other than sexual contact.

Nursing Process

Sexually Transmitted Diseases

• Nurses need to be sensitive to clients' reasons for seeking or avoiding care for sexually transmitted diseases (STDs). Psychosocial reactions to a diagnosis of an STD may include feelings of anger, depression, shame, guilt, hurt, fear, and concern. Clients need privacy during the interview and examination, with attention to their comfort, such as warming the speculum before a pelvic examination. A second health professional should be present in the examination room during the physical examination of a female client.

ASSESSMENT

■ Before physical data are gathered, a history is elicited. Less sensitive issues are addressed first so that trust can be established. The term "partners" is used when discussing sexual activity rather than value-laden terms such as "wife" or "boyfriend."

■ The history includes the chief complaint, a description of the course of illness, a review of systems and general health history, a reproductive history, a sexual history, a review of lifestyle and social habits, and identification of allergies.
■ Physical examination includes inspection and palpation of the genitalia and other points of inoculation.
■ Laboratory tests include wet slides with microbe-specific setting agents, urinalysis, cultures, Papanicolaou smear, a complete blood count, syphilis serology, and herpes simplex virus types 1 and 2 antibodies.

NURSING DIAGNOSES

■ Actual as well as potential infection
■ Deficient knowledge with regard to transmission and prevention as well as treatment
■ Noncompliance with known prevention strategies
■ Pain
■ Situational low self-esteem
■ Ineffective sexuality patterns
   A medical diagnosis of HIV disease would bring with it these additional nursing diagnoses:
■ Fatigue
■ Anxiety
■ Anticipatory grieving
■ Risk for loneliness
■ Ineffective therapeutic regimen management/health maintenance

PLANNING

■ Short-term goals include client's adherence to the treatment regimen and avoidance of adverse effects.
■ Long-term goals include client's return for follow-up evaluation and adoption of risk-reducing sexual behaviors.

NURSING INTERVENTIONS

■ Client needs to understand procedures performed during evaluation and how to administer prescribed medications and treatments. Side effects and adverse reactions that require immediate intervention are reviewed.

■ Specific interventions include providing needed support as client deals with the fact that the infection is sexually transmitted.

■ Client needs to notify sexual partners so that they can be evaluated and treated.

■ Ideally, sexual contact is avoided during treatment. At the least, condoms should be used until both partners are shown to be clear of infection.

■ Individuals are scheduled for follow-up visits from 4 days to 4 weeks, depending on the type of infection and treatment.

■ Individuals with any STD are counseled about being tested for HIV infection.

Client Teaching

• The mode of transmission of STDs, the relationship of all STDs with HIV infection, and how HIV risk is avoided should all be reviewed.

• Individuals are advised to plan periodic reproductive health check-ups.

Cultural Considerations ⊕

• Because of their modesty, many Asian and Middle Eastern women will only be examined by a female health care provider.

• Use an interpreter as appropriate; one of same gender and culture is preferred for sensitive topics.

• In male-dominated cultures, the male may be unwilling to undergo testing or treatment.

EVALUATION

■ Intervention has been successful if the individual's infection is clear on reevaluation or, in the case of viral infections, the individual experiences quiescence of the virus.

■ One important outcome to evaluate is that the infection is not transmitted to other individuals. Another is that the individual is able to avoid sexual practices that carry risk for acquiring STDs, including promiscuity, intercourse without the use of a condom, and traumatic sexual practices.

Summary

Reproductive health and fertility require integrity of hormonal mechanisms and reproductive anatomy. Infertility can be caused by male, female, or couple factors. Often the use of drugs to stimulate ovulation is effective treatment. Clients need to understand the treatment regimen, and they need support in dealing with the psychologic impact of this condition.

Because STDs can threaten reproductive health, neonatal health, fertility, and even life, early diagnosis and treatment are crucial but less effective than prevention. Numerous opportunistic infections and autoimmune processes complicate HIV and AIDS. For some, drug therapies may offer relief, although ultimately death is the result.

WEBSITES

For further information on Drugs Related to Reproductive Health: Infertility and Sexually Transmitted Diseases, visit these Internet resources:

Sexually Transmitted Diseases Treatment Guidelines: *www.cdc.gov/STD/treatment/*

InterNational Council on Infertility Information Dissemination: *www.inciid.org/bastest.html*

Critical Thinking Case Study

T.D. married D.D., age 32, 3 years ago. D.D. is the only sexual partner T.D. has ever had. For the last year, they have been trying to conceive without success. D.D.'s nurse practitioner learns when taking D.D.'s history that she had multiple sexual partners while in college and that she was once treated for gonorrhea. D.D.'s menstrual history reveals an erratic pattern of unpredictable periods, about every 2 or 3 months. The nurse practitioner reviews the relationship between timing of coitus and conception, instructs D.D. to take her temperature each morning before she gets out of bed, and to maintain an ovulation record. She also suggests that a home test kit be used to identify when ovulation has occurred. D.D. and T.D. are referred to an infertility specialist.

1. What is the relevance of D.D.'s past sexual history to the current complaint?

2. Why would the infertility specialist consider cultures for *Chlamydia trachomatis* and *Neisseria gonorrhoeae* years after exposure?

3. What other tests would reveal damage resulting from STDs?

4. What is positive about D.D.'s menstrual history? What about her menstrual pattern makes conception difficult?

5. How can D.D. predict when she will ovulate?

After a complete evaluation of T.D. and D.D., a course of clomiphene citrate is prescribed.

6. What side effects can D.D. expect?

7. When should D.D. take the medication?

8. When should T.D. and D.D. have sexual intercourse?

9. D.D. experiences midcycle abdominal pain. What should she do when this occurs? How will her infertility specialist interpret this?

10. D.D. becomes pregnant after four cycles on clomiphene citrate. What is one potential risk factor with this pregnancy?

D.D. becomes pregnant and gives birth to a boy following an uneventful pregnancy. The infant has numerous upper respiratory infections during his first 4 months of life—twice requiring hospitalization—and gains weight slowly. When the family is referred to a tertiary pediatric medical center, the medical staff asks D.D. if she would consider being tested for HIV.

11. What in her history puts D.D. at risk for HIV infection?

12. Why is it possible that D.D. could test positive for HIV when she has shown no signs of infection for nearly a decade after her high-risk behavior?

Study Questions

1. What is the relationship between STDs and infertility?

2. How should couples determine the timing of coitus when trying to conceive?

3. What should be the timing of coitus in relation to ovarian stimulation therapy?

4. What are some adverse reactions of clomiphene citrate therapy?

5. What are some psychosocial effects of infertility therapy?

6. Which STDs cannot be cured?

7. Which STDs are associated with life-threatening illness?

8. Whenever an individual is successfully treated for an STD, what should the nurse emphasize in client teaching?

9. What reproductive tract infections may or may not be sexually transmitted? What should the client tell his or her partner when such an infection occurs?

10. Why do ulcerative STDs place an individual at risk for HIV infection?

11. What are cultural considerations related to caring for clients with STDs and infertility?

12. What is the nurse's role in each step of the nursing process when caring for clients with STDs and infertility?

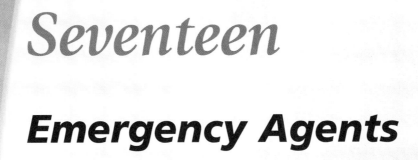

Seventeen

Emergency Agents

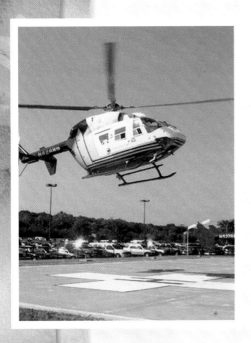

This final unit focuses on adult and pediatric emergency drugs. Chapter 57 considers oxygen as an emergency drug and pharmacologic treatment for five categories of emergency situations: (1) cardiac, (2) neurosurgical, (3) poisoning, (4) shock, and (5) hypertensive crisis. Specific drug protocols and dosages for the pediatric client are included.

Photo courtesy Christiana Care Health System, Wilmington, Delaware.

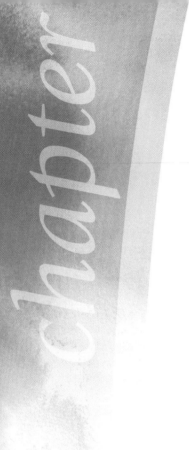

57 Adult and Pediatric Emergency Drugs

LINDA LASKOWSKI-JONES

> **ELECTRONIC RESOURCES**   *evolve*
>
> Additional information can be found on the companion website at *http://evolve.elsevier.com/KeeHayes/pharmacology/* or on the companion CD-ROM, which includes:
> - *NCLEX-style examination review questions*
> - *Pharmacology animations*
> - *Medication error and IV therapy checklists*
> - *Medication calculation problems*
> - *Electronic calculators*

OUTLINE

OBJECTIVES

- Describe indications for the emergency drugs listed in this chapter.
- Define the basic mechanism of action for each emergency drug.

TERMS

anaphylactic shock	cathartic	hypertensive crisis	preload
angina pectoris	dysrhythmias	hypomagnesemia	pulse oximetry
asthma	extravasation	hypovolemic shock	tachycardia
asystole	glycogenolysis	hypoxemia	torsades de pointes
bradycardia	heart block	myocardial infarction	

Introduction

The drugs described in this chapter are first-line agents commonly used to treat various medical emergencies. Nurses must have a ready knowledge of the indications and actions of these agents because medical and surgical emergencies can occur in virtually any area of nursing practice. Learning key nursing implications *before* a crisis situation enables the nurse to function at the highest possible level when the client requires life-saving intervention.

At the end of each discussion of a group of emergency drugs is a summary prototype drug chart of the drugs that contains the drugs' dosages and indications. Common adult doses are listed in the drug charts; pediatric dosages may vary widely depending on the child's age and weight. The drug charts list only the most common indications and dosages for the emergency drugs discussed; they *do not* describe all possible uses and dosing regimens for the agents.

Oxygen as an Emergency Drug

Oxygen can be classified as a drug because it can have both beneficial and adverse effects on the body based on the amount and manner in which it is administered. Oxygen is essential to life—without it, brain death begins within 6 minutes. Inadequate oxygenation produces **hypoxemia** (inadequate oxygen in the blood) and significant physiologic sequelae to all body systems; therefore oxygen is a first-line drug for all emergency situations. Depending on the circumstances, adequate oxygenation may be all that is necessary to effectively treat physiologic disturbances such as chest pain, bradycardia, and cardiac dysrhythmias.

Before the other pharmacologic agents discussed in this chapter are administered, ensure that the client's airway and breathing are addressed to promote optimal oxygenation and ventilation. Giving a drug to treat a disorder brought on by hypoxemia without effectively correcting the cause of the hypoxemia is ineffective and ultimately does not produce the desired outcome. **Pulse oximetry,** which provides a digital display of oxygen saturation, is an essential monitoring tool that should be used in emergency situations to assess the adequacy of oxygenation and guide further interventions. Ideally, oxygen saturation should be kept at or above 95%.

In general, clients suffering from severe physiologic stress such as shock states, traumatic injury, acute myocardial infarction (AMI) with hemodynamic instability, and cardiac arrest initially require oxygen in high concentrations (i.e., the fraction of inspired oxygen [FiO_2] close to 100%). The oxygen devices of choice for these conditions include a non-rebreather mask with an oxygen reservoir (oxygen flow rate set at 10 to 15 L/min) for spontaneously breathing clients and a bag-valve-mask device attached to an oxygen source at a flow rate of 15 L/min for clients who require assisted ventilation. Although caution must be exercised for clients with chronic obstructive pulmonary disease (COPD) (they may lose their hypoxic respiratory drive when given oxygen in high concentration), oxygen should never be denied to a client who needs it. In the case of COPD, the nurse should be prepared to ventilate the client manually with a bag-valve-mask if respiratory depression or arrest occurs. As the client's condition stabilizes, the oxygen concentration should be decreased. An FiO_2 above 50% for a prolonged period can lead to oxygen toxicity and other detrimental effects to the pulmonary system in adults and children.

For emergency situations that do not involve severe physiologic stress (e.g., angina, dysrhythmias, pulmonary disease), supplemental oxygen delivered by nasal cannula at 1 to 6 L/min or by simple face mask at 6 to 10 L/min may have significant physiologic benefit. Children may tolerate a face tent with a high oxygen flow of 10 to 15 L better than a nasal cannula or face mask.

Emergency Drugs for Cardiac Disorders

Drugs described in this section are indicated for cardiac emergencies such as angina, MI, disturbances of cardiac rate or rhythm, and cardiac arrest. These drugs often must be prepared and administered rapidly. A sound knowledge base as well as easy access to the drugs and necessary equipment is essential for the best client outcome in a cardiac emergency. Usually in an emergency, detailed personal, medical, drug, and herbal histories are unavailable (see Herbal Alert 57–1). Treatment is based on client presentation. Drugs for cardiac emergencies are cross-referenced to the specialty chapter.

Nitroglycerin

Nitroglycerin dilates coronary arteries and improves blood flow to an ischemic myocardium. It is therefore the treatment of choice for **angina pectoris** (chest pain) and **myocardial infarction** (heart attack). Nitroglycerin is available in sublingual, translingual aerosol spray, oral, topical, and intravenous (IV) forms. Only the sublingual and translingual aerosol spray preparations are discussed.

Sublingual nitroglycerin (0.3-0.4 mg) and the translingual aerosol spray (0.4 mg-metered dose) preparations are indicated for clients experiencing an acute anginal attack. The client is taught to sit or lie down and place one sublingual nitroglycerin tablet under the tongue and to allow it to dissolve slowly. Not all sublingual nitroglycerin preparations cause a burning sensation under the tongue, so a lack of burning sensation should not be relied on to indicate potency. If the chest pain is not relieved, sublingual nitroglycerin may be repeated at 5-minute intervals until a total of three tablets has been taken. Clients prescribed the translingual aerosol preparation should be reminded that the spray should not be inhaled. Instead, it should be sprayed onto or under the tongue. The client should be instructed not to swallow for approximately 10 seconds to allow absorption of the drug. As with sublingual nitroglycerin, up to three doses may be taken within 15 minutes. If pain persists despite three doses of the sublingual or aerosol forms, further interventions are necessary in an emergency or critical care setting. An ambulance should be called if the client is outside the hospital. Blood pressure and heart rate must be monitored closely. Hypotension is a common adverse effect, especially the first time a client takes nitroglycerin. Tachycardia or, uncommonly, bradycardia also may occur. If nitroglycerin preparations are given to clients taking drugs for erectile dysfunction, such as Viagra, profound hypotension can result. This combination is contraindicated.

IV nitroglycerin is reserved for clients with unstable angina or an AMI. A continuous infusion is usually initiated at a rate of 10 to 20 mcg/min and increased by 5 to 10 mcg/min every 5 to 10 minutes based on chest pain and blood pressure response. Continuous blood pressure and heart monitoring are required because hypotension is a common adverse effect. Hypotension usually is treated by reducing or discontinuing the nitroglycerin infusion (see Chapter 40, Cardiac Glycosides, Antianginals, and Antidysrhythmics) and by placing the client in a supine position with legs elevated if tolerated.

Morphine Sulfate

Morphine sulfate, a narcotic analgesic, is used to treat the chest pain associated with an AMI. It also is indicated for acute pulmonary edema. Morphine relieves pain, dilates venous vessels, and reduces the workload on the heart. The standard dosage of morphine sulfate is 1 to 4 mg IV over 1 to 5 minutes repeated every 5 to 30 minutes until chest pain is relieved. The nurse must be aware that respiratory depression and hypotension are common adverse effects; close client monitoring is essential. The narcotic antagonist naloxone (Narcan) may be ordered to reverse the action of morphine if adverse effects pose a significant risk to the client. The dose is 0.4 to 2 mg every 2 minutes as indicated (see Chapter 21, Drugs for Pain Management: Nonnarcotic and Narcotic Analgesics).

Atropine Sulfate

Atropine sulfate is indicated in the treatment of hemodynamically significant **bradycardia** (slow heart rate) and some types of **heart block** (e.g., atrioventricular (AV) block at nodal level), as well as asystole. Atropine acts to increase heart rate by inhibiting the action of the vagus nerve (parasympatholytic effect). Atropine sulfate is also used as an emergency drug to reverse the toxic effects of organophosphate pesticide exposure, which include bradycardia and excessive secretions. In symptomatic bradycardia, atropine is administered IV in 0.5- to 1-mg doses at 3- to 5-minute intervals until the desired heart rate is achieved or until 0.04 mg/kg (generally not more than 3 mg) is given. In **asystole** (cardiac arrest), atropine is given as a 1-mg bolus dose IV, which may be repeated up to the dosing limits every 3 to 5 minutes.

The adult IV atropine dose should not be less than 0.5 mg or exceed 0.04 mg/kg (usually not more than 3 mg IV). Doses below 0.5 mg can produce a paradoxical bradycardia; at doses of 0.04 mg/kg or greater, vagal activity is considered completely blocked and further atropine administration may have no benefit. Atropine sulfate can be administered through an endotracheal tube (ETT) if no venous access exists; 2 to 3 mg should be diluted in 10 ml of normal saline and instilled deep into the ETT via a feeding tube attached to a syringe. After endotracheal administration, the client should be ventilated vigorously with a bag-valve device to enhance absorption of the drug.

Continuous cardiac and blood pressure monitoring is essential for the client who receives IV atropine sulfate. Significant adverse effects include cardiac dysrhythmias, tachycardia, myocardial ischemia, restlessness, anxiety, mydriasis, thirst, and urinary retention.

Pediatric Implications

Because cardiac output is dependent on heart rate in infants younger than 6 months, bradycardia (heart rate <60 beats per minute [beats/min]) must be treated. Before administration of drugs, efforts should be targeted toward restoring adequate ventilation and oxygenation. If these maneuvers do not produce the desired clinical response, then atropine is indicated.

The pediatric dose of atropine is 0.02 mg/kg IV or via ETT or intraosseous route. It is important to be cognizant that the minimum single pediatric dose is 0.1 mg and the maximum single child dose is 0.5 mg IV. The maximum total pediatric dose is 1 mg in a child and 2 mg in an adolescent. For the neonate in cardiac arrest or with a spontaneous heart rate of less than 80 beats/min, epinephrine 0.01 to 0.03 mg/kg IV or via ETT every 3 to 5 minutes as indicated may be preferred to elevate the heart rate because stressed neonates quickly deplete their own stores of catecholamines (see Chapter 18, Cholinergics and Anticholinergics).

Isoproterenol

Isoproterenol is a beta-adrenergic drug given to increase the heart rate. Typically, isoproterenol is considered only after the maximum dose of atropine (3 mg), dopamine and epinephrine infusions, and a transcutaneous pacemaker have failed to produce the desired clinical response in clients with hemodynamically significant bradycardia. Thus the client who exhibits symptomatic refractory bradycardia is a candidate for isoproterenol. Isoproterenol is administered as an IV infusion, generally 1 mg diluted in 250 ml of 5% dextrose in water or normal saline, at 2 to 10 mcg/min titrated to heart rate (usually 60 beats/min). An electronic infusion device must be used to provide precise infusion control.

Myocardial oxygen consumption is greatly increased with isoproterenol administration; therefore the nurse must carefully monitor the client receiving isoproterenol. Significant adverse effects include myocardial ischemia, tachycardia, and life-threatening dysrhythmias such as ventricular tachycardia and ventricular fibrillation. The nurse should alert the physician promptly if any increase in premature ventricular contractions is noted on the cardiac monitor or if the heart rate exceeds 100 beats/min because the dosage may need to be decreased or the infusion stopped.

Pediatric Implications

Epinephrine infusions are preferable to isoproterenol infusions to increase heart rate above 60 beats/min in pediatric clients. Isoproterenol can cause a large decrease in diastolic blood pressure. Isoproterenol infusions are no longer recommended for treating bradycardia in children. As in the adult client, isoproterenol should never be used in clients experiencing cardiac arrest (see Chapter 17, Adrenergics and Adrenergic Blockers).

Adenosine

Adenosine is the first-line drug of choice to treat paroxysmal supraventricular tachycardia (PSVT), a sudden, uncontrolled, rapid rhythm. A natural substance found in all body cells, adenosine slows impulse conduction through the heart's atrioventricular (AV) node, interrupts dysrhythmia-producing reentry pathways, and restores a normal rhythm in clients with PSVT. Because the half-life is less than 5 seconds, adenosine is administered rapidly as a 6-mg IV bolus over 1 to 3 seconds followed by a 20-ml saline flush. A 12-mg bolus may be given 1 to 2 minutes after the initial dose if PSVT persists. A third dose of 12 mg may be considered after 1 to 2 minutes if needed. Higher doses are not recommended.

Nursing considerations include continuous cardiac monitoring and frequent assessment of vital signs. Adenosine is inhibited by methylxanthines such as caffeine and theophylline. Although few adverse reactions have been reported, hypotension and dyspnea may occur. In addition, a short period of asystole may follow administration (up to 15 seconds). Spontaneous cardiac activity resumes. Adenosine is contraindicated in clients with second- and third-degree heart block and in clients with sick sinus syndrome, except those with functioning pacemakers. Clients should be placed in a mild reverse Trendelenburg position before drug administration to guard against hypotension (see Chapter 40, Cardiac Glycosides, Antianginals, and Antidysrhythmics).

Verapamil

Verapamil, a calcium channel blocker, is indicated for the treatment of **tachycardia** (rapid heart rate) originating above the ventricles (narrow complex PSVT). Such heart rates generally exceed 150 beats/min. Verapamil slows conduction (negative chronotropic) through the heart and has negative inotropic and vasodilating effects. In emergency situations, verapamil is administered as an IV bolus in variable age- and weight-dependent dosages, which should not exceed 2.5 to 5 mg given slowly over 2 minutes. Repeat doses of 5 to 10 mg may be ordered in 15 to 30 minutes. The maximum total dose with this regimen is 20 mg. The nurse must carefully monitor heart rate and rhythm as well as blood pressure. Cardiac conduction disturbances and profound hypotension can occur, especially with concurrent use of beta-blockers. An IV injection of calcium may be ordered to prevent or treat calcium channel blocker-induced hypotension (see Chapters 40, Cardiac Glycosides, Antianginals, and Antidysrhythmics, and 42, Antihypertensive Drugs).

Diltiazem

Diltiazem is a calcium channel blocker like verapamil and is administered as an IV bolus to treat PSVT and to slow the ventricular response rate in atrial fibrillation or flutter. Diltiazem has less of a negative inotropic effect than verapamil, but it has strong negative chronotropic actions.

Therefore IV diltiazem is less likely to cause cardiac depression but is very effective in controlling heart rate.

The usual initial bolus dose of IV diltiazem is 0.25 mg/kg given over 2 minutes. If the supraventricular tachycardia does not convert to a normal sinus rhythm in 15 minutes, a second IV bolus of 0.35 mg/kg over 2 to 5 minutes may be necessary. For ongoing control of the ventricular rate in clients with atrial fibrillation or flutter, a continuous infusion of diltiazem is indicated at a dose range of 5 to 15 mg/hour, titrated according to the desired heart rate for not longer than 24 hours.

The nurse must carefully monitor blood pressure and heart rate after administering IV diltiazem. Although mild, transient hypotension is common; significant hypotension may be treated with injection of IV calcium to elevate blood pressure. In clients who are hypotensive before calcium channel blocker administration, IV calcium may be ordered as a pretreatment to prevent the hypotensive response to the drug.

Diltiazem can elevate serum digoxin levels, predisposing the client to digitalis toxicity. Simultaneous use of calcium channel blockers and beta-blockers is contraindicated because their negative inotropic and negative chronotropic effects are synergistic, causing myocardial depression and bradycardia. Other contraindications include heart block or sick sinus syndrome in the client without a pacemaker and severe heart failure. The nurse should be especially careful when administering calcium channel blockers to pediatric clients because they may have preexisting myocardial dysfunction.

Lidocaine

Lidocaine is commonly used to treat significant ventricular **dysrhythmias** (irregular heartbeats), such as frequent premature ventricular contractions (PVCs), ventricular tachycardia, and ventricular fibrillation. Lidocaine exerts a local anesthetic effect on the heart thus decreasing myocardial irritability. Typically a client with ventricular dysrhythmias is given a 1- to 1.5-mg/kg bolus of lidocaine, followed by 0.5 mg/kg to 0.75 mg/kg every 5 to 10 minutes until the dysrhythmia is controlled or a total dose of 3 mg/kg has been administered. A continuous lidocaine infusion is initiated at a rate of 1 mg to 4 mg/min to maintain a therapeutic serum level. Lidocaine may also be administered via the endotracheal route in doses of 2 to 4 mg/kg.

Important nursing considerations for the client receiving lidocaine include continuous cardiac monitoring and assessment for signs and symptoms of lidocaine toxicity (confusion, drowsiness, hearing impairment, cardiac conduction defects, myocardial depression, muscle twitching, and seizures). Because lidocaine is metabolized by the liver, clients with hepatic impairment, congestive heart failure, shock, and advanced age (older than 70 years) are at higher risk for toxicity. In these clients, the lidocaine dose may need to be reduced by as much as 50%.

Pediatric Implications

Ventricular ectopy is uncommon in children. Metabolic causes should be suspected if ventricular dysrhythmias occur. The pediatric dose of lidocaine is 1 mg/kg IV via ETT or the intraosseous route. A maintenance infusion of 20 to 50 mcg/kg/min is recommended following the bolus dose (see Chapter 40, Cardiac Glycosides, Antianginals, and Antidysrhythmics). Drug data for lidocaine are presented in Prototype Drug Chart 57–1.

Amiodarone

The IV form of amiodarone recently has been incorporated into advanced cardiac life support algorithms for the treatment of atrial and ventricular dysrhythmias. It has alpha- and beta-adrenergic blocking effects and acts on sodium, potassium, and calcium channels. Indications for use include pulseless ventricular tachycardia and ventricular fibrillation (after defibrillation and epinephrine), hemodynamically stable ventricular tachycardia, PSVT refractory to adenosine, ventricular rate control in atrial fibrillation, and for pharmacologic treatment of atrial fibrillation.

Amiodarone is especially good for clients with impaired heart function who have atrial and ventricular dysrhythmias. It has been found to be more effective and to have fewer proarrhythmic properties than other agents with similar actions.

For clients who have a pulse (e.g., not in cardiac arrest), amiodarone 150 mg IV is given over 10 minutes followed by a continuous infusion of 1 mg/min for 6 hours, then 0.5 mg/min. For clients in cardiac arrest because of pulseless ventricular tachycardia or ventricular fibrillation, a dose of 300 mg diluted in 20 to 30 ml dextrose 5% in water (D_5W) or normal saline is given as a rapid infusion followed by a continuous infusion as described earlier. Additional doses of 150 mg may be given by rapid infusion if ventricular fibrillation or ventricular tachycardia recurs. The maximum daily dose is 2.2 grams per 24-hour period.

Significant adverse effects include hypotension and bradycardia. The nurse should slow the infusion rate to prevent or treat these effects as well as be prepared to administer IV fluids, vasopressors, and agents to increase heart rate. A temporary pacemaker may be needed.

Pediatric Implications

Amiodarone is given for pulseless ventricular tachycardia and ventricular fibrillation as a 5 mg/kg rapid IV/intraosseous bolus. For responsive children who have supraventricular (junctional and atrial) tachycardia and ventricular dysrhythmias with pulses present, amiodarone is given as a 5 mg/kg IV/intraosseous loading dose over 20 to 60 minutes and repeated to a maximum daily IV dose of 15 mg/kg per 24-hour period.

PROTOTYPE DRUG CHART 57–1

LIDOCAINE HCl

Drug Class

Antidysrhythmic, class IB
Trade Name: Xylocaine
Pregnancy Category: C

Dosage

A: IV: ETT*: 1-1.5 mg/kg; may repeat 0.5 mg/kg q 5-10 min
    up to 3 mg/kg *(max)*
Drip: 1-4 mg/min
C: IV: ETT* or IO: Initially: 1 mg/kg; maint: 20-50 mcg/kg/
    min is recommended after bolus
Therapeutic range: 1.5-5 mcg/ml

Contraindications

Hypersensitivity, advanced atrioventricular block
Caution: Liver disease, congestive heart failure, elderly

Drug-Lab-Food Interactions

Drug: Increase effects with phenytoin, quinidine,
    procainamide, propranolol; *increase* risk of toxicity
    with cimetidine, beta-adrenergic blockers

Pharmacokinetics

Absorption: IV
Distribution: PB: 60%-80%; concentrates in adipose tissue
Metabolism: $t\frac{1}{2}$: Initial: 7-30 min; terminal: 9-120 min
Excretion: Through the liver

Pharmacodynamics

PO: Onset: 45-60 sec
    Peak: 45-60 sec
    Duration: 10-20 min

Therapeutic Effects/Uses

Antiarrhythmic drug to treat ventricular dysrhythmias such as premature ventricular contractions (PVCs), ventricular
    tachycardia, and ventricular fibrillation
Mode of Action: Decreases automaticity; increases electrical threshold of ventricle

Side Effects

Drowsiness, confusion, dyspnea, lethargy, hypotension,
    nausea, vomiting

Adverse Reactions

Life-threatening: Seizures, cardiac arrest

A, Adult; *C,* child; *ETT,* endotracheal tube; *IO,* intraosseous; *IV,* intravenous; *PB,* protein-binding; *maint,* maintenance; *max,* maximum;
min, minute; *sec,* seconds; $t\frac{1}{2}$, half-life.
*Note: For endotracheal drug administration, dose should be 2 to 4 mg/kg in adults.

Procainamide

Procainamide is an antidysrhythmic agent prescribed for ventricular tachycardia, PVCs, and rapid supraventricular dysrhythmias. The typical IV loading dose of procainamide is 20 mg/min until the dysrhythmia is successfully treated. Other endpoints to procainamide administration include a total administration of 17 mg/kg of the drug, the development of hypotension, and specific changes on the electrocardiogram (ECG) (e.g., widening of the QRS complex by 50% or more). A continuous maintenance infusion of 1 to 4 mg/min may be ordered following the loading dose.

Procainamide administration can cause severe hypotension. Heart block, rhythm disturbances, and cardiac arrest can occur. Procainamide is contraindicated in clients with torsades de pointes. The drug is eliminated via the kidneys; therefore clients with renal failure are at higher risk of adverse effects and often require a lower dosage (see Chapter 40, Cardiac Glycosides, Antianginals, and Antidysrhythmics).

Magnesium Sulfate

Magnesium is an essential element in multiple enzymatic reactions in the body, including function of the sodium-potassium adenosine triphosphatase (ATPase) pump. Its physiologic effects can be likened to a calcium channel blocker with neuromuscular blocking properties. Hypomagnesemia is associated with the development of atrial and ventricular dysrhythmias.

The primary indications for emergency administration of magnesium sulfate are refractory ventricular tachycardia, refractory ventricular fibrillation, cardiac arrest associated with **hypomagnesemia** (low serum magnesium level), and life-threatening ventricular dysrhythmias from digitalis toxicity. It is also the drug of choice for the treatment of **torsades de pointes,** an unusual polymorphic ventricular tachycardia often associated with a prolonged Q-T interval.

Magnesium is administered by diluting 1 to 2 g (2 to 4 ml of a 50% solution) in 10 ml of D_5W. For cardiac arrest caused by hypomagnesemia or torsades de pointes, magnesium is given by direct IV push. For clients experiencing torsades de pointes who are not in cardiac arrest, a magnesium infusion of 1 to 2 g diluted in 50 to 100 ml of D_5W can be given IV over 5 to 60 minutes followed by a continuous infusion of 0.5 to 1 g/hour.

Although magnesium toxicity is rare, the nurse should monitor the client's response to magnesium administration. Hypotension is the most common adverse effect when magnesium is given by rapid IV push. Other effects include mild bradycardia, flush, and sweating. True hypermagnesemia can cause diarrhea, respiratory depression, deep tendon reflex impairment, flaccid paralysis, and circulatory collapse. Because magnesium is eliminated via the kidneys, it should be administered with caution in clients with renal impairment.

Epinephrine

Epinephrine is a catecholamine with alpha- and beta-adrenergic effects. Indications for administration of IV epinephrine include profound bradycardia, asystole, pulseless ventricular tachycardia, and ventricular fibrillation. Epinephrine is thought to improve perfusion of the heart and brain in cardiac arrest states through constriction of peripheral blood vessels. In addition, epinephrine increases the chances for successful electrical countershock (defibrillation) in ventricular fibrillation. For bradycardia, an epinephrine infusion may be ordered at 2 to 10 mcg/min. For asystole, pulseless ventricular tachycardia, and ventricular fibrillation, epinephrine is administered in 1-mg doses IV every 3 to 5 minutes until the desired clinical response is achieved (usually, return of effective cardiac activity). Epinephrine also may be given via the ETT route in doses of 2 to 2.5 mg diluted in 10 ml of normal saline.

Nursing implications for clients receiving epinephrine include constant cardiac and hemodynamic monitoring. Epinephrine can cause myocardial ischemia and cardiac dysrhythmias. Epinephrine should never be administered in the same site as an alkaline solution such as sodium bicarbonate because alkaline solutions inactivate epinephrine. In addition, the presence of metabolic or respiratory acidosis decreases the effectiveness of epinephrine. All efforts should be made to correct acid-base imbalances in the client.

Pediatric Implications

The pediatric dose of epinephrine is 0.01 mg/kg (1:10,000 solution) given every 3 to 5 minutes IV or via the intraosseous route for cardiac arrest (see Chapter 17, Adrenergics and Adrenergic Blockers). The ETT dose of 0.1 mg/kg should be given using the 1:1000 solution.

Vasopressin

Vasopressin is indicated for the treatment of ventricular fibrillation that is refractory to defibrillation. It is found in the human body as endogenous antidiuretic hormone. The therapeutic dose is significantly higher than the amount normally present in humans. The effects of vasopressin as a cardiac emergency drug include nonadrenergic peripheral vasoconstriction. When used as an emergency agent, it ap-

pears to increase coronary artery perfusion during cardiopulmonary resuscitation (CPR) and to exhibit vasopressor effects. It is given to clients in cardiac arrest after epinephrine administration as a single 40 units IV, intraosseous, or ETT dose. Vasopressin is considered an adjunct to epinephrine in this situation. Because vasopressin can induce myocardial ischemia and angina, it is contraindicated in responsive clients who have coronary artery disease (CAD) (e.g., clients with CAD who are not in cardiac arrest).

Pediatric Implications

Vasopressin administration is not recommended for the treatment of pediatric cardiac arrest at this time.

Sodium Bicarbonate

Sodium bicarbonate is prescribed to treat the metabolic acidosis that may accompany cardiac arrest. The current standard is to give sodium bicarbonate only after adequate ventilation, chest compressions, IV fluids, and drug therapy fail to correct the acidotic state. Sodium bicarbonate is rarely a first-line drug used for cardiac arrest situations; it is preferentially given based on results of arterial blood gas analysis when acidosis is severe. If a client has been in arrest for a prolonged period and blood gas analysis is not available, sodium bicarbonate may be ordered as part of the ongoing resuscitation attempt. The standard initial IV dose of sodium bicarbonate is 1 mEq/kg. The drug may be repeated at 0.5 mEq/kg every 10 minutes as needed.

Important nursing considerations relevant to sodium bicarbonate include careful monitoring of arterial blood gas analysis results. Sodium bicarbonate administration can lead to metabolic alkalosis. In addition, catecholamines such as epinephrine, norepinephrine, and dopamine should not be infused in the same site as sodium bicarbonate because they are inactivated by solutions containing sodium bicarbonate.

Pediatric Implications

If severe metabolic acidosis persists after attention has been directed at maintaining optimal ventilation and oxygenation, sodium bicarbonate may be given to the pediatric client in a 1-mEq/kg dose via the IV or intraosseous route. Subsequent doses of 0.5 mEq/kg may be given every 10 minutes if blood gases are not available. Sodium bicarbonate is hyperosmolar and should be diluted from an 8.4% solution (1 mEq/ml) to a 4.2% solution (0.5 mEq/ml) for infants younger than 3 months of age (see Chapter 14, Vitamin and Mineral Replacement).

Table 57–1 lists emergency cardiac drugs and their dosages and indications.

Emergency Drugs for Neurosurgical Disorders

The neurosurgical drugs discussed in this section are commonly administered in emergency, trauma, and critical care settings. For maximum benefit, these agents must be given as early as possible when clinically indicated. Knowl-

Table 57-1

Cardiac Emergency Drugs

Generic (Brand)	Route and Dosage	Uses and Considerations
adenosine	A: Initially: 6 mg; then 12 mg in 1-2 min if needed; may repeat 12 mg × 1	Paroxysmal supraventricular tachycardia. *Pregnancy category:* C; PB: UK; t½: <10 sec
amiodarone IV	A: IV: *with pulse:* 150 mg over 10 min; then continuous infusion 1 mg/min for 6 h; then 0.5 mg/min. *Cardiac arrest:* 300 mg diluted in 20-30 ml D₅W or normal saline rapidly followed by continuous infusion as above; *max:* 2.2 g/d. C: IV: *without pulse:* 5 mg/kg rapid IV/IO bolus. *With pulse:* 5 mg/kg IV/IO loading dose over 20-60 min; repeated to max daily dose of 15 mg/kg	Part of ACLS algorithm for treatment of both atrial and ventricular dysrhythmias. *Pregnancy category:* C; PB: UK; t½: 26-107 d
atropine sulfate	IV: 0.5-1 mg; can repeat up to 0.04 mg/kg or 3 mg *(max)* ETT: 2-3 mg diluted in 10 ml normal saline	Symptomatic bradycardia; asystole. *Pregnancy category:* C; PB: 60%-80%; t½: 2-3 h
diltiazem	IV: 0.25 mg/kg; repeat in 15 min at 0.35 mg/kg IV: drip 5-15 mg/h	Supraventricular tachycardia, atrial fibrillation and flutter. *Pregnancy category:* C; PB: 80%; t½: 2-5 h
epinephrine	IV: 0.5-1 mg; may be repeated q3-5min ETT: 2.0-2.5 mg diluted in 10 ml normal saline	Cardiac arrest. *Pregnancy category:* C; PB: UK; t½: UK
lidocaine	See Prototype Drug Chart 57-1.	
magnesium sulfate	Dilute 1-2 g (2-4 ml of a 50% solution) in 10 ml of D₅W. Give IV push in cardiac arrest; for torsades de pointes, 1-2 g diluted in 50-100 ml of D₅W given IV over 5-60 min followed by a continuous infusion of 0.5-1 g	Used for hypomagnesemia, treatment of ventricular tachycardia and ventricular fibrillation. Drug of choice for torsades de pointes. Rapid infusion can cause hypotension. *Pregnancy category:* D; PB: 25%-35%; t½: 30 min
morphine sulfate	IV: 1-4 mg q5-30min	Chest pain, unstable angina, pulmonary edema. *Pregnancy category:* C; PB: 35%; t½: 2-2.5 h
nitroglycerin	SL: 0.3-0.4 mg; Translingual aerosol spray: 0.4 mg-metered dose, up to 3 sprays in 15 min onto or under the tongue IV: Drip: 10-20 mcg/min, increased 5-10 mcg/min q 5-10 min (titrated)	Chest pain, angina, unstable angina, MI. Hypotension/contraindicated in clients taking drugs for erectile dysfunction (e.g., Viagra) *Pregnancy category:* C; PB: 60%; t½: 1-4 min
procainamide HCl	IV: 20 mg/min; *max:* 17 mg/kg *Recognize endpoints:* • Hypotension • QRS widens >50% • Total dose of 17 mg/kg given Drip: 1-4 mg/min	PVCs, ventricular tachycardia, ventricular fibrillation, atrial dysrhythmias. *Pregnancy category:* C; PB: 20%; t½: 3-4 h
sodium bicarbonate	IV: Initially: 1 mEq/kg; then 0.5 mEq/kg if needed q10min	Metabolic acidosis. *Pregnancy category:* C; PB: UK; t½: UK
vasopressin	A: IV/IO/ETT: single 40 U dose after epinephrine administration	Ventricular fibrillation refractory to defibrillation. Contraindicated in responsive clients with CAD. *Pregnancy category:* C; PB: UK; t½: 10-20 min
verapamil HCl	IV: Age- and weight-dependent dosages; should not exceed 5 mg; repeat doses may be needed to max of 20 mg	Paroxysmal supraventricular tachycardia. *Pregnancy category:* C; PB: 90%; t½: 3-8 h

A, Adult; *ACLS,* Advanced Cardiac Life Support; *C,* child; *CAD,* coronary artery disease; *d,* day; *ETT,* endotracheal tube; *h,* hour; *IO,* intraosseous; *IV,* intravenous; *max,* maximum; *MI,* myocardial infarction; *min,* minute; *PB,* protein-binding; *PVC,* premature ventricular contraction; *sec,* second; *SL,* sublingual; *t½,* half-life; *UK,* unknown; >, greater than; <, less than.

edge of proper administration techniques and guidelines enhances therapeutic effectiveness. These drugs are cross-referenced to their specialty chapters.

Mannitol

Mannitol is an osmotic diuretic used in the emergency and neurosurgical setting to treat cerebral edema and increased intracranial pressure, which may occur following head trauma, neurosurgery, and other types of intracranial pathology. Mannitol may be given as an IV bolus or via a continuous drip. The usual initial bolus dose of mannitol is 0.5 to 1 g/kg IV of a 25% solution. Subsequent dosing is highly variable and is influenced by serum osmolality. In general, mannitol is held when serum osmolality exceeds 310 to 320. Mannitol is highly irritating to veins. The nurse must use a filter needle when administering mannitol because crystals may form in the solution and syringe and thus be inadvertently injected. When a filter needle is used to draw up the mannitol, a *new* filter needle *must* be used to administer the mannitol IV. In addition, the nurse

PROTOTYPE DRUG CHART 57–2

MANNITOL

Drug Class	Dosage
Osmotic diuretic Trade Name: Osmitrol *Pregnancy Category:* C	**A: IV:** Initially 0.5-1 g/kg of 25% sol as a bolus Highly individualized

Contraindications	Drug-Lab-Food Interactions
Hypersensitivity, severe dehydration *Caution:* Pregnancy, breastfeeding, current intracranial bleeding	*Drug:* May *decrease* effectiveness with lithium

Pharmacokinetics	Pharmacodynamics

Absorption: IV
Distribution: PB: Confined to extracellular space
Metabolism: t½: 100 min
Excretion: In urine
	Decrease in Intracranial Pressure:
	IV: Onset: 30-60 min
	    Peak: 1 h
	    Duration: 6-8 h
	Diuresis: Onset: 1-3 h
	    Peak: 1 h
	    Duration: 6-8 h

Therapeutic Effects/Uses

To treat increased intracranial pressure, cerebral edema
Mode of Action: Inhibition of reabsorption of electrolytes and water by affecting pressure of glomerular filtrate

Side Effects	Adverse Reactions
Temporary volume expansion, hypo/hypernatremia, hypo/ hyperkalemia, dehydration, blurred vision, dry mouth	Pulmonary congestion, fluid/electrolyte imbalances **Life-threatening:** Convulsions

A, Adult; *h,* hour; *IV,* intravenous; *min,* minute; *PB,* protein-binding; *sol,* solution; *t½,* half-life.

should carefully assess the client's neurologic status; monitor laboratory studies, including serum osmolality; and keep accurate intake and output records to assess fluid volume status because diuresis may be substantial (see Chapters 15, Fluid and Electrolyte Replacement, and 41, Diuretics). Drug data for mannitol are presented in Prototype Drug Chart 57–2.

Methylprednisolone

High-dose methylprednisolone may be administered as an option to clients with traumatic spinal cord injuries. Its efficacy is currently under question in regard to reducing sensory/motor deficits. A strict pharmacologic protocol must be followed. Methylprednisolone must be administered in the following manner within 8 hours of acute spinal cord injury: A bolus dose of 30 mg/kg of client's body weight is given IV over 15 minutes (mixed in 100 ml of normal saline solution); a maintenance infusion of 5.4 mg/kg/hour is then initiated within 45 minutes of the bolus and continued for 23 hours if the injury is less than 3 hours old. If the injury is between 3 and 8 hours old, the maintenance infusion must run for 48 hours.

Contraindications include allergy to the drug, penetrating trauma to the spinal cord or spinal lesions below L2,

human immunodeficiency virus (HIV) infection, severe infection, and a spinal cord injury more than 8 hours old. Relative contraindications include pregnancy and uncontrolled diabetes mellitus. Adverse effects include transient hypertension with administration of the loading dose and elevation of blood sugar during the infusion. The nurse must monitor vital signs and blood sugar and perform frequent and accurate neurologic assessments pertinent to spinal cord injury.

Table 57–2 lists neurosurgical emergency drugs and their dosages and indications (see Chapters 25, Antipsychotics and Anxiolytics, and 48, Drugs for Dermatologic Disorders).

Emergency Drugs for Poisoning

Although there are numerous antidotes for specific types of poisoning, the drugs presented in this section are the most commonly prescribed agents in cases of drug overdose and ingestion of toxic substances, with pertinent exceptions noted. Particular attention must be given to administration guidelines to achieve the best possible clinical outcome for the client. These drugs are cross-referenced to their specialty chapters.

Table 57–2

Neurosurgical Emergency Drugs

Generic (Brand)	Route and Dosage	Uses and Considerations
mannitol methylprednisolone (Solu-Medrol)	See Prototype Drug Chart 57–2. IV: bolus dose: 30 mg/kg in 100 ml NSS; then 5.4 mg/kg/h (23 h) or 48 h for SCI >3 h but <8 h old	For treatment of acute SCI (within 8 h of injury). Contraindicated in penetrating spinal cord trauma. *Pregnancy category*: C; PB: 80%-90%; $t^{1}/_{2}$: 2-4 h

h, Hour; *IV*, intravenous; *NSS*, normal saline solution; *PB*, protein-binding; *SCI*, spinal cord injury; $t^{1}/_{2}$, half-life; <, less than; >, greater than.

Naloxone

Naloxone is classified as an opiate antagonist. It reverses the effects of all opiate drugs (e.g., morphine, meperidine, codeine, propoxyphene, heroin) by competitively binding to opiate receptor sites in the body. Naloxone is indicated for individuals who have taken an overdose of opiate drugs, those experiencing respiratory or cardiovascular depression from therapeutic doses of opiates given in a health care setting, and those brought to the emergency department in a coma of unknown etiology (which may be drug induced).

The typical dose of naloxone for actual or suspected opiate overdose in adults is 0.4 to 2 mg IV administered every 2 minutes until the client's condition improves to an acceptable level. If there is no improvement within 10 minutes after 10 mg of the drug has been injected, nonopiate drugs or disease must be suspected. Although naloxone should be administered IV in emergency situations, it also may be given intramuscularly (IM) or subQ if IV access is not readily obtainable.

Because most opiate drugs have a longer duration of action than naloxone, the nurse must monitor the client closely for signs and symptoms of recurrent opiate effects such as respiratory depression and hypotension. In this situation, naloxone administration may need to be repeated several times or a continuous IV infusion ordered. Naloxone has no major adverse effects but can precipitate withdrawal symptoms in clients addicted to opiate drugs and, rarely, cause anaphylaxis. In addition, pulmonary edema has been reported following naloxone administration in clients who have had an overdose of morphine (see Chapter 21, Drugs for Pain Management: Nonnarcotic and Narcotic Analgesics). Drug data for naloxone are presented in Prototype Drug Chart 57–3.

For total narcotic reversal in children up to 5 years old and less than 20 kg, give 0.1 mg/kg. For children older than 5 years and more than 20 kg, give 2 mg. Repeat as necessary. Naloxone can be administered either IV or via the intraosseous route in children.

Flumazenil

Flumazenil is the reversal agent for the respiratory depressant and sedative effects of benzodiazepine medications (e.g., diazepam [Valium], midazolam [Versed], chlordiazepoxide [Librium]). It is administered to counteract the effects of benzodiazepines given as sedative or anesthetic agents as well as to treat accidental or intentional benzodiazepine overdose. Flumazenil does not reverse the central nervous system (CNS) depressant effects of nonbenzodiazepine agents such as alcohol, opiates, and barbiturates. In addition, flumazenil may not reverse amnesia induced by benzodiazepines.

Flumazenil is given IV in an initial dose of 0.2 mg over 15 seconds. A second dose of 0.3 mg may be given over 30 seconds. A third dose and subsequent doses of 0.5 mg IV may be given every minute until the desired clinical response is achieved or until a total dose of 3 mg is given. If sedation occurs again, doses of flumazenil may be repeated at 20-minute intervals (not to exceed 1 mg at a time) to a total hourly dose of no more than 3 mg IV.

Nursing considerations include careful assessment of respiratory rate and effort, blood pressure, and mental status. If the benzodiazepine is reversed too rapidly, clients may have emergent reactions in which they become agitated and confused and experience perceptual distortions. Because seizures are precipitated by benzodiazepine withdrawal, seizure precautions must be implemented for clients at risk (those with long-standing benzodiazepine use or abuse) or for those who have a known seizure disorder.

Activated Charcoal

Activated charcoal is prescribed for poisoning because it adsorbs ingested toxins in the gastrointestinal (GI) tract and prevents their absorption into the body. In cases of known or suspected poisoning, activated charcoal is prepared as a slurry and given orally or via a gastric tube following gastric lavage. The dose is dependent on the amount of poison ingested; the typical adult and pediatric dose is 1 to 2 g/kg.

Vomiting is a common adverse reaction, and the nurse should use activated charcoal with extreme caution in the client with an impaired gag reflex or altered level of consciousness because there is risk of aspiration. Activated charcoal should not be administered with milk products because they decrease its adsorptive properties. A **cathartic** is often ordered following administration of activated charcoal to speed elimination of the charcoal-toxin complex from the body. The client should be told that charcoal produces black stools (see Chapter 45, Drugs for Gastrointestinal Tract Disorders).

PROTOTYPE DRUG CHART 57–3

NALOXONE HCl

Drug Class	Dosage
Narcotic antagonist Trade Name: Narcan *Pregnancy Category:* B	IV/IM/subQ: 0.4-2 mg; repeat every 2-3 min, as indicated

Contraindications	Drug-Lab-Food Interactions
Hypersensitivity, respiratory depression *Caution:* Opiate-dependent clients, cardiac disease, breastfeeding neonates of opiate-dependent mothers	*Drug:* Naloxone can precipitate withdrawal in a client dependent on narcotic analgesics *Lab:* Urine vanillylmandelic acid (VMA), 5-hydroxyheptadecatrienoic acid (5-HIAA), urine glucose

Pharmacokinetics	Pharmacodynamics
Absorption: IM/subQ: Well absorbed Distribution: PB: UK Metabolism: $t^{1/2}$: Adults: 1-4 h; neonates: 1-3 h Excretion: In urine metabolites	subQ/IM: Onset: 2-5 min Peak: UK Duration: 1-4 h IV: Onset: 1-2 min Peak: UK Duration: 1-4 h

Therapeutic Effects/Uses

To treat respiratory depression caused by narcotics; to treat narcotic-induced depressant effects and narcotic overdose
Mode of Action: Blocks effects of narcotics by competing for the receptor sites

Side Effects	Adverse Reactions
Negligible pharmacologic effect without narcotics in body	Nausea, vomiting, tremulousness, sweating, tachycardia, elevated blood pressure **Life-threatening:** Atrioventricular fibrillation, pulmonary edema (with overdose of morphine)

h, Hour; *IV,* intravenous; *IM,* intramuscular; *min,* minute; *PB,* protein-binding; *subQ,* subcutaneous; $t^{1/2}$, half-life; *UK,* unknown.

Table 57–3 lists the emergency drugs for poisoning and their dosages and indications.

Emergency Drugs for Shock

Drugs may be required to elevate blood pressure and to improve cardiac performance in various types of shock states. Therapeutic agents described in this section are indicated in conditions such as cardiogenic shock, neurogenic shock, septic shock, anaphylactic shock, and insulin shock. A noteworthy exception to the list of shock states is **hypovolemic shock** (shock resulting from loss of blood or fluid volume); drugs should not be used in an attempt to correct the hypotension associated with this condition. Administration of fluids or blood products or both is the only acceptable means to treat hypovolemic shock. These drugs are cross-referenced to their specialty chapters.

Dopamine

Dopamine is a sympathomimetic agent often used to treat hypotension in shock states that are *not* caused by hypovolemia. Dopamine may also be used to increase heart rate (beta$_1$ effect) in bradycardic rhythms when atropine has not been effective. The dose range is 1 to 20 mcg/kg/min.

The actions of dopamine are dose dependent. At low doses (1 to 2 mcg/kg/min), dopamine dilates renal and mesenteric blood vessels, producing an increase in urine output (dopaminergic effect). At doses of 2 to 10 mcg/kg/min, dopamine enhances cardiac output by increasing myocardial contractility and increasing heart rate (beta$_1$ effect) and elevates blood pressure through vasoconstriction (alpha-adrenergic effect). Alpha effects predominate at doses of 10 mcg/kg/min and above—vasoconstriction of renal, mesenteric, and peripheral blood vessels occurs. Such vasoconstriction, although sometimes necessary to maintain adequate blood pressure in severe shock, can lead to poor organ and tissue perfusion, decreased cardiac performance, and reduction of urine output. The lowest effective dose of dopamine should be used. Clients must be weaned gradually from dopamine; abrupt discontinuation of the infusion can cause severe hypotension.

Dopamine is typically mixed as a concentration of 400 to 800 mg in 250 ml D$_5$W and administered IV by a volumetric infusion pump for precision, preferably in a central vein. Sodium bicarbonate will inactivate dopamine; therefore do not infuse dopamine in the same IV line. Continuous heart and blood pressure monitoring is essential. The nurse must carefully document vital signs and intake and

Table 57–3

Emergency Drugs for Poisoning

Generic (Brand)	Route and Dosage	Uses and Considerations
flumazenil	IV: Initial dose 0.2 mg over 15 sec. Additional doses of 0.3-0.5 mg over 30 sec every 1 min as indicated. For re-sedation, may be repeated at 20-min intervals to a total dose of no more than 3 mg.	Reversal agent for benzodiazepine overdose; may precipitate seizures in clients with long-term use or abuse of benzodiazepines and those with seizure disorders; may precipitate emergent reactions. *Pregnancy category:* C; PB: 50%; $t^{1}/_{2}$: Variable (40-80 min)
naloxone (Narcan)	See Prototype Drug Chart 57–3.	
activated charcoal	A & C: 1-2 g/mg PO	To treat poisoning. Onset: <1 min. *Pregnancy category:* C; PB: NA; $t^{1}/_{2}$: NA

A, Adult; *C,* child; *IV,* intravenous; *min,* minute; *NA,* not applicable; *PB,* protein-binding; *PO,* by mouth; *sec,* second; $t^{1}/_{2}$, half-life; <, less than.

PROTOTYPE DRUG CHART 57–4

DOPAMINE HCl

Drug Class
Adrenergic
Trade Name: Intropin
Pregnancy Category: C

Dosage
A: IV: Drip: 1-20 mcg/kg/min (>10 mcg/kg/min may be ordered if lower doses are ineffective)

Contraindications
Hypersensitivity, tachydysrhythmias, ventricular fibrillation, pheochromocytomas
Caution: Safety in children is not known.

Drug-Lab-Food Interactions
Drug: Use within 2 wk of MAOIs may result in hypertensive crisis; concurrent IV administration of phenytoin may result in hypotension and bradycardia; sodium bicarbonate solutions inactivate dopamine—do *not* administer through the same IV line

Pharmacokinetics
Absorption: IV
Distribution: PB: UK
Metabolism: $t^{1}/_{2}$: 2 min
Excretion: In urine

Pharmacodynamics
IV: Onset: 1-2 min
Peak: <5 min
Duration: <10 min

Therapeutic Effects/Uses
To treat hypotension in shock states *not* caused by hypovolemia; to increase heart rate in atropine-refractory bradycardia; to increase urine output at a "renal dose" (<5 mg/kg/min)
Mode of Action: Stimulates receptors to cause cardiac stimulation and renal vasodilation; increases systemic vascular resistance at higher dose ranges

Side Effects
Palpitations, tachycardia, hypertension, ectopic beats, angina, IV line site irritation, piloerection, nausea, vomiting

Adverse Reactions
Cardiac dysrhythmias, azotemia, tissue sloughing (from extravasation)
Life-threatening: MI, gangrene in extremities (from vasoconstriction)

A, Adult; *IV,* intravenous; *MAOIs,* monoamine oxidase inhibitors; *MI,* myocardial infarction; *min,* minute; *PB,* protein-binding; $t^{1}/_{2}$, half-life; *UK,* unknown; *wk,* week; >, greater than; <, less than.

output as ordered. Significant adverse effects include tachycardia, dysrhythmias, myocardial ischemia, nausea, and vomiting. The IV site must be assessed hourly for signs of drug infiltration: **extravasation** (escape into tissues) of dopamine can produce tissue necrosis that can necessitate surgical debridement and skin grafting. If extravasation occurs, the site should be injected in multiple areas with phentolamine (Regitine), 5 to 10 mg diluted in 10 to 15 ml of normal saline to reduce or prevent tissue damage (see Chapter 17, Adrenergics and Adrenergic Blockers). Drug data for dopamine are presented in Prototype Drug Chart 57–4.

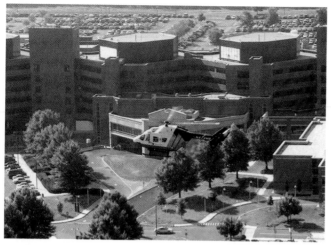

FIGURE 57–1 Most severe injury-related emergencies are best managed at a level I trauma center. (Courtesy Christiana Care Health System, Wilmington, Delaware.)

Dobutamine

Dobutamine is a sympathomimetic drug with beta$_1$-adrenergic activities. The beta$_1$ effects include enhancing the force of myocardial contraction (positive inotropic effect) and increasing heart rate (positive chronotropic effect). Dobutamine is indicated in shock states when improvement in cardiac output and overall cardiac performance is desired. Blood pressure is elevated only through the increase in cardiac output; dobutamine has no vasoconstriction effects and may produce a mild vasodilation. The usual IV dose range of dobutamine is 2 to 20 mcg/kg/min administered via a volumetric infusion pump for precision. A typical concentration of dobutamine is 250 mg to 1000 mg mixed in 250 ml of D$_5$W or normal saline. Like dopamine, dobutamine administration should be tapered gradually as the client's condition warrants.

Continuous cardiac and blood pressure monitoring are required for clients receiving dobutamine infusions. Adverse effects are dose related and include myocardial ischemia, tachycardia, dysrhythmias, headache, nausea, and tremors. The nurse must carefully monitor vital signs and intake and output and assess for any signs or symptoms of myocardial ischemia such as chest pain or development of dysrhythmias (see Chapter 23, Drugs for Neurologic Disorders: Parkinsonism and Alzheimer's Disease).

Norepinephrine

Norepinephrine is a catecholamine with extremely potent vasoconstrictor actions (alpha-adrenergic effect). It is used in shock states, often when drugs such as dopamine and dobutamine have failed to produce adequate blood pressure. Like high-dose dopamine, the peripheral vasoconstriction that results has the potential to impair cardiac performance and decrease organ and tissue perfusion. In general, 4 to 8 mg of norepinephrine are added to 250 ml D$_5$W or normal saline solution and infused at 0.5 to 30 mcg/min (titrated) for adults. Continuous cardiac monitoring and precise blood pressure monitoring are required. The drug

must be tapered slowly; abrupt discontinuation can result in severe hypotension.

Nursing actions and considerations are the same as those for dopamine. Norepinephrine should not be used to treat hypotension in hypovolemic clients; fluid, blood, or both must be administered to restore adequate volume first. Adverse effects of norepinephrine include myocardial ischemia, dysrhythmias, and impaired organ perfusion. Extravasation of norepinephrine causes tissue necrosis; therefore attention to the IV site is essential. If extravasation occurs, the area should be infiltrated with phentolamine, as described for dopamine (see Chapter 17, Adrenergics and Adrenergic Blockers).

Epinephrine

Epinephrine is the drug of choice in the treatment of **anaphylactic shock**, an allergic response of the most serious type brought about by an antibody-antigen reaction. Anaphylactic shock can be fatal if prompt treatment is not initiated. Severe bronchoconstriction and hypotension resulting from cardiovascular collapse are its hallmarks. Epinephrine is also indicated for an acute, severe asthmatic attack.

Administration of epinephrine causes bronchodilation, enhanced cardiac performance, and vasoconstriction to increase blood pressure. In severe **asthma** and anaphylactic shock, epinephrine is given in a 0.2- to 0.5-mg dose range IM or subQ for adults via a tuberculin syringe for accuracy (1:1000 solution). IM administration is preferable to subQ administration because the IM route has a more predictable pattern of absorption. As an alternative, epinephrine can be given in a dose of 0.1 to 0.25 mg IV over 5 to 10 minutes (1:10,000 solution). Epinephrine administration can be repeated every 5 to 15 minutes if necessary.

The nurse must carefully monitor the client who receives epinephrine for tachycardia, cardiac dysrhythmias, hypertension, and angina. Clients who are given IV epinephrine must be on a cardiac monitor, with resuscitation equipment immediately available. Other adverse effects include excitability, fear, anxiety, and restlessness. In addition, the nurse should be alert to the possibility that the anaphylactic response may recur and necessitate repeated treatment. For this reason, steroids are commonly ordered and are slowly tapered over days to weeks to prevent recurrence. Examples of steroids are hydrocortisone sodium succinate, prednisone, and methylprednisolone. Client education should include strict avoidance of the agents responsible for the anaphylactic reaction and follow-up care with a physician. For some clients, such as those with severe allergic responses to bee stings, the physician may prescribe an epinephrine kit or pen to be carried with the client for self-medication in the event of contact with the antigen. Proper client education regarding the use of the kit or pen is essential (see Chapters 17, Adrenergics and Adrenergic Blockers, and Chapter 39, Drugs for Acute and Chronic Lower Respiratory Disorders).

Albuterol

Albuterol is a beta-adrenergic bronchodilator used to reverse bronchoconstriction in anaphylactic shock, asthma, and COPD. In emergency situations, it is administered via a nebulizer (adults: 0.5 ml of 0.5% inhalation solution in 2.5 ml saline). The nurse should assess breath sounds before and after administration; effectiveness is evidenced by relief of bronchospasm. In severe bronchospasm, wheezing may not be audible. As the bronchospasm is relieved, wheezing may become more pronounced, indicating that the drug is producing the desired therapeutic effect. Assessment of the client's subjective feelings of respiratory distress before and after administration is especially important. Adverse effects of albuterol include tachycardia, tremor, nervousness, cardiac dysrhythmias, and hypertension.

Diphenhydramine Hydrochloride

Diphenhydramine, an antihistamine, is often administered with epinephrine in anaphylactic shock. This agent is effective for treating the histamine-induced tissue swelling and pruritus common to severe allergic reactions. The standard adult dose is 25 to 50 mg administered IV or deep IM. An oral form of the drug exists, but the parenteral form is preferred in emergencies. Adverse effects include drowsiness, sedation, confusion, vertigo, excitability, hypotension, tachycardia, GI disturbances, and dry mouth (see Chapter 38, Drugs for Common Upper Respiratory Disorders).

Dextrose 50%

Dextrose 50% is a concentrated, high-carbohydrate solution given to treat insulin-induced hypoglycemia or insulin shock. When insulin shock is known or suspected and the client's state of consciousness is impaired such that oral administration of sugar solutions is contraindicated, 50 ml of dextrose 50% is commonly ordered and given as an IV bolus. Dextrose 50% is highly irritating to veins and should be administered in a large peripheral or central vein whenever possible. Phlebitis can occur. Extravasation of the solution can cause tissue sloughing and necrosis. The nurse must monitor the client's blood sugar carefully; hyperglycemia is common, especially after rapid injection. Urine output should be accurately recorded because osmotic diuresis can occur when blood sugar is elevated, and a hyperosmolar state can result. Client education must be centered on teaching about diabetes and insulin administration.

Pediatric Implications

Glycogen stores in infants and children may be quickly depleted in stress states produced by severe illness. Because adequate amounts of glucose are essential to strong myocardial function, hypoglycemia must be corrected to provide the greatest chance for successful resuscitation. After determining that hypoglycemia is present by the finger- or heel-stick method of rapid blood glucose testing, dextrose 25% or less may be administered per physician order. Because glucose is supplied in a 50% concentration, it must be diluted 1:1 in sterile water before administration to reduce its osmolarity and prevent sclerosis of peripheral veins. The standard dose is 0.5 to 1 g/kg IV (see Chapter 50, Antidiabetic Drugs).

Glucagon

Glucagon is a hormone produced by the pancreas that elevates blood sugar by stimulating glycogen breakdown (**glycogenolysis**). Glucagon, like dextrose 50%, is indicated in the treatment of severe insulin-induced hypoglycemia or insulin shock. In an emergency when dextrose 50% is unavailable or cannot be administered IV, glucagon is an effective agent. Glucagon may be given subQ, IM, or IV. The standard dose for adults and children is 0.5 to 1 mg, which can be repeated in 20 minutes for persistent coma. If the coma has not resolved after two doses, dextrose 50% should be administered. Adverse effects from glucagon are uncommon but can include nausea and vomiting. Glucagon can also be used as an agent to reverse the effects of calcium channel blocker and beta-blocker overdose with an IV infusion of 1 to 5 mg given over 2 to 5 minutes.

Table 57–4 lists the emergency drugs for shock and their dosages and indications (see Chapter 50, Antidiabetic Drugs).

Emergency Drugs for Hypertensive Crises and Pulmonary Edema

A variety of pharmacologic agents may be prescribed to treat **hypertensive crisis**, generally defined as a diastolic blood pressure that exceeds 110 to 120 mm Hg, and pulmonary edema. Three of the most commonly prescribed drugs are discussed in this section. The drugs are cross-referenced to their specialty chapter.

Labetalol

Labetalol is a beta-adrenergic blocker that acts by inhibiting the effects of the sympathetic nervous system. Its pharmacologic actions include lowering heart rate, blood pressure, myocardial contractility, myocardial oxygen consumption, and reducing the vasoconstriction that results from sympathetic nervous system stimulation. This agent is indicated for the acute management of clinically significant hypertension in the presence of ischemic and hemorrhagic stroke as well as for hypertensive crisis.

Initially 10 mg of labetalol is administered IV push over 1 to 2 minutes. This starting dose can be repeated or doubled every 10 minutes until the desired clinical response is achieved, to a maximum dose of 150 mg. A continuous infusion mixed with D_5W or normal saline can then be prepared to deliver 2 to 8 mg/min of labetalol.

Important nursing considerations during the administration of labetalol include the use of a volumetric infusion pump for accurate continuous infusion medication delivery, cardiac monitoring, and frequent blood pressure measurement. Documentation of blood pressure may need to be as often as every 5 minutes during the IV push phase

Table 57–4

Agents for Emergency Treatment of Shock

Generic	Route and Dosage	Uses and Considerations
albuterol	A: nebulizer: 0.5 ml of 0.5% inhalation solution in 2.5 ml saline	Bronchoconstriction secondary to anaphylactic shock, asthma, and COPD. Tachycardia, tremor, nervousness, cardiac dysrhythmias, and hypertension. *Pregnancy category:* C; PB: UK; $t^{1}/_{2}$: 3.7-5 h
dextrose 50%	A: IV: 50 ml C: 0.5-1.0 g/kg IV of a D 25% sol	Insulin shock; severe hypoglycemia. *Pregnancy category:* C; PB: UK; $t^{1}/_{2}$: UK
diphenhydramine	IM/IV: 25-50 mg	Anaphylactic shock; acute allergic reaction. *Pregnancy category:* C; PB: 98%-99%; $t^{1}/_{2}$: 3-8 h
dobutamine	IV: Drip: 2-10 mcg/kg/min	Low cardiac output. Effects antagonized by beta-blockers. *Pregnancy category:* C; PB: UK; $t^{1}/_{2}$: 2 min
dopamine HCl	See Prototype Drug Chart 57–4.	
epinephrine	IM/subQ: 0.2-0.5 mg (1:1000 sol) IV: 0.1-0.25 mg (1:10,000 sol) ETT: 2.0-2.5 mg diluted in 10 ml normal saline	Anaphylactic shock; severe acute asthmatic attack. Hypertensive crisis with MAOIs; increased dysrhythmias with cardiac glycosides. *Pregnancy category:* C; PB: UK; $t^{1}/_{2}$: UK
glucagon	subQ/IM/IV: 0.5-1 mg; may repeat × 1	Insulin shock; severe hypoglycemia; beta-blocker overdose (reverses effects of beta-blockers). *Pregnancy category:* B; PB: UK; $t^{1}/_{2}$: 3-10 min
norepinephrine	IV: Drip: 0.1-30 mcg/min (titrated)	Hypotension not responsive to other therapies. *Pregnancy category:* D; PB: UK; $t^{1}/_{2}$: UK

A, Adult; *C*, child; *COPD*, chronic obstructive pulmonary disease; *ETT*, endotracheal tube; *h*, hour; *IM*, intramuscular; *IV*, intravenous; *MAOIs*, monoamine oxidase inhibitors; *min*, minute; *PB*, protein-binding; *sol*, solution; *subQ*, subcutaneous; $t^{1}/_{2}$, half-life; *UK*, unknown.

of dosing and at the initiation of the continuous infusion. Serious adverse effects include hypotension, ventricular dysrhythmias, and bronchospasm. Labetalol is contraindicated in clients with bronchial asthma or COPD because of the risk of bronchospasm and in clients with severe bradycardia or apparent heart failure.

Sodium Nitroprusside

Sodium nitroprusside is an IV agent used to reduce arterial blood pressure in hypertensive emergencies. The mechanism of action is immediate direct arterial and venous vasodilation. Antihypertensive effects end when sodium nitroprusside is discontinued; blood pressure increases as soon as drug administration is stopped. Continuous and accurate blood pressure measurement is required. In general, 50 mg of sodium nitroprusside is mixed in 250 ml D_5W. The typical dose range for adults is 0.1 to 5 mcg/kg/min, titrated to the desired clinical response.

There are several important nursing considerations:
1. Sodium nitroprusside is rapidly inactivated by light; the IV bottle or bag must be wrapped with aluminum foil or another opaque material to protect the solution from degradation.
2. Although a faint brown tint is typical, blue or brown discoloration of the solution indicates degradation and necessitates that the solution be discarded.
3. When sodium nitroprusside therapy is prolonged, clients are at risk for toxicity resulting from elevated serum thiocyanate or cyanide levels (byproducts of drug metabolism). Signs and symptoms include metabolic acidosis, profound hypotension, dizziness, and vomit-

ing. Serum thiocyanate levels should be monitored at least every 24 hours for clients receiving prolonged infusions of more than 3 mcg/kg/min. Clients with renal insufficiency or failure are at a higher risk because the metabolites are excreted in the urine.
4. Clients should be placed on an oral antihypertensive agent as soon as possible so that sodium nitroprusside can be tapered slowly (see Chapters 41, Diuretics; and Chapter 42, Antihypertensive Drugs). Drug data for sodium nitroprusside are presented in Prototype Drug Chart 57–5.

Furosemide

Furosemide is classified as a loop diuretic that acts by inhibiting sodium and chloride reabsorption from the ascending loop of Henle. It promotes the renal excretion of water, sodium, chloride, magnesium, hydrogen, and calcium and depletes potassium. Furosemide also has peripheral and renal vasodilating effects that can lower blood pressure. The main indications for use of furosemide as an emergency drug are acute pulmonary edema from left ventricular dysfunction and hypertensive crisis.

Furosemide is given as an initial bolus of 0.5 to 1 mg/kg IV over 1 to 2 minutes. For clients who take furosemide on a regular basis, the effective dose may be much higher (up to 2 mg/kg). The vasodilatory effects occur *before* diuresis begins and act to lower blood pressure. Central venous pressure is reduced through a decrease in venous return to the heart from venodilation. Diuresis should start within 10 minutes of drug administration and may continue for approximately 6 hours.

PROTOTYPE DRUG CHART 57-5

SODIUM NITROPRUSSIDE

Drug Class Vasodilator Trade Name: Nipride *Pregnancy Category:* C	**Dosage** **A: IV: Drip:** 0.5-5 mcg/kg/min; begin at 0.1 mg/kg/min and titrate to desired effect up to 5 mcg/kg/min
Contraindications Hypersensitivity, hypertension (compensatory), decreased cerebral perfusion, coarctation of aorta *Caution:* Increased intracranial pressure	**Drug-Lab-Food Interactions** *Drug:* Antihypertensives, general anesthetics Do not mix with any other drug in syringe or solution. *Lab:* Decrease in P_{CO_2}, pH
Pharmacokinetics **Absorption:** IV only **Distribution:** PB: UK **Metabolism:** t½: <10 min **Excretion:** In urine	**Pharmacodynamics** **IV:** Onset: 1-2 min Peak: Rapid Duration: 1-10 min

Therapeutic Effects/Uses

To treat hypertensive crisis; and to decrease systemic vascular resistance to improve cardiac performance
Mode of Action: Stimulates smooth muscle of veins and arteries; produces peripheral vasodilation

Side Effects Dizziness, headache, nausea, abdominal pain, sweating, palpitations, weakness, vomiting	**Adverse Reactions** Thiocyanate toxicity: tinnitus, dyspnea, blurred vision, metabolic acidosis **Life-threatening:** Severe hypotension, loss of consciousness, profound cardiovascular depression

A, Adult; *IV,* intravenous; *min,* minute; *PB,* protein-binding; P_{CO_2}, partial pressure of carbon dioxide; *t½,* half-life; *UK,* unknown; <, less than.

The most significant adverse effects are severe hypovolemia, dehydration, and electrolyte disturbances (hypokalemia, hypomagnesemia, hyponatremia, and hypochloremia). Clients on digitalis preparations are at an increased risk of digitalis toxicity from hypokalemia. The client's fluid and electrolyte status must be carefully assessed before and after furosemide administration, including auscultation of breath sounds for rales, strict surveillance of intake and output, and review of laboratory data when available. Electrolyte and careful fluid replacement may be required during furosemide therapy to prevent physiologic consequences. The nurse must also exercise caution in administering the drug to clients with sulfonamide sensitivity because furosemide is a sulfonamide derivative and can produce an allergic reaction.

Morphine Sulfate

Like furosemide, morphine sulfate is also indicated for acute pulmonary edema because it produces venous vasodilation that decreases cardiac **preload** (the amount of blood returning to the right ventricle). The net effect is a decrease in pulmonary venous congestion. Morphine has been discussed previously in this chapter.

Table 57–5 lists the emergency drugs for hypertensive crises and pulmonary edema and their dosages and considerations.

WEBSITES

For further information on *Adult and Pediatric Emergency Drugs,* visit these Internet resources:

American Association of Critical Care Nurses:
www.aacn.org

American Heart Association:
www.americanheart.org/cpr

Emergency Nurses Association:
www.ena.org

Table 57-5

Emergency Drugs for Hypertensive Crises and Pulmonary Edema

Generic (Brand)	Route and Dosage	Uses and Considerations
sodium nitroprusside (Nipride)	See Prototype Drug Chart 57-5.	
furosemide (Lasix)	IV: initial bolus of 0.5-1.0 mg/kg over 1-2 min, up to 2 mg/kg	Acute pulmonary edema from left ventricular dysfunction; hypertensive crisis. *Adverse effects:* hypovolemia, dehydration, electrolyte disturbances
morphine	IV: 1-4 mg q5-30min	Pulmonary edema, chest pain, unstable angina, MI
labetalol hydrochloride	IV: Initial push 10 mg over 1-2 min, repeated or doubled q10 min up to a max of 150 mg; continuous infusion 2-8 mg/min	Uses: Hypertension in CVA and hypertensive crisis. *Adverse effects:* ventricular dysrhythmias, hypotension, bronchospasm. Contraindications: bronchial asthma, COPD, severe bradycardia, heart failure

COPD, Chronic obstructive pulmonary disease; *CVA,* cerebrovascular accident; *IV,* intravenous; *max,* maximum; *min,* minute; *MI,* myocardial infarction.

Critical Thinking Case Study

J.S., age 23, was assaulted during a gang fight 1 hour ago. He was stabbed in the back and suffered blows to the head with a baseball bat. The knife penetrated the spinal cord at the T4 level. At this time, J.S. opens his eyes spontaneously, is agitated, and does not follow commands. He moans and localizes to pain with his upper extremities only. His lower extremities exhibit no movement. His admitting diagnoses include penetrating spinal cord injury with paraplegia at the T4 level and a closed head injury with cerebral edema diagnosed by computed tomography (CT) scan at the trauma center.

J.S. is HIV-positive and addicted to heroin. He also abuses oral diazepam (Valium) and other street drugs. His current vital signs are BP 88/56, HR 56, RR 24, temp 96.8° F (36° C). He has two functional IV catheters (one peripheral line in the right forearm and one central line in the left femoral vein), an oral gastric tube, and an indwelling urinary catheter.

1. On arrival to the trauma center, should J.S. have received supplemental oxygen based on his mechanism of injury? What type of oxygen device would be appropriate for J.S. upon initial presentation?

2. The physician orders 50 g of mannitol to be given now, IV push. On hand are several 50-ml vials of "mannitol, 25%" solution. How many milliliters of mannitol are needed to draw up in the syringe to administer 50 g?

3. Describe the type of needle that must be used when administering mannitol and why. What size syringe should be used? Which IV line should be used to administer the mannitol to J.S.?

4. Based on the case study, what are the indications for mannitol administration? List at least three nursing considerations when giving mannitol.

5. J.S. has a T4 spinal cord injury with paralysis. Should methylprednisolone be administered within 8 hours of injury in his case? Why or why not?

6. J.S. has a history of heroin and diazepam abuse. List the reversal agents that could be used if the trauma team believes recent illicit drug use may be a contributing factor to his altered mental state.

7. Because of J.S.'s spinal cord injury, he is exhibiting signs of neurogenic shock: bradycardia, warm skin, hypotension. What is the drug of choice that the nurse should keep at the bedside in case J.S. requires emergency treatment for symptomatic bradycardia? Name the drug, its mechanism of action, and dosing considerations.

8. The physician orders a dopamine infusion, 800 mg/250 ml D₅W, to be titrated to maintain systolic BP >110 mmHg. Which IV site would be the best choice for a continuous dopamine infusion in J.S.? What is the consequence of dopamine extravasation? What is the treatment for dopamine extravasation?

9. What vital sign parameters must be monitored while J.S. receives dopamine? Name at least four adverse effects of dopamine.

Antibiotics are initiated to address the potential for infection in J.S.'s stab wound because the stab wound communicates with his spinal cord. Upon infusion of the antibiotic, a body-wide rash, swelling of the lips and tongue, wheezing, and hypotension develop.

10. After antibiotic administration, what condition has developed in J.S.?

11. What are the drugs of choice to treat J.S.'s condition now?

12. How can the nurse evaluate the effectiveness of these drugs?

Study Questions

1. What is the minimum dose of atropine that should be given to an adult with bradycardia?

2. Explain the actions of epinephrine and diphenhydramine for clients in anaphylactic shock. How are these drugs administered in this situation?

3. What are the signs and symptoms of lidocaine toxicity?

4. Why is activated charcoal given for poisoning? List the actions of activated charcoal.

5. What are the similarities and dissimilarities in dextrose 50% and glucagon?

6. For what class of drug overdose is naloxone effective? What important precautions must be taken?

7. Describe the protocol for administering methylprednisolone to a client with an acute spinal cord injury. Would you expect the drug to produce a noticeable effect immediately?

8. What are the emergency indications for mannitol in the neurosurgical setting? Describe pertinent nursing considerations for its administration.

9. What are the adverse effects of isoproterenol and the pertinent nursing considerations and actions?

10. What are the endpoints of procainamide administration?

11. What is the antidote for extravasation of both norepinephrine and dopamine? How should it be administered?

12. What are the signs and symptoms of thiocyanate toxicity in clients receiving sodium nitroprusside?

13. How does dobutamine increase blood pressure compared with dopamine?

14. What are the dose-dependent effects of dopamine?

15. What are the relevant nursing considerations and actions when administering verapamil?

16. Discuss indications for adenosine. What are pertinent nursing considerations when administering adenosine?

17. What are the similarities and dissimilarities in IV diltiazem and verapamil?

18. What is the maximum total adult dose of IV atropine for the treatment of bradycardia? Why will additional doses of atropine be ineffective?

19. What are at least three contraindications to methylprednisolone administration in acute spinal cord injury?

20. What are the relevant nursing considerations when administering sodium nitroprusside?

21. After administering the initial dose of adenosine, the nurse observes a short period of asystole. Does this represent an adverse drug effect?

22. How are sublingual nitroglycerin tablets administered to the client experiencing chest pain?

23. What teaching points should be emphasized when a client is discharged to home with a prescription for sublingual nitroglycerin?

24. What drug is indicated to reverse significant respiratory depressant effects of morphine sulfate?

25. What is the typical dose range of IV morphine?

26. How should 50% dextrose solution be diluted for safe administration to pediatric clients?

27. What is the reversal agent for benzodiazepine overdose and what are two key nursing considerations when administering this drug?

28. What are the uses and indications for magnesium sulfate as they relate to clients with cardiac disorders?

29. What is the mechanism of action for furosemide (Lasix) in relation to pulmonary edema and hypertensive crisis?

30. What is the drug of choice for treatment of hypoxemia?

Appendix A — Generic Drugs with Corresponding Canadian Trade Drug Names*

Generic Drug Names	Canadian Trade/Brand Names	Generic Drug Names	Canadian Trade/Brand Names
acebutolol	Monitan	chlordiazepoxide hydrochloride	Medilium, Novopoxide, Solium
acetaminophen	Abenol, Apo-Acetaminophen, Atasol, Exdol, Robigesic, Rounox	chloroprocaine hydrochloride	Nesacaine-CE
acetazolamide	Acetazolam, Apo-Acetazolamide	chlorpheniramine maleate	Chlor-Tripolon, Novo-Pheniram
acetohexamide	Dimelor	chlorpromazine hydrochloride	Chlorpromanyl, Largactil, Novo-Chlorpromazine
acetylcysteine	Airbron, Parvolex	chlorpropamide	Apo-Chlorpropamide, Chloronase, Novopropamide
albuterol	Novo-Salmol, Airomir		
allopurinol	Alloprin, Apo-Allopurinol, Novopurinol, Purinol	chlorprothixene	Tarasan
aminophylline	Gorophyllin, Paladron	chlorthalidone	Novothalidone, Uridon
aminosalicylate sodium	Parasal Sodium	cimetidine	Novo-Cimetine, Peptol
amitriptyline hydrochloride	Apo-Amitriptyline, Levate, Novotriptyn	cisplatin	Abiplatin
		clindamycin	Dalacin C
amoxicillin	Apo-Amoxi, Novamoxin	clofibrate	Claripex, Novofibrate
amoxicillin clavulanate K	Clavulin	clonazepam	Rivotril
ampicillin	NovoAmpicillin, Apo-Ampi, Nu-Ampi	clonidine hydrochloride	Dixarit
		clorazepate dipotassium	Novo-Clopate
ascorbic acid	Apo-C, Ce-Vi-Sol, Redoxon	clotrimazole	Canesten
asparaginase	Kidrolase	cloxacillin sodium	Apo-Cloxi, Novo-Cloxin, Orbenin
aspirin	Astrin, Entrophen, Novasen, Supasa, Triaphen-10		
		codeine phosphate	Paveral
atenolol	Apo-Atenol	colchicine	Novocolchine
atropine sulfate	Atropair	colestipol hydrochloride	Cholestabyl, Lestid
bacampicillin hydrochloride	Penglobe	co-trimoxazole	Apo-Sulfatrim
benzalkonium chloride	Pharmatex	cromolyn sodium	Fivent, Rynacrom, Vistacrom
benztropine mesylate	Apo-Benztropine, Bensylate, PMS Benzotropine	cyanocobalamin	Anacobin, Bedoz, Cyanabin, Rubion
betamethasone	Beban, Betaderm, Betnelan, Betnesol, Betnovate, Celestoderm, Novobetamet	cyclizine hydrochloride	Marzine
		cyclophosphamide	Procytox
bisacodyl	Apo-Bisacodyl, Bisco-Lax, Laxit	cyproheptadine hydrochloride	Vimicon
		danazol	Cyclomen
bretylium tosylate	Bretylate	dapsone	Avlosulfon
calcium carbonate	Apo-Cal, Calsan, Caltrate	dexamethasone	Deronil, Dexasone, Oradexon
carbamazepine	Apo-Carbamazepine, Mazepine, PMS Carbamazepine	dextroamphetamine sulfate	Oxydess II
		dextromethorphan	Balminil DM, Koffex, Ornex DM, Robidex, Sedatuss
carbenicillin indanyl sodium	Geopen oral		
carvedilol	Kredex	diazepam	Apo-Diazepam, Diazemuls, Novodipam, Vivol
cephalexin	Ceporex, Novo-Lexin		
cephalothin sodium	Ceporacin	dicyclomine hydrochloride	Bentylol, Formulex, Lomine, Protylol, Spasmoban, Viscerol
cetirizine	Reactine		
chloral hydrate	Novo-Chlorhydrate		
chloramphenicol	Novochorocap, Pentamycetin	diethylpropion hydrochloride	Nobesine

*Many of the trade or brand names are used in both the United States and Canada. This appendix lists selected trade or brand names specific to Canada.

Generic Drug Names	Canadian Trade/Brand Names	Generic Drug Names	Canadian Trade/Brand Names
diethylstilbestrol	Honval, Stilboestrol	iodoquinol	Diodoquin
dimenhydrinate	Apo-Dimenhydrinate, Gravol, Nauseatol, Novo-Dimenate, Travamine	isoniazid (INH)	Isotamine
		isosorbide dinitrate	Coronex, Novosorbide
		kaolin/pectin	Donnagel-MB, Kao-Con
diphenhydramine hydrochloride	Allerdryl	ketoprofen	Rhodis, Orudis E
		lactulose	Lactulax
dipyridamole	Apo-Dipyridamole	levothyroxine sodium (T_4)	Eltroxin
disopyramide	Rythmodan-LA	lidocaine hydrochloride	Xylocard
docusate sodium	Regulax	lithium carbonate	Carbolith, Duralith, Lithizine
dopamine hydrochloride	Revimine	lorazepam	Apo-Lorazepam, Novolorazepam
doxepin hydrochloride	Triadapin		
doxycycline hyclate	Apo-Doxy, Doxycin, Novodoxylin	loxapine hydrochloride	Loxapac
		meclizine hydrochloride	Bonamine
dyphylline	Protophylline	meperidine hydrochloride	Pethadol, Pethidine Hydrochloride
econazole nitrate	Ecostatin		
epinephrine hydrochloride	Sus-Phrine, Eppy	meprobamate	Apo-Meprobamate, Novomepro
epinephrine racemic	Vaponefrin		
ergocalciferol	Ostoforte, Radiostol	mesalamine	Salofalk
ergotamine tartrate	Gynergen	methohexital	Brietal
erythromycin	Apo-Erythro Base, Erythromid, Novo-Rythro, Ro-Mycin	methotrimeprazine	Nozinan
		methylclothiazide	Duretic
		methyldopa	Apo-Methyldopa, Dopamet, Novo-Medopa
estradiol	Delestrogen		
estrogen, conjugated	C.E.S.	methyltestosterone	Metandren
estrogen, esterified	Neo-Estrone	metoclopramide	Maxeran
estrone	Femogen Forte	metoprolol	Apo-Metoprolol, Betaloc, Novometoprol
ethambutol hydrochloride	Etibi		
ferrous fumarate	Neo-Fer-50, Novofumar, Palafer	metronidazole	Novonidazol, PMS Metronidazole
ferrous gluconate	Fertinic, Novoferrogluc	miconazole	Monistat
ferrous sulfate	Novoferrosulfa	mineral oil	Kondremul, Lansoyl
flucytosine	Ancotil	modafinil	Alertec
flumazenil	Mazicon	morphine sulfate	Epimorph, Statex
fluocinolone acetonide	Fluoderm	naphazoline	Vasocon
fluoxymesterone	Ora Testryl	naproxen	Apo-Naproxen, Naxen, Novo-Naprox
fluphenazine decanoate	Modecate, Decanoate		
fluphenazine enanthate	Moditen Enanthate	niacin (vitamin B_3, nicotinic acid)	Novo-Niacin, Tri-B3
fluphenazine hydrochloride	Moditen HCl		
flurandrenolide	Drenison	nifedipine	Adalat P.A., Apo-Nifed, Novo-Nifedin
flurazepam	Apo-Flurazepam, Novoflupam, Somnol		
		nitrofurantoin	Apo-Nitrofurantoin, Nephronex, Novofuran
folic acid	Apo-Folic, Novofolacid		
furosemide	Fumide, Furomide, Luramide, Uritol	norethindrone acetate	Aygestin, Norlutate
		nystatin	Nadostine, Nyaderm
gentamicin sulfate	Alcomicin, Cidomycin	omeprazole	Losec
glyburide	DiaBeta, Euglucon	oxazepam	Apo-Oxazepam, Novoxapam
griseofulvin, microsize	Grisovin-FP	oxtriphylline	Apo-Oxtriphylline, Novotriphyl
guaifenesin	Resyl		
guanethidine sulfate	Apo-Guanethidine	oxycodone	Roxicodone Supeudol
haloperidol	Apo-Haloperidol LA, Novoperidol, Peridol	oxymetazoline hydrochloride	Nafrine
		oxymetholone	Anapolon
heparin calcium	Calcilean, Calciparine	penicillin G potassium	Megacillin, NovoPen-G, Crystapen
heparin sodium	Hepalean		
hydrochlorothiazide	Apo-Hydro, Hydrozide, Neo-Codema, Urozide	penicillin G procaine	Ayercillin
		penicillin G sodium	Crystapen
hydrocodone bitartrate	Robidone	penicillin V	Apo-Pen-VK, Nadopen-V, Novopen-VK
hydrocortisone	Cortamed, Cortiment, Rectocort		
		pentamidine isethionate	Pentacarinat
hydroxocobalamin	Acti-B_{12}	pentobarbital	Novopentobarb
ibuprofen	Amersol	perphenazine	Apo-Perphenazine
imipramine hydrochloride	Impril, Novo Pramine	phenazopyridine hydrochloride	Phenazo, Pyronium
indapamide	Lozide	phentolamine mesylate	Rogitine
indomethacin	Indocid	pilocarpine hydrochloride	Pilocarpine, Miocarpine

Generic Drug Names	Canadian Trade/Brand Names	Generic Drug Names	Canadian Trade/Brand Names
piroxicam	Apo-Piroxicam	sodium fluoride	Fluor-A-Day
potassium chloride	Apo-K, Kalium Durules, K-Long, Novolente K, Roychlor 10% and 20%, Slo-Pot	sotalol	Sotacar
		spironolactone	Novo-Spiroton
		sucralfate	Sulcrate
		sulfasalazine	PMS-Sulfasalazine, Salazopyrin, SAS-Enema, SAS Enteric-500, S.A.S.-500
potassium gluconate	Potassium-Rougier, Royonate		
potassium iodide	Thyro-Block	sulfinpyrazone	Antazone, Anturan, Apo-Sulfinpyrazone, Novopyrazone
pramoxine hydrochloride	Tronothane		
prednisone	Apo-Prednisone		
primidone	Apo-Primidone, Sertan	sulfisoxazole	Novo-Soxazole
probenecid	Benuryl	tamoxifen citrate	Nolvadex-D, Tamofen
procarbazine hydrochloride	Natulan	testosterone	Malogen
prochlorperazine maleate	Stemetil	testosterone enanthate	Malogex
procyclidine hydrochloride	Procyclid	testosterone propionate	Malogen in oil
promethazine hydrochloride	Histantil	tetracycline hydrochloride	Novotetra, Apo-Tetra
propantheline bromide	Propanthel	theophylline	PMS Theophylline, Pulmophylline, Somophyllin-12
propoxyphene hydrochloride	642, Novopropoxyn		
propranolol hydrochloride	Apo-Propranolol, Detensol, Novo-Pranol		
propylthiouracil (PTU)	Propyl-Thyracil	thiamine HCl (vitamin B_1)	Bewon, Betaxin
protriptyline hydrochloride	Triptil	thioguanine (TG, 6-thioguanine)	Lanvis
pseudoephedrine hydrochloride	Eltor, Eltor 120, Pseudofrin, Robidrine	thioridazine hydrochloride	Novo-Ridazine
		timolol maleate	Apo-Timol
psyllium hydrophilic mucilloid	Karasil	tolbutamide	Mobenol, Novobutamide
pyrantel pamoate	Combantrin	tolnaftate	Pitrex
pyrazinamide	PMS Pyrazinamide, Tebrazid	tramadole hydrochloride	Zydol
pyridostigmine	Mestinon, Regonol	trifluoperazine hydrochloride	Novoflurazine, Solazine, Terfluzine
quinidine sulfate	APO-Quinidine, Novoquinidin		
quinine sulfate	Novoquinine	trihexyphenidyl hydrochloride	Aparkane, Apo-Trihex, Novohexidyl
reserpine	Novoreserpine, Reserfia		
rifampin	Rofact	trimeprazine tartrate	Panectyl
scopolamine	Transderm-V	tripelennamine hydrochloride	Pyribenzamine
secobarbital	Novosecobarb	valproic acid (divalproex sodium, sodium valproate)	Epival
silver sulfadiazine	Flamazine		
simethicone	Ovol	vinblastine sulfate	Velbe
		warfarin sodium	Warfilone

Appendix B Therapeutic Drug Monitoring (TDM)*

Selected drugs are monitored by serum and urine to achieve and maintain therapeutic drug effect and to prevent drug toxicity. Drugs with a wide therapeutic range (window), the difference between effective dose and toxic dose, are not usually monitored. Drug monitoring is important in maintaining a drug concentration–response relationship, especially when the serum drug range (window) is narrow, such as with digoxin and lithium. Therapeutic drug monitoring (TDM) is the process of following drug levels and adjusting them to maintain a therapeutic level. Not all drugs can be dosed and/or monitored by their blood levels alone.

Drug levels are obtained at peak time and trough time after a steady state of the drug has been achieved in the client. Steady state is reached after four to five half-lives of a drug and can be reached sooner if the drug has a short half-life. Once steady state is achieved, the serum drug level is checked at the peak level (maximum drug concentration) and/or at trough/residual level (minimum drug concentration). If the trough or residual level is at the high therapeutic point, toxicity might occur. Careful assessment is needed by both physical and laboratory means.

TDM is required for the following:
- Drugs with a narrow therapeutic index or range (window)
- When other methods for monitoring drugs are non-effective, such as blood pressure (BP) monitoring
- To determine when adequate blood concentrations are reached
- To evaluate a client's compliance to drug therapy
- To determine whether other drugs have altered serum drug levels (increased or decreased) that could result in drug toxicity or lack of therapeutic effect
- To establish a new serum-drug level when the dosage is changed

Drug groups for TDM include analgesics, antibiotics, anticonvulsants, antineoplastics, bronchodilators, cardiac drugs, hypoglycemics, sedatives, and tranquilizers. To effectively conduct TDM, the laboratory must be provided with the following information: the drug name and daily dosage, time and amount of last dose, time blood was drawn, route of administration, and client's age. Without complete information, serum drug reporting might be incorrect.

*Revised by Ronald J. LeFever, RPh, Pharmacy Services, Medical College of Virginia, Richmond, Va.

Drug	Therapeutic Range	Peak Time	Toxic Level
acetaminophen (Tylenol)	10-20 mcg/ml	1-2.5 hours	>50 mcg/ml Hepatotoxicity: >200 mcg/ml
acetohexamide (Dymelor)	20-70 mcg/ml (should be dosed according to blood glucose levels)	2-4 hours	>75 mcg/ml
alcohol	Negative		Mild toxic: 150 mg/dl Marked toxic: >250 mg/dl
alprazolam (Xanax)	10-50 ng/ml	1-2 hours	>75 ng/ml
amikacin (Amikin)	Peak: 20-30 mcg/ml Trough: ≤ 10 mcg/ml	Intravenously: 0.5 hour Intramuscular: 0.5-1.5 hours	Peak: >35 mcg/ml Trough: >10 mcg/ml

Continued

927

Drug	Therapeutic Range	Peak Time	Toxic Level
aminocaproic acid (Amicar)	100-400 mcg/ml	1 hour	>400 mcg/ml
aminophylline (see theophylline)			
amiodarone (Cordarone)	0.5-2.5 mcg/ml	2-10 hours	>2.5 mcg/ml
amitriptyline (Elavil) + nortriptyline (parent and active metabolite)	110-225 ng/ml	2-4 hours (and up to 12 hours)	>500 ng/ml
amobarbital (Amytal)	1-5 mcg/ml	2 hours	>15 mcg/ml Severe toxicity: >30 mcg/ml
amoxapine (Asendin)	200-400 ng/ml	1.5 hours	>500 ng/ml
amphetamine: Serum urine	20-30 ng/ml	Detectable in urine after 3 hours; positive for 24-48 hours	0.2 mcg/ml >30 mcg/ml urine
aspirin (see salicylates)			
atenolol (Tenormin)	200-500 ng/ml	2-4 hours	>500 ng/ml
beta carotene	48-200 mcg/dl	Several weeks	>300 mcg/dl
bromide	20-80 mg/dl		>100 mg/dl
butabarbital (Butisol)	1-2 mcg/ml	3-4 hours	>10 mcg/ml
butalbital	10-20 mcg/ml		>40 mcg/ml
caffeine	Adult: 3-15 mcg/ml Infant: 8-20 mcg/ml	0.5-1 hour	>50 mcg/ml
carbamazepine (Tegretol)	4-12 mcg/ml	6 hours (range 2-24 hours)	>9-15 mcg/ml
chloral hydrate (Noctec)	2-12 mcg/ml	1-2 hours	>20 mcg/ml
chloramphenicol (Chloromycetin)	10-20 mg/L		>25 mg/L
chlordiazepoxide (Librium)	1-5 mcg/ml	2-3 hours	>5 mcg/ml
chlorpromazine (Thorazine)	50-300 ng/ml	2-4 hours	>750 ng/ml
chlorpropamide (Diabinese)	75-250 mcg/ml	3-6 hours	>250-750 mcg/ml
clonidine (Catapres)	0.2-2.0 ng/ml (hypotensive effect)	2-5 hours	>2.0 ng/ml
clorazepate (Tranxene)	0.12-1.0 mcg/ml	1-2 hours	>1.0 mcg/ml
cimetidine (Tagamet)	Trough: 0.5-1.2 mcg/ml	1-1.5 hours	Trough: >1.5 mcg/ml
clonazepam (Klonopin)	10-60 ng/ml	2 hours	>80 ng/ml
codeine	10-100 ng/ml	1-2 hours	>200 ng/ml
cyclosporine	100-300 ng/ml	3-4 hours	>400 ng/ml
dantrolene (Dantrium)	1-3 mcg/ml	5 hours	>5 mcg/ml
desipramine (Norpramin)	125-300 ng/ml	4-6 hours	>500 ng/ml
diazepam (Valium)	0.5-2 mg/L 400-600 ng/ml therapeutic	1-2 hours	>3 mg/L >3000 ng/ml
digitoxin (rarely administered)	10-25 ng/ml	Noticeable: 2-4 hours Peak: 12-24 hours	>30 ng/ml
digoxin	0.5-2 ng/ml	PO: 6-8 hours IV: 1.5-2 hours	2-3 ng/ml
Dilantin (see phenytoin)			
diltiazem (Cardizem)	50-200 ng/ml	2-3 hours	>200 ng/ml
disopyramide (Norpace)	2-4 mcg/ml	2 hours	>4 mcg/ml
doxepin (Sinequan)	150-300 ng/ml	2-4 hours	>500 ng/ml
ethchlorvynol (Placidyl)	2-8 mcg/ml	1-2 hours	>20 mcg/ml
ethosuximide (Zarontin)	40-100 mcg/ml	2-4 hours	>150 mcg/ml
flecainide (Tambocor)	0.2-1.0 mcg/ml	3 hours	>1.0 mcg/ml
5-Flucytosine	Peak: 100 mcg/ml Trough: 50 mcg/ml		125 mcg/ml 125 mcg/ml
fluoride			>15 μmol/L
fluoxetine	90-300 ng/ml	2-4 hours	>500 ng/ml
flurazepam (Dalmane)	20-110 ng/ml	0.5-1 hour	>1500 ng/ml

Drug	Therapeutic Range	Peak Time	Toxic Level
folate	>3.5 mcg/ml	1 hour	
gentamicin (Garamycin)	Peak: 6-12 mcg/ml Trough: <2 mcg/ml	IV: 15-30 minutes	Peak: >12 mcg/ml Trough: >2 mcg/ml
glutethimide (Doriden)	2-6 mcg/ml	1-2 hours	>20 mcg/ml
gold	1.0-2.0 mcg/ml	2-6 hours	>5.0 mcg/ml
haloperidol (Haldol)	5-15 ng/ml	2-6 hours	>50 ng/ml
hydromorphone (Dilaudid)	1-30 ng/ml	0.5-1.5 hours	>100 ng/ml
ibuprofen (Motrin, etc.)	10-50 mcg/ml	1-2 hours	>100 mcg/ml
imipramine (Tofranil) + desipramine (parent and active metabolite)	200-350 ng/ml	PO: 1-2 hours IM: 30 minutes	>500 ng/ml
isoniazid (INH, Nydrazid)	1-7 mcg/ml (dose usually adjusted based on liver function tests)	1-2 hours	>20 mcg/ml
kanamycin (Kantrex)	Peak: 15-30 mcg/ml	PO: 1-2 hours IM: 30 minutes- 1 hour	Peak: >35 mcg/ml Trough: >10 mcg/ml
lead	<20 mcg/dl Urine: <80 mcg/24 hours		>80 mcg/dl Urine: >125 mcg/24 hours
lidocaine (Xylocaine)	1.5-5 mcg/ml	IV: 10 minutes	>6 mcg/ml
lithium	0.8-1.2 mEq/L	0.5-4 hours	>1.5 mEq/L
lorazepam (Ativan)	50-240 ng/ml	1-3 hours	>300 ng/ml
maprotiline (Ludiomil)	200-300 ng/ml	12 hours	>500 ng/ml
meperidine (Demerol)	0.4-0.7 mcg/ml	2-4 hours	>1.0 mcg/ml
mephenytoin (Mesantoin)	15-40 mcg/ml	2-4 hours	>50 mcg/ml
meprobamate (Equanil, Miltown)	15-25 mcg/ml	2 hours	>50 mcg/ml
methadone (Dolophine)	100-400 ng/ml	0.5-1 hour	>2000 ng/ml or >0.2 mcg/ml
methaqualone	1-5 mcg/ml		>10 mcg/ml
methotrexate	<0.1 μmol/L after 48 h	1-2 hours	1.0×10^6 at 48 h
methsuximide	<1.0 mcg/ml	1-4 hours	>40 mcg/ml
methyldopa (Aldomet)	1-5 mcg/ml	3-6 hours	>7 mcg/ml
methyprylon (Noludar)	8-10 mcg/ml	1-2 hours	>50 mcg/ml
metoprolol (Lopressor)	75-200 ng/ml	2-4 hours	>225 ng/ml
mexiletine (Mexitil)	<0.5-2 mcg/ml	2-3 hours	>2 mcg/ml
morphine	10-80 ng/ml	IV: Immediately IM: 0.5-1 hour subQ: 1-1.5 hours	>200 ng/ml
netilmicin (Netromycin)	Peak: 0.5-10 mcg/ml Trough: <4 mcg/ml	IV: 30 minutes	Peak: >16 mcg/ml Trough: >4 mcg/ml
nifedipine (Procardia)	50-100 ng/ml	0.5-2 hours	>100 ng/ml
nortriptyline (Aventyl)	50-150 ng/ml	8 hours	>200 ng/ml
oxazepam (Serax)	0.2-1.4 mcg/ml	1-2 hours	
oxycodone (Percodan)	10-100 ng/ml	0.5-1 hour	>200 ng/ml
pentazocine (Talwin)	0.05-0.2 mcg/ml	1-2 hours	>1.0 mcg/ml Urine: >3.0 mcg/ml
pentobarbital (Nembutal)	1-5 mcg/ml	0.5-1 hour	>10 mcg/ml Severe toxicity: >30 mcg/ml
phenmetrazine (Preludin)	5-30 mcg/ml (urine)	2 hours	>50 mcg/ml (urine)
phenobarbital (Luminal)	15-40 mcg/ml	6-18 hours	>40 mcg/ml Severe toxicity: >80 mcg/ml
phenytoin (Dilantin)	10-20 mcg/ml	4-8 hours	>20-30 mcg/ml Severe toxicity: >40 mcg/ml
pindolol (Visken)	0.5-6.0 ng/ml	2-4 hours	>10 ng/ml
primidone (Mysoline)	5-12 mcg/ml	2-4 hours	>12-15 mcg/ml
procainamide (Pronestyl)	4-10 mcg/ml	1 hour	>10 mcg/ml
procaine (Novocain)	<11 mcg/ml	10-30 minutes	>20 mcg/ml

Drug	Therapeutic Range	Peak Time	Toxic Level
prochlorperazine (Compazine)	50-300 ng/ml	2-4 hours	>1000 ng/ml
propoxyphene (Darvon)	0.1-0.4 mcg/ml	2-3 hours	>0.5 mcg/ml
propranolol (Inderal)	>100 ng/ml	1-2 hours	>150 ng/ml
protriptyline (Vivactil)	50-150 ng/ml	8-12 hours	>200 ng/ml
quinidine	2-5 mcg/ml	1-3 hours	>6 mcg/ml
ranitidine (Zantac)	100 ng/ml	2-3 hours	>100 ng/ml
reserpine (Serpasil)	20 ng/ml	2-4 hours	>20 ng/ml
salicylates (Aspirin)	10-30 mg/dl	1-2 hours	Tinnitus: 20-40 mg/ml Hyperventilation: >35 mg/dl Severe toxicity: >50 mg/dl
secobarbital (Seconal)	2-5 mcg/ml	1 hour	>15 mcg/ml Severe toxicity: >30 mcg/ml
streptomycin	Peak: 5-20 mcg/ml Trough: <5 mcg/ml		>40 mcg/ml >40 mcg/ml
sulfadiazine	100-120 mcg/ml		>300 mcg/ml
sulfamethoxazole	90-100 mcg/ml		>300 mcg/ml
sulfapyridine	75-90 mcg/ml		>300 mcg/ml
sulfisoxazole	90-100 mcg/ml		>300 mcg/ml
theophylline (Theo-Dur)	10-20 mcg/ml	PO: 2-3 hours IV: 15 minutes (depends on smoking or nonsmoking)	>20 mcg/ml
thiocyanate	4-20 mcg/ml		>60 mcg/ml
thioridazine (Mellaril)	100-600 ng/ml 1.0-1.5 mcg/ml	2-4 hours	>2000 ng/ml >10 mcg/ml
timolol (Blocadren)	3-55 ng/ml	1-2 hours	>60 ng/ml
tobramycin (Nebcin)	Peak: 5-10 mcg/ml Trough: 1-1.5 mcg/ml	IV: 15-30 minutes IM: 0.5-1.5 hours	Peak: >12 mcg/ml Trough: >2 mcg/ml
tocainide (Tonocard)	4-10 mcg/ml	0.5-3 hours	>12 mcg/ml
tolbutamide (Orinase)	80-240 mcg/ml	3-5 hours	>640 mcg/ml
trazodone (Desyrel)	500-2500 ng/ml	1-2 weeks	>4000 ng/ml
trifluoperazine (Stelazine)	50-300 ng/ml	2-4 hours	>1000 ng/ml
trimethoprim/ sulfamethoxazole (TMP/SMX)	Peak: trimethoprim: >5 mcg/ml Peak: sulfamethoxazole >100 mcg/ml		
valproic acid (Depakene)	50-100 mcg/ml	0.5-1.5 hours	>100 mcg/ml Severe toxicity: >150 mcg/ml
vancomycin (Vancocin)	Peak: 20-40 mcg/ml Trough: 5-10 mcg/ml	IV: Peak: 5 minutes IV: Trough: 12 hours	Peak: >80 mcg/ml
verapamil (Calan)	100-300 ng/ml	PO: 1-2 hours IV: 5 minutes	>500 ng/ml
warfarin (Coumadin)	1-10 mcg/ml (dose usually adjusted by patient: 1 to 2.5 × control) or INR: 2.0-3.0	1.5-3 days	>10 mcg/ml INR: >4.0

HIV drugs are primarily dosed based on the clients' viral load or CD4 counts. Many of these drugs have dosage adjustments for renal and/or hepatic impairment.

	Peak Time	Half-Life
Combination HIV Drugs for Monitoring Antiretroviral Protease Inhibitors		
lopinavir/ritonavir (Kaletra)	4 hours	5 to 6 hours
Nucleoside Analog Reverse Transcriptase Inhibitors (NARTIs)		
abacavir/lamivudine/zidovudine (Trizivir) lamivudine/zidovudine (Combivir)		
Single HIV Drugs For Monitoring Protease Inhibitors		
amprenavir (Agenerase)	1-2 hours	7 to 9.5 hours
indinavir (Crixivan)	0.8 hour	2 hours (hepatic impairment, 3 hours)
Antiretroviral		
stavudine (Zerit)	1 to 1.5 hours	1.5 hours (8 hours in renal impairment)
Antiretroviral Protease Inhibitors		
ritonavir (Norvir)	2 to 4 hours	3 to 5 hours
Guanosine Nucleoside Reverse Transcriptase Inhibitor		
abacavir (Ziagen)		1.5 hours
Nucleoside Reverse Transcriptase Inhibitors (NRTIs)		
didanosine (Videx)	0.25 to 1.5 hours	1.5 hours
lamivudine (Epivir)		5 to 7 hours (dose adjustment in renal impairment)
zidovudine (Retrovir)	0.5 to 1.5 hours	1 hour (1.4 to 2.9 hours in renal impairment)
Nonnucleoside Reverse Transcriptase Inhibitors (NNRTIs)		
efavirenz (Sustiva)	3 to 5 hours	40 to 55 hours
nevirapine (Viramune)	4 hours	25 to 30 hours

From Kee JL: *Laboratory and diagnostic tests with nursing implications,* ed 5, Upper Saddle River, NJ, 2002, Prentice Hall Health, pp. 738-746.

Appendix C   Selected Drug-Drug Interactions

Drugs and Drug Categories	Interacting Effects with Drugs
Acyclovir	IV incompatible with dobutamine, dopamine, and morphine.
Alteplase	IV incompatible with dobutamine, dopamine, heparin, morphine, and nitroglycerin.
Aminoglycosides	Cephalosporins, ethacrynic acid, furosemide, polymyxin, and vancomycin can increase the risk of nephrotoxicity and ototoxicity. This is especially true with the young and older adults.
Aminophylline	IV incompatible with dobutamine, dopamine, meperidine, and ondansetron.
Angiotensin-converting enzyme (ACE) inhibitors example: captopril	Antacids will decrease absorption of ACE inhibitors. Potassium-sparing diuretics will decrease potassium excretion, and lithium use will decrease lithium excretion. Antihypertensives, nitrates, and diuretics enhance hypotensive effects.
Anticoagulants example: warfarin (Coumadin)	Drugs that may enhance anticoagulant effects include acetaminophen (high doses), alcohol, antiplatelet drugs, aspirin, aminoglycosides, cephalosporins, erythromycins, furosemide, fluoroquinolones, isoniazid, NSAIDs, sulfonamides, thiazides, tricyclic antidepressants, and vitamin E.
Anticonvulsants example: phenytoin (Dilantin)	Alcohol decreases phenytoin effect. Warfarin absorption may be decreased. Oral contraceptives' and corticosteroids' effectiveness may be decreased. Isoniazid increases phenytoin levels.
Antipsychotic agents example: phenothiazines	Alcohol increases CNS depression. Antacids and antidiarrheals decrease drug absorption. Tricyclic antidepressants may increase the risk of hypotension. Anticonvulsant dose may need to be increased because phenothiazines can decrease seizure threshold.
Antitubercular agents example: isoniazid	Alcohol increases risk of hepatotoxicity. Antacids decrease absorption of isoniazid. Phenytoin levels can increase and could result in phenytoin toxicity.
Aspirin (salicylates)	Anticoagulants can increase the risk of bleeding when taken with aspirin. Oral antidiabetic agents may increase the risk of hypoglycemia.
Benzodiazepines example: diazepam, lorazepam	Alcohol, narcotics, and anticonvulsants can increase CNS depression. Cimetidine can increase diazepam and lorazepam toxicity. Levodopa effects may be decreased. Phenytoin serum levels may be increased.
Beta (adrenergic) blockers example: propranolol (Inderal)	Diuretics, antihypertensives, and phenothiazines can increase the state of hypotension. Atropine can correct bradycardia. Antacids decrease propranolol absorption. Cimetidine decreases drug clearance and increases beta blocker effects.
Calcium channel blockers example: nifedipine (Procardia)	Digoxin levels may be increased. Beta blockers have an additive effect and can cause bradycardia. H_2 blockers decrease drug clearance, thus calcium blocker levels could be elevated.
Cardiac glycosides example: digoxin (Lanoxin)	Thiazide and loop diuretics, corticosteroids, laxatives, and amphotericin B can cause hypokalemia, which could cause digitalis toxicity. Antacids, antidiarrheals, and colestipol decrease absorption of digoxin. Quinidine, verapamil, and erythromycin increase digoxin levels.

Drugs and Drug Categories	Interacting Effects with Drugs
Diazepam	IV incompatible with dobutamine, heparin, meperidine, and potassium in D_5W.
Diuretics (potassium-wasting) (thiazide and loop)	Digoxin toxicity may result from hypokalemia because of loop or thiazide diuretics. Corticosteroids increase potassium loss. Lithium levels may be increased.
Fluoroquinolones example: ciprofloxacin (Cipro)	Theophylline levels and warfarin (Coumadin) levels may be increased. Antacids and iron products can decrease ciprofloxacin absorption.
Furosemide	IV incompatible with dobutamine, meperidine, morphine, and ondansetron.
Lithium carbonate	Diuretics, NSAIDs, tetracyclines, and methyldopa can increase lithium toxicity. Theophylline, sodium bicarbonate, and potassium or sodium citrate can promote lithium excretion.
Narcotics example: morphine and meperidine (Demerol)	Alcohol, sedatives, benzodiazepines, barbiturates, and tricyclic antidepressants can increase CNS depression. Monoamine oxidase inhibitors (MAOIs) may cause a hypertensive crisis.
Nonsteroidal antiinflam-matory drugs (NSAIDs) example: ibuprofen (Motrin)	Warfarin, heparin, and alcohol may prolong bleeding time. Lithium and methotrexate levels may increase; lithium toxicity may result. Corticosteroids may cause a peptic ulcer.
Penicillins	Warfarin effects may be decreased. NSAIDs prolong the effects of penicillin. Diuretics with penicillin G-K may cause hyperkalemia. Oral contraceptives' effectiveness may be decreased. Rifampin inhibits the action of penicillin.
Phenytoin	IV incompatible with dobutamine, heparin, meperidine, morphine, nitroglycerin, and potassium in D_5W.
Sulfonylureas	Alcohol, aspirin, anticoagulants, some NSAIDs, anticonvulsants, sulfonamides, and oral contraceptives may increase the risk of hypoglycemia. Corticosteroids, thiazide diuretics, estrogen, calcium channel blockers, phenytoin, and thyroid drugs may increase the blood sugar level.
Tetracyclines	Milk, antacids, and iron supplements decrease tetracycline absorption. Oral contraceptive effects can be decreased.
Theophylline	Erythromycins, fluoroquinolones, and tacrine can increase theophylline levels. Lithium excretion may be increased. Cigarette smoking decreases theophylline levels.
Tricyclic antidepressants example: amitriptyline	Warfarin's anticoagulant effects can be increased. Alcohol, narcotics, and sedatives increase CNS depression. MAOIs should not be taken with tricyclics. Antihypertensive drug effects may be reduced. Cimetidine may increase tricyclic serum levels.

Appendix D   Selected Herb-Drug Interactions

Herbal Ingredient	Documented Drug Interaction	Comment	Potential Drug Interaction	Comment
Alfalfa (*Medicago sativa*)	—	—	Anticoagulants	⇓ Drug effect
			Oral contraceptives	⇓ Drug effect
Aloe (*Aloe vera*)	—	—	Antidiabetics	⇑ Drug effect
			Digoxin	⇑ Drug effect
			Diuretics	⇑ Hypokalemia
Bilberry (*Vaccinium myrtillus*)	—	—	Anticoagulants	⇑ Drug effect
			Antidiabetics	⇑ Drug effect
Black cohosh (*Cimicifuga racemosa*)	—	—	Antihypertensives	⇑ Drug effect
			Iron salts	⇓ Drug absorption
Cascara (*Rhamnus purshiana*) – and – Senna (*Cassia senna*)	—	—	Corticosteroids	⇑ Hypokalemia
			Digoxin	⇑ Drug effect
Chamomile (*Matricaria chamomilla*)	—	—	Sedatives	⇑ Drug effect
Cocoa (*Theobroma cacao*)	—	—	Antidiabetics	⇓ Drug effect
Dandelion (*Taraxacum officinale*)	—	—	Antidiabetics	⇑ Drug effect
			Diuretics	⇑ Drug effect
			Lithium	⇑ Drug levels
Danshen (*Salvia bowelyana*)	Warfarin	⇑ INR & bleeding risk	Antiplatelet agents	⇑ Drug effect
Echinacea (*Echinacea* spp.)	—	—	Immunomodulators	Altered drug effect
Evening primrose (*Oenothera biennis*)	—	—	Anticoagulants	⇑ Drug effect
			Antiplatelet agents	⇑ Drug effect
			Phenothiazines	⇑ Seizure risk
Feverfew (*Tanacetum parthenium*)	—	—	Antiplatelet agents	⇑ Drug effect
Garlic (*Allium sativum*)	Protease inhibitors	⇓ Drug levels	Anticoagulants	⇑ Drug effect
	Warfarin	⇑ Drug effect	Antidiabetics	⇑ Drug effect
			Antiplatelet agents	⇑ Drug effect
			Cyclosporine	⇓ Drug effect
			Non-nucleoside RTIs	⇓ Drug effect
Ginger (*Zingiber officinale*)	—	—	Anticoagulants	⇑ Drug effect
			Antiplatelet agents	⇑ Drug effect
Ginkgo (*Ginkgo biloba*)	Trazodone	⇑ Drug effect	Anticoagulants	⇑ Drug effect
	Antiplatelet agents	⇑ Bleeding risk	MAO inhibitors	⇑ Drug effect
Ginseng (*Panax ginseng, Panax quinquefolius*)	Warfarin	⇓ Drug effect	Anticoagulants	Altered drug effect
			Antidiabetics	⇑ Drug effect
			Antiplatelet agents	Altered drug effect
			Immunomodulators	Altered drug effect
			MAO inhibitors	⇑ Drug effect

Herbal Ingredient	Documented Drug Interaction	Comment	Potential Drug Interaction	Comment
Goldenseal (*Hydrastis canadensis*)	—	—	Anticoagulants	⇓ Drug effect
			Antihypertensives	⇓ Drug effect
			Immunomodulators	Altered drug effect
Hawthorn (*Crataegus laevigata*)	—	—	CNS depressants	⇑ Drug effect
			Cardiovasculars	Altered drug effect
			Digoxin	⇑ Drug effect
Juniper (*Juniperus communis*)	—	—	Antidiabetics	⇓ Drug effect
			Diuretics	⇑ Drug effect
			Lithium	⇑ Drug levels
Kava (*Piper methysticum*)	Alprazolam	⇑ Drug effect	CNS depressants	⇑ Drug effect
	Levodopa	⇓ Drug effect		
Licorice (*Glycyrrhiza glabra*)	—	—	Antihypertensives	⇓ Drug effect
			Antiplatelet agents	⇑ Drug effect
			Corticosteroids	⇑ Drug effect
			Digoxin	⇑ Drug effect
			Diuretics	⇑ Hypokalemia
Peppermint (*Mentha piperita*)	—	—	Iron salts	⇓ Drug absorption
Psyllium (*Plantago* spp.)	Lithium	⇓ Drug absorption	Digoxin	⇓ Drug effect
Rosemary (*Rosmarinus officinalis*)	—	—	Antidiabetics	⇓ Drug effect
St. John's wort (*Hypericum perforatum*)	Alprazolam	⇓ Drug effect	Etoposide	⇓ Drug effect
	Amitriptyline	⇓ Drug level & effect	Omeprazole	⇑ Photosensitivity risk
	Cyclosporine	⇓ Drug level & effect		
	Digoxin	⇓ Drug level & effect		
	Indinavir	⇓ Drug level & effect		
	Oral contraceptives	⇓ Drug effect		
	SSRIs	Serotonin syndrome		
	Tacrolimus	⇓ Drug level & effect		
	Theophylline	⇓ Drug level		
	Warfarin	⇓ Drug effect		
Saw Palmetto (*Serenoa repens*)	—	—	Hormone therapy	⇓ Drug effect
Valerian (*Valeriana officinalis*)	—	—	CNS depressants	⇑ Drug effect
Yohimbe (*Pausinystalia yohimbe*)	—	—	Antihypertensives	⇓ Drug effect
			MAO inhibitors	⇑ Hypertension

Appendix E   Selected Sugar-Free Products*

Product	Therapeutic Category
Acetaminophen Oral Solution, USP, Cherry	Analgesic
Alka-Seltzer Original	Antacid
Alka-Seltzer, Lemon Lime	Antacid
Aluminum Hydroxide Gel	Antacid
Arthritis Pain Formula	Analgesic
Aspirin, Delayed Release	Analgesic
Bayer Aspirin	Analgesic
Benadryl Dye-Free	Antihistamine
Benylin Adult Cough Formula	Antitussive
Benylin Expectorant Cough Formula	Antitussive
Bufferin Arthritis Strength	Analgesic
Bufferin Extra Strength	Analgesic
Cheracol Sore Throat	Analgesic
Diabetic Tussin Allergy Relief	Antihistamine
Diabetic Tussin DM	Antitussive
Doxidan	Laxative
Dulcolax	Laxative
Excedrin Aspirin Free	Analgesic
Feverall Sprinkle Caps	Analgesic
Fiberall, Natural	Laxative
Gaviscon Liquid	Antacid
Gelusil Liquid	Antacid
Guaifenesin CF, Guaifenesin DM	Expectorant
Haley's M-O	Laxative
Konsyl	Laxative
Maalox, Maalox HRF	Antacid
Metamucil Sugar Free	Laxative
Milk of Magnesia	Laxative
Motrin IB	Analgesic
Mucinex	Expectorant
Nuprin	Analgesic
Riopan, Riopan Plus	Antacid
Robitussin Pediatric Cough	Antitussive
Surfak	Laxative
Tempra	Analgesic
Tussar SF	Antitussive
Tylenol	Analgesic

*ALERT: Read the label before use. Some of these products may contain other carbohydrate sources.

Appendix F **Selected Alcohol-Free Products***

Product	Therapeutic Category
Acetaminophen	Analgesic
Aerolate Oral Solution	Antiasthmatic
Alupent Syrup	Antiasthmatic
Benadryl Allergy Decongestant Liquid	Decongestant
Benylin Adult Liquid, Benylin Pediatric Liquid	Antitussive
Benylin Expectorant	Antitussive, expectorant
Chloroseptic Gly-Oxide Liquid	Gargle/mouthwash
Diabetic Tussin DM, Diabetic Tussin EX	Antitussive
Dilor G Liquid	Antiasthmatic
Dimetapp Elixir, Dimetapp DM Elixir	Antitussive
Drixoral Cough & Congestion Cough Caps	Antitussive
Haldol Concentrate	Psychotropic
Liquiprin Drops	Analgesic
Mapap Infant Drops	Analgesic
Orobase-O, Orabase Plan	Gargle/mouthwash
Oral-B Anti-Cavity Rinse	Gargle/mouthwash
PediaCare Cough-Cold Liquid	Antitussive
Robitussin Pediatric Cough & Cold Liquid	Antitussive
Robitussin Night Relief	Antitussive
Silapap, Infants'	Analgesic, antipyretic
Slo-Phyllin Syrup, Slo-Phyllin GC Syrup	Antiasthmatic
Stelazine Concentrate	Psychotropic
Theolair Liquid	Antiasthmatic
Thorazine Syrup	Psychotropic
Triaminic AM Cough & Decongestant Formula	Antitussive
Triaminic Expectorant Liquid	Expectorant
Tussar-DM Syrup	Antitussive
Tylenol Children's Cold Multi-Symptom	Decongestant, antipyretic
Tylenol, Children's Cherry Flavor; Tylenol, Children's Liquid; Tylenol, Infants'	Analgesic, antipyretic
Vick's Pediatric Formula 44E	Antitussive, decongestant
Vick's DayQuil Liquid	Antitussive, decongestant

*ALERT: Read label before use.

Appendix G Potential Weapons of Bioterrorism

Note: Refer to online resources for the most current information.

Agent/Etiology	Transmission/Clinical Manifestations	Drug Treatment/Considerations
Bacteria and Viruses		
Anthrax, pulmonary/ *Bacillus anthracis*	Inhalation of spores; incubation up to 60 d. Initially ILS: fever, malaise, fatigue, non-productive cough, chest discomfort; later, severe respiratory distress, stridor, cyanosis, septicemia, and hemorrhagic meningitis	Early treatment with antibiotics IMPORTANT; IV route preferred; ciprofloxacin and doxycycline drugs of choice; use of additional antibiotics to avoid drug resistance; duration for IV and PO 60 d; low morbidity when treated early; with onset of respiratory distress, morbidity near 100%
Anthrax, cutaneous/ *Bacillus anthracis*	Spores enter through non-intact skin; incubation up to 60 d; papule becomes fluid-filled vesicle that dries and forms dark eschar	Ciprofloxacin or doxycycline, PO for 7-10 d; with systemic symptoms or risk of inhalation, treat as above; morbidity up to 24% if untreated; treated <1%
Smallpox/variola virus	Respiratory droplets and pustule drainage; incubation 7-17 d; prodrome 2-4 d of ILS; papular rash that becomes deep vesicles, then scabs; mostly face and extremities; does involve palms and soles	Supportive; gancyclovir may help; other antiviral effects unknown; vaccinate client, all contacts, and health care workers in facility; morbidity: 30% likely; in rare hemorrhagic form: up to 90%
Plague, pneumonic/ *Yersinia pestis*	Inhaled droplets; incubation: 2-3 d; begins as ILS; rapid 24 h progression to severe pneumonia, hemoptysis, and then respiratory distress and failure	IV doxycycline or gentamycin; morbidity 100% untreated; unknown when treated
Tularemia/*Francisella tularensis*	Inhaled or through skin; incubation 2-5 d (up to 14 d); begins as ILS; progresses over days to pneumonia with dyspnea and hilar adenopathy	IV streptomycin, gentamycin, or ciprofloxacin; morbidity <5%
Viral hemorrhagic fevers; ebola	Blood or secretions; incubation 2-10 d; prodrome of ILS; bleeding day 3; desquamation day 5; progresses rapidly to multisystem organ failure and delirium	Supportive care; transfusions and fresh frozen plasma; dialysis
Biotoxins		
Botulinum	Inhaled; incubation of 24-72 h; symmetric descending flaccid paralysis; eyes, bulbar muscles, then respiratory and skeletal effects	Supportive; antitoxin (from Centers for Disease Control or Public Health) may decrease progress; no antibiotics; morbidity uncertain; long recovery

Adapted from Lehne R: *Pharmacology for nursing care,* ed 5, Philadelphia, 2004, Saunders.

ARDS, Adult respiratory distress syndrome; *d,* day; *FDA,* Food and Drug Administration; *GI,* gastrointestinal; *h,* hour; *ILS,* influenza-like syndrome; *IM,* intramuscular; *IV,* intravenous; *min,* minute; *mo,* month; *PEEP,* positive end-expiratory pressure; *PO,* by mouth; *PRN,* as needed; *y,* year; >, greater than; <, less than.

Note: All clients exposed to chemical agents should be decontaminated. Removal of clothing will remove up to 90% of contamination. Further decontamination should be performed with soap and water. All health care providers treating clients **PRIOR** to decontamination should wear protective equipment to prevent skin, mucous membrane, or respiratory exposure (i.e., impervious suit, gloves, boots, protective face shield with respirator).
Websites:
www.bt.cdc.gov
www.fda.gov/oc/opacom/hottopics/bioterrorism.html
www.idsociety.org/bt/toc.htm
www.hopkins-biodefense.org/
Jama.ama-assn.org/cgi/collection/bioterrorism
Medicalletter.com/html/prm.htm#Reprints
www.who.int/ionizing_radiation/a_e/terrorism/en/

Agent/Etiology	Transmission/Clinical Manifestations	Drug Treatment/Considerations
Biotoxins—cont'd		
Ricin/*Ricinus communis*	Inhalation: onset within hours with coughing, chest tightness, dyspnea, nausea, and muscle ache; later, edematous airway; cyanosis and death may follow Ingested: GI hemorrhage, vomiting and diarrhea; later, liver and kidney failure; may die within 10-12 d; injection: severe symptoms and death; route not available to terrorists	Supportive; no antidote for ricin
Chemical Weapons		
Nerve agents (e.g., Sarin, VX, GA, GB)	Absorbed through skin and mucous membranes and inhaled; onset rapid when inhaled; skin or mucous membrane onset 30 min to 18 h; early signs: eye pain, rhinorrhea, and local sweating if droplet; classic toxidrome: diarrhea, urination, miosis, bronchospasm, bronchorrhea, bradycardia, emesis, lacrimation, and salivation	Atropine IV or IM in high doses: 2 mg q3-5min; pralidoxime chloride (2-PAM) 1-2 g IV over 30-60 min; may need drip of 500 mg over 24 h; valium or Versed PRN for seizures; homatropine for ciliary spasm; morbidity potentially high depending on concentration and duration of exposure
Chlorine or phosgene	Inhaled, mucous membranes, and eyes; rapid irritant effects; pulmonary effects (distress and edema) may be seen in 6 to 24 h	Humidified oxygen; bronchodilators; ventilatory support with PEEP for ARDS; monitor for 24 h if suspected significant exposure; morbidity depends on exposure level; phosgene higher than chlorine
Mustard gas (sulfur mustard)	Mainly absorbed through skin; can affect airway & eyes; delayed onset of >6 h with few warning symptoms of contact; blistering of affected areas; later, seizures and dysrhythmias	Wash with dilute sodium thiosulfite (2.5% solution); prednisone may have antidote effects; neupogen for later leukopenia; morbidity under 5%-10%
Cyanide	Absorbed in GI tract via contaminated products; inhaled vapors or via skin; generally rapid onset of symptoms; delayed if low concentration; sudden loss of consciousness with high concentration; cyanosis and severe respiratory distress	Inhaled amyl nitrite, sodium nitrite IV, sodium thiosulfate; morbidity varies by exposure level
Radiologic Agents		
Nuclear bombs	Immediate threat: blast; delayed threat: radioactive fallout	Potassium iodide blocks uptake by thyroid of radioactive iodine, thus reducing risk of cancer; tablets for this purpose are released by public health after determining presence of iodine-131. FDA recommended doses: Birth to 1 m: 16 mg >1 mo to 3 y: 32 mg >3 y to 18 y: 65 mg >18 y: 130 mg Pregnant or lactating: 65 mg

Appendix H Abbreviations

Selected abbreviations are listed in three categories: drug measurements and drug forms, routes of drug administration, and times of administration. These are frequently used in drug therapy and must be known by the nurse.

Drug Measurements and Drug Forms

Abbreviation	Meaning	Abbreviation	Meaning
cap	capsule	♏, min	minim
cc	cubic centimeter	oz	ounce
dr	dram	pt	pint
elix	elixir	qt	quart
fl dr	fluid dram (fl ℨ)	SR	sustained release
fl oz	fluid ounce (fl ℥)	s̄s̄	one half
g, gm, G, GM	gram	supp	suppository
gr	grain	susp	suspension
gtt	drops	T.O.	telephone order
kg	kilogram	T, tbsp	tablespoon
l, L	liter	t, tsp	teaspoon
m²	square meter	U	unit
mcg, μg	microgram	V.O.	verbal order
mEq	milliequivalent	>	greater than
mg	milligram	<	less than
mL, ml	milliliter		

Routes of Drug Administration

Abbreviation	Meaning	Abbreviation	Meaning
A.D., ad	right ear	O.D., od	right eye
A.S., as	left ear	O.S., os	left eye
A.U., au	both ears	O.U., ou	both eyes
ID	intradermal	PO, po, os	by mouth
IM	intramuscular	Ⓡ	right
IV	intravenous	SC, subc, sc, SQ, subQ	subcutaneous
IVPB	intravenous piggyback		
KVO	keep vein open	SL, sl, subl	sublingual
Ⓛ	left	TKO	to keep open
NGT	nasogastric tube	Vag	vaginal

Times of Administration

Abbreviation	Meaning	Abbreviation	Meaning
AC, ac	before meals	qh	every hour
ad lib	as desired	q2h	every 2 hours
B.i.d., b.i.d.	twice a day	q4h	every 4 hours
c̄	with	q6h	every 6 hours
hs	hour of sleep	q8h	every 8 hours
noct	at night	Q.i.d., q.i.d.	four times a day
NPO	nothing by mouth	q.o.d.	every other day
PC, pc	after meals	s̄	without
PRN, p.r.n.	whenever necessary, as needed	SOS	once if necessary: if there is a need
q	every	Stat	immediately
qAM	every morning	T.i.d., t.i.d.	three times a day
qd, od	every day		

Disclaimer: The newest abbreviation guidelines from the Joint Commission on Accreditation of Healthcare Organization (JCAHO) *2004 National Patient Safety Goals* have been developed for the prevention of medication errors. It is suggested that some of the abbreviations should not be used to avoid misinterpretation. These abbreviations are as follows:

Abbreviation	Preferred	Abbreviation	Preferred
q.d., Q.D.	Write "daily" or "every day."	D/C	Write "discharge" or "discontinued."
o.d., O.D.	Write "once a day."	MS, MSO$_4$	Write "morphine sulfate."
q.o.d., Q.O. D.	Write "every other day."	MgSO$_4$	Write "magnesium sulfate."
μg	Use "mcg."	HCT	Write "hydrochlorothiazide" or "hydrocortisone."
c.c.	Use "ml" (milliliter).		
O.S., O.D., O.U.	Write "left eye," "right eye," and "both eyes."	>	Write "greater than."
		<	Write "less than."
A.S., A.D., A.U.	Write "left ear," "right ear," and "both ears."	/	Write "per" instead of a slash mark.
		0.5 mg	Use zero before a decimal point when the dose is less than a whole.
h.s.	Write "hour of sleep or bedtime."		
ss	Write "one-half" or "¹/₂."	1.0 mg	Use a decimal point after a whole number when a zero is used following a whole number.
U	Write "unit."		
IU	Write "international unit."		
SC	Write "subcut" or "subcutaneous."		

Appendix I Examples of Internet Sites

The following are examples of available Internet sites that provide drug information.

http://www.nlm.nih.gov/medlineplus/
http://www.nlm.nih.gov/
http://virtualnurse.com
http://www.nursingethics.ca/
http://healthweb.org/index.cfm
http://www.rxlist.com/
www.fda.gov/cder/drug
http://www.drugs.com/
www.druginfonet.com/drug.htm
www.nida.nih.gov

www.healthtouch.com
www.coreynahman.com/druginfopage.html
www.medscape.com/druginfo
www.healthsquare.com/drugmain.htm
www.intmed.mcw.edu/drug.html
www.safemedication.com
www.drugs.com/xq/cfm/pageID_1146/qx
www.psyweb.com/Drughtm/xanax.html
dir.yahoo.com/health/pharmacy/drugs_and_medications
pharmacy.dal.ca/druginfo/table.html

Top Prescribed Drugs in 2004

The drugs illustrated in this appendix represent those most frequently prescribed as identified by *RxList: The Internet Drug Index* found at *www.rxlist.com/top200.htm*. The data are furnished by NDC Health and based upon more than three billion prescriptions. The drugs are listed in order of frequency. Duplicates are present in the list because some drugs are prescribed by generic name as well as trade name.

	Generic Name and Pronunciation	Brand Name
1	hydrocodone w/ APAP (high-drow-**koe**-doan)	Hydrocodone w/APAP
2	atorvastatin (ah-tore-vah-**stat**-in)	Lipitor
3	lisinopril (lye-**sin**-oh-pril)	Lisinopril
4	atenolol (a-**ten**-oh-lol)	Atenolol
5	levothyroxine (**lee**-voe-thigh-**rocks**-in)	Synthroid
6	amoxicillin (a-**mox**-ih-**sill**-in)	Amoxicillin
7	hydrochlorothiazide (**high**-drow-**klor**-oh-**thigh**-ah-zide)	Hydrochlorothiazide
8	azithromycin (a-**zith**-row-**my**-sin)	Zithromax
9	furosemide (fur-**oh**-se-mide)	Furosemide
10	amlodipine (am-**low**-dih-peen)	Norvasc
11	metoprolol (meh-**toe**-proe-lol)	Toprol XL
12	alprazolam (al-**pray**-zoe-lam)	Alprazolam
13	albuterol (al-**byoo**-ter-all)	Albuterol
14	sertraline (**sir**-trah-leen)	Zoloft
15	simvastatin (sim-vah-**stat**-in)	Zocor
16	metformin (met-**for**-min)	Metformin HCl
17	ibuprofen (eye-**byoo**-pro-fen)	Ibuprofen
18	triamterene/HCTZ (try-**am**-ter-een)	Triamterene/HCTZ
19	zolpidem (**zol**-pi-dem)	Ambien
20	cephalexin (sef-ah-**lex**-in)	Cephalexin
21	esomeprazole (es-oh-**mep**-rah-zole)	Nexium
22	lansoprazole (lan-**soe**-pra-zole)	Prevacid
23	escitalopram (es-sih-**tail**-oh-pram)	Lexapro
24	prednisone (**pred**-nih-sewn)	Prednisone
25	cetirizine (sih-**tier**-eh-zeen)	Zyrtec
26	montelukast (mon-tee-**leu**-cast)	Singulair
27	celecoxib (sell-eh-**cox**-ib)	Celebrex
28	fluoxetine (flu-**ox**-eh-teen)	Fluoxetine
29	alendronate (ah-**len**-drew-nate)	Fosamax
30	metoprolol (meh-**toe**-proe-lol)	Metoprolol Tartrate
31	conjugated estrogens (**kan**-ji-gate-ed **ess**-tro-jenz)	Premarin
32	levothyroxine (**lee**-voe-thigh-**rocks**-in)	Levoxyl
33	lorazepam (lor-az-e-pam)	Lorazepam
34	fexofenadine (fex-oh-**fen**-ah-deen)	Allegra
35	clopidogrel (klo-**pid**-eh-grel)	Plavix
36	venlafaxine (ven-lah-**fax**-een)	Effexor XR
37	potassium chloride (poe-**tass**-ee-um **klor**-ide)	Potassium Chloride
38	pantoprazole (pan-**tow**-pra-zoll)	Protonix
39	propoxyphene N/APAP (pro-**pox**-ih-feen)	Propoxyphene Nap/APAP
40	salmeterol/fluticasone (sal-**met**-er-all flu-**tick**-ah-sewn)	Advair Diskus
41	warfarin (**war**-fair-in)	Warfarin Sodium
42	acetaminophen/codeine (ah-see-tah-**min**-oh-fen/**koe**-deen)	Acetaminophen/Codeine
43	clonazepam (klo-**naz**-e-pam)	Clonazepam
44	gabapentin (gab-ah-**pen**-tin)	Neurontin
45	fluticasone (flu-**tick**-ah-sewn)	Flonase

Continued

Generic Name and Pronunciation	Brand Name
46	amitriptyline (am-ih-**trip**-tih-leen)	Amitriptyline HCl
47	ranitidine (rah-**nih**-tih-deen)	Ranitidine HCl
48	trazodone (**tray**-zah-doan)	Trazodone HCl
49	naproxen (nah-**prox**-en)	Naproxen
50	amoxicillin/clavulanate (a-mox-i-**sill**-in/**klav**-u-la-nate)	Amox Tr-Potassium/Clavulanate
51	enalapril (en-**al**-ah-prill)	Enalapril Maleate
52	paroxetine (pear-**ox**-eh-teen)	Paroxetine HCl
53	pravastatin (**prav**-ah-stat-in)	Pravachol
54	sildenafil citrate (sil-**den**-ah-fill **ci**-trate)	Viagra
55	cyclobenzaprine (ci-klo-**ben**-zah-preen)	Cyclobenzaprine HCl
56	rofecoxib (row-feh-**cox**-ib)	Vioxx
57	ramipril (**ram**-ih-prill)	Altace
58	valsartan (val-**sar**-tan)	Diovan
59	amlodipine/benazepril (am-**low**-dih-peen/ben-**ayz**-ah-prill)	Lotrel
60	levofloxacin (leave-oh-**flocks**-ah-sin)	Levaquin
61	levothyroxine (**lee**-voe-thigh-**rocks**-in)	L-Thyroxine Sodium
62	valdecoxib (val-de-**cox**-ib)	Bextra
63	oxycodone/APAP (ox-ih-**koe**-doan)	Oxycodone/APAP
64	diazepam (dye-**az**-eh-pam)	Diazepam
65	tramadol (**tray**-mah-doll)	Tramadol HCl
66	verapamil (ver-**ap**-ah-mill)	Verapamil HCl
67	valsartan/HCTZ (val-**sar**-tan)	Diovan HCT
68	albuterol (al-**byoo**-ter-ole)	Albuterol Sulfate
69	lisinopril/HCTZ (lye-**sin**-oh-prill)	Lisinopril/HCTZ
70	norelgestromin/ethinyl estradiol (nor-el-**jes**-tro-min/**eth**-ih-nal es-tra-**dye**-ol)	Ortho Evra
71	citalopram (si-**tal**-o-pram)	Celexa
72	quinapril (**quin**-ah-prill)	Accupril
73	carisoprodol (kar-i-so-**pro**-dol)	Carisoprodol
74	pioglitazone (pie-oh-**glit**-ah-zone)	Actos
75	promethazine (pro-**meth**-ah-zeen)	Promethazine HCl
76	risedronate (ris-**ed**-ron-ate)	Actonel
77	isosorbide mononitrate S.A. (eye-so-**sore**-bide **mon**-oh-**nigh**-trate)	Isosorbide Mononitrate
78	allopurinol (al-low-**pure**-ih-nawl)	Allopurinol
79	paroxetine (pear-**ox**-eh-teen)	Paxil CR
80	losartan (low-**sar**-tan)	Cozaar
81	clonidine (**klon**-ih-deen)	Clonidine HCl
82	ciprofloxacin (sip-row-**flocks**-ah-sin)	Ciprofloxacin HCl
83	bupropion HCl (bu-**pro**-pe-on)	Wellbutrin XL
84	glyburide (**glye**-byoor-ide)	Glyburide
85	rosiglitazone maleate (rose-ih-**glit**-ah-zone **mal**-ee-ate)	Avandia
86	penicillin VK (pen-ih-**sill**-in)	Penicillin VK
87	ezetimibe (eh-**zeh**-tih-myb)	Zetia
88	amoxicillin (a-mox-i-**sill**-in)	Trimox
89	methylprednisolone (**meth**-ill-pred-**niss**-oh-lone)	Methylprednisolone
90	folic acid (**fol**-ic **as**-id)	Folic Acid
91	rabeprazole (rah-**bep**-rah-zole)	Aciphex
92	glipizide (**glip**-ih-zide)	Glipizide ER
93	tamsulosin (tam-**soo**-low-sin)	Flomax
94	diltiazem (dill-**tie**-ah-zem)	Diltiazem HCl
95	risperidone (ris-**pear**-ih-doan)	Risperdal
96	omeprazole (oh-**mep**-rah-zole)	Omeprazole
97	drospirenone/ethinyl estradiol (draw-**speer**-a-none/**eth**-ih-nal ess-tra-**dye**-ole)	Yasmin 28
98	doxycycline (dock-see-**sigh**-clean)	Doxycycline Hyclate
99	fenofibrate (fen-oh-**fi**-brate)	Tricor
100	quetiapine (kwe-**tie**-ah-peen)	Seroquel
101	warfarin (**war**-fair-in)	Coumadin
102	amphetamine mixed salts (am-**fet**-ah-meen)	Adderall XR
103	methylphenidate XR (meh-thyl-**fen**-ih-date)	Concerta
104	mometasone (mo-**met**-ah-sone)	Nasonex
105	desloratadine (des-low-**rah**-tah-deen)	Clarinex
106	lovastatin (low-vah-**stat**-in)	Lovastatin
107	losartan/HCTZ (lo-**sar**-tan)	Hyzaar
108	spironolactone (**spear**-on-oh-**lack**-tone)	Spironolactone
109	glimepiride (gli-**mep**-ih-ride)	Amaryl
110	digoxin (di-**jox**-sin)	Digitek

	Generic Name and Pronunciation	Brand Name
111	temazepam (te-**maz**-eh-pam)	Temazepam
112	fluconazole (flu-**con**-ah-zole)	Diflucan
113	raloxifene (ra-**lox**-ih-feen)	Evista
114	latanoprost (la-**tan**-oh-prost)	Xalatan
115	insulin glargine (**in**-sull-in **glar**-jean)	Lantus
116	carvedilol (car-**veh**-dih-lol)	Coreg
117	ipratropium/albuterol (ih-pra-**trow**-pee-um/al-**byoo**-ter-ole)	Combivent
118	rosuvastatin (ross-uh-vah-**stat**-in)	Crestor
119	trimethoprim/sulfamethoxazole (try-**meth**-oh-prim/sul-fah-meth-**ox**-ah-zole)	Cotrim
120	valacyclovir (val-ah-**sigh**-klo-veer)	Valtrex
121	olanzapine (oh-**lan**-za-peen)	Zyprexa
122	doxazosin (docks-ah-**zoe**-sin)	Doxazosin Mesylate
123	oxycodone (ox-ih-**koe**-doan)	Oxycontin
124	triamcinolone acetonide (**try**-am-**sin**-oh-lone **as**-eh-toe-nide)	Triamcinolone Acetonide
125	estradiol (ess-tra-**dye**-ole)	Estradiol
126	aspirin (**as**-purr-in)	Aspirin
127	fexofenadine/pseudoephedrine (fex-oh-**fen**-ah-deen/soo-doe-eh-**fed**-rin)	Allegra-D 12 Hour
128	oxycodone/APAP (ox-ih-**koe**-doan)	Endocet
129	gemfibrozil (gem-**fib**-row-zil)	Gemfibrozil
130	norgestimate/ethinyl estradiol (nor-**jess**-ti-mate/**eth**-ih-nal ess-tra-**dye**-ole)	Ortho Tri-Cyclen
131	metoclopramide (meh-tah-**klo**-prah-mide)	Metoclopramide HCl
132	hydroxyzine (high-**drox**-ih-zeen)	Hydroxyzine HCl
133	irbesartan (ir-beh-**sar**-tan)	Avapro
134	norgestimate/ethinyl estradiol (nor-**jess**-ti-mate/**eth**-ih-nal ess-tra-**dye**-ole)	Ortho Tri-Cyclen Lo
135	topiramate (toe-**pie**-rah-mate)	Topamax
136	sumatriptan (sue-mah-**trip**-tan)	Imitrex
137	atomoxetine (ah-toe-**mocks**-eh-teen)	Strattera
138	metformin (met-**for**-min)	Metformin HCl ER
139	tolterodine (toll-**tear**-oh-deen)	Detrol LA
140	cefdinir (**cef**-din-ur)	Omnicef
141	meclizine (**mek**-li-zin)	Meclizine HCl
142	norgestimate/ethinyl estradiol (nor-**jess**-ti-mate/**eth**-ih-nal ess-tra-**dye**-ole)	TriNessa
143	fluticasone propionate (flu-**tick**-ah-sewn **pro**-pee-oh-nate)	Flovent
144	glipizide (**glip**-ih-zide)	Glipizide
145	propoxyphene (pro-**pox**-ih-feen)	Propoxyphene Napsylate/APAP
146	tramadol/acetaminophen (**tray**-mah-doal/ah-see-tah-**min**-oh-fen)	Ultracet
147	clindamycin (klin-da-**my**-sin)	Clindamycin HCl
148	metronidazole (meh-trow-**nye**-dah-zole)	Metronidazole
149	digoxin (di-**jox**-sin)	Lanoxin
150	nystatin (nigh-**stat**-in)	Nystatin
151	bisoprolol fumarate/HCTZ (bye-**sew**-pro-lol **fum**-ah-rate)	Bisoprolol Fumarate/HCTZ
152	valproic acid (val-**pro**-ick **as**-id)	Depakote
153	potassium chloride (poe-**tass**-ee-um **klor**-ide)	Klor-Con
154	trimethoprim/sulfamethoxazole (try-**meth**-oh-prim/sul-fah-meth-**ox**-ah-zole)	SMZ-TMP
155	benazepril (ben-**ah**-za-prill)	Benazepril HCl
156	minocycline (min-know-**sigh**-clean)	Minocycline HCl
157	triamcinolone acetonide (**try**-am-**sin**-oh-lone **as**-eh-toe-nide)	Nasacort AQ
158	diltiazem (dill-**ti**-ah-zem)	Cartia XT
159	mirtazapine (murr-**taz**-ah-peen)	Mirtazapine
160	bupropion (bu-**pro**-pe-on)	Wellbutrin SR
161	budesonide (bu-**des**-oh-nide)	Rhinocort Aqua
162	propranolol (pro-**pran**-oh-lol)	Propranolol
163	promethazine/codeine (pro-**meth**-ah-zeen/**koe**-deen)	Promethazine/Codeine
164	terazosin (tear-**aye**-zoe-sin)	Terazosin HCl
165	bupropion (bu-**pro**-pe-on)	Bupropion HCl
166	conj. estrogen/medroxyprogesterone (**es**-tro-jen/med-**rok**-se-pro-**jes**-ter-own)	Prempro
167	donepezil (doh-**neh**-peh-zil)	Aricept
168	levothyroxine (**lee**-voe-thigh-**rocks**-in)	Levothroid
169	buspirone (**byoo**-spear-own)	Buspirone HCl
170	metaxalone (meh-**tacks**-eh-lon)	Skelaxin
171	meloxicam (mel-**ox**-ih-cam)	Mobic
172	fentanyl (**fen**-tah-nil)	Duragesic
173	acyclovir (ay-**sigh**-klo-veer)	Acyclovir
174	famotidine (fah-**mow**-tih-deen)	Famotidine
175	human insulin NPH (**in**-sull-in)	Humulin N

Continued

Generic Name and Pronunciation	Brand Name
176 niacin (**nye**-ah-sin)	Niaspan
177 digoxin (di-**jox**-sin)	Digoxin
178 ferrous sulfate (**fair**-us sul-fate)	Ferrous Sulfate
179 norethindrone (nor-eth-**in**-drone)	Necon
180 levonorgestrel/ethinyl estradiol (**lee**-voe-nor-**jes**-trel eth-ih-nal ess-tra-**dye**-ole)	Aviane
181 diclofenac (dye-**klo**-fen-ak)	Diclofenac Sodium
182 insulin lispro (**in**-sull-in **lis**-pro)	Humalog
183 pimecrolimus (pim-eh-**crow**-leh-mus)	Elidel
184 fluconazole (flu-**con**-ah-zole)	Fluconazole
185 loratadine (low-**rah**-tah-deen)	Loratadine
186 olopatadine (oh-loe-**pa**-ta-deen)	Patanol
187 olmesartan medoxomil (ol-me-**sar**-tan)	Benicar
188 clotrimazole/betamethasone (kloe-**try**-mah-zole/bay-tah-**meth**-ah-sone)	Clotrimazole/Betamethasone
189 potassium chloride (poe-**tass**-ee-um **klor**-ide)	Klor-Con M20
190 clarithromycin (clair-**rith**-row-**my**-sin)	Biaxin XL
191 norgestimate/ethinyl estradiol (nor-**jess**-ti-mate/**eth**-ih-nal ess-tra-**dye**-ole)	Tri-Sprintec
192 methotrexate (meth-oh-**trex**-ate)	Methotrexate
193 lamotrigine (lam-**oh**-trih-geen)	Lamictal
194 quinine sulfate (**kwye**-nine **sul**-fate)	Quinine Sulfate
195 phenytoin (**phen**-ih-toyn)	Dilantin
196 fosinopril (fo-**sin**-oh-pril)	Fosinopril Sodium
197 amoxicillin (a-mox-ih-**sill**-in)	Amoxil
198 polyethylene glycol 3350 (pol-ee-**eth**-ih-leen **gli**-kol)	Miralax
199 budesonide (bu-**des**-o-nide)	Pulmicort
200 ketoconazole (key-toe-**con**-ah-zole)	Ketoconazole
201 nortriptyline (nor-**trip**-tih-leen)	Nortriptyline HCl
202 irbesartan/HCTZ (ir-beh-**sar**-tin)	Avalide
203 oxybutynin (ox-ee-**byoo**-tih-nin)	Ditropan XL
204 cetirizine/pseudoephedrine (sih-**tier**-eh-zeen/soo-doe-eh-**fed**-rin)	Zyrtec-D
205 nitrofurantoin (ny-tro-feur-**an**-twon)	Nitrofurantoin Monodyd Macro
206 tizanidine (tih-**zan**-ih-deen)	Tizanidine HCl
207 medroxyprogesterone (meh-**drocks**-ee-pro-**jes**-ter-own)	Medroxyprogesterone
208 glyburide/metformin (**glye**-byoor-ide/met-**for**-min)	Glucovance
209 timolol (**tim**-oh-lol)	Timolol Maleate
210 phenytoin (**phen**-ih-toyn)	Phenytoin Sodium
211 captopril (**cap**-toe-prill)	Captopril
212 nifedipine (nye-**fed**-ih-peen)	Nifedipine ER
213 carbidopa/levodopa (**kar**-bih-**doe**-pa/**lev**-oh-**doe**-pa)	Carbidopa/Levodopa
214 amoxicillin/clavulanate (a-mox-ih-**sill**-in/**klav**-u-la-nate)	Augmentin ES-600
215 human insulin 70/30 (**in**-sull-in)	Humulin 70/30
216 norethindrone/ethinyl estradiol w/ferrous fumarate (nor-eth-**in**-drone/**eth**-in-il es-tra-**dye**-ole)	Microgestin Fe
217 nabumetone (nah-**byoo**-meh-tone)	Nabumetone
218 hydrocortisone (**high**-droe-**core**-tah-sewn)	Hydrocortisone
219 indomethacin (in-doe-**meth**-ah-sin)	Indomethacin
220 propranolol (pro-**pran**-oh-lol)	Inderal LA
221 lithium carbonate (**lith**-ee-um)	Lithium Carbonate
222 valproic acid (val-**pro**-ick **as**-id)	Depakote ER
223 glyburide/metformin (**glye**-byoor-ide/met-**for**-min)	Glyburide-Metformin HCl
224 benzonatate (ben-**zow**-nah-tate)	Benzonatate
225 atenolol/clorthalidone (a-**ten**-oh-lol/klor-**thal**-ih-doan)	Atenolol w/Clorthalidone
226 phenobarbital (feen-oh-**bar**-bih-tall)	Phenobarbital
227 amphetamine (am-**fet**-ah-meen)	Amphetamine Salt Combo
228 hyoscyamine (high-oh-**sigh**-ah-meen)	Hyoscyamine Sulfate
229 phenazopyridine HCl (feen-ah-zoe-**peer**-ih-deen)	Phenazopyridine HCl
230 desogestrel/ethinyl estradiol (des-oh-**jes**-trel/**eth**-in-il es-tra-**dye**-ole)	Apri
231 desogestrel/ethinyl estradiol (des-oh-**jes**-trel/**eth**-in-il es-tra-**dye**-ole)	Kariva
232 tamoxifen citrate (tam-**ox**-ih-fen)	Tamoxifen Citrate
233 moxifloxacin (mox-ih-**flocks**-ah-sin)	Avelox
234 fluvastatin (flu-vah-**stat**-in)	Lescol XL
235 finasteride (fin-**ah**-stir-eyd)	Proscar
236 methocarbamol (meth-oh-**kar**-bah-mole)	Methocarbamol
237 levonorgestrel/ethinyl estradiol (**le**-vo-nor-**jes**-trel/**eth**-in-il es-tra-**dye**-ole)	Trivora-28
238 nitroglycerin (nigh-tro-**glih**-sir-in)	Nitroquick
239 oxycodone (ox-ih-**koe**-doan)	Oxycodone HCl

	Generic Name and Pronunciation	Brand Name
240	cefprozil (**sef**-proz-ill)	Cefzil
241	oxcarbazepine (ox-kar-**bah**-zeh-peen)	Trileptal
242	dicyclomine (dye-**sigh**-klo-meen)	Dicyclomine HCl
243	phentermine (fen-**ter**-ah-meen)	Phentermine HCl
244	chlorhexidine gluconate (klor-**hex**-ih-deen **glue**-con-ate)	Chlorhexidine Gluconate
245	tetracycline (tet-rah-**sigh**-clean)	Tetracycline
246	metformin/rosiglitazone (met-**for**-min rose-ih-**glit**-ah-zone)	Avandamet
247	candesartan (can-deh-**sar**-tan)	Atacand
248	hydrocodone/chlorpheniramine (hi-dro-**koe**-doan/klor-fen-**eer**-ah-meen)	Tussionex
249	nitroglycerin (nigh-tro-**glih**-sir-in)	Nitroglycerin
250	brimonidine tartrate (bri-**moe**-nih-deen)	Alphagan P
251	amoxicillin/clavulanate (a-**mox**-ih-sill-in **klav**-u-la-nate)	Augmentin XR
252	carbamazepine (kar-bah-**maz**-eh-peen)	Carbamazepine
253	hydroxychloroquine sulfate (high-drocks-ee-**klor**-oh-kwin)	Hydroxychloroquine Sulfate
254	morphine sulfate (**mor**-feen **sul**-fate)	Morphine Sulfate
255	clarithromycin (clair-**rith**-row-**my**-sin)	Biaxin
256	theophylline (thee-**off**-ih-lin)	Theophylline
257	docusate sodium (**dock**-cue-sate)	Docusate Sodium
258	naproxen (nah-**prox**-en)	Naproxen Sodium
259	amiodarone (ah-mee-**oh**-dah-rone)	Amiodarone HCl
260	terbinafine (ter-**bin**-ah-feen)	Lamisil
261	norgestrel/ethinyl estradiol (nor-**jes**-trel/**eth**-ih-nal es-tra-**dye**-ol)	Low-Ogestrel
262	bupropion (bu-**pro**-pe-on)	Budeprion SR
263	clindamycin phosphate (klin-da-**my**-sin)	Clindamycin Phosphate
264	clobetasol propionate (kloe-**bay**-tah-sole)	Clobetasol Propionate
265	baclofen (**back**-low-fin)	Baclofen
266	tadalafil (tah-**dah**-ah-fil)	Cialis
267	tobramycin/dexamethasone (**toe**-bra-**my**-sin/dex-ah-**meth**-ah-sone)	Tobradex
268	erythromycin (eh-**rith**-row-**my**-sin)	Erythromycin
269	timolol/dorzolamide (**tim**-oh-lol/dor-**zole**-ah-mide)	Cosopt
270	calcitonin (kal-si-**toe**-nin)	Miacalcin
271	multivitamins w/fluoride	Multivitamins w/Fluoride
272	colchicine (**coal**-cheh-seen)	Colchicine
273	doxepin (**dox**-eh-pin)	Doxepin HCl
274	levalbuterol (lev-ah-**bwet**-err-all)	Xopenex
275	thyroid (**thigh**-roid)	Armour Thyroid
276	aripiprazole (air-ee-**pip**-rah-zole)	Abilify
277	labetalol (la-**bet**-ah-lol)	Labetalol HCl
278	benztropine mesylate (**benz**-trow-peen)	Benztropine Mesylate
279	butalbital w/APAP/caffeine (byoo-**tal**-bi-tall)	Butalbital w/APAP/Caffeine
280	diphenoxylate (dye-fen-**ox**-e-late)	Diphenoxylate w/Atropine
281	methylphenidate (meth-ill-**fen**-ih-date)	Methylphenidate HCl
282	nystatin-triamcinolone (nigh-**stat**-in try-am-**sin**-oh-lone)	Nystatin-Triamcinolone
283	mupirocin (mew-**pir**-oh-sin)	Bactroban
284	etodolac (eh-**toe**-doe-lack)	Etodolac
285	felodipine (feh-**low**-dih-peen)	Plendil
286	estradiol (ess-tra-**dye**-ole)	Vivelle-Dot
287	salmeterol (sal-**met**-er-all)	Serevent Diskus
288	gabapentin (gab-ah-**pen**-tin)	Gabapentin
289	indapamide (in-**dap**-ah-mide)	Indapamide
290	moxifloxacin (mox-ih-**flocks**-ah-sin)	Vigamox
291	oxybutynin (ox-ee-**byoo**-tih-nin)	Oxybutynin Chloride
292	progesterone (proe-**jess**-ter-one)	Prometrium
293	hydrochlorothiazide/olmesartan (**high**-drow-**klor**-oh-**thigh**-ah-zide/ol-**mess**-er-tan)	Benicar HCT
294	nifedipine (nye-**fed**-ih-peen)	Nifedical XL
295	hydrocodone/ibuprofen (high-drow-**koe**-doan eye-**byoo**-pro-fen)	Hydrocodone Bit-Ibuprofen
296	azelastine (aye-zeh-**las**-teen)	Astelin

References

Abernathy E: Biological response modifiers, *Am J Nurs* 87(4):458-459, 1987.

Abraham WT, Schrier RW: Body fluid volume regulation in health and disease, *Adv Intern Med* 39(23-47k):1994.

Adler CH et al: Parkinson's disease: process along the continuum of care, *Patient Care Nurse Pract* 26:45, 46, December 2000.

Aggrenox: A combination of antiplatelet drugs for stroke prevention, *The Medical Letter* 42(1071):11-12, 2000.

Aldosterone, *Mayo Clinic Health Letter* 22(7):6, 2004.

Alexander SE, Aksel S: Estrogen replacement therapy: which regimen to choose? In Cefalo RC: *Clinical decisions in obstetrics and gynecology*, Rockville, Md, 1990, Aspen, pp 226-278.

Alschuler L et al: Herbal medicine: what works, what's safe, *Patient Care* 31(16):49, 1997.

American Academy of Pediatrics and American Heart Association: *PALS provider manual*, Dallas, 2002, American Heart Association.

American College of Obstetricians and Gynecologists: *Antenatal corticosteroid therapy for fetal maturation*, ACOG Committee opinion, No 147, Washington, DC, 1994, The College.

American College of Obstetricians and Gynecologists: Menopause: emerging issues, *ACOG Update: An Approved System for Continuing Medical Education* 21(3):1-9, 1995.

American College of Obstetricians and Gynecologists: *Nausea and vomiting of pregnancy practice bulletin*, 2004, Washington, DC, The College.

American Heart Association: Guidelines for emergency cardiac care, *J Am Med Assoc* 268:16, October 28, 1992.

American Heart Association: *Textbook of advanced cardiac life support*, Dallas, 1997, The Association.

American Heart Association: *Guidelines 2003 for cardiopulmonary resuscitation and emergency cardiovascular care—International Consensus on Science*, Philadelphia, 2003, Lippincott, Williams & Wilkins.

American Medical Association, Division of Drugs and Toxicology: *Drug evaluations annual*, Chicago, 1993, The Association.

American Society of Hospital Pharmacists: *AHFS drug information*, Bethesda, Md, 1995, The Society.

Amgen: *Neupogen (Filgrastim)* (product monograph), Thousand Oaks, Calif, 1991, Amgen.

Amgen: *Procrit: epoetin alpha for injections* (product monograph), Thousand Oaks, Calif, 1992, Amgen.

Anderson RJ: Hypopituitarism. In Rakel RE, editor: *Conn's current therapy 2000*, Philadelphia, 2000, Saunders, pp 638-639.

A new ACE inhibitor and two new angiotensin receptor blockers for hypertension, *The Medical Letter* 41(1065): 105-107, 1999.

Anticoagulants, *Mayo Clinic Health Letter* 22(6):6, 2004.

Anttila T et al: Serotypes of *Chlamydia trachomatis* and risk for development of cervical squamous cell carcinoma, *JAMA* 285(1):47-51, 2001.

Aral SO, Holmes KK: Sexually transmitted diseases in the AIDS era, *Scientific Am* 264(2):62-68, 1991.

Aronow WS: Hypertension in elderly patients; treatment reduces mortality, but is underused, *Cleveland Clinic J Med* 66(8):487-493, 1999.

Aschenbrenner DS: Drug watch: addiction treatment discontinued, *Am J Nurs* 103(12):65, 2003.

Aspirin for primary prevention of cardiovascular disease, *The Medical Letter* 42(1079):18, 2000.

Association of Women's Health, Obstetrics, and Neonatal Nursing: *Cervical ripening and induction and augmentation of labor* (practice resource), December 1993, The Association.

Association of Women's Health, Obstetrics, and Neonatal Nursing: *Issues in contraceptive method selection* (independent study), monograph(module 2):4-30, 1994.

AstraZeneca's Exanta fails to get OK: *DE/The News Journal*, A-1, A-5, Sept 11, 2004.

Atovaquone/Proquanil (Malarone) for malaria, *The Medical Letter* 42(1093):109-111, 2000.

Avoid the risks of mixed medications, *The Cleveland Clinic Heart Advisor* 7(5):3, 2004.

AWHONN, Mattson S, Smith JE, editors: *Core curriculum for maternal newborn nursing*, ed 3, Philadelphia, 2004, Saunders.

Bachmaier K et al: Chlamydia infections and heart disease linked through antigenic mimicry, *Science* 283(5406):1335, 1999.

Banahan BF, Bonnarens, JK, Bentley JP: Generic substitution of NTI drugs: issues for formulary committee consideration, *Formulary*, cover article, November 1998.

Baquiran DC, Gallagher J: *Lippincott's cancer chemotherapy handbook*, Philadelphia, 1998, Lippincott.

Barbieri RL: The use of danazol as a treatment of endometriosis. In Thomas E, Rock J, editors: *Modern approaches to endometriosis*, Dordrecht, The Netherlands, 1991, Kluwer Academic, pp 239-255.

Barbieri RL: Management of infertility caused by ovulatory dysfunction, ACOG practice bulletin, No 34, *Obstetrics and Gynecology*, 99(2): 347-358, 2002.

Barkauskas V et al: *Quick reference to health and physical assessment*, St Louis, 1994, Mosby.

Barnhart ER: *Physician's desk reference*, ed 55, Oradell, NJ, 2001, Medical Economics Company.

Bartlett JG: *1998 Medical management of HIV infection*, Baltimore, 1998, Port City Press.

Basaria S, Dobs AS: Risks versus benefits of testosterone therapy in elderly men, *Drugs and Aging* 15(2):131-142, 1999.

Baylor College of Medicine: Weighing the risks and benefits of hormone replacement therapy after menopause, *The Contraceptive Report* VI(4):4-14, 1995.

Bedell C: Pegfilgrastim for chemotherapy-induced neutropenia, *Clinical Journal of Oncology Nursing* 7(1):55-56, 63-64, 2003.

Belew C: Herbs and the childbearing woman: guidelines for midwives, *Journal of Nurse-Midwifery* 44(3):231-252, 1999.

Bender S: Personal communication, letter from Professional Service Manager, Amgen, February 20, 1991.

Benenson AS: *Control of communicable disease in man,* ed 17, Washington, DC, 2000, American Public Health Association.

Benson MD: *Obstetrical pearls: a practical guide for the efficient resident,* ed 2, Philadelphia, 1994, FA Davis.

Besinger RE, Niebyl JR: Tocolytic agents for the treatment of preterm labor. In Niebyl JR, editor: *Drug use in pregnancy,* ed 2, Philadelphia, 1988, Lea & Febiger, pp 127-172.

Bindler RM, Howry LB: *Pediatric drugs and nursing implications,* Stamford, Conn, 1997, Appleton & Lange.

Biological Therapy Nurses of University of Chicago Hospital: *Interleukin-2: a patient handbook,* Chicago, 1989, University of Chicago Hospital.

Blake DA, Niebyl JR: Requirements and limitations in reproductive and teratogenic risk assessment. In Niebyl JR, editor: *Drug use in pregnancy,* ed 2, Philadelphia, 1988, Lea & Febiger, pp 1-9.

Blenner JL: Clomiphene-induced mood swings, *J Obstetric Gyn Neonatal Nurs* 20(4):321-327, 1991.

Blood pressure, *Mayo Clinic Health Letter* 21(9):7, 2003.

Bobak IM, Jensen MO, Zalar MK: *Maternity and gynecologic care: the nurse and the family,* ed 4, St Louis, 1989, Mosby.

Bobak IM, Lowdermilk DL, Jensen MD: *Maternity nursing,* ed 4, St Louis, 1995, Mosby.

Bonapace C, Fisher J, Steele R: New developments in antibiotics, *Patient Care Nurs Pract,* 25-43, August 2000.

Bond L: Physiological changes. In Mattson S, Smith JE, editors: *NAACOG core curriculum for maternal newborn nursing,* Philadelphia, 1993, Saunders, pp 315-324.

Bortenschlager L, Zaloga GP: Vitamins. In Chernow B, editor: *The pharmacologic approach to the critically-ill patient,* ed 3, Baltimore, 1994, Williams & Wilkins, pp 3-17.

Bozzette SA et al: Randomized trial of three antipneumocystis agents in patients with advanced human immunodeficiency virus infection, *New Engl J Med* 332(11):593-639, 1995.

Brensilver JM, Goldberger E: *Water, electrolyte, and acid-base syndromes,* ed 8, Philadelphia, 1996, FA Davis.

Briggs GG, Freeman RK, Yaffe SJ: *Drugs in pregnancy and lactation: a reference guide to fetal and neonatal risk,* ed 4, Baltimore, 1994, Williams & Wilkins.

Buck ML: Impact of new regulations for pediatric labeling by the Food and Drug Administration, *Pediatric Nurs* 26(1):95-96, 2000.

Buffum M, Buffum JC: Nonsteroidal anti-inflammatory drugs in the elderly, *Pain Manag Nurs* 1(2):40-50, 2000.

Bullock BL, Rosendahl DP: *Pathophysiology: adaptations and alterations in function,* ed 2, Glenview, Ill, 1988, Scott, Foresman.

Buprenorphine, 2003, Washington, DC, Substance Abuse and Mental Health Services Administration (SAMHSA), Office of Applied Studies, US Department of Health and Human Services.

Campinha-Bacote J: African-Americans. In Purnell L, Paulanka B, editors: *Transcultural health care: a culturally competent approach,* ed 2, Philadelphia, 2003, FA Davis, pp 53-73.

Camp-Sorrell D: Chemotherapy: toxicity management. In Groenwald SL, editor: *Cancer nursing: principles and practice,* Boston, 2000, Jones and Bartlett, pp 444-486.

Candesartan for hypertension, *The Medical Letter* 40(1040):109-110, 1998.

Cargill JM: Medication compliance in elderly people: influencing variables and interventions, *J Adv Nurs* 17:422-426, 1992.

Carotid artery disease: a red flag for strike, *The Cleveland Clinic Men's Health Advisor* 6(1):1-2, 2004.

Caudle P: Providing culturally sensitive health care to Hispanic clients, *Nurse Pract* 18(12):40-51, 1993.

Cefdinir—a new oral cephalosporin, *The Medical Letter* 40(1034):85-87, 1998.

Centers for Disease Control and Prevention: Guidelines for prophylaxis against *Pneumocystis carinii* pneumonia for children infected with human immunodeficiency virus, *MMWR Morbid Mortal Wkly Rep* 40(RR-2):1-13, 1991.

Centers for Disease Control and Prevention (CDC): *1992 revised classification system for HIV infection and expanded AIDS surveillance case definition for adolescents and adults,* draft of November 15, 1991, Atlanta, 1992, US Department of Health and Human Services, Public Health Service, The Center.

Centers for Disease Control and Prevention: Recommendations of the US Public Health Service task force on the use of zidovudine to reduce perinatal transmission of human immunodeficiency virus, *MMWR Morbid Mortal Wkly Rep* 43(RR-11):1-20, 1994.

Centers for Disease Control and Prevention: Sexually transmitted diseases treatment guidelines, *MMWR Morbid Mortal Wkly Rep,* 51, 2002, *www.cdc.gov/STD/treatment/.*

Cerivastatin for hypercholesterolemia, *The Medical Letter* 40(1018):13-14, 1998.

Chameides L, Hazinski MF, editors: *Textbook of pediatric advanced life support,* Dallas, 1994, American Heart Association.

Chan PD, Johnson SM: *Gynecology and obstetrics,* California, 2004, Current Clinical Strategies Publishing.

Chasse R: Diuretics, erythropoietin, and other medications used in renal failure. In Chernow B, editor: *The pharmacologic approach to the critically-ill patient,* ed 3, Baltimore, 1994, Williams & Wilkins, pp 632-637.

Chernow B, editor: *The pharmacologic approach to the critically-ill patient,* ed 3, Baltimore, 1994, Williams & Wilkins.

Chevalier C: *The encyclopedia of medicinal plants,* England, 1996, Dorling Kindersley, pp 289-319.

Chin JE, editor: *Control of communicable disease manual,* ed 17, Washington, DC, 2000, American Public Health Association.

Chiron Cetus Oncology: *Drug package insert for Proleukin,* Emeryville, Calif, 1994, Chiron.

Chlebowski RT: Reducing the risk of breast cancer, *New Engl J Med* 343(3):191-198, 2000.

Chohan N, Doyle RM, Nale A, editors: *Nursing 2001 drug handbook,* ed 21, Springhouse, Penn, 2001, Springhouse.

Choice of antibacterial drugs, *The Medical Letter* 40(1023):33-42, 1998.

Cholesterol: the good, the bad, and the balanced, *Nursing Spectrum* 13(10):1, 7, 2003.

Chu SY, Barker LE, Smith PJ: Racial/ethnic disparities in preschool immunizations: United States, 1996-2001, *American Journal of Public Health* 94:6, 973-977.

Clark J, Longo D: Biological response modifiers, *Mediguide to Oncology* 6(2):1-5, 9, 10, 1986.

Clark J, Queener S, Karb V: *Pharmacologic basis of nursing practice,* ed 6, St Louis, 2000, Mosby.

Colditz GA et al: The uses of estrogens and progestins and the risk of breast cancer in postmenopausal women, *New Engl J Med* 332(24):1589-1593, 1995.

Colfosceril: Drug evaluation monographs, 1974-1995, *Micromedex* 85, August 31, 1995.

Colucci RD, Somberg JC: Treatment of cardiac arrhythmias. In Chernow B, editor: *The pharmacologic approach to the critically-ill patient,* ed 3, Baltimore, 1994, Williams & Wilkins, pp 445-463.

Community Program for Clinical Research on AIDS: *The human immunodeficiency virus (HIV) and protocol synopses*, Wilmington, Del, 1991, Mid-Atlantic Regional Education and Training Center, HIV Grant Program, Medical Center of Delaware.

Compendium of pharmaceutical and specialties, ed 33, Canadian Pharmacists Association, Toronto, 1998, Webcom Limited.

Compton P, McCaffery M: Treating acute pain in addicted patients, *Nursing* 31:17, 2001.

Conte JE: *Manual of antibiotics and infectious disease*, ed 9, Baltimore, 2001, Williams & Wilkins.

Costello CA: The varicella vaccine, *Adv Nurse Pract*, 47-48, December 1999.

Cotran RS, Kumar V, Robbins SL: *Robbins' pathologic basis of disease*, ed 5, Philadelphia, 1994, Saunders.

Cott J, Fugh-Berman AJ, Rakel D: Drug-herb interactions: how vigilant should you be? *Patient Care Nurse Pract*, 17-46, October 2000.

Craig CR, Stitzel RE: *Modern pharmacology with clinical application*, ed 5, Boston, 1997, Little, Brown.

Crestor (rosuvastatin calcium), 2004, *http://crestor@crestor.com*.

Cummins RO, editor: *ACLS: principles and practice*, Dallas, 2003, American Heart Association.

Cunningham FG et al: *Williams obstetrics*, ed 21, 361-383, New York, McGraw-Hill.

Davies K: Genital herpes: an overview, *J Obstet Gyn Neonatal Nurs* 19(5):401-406, 1990.

Davis JR, Sherer K: *Applied nutrition and diet therapy for nurses*, ed 2, Philadelphia, 1994, Saunders.

Dayer-Berenson L: Polypharmacology in the elderly, *Nursing Spectrum*, 14, 16, December 13, 1999.

Department of Health and Human Services, The Henry J. Kaiser Family Foundation: *Guidelines for the use of antiretroviral agents in HIV-infected adults and adolescents*, Panel on Clinical Practices for Treatment of HIV-Infection, 1998.

Deraps RK: Migraines, *Adv for Nurses*, 13-16, February 28, 2000.

Derby SA: Opioid conversion guidelines for managing adult cancer pain, *AJN* 99(10):62-65, 1999.

Detrol LA and ditropan XL for overactive bladder, *The Medical Letter* 43(1101):28, 2001.

DeVane CL: Brief comparison of the pharmacokinetics and pharmacodynamics of the traditional and newer antipsychotic drugs, *Am J Health-Systems Pharm* 52(3):S15-S19, 1995.

DeVries C: Reflections:deception, *Am J Nurs* 104(2):39, 2004.

Dion B: Hypertensive disorders in pregnancy, *Intl J Childbirth Educ* 4(1):29-30, 1989.

Ditropano C: Arrival of ARBs: potential drugs in the treatment of hypertension and heart failure, *Adv for Nurses*, 40, March 17, 2003.

Dofetilide for atrial fibrillation, *The Medical Letter* 42(1078):41-42, 2000.

Dombrowski KJ, Lantz PM, Freed GL: Risk factors for delay in age-appropriate vaccination, *Public Health Reports* 119:2, 144-155.

Dorr RT: *Hematopoietic colony stimulating factors*, Amgen teleconference, February 21, 1992, Amgen, Rockville, Md.

Douglas MJ, Levinson G: Systemic medication for labor and delivery. In Hughes S et al: *Shnider and Levinson's anesthesia for obstetrics*, Philadelphia, 2002, Lippincott, Williams & Wilkins, p 115.

Dream of a do-it-all "polypill," *The Cleveland Clinic Men's Health Advisor* 10(6):1, 7, 2003.

Drugs for asthma, *The Medical Letter* 42(1073):19-24, 2000.

Drugs for depression and anxiety, *The Medical Letter* 41(1050):33-38, 1999.

Drugs for HIV infection, *The Medical Letter* 39(1015):111-116, 1997.

Drugs for hypertension, *The Medical Letter* 43(1099):17-22, 2001.

Drugs for intermittent claudication, *The Medical Letter* 46(1176):13-15, February 16, 2004.

Drugs for non-HIV viral infections, *The Medical Letter* 41(1067):113-120, 1999.

Drugs for pain, *The Medical Letter* 42(1085):73-78, 2000.

Drugs for rheumatoid arthritis, *The Medical Letter* 42(1082):57-64, 2000.

Drugs for sexually transmitted infections, *The Medical Letter* 41(1062):85-90, 1999.

Drugs for treatment of peptic ulcers, *The Medical Letter* 39(991):1-4, 1997.

Drugs of choice for cancer chemotherapy, *The Medical Letter* 42(1087-1088):83-92, 2000.

Dudjak L: New roles of interferon-alpha, *AJN* 92(2):16, 1992.

Engel NS: Anabolic steroid use among high school athletes, *MCN Am J Matern Child Nurs* 14(6):417, 1989.

Entacapone for Parkinson's disease, *The Medical Letter* 42(1070):7-8, 2000.

Epilepsy: two new drugs, *The Medical Letter* 42(1076):33-35, 2000.

Epirubicin for adjuvant therapy in node-positive breast cancer, *The Medical Letter* 42(1071):12-13, 2000.

Eyre H, Kahn R, Robertson RM: Preventing cancer, cardiovascular disease, and diabetes: a common agenda for the American Cancer Society, the American Diabetes Association, and the American Heart Association, *CA—A Cancer Journal for Clinicians* 54(4):190-207, 2004.

Ezekial MR: *Handbook of anesthesiology*, 2004-2005 ed, Laguna Hills, Calif, 2004, Current Clinical Strategies Publishing, pp 81-109.

Fenofibrate for hypertriglyceridemia, *The Medical Letter* 40(1030):68-69, 1998.

Fernando R, Collis R: Mobile epidural techniques and new drugs in labour. In Reynolds R, editor: *Regional alegesia in obstetrics: a millennium update*, New York, 2001, Springer, p 115.

Fetro CW: *Professional's handbook of complementary and alternative medicines*, Springhouse, Penn, 1999, Springhouse.

Fielo SB: The mystery of sleep: how nurses can help the elderly, *Nursing Spectrum* 9(18PA):15-18, 2000.

Findling RL, Dogin JW: Psychopharmacology of ADHD: children and adolescents, *J Clin Psychiatry* 59(suppl 7):42-49, 1998.

Finn P: Addressing the needs of cultural minorities in drug treatment, *J Sub Abuse Treat* 11(4):325-337, 1994.

Fitzgerald MA: Prescribing for the neonate and young child: a focus on special situations, *Clin Excellence Nurse Pract* 1(2):89-94, 1997.

Fitzpatrick A, Frank L: An integrative approach to female sexual dysfunction, *Intl J Integrative Med* 3(2):8-18, 2001.

Fleming DR: Mightier than the syringe, *AJN* 100(11):44-48, 2000.

Formulary and drug therapy guide, 1998-1999, Hudson, Ohio, 1999, Lexi-Comp.

Frate DA et al: Intelligent prescribing in disease populations, *Patient Care Nurse Pract*, 47-67, May 2000.

Fujisawa: *Adenocard (adenosine) for rapid bolus intravenous use*, product insert No 45514A, Deerfield, Ill, 1990, Fujisawa.

Garner CH: The climacteric, menopause, and the process of aging. In EQ Youngkin, MS Davis, editors: *Women's health: a primary care clinical guide,* Norwalk, Conn, 1994, Appleton & Lange, pp 309-343.

Garner CH: Uses of GRH agonists, *J Obstet Gyn Neonatal Nurs* 23(7):563-570, 1994.

Gatifloxacin and moxifloxacin: two new fluoroquinolones, *The Medical Letter* 42(1072):15-18, 2000.

Geissler EM: *Pocket guide to cultural assessments,* St Louis, 1994, Mosby.

Gelone S: *Therapy of opportunistic infections associated with the human immunodeficiency virus,* Philadelphia, 1995, Temple University Hospital.

Gene M, Ledger WJ: Syphilis in pregnancy, *Sexual Transmission of Infections* 76(2):73-79, 2000.

Generic drugs, *The Medical Letter* 41(1053):47-48, 1999.

George TP, O'Malley SS: Current pharmacological treatments for nicotine dependence, *Trends Pharmacol Sci* 25(1):42-48, 2004.

Giaccone G, Pinedo HM: Drug resistance, *The Oncologist* 1:82-87, 1996.

Giamarellou H: Empiric therapy for infections in the febrile, neutropenic compromised host, *Med Clin North Am* 79(3):559-571, 1995.

Gilman AG, Goodman LS, Gilman A: *Goodman and Gilman's the pharmacologic basis of therapeutics,* ed 10, New York, 1999, Pergamon Press.

Gliashan R: A randomized controlled study of intravesicular alpha 2b-interferon in carcinoma in situ of the bladder, *J Urology* 144:658-661, 1990.

Glyburide/metformin (Glucovance) for type 2 diabetes, *The Medical Letter* 42(1092):105-106, 2000.

Goldfien A: The gonadal hormones and inhibitors. In BG Katzung, editor: *Basic and clinical pharmacology,* ed 6, Norwalk, Conn, 1995, Appleton & Lange, pp 608-636.

Gonsalves MY: Coordinating care for patients with type 2 diabetes, *Patient Care Nurse Pract,* 15-31, September 2000.

Goodman M: Chemotherapy: principles of administration. In Groenwald SL, editor: *Cancer nursing: principles and practice,* Boston, 2000, Jones and Bartlett, pp 385-443.

Gordon S: Hispanic cultural health beliefs and folk remedies, *J Holistic Nurs* 12(3):307-322, 1994.

Gorman C: Aspirin without ulcers, *Time* 73, July 13, 1998.

Green MR: *The role of colony-stimulating factors in chemotherapy-induced neutropenia,* Seattle, 1991, Immunex.

Green MR: Targeting targeted therapy, *New Engl J Med* 350(21): 2191-2193, 2004.

Griffin JE, Wilson JD: Disorders of the testes and the male reproductive tract. In Wilson JD, Foster DW, editors: *Williams' textbook of endocrinology,* ed 8, Philadelphia, 1992, Saunders, pp 799-852.

Groopman J: Clinical experience with hematopoietic growth factors, *Biotherapy and Cancer* 2(4):1, 4, 5, 1989.

Gross KM, Ponte CD: New strategies in the medical management of asthma, *Am Fam Physician* 58(1):89-100, 1998.

Gullatte MM, Graves T: Advances in antineoplastic therapy, *Oncol Nurs Forum* 17(6):867-876, 1990.

Gurevich I: AIDS in critical care, *Heart and Lung* 18(2):107-112, 1989.

Guyton AC, Hall JE: *Human physiology and mechanisms of disease,* ed 7, Philadelphia, 2000, Saunders.

Haeuber D: Recent advances in the management of biotherapy-related side effects: flu-like syndrome, *Oncol Nurs Forum* 16(6):35-41, 1989.

Haeuber D, Dijulio JE: Hematopoietic colony-stimulating factors: an overview, *Oncol Nurs Forum* 16(2):247-255, 1989.

Haifizi H, Lipson J: People of Iranian heritage. In Purnell L, Paulanka B, editors, *Transcultural health care: a culturally competent approach,* Philadelphia, 2003, FA Davis, pp 177-193.

Handley DA, Graff F: A look ahead, third-generation antihistamines, *Adv Nurse Pract,* 53, 54, 71, 72, April 1998.

Haney AF: The pathogenesis and aetiology of endometriosis. In Thomas E, Rock J, editors: *Modern approaches to endometriosis,* Dordrecht, The Netherlands, 1991, Kluwer Academic, pp 3-19.

Hardman JG et al: *Goodman and Gilman's The pharmacological basis of therapeutics,* ed 9, New York, 1996, McGraw-Hill.

Hatcher RA et al: *Contraceptive technology,* ed 18 rev, New York, 2005, Irvington.

Hatcher T: The proverbial herb, *AJN* 101(2):36-43, 2001.

Hayden FG et al: Inhaled Zanamivir for the prevention of influenza in families, *New Engl J Med,* 1282, 2000.

Hayes ER, Kee JL: *Pharmacology: pocket companion for nurses,* Philadelphia, 1996, Saunders.

Hazinsky MF, Cummins RO, Field JM, editors: *2003 Handbook of emergency cardiovascular care for healthcare providers,* 2003, American Heart Association.

Healthy heart checklist: are you doing all you can?, *Men's Health Advisor* 5(12):7, 2003.

Heart failure: a growing problem with age, *Mayo Clinic Health Letter* 20(12):1-3, December 2002.

Hellerstein DK, Lipshultz LI: Male infertility. In Copeland LJ, editor: *Textbook of gynecology,* Philadelphia, 1993, Saunders, pp 347-368.

Henke-Yarbro C, editor: Management of patients receiving interleukin-2 therapy, *Sem Oncol Nurs* 9(3, suppl 1):1-35, 1994.

High triglycerides: a red flag, *Mayo Clinic Health Letter* 20(9):7, 2002.

Hill P, Lipson J, Meleis AI: *Caring for women cross-culturally,* Philadelphia, 2003, FA Davis.

Hillis LB: Low molecular weight heparins, *Adv Nurse Pract,* 53-56, October 1997.

Hine S: Intelligent prescribing in diverse populations, *Patient Care* 9:133-149, 2000.

Hirsch MS: The treatment of cytomegalovirus in AIDS—more than meets the eye, *New Engl J Med* 326:264-266, January 23, 1992.

Hirschel B et al: A controlled study of inhaled pentamidine for primary prevention of *Pneumocystis carinii* pneumonia, *New Engl J Med* 324:1079-1083, April 18, 1991.

HIV Digest: Update: HIV infection among health care workers in 1991, publication of the Pennsylvania AIDS Education and Training Center, *HIV Digest* 1(1):1, 6, 1991.

Hobbs C: *Handmade medicines—simple recipes for herbal health,* Loveland, Colo, 1998, Interweave Press.

Hodgson BB, Kizior RJ: *Saunders' nursing drug handbook 2005,* Philadelphia, 2005, Saunders.

Hoechst-Roussel Pharmaceuticals: *Myeloid growth factors,* Somerville, NJ, 1991, Hoechst-Roussel Pharmaceuticals.

Hoechst-Roussel Pharmaceuticals: *Prokine (Sargramostim),* product monograph, Somerville, NJ, 1991, Hoechst-Roussel Pharmaceuticals.

Holgate ST, Bradding P, Sampson AP: Leukotriene antagonists and synthesis inhibitors: new directions in asthma therapy, *J Allergy Clin Immunol* 98(1):1-13, 1996.

Holland N: Multiple sclerosis: new options for care, *Nursing Spectrum* 9(18 PA):15-18, 2000.

Homocysteine, *Mayo Clinic Health Letter* (20)9:6, 2002.

Hood LE: Interferon, *AJN* 87(4):459-464, 1987.

Hostetler J: *Amish society*, ed 4, Baltimore, 1993, The Johns Hopkins University Press.

Howards SS: Treatment of male infertility, *New Engl J Med* 332(5):312-317, 1995.

Human Nutrition Information Service: USDA's food guide pyramid, 2005.

Hypertension prevalence rising, *The Cleveland Clinic Heart Advisor* 6(11):6, 2003.

Immunex: *Leukine (Sargramostim)*, product monograph, Seattle, 1991, Immunex.

Inflammation and the heart, *The Cleveland Clinic Heart Advisor* 7(6):4-5, 2004.

InterNational Council on Infertility Information Dissemination: *The infertility Q&A: Basic testing with a reproductive endocrinologist*, InterNational Council in Infertility Information Dissemination, Inc, *http://www.inclid.org/bastest.html* (accessed May 4, 2004), 2002.

Intramuscular injections: a guide to sites technique, Philadelphia, 1989, Wyeth-Ayerst Laboratories.

Irbesartan for hypertension, *The Medical Letter* 40(1019):18-19, 1998.

Irwin MM: Patients receiving biologic response modifiers: overview of nursing care, *Oncol Nurs Forum* 14(6, suppl):32-37, 1987.

Irwin RP, Nutt JG: Principles of neuropharmacology: I. Pharmacokinetics and pharmacodynamics. In Klawans HL et al, editors: *Textbook of clinical neuropharmacology and therapeutics*, ed 2, New York, 1992, Raven Press, pp 1-28.

Is it the "new cholesterol"? What you should know about homocysteine, *The Cleveland Clinic Men's Health Advisor* 2(6):4-5, 2000.

Jackson B et al: Longterm biopsychosocial effects of interleukin-2 therapy, *Oncol Nurs Forum* 18(4):683-690, 1991.

Jamerson L, DeQuattro V: The impact of ethnicity on response to antihypertensive therapy, *American Journal of Medicine* (suppl, 3A): 22S-32S, 1996.

Jawetz E: Penicillins and cephalosporins. In Katzung BG, editor: *Basic and clinical pharmacology*, ed 6, Norwalk, Conn, 1995, Appleton & Lange, pp 680-692.

Jemal A et al: Annual report for the nation on the status of cancer 1975-2001, with a special feature regarding survival. *Cancer* 101(1):3-27, 2004.

Jemal A et al: Cancer statistics, 2004, *CA—A Cancer Journal for Clinicians* 54:8-29, 2004.

Johnson BA: The biologic basis of alcohol dependence, *Advanced Studies in Nursing* 2(2):48-52, 2004.

Johnson J: Influence of race or ethnicity on pharmacokinetics of drugs, *J Pharm Science* 86(12):1328-1333, 1997.

Johnson ST: Antipsychotics, *RN*, 45-50, August 1997.

Karig AW, Murray JL, Pray WS: Trends for self-care, *Patient Care Nurse Pract*, 9-23, August 2000.

Katz R: Addressing the health care needs of American Indians and Alaskan natives, *American Journal of Public Health* 94(1): 13-14, 2004.

Kee JL: *Handbook of laboratory and diagnostic tests*, ed 5, New Jersey, 2004, Prentice Hall.

Kee JL: *Laboratory and diagnostic tests*, ed 7, Upper Saddle River, NJ, 2005, Prentice Hall Health.

Kee JL, Hayes ER: Assessment of patient laboratory data in the acutely ill, *Nurs Clin North Am* 25(4):751-759, 1990.

Kee JL, Marshall SM: *Clinical calculations*, ed 5, Philadelphia, 2004, Saunders.

Kee JL, Paulanka B, Purnell L: *Fluids and electrolytes with clinical applications*, ed 7, New York, 2004, Delmar.

Kelley WN, editor: *Textbook of internal medicine*, vols I and II, ed 2, Philadelphia, 1992, JB Lippincott.

Kellick KA: Pharmacologic considerations in statin use, *Clinician Reviews (supplement)*, *Therapeutic Spotlight*, 10-13, April 2001.

Kelly AW Saucier J: Is your patient suffering from alcohol withdrawal?, *RN* 67(2):27-31, 2004.

Kern KB, Halperin HR, Field J: New Guidelines for cardiopulmonary resuscitation and emergency cardiac care: changes in the management of cardiac arrest, *JAMA* 285:1267-1269, 2001.

Keyler DE et al: Monitoring blood levels of selected drugs, *Postgrad Med* 103(3):209-219, 1998.

Kittler P, Sucher K: *Food and culture in America*, New York, 1989, Reinhold.

Knudson M: The hunt is on, *Technology Rev*, 23-29, January-February 1998.

Koll BS, Armstrong D: Acquired immune deficiency syndrome (AIDS). In Rakel RE, editor: *1995 Conn's current therapy*, Philadelphia, 1995, Saunders, pp 42-52.

Kosnik L: Retavase (reteplase): treatment option for myocardial infarction, *Adv Nurses*, 37-39, January 29, 2001.

Kosten TR, Biegel D: Therapeutic vaccines for substance dependence, *Expert Rev Vaccines* 1(3):363-371, 2002.

Kreek MG, LaForge KS, Butelman E: Pharmacology of addictions, *Nat Rev Drug Discov* 1(9):710-726, 2002.

Krozely P: Epidermal growth factor receptor tyrosine kinase inhibitors: evolving role in the treatment of solid tumors, *Clinical Journal of Oncology Nursing* 8(2):163-168, 2004.

Kulwicki A: People of Arab ancestry. In Purnell L, Paulanka B, editors: *Transcultural health care: A culturally competent approach*, ed 2, Philadelphia, 2003, FA Davis, pp 90-105.

LaGodna G, Hendrix M: Impaired nurses: a cost analysis, *J Nurs Admin* 19(9):13-18, 1989.

Lambrecht JE, Hamilton W, Rabinovich A: A review of drug-herb interactions: documented and theoretical, *Pharmacist*, 42-53, August 2000.

Languages spoken at home, *www.census.gov/population/cen2000/phc-t20/tab06.xls* (accessed February 28, 2004), 2002.

Lantus (insulin glargine), 2001, American Pharmaceutical Association, pp 1-13.

Lauver D, Welch MB: Sexual response cycle. In Fogel CI, Lauver D, editors: *Sexual health promotion*, Philadelphia, 1990, Saunders, pp 39-52.

Lawler S: Bacteria linked to colon cancer, *The Scientist*, *http://www.biomedcentral.com/news/20031119/01* (accessed August 8, 2004), 2004.

Lefever RJ: Therapeutic Drug Monitoring (TDM). In Kee JL: *Laboratory and diagnostic tests with nursing implications*, ed 7, Upper Saddle River, NJ, 2005, Prentice Hall Health, pp 725-731.

Lehne RA: *Pharmacology for nursing care*, ed 5, Philadelphia, 2004, Saunders.

Leibowitz D, Hoffman J: *Control of communicable disease manual*, ed 17, Washington, DC, 2000, American Public Health Association.

Levalbuterol for asthma, *The Medical Letter* 41(1054):51-53, 1999.

Levy R: *Ethnic and racial differences in response to medicines,* Reston, Va, 1993, National Pharmaceutical Council.

Levy R: Multicultural medicine and pharmacy management: Part II: compliance with medications, *Drug Benefit Trends* 7(4):13-14, 24, 1995.

Levy SB: Multidrug resistance—a sign of the times, *New Engl J Med* 338(19):1376-1378, 1998.

Lewis G: Drug therapy in diabetes management, *Nurse Pract Forum* 9(2):58-60, 1998.

Lieberman J et al: HLA-B38, DR4, DQW3 and clozapine-induced agranulocytosis in Jewish patients with schizophrenia, *Arch Psychiatry* 47:945-948, 1991.

Linezolid, *The Medical Letter* 42(1079):45-46, 2000.

Lipp F: *Herbalism,* New York, 1996, Little, Brown.

Lipson J, Haifizi H: Iranians. In Purnell L, Paulanka B, editors: *Transcultural health care: a culturally competent approach,* Philadelphia, 1998, FA Davis, pp 323-351.

Lipton SA, Gendelman HE: Dementia associated with the acquired immunodeficiency syndrome. *New Engl J Med* 332(14):934-940, 1995.

Lloyd M, Matthews M, Mulholland H: Parkinson's disease; what a nurse should know, *Nursing Spectrum* 8(24):12-14, 1999.

Lowdermilk DL, Piotrawski KA, editors: *Maternity nursing,* ed 7, St Louis, 2005, Mosby, pp 221-245.

Luckmann J. *Transcultural communication in nursing,* New York, 1999, Delmar.

Lueckenotte AG: *Gerontologic nursing,* ed 2, St Louis, 2000, Mosby.

Lynch JS: Prescribing medications for mood disorders, *Adv Nurse Pract,* 23, 26, March 1998.

Lynn MM: Primary and secondary prevention of coronary heart disease, *Adv Nurse Pract,* 37-42, June 2000.

Management of COPD, *Postgrad Med* 103(4):131-132, 136, 192, 1998.

March of Dimes: Caffeine in pregnancy, March of Dimes Fact Sheet, *http://www.marchofdimes.com/printableArticles/681_1148. asp* (accessed August 17, 2004).

Marcus AO, Fernandez MP: Insulin pump therapy, *Postgrad Med* 99(3):1, 1996.

Marshall C: The art of induction/augmentation of labor, *J Obstet Gyn Neonatal Nurs* 14(1):22-28, 1985.

Masten Y: *The Skidmore-Roth outline series: obstetric nursing,* El Paso, Texas, 1993, Skidmore Roth Publishing.

Mathias R: Blood pressure medication can improve cocaine treatment results in patients with severe withdrawal symptoms, *NIDA Notes* 16(6), 2002.

Matocha L: Chinese-Americans. In Purnell L, Paulanka B, editors: *Transcultural health care: a culturally competent approach,* ed 2, Philadelphia, 2003, FA Davis, pp 163-188.

Matthews H: Racial, ethnic, and gender differences in response to medicines, *Drug Metabolism: Drug Interaction* 12(2):77-91, 1995.

Mattison D: Herbal supplements: their safety: a concern for health care providers, *March of Dimes Fact Sheet, http://www/marchofdimes.com/professionals/681_1815.asp* (accessed August 17, 2004).

Mazanec P, Tyler MK: Cultural considerations in end-of-life care: how ethnicity, age, and spirituality affect decisions when death is imminent, *American Journal of Nursing* 103(3):50-58, 2003.

McCance KL, Huether SE: *Pathophysiology: the biologic basis for disease in adults and children,* St. Louis, 1990, Mosby.

McCaul ME: Pharmacotherapy strategies for alcoholism treatment, *Advanced Studies in Nursing* 2(2):54-59, 2004.

McDonald K: Tamiflu, a flu fighter for the new millennium, *Adv for Nurses,* 19-20, December 20, 1999.

McDonald K: New treatment for diabetes: Humalog mix 75/25, *Adv for Nurses,* 27, July 2000.

McDonald LY: Personal communication regarding IL-2 administration, Emeryville, Calif, 1994, The Cetus Oncology Corporation.

McEvoy GK: *AHFS Drug Information 2000,* Bethesda, Md, 2000, American Society of Health-System Pharmacists, pp 2774, 2818.

McFarlin B et al: A national survey of herbal preparation use by nurse-midwives for labor stimulation: review of the literature and recommendations for practice, *Journal of Nurse-Midwifery* 44(3):205-216, 1999.

McGregor JA: Trichomoniasis: a continuing challenge. In Cefalo RC, editor: *Clinical decisions on obstetrics and gynecology,* Rockville, Md, 1990, Aspen, pp 289-295.

McIntyre A: *Herbs for common ailments,* New York, 1992, Fireside.

McIntyre A: *The medicinal garden,* New York, 1997, Henry Holt.

McKenry LM, Salerno E: *Mosby's pharmacology in nursing,* ed 21, St Louis, 2001, Mosby.

McKeon VA: Hormone replacement therapy: evaluating the risks and benefits, *J Obstet Gyn Neonatal Nurs* 23(8):647-657, 1993.

McMurdo MET et al: A novel approach to the assessment of drug compliance in the elderly, *Gerontology* 37:339-344, 1991.

Miglitol for type 2 diabetes mellitus, *The Medical Letter* 41(1053):49-50, 1999.

Miller EP, Armstrong CL: Surfactant replacement therapy: innovative care for the premature infant, *J Obstet Gyn Neonatal Nurs* 19(1):14-17, 1990.

Miller S, Fiorvanti J: *Pediatric medications: a handbook for nurses,* St Louis, 1997, Mosby.

Minoff H: HIV infection in pregnancy. In Cefalo RC, editor: *Clinical decisions in obstetrics and gynecology,* Rockville, Md, 1990, Aspen, pp 34-36.

Monahan FD, Neighbors M: *Medical-surgical nursing,* ed 2, Philadelphia, 1998, Saunders.

Montelukast for persistent asthma, *The Medical Letter* 40(1031):71-73, 1998.

Morbidity and Mortality Weekly Reports, 43(RR-11), August 5, 1994.

Morbidity and Mortality Weekly Reports, 47(RR-7), May 15, 1998.

Mosby's drug consult, St Louis, 2004, Mosby.

Moss A: *HIV and AIDS: management by the primary team,* Oxford, 1992, Oxford University Press.

Murphy P, Kronenburg F, Wade C: Complementary and alternative medicine in women's health: Developing a research agenda, *Journal of Nurse-Midwifery* 44(3):192-202, 1999.

Nadeau C et al: The challenges of oral anticoagulation, *Patient Care Nurse Pract,* 17-22, December 2000.

Nadler JL, Rude RK: Disorders of magnesium metabolism, *Endocrinol Metab Clin North Am* 24(3):623-637, 1995.

Nateglinide for type 2 diabetes, *The Medical Letter* 43(1101):29-30, 2001.

National Academies Press: Folate in dietary reference intakes for thiamin, riboflavin, niacin, vitalin B$_6$, folate, vitamin B$_{12}$, pantothenic acid, biotin, and choline, *http://www.nap.ecu/openbook/0309072794/html/196.html#pagetop,* pp 196-305, 1998.

National Academies Press: Iron in dietary reference intakes for vitamin A, vitamin K, arsenic, boron, chromium, copper, iodine, iron, manganese, molybdenum, nickel, silicon, vanadium, and zinc, *http://www.nap.ecu/openbook/0309072794/html/290.html#pagetop*, pp 290-393, 2000.

National Academies Press: *Improving birth outcomes: meeting the challenge in the developing world, http://www.nap.ecu/openbook/0309086140/html/243.html*, p 243, 2003.

National Institute of Allergy and Infectious Diseases: *Understanding vaccines*, NIH Publication No 98-4219, Washington, DC, 1998, US Department of Health and Human Services.

National Institute on Drug Abuse: Gender differences in drug abuse risks and treatment, *NIDA Notes* 15:4, 2000.

National Institute on Drug Abuse: Bridging science and culture to improve drug abuse research in communities, conference held Sept 24-26, 2001, Philadelphia, *http://165.112.78.61/Meetings/Bridging/BridgeAbs1.html* (accessed June 2004).

National survey on drug use and health, Washington DC, 2002, Substance Abuse and Mental Health Services Administration (SAMHSA), Office of Applied Studies, US Department of Health and Human Services.

Nayduch D, Lee A, Butler D: High-dose methyl-prednisolone after acute spinal injury, *Critical Care Nurse* 14(4):69-78, 1994.

New cholesterol-lowering drug makes its mark, *Mayo Clinic Health Letter* 21(3):4, 2003.

New drug fights fluid build-up, *The Cleveland Clinic Heart Advisor* 7(4):3, 2003.

New hypertension guidelines, *The Cleveland Clinic Men's Health Advisor* 6(8):5, 2003.

New triptans and other drugs for migraine, *The Medical Letter* 40(1037):97-100, 1998.

Newberry L, editor: *Sheehy's emergency nursing principles and practice*, ed 5, St. Louis, 2003, Mosby.

Newman V, Fullerton JT, Anderson PO: Clinical advances in the management of severe nausea and vomiting during pregnancy, *J Obstet Gyn Neonatal Nurs* 22(6):483-490, 1993.

Nichols R: Pain management in patients with addictive disease, *Am J Nurs* 103(3):87-90, 2003.

Nicolau DP, Quintiliani R, Nightingale CH: Antibiotic kinetics and dynamics for the clinician, *Med Clinics North Am* 79(3):477-493, 1995.

Niederhauser V: Prescribing for children: issues in pediatric pharmacology, *The Nurse Practitioner* 22(3):16-18, 23-26, 28, 30, 1997.

Noble SL, Forbes RC, Stamm PL: Diagnosis and management of common tinea infections, *Am Fam Physician* 58(1):163-174, 1998.

Noronha S, Arnason BGW: Multiple sclerosis. In Klawans HL: *Textbook of clinical neuropharmacology and therapeutics*, ed 2, New York, 1992, Lippincott-Raven, pp 287-296.

North American Nursing Diagnosis Association: *Nursing diagnoses: definitions and classifications 2003-2004*, Philadelphia, 2003, The Association.

Notterman DA: Pediatric pharmacotherapy. In Chernow B, editor: *The pharmacologic approach to the critically-ill patient*, ed 3, Baltimore, 1994, Williams & Wilkins, pp 139-151.

Nowak T: Vietnamese-Americans. In Purnell L, Paulanka B, editors: *Transcultural health care: a culturally competent approach*, ed 2, Philadelphia, 2003, FA Davis, pp 449-477.

Nurse practitioner prescribing reference—fall 2004, spring 2005, New York, 2004, Prescribing Reference.

Nyerges C: A better way to heal, *Mother Earth News* 161:22, 1997.

O'Brien P: Addictive behaviors. In Lewis S et al, editors: *Medical-surgical nursing: assessment and management of clinical problems*, ed 6, St Louis, 2004, Mosby.

Olds SB, London ML, Ladewig PW: *Maternal-newborn nursing: a family-centered approach*, Menlo Park, Calif, 1996, Addison-Wesley.

Olin BR, editor: *Drug facts and comparisons*, St Louis, 1994, Facts and Comparisons.

Oncology Education Services: *Molecular and targeted therapies in cancer care: from concept to chairside*, Pittsburgh, 2003, Oncology Education Services.

Oncology Nursing Society: *Biologic response modifier guidelines: recommendations for nursing education and practice*, Pittsburgh, 1989, The Society.

Ott MJ: Imagine the possibilities: guided imagery with toddlers and preschoolers, *Pediatric Nursing* 12(1):34-38, 1996.

Over-the-counter (OTC) cough remedies, *The Medical Letter* 43(1100):23-25, 2001.

Pacquiao D: People of Filipino ancestry. In Purnell L, Paulanka B, editors: *Transcultural health care: a culturally competent approach*, Philadelphia, 2003, FA Davis, pp 138-159.

Pain killers appear to weaken aspirin's primary protection, *The Cleveland Clinic Heart Advisor* 6(11):7, 2003.

Pantoprazole (Protonix), *The Medical Letter* 42(1083):65-66, 2000.

Pepping PB: Endometriosis: a nursing perspective, *Innovations in Women's Health Nursing* 1(1):2-8, 1994.

Pepping PB, Fitzgerald K: Treating endometriosis, *Innovations in Women's Health Nursing* 1(1):11-12, 1994.

Perry PJ, Alexander B, Liskow BI: *Psychotropic drug handbook*, ed 7, Washington, DC, 1997, American Psychiatric Press.

Peter G, editor: *1997 Red book: report of the committee of infectious diseases*, ed 24, Elk Grove Village, Ill, 1997, American Academy of Pediatrics.

Phair JP, Chadwick EG: Human immunodeficiency virus infection and AIDS. In Shulman ST, Phair JP, Somers HM, editors: *The biologic and chemical basis of infectious diseases*, Philadelphia, 1992, Saunders, pp 380-393.

Phenylpropanolamine and other OTC alpha-adrenergic agonists, *The Medical Letter* 42(1094):113, 2000.

Phipps WJ, Long BC, Woods NF: *Medical-surgical nursing*, ed 7, St Louis, 2002, Mosby.

Porth CM: *Pathophysiology*, ed 4, Philadelphia, 1994, JB Lippincott.

Prendergast MR et al: Massive steroids do not reduce the zone of injury after penetrating spinal cord injury, *J Trauma* 37(4):576-580, 1994.

Prevention of malaria, *The Medical Letter* 42(1070):8-9, 2000.

Prozac weekly, *The Medical Letter* 43(1101):27, 2001.

Purnell L: Mexican-Americans. In Purnell L, Paulanka B, editors: *Transcultural health care: a culturally competent approach*, ed 2, Philadelphia, 2003, FA Davis, pp 371-395.

Purnell L: Panamanian and Panamanian-American health beliefs and the meaning of respect afforded them by healthcare providers, *National J Wellness* 2(2):17-27, 1998.

Purnell L: Guatemalans' practices for health promotion and wellness and the meaning of respect afforded them by healthcare providers, *Journal of Transcultural Nursing* 11(3):40-46, 2000.

Purnell L: People of Appalachian heritage. In Purnell L, Paulanka B, *Transcultural health care: a culturally competent approach,* ed 2, pp. 73-89, Philadelphia, 2003a, FA Davis.

Purnell L: People of Brazilian heritage. In Purnell L, Paulanka B, editors: *Transcultural health care: a culturally competent approach* (chapter on CD-ROM), ed 2, Philadelphia, 2003b, FA Davis.

Purnell L: People of Cuban heritage. In Purnell L, Paulanka B: *Transcultural health care: a culturally competent approach,* ed 2, Philadelphia, 2003c, FA Davis, pp 122-137.

Purnell L: People of Egyptian heritage. In Purnell L, Paulanka B: *Transcultural health care: a culturally competent approach* (chapter on CD-ROM), ed 2, Philadelphia, 2003d, FA Davis.

Purnell L: The Purnell model for cultural competence. In Purnell L, Paulanka B, editors: *Transcultural health care: a culturally competent approach,* ed 2, Philadelphia, 2003e, FA Davis, pp 7-52.

Purnell L, Kim S: People of Korean heritage. In Purnell L, Paulanka B, editors: *Transcultural health care: a culturally competent approach* (chapter on CD-ROM), ed 2, Philadelphia, 2003, FA Davis.

Purnell L, Papadopoulos I: People of Greek heritage. In Purnell L, Paulanka B, editors: *Transcultural health care: a culturally competent approach,* ed 2, Philadelphia, 2003, FA Davis, pp 249-263.

Purnell L, Paulanka B, editors: *Transcultural health care: a culturally competent approach,* ed 3, Philadelphia, 2003, FA Davis.

Purohit SK, Hellstrom WJG: Erectile dysfunction. In Rakel RE, editor: *Conn's current therapy 2000,* Philadelphia, 2000, Saunders, pp 691-694.

Quetiapine for schizophrenia, *The Medical Letter* 39(1016):117-119, 1997.

Quinupristin/Dalfopristin, *The Medical Letter* 41(1066):109-110, 1999.

Rabeprazole, *The Medical Letter* 41(1066):110-112, 1999.

Rainey TG, Read CA: Pharmacology of colloids and crystalloids. In Chernow B, editor: *The pharmacologic approach to the critically-ill patient,* ed 3, Baltimore, 1994, Williams & Wilkins, pp 272-288.

Raise your "good" cholesterol, *The Cleveland Clinic Heart Advisor* 7(5):3, 2003

Rakel RE, editor: *Conn's current therapy 2000,* Philadelphia, 2000, Saunders.

Rapp CJ, Gordon DB: Understanding equianalgesic dosing, *Orthopaedic Nursing* 19(3):65-70, 2000.

Recommended childhood immunization schedule, United States, *Clinician Reviews* 11(3):31-32, January-December 2001, *http://www.cdc.gov/nip.*

Redeker NS: Provigil (modafinil): a new wake-promoting drug, *Adv for Nurses,* 19-20, November 22, 1999.

Repaglinide for type 2 diabetes mellitus, *The Medical Letter* 40(1027):55-58, 1998.

Rheinstein PH, Albari B: Significant FDA approvals in 1997, *Am Fam Physician* 57(11):2865-2868, 1998.

Rittenberg C, Grallo R, Rehmeyer T: Assessing managing venous irritation associated with vinorelbine tartrate (Navelbine), *Oncol Nurs Forum* 22(4):707-710, 1995.

Rituximab for non-Hodgkins lymphoma, *The Medical Letter* 40(1029):65-66, 1998.

Rivastigmine (Exelon) for Alzheimer's disease, *The Medical Letter* 42(1089):93-94, 2000.

Roark D: Bar codes and drug administration, *Am J Nurs* 104(1):63-66, 2004

Robbins DC: Management of dyslipidemia, *Clinician Rev (suppl): Therapeutic Spotlight,* 4-9, April 2001.

Robinson W: Clinical use of colony-stimulating factors, *Mediguide to Oncology* 8(3):1-4, 1988.

Rogers A: Drugs and disturbed sexual functioning. In Fogel CI, Lauver D, editors: *Sexual health promotion,* Philadelphia, 1990, Saunders, pp 485-497.

Rogove HJ, Moore KA: *Critical care medicines: handbook of intravenous pharmacotherapeutics,* Columbus, Ohio, 1993, Contemporary Critical Care Resources.

Rosen MA, Hughes SC, Levinson G: Regional anesthesia for labor and delivery. In Hughes S et al, editors: *Shnider and Levinson's anesthesia for obstetrics,* Philadephia, 2002, Lippincott, Wiliams & Wilkins, pp 123-154.

Rowland M, Tozer TN: *Clinical pharmacokinetics: concepts and applications,* ed 4, Philadelphia, 1999, Lea & Febiger.

Rudy AC, Brater DC: Drug interactions. In Chernow B, editor: *The pharmacologic approach to the critically-ill patient,* ed 3, Baltimore, 1994, Williams & Wilkins, pp 18-32.

Rudy AC, Brater DC: Pharmacokinetics. In Chernow B, editor: *The pharmacologic approach to the critically-ill patient,* ed 3, Baltimore, 1994, Williams & Wilkins, pp 3-17.

Ruhl JM: Myasthenia gravis: a baffling neuromuscular disorder, *Nursing Spectrum* 9(12 PA):14-16, 2000.

Santos AC, Pedersen H: Local anesthetics in obstetrics. In Petrie RH, editor: *Perinatal pharmacology,* Oradell, NJ, 1989, Medical Economics Books, pp 371-383.

Sautter U: The new spice trade: a chemist's faith in garlic led to a big business in alternative medicine; scientific credibility is key, *Time Intl* 150(32):48, 1998.

Scavone JM: Pharmacotherapy in the elderly. In Chernow B, editor: *The pharmacologic approach to the critically-ill patient,* ed 3, Baltimore, 1994, Williams & Wilkins, pp 202-219.

Schwertz DW: Basic principles of pharmacologic action, *Nurs Clin North Am* 26(2):245-262, 1991.

Schwertz DW, Buschmann MGT: Pharmacogeriatrics, *Crit Care Nurs Quarterly* 12(1):26-37, 1989.

Science vs. a fabled heart threat, *The Cleveland Clinic Heart Advisor* 7(8):6-7, 2004.

Second opinion, *Mayo Clinic Health Letter* 22(5):8, 2004.

Segraves R: Pediatric dosing information for health care providers, *J Ped Health Care* 9:272, 277, 1995.

Selekman J: Jewish-Americans. In Purnell L, Paulanka B, editors: *Transcultural health care: a culturally competent approach,* Philadelphia, 1998, FA Davis, pp 371-395.

Seligman M: Bronchodilators. In Chernow B, editor: *The pharmacologic approach to the critically-ill patient,* ed 3, Baltimore, 1994, Williams & Wilkins, pp 567-575.

Seymour FJ: *A new program for the management of the chemically impaired nurse in Delaware,* unpublished manuscript, executive position paper, 1991.

Sharts-Engel NC: Syphilis in pregnancy: Centers for Disease Control guidelines, *MCN Am J Matern Child Nurs* 15(6):342, 1990.

Shaw RW: GrRH analogues in the treatment of endometriosis: rationale and efficacy. In Thomas E, Rock J, editors: *Modern approaches to endometriosis,* Dordrecht, The Netherlands, 1991, Kluwer Academic, pp 257-274.

Sheehan DV: Venlafaxine extended release (XR) in the treatment of generalized anxiety disorder, *J Clin Psychiatry* 60(22):23-28, 1999.

Shelton BK, Ziegfeld CR, Olsen MM: *The Sydney Kimmel Comprehensive Cancer Center at John's Hopkins manual of cancer nursing*, Philadelphia, 2004, Lippincott, Williams & Wilkins.

Sibai BM, Armon EA: Aspirin safety during pregnancy. In Petric RH, editor: *Perinatal pharmacology*, Oradell, NJ, 1989, Medical Economics Books, pp 53-60.

Simchak M: Medications for labor pain, *Intl J Childbirth Educ* 4(4):15-17, 1989.

Simpson C, Seipp D, Rosenberg S: The current status and future application of interleukin-2 and adaptive immunotherapy in cancer treatment: seminars, *Oncology Nursing* IV(2):132-141, 1988.

Skidmore-Roth L: *Mosby's handbook of herbs and natural supplements*, St Louis, 2001, Mosby.

Smeltzer SC, Kelley L: Multiple sclerosis, *Adv for Nurses*, 10-12, July 31, 2001.

Sohn M et al: Tobacco use and dependence, *Semin Oncol Nurs* 19(4):250-260, 2003.

Some drugs that cause psychiatric symptoms, *The Medical Letter* 40(1020):21-24, 1998.

Soo-Jin Lee S: Mountain J, Koenig A: New genomics: implications for health disparities research, *Yale Journal of Public Health, Law and Ethics* 102:33-68, 2001.

Sorting through *H. pylori* ulcer therapy options, *Clinician Rev* 8(6):45-48, 1998.

Soules MR: Endometriosis: new facets of treatment for an old disease. In Cefalo RC, editor: *Clinical decisions in obstetrics and gynecology*, Rockville, Md, 1990, Aspen, pp 208-212.

Spector RE: *Cultural diversity in health and illness*, ed 4, Norwalk, Conn, 2002, Appleton & Lange.

Speroff L, Glass RH, Kase NG: *Clinical gynecologic endocrinology and infertility*, ed 6, Philadelphia, 1999, Lippincott Williams & Wilkins, p 1082.

Spironolactone for heart failure, *The Medical Letter* 41(1061):81, 82, 1999.

Spratto GR, Woods AL: *Nurse's drug reference*, New York, 2004, Delmar.

St. John's wort, *The Medical Letter* 39(1014):107-108, 1997.

Starr C: The essentials of pediatric dosing, *Patient Care Nurse Pract*, 48-51, 62-66, 68, 72, 75, 2000.

Statin safety, *The Cleveland Clinic* 5(1):4-5, 2003.

Steckel L: Antiplatelet agents in acute coronary syndromes, *Adv Nurse Pract*, 41-44, December 1999.

Steckler J: German-Americans. In Purnell L, Paulanka B, editors: *Transcultural health care: a culturally competent approach* (electronic chapter), Philadelphia, 2003, FA Davis.

Steefel L: Epilepsy poses unique issues for women, *Nursing Spectrum* 9(2PA):6-7, January 24, 2000.

Stevens DA: Coccidioidomycosis, *New Engl J Med* 332(16):1077-1082, 1995.

Stevenson AM: Pharmacokinetics in pregnant women and children, *MCN Am J Matern Child Nurs* 23(3):157, 1998.

Stewart GK: Impaired fertility. In Hatcher RA et al, editors: *Contraceptive technology*, ed 17 rev, New York, 1998, Ardent Media, pp 653-678.

Stockley IH: *Drug interactions*, ed 3, Oxford, 1994, Blackwell Scientific Publications.

Stone JT, Wyman JF, Salisbury SA: *Clinical gerontological nursing*, ed 2, Philadelphia, 1999, Saunders.

Stratton P, McGregor JA: Human immunodeficiency virus infection in women. In Copeland LJ, editor: *Textbook of gynecology*, Philadelphia, 1993, Saunders, pp 576-585.

Streptococcal pharyngitis, assessment and treatment, *Emergency Med Abstracts* 21(12), 1997.

Suggs DM: Pharmacokinetics in children: history, considerations, and applications, *J Am Academy Nurse Pract* 12(6):236-239, 2000.

Swan N: The long road to medication development: cocaine treatment moves to clinical trials, *NIDA Notes* 18(6), 2004.

Systemic candidiasis. In *The Merck manual*, chapter 158:1-3, 2000.

Tape S: Have targeted therapies lived up to their promise? *Hematology Oncology* 395:15-19, 26-27, 2004.

Targeted cancer therapies: questions and answers, National Cancer Institute, http://cis.nci.nih.gov/fact/7_49.htm (accessed August 5, 2004), 2004.

Taylor PJ, Kredenster JV: Investigation of the infertile couple. In Copeland LJ, editor: *Textbook of gynecology*, Philadelphia, 1993, Saunders, pp 261-275.

The choice of antibacterial drugs, *The Medical Letter* 41(1064):95-104, 1999.

Thomas H: Overcoming mutidrug resistance in cancer: an update on the clinical strategy of inhibiting p-glycoprotein, Cancer-Consultants.com, http://professional.cancerconsultants.com/print/aspx?id123711 (accessed August 3, 2004), 2004.

Timmons MC: The use of estrogen replacement therapy. In Cefalo RC, editor: *Clinical decisions in obstetrics and gynecology*, Rockville, Md, 1990, Aspen, pp 229-231.

Tinzaparin: a low molecular-weight heparin for treatment of deep vein thrombosis, *The Medical Letter* 43(1098):14-16, 2001.

Top 10 ways to avoid a heart attack, *The Cleveland Clinic Men's Health Advisor* 2(6):6-7, 2000.

Toremifene and letrozole for advanced breast cancer, *The Medical Letter* 40(1024):43-46, 1998.

Tortorice PV: Chemotherapy: principles of therapy. In Groenwald SL, editor: *Cancer nursing: principles and practice*, Boston, 2000, Jones and Bartlett, pp 352-384.

Towers PM: Urinary tract infections, *J Am Academy Nurses* 12(4):149-154, 2000.

Treatment of lyme disease, *The Medical Letter* 42(1077):37-39, 2000.

"Trojan Horse" to fight clots, *The Cleveland Heart Advisor* 6(11):4-5, 2003.

Trossman S: Nurses' addictions, *Am J Nurs* 103(9):27-28, 2003.

Twedell D: Genomics offer opportunities for nurses, *Journal of Continuing Education in Nursing* 34(5):195-196, 2003.

Two neuraminidase inhibitors for treatment of influenza, *The Medical Letter* 41(1063):91-93, 1999.

Umland EM: Applying pharmacokinetics; absorption, distribution, metabolism, and excretion of drugs, *Adv for Nurses* 29, 30, May 22, 2000.

Understanding lung medications: how they work—how to use them, New York, 1993, American Lung Association.

Understanding the immune system, NIH Publication No 88-529, 1991.

United States Pharmacopeia drug information (USP-DI) for the health care professional, vol I, ed 18, Rockville, Md, 1998, US Pharmacopeia Convention.

Upton R: Herbal monographs push natural medicines into the 21st century, *J Alternative Complementary Med* 3(4):397-399, 1997.

US Department of Health and Human Services: Final regulations amending basic HHS policy for the protection of human subjects: final rule: 45 CFR 46. *Federal register: rules and regulations* 46(No 16):8366-8392, January 26, 1981.

US Department of Health and Human Services: *Understanding the immune system,* Bethesda, Md, 1989, National Cancer Institute.

US Department of Health and Human Services: *1992 Revised classification system for HIV infection and expanded AIDS surveillance case definition for adolescents and adults,* Centers for Disease Control and Prevention, Bethesda, Md, November 15, 1991.

US Public Health Service Task Force on Antipneumocystis Prophylaxis for the Patient with Human Immunodeficiency Virus Infection: *Recommendations for prophylaxis against* Pneumocystis carinii *pneumonia for adults and adolescents infected with human immunodeficiency virus,* Washington, DC, 1992, US Public Health Service.

Vaccine-preventable diseases: improving vaccination coverage in children, adolescents, and adults, *MMWR Morbid Mortal Wkly Rep* 48:577-581, 1999.

Valproate and other anticonvulsants for psychiatric disorders, *The Medical Letter* 42(1094):114-115, 2000.

Vaughn CJ, Gott AM: Update on statins, *Circulation* 110: 886-892, 2003.

Vytorin: A combination of ezetimibe and simvastatin, *The Medical Letter* 46(1191):73-74, 2004.

Waitman J, McCaffery M, Pasero C: Meperidine—a liability, *AJN* 101(1):57-58, 2001.

Wang Y: People of Chinese heritage. In Purnell L, Paulanka B, editors: *Transcultural health care: a culturally competent approach,* ed 2, pp 106-121, Philadelphia, 2003, FA Davis.

What readers say about statins, *The Cleveland Clinic Heart Advisor* 7(8):4-5, 2004.

Where most heart attacks begin, *The Cleveland Clinic Heart Advisor* 7(6):4-5, 2004.

Which beta-blocker? *The Medical Letter* 43(1097):9-12, 2001.

Which medication is best for newly diagnosed hypertension? *The Cleveland Clinic Men's Health Advisor* 5(5):4-5, 2003.

Whooley MA, Simon GE: Managing depression in medical outpatients, *New Engl J Med* 343(26):1942-1949, 2000.

Wilcox SM, Himmelstein DU, Woolhandler S: Inappropriate drug prescribing for the community-dwelling elderly, *J Am Med Assoc* 272(4):292-296, 1994.

Wilkes GM, Ingwersen K, Burke MB: *Oncology nursing drug reference,* Boston, 1994, Jones and Bartlett.

Williams JS: Cognitive deficits in marijuana smokers persist after use stops, *NIDA Notes* 18(5), 2003.

Wilson BA, Shannon MT, Stang CL: *Nurses drug guide 2001,* Stamford, Conn, 2001, Appleton & Lange.

Winter ME: *Basic clinical pharmacokinetics,* ed 3, Vancouver, Wash, 1994, Applied Therapeutics.

Wittert DD: Cholesterol: the good, the bad, and the balanced, *Nursing Spectrum* 13:16, 17, 2004.

Wong DL: *Whaley & Wong's nursing care of infants and children,* ed 6, St Louis, 1999, Mosby.

Woods NF, Olshansky E, Draye MA: Infertility: women's experiences, *Health Care for Women International* 12:179-190, 1991.

Yasko J, Dudjak L: *Biological response modifier therapy-symptom management,* Pittsburgh, 1990, Park Row.

Young TE, Manqum OB: *NeoFax '94: a manual of drugs used in neonatal care,* ed 7, Columbus, Ohio, 1994, Ross Products Division, Abbott Laboratories.

Youngkin EQ, Israel D: A review and critique of common herbal alternative therapies, *Nurse Pract* 21(10):10, 39, 43-44, 49-52, 54-56, 59-62, 1996.

Zaloga GP: Enteral nutrition in the critically ill. In Chernow B, editor: *The pharmacologic approach to the critically ill patient,* ed 3, Baltimore, 1994, Williams & Wilkins, pp 1034-1046.

Zaloga GP, Chernow B: Insulin and oral hypoglycemics. In Chernow B, editor: *The pharmacologic approach to the critically ill patient,* ed 3, Baltimore, 1994, Williams & Wilkins, pp 758-771.

Zannad F: Trandolapril: how does it differ from other angiotensin-converting enzyme inhibitors, *Drugs* 46(2): 172-182, 1993.

Zickler P: Nicotine medication also reduces craving in cocaine addicts, *NIDA Notes* 15(1), 2002.

Zickler P: In chronic drug abuse, acute dopamine surge may erode resolve to abstain, *NIDA Notes* 19(1), 2004.

Ziegler MG, Ruiz-Ramon PF: Antihypertensive therapy. In Chernow B, editor: *The pharmacologic approach to the critically ill patient,* ed 3, Baltimore, 1994, Williams & Wilkins, pp 405-425.

Zonisamide for epilepsy, *The Medical Letter* 42(1089):94-95, 2000.

Zoucha R, Purnell L: People of Mexican heritage. In Purnell L, Paulanka B, editors: *Transcultural health care: a culturally competent approach,* ed 2, Philadelphia, 2003, FA Davis, pp 264-278.

Zurlinden J: St. John's wort popularity grows, but so do concerns, *Nursing Spectrum* 9(7PA):18, 19, 2000.

Zurlinden J: Research deflates value of vitamin E for heart disease, *Nursing Spectrum* 11(3 PA):26, February 11, 2002.

Zurlinden J: New lab tests for CHF, kidney function, *Nursing Spectrum* 12(16 PA):25, August 11, 2003.

Zurlinden J: FDA bans importing certain high-risk prescription drugs using the Internet, *Nursing Spectrum* 12(3 PA):19, February 10, 2004.

Index

Page numbers followed by *t* and *b* refer to tables and boxes, respectively.

List of Features—cont'd

List of Features

Prototype Drug Charts